W9-BXG-336

Become a better student and a BETTER NURSE

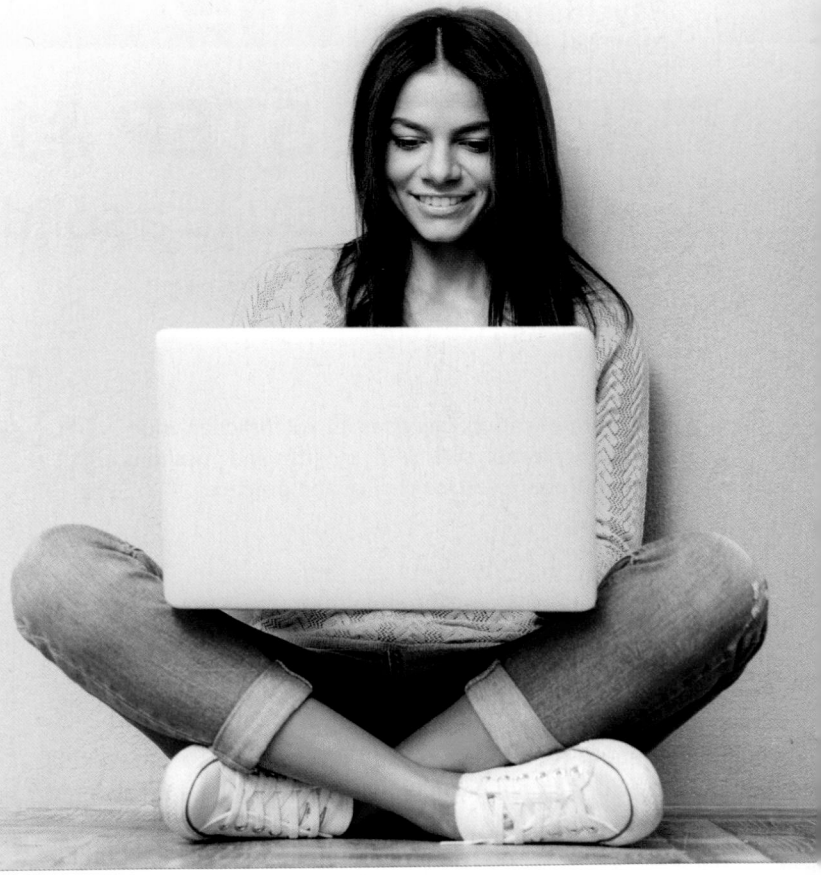

Davis Advantage offers a personalized, interactive learning platform with proven results to help you succeed in your course.

94% of students said Advantage improved their test scores.

"My grades have improved; my understanding about topics is much clearer; and overall, it has been the total package for what a nursing student needs to succeed."

— Hannah, Student, Judson University

Your journey to success BEGINS HERE!

Redeem your access code on the inside front cover of your text to access the tools you need to succeed in your course. Need a code? Visit FADavis.com to purchase access.

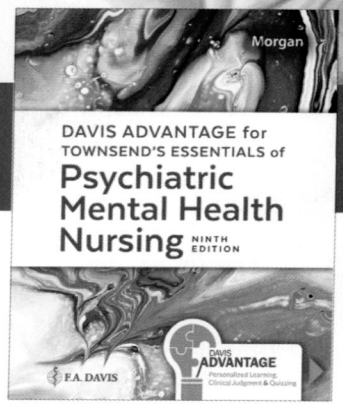

TEXT

STEP #1

Build a solid foundation.

Communication Exercises let you practice your communication skills with vignettes and questions that prepare you for clinical and practice.

Communication Exercises

1. Hal, a patient on the psychiatric unit, has a diagnosis of schizophrenia. He lives in a halfway house, where last evening he began yelling that "aliens were on the way to take over our bodies! The message is coming through loud and clear!" The residence supervisor became frightened and called 911. As Hal was being admitted to the psychiatric unit, he told the nurse, "I'm special! I get messages from a higher being! We are in for big trouble!" How would the nurse respond appropriately to this statement by Hal?

One of the Quality and Safety in Nursing Education (QSEN) criteria identified by the Institute of Medicine (IOM) (2003) stresses that the patient must be at the center of decisions about treatment (patient-centered care), and this type of assessment tool provides an opportunity to actively engage the patient in describing what medications have been effective or ineffective and identifying side effects that may impact willingness to adhere to a medication regimen.

Quality and Safety Education for Nurses (QSEN) activities and content, highlighted with a special icon, help you attain the knowledge, skills, and attitudes required to fulfill the initiative's quality and safety competencies.

Real Nurses, Real Advice shares helpful tips from practicing nurses to help you navigate clinical situations and provide the best possible care to your patients.

Real Nurses, Real Advice

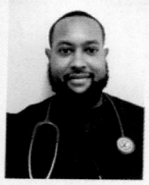

"The anhedonia, psychomotor retardation, and anergia in acute depression can make assessment a challenge. It's important to offer hope to a client who may be uncertain about how to navigate their present state of deep depression and to remain diligent while not making the patient feel pressured to speak. Paraphrasing what the patient has said to you conveys understanding and provides validation. Open-ended questions encourage the patient to elaborate rather than just answer 'yes' or 'no.'"

—Larry Johnson, RN

Real People, Real Stories features interviews with patients and provides a model for effective therapeutic communication.

Real People, Real Stories: Dr. Fred Frese

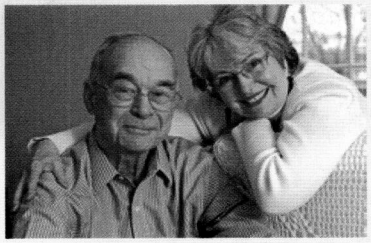

People with schizophrenia continue to be disenfranchised, misunderstood, and stigmatized. Even within healthcare, evidence has shown that some settings have been very hostile to people with severe mental illnesses. One way to begin combating stigmatization of people with mental illness is to get to know them personally. Dr. Fred Frese is a licensed psychologist and an internationally renowned speaker, writer, and advocate in the field of mental illness.

Karyn: Could you share a little bit about your history with the illness of schizophrenia?

Dr. Frese: I was 25 when I had my first episode. I was in the Marines and—I know I had seen the movie *The Manchurian Candidate* previously—and I began to think that the Vietnamese were using the same strategies from the movie to control us. When I let my commanding officer me. During the last attempt to hospitalize me, I actually escaped and ran away, even though I was in pretty bad shape.

Karyn: So since you were knowledgeable about the laws, you could essentially be your own self-advocate and argue your case, so to speak?

Dr. Frese: Yes, and by that time, I was in grad school and had secured a job at what is now the Department of Mental Health and Addiction Services. I remember I was living in the hallway of some university housing, and one of the students, who saw me day after day just hanging around and not really doing anything, suggested that I might be eligible for a government job because of my military background. When I applied, the receptionist saw my history of mental health commitments and said I would never get the job, but I did. The last time I went to the hospital, I went voluntarily because I knew I needed more medication, but they thought I needed to be hospitalized and I didn't; so I ran away.

Karyn: Sounds like you were managing a lot of stuff—grad school, working—and, at the same time, episodically struggling with symptoms of illness. You were working in the field of mental health, too. Was the work environment supportive?

Dr. Frese: Not always. It seemed like even among my coworkers, when something strange happened, they thought it was something wrong with me.

Karyn: What do you mean by "something strange"?

Dr. Frese: Like one time when they perceived I was spending too much time interacting with patients, they assumed I was "going off again," and next thing I knew, they called a "blue alert" and wanted to hospitalize me. But that time, the medical director just told me to take some time off. I never did find out why they called that blue alert.

Karyn: So you haven't been hospitalized for a very long time, and you are internationally renowned for all of your work and advocacy in the field of mental health. What do you think has contributed most to your recovery?

Dr. Frese: No, I haven't been hospitalized since I got married. I think that has been central in my recovery: having a person who you trust to give you feedback and let me know when I need more medication.

Karyn: What role do medications play in recovery?

Dr. Frese: It's very individual. We need more research to identify who, among people with schizophrenia, will benefit most by continuous medication versus episodic, reduced doses, or no medication. Genetic research is hopeful, but we're not there yet. It's hard to advise any individual what to do without knowing their individual circumstances, and even knowing, it can be very hard.

TABLE 15–2 | CARE PLAN FOR THE PATIENT WITH SCHIZOPHRENIA–cont'd

NURSING DIAGNOSIS: DISTURBED THOUGHT PROCESSES

RELATED TO: Inability to trust, panic anxiety, possible hereditary or biochemical factors

EVIDENCED BY: Delusional thinking; inability to concentrate; impaired volition; inability to problem solve, abstract, or conceptualize; extreme suspiciousness of others

OUTCOME CRITERIA	NURSING INTERVENTIONS	RATIONALE
Short-Term Goal ■ By the end of 2 weeks, patient will recognize and verbalize that false ideas occur at times of increased anxiety. **Long-Term Goals** ■ By time of discharge from treatment, patient's verbalizations will reflect reality-based thinking with no evidence of delusional ideation. ■ By time of discharge from treatment, the patient will be able to differentiate between delusional thinking and reality.	1. Convey acceptance of patient's need for the false belief but indicate that you do not share the belief. 2. Do not argue or deny the belief. Use "reasonable doubt" as a therapeutic technique: "I understand that you believe this is true, but I personally find it hard to accept." 3. Reinforce and focus on reality. Discourage long ruminations about the irrational thinking. Talk about real events and real people. 4. If patient is highly suspicious, the following interventions may be helpful: a. Use same staff as much as possible; be honest and keep all promises.	1. Patient must understand that you do not view the idea as real. 2. Arguing with the patient or denying the belief serves no useful purpose, because delusional ideas are not eliminated by this approach, and the development of a trusting relationship may be impeded. 3. Discussions that focus on the false ideas are purposeless and useless and may even aggravate the psychosis. 4. To decrease patient's suspiciousness: a. Familiar staff and honesty promotes trust.

Therapeutic Communication Icon identifies helpful interventions and guidance on how to speak with your patients. Look for this icon in Care Plan sections.

Movie Connections list films that demonstrate conditions and behaviors you may not encounter in clinical.

MOVIE CONNECTIONS

I Never Promised You a Rose Garden (schizophrenia) • *A Beautiful Mind* (schizophrenia) • *The Fisher King* (schizophrenia) • *Bennie & Joon* (schizophrenia) • *Out of Darkness* (schizophrenia) • *Conspiracy Theory* (delusional disorder) • *The Fan* (delusional disorder)

Personalized Learning

LEARN

DAVIS ADVANTAGE

STEP #2

Make the connections to key topics.

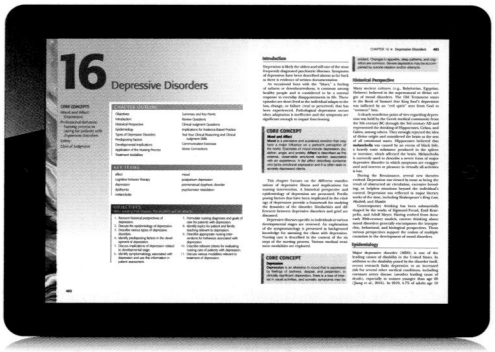

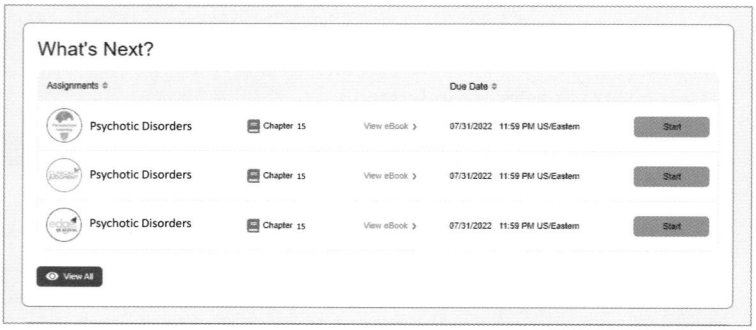

Assignments in Davis Advantage correspond to key topics in your book. Begin by reading from your printed text or click the eBook button to be taken to the **FREE, integrated eBook.**

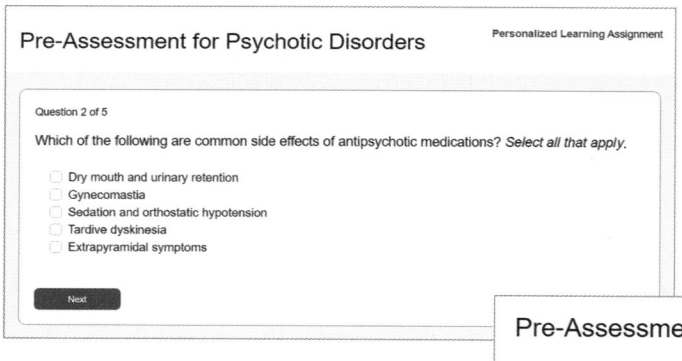

You'll receive **immediate feedback** that identifies your strengths and weaknesses using a thumbs up, thumbs down approach. *Thumbs up* indicates competency, while *thumbs down* signals an area of weakness that requires further study.

Following your reading, take the **Pre-Assessment** quiz to evaluate your understanding of the content. Questions feature single answer, multiple-choice, and select-all-that-apply formats.

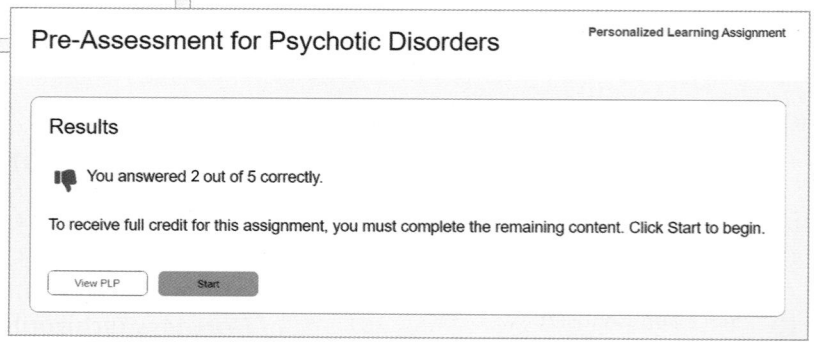

Content subject to change upon publication.

Psychotic Disorders

Personalized Learning Assignment

VIDEO

ACTIVITY

POST-ASSESSMENT

Premorbid Phase

- Subtle signs and symptoms
- Usually occurs in early adolescence
- Individual appears very shy or withdrawn
- Not having a lot of friends

Animated mini-lecture videos make key concepts easier to understand, while interactive learning activities allow you to expand your knowledge and make the connections to important topics.

Post-Assessment for Psychotic Disorders

Personalized Learning Assignment

Question 4 of 5

The RAISE approach stands for *R*ecovery *A*fter an *I*nitial *S*chizophrenia *E*pisode. What are the approaches used in RAISE? *Select all that apply.*

- Personalized treatment plan
- Vocational support
- Case management
- Cognitive remediation
- Family education and support

Next

After working through the video and activity, a **Post-Assessment** quiz tests your mastery.

Personalized Learning at a Glance

Personalized Learning Assignments

Average

Performance	Time Spent	Participation
82% Average Score	18 min	15 / 36

Performance Summary

Congratulations! You have demonstrated competency in 13 of the Personalized Learning topics.

The following topics could use further study and review. Focus study time on:

- Depressive Disorders
- Bereaved Individual

Clinical Judgment Assignments

Average

Performance	Time Spent	Participation
75% Average Score	25 min	2 / 3

Quizzing Assignments

Average

Performance	Time Spent	Participation
83% Average Score	15 min	13 / 63

Your dashboard provides **snapshots of your performance**, time spent, participation, and strengths and weaknesses at a glance.

NF Personalized Learning Plan

Psych

Start Date: 10/01/2020 • End Date: 12/31/2020

DISPLAY | PERSONALIZED LEARNING | CLINICAL JUDGMENT | QUIZZING

Personalized Learning Assignments

Assignments	Pre-Assessment	Video	Activity	Post-Assessment	Date Complete		
Recovery Models Chapter 10					10/05/2020	10:10 AM US/Eastern	Review
Suicide Prevention Chapter 11				3x	10/10/2020	10:30 AM US/Eastern	Review
Neurocognitive Disorders Chapter 13					10/12/2020	10:36 PM US/Eastern	Review
Bipolar and Related Disorders Chapter 17					10/14/2020	10:44 PM US/Eastern	Review
Eating Disorders Chapter 21							Continue
Personality Disorders Chapter 22							Continue

Your **Personalized Learning Plan** is tailored to your individual needs and tracks your progress **across all your assignments**, helping you to identify the exact areas that require additional study.

CLINICAL JUDGMENT

APPLY

STEP #3

Develop critical-thinking skills & prepare for the Next Gen NCLEX®

Psychotic Disorders

Clinical Judgment Assignment

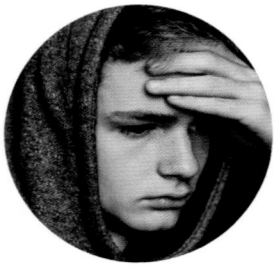

Psychotic Disorders

The nurse is caring for a 16-year-old boy presenting to the behavioral health provider's office with his mother for withdrawn behavior.

This case consists of six clinical judgment questions. Read each question carefully and select the best answer(s). Use the chart to help answer the question. The chart is dynamic and may change as the case progresses.

Real-world cases mirror the complex clinical challenges you will encounter in a variety of healthcare settings. Each **case study** begins with a patient photograph and a brief introduction to the scenario.

Scenario

The nurse is caring for a 16-year-old boy presenting to the behavioral health provider's office with his mother for withdrawn behavior. Use the chart to answer the questions. *The chart may update as the scenario progresses.*

History and Physical Assessment | **Nurses' Notes** | **Vital Signs** | **Laboratory Results**

to no interest in things that he used to like to do.

Family History: Paternal aunt with bipolar disorder. Maternal grandmother with depression.

Assessment: Client is a 16-year-old male who appears very withdrawn and disheveled. Only answers questions with one word and does not make eye contact. His movements are very slowed. He states that he feels like there is no hope for the future but denies suicidal ideation. Mother states that over the last 2 years, he has gotten progressively worse with hygiene, not completing schoolwork, and staying in his room all the time with the door locked. Mother states that more recently, he started to exhibit repetitive behaviors such as turning lights on and off seven times when entering the bathroom. Client states that "it's just something I need to do."

Medications: No current medications.

The Patient Chart displays tabs for History & Physical Assessment, Nurses' Notes, Vital Signs, and Laboratory Results. As you progress through the case, the chart expands and populates with additional data.

Psychotic Disorders

Clinical Judgment Assignment

Scenario

The nurse is caring for a 16-year-old boy presenting to the behavioral health provider's office with his mother for withdrawn behavior. Use the chart to answer the questions. *The chart may update as the scenario progresses.*

History and Physical Assessment | Nurses' Notes | Vital Signs | Laboratory Results

Medical/Surgical history: No significant medical history. Had a broken arm when he was 8 from a skateboarding accident.
Social history: Client has always been shy and withdrawn with few friends. He has always struggled in school, but more recently his grades have gone from Cs to Ds and Fs. He is more withdrawn and has stopped talking to all of his friends. More recently he has started some repetitive behaviors. He is also not showering or washing his clothes and has little to no interest in things that he used to like to do.
Family History: Paternal aunt with bipolar disorder. Maternal grandmother with depression.
Assessment: Client is a 16-year-old male who appears very withdrawn and disheveled. Only answers questions with one word and does not make eye contact. His movements are very slowed. He states that he

Question 3 of 6

The nurse is reviewing the client's information. Drag to the box on the right each potential criterion that the client is exhibiting that fits the *DSM-5* diagnosis of schizophrenia. *Be sure to drag all that apply.*

- Appears withdrawn
- Performs repetitive behaviors
- Thinks people are out to get him
- Fails to complete schoolwork
- Displays blunted affect

- Hears people laughing at him
- Appears disheveled
- Lacks interest in activities

Next

Complex questions that mirror the format of the Next Gen NCLEX® require careful analysis, synthesis of the data, and multi-step thinking.

Psychotic Disorders

Clinical Judgment Assignment

Results

You answered 2 out of 6 questions correctly.

Review the questions, answers and rationales below to improve your understanding. Identify which questions you answered correctly (indicated by a green check mark) and incorrectly (identified by a red x). Remember, you must choose all correct options and only the correct options to get a question correct. Expand the questions to review your individual answer choices, the correct answers (indicated by green shading), and complete rationales.

Hide All Details | Return to Assignments

Question 1 of 6 — Hide

The nurse is reviewing the signs of schizophrenia. For each client finding below, specify whether it is consistent with the premorbid phase, prodromal phase, or both. *Select one option in each row.*

	Premorbid Phase	Prodromal Phase	Both Phases
Shy and withdrawn	●	○	○
Poor relationships with friends	●	○	○
Repetitive behaviors	○	●	○
Poor school performance	○	○	●
Not showering	○	○	●
Stays in room all day	○	●	○
No interest in activities	●	○	○

Rationale

The premorbid phase of schizophrenia is characterized by being shy and withdrawn and having poor peer relationships, poor school performance, and antisocial behavior. These signs occur before there is clear evidence to suggest a diagnosis of schizophrenia.

The prodromal phase of schizophrenia has more clearly manifested signs and symptoms and is a worsening of the premorbid phase. This phase can last from a few weeks to 5 years and the person shows significant deterioration in functioning. Half will have depressive symptoms and some will develop symptoms of OCD.

There is overlap in some of the signs and symptoms, but the prodromal phase is significantly worse than premorbid functioning.

Clinical Judgment Cognitive Skill: Analyze Cues Page Reference: p. 341

Test-Taking Tip Make a chart for yourself to distinguish among the four phases of schizophrenia.

Immediate feedback with **detailed rationales** encourages you to consider what data is important and how to prioritize the information to ensure safe and effective nursing care.

Test-taking tips provide important context and strategies for how to consider the structure of each question type when answering.

edge QUIZZING

ASSESS

STEP #4

Improve comprehension & retention.

Comprehensive rationales explain why your responses are correct or incorrect. Page-specific references direct you to the relevant content in your text, while test-taking tips improve your test-taking skills.

High-quality questions, including more difficult question types like **select-all-that-apply**, assess your understanding and challenge you to think at a higher cognitive level.

PLUS! Brand-new Next Gen NCLEX® stand-alone questions provide you with even more practice answering the new item types and help build your confidence.

Feedback

You answered 9 out of 10 correctly.
Review the questions, answers and rationales below.

Hide All Details | Return to Assignments

Question 1 — Hide

Which finding in the client in the psychiatric ward enables the nurse to reach the conclusion that the client is in the premorbid phase of schizophrenia?

- The client is anxious and irritable.
  Rationale: The client in the prodromal phase exhibits nonspecific symptoms such as anxiety and
- The client has disorganized speech.
  Rationale: The client in the schizophrenia phase may show symptoms such as disorganized spee
- The client is very shy and withdrawn.
  Rationale: The client in the premorbid phase of schizophrenia exhibits symptoms such as being v withdrawn.
- The client has diminished emotional expression.
  Rationale: The client in the schizophrenia phase may show negative symptoms such as diminishe expression.

Psychotic Disorders — Quizzing: Assignment

Question 3 of 15

Which symptoms in a client indicate the persecutory type of delusional disorder? Select all that apply.

- [ ] The feeling of being spied on
- [ ] The feeling of being poisoned
- [ ] The feeling of being plotted against
- [ ] The feeling of a famous person being in love with him or her
- [ ] The feeling of being in a relationship with a religious leader

Practice Quizzes — Create Practice Quiz

You may generate their own practice quizzes (NCLEX®-style assessments) to test or expand your understanding of topics).

Assignments		Competency	Percent Correct	Date Complete	
Crisis Intervention	15 Questions		85%	09/11/2020 10:40 PM US/Eastern	Review
Ethical and Legal Issues	15 Questions		79%	09/25/2020 10:45 PM US/Eastern	Review

Create your own **practice quizzes** to focus on topic areas where you are struggling, or use as a study tool to review for an upcoming exam.

GET STARTED TODAY!

Use the access code on the inside front cover to unlock **Davis Advantage** for **Townsend's Essentials of Psychiatric Mental Health Nursing!**

PERFECT | Anytime Anywhere

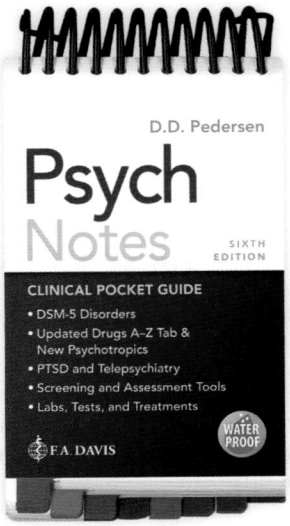

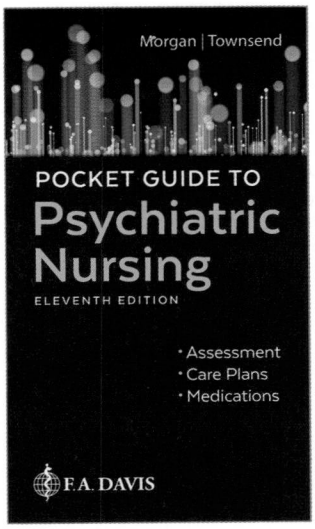

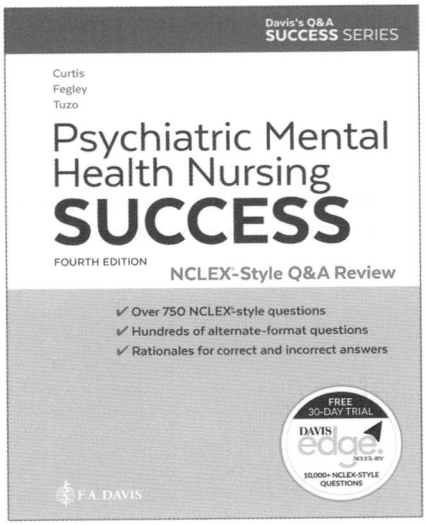

Quick Reference Guide

"Great for review or quick reference in clinical practice. Easy to carry with you and useful as a quick reference as no one can remember everything."

Practical Diagnoses & the Latest Psychotropics

"Great book.... Helped me to do my concept maps in less than 5 minutes... Well worth the money..."

Q&A Course Review & NCLEX® prep

"Great book with tough questions that was very helpful for Mental Health Nursing course and NCLEX® prep. Definitely worth the extra purchase."

—Online Student Reviewers

SAVE 20% + FREE SHIPPING

Use Promo Code: **DAVIS20**

ORDER TODAY!

at FADavis.com

Promotion subject to change without notice. Offer valid for individual purchases from FADavis.com in the U.S. only.

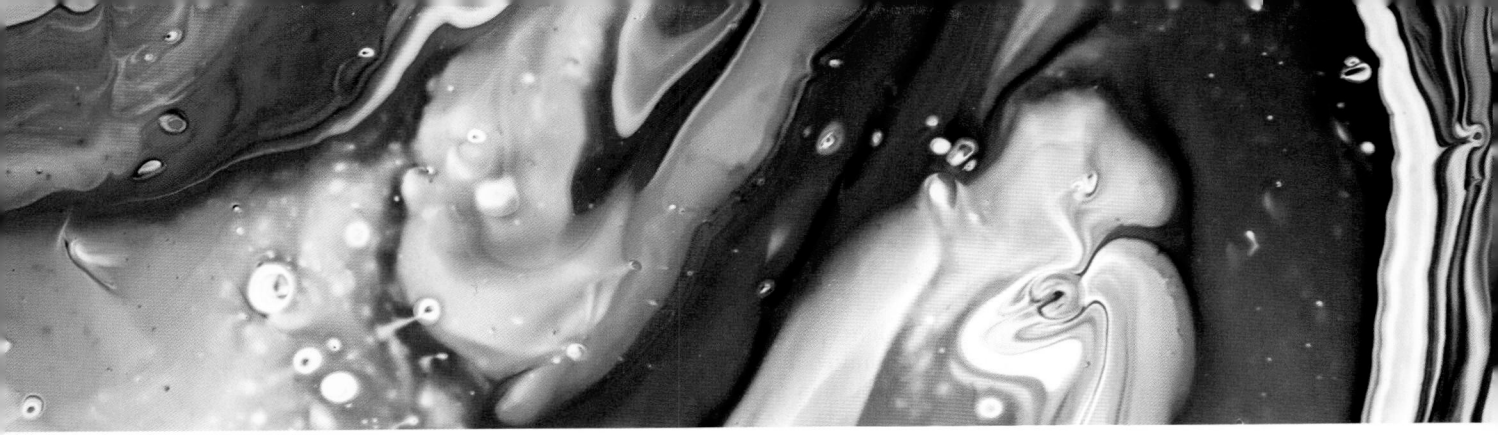

DAVIS ADVANTAGE for TOWNSEND'S ESSENTIALS of Psychiatric Mental Health Nursing

NINTH EDITION

Concepts of Care in Evidence-Based Practice

Karyn I. Morgan, RN, MSN, APRN-CNS
Psychiatric Clinical Nurse Specialist
Professor Emerita, Psychiatric Mental Health Nursing
The University of Akron
Akron, Ohio

F.A. DAVIS
Philadelphia

F. A. Davis Company
1915 Arch Street
Philadelphia, PA 19103
www.fadavis.com

Copyright © 2023 by F. A. Davis Company

Copyright © 2023 by F. A. Davis Company. All rights reserved. This book is protected by copyright. No part of it may be reproduced, stored in a retrieval system, or transmitted in any form or by any means, electronic, mechanical, photocopying, recording, or otherwise, without written permission from the publisher.

Printed in the United States of America

Last digit indicates print number: 10 9 8 7 6 5 4 3 2 1

Publisher, Nursing: Susan R. Rhyner
Senior Content Project Manager: Amy M. Romano
Design and Illustrations Manager: Carolyn O'Brien

As new scientific information becomes available through basic and clinical research, recommended treatments and drug therapies undergo changes. The author(s) and publisher have done everything possible to make this book accurate, up to date, and in accord with accepted standards at the time of publication. The author(s), editors, and publisher are not responsible for errors or omissions or for consequences from application of the book, and make no warranty, expressed or implied, in regard to the contents of the book. Any practice described in this book should be applied by the reader in accordance with professional standards of care used in regard to the unique circumstances that may apply in each situation. The reader is advised always to check product information (package inserts) for changes and new information regarding dose and contraindications before administering any drug. Caution is especially urged when using new or infrequently ordered drugs.

Library of Congress Cataloging-in-Publication Data

Names: Morgan, Karyn I., author.
Title: Davis advantage for Townsend's essentials of psychiatric mental health nursing : concepts of care in evidence-based practice / Karyn I. Morgan.
Other titles: Essentials of psychiatric mental health nursing
Description: Ninth edition. | Philadelphia, PA : F.A. Davis, [2023] | Preceded by Essentials of psychiatric mental health nursing : concepts of care in evidence-based practice / Karyn I. Morgan, Mary C. Townsend. 8th edition. 2020. | Includes bibliographical references and index.
Identifiers: LCCN 2021051692 (print) | LCCN 2021051693 (ebook) | ISBN 9781719645768 (paperback) | ISBN 9781719647571 (ebook)
Subjects: MESH: Psychiatric Nursing--methods | Evidence-Based Nursing--methods | Mental Disorders--nursing
Classification: LCC RC440 (print) | LCC RC440 (ebook) | NLM WY 160 | DDC 616.89/0231--dc23/eng/20220110
LC record available at https://lccn.loc.gov/2021051692
LC ebook record available at https://lccn.loc.gov/2021051693

Authorization to photocopy items for internal or personal use, or the internal or personal use of specific clients, is granted by F. A. Davis Company for users registered with the Copyright Clearance Center (CCC) Transactional Reporting Service, provided that the fee of $.25 per copy is paid directly to CCC, 222 Rosewood Drive, Danvers, MA 01923. For those organizations that have been granted a photocopy license by CCC, a separate system of payment has been arranged. The fee code for users of the Transactional Reporting Service is: 978-1-7196-4576-8/22 0 + $0.25.

In memory of Dr. Fred Frese, who relentlessly shared his knowledge and experience and will always be remembered as a fierce advocate for those with mental illness. In appreciation of his wife, Penny Frese, who, through her work as the founder of Red Flags National, continues to promote the need for education and institutional protocols within schools to build skills in resilience, recognition of early symptoms of mental illness, and informed support networks for responding to individual needs.

—Karyn Morgan

Contributors

Lois Angelo, MSN, APRN, BC
ED Care Manager
Newton Wellesley Hospital
Newton, Massachusetts

Cathy Melfi Curtis, MSN, RN-BC
Nursing Educator Consultant
Charleston, South Carolina

Tona Leiker, PhD, APRN, CNE
Assistant Dean, Nursing Curriculum and Assessment
American Sentinel University
Aurora, Colorado

Mary Jean Thompson, RN, BN, MHS, MPC
Instructor, MHC
University of Calgary
Medicine Hat, Alberta, Canada

Carol Norton Tuzo, MSN, RN-BC
Nursing Educator Consultant
Charleston, South Carolina

Reviewers

Lois Angelo, MSN, APRN, BC
ED Care Manager
Newton Wellesley Hospital
Newton, Massachusetts

Linda Blair, BSN, RN
Nursing Instructor
Central Carolina Community College
Sanford, North Carolina

Debra DeVoe, RN, MSN, NE-BC
Nursing Instructor
Thomas Edison State University
Trenton, New Jersey

Donna A. Enrico, MBS, BSN, RN
Clinical Instructor
College of Southern Nevada
Las Vegas, Nevada

Elizabeth Fife, MSN, RN, CNS, CPN
Associate Professor
Louisiana Tech University
Ruston, Louisiana

Wanda Golden, RN, MSN, CCRN, PhD(c)
Dean and Associate Professor of Nursing
Abraham Baldwin Agricultural College
Tifton, Georgia

Sandra Gustafson, MA, RN, CNE
Nursing Faculty
Hibbing Community College
Hibbing, Minnesota

Patricia J. Hefner, MSN, RN-BC
Faculty; Course Coordinator of Psychiatric Mental Health Nursing
Heritage Valley Sewickley
Moon, Pennsylvania

Sharon A. Henle, EdD, ANP, RHIA, CNE
Assistant Professor of Nursing
Farmingdale State College
Farmingdale, New York

Jennifer E. Herrold, RN, MSN, CRNP
Instructor
Thomas Jefferson University
Danville, Pennsylvania

Beverly J. Howard, MSN, RN, FNP
Instructor
Alvin Community College
Alvin, Texas

Katherine M. Howard, MS, RN-BC
Nursing Instructor
Middlesex County College Nursing Program, Raritan Bay Medical Center
Edison, New Jersey

JoAnna Johns, MSN, RN, BA
Assistant Professor of Nursing
Atlantic Cape Community College
Mays Landing, New Jersey

Janet K. Johnson, MBA, MSN, RN
Nursing Coordinator
Fort Berthold Community College
New Town, North Dakota

Rebecca King, RN, MSN, PMHCNS-BC
Division Chair for Nursing and Allied Health
University of Arkansas, Community College of Batesville
Batesville, Arkansas

Brenda Kucirka, PhD, RN, PMHCNS-BC, CNE
Clinical Instructor
Widener University
Chester, Pennsylvania

Jan E. Lawrenz Blasi, MSN, RN
Nursing Instructor
Chandler School of Nursing and Allied Health, Pratt Community College
Pratt, Kansas

Anne Marie Leveille, RN, MSN, MPH
Assistant Professor
Medgar Evers College
Brooklyn, New York

Mark Longshore, JD, MSN, RN
Nursing Department Chair
Front Range Community College
Fort Collins, Colorado

Dimitra Loukissa, PhD, RN
Professor
North Park University
Chicago, Illinois

Tamar Lucas, EdD, MSN, RN-BC
Nursing Instructor
Itawamba Community College
Tupelo, Mississippi

Jana S. Martin, MS, RN, CNE
Division Chair, Allied Health Services
OSU Institute of Technology
Okmulgee, Oklahoma

Renee Menkens, RN, MS
Assistant Professor
Southwestern Oregon Community College
Coos Bay, Oregon

Bonnie Parker, DNP, RN, CRRN
Assistant Professor of Nursing, Malek School of Health Professions
Marymount University
Arlington, Virginia

Norma Perez, MSN/Ed, RN
Assistant Professor
Ivy Tech Community College Northwest
Valparaiso, Indiana

Larry Purnell, PhD, RN, FAAN
Professor Emeritus, University of Delaware
Adjunct Professor, Florida International University
Adjunct Professor, Excelsior College

Susan M. Reading-Martin, MS, RN, CS, FNP, ARNP-BC
Nursing Faculty
Western Nebraska Community College
Scottsbluff, Nebraska

Donna F. Rye, MSN, RN
Assistant Professor
Cox College
Springfield, Missouri

Karen B. Silva, RN, MSN, MFN, BC
Nursing Faculty
Keiser University
Sarasota, Florida

Alexandra Winter, RN, MSN
Assistant Director of Nursing
Metropolitan Community College
Omaha, Nebraska

Jordon D. Bosse, PhD, RN
Assistant Professor, Bouvé College of Health Sciences, School of Nursing
Faculty Scholar, Institute for Health Equity and Social Justice Research
Northeastern University
External Faculty Nurse Scientist, Massachusetts General Hospital (MGH)
Boston, MA

Acknowledgments

Sincere thanks go to:

Susan Rhyner, for your skills, your integrity, and your gift of encouragement.

Amy Romano and Laura Horowitz for all your support, accessibility, and assistance in preparing the manuscript.

The nursing educators, students, and clinicians, who provide critical information about the usability of the textbook and offer suggestions for improvements. Many changes have been made based on your input.

The individuals who critiqued the manuscript for this edition and shared your ideas, opinions, and suggestions for enhancement. I sincerely appreciate your contributions to the final product.

Special thanks also to Erin Barnard, Alan Brunner, Vic Farracone, Fred Frese, Bridget Hutchens, Myrle Weems, and the others who courageously allowed their stories to be told and to Jennifer Feldman for research assistance.

I appreciate each of you more than I can say.

Karyn I. Morgan

To the Instructor

The impact of the COVID-19 global pandemic put a spotlight on psychiatric and mental health concerns in ways we could not even imagine just a few short years ago. The need for confident nurses—well versed in assessment and intervention across a broad spectrum of mental health disorders—remains higher than ever. To that end, the 9th edition of *Essentials of Psychiatric Mental Health Nursing* includes changes associated with the latest edition and update to the *American Psychiatric Association's Diagnostic and Statistical Manual of Mental Disorders (DSM-5-TR).* Also, in the 8th edition of *Essentials of Psychiatric Mental Health Nursing,* we felt it was imperative to present a new chapter, **Caring for Patients With Mental Illness and Substance Use Disorders in General Practice Settings,** to highlight why every nurse—regardless of the care setting—needs the knowledge and skills necessary to support and treat patients with mental health disorders, wherever they are encountered. We are pleased that faculty have responded so positively to the addition of that chapter.

Additionally, the onset of COVID-19 challenged faculty and students across the globe to migrate almost overnight from in-person, "brick-and-mortar" classroom settings to online and distance education. Recognizing those challenges, *Townsend's Essentials* expanded the array of faculty and student resources to provide a complete teaching and learning package, including the online resource, *Davis Advantage for Essentials of Psychiatric Mental Health Nursing.* Davis Advantage provides a wide variety of online activities, animations, and assessments, designed specifically for distance learning, with a dashboard of metrics delivered seamlessly to faculty and students alike.

Prior to COVID-19, as faculty we were already aware of dangerous trends related to suicide and addiction, especially opioids. Current federally endorsed initiatives, such as the Zero Suicide Initiative (2012) and HEAL (Helping to End Addiction Long-term) (2018), underscore the magnitude of these two mental health issues and make clear that nurses practicing in any arena need a strong foundation in psychiatric mental health nursing care. Perhaps as never before, many nurse leaders see this period of mental health-care reform as an opportunity for nurses to expand their roles and assume key positions in education, prevention, assessment, and referral. Nurses are, and will continue to be, in key positions to assist individuals to attain, maintain, or regain optimal emotional wellness.

As it has been with each new edition of *Essentials of Psychiatric Mental Health Nursing* the goal of this ninth edition is to bring to practicing nurses and nursing students the most up-to-date information related to neurobiology, psychopharmacology, and evidence-based nursing interventions. This edition includes changes associated with the latest (fifth) edition, text revision of the American Psychiatric Association's *Diagnostic and Statistical Manual of Mental Disorders (DSM-5-TR).*

The Teaching and Learning Package

How students learn is evolving. In this digital age, we consume information in new ways. The possibilities to interact and connect with content in new, dynamic ways are enhancing students understanding and retention of complex concepts.

In order to meet the needs of today's learners, how faculty teach is also evolving. Classroom (traditional or online) time is valuable for active learning. This approach makes students responsible for the key concepts, allowing faculty to focus on clinical application. Relying on the textbook alone to support an active classroom leaves a gap. ***Davis Advantage*** is designed to fill that gap and help students and faculty succeed in core courses. It is composed of the following:

- **A Strong Core Textbook** that provides the foundation of knowledge that today's nursing students need to pass the NCLEX® and enter practice prepared for success.
- **An Online Solution** that provides resources for each step of the learning cycle: learn, apply, assess.
  - **Personalized Learning** assignments are the core of the product and are designed to prepare students for classroom (live or online) discussion. They provide directed learning based on needs. After completing text reading assignments, students take a pre-assessment for each ***topic.*** Their results feed into their *Personalized Learning Plan.* If students do not pass the pre-assessment, they are required to complete further work within the topic: watch an animated mini-lecture, work through an activity and take the post-assessment.

    The personalized learning content is designed to connect students with the foundational information about a given topic or concept. It provides the gateway to helping make the content accessible to all students and complements different learning styles.
  - **Clinical Judgment** assignments are case-based and build off key Personalized Learning topics. These cases help students develop Clinical Judgment skills through exploratory learning. Students will link their knowledge base (developed through the text and personalized learning) to new data and patient situations. Cases include dynamic charts that expand as the case progresses and use complex question types that require students to analyze data, synthesize conclusions, and make judgments. Each case will end with comprehensive feedback, which provides detailed rationales for the correct and incorrect answers.
  - **Quizzing** assignments build off Personalized Learning Topics (and are included for every topic) and help assess students' understanding of the broader scope and increased depth of that topic. The quizzes use NCLEX®-style questions to assess understanding and synthesis of content. Quiz results include comprehensive feedback for correct and incorrect answers to help students understand why their answer choices were right or wrong.
- **Online Instructor Resources** are aimed at creating a dynamic learning experience that relies heavily on interactive participation and is tailored to students' needs. Results from the post-assessments are available to faculty, in aggregate or by student, and inform a **Personalized Teaching Plan** that faculty can use to deliver a targeted classroom experience. Faculty will know students' strengths and weaknesses *before* they come to class and can spend class time focusing on where students are struggling. Suggested in-class activities are provided to help create an interactive, hands-on learning environment that helps students connect more deeply with the content. NCLEX®-style questions are from the **Instructor Test Bank** and **PowerPoint** slides that correspond to the textbook chapters are referenced in the Personalized Teaching Plans. New to the 9th edition, we are excited to include a special set of NCLEX questions using the new "NCLEX Next Gen" question types. These include Extended Multiple Response, Extended Drag and Drop, Matrix/Grid, Cloze (Drop-Down), Enhanced Hot Spot (Highlighting), Bowtie, and Trend. We hope faculty can use these questions–in addition to those provided in the Instructor Test Bank–to specifically help provide students with more practice with the new question types.
- **Davis Edge** online quizzing assesses understanding, using an adaptive format with NCLEX®-style questions. Faculty can set up a review and remediation system to take a constant pulse of classroom performance, with student results available in real-time to easily identify areas of weakness. Comprehensive rationales for all answer options are provided for students and explain why an answer is correct or incorrect.

Updated or New Content in the 9th Edition Text

All content has been updated to reflect the current state of the discipline of nursing.

- All nursing diagnoses are current with the NANDA-I, Inc., *Nursing Diagnoses: Definitions and Classification 2021–2023.*
- Each chapter features review questions that have been updated to reflect the next generation NCLEX test plan's focus on clinical judgment (the term *client* has been retained in these questions to reflect terminology consistent with the test plan).
- "Real People, Real Stories" appear in Chapter 11, "Suicide Prevention"; Chapter 14, "Substance Use and Addiction Disorders"; Chapter 15, "Schizophrenia Spectrum and Other Psychotic Disorders"; Chapter 16, "Depressive Disorders"; Chapter 17, "Bipolar and Related Disorders"; Chapter 21, "Eating Disorders"; Chapter 23, "Children and Adolescents"; Chapter 25, "Survivors of Abuse or Neglect"; Chapter 28, "Military Families"; and Chapter 32 (online), "Issues Related to Human Sexuality and Gender Dysphoria". This popular feature is written in an interview format as author Karyn Morgan speaks with real individuals about their mental health challenges. This feature provides examples of a therapeutic communication process, promotes an understanding of the experience of having a mental illness from the individual's perspective, and gives real patient perspectives on what is needed from the nurses they encounter. They may be used by the instructor as exercises geared toward destigmatizing those with mental illnesses.
- A new feature, "Real Nurses, Real Advice," provides brief, key interventions on selected topics from nurses who are practicing in psychiatric care settings. They appear in Chapter 5, "Relationship Development and Therapeutic Communication"; Chapter 15 "Schizophrenia Spectrum and Other Psychotic Disorders"; and Chapter 16, "Depressive Disorders."
- Chapter 30, "Complementary Therapies and Integrative Care," and Chapter 31, "Cultural Concepts Relevant to Psychiatric Mental Health Nursing," are maintained as online chapters but content about psychosocial therapies and spiritual care have been relocated to Chapter 7 ("Psychosocial Interventions and Spiritual Care"). Milieu therapy content, which was a complete chapter in the last edition, has been incorporated in Chapter 7.
- Content has been added to several chapters to integrate concepts on trauma-informed care. Content on Forensic Nursing has been added to Chapter 25, "Survivors of Abuse or Neglect."
- The term *patient* is used to refer to the recipient of nursing care and the term *client* is used to describe individuals in the broader context of the individual who accesses a variety of mental health-related services. The purpose is to add consistency, particularly with concepts such as "patient-centered care," one of the six Quality and Safety Education for Nurses (QSEN) criteria.
- QSEN icons in many chapters highlight when specific content represents an application of one of the six QSEN criteria.

Features That Have Been Retained in the Ninth Edition

The concept of holistic nursing is retained in the ninth edition of *Essentials of Psychiatric Mental Health Nursing.* An attempt has been made to ensure that the physical aspects of psychiatric mental health nursing are not overlooked. In all relevant situations, the mind/body connection is addressed.

Nursing process is retained in the ninth edition as the tool for delivery of care to the individual with a psychiatric disorder or to assist in the primary prevention or exacerbation of mental illness symptoms. The six steps of the nursing process, as described in the American Nurses Association *Standards of Clinical Nursing Practice,* are used to provide guidelines for the nurse. These standards of care are included for the *DSM-5-TR* diagnoses featured in specific chapters as well as for the aging individual, the bereaved individual, victims of abuse and neglect, and as examples in several of the therapeutic approaches. The six steps are:

- **Assessment:** Background assessment data, including a description of symptomatology, provides an extensive knowledge base from which the nurse may draw when performing an assessment. Several assessment tools are also included.
- **Diagnosis:** Analysis of the data is included from which nursing diagnoses common to specific psychiatric disorders are derived.
- **Outcome identification:** Outcomes are derived from the nursing diagnoses and stated as measurable goals.

- **Planning:** A plan of care is presented with selected nursing diagnoses for the selected *DSM-5-TR* diagnoses as well as for the elderly client, the bereaved individual, survivors of abuse and neglect, the elderly homebound client, and the primary caregiver of the client with a chronic mental illness. The planning standard also includes tables that list topics for educating clients and families about mental illness. Concept map care plans are included for all major psychiatric diagnoses.
- **Implementation:** The interventions that have been identified in the plan of care are included along with rationale for each. Case studies at the end of each *DSM-5-TR* chapter assist the student in the practical application of theoretical material. Also included as a part of this particular standard, "Psychiatric Mental Health Nursing Interventions," located in Unit 2 of the following textbook. This section addresses psychiatric nursing intervention in depth and frequently speaks to the differentiation in scope of practice between the basic psychiatric nurse and advanced-practice psychiatric nurse.
- **Evaluation:** The evaluation standard includes a set of questions that the nurse may use to assess whether the nursing actions have been successful in achieving the objectives of care.

Other Features

Each chapter on psychiatric disorders is structured to first describe the disorder, followed by *DSM-5-TR* (2022) diagnostic criteria, then nursing care, and finally, evidence-based treatment strategies.

- All psychiatric diagnostic content is reflective of the American Psychiatric Association's *Diagnostic and Statistical Manual of Mental Disorders, Fifth Edition, Text Revision* (2022).
- Communication Exercises boxes are presented in Chapter 10, "The Recovery Model"; Chapter 13, "Neurocognitive Disorders"; Chapter 14, "Substance Use and Addiction Disorders"; Chapter 15, "Schizophrenia Spectrum and Other Psychotic Disorders"; Chapter 16, "Depressive Disorders"; Chapter 17, "Bipolar and Related Disorders"; Chapter 21, "Eating Disorders"; Chapter 22, "Personality Disorders"; Chapter 25, "Survivors of Abuse or Neglect"; Chapter 27, "The Bereaved Individual"; and in the eBook bonus chapter, Chapter 32, "Issues Related to Human Sexuality and Gender Dysphoria." These exercises portray clinical scenarios that allow the student to practice communication skills with clients. Answers appear in Appendix D at the back of the book.
- An updated list of movies at the end of most diagnostic chapters may be used to visually reinforce material discussed in the textbook. These movies may be used as learning tools to allow students to see on-screen the behaviors that they may only read about.
- Tables that list topics for patient and family education are included in the clinical chapters.
- Boxes that highlight current research studies with implications for evidence-based nursing practice are included in the clinical chapters.
- Assigning nursing diagnoses to patient behaviors is addressed in each of the disorder-specific chapters found in Unit 3, "Care of Patients With Psychiatric Disorders."
- Taxonomy and diagnostic criteria from the *DSM-5-TR* (2022) are used throughout the text.
- References throughout the text have been updated, and classical references are distinguished from general references.
- Boxes with core definitions are presented throughout the text.
- Core concepts have been updated to reflect a consistent taxonomy of concepts that occurs in all F. A. Davis nursing titles. The purpose is to facilitate incorporation in a concept-based curriculum.
- Appendix B provides a comprehensive glossary.
- Answers to end-of-chapter review questions are presented in Appendix C.
- Answers to communication exercises are presented in Appendix D.

It is hoped that the revisions and additions to this ninth edition of *Davis Advantage for Essentials of Psychiatric Mental Health Nursing* continue to satisfy a need in psychiatric mental health nursing practice. The mission of this textbook has been, and continues to be, to provide both students and clinicians with up-to-date information about psychiatric mental health nursing. The user-friendly format and easy-to-understand language, for which we have received many positive comments, have been retained in this edition. We hope that this ninth edition continues to promote and advance the commitment to psychiatric mental health nursing.

Karyn Morgan

Contents in Brief

UNIT 1
Introduction to Psychiatric Mental Health Concepts 1

Chapter 1 **Mental Health and Mental Illness** 2
Chapter 2 **Biological Implications** 12
Chapter 3 **Ethical and Legal Issues** 38
Chapter 4 **Psychopharmacology** 59

UNIT 2
Psychiatric Mental Health Nursing Interventions 99

Chapter 5 **Relationship Development and Therapeutic Communication** 100
Chapter 6 **The Nursing Process in Psychiatric Mental Health Nursing** 125
Chapter 7 **Psychosocial Interventions and Spiritual Care** 149
Chapter 8 **Intervention in Groups** 170
Chapter 9 **Crisis Intervention** 182
Chapter 10 **The Recovery Model** 205
Chapter 11 **Suicide Prevention** 219

UNIT 3
Care of Patients With Psychiatric Disorders 247

Chapter 12 **Caring for Patients With Mental Illness and Substance Use Disorders in General Practice Settings** 248
Chapter 13 **Neurocognitive Disorders** 263
Chapter 14 **Substance Use and Addiction Disorders** 299
Chapter 15 **Schizophrenia Spectrum and Other Psychotic Disorders** 362
Chapter 16 **Depressive Disorders** 402
Chapter 17 **Bipolar and Related Disorders** 445
Chapter 18 **Anxiety, Obsessive-Compulsive, and Related Disorders** 475
Chapter 19 **Trauma- and Stressor-Related Disorders** 508
Chapter 20 **Somatic Symptom and Dissociative Disorders** 533
Chapter 21 **Eating Disorders** 561
Chapter 22 **Personality Disorders** 587

UNIT 4
Psychiatric Mental Health Nursing of Special Populations 623

Chapter 23 **Children and Adolescents** 624
Chapter 24 **The Aging Individual** 669
Chapter 25 **Survivors of Abuse or Neglect** 700
Chapter 26 **Community Mental Health Nursing** 725
Chapter 27 **The Bereaved Individual** 756
Chapter 28 **Military Families** 775

Appendix A Mental Status Assessment A-1
Appendix B Glossary A-5
Appendix C Answers to Review Questions A-29
Appendix D Examples of Answers to Communication Exercises A-31
Index I-1

Online Chapters

Chapter 29 **Concepts of Personality Development** 795
Chapter 30 **Complementary and Integrative Therapies** 812
Chapter 31 **Cultural Concepts Relevant to Psychiatric Mental Health Nursing** 835
Chapter 32 **Issues Related to Human Sexuality and Gender Dysphoria** 847

Contents

UNIT 1
Introduction to Psychiatric Mental Health Concepts 1

Chapter 1 **Mental Health and Mental Illness** 2
Introduction 2
Mental Health 3
Mental Illness 3
Physical and Psychological Responses to Stress 4
Physical Responses 4
Psychological Responses 5
Summary and Key Points 9

Chapter 2 **Biological Implications** 12
Introduction 13
The Nervous System: An Anatomical Review 13
The Brain 13
Nerve Tissue 17
Autonomic Nervous System 19
Neurotransmitters 19
Neuroendocrinology 24
Pituitary Gland 24
Circadian Rhythms 28
Genetics 29
Psychoneuroimmunology (PNI) 30
Normal Immune Response 30
Implications of the Immune System in Psychiatric Illness 30
Psychopharmacology and the Brain 33
Implications for Nursing 33
Summary and Key Points 33

Chapter 3 **Ethical and Legal Issues** 38
Introduction 39
Ethical Considerations 40
Theoretical Perspectives 40
Ethical Dilemmas 40
Ethical Principles 41
A Model for Making Ethical Decisions 42
Ethical and Legal Issues in Psychiatric Mental Health Nursing 42
Legal Considerations 45
Patient Rights 45
Nurse Practice Acts 45
Types of Law 46
Classifications Within Statutory and Common Law 46
Legal Issues in Psychiatric Mental Health Nursing 46
Hospitalization 51
Nursing Liability 53
Summary and Key Points 55

Chapter 4 **Psychopharmacology** 59
Introduction 60
Historical Perspectives 60
The Role of the Nurse in Psychopharmacology 60
Ethical and Legal Implications 60
Assessment 61
Medication Administration and Evaluation 63
Patient Education 63
How Do Psychotropics Work? 64
Applying the Nursing Process in Psychopharmacological Therapy 66
Antianxiety Agents 67
Antidepressants 68
Mood-Stabilizing Agents 73
Antipsychotic Agents 79
Sedative-Hypnotics 87
Agents for Attention Deficit-Hyperactivity Disorder (ADHD) 89
Summary and Key Points 92

UNIT 2
Psychiatric Mental Health Nursing Interventions 99

Chapter 5 **Relationship Development and Therapeutic Communication** 100
Introduction 101
The Therapeutic Nurse-Patient Relationship 101
Therapeutic Use of Self 101
Conditions Essential to Development of a Therapeutic Relationship 102
Rapport 102
Trust 102
Respect 103
Genuineness 103
Empathy 103

Phases of a Therapeutic Nurse-Patient Relationship 104
The Preinteraction Phase 104
The Orientation (Introductory) Phase 105
The Working Phase 105
The Termination Phase 106
Boundaries in the Nurse-Patient Relationship 106
Interpersonal Communication 108
The Impact of Pre-existing Conditions 108
Nonverbal Communication 109
Therapeutic Communication Techniques 111
Nontherapeutic Communication Techniques 111
Active Listening 111
Process Recordings 119
Feedback 119
Summary and Key Points 121

Chapter 6 **The Nursing Process in Psychiatric Mental Health Nursing** 125
Introduction 126
The Nursing Process 126
Definition 126
Standards of Practice 126
Why Nursing Diagnosis? 136
Nursing Case Management 137
Critical Pathways of Care 138
Applying the Nursing Process in the Psychiatric Setting 138
Concept Mapping 140
Documentation of the Nursing Process 141
Types of Documentation Methods 141
Electronic Documentation 145
Summary and Key Points 146

Chapter 7 **Psychosocial Interventions and Spiritual Care** 149
Introduction 149
Individual Psychosocial Therapies 150
Psychoanalysis and Psychoanalytic Psychotherapy 150
Interpersonal Psychotherapy 150
Reality Therapy 151
Cognitive Behavior Therapy 151
Dialectical Behavior Therapy 152
Psychosocial Interventions in Nursing Practice 152
Milieu Therapy: The Therapeutic Community 152
Relaxation Therapy 156
Assertiveness Training 157
Spiritual Care 157
Spiritual Needs 159
Religion 161
Addressing Spiritual and Religious Needs Through the Nursing Process 162
Assessment 162
Diagnoses/Outcome Identification 162
Planning and Implementation 162
Evaluation 162
Summary and Key Points 166

Chapter 8 **Intervention in Groups** 170
Introduction 170
Functions of a Group 171
Types of Groups 171
Task Groups 171
Teaching Groups 171
Supportive/Therapeutic Groups 171
Self-Help Groups 172
Physical Conditions That Influence Group Dynamics 172
Seating 172
Size 172
Membership 173
Therapeutic Factors 173
Phases of Group Development 173
Phase I. Initial or Orientation Phase 174
Phase II. Middle or Working Phase 174
Phase III. Final or Termination Phase 174
Leadership Styles 174
Autocratic 175
Democratic 175
Laissez-Faire 175
Member Roles 175
Psychodrama 175
The Family as a Group 177
The Role of the Nurse in Therapeutic Groups 177
Summary and Key Points 178

Chapter 9 **Crisis Intervention** 182
Introduction 182
Characteristics of a Crisis 183
Phases in the Development of a Crisis 183
Types of Crises 184
Class 1: Dispositional Crises 184
Class 2: Crises of Anticipated Life Transitions 185
Class 3: Crises Resulting From Traumatic Stress 185
Class 4: Maturational and Developmental Crises 185
Class 5: Crises Reflecting Psychopathology 186
Class 6: Psychiatric Emergencies 186

Crisis on the Inpatient Unit: Anger and Aggression Management 186
Assessment 186
Symptoms Associated With Anger and Aggression 187
Diagnosis and Outcome Identification 188
Planning and Implementation 189
Evaluation 192
Crisis Intervention 192
Phases of Crisis Intervention: The Role of the Nurse 193
Phase 1. Assessment 193
Phase 2. Planning of Therapeutic Intervention 193
Phase 3. Intervention 193
Phase 4. Evaluation of Crisis Resolution and Anticipatory Planning 194
Disaster Nursing 194
Application of the Nursing Process to Disaster Nursing 194
Background Assessment Data 194
Nursing Diagnoses and Outcome Identification 195
Planning and Implementation 195
Evaluation 195
Summary and Key Points 201

Chapter 10 **The Recovery Model** 205
Introduction 205
What Is Recovery? 206
Guiding Principles of Recovery 206
Models of Recovery 208
The Tidal Model 208
The Wellness Recovery Action Plan (WRAP) 210
The Psychological Recovery Model 212
Nursing Interventions That Assist With Recovery 214
Summary and Key Points 216

Chapter 11 **Suicide Prevention** 219
Introduction 219
Historical Perspectives 220
Epidemiology 220
Risk Factors 222
Marital Status 222
Sex 222
Age 222
Religion 223
Socioeconomic Influences 223
Ethnicity 223
Other Risk Factors 223
Predisposing Factors: Theories of Suicide 224
Psychological Theories 224
Sociological Theories 225
Biological Theories 226
Application of the Nursing Process With the Suicidal Patient 226
Assessment 226
Diagnosis and Outcome Identification 232
Planning and Implementation 232
Evaluation 241
Summary and Key Points 241

UNIT 3
Care of Patients With Psychiatric Disorders 247

Chapter 12 **Caring for Patients With Mental Illness and Substance Use Disorders in General Practice Settings** 248
Introduction 248
The Need for Education of Health-Care Providers 249
Screening 250
Priority Issues for Screening in Any Health-Care Setting 251
Trauma History 252
Risk for Suicide 252
Substance Use Disorders 253
Referral 254
Stigma 257
The Role of the Nurse in Caring for Patients With Psychiatric and Substance Use Disorders in Nonpsychiatric Settings 258
Summary and Key Points 258

Chapter 13 **Neurocognitive Disorders** 263
Introduction 263
Delirium 264
Clinical Findings and Course 264
Predisposing Factors 264
Neurocognitive Disorder 265
Clinical Findings, Epidemiology, and Course 265
Predisposing Factors 268
Application of the Nursing Process 274
Background Assessment Data 274
Nursing Diagnosis and Outcome Identification 278
Planning and Implementation 280
Concept Care Mapping 280
Patient and Family Education 280
Evaluation 280
Quality and Safety Education for Nurses (QSEN) 284

Treatment Modalities 287
Delirium 287
Neurocognitive Disorder (NCD) 287
Summary and Key Points 294

Chapter 14 **Substance Use and Addiction Disorders** 299
Introduction 300
Substance Use Disorder, Defined 300
Substance Addiction 300
Substance-Induced Disorder, Defined 301
Substance Intoxication 301
Substance Withdrawal 301
Classes of Psychoactive Substances 301
Predisposing Factors to Substance-Related Disorders 301
Biological Factors 301
Psychological Factors 302
Sociocultural Factors 303
The Dynamics of Substance-Related Disorders 303
Alcohol Use Disorder 303
Sedative, Hypnotic, or Anxiolytic Use Disorder 309
Stimulant Use Disorder 312
Inhalant Use Disorder 319
Opioid Use Disorder 320
Hallucinogen Use Disorder 323
Cannabis Use Disorder 326
Application of the Nursing Process 329
Background Assessment Data 329
Diagnosis and Outcome Identification 337
Planning and Implementation 338
Concept Care Mapping 342
Patient and Family Education 342
Evaluation 342
The Chemically Impaired Nurse 344
Codependency 345
The Codependent Nurse 346
Treating Codependency 346
Treatment Modalities 346
Self-Help Groups: Alcoholics Anonymous 346
Pharmacotherapy 347
Counseling 351
Group Therapy 352
Nonsubstance Addictions 352
Gambling Disorder 352
Summary and Key Points 355

Chapter 15 **Schizophrenia Spectrum and Other Psychotic Disorders** 362
Introduction 363
Nature of the Disorder 363
Phases of Schizophrenia 363
Prognosis 364
Predisposing Factors 365
Biological Factors 365
Psychological Factors 370
Environmental Influences 370
Theoretical Integration 371
Other Schizophrenia Spectrum and Psychotic Disorders 371
Delusional Disorder 372
Brief Psychotic Disorder 372
Substance- and Medication-Induced Psychotic Disorder 372
Psychotic Disorder Due to Another Medical Condition 372
Catatonic Disorder Due to Another Medical Condition 373
Schizophreniform Disorder 373
Schizoaffective Disorder 373
Application of the Nursing Process 373
Background Assessment Data 373
Diagnosis and Outcome Identification 376
Planning and Implementation 377
Concept Care Mapping 383
Patient and Family Education 383
Evaluation 383
Quality and Safety Education for Nurses (QSEN) 385
Treatment Modalities 386
Psychological Treatments 387
Social Treatments 388
Psychopharmacological Treatment 390
Smoking Cessation 394
Summary and Key Points 395

Chapter 16 **Depressive Disorders** 402
Introduction 403
Historical Perspective 403
Epidemiology 403
Age and Sex 404
Socioeconomic Factors 404
Race and Culture 404
Marital Status 404
Seasonality 405
Types of Depressive Disorders 405
Major Depressive Disorder 405
Persistent Depressive Disorder (Dysthymia) 405
Premenstrual Dysphoric Disorder 405
Substance/Medication-Induced Depressive Disorder 408
Depressive Disorder Due to Another Medical Condition 408
Predisposing Factors 409
Biological Theories 409
Psychosocial Theories 413

Developmental Implications 414
Childhood 414
Adolescence 415
Senescence 416
Postpartum Depression 417
Application of the Nursing Process 418
Background Assessment Data 418
Diagnosis and Outcome Identification 421
Planning and Implementation 422
Concept Care Mapping 422
Patient and Family Education 422
Evaluation of Care for the Depressed Patient 422
Treatment Modalities 422
Interpersonal Psychotherapy 422
Group Therapy 428
Family Therapy 430
Cognitive Behavior Therapy 430
Electroconvulsive Therapy 431
Repetitive Transcranial Magnetic Stimulation (rTMS) 432
Vagus Nerve Stimulation and Deep Brain Stimulation 433
Bright Light Therapy 433
Psychopharmacology 434
Summary and Key Points 439

Chapter 17 **Bipolar and Related Disorders** 445
Introduction 446
Historical Perspective 446
Epidemiology 446
Types of Bipolar Disorders 447
Bipolar I Disorder 447
Bipolar II Disorder 448
Cyclothymic Disorder 448
Substance/Medication-Induced Bipolar Disorder 448
Bipolar Disorder Due to Another Medical Condition 449
Predisposing Factors 449
Biological Theories 449
Developmental Implications 451
Treatment Strategies 451
Application of the Nursing Process to Bipolar Disorder (Mania) 452
Background Assessment Data 452
Diagnosis and Outcome Identification 453
Planning and Implementation 453
Concept Care Mapping 457
Patient and Family Education 457
Evaluation of Care for the Patient Experiencing a Manic Episode 457
Treatment Modalities 459
Individual Psychotherapy 459
Group Therapy 459
Family Therapy 460
Cognitive Behavior Therapy 460
The Recovery Model 460
Electroconvulsive Therapy 462
Psychopharmacology With Mood-Stabilizing Agents 463
Summary and Key Points 470

Chapter 18 **Anxiety, Obsessive-Compulsive, and Related Disorders** 475
Introduction 476
Historical Perspectives 476
Epidemiology 478
How Much Is Too Much? 478
Application of the Nursing Process 479
Background Assessment Data 479
Diagnosis and Outcome Identification 488
Planning and Implementation 489
Concept Care Mapping 489
Patient and Family Education 489
Evaluation 495
Treatment Modalities 495
Individual Psychotherapy 495
Cognitive Behavior Therapy (CBT) 497
Behavior Therapy 498
Psychopharmacology 499
Summary and Key Points 503

Chapter 19 **Trauma- and Stressor-Related Disorders** 508
Introduction 508
Historical Perspectives and Epidemiology 509
Application of the Nursing Process—Trauma-Related Disorders 510
Trauma-Informed Care 510
Background Assessment Data 510
Predisposing Factors Related to Trauma-Related Disorders 511
Diagnosis and Outcome Identification 514
Planning and Implementation 515
Patient and Family Education 515
Evaluation 517
Application of the Nursing Process—Stressor-Related Disorders 518
Background Assessment Data 518
Predisposing Factors to Adjustment Disorders 519
Diagnosis and Outcome Identification 519
Planning and Implementation 520
Evaluation 520
Treatment Modalities 523
Trauma-Related Disorders 523
Adjustment Disorders 526
Summary and Key Points 528

Chapter 20 **Somatic Symptom and Dissociative Disorders** 533
Introduction 534
Historical Perspectives 534
Epidemiology 535
Application of the Nursing Process 536
Background Assessment Data for Somatic Symptom Disorders 536
Predisposing Factors Associated With Somatic Symptom and Related Disorders 539
Background Assessment Data for Dissociative Disorders 540
Predisposing Factors Associated With Dissociative Disorders 542
Diagnosis and Outcome Identification 543
Planning and Implementation 544
Concept Care Mapping 544
Patient and Family Education 552
Evaluation 553
Treatment Modalities 553
Somatic Symptom Disorders 553
Dissociative Amnesia 554
Dissociative Identity Disorder 554
Depersonalization-Derealization Disorder 554
Summary and Key Points 556

Chapter 21 **Eating Disorders** 561
Introduction 561
Epidemiology 562
Application of the Nursing Process 564
Background Assessment Data 564
Predisposing Factors and Theories of Etiology Associated With AN, BN, and BED 566
Diagnosis and Outcome Identification 568
Planning and Implementation 568
Concept Care Mapping 576
Patient and Family Education 576
Evaluation 576
Treatment Modalities 579
Behavior Modification 580
Family Treatment: The Maudsley Approach 580
Individual Therapy 580
Psychopharmacology 580
Summary and Key Points 582

Chapter 22 **Personality Disorders** 587
Introduction 588
Historical Perspectives 590
Types of Personality Disorders 590
Paranoid Personality Disorder 590
Schizoid Personality Disorder 591
Schizotypal Personality Disorder 591
Antisocial Personality Disorder 592
Borderline Personality Disorder 592
Histrionic Personality Disorder 592
Narcissistic Personality Disorder 593
Avoidant Personality Disorder 594
Dependent Personality Disorder 594
Obsessive-Compulsive Personality Disorder 595
Application of the Nursing Process: Borderline Personality Disorder 596
Background Assessment Data 596
Diagnosis and Outcome Identification 599
Planning and Implementation 599
Concept Care Mapping 600
Evaluation 604
Application of the Nursing Process: Antisocial Personality Disorder 604
Background Assessment Data 604
Diagnosis and Outcome Identification 608
Planning and Implementation 608
Concept Care Mapping 608
Evaluation 608
Treatment Modalities 613
Individual Psychotherapy 613
Milieu or Group Therapy 614
Cognitive Behavior Therapy (CBT) 614
Dialectical Behavior Therapy (DBT) 614
Psychoanalytic Therapies 614
Psychopharmacology 614
Summary and Key Points 616

UNIT 4
Psychiatric Mental Health Nursing of Special Populations 623

Chapter 23 **Children and Adolescents** 624
Introduction 625
Neurodevelopmental Disorders 625
Intellectual Developmental Disorder (Intellectual Disability) 625
Autism Spectrum Disorder 627
Attention Deficit-Hyperactivity Disorder 635
Tourette's Disorder 644
Disruptive Behavior Disorders 649
Oppositional Defiant Disorder 649
Conduct Disorder 652
Anxiety Disorders 656
Separation Anxiety Disorder 656
Treatment Modalities 660
Behavior Therapy 660
Family Therapy 662

Group Therapy 662
Psychopharmacology 663
Summary and Key Points 663

Chapter 24 **The Aging Individual** 669
Introduction 669
How Old Is *Old*? 670
Epidemiology 670
The Population 670
Marital Status 671
Living Arrangements 671
Economic Status 671
Employment 671
Health Status 672
Theories of Aging 672
Biological Theories 672
Psychosocial Theories 673
The Normal Aging Process 674
Biological Aspects of Aging 674
Psychological Aspects of Aging 677
Sociocultural Aspects of Aging 680
Sexual Aspects of Aging 680
Special Concerns of the Older Population 682
Retirement 682
Long-Term Care 683
Elder Abuse 683
Suicide 685
Application of the Nursing Process 686
Background Assessment Data 686
Diagnosis and Outcome Identification 686
Planning and Implementation 688
Evaluation 688
Summary and Key Points 688

Chapter 25 **Survivors of Abuse or Neglect** 700
Introduction 701
Predisposing Factors 702
Biological Theories 702
Psychological Theories 702
Sociocultural Theories 704
Application of the Nursing Process 704
Background Assessment Data 704
Diagnosis and Outcome Identification 713
Planning and Implementation 714
Evaluation 714
Forensic Nursing 714
Treatment Modalities 718
Trauma-Informed Care 718
Crisis Intervention 718
The Safe House or Shelter 719
Family-Based Interventions 719
Summary and Key Points 720

Chapter 26 **Community Mental Health Nursing** 725
Introduction 725
Historical Perspective 726
The Public Health Model 727
The Community as Client 729
Primary Prevention 729
Secondary Prevention 734
Tertiary Prevention 735
Summary and Key Points 750

Chapter 27 **The Bereaved Individual** 756
Introduction 757
Theoretical Perspectives on Loss and Bereavement 757
Stages of Grief 757
Length of the Grief Process 761
Anticipatory Grief 762
Maladaptive Responses to Loss 762
Delayed or Inhibited Grief 762
Distorted (Exaggerated) Grief Response 762
Chronic or Prolonged Grieving 763
Normal Versus Maladaptive Grieving 763
Application of the Nursing Process 764
Background Assessment Data 764
Nursing Diagnosis and Outcome Identification 765
Planning and Implementation 766
Evaluation 766
End-of-Life Resources 766
Hospice 766
Advance Directives 770
Summary and Key Points 770

Chapter 28 **Military Families** 775
Introduction 775
Historical Perspective 775
Epidemiology 776
Application of the Nursing Process 776
Background Assessment Data 776
Diagnosis and Outcome Identification 785
Planning, Implementation, and Evaluation 785
Treatment Modalities 785
Post-traumatic Stress Disorder 785
Traumatic Brain Injury 790
Summary and Key Points 790

Appendix A Mental Status Assessment A-1

Appendix B Glossary A-5

Appendix C Answers to Review Questions A-29

Appendix D Examples of Answers to Communication Exercises A-31

Index I-1

Ebook Bonus Chapters

Chapter 29 **Concepts of Personality Development** 795

Introduction 795
Psychoanalytic Theory 796
Structure of the Personality 796
Topography of the Mind 797
Dynamics of the Personality 797
Freud's Stages of Personality Development 798
Relevance of Psychoanalytic Theory to Nursing Practice 799
Interpersonal Theory 799
Sullivan's Stages of Personality Development 800
Relevance of Interpersonal Theory to Nursing Practice 801
Theory of Psychosocial Development 801
Erikson's Stages of Personality Development 801
Relevance of Psychosocial Development Theory to Nursing Practice 804
Theory of Object Relations 804
Mahler's Phases of Infant Development 804
Relevance of Object Relations Theory to Nursing Practice 805
A Nursing Model—Hildegard E. Peplau 805
Phases of the Nurse-Patient Relationship 806
Peplau's Stages of Personality Development 806
Relevance of Peplau's Model to Nursing Practice 809
Summary and Key Points 809

Chapter 30 **Complementary and Integrative Therapies** 812

Introduction 812
Differences Between Complementary and Conventional Health Care 818
Types of Complementary Therapies 818
Herbal Medicine 818
Acupressure and Acupuncture 819
Diet and Nutrition 822
Chiropractic Medicine 823
Therapeutic Touch 828
Massage 828
Yoga 829
Animal-Assisted Therapy and Pets 829
Summary and Key Points 831

Chapter 31 **Cultural Concepts Relevant to Psychiatric Mental Health Nursing** 835

Cultural Concepts 835
How Do Cultures Differ? 837
Communication 837
Space 837
Social Organization 838
Time 838
Environmental Control 838
Biological Variations 839
Changing Trends in American Culture and Nurse Self-Awareness 839
Health-Care Disparities 840
Cultural Syndromes 840
Application of the Nursing Process 840
Background Assessment Data 840
Diagnosis and Outcome Identification 842
Planning and Implementation 842
Evaluation 844
Summary and Key Points 844

Chapter 32 **Issues Related to Human Sexuality and Gender Dysphoria** 847

Introduction 848
Gender Dysphoria 848
Course and Epidemiology 849
Predisposing Factors 849
Application of the Nursing Process to Gender Dysphoria in Children 849
Background Assessment Data 849
Diagnosis and Outcome Identification 849
Planning and Implementation 850
Evaluation 850
Treatment Issues 850
Gender Dysphoria in Adolescents and Adults 850
Treatment Issues 852
Paraphilic Disorders 853
Epidemiology 853
Types of Paraphilic Disorders 855
Predisposing Factors and Theories of Etiology 857
Treatment Modalities 857
Role of the Nurse in the Treatment of Persons With Paraphilias 858
Sexual Dysfunctions 858
The Human Sexual Response Cycle 858
Historical Perspectives and Epidemiology 859
Types of Sexual Dysfunction 859
Predisposing Factors 860
Application of the Nursing Process to Sexual Dysfunctions 862
Background Assessment Data 862
Diagnosis and Outcome Identification 862
Planning and Implementation 864
Concept Care Mapping 864
Patient and Family Education 864
Evaluation 864
Treatment Modalities 864
Summary and Key Points 871

UNIT 1

Introduction to Psychiatric Mental Health Concepts

1 Mental Health and Mental Illness

CORE CONCEPTS
Stress and Coping
Grief and Loss

CHAPTER OUTLINE

Objectives
Introduction
Mental Health
Mental Illness
Physical and Psychological Responses to Stress
Summary and Key Points
Review Questions
Clinical Judgment Questions

KEY TERMS

anosognosia
anxiety
coping skills
ego defense mechanisms
fight-or-flight syndrome
grief
mental health
mental illness
neurosis
psychosis

OBJECTIVES

After reading this chapter, the student will be able to:

1. Define *mental health* and *mental illness*.
2. Discuss cultural elements that influence attitudes toward mental health and mental illness.
3. Identify physiological responses to stress.
4. Discuss the concepts of anxiety and grief as psychological responses to stress.

Introduction

The concepts of mental health and mental illness are rooted in the culture of one's society. Some cultures are quite liberal in the range of behaviors that are considered acceptable, whereas others have very little tolerance for behaviors that deviate from the cultural norms (Abdullah & Brown, 2011). A study of the history of psychiatric care reveals some shocking truths about past treatment of mentally ill individuals. Many were kept in control by means that were cruel and inhumane because of erroneous views of mental illness that we now know to be incorrect.

Older beliefs regarding mental disturbances took several views. Some thought that individuals with mental illness had been dispossessed of their souls and that the only way wellness could be achieved was if the souls returned. Others believed that evil spirits or supernatural or magical powers had entered the body. The "cure" for these individuals involved a ritualistic exorcism that often consisted of brutal beatings, starvation, or other harsh means to purge the body of these unwanted forces. Still others considered that the mentally ill individual may have broken a taboo or sinned against another individual or God, for which ritualistic purification was required or various types of retribution were demanded. The correlation of mental illness to demonology or witchcraft led to some mentally ill individuals being executed.

This chapter defines *mental health* and *mental illness* and describes physical and psychological responses to stress. Symptoms associated with anxiety and grief are presented as major psychological responses in the adaptation to stress.

Mental Health

A number of theorists have attempted to define the concept of mental health. Many of these concepts focus on how well the individual is able to function. Maslow (1970) emphasized that mental health is associated with an individual's motivation toward self-actualization. He identified a "hierarchy of needs," with the lower needs requiring fulfillment before those at higher levels can be achieved, and self-actualization being fulfillment of one's highest potential. An individual's position within the hierarchy may fluctuate on the basis of life circumstances. For example, an individual facing major surgery who has been working on tasks to achieve self-actualization may become preoccupied, if only temporarily, with the need for physiological safety. A representation of this needs hierarchy is presented in Figure 1–1.

Maslow described self-actualization as the state of being "psychologically healthy, fully human, highly evolved, and fully mature" (p. 149). He believed that healthy, or self-actualized, individuals possessed the following characteristics:

- An appropriate perception of reality
- The ability to accept oneself, others, and human nature
- The ability to manifest spontaneity
- The capacity for focusing concentration on problem-solving
- A need for detachment and desire for privacy
- Independence, autonomy, and a resistance to enculturation
- An intensity of emotional reaction
- A frequency of "peak" experiences that validate the worthwhileness, richness, and beauty of life
- An identification with humankind
- The ability to achieve satisfactory interpersonal relationships
- A democratic character structure and strong sense of ethics

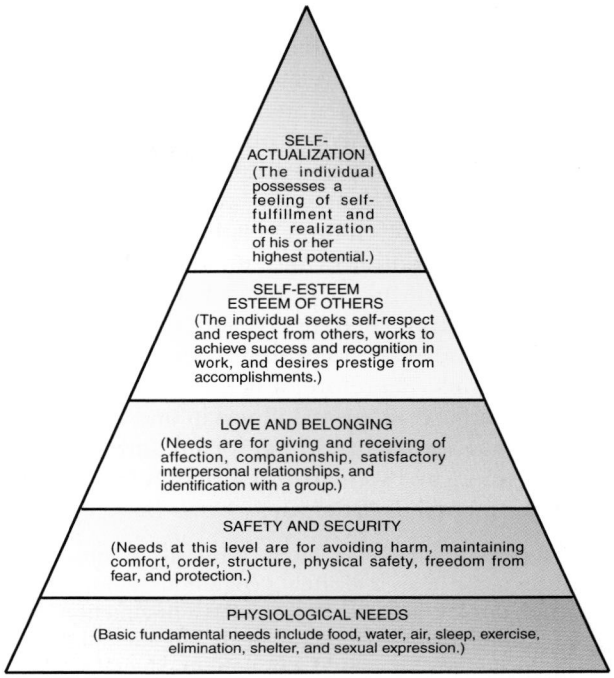

FIGURE 1–1 Maslow's hierarchy of needs.

- Creativity
- A degree of nonconformance

Expanding on this model, mental health may be viewed as a relative state that occurs along a continuum of thoughts, feelings, and behaviors that are all part of the human psychological experience and are influenced by the perceived magnitude of stressors in interaction with adaptive capabilities. For example, everyone experiences angry feelings or paranoid thoughts from time to time, but whether those thoughts and feelings result in significant or sustained distress is influenced by the individual's perceived degree of stress and their ability to adapt in healthy ways to decrease distress. In this text, we define **mental health** as "the successful adaptation to stressors from the internal or external environment, evidenced by thoughts, feelings, and behaviors that are age appropriate and congruent with local and cultural norms" (Morgan & Townsend, 2021, p. 15).

Mental Illness

Mental illness is difficult to define because of the many cultural factors that influence this concept. Horwitz (2010) attempts to define mental illness from a sociocultural perspective characterized by two elements: incomprehensibility and cultural relativity.

Incomprehensibility relates to the inability of the general population to understand the motivation behind the behavior. When observers are unable to find meaning or comprehensibility in behavior, they are likely to label that behavior as mental illness.

The element of cultural relativity considers that the rules, conventions, and understanding about behavior are conceived within an individual's own particular culture. Behavior is categorized as "normal" or "abnormal" according to one's cultural or societal norms. Therefore, a behavior that is recognized as evidence of mental illness in one society may be viewed as normal in another society and vice versa.

The American Psychiatric Association (APA, 2022) defines a mental disorder as:

> a syndrome characterized by clinically significant disturbance in an individual's cognitions, emotional regulation, or behavior that reflects a dysfunction in the psychological, biological, or developmental processes underlying mental functioning. Mental disorders are usually associated with significant distress or disability in social, occupational, or other important activities. An expected or culturally approved response to a common stressor or loss such as the death of a loved one is not a mental disorder. (p. 14)

In this text, we define **mental illness** as "maladaptive responses to stressors from the internal or external environment, evidenced by thoughts, feelings, and behaviors that are incongruent with the local and cultural norms, and interfere with the individual's social, occupational, and/or physical functioning" (Morgan & Townsend, 2021, p. 16).

An individual's experience of mental health or mental illness fluctuates along a continuum throughout life and is influenced by one's coping mechanisms in response to stress and loss.

Physical and Psychological Responses to Stress

Physical Responses

In 1956, Hans Selye published the results of his research concerning the physiological response of a biological system to a change imposed on it. After the initial publication of his findings, he revised his definition of stress as "the state manifested by a specific syndrome which consists of all the nonspecifically-induced changes within a biologic system" (Selye, 1976, p. 64). This syndrome of symptoms has come to be known as the **fight-or-flight syndrome.** Selye called the reactions of the body to stress the *general adaptation syndrome.* He described the reaction in three distinct stages:

1. ***Alarm reaction stage:*** During this stage, the responses of the fight-or-flight syndrome are initiated.
2. ***Stage of resistance:*** The individual uses the physiological responses of the first stage as a defense in an attempt to adapt to the stressor. If adaptation occurs, the third stage is prevented or delayed. Physiological symptoms may disappear.
3. ***Stage of exhaustion:*** This stage occurs when there is a prolonged exposure to the stressor to which the body has become adjusted. The adaptive energy is depleted, and the individual can no longer draw from the resources for adaptation described in the first two stages. Diseases of adaptation (e.g., headaches, mental disorders, coronary artery disease, ulcers, colitis) may occur. Without intervention for reversal, exhaustion or even death ensues (Selye, 1956, 1974).

Biological responses associated with the fight-or-flight syndrome include the following:

- ***The immediate response:*** The hypothalamus stimulates the sympathetic nervous system, which results in the following physical effects:
  - The adrenal medulla releases norepinephrine and epinephrine into the bloodstream.
  - The pupils of the eyes dilate.
  - In the lungs, the bronchioles dilate, and the respiration rate is increased.
  - The force of cardiac contraction increases, as does cardiac output, heart rate, and blood pressure.
  - Gastrointestinal motility and secretions decrease, and sphincters contract.
  - In the liver, there is increased glycogenolysis and gluconeogenesis and decreased glycogen synthesis.
  - The bladder muscle contracts, and the sphincter relaxes; there is increased ureter motility.
  - Secretion from the sweat glands is increased.
  - Lipolysis occurs in the fat cells.
- ***The sustained response:*** When the stress response is not relieved immediately and the individual remains under stress for a long period, the hypothalamus stimulates the pituitary gland to release hormones that produce the following effects:
  - Adrenocorticotropic hormone stimulates the adrenal cortex to release glucocorticoids and mineralocorticoids, resulting in increased gluconeogenesis and retention of sodium and

water and decreased immune and inflammatory responses.
- Vasopressin (antidiuretic hormone) increases fluid retention and also increases blood pressure through constriction of blood vessels.
- Growth hormone has a direct effect on protein, carbohydrate, and lipid metabolism, resulting in increased serum glucose and free fatty acids.
- Thyrotropic hormone stimulates the thyroid gland to increase the basal metabolic rate.
- Gonadotropins cause a decrease in secretion of sex hormones, resulting in decreased libido and impotence.

This fight-or-flight response undoubtedly served our ancestors well. When *Homo sapiens* had to face the giant grizzly bear or the saber-toothed tiger as part of their struggle for survival, these adaptive resources were advantageous. The response was elicited in emergencies, used in the preservation of life, and followed by restoration of the compensatory mechanisms to the pre-emergent condition (homeostasis).

Selye performed his extensive research in a controlled setting with laboratory animals as subjects. He elicited physiological responses with physical stimuli, such as exposure to heat or extreme cold, electric shock, injection of toxic agents, restraint, and surgical injury. Since the publication of Selye's original research, it has become apparent that the fight-or-flight syndrome occurs in response to psychological or emotional stimuli just as it does to physical stimuli. The psychological or emotional stressors are often not resolved as rapidly as some physical stressors; therefore, the body may be depleted of its adaptive energy more readily than it is from physical stressors. The fight-or-flight response may be inappropriate or even dangerous to the lifestyle of today, wherein stress has been described as a psychosocial state that is pervasive, chronic, and relentless. It is this chronic response that maintains the body in the aroused condition for extended periods that promotes susceptibility to diseases of adaptation.

Psychological Responses

Anxiety and grief have been described as two major, primary psychological response patterns to stress. Various thoughts, feelings, and behaviors are associated with each of these response patterns. Adaptation is determined by the degree to which the thoughts, feelings, and behaviors interfere with an individual's functioning.

CORE CONCEPT

Anxiety

Anxiety is a feeling of discomfort and apprehension related to fear of impending danger. Individuals may be unaware of the source of their anxiety, which is often accompanied by feelings of uncertainty and helplessness.

Anxiety

Feelings of anxiety are so common in our society that they are almost considered universal. Anxiety arises from the chaos and confusion that exists in the world today. Fears of the unknown and conditions of ambiguity offer a perfect breeding ground for anxiety to take root and grow. Low levels of anxiety are adaptive and can provide the motivation required for survival. Anxiety becomes problematic when the individual is unable to prevent the anxiety from escalating to a level that interferes with the ability to meet basic needs.

Peplau (1963) described four levels of anxiety: mild, moderate, severe, and panic. A variety of psychological and behavioral responses occur at each level of anxiety. Figure 1–2 depicts these responses

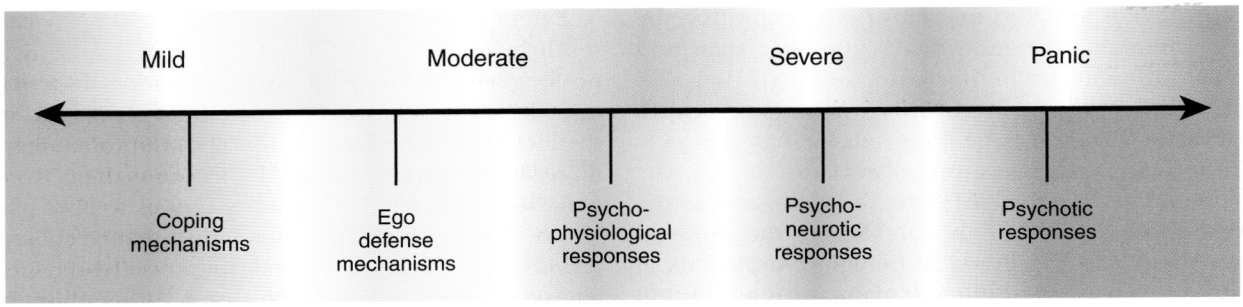

FIGURE 1–2 Adaptation responses on a continuum of anxiety.

on a continuum of anxiety ranging from mild to panic. Nurses must be able to recognize the symptoms associated with each level to plan for appropriate intervention with anxious individuals.

Mild Anxiety

Mild anxiety is seldom a problem for the individual. It is associated with the tension experienced in response to the events of day-to-day living. Mild anxiety prepares people for action. It sharpens the senses, increases motivation for productivity, increases the perceptual field, and results in a heightened awareness of the environment. Learning is enhanced, and the individual is able to function at an optimal level.

At the mild level, individuals may use a number of behaviors that satisfy their needs for comfort. Menninger (1963) described the following types of coping mechanisms that individuals use to relieve anxiety in stressful situations:

- Crying
- Cursing
- Daydreaming
- Drinking
- Eating
- Foot swinging
- Fidgeting
- Finger tapping
- Laughing
- Nail biting
- Pacing
- Physical exercise
- Sleeping
- Smoking
- Talking to someone with whom one feels comfortable
- Yawning

Undoubtedly, there are many more coping mechanisms, too numerous to mention here, considering that individuals develop their own unique ways to relieve anxiety at the mild level. Some of these behaviors are more adaptive than others. The term **coping skills** is used to describe those coping behaviors that enhance one's adaptation. These include enhancing knowledge, social affiliation with others, and problem-solving.

Mild to Moderate Anxiety

As the level of anxiety increases, the extent of the perceptual field diminishes. The moderately anxious individual is less alert to events occurring within the environment. The individual's attention span and ability to concentrate decrease, although they may still attend to needs with direction. Assistance with problem-solving may be required. Increased muscular tension and restlessness are evident.

Sigmund Freud (1961) identified the ego as the reality component of the personality that governs problem-solving and rational thinking. As the level of anxiety increases, the strength of the ego is tested, and energy is mobilized to confront the threat. Anna Freud (1953) identified a number of defense mechanisms employed by the ego in the face of threat to biological or psychological integrity (Table 1–1). Some of these **ego defense mechanisms** are more adaptive than others, but all are used either consciously or unconsciously as protective devices for the ego in an effort to relieve mild to moderate anxiety. They become maladaptive when an individual uses them to such a degree that the defense mechanism interferes with the ability to deal with reality, with interpersonal relations, or with occupational performance.

Moderate to Severe Anxiety

Anxiety at the moderate to severe level that remains unresolved over an extended period can contribute to a number of physiological disorders. The *Diagnostic and Statistical Manual of Mental Disorders, Fifth Edition, Text Revision (DSM-5-TR)* (APA, 2022) describes these disorders under the category "Psychological Factors Affecting Other Medical Conditions." The psychological factors may exacerbate symptoms of, delay recovery from, or interfere with treatment of the medical condition. The condition may be initiated or exacerbated by an environmental situation that the individual perceives as stressful. Measurable pathophysiology can be demonstrated. It is thought that psychological and behavioral factors may affect the course of almost every major category of disease, including, but not limited to, cardiovascular, gastrointestinal, neoplastic, neurological, and pulmonary conditions.

Severe Anxiety

The perceptual field of the severely anxious individual is so greatly diminished that concentration centers on only one particular detail or on many extraneous details. Attention span is extremely limited, and the individual has much difficulty completing even the simplest task. Physical symptoms (e.g., headaches, palpitations, insomnia) and emotional symptoms (e.g., confusion, dread, horror) may be evident. Discomfort is experienced to the degree that virtually all overt behavior is aimed at relieving the anxiety.

Extended periods of repressed severe anxiety can result in neurotic patterns of behaving. Neurosis is no longer considered a separate category of mental disorder. However, the term sometimes is still used in the literature to further describe the symptomatology of certain disorders and to differentiate them from behaviors that occur at the more serious level of psychosis. A **neurosis** is a psychiatric disturbance characterized by excessive anxiety that is expressed directly or altered through defense mechanisms. Although there is no gross distortion of reality or severe personality disorganization, the symptoms are significant enough

TABLE 1–1 **Ego Defense Mechanisms**

DEFENSE MECHANISM	EXAMPLE	DEFENSE MECHANISM	EXAMPLE
COMPENSATION		**RATIONALIZATION**	
Covering up a real or perceived weakness by emphasizing a trait one considers more desirable	A teenage boy with cerebral palsy is unable to participate in football, so he compensates by becoming a great student.	Attempting to make excuses or formulate logical reasons to justify unacceptable feelings or behaviors	A patient tells the rehab nurse, "I drink because it's the only way I can deal with my bad marriage and my worse job."
DENIAL		**REACTION FORMATION**	
Refusing to acknowledge the existence of a real situation or the feelings associated with it	A woman drinks alcohol every day, cannot stop, and does not acknowledge that she has a problem.	Preventing unacceptable or undesirable thoughts or behaviors from being expressed by exaggerating opposite thoughts or types of behaviors	A student attended nursing school to please her parents, but she hates nursing. During career day, she speaks to prospective students about the excellence of nursing as a career.
DISPLACEMENT		**REGRESSION**	
The transfer of feelings from one target to another that is considered less threatening or that is neutral	A patient is angry at his doctor and does not express it but becomes verbally abusive with the nurse.	Responding to stress by retreating to an earlier level of development and the comfort measures associated with that level of functioning	When a 2-year-old is hospitalized for tonsillitis, he will drink only from a bottle, although his mother states he has been drinking from a cup for 6 months.
IDENTIFICATION		**REPRESSION**	
An attempt to increase self-worth by acquiring certain attributes and characteristics of an individual one admires	A teenager who required lengthy rehabilitation after an accident decides to become a physical therapist as a result of his experiences.	Involuntarily blocking unpleasant feelings and experiences from one's awareness	A trauma victim is unable to remember anything about the traumatic event.
INTELLECTUALIZATION		**SUBLIMATION**	
An attempt to avoid expressing actual emotions associated with a stressful situation by using the intellectual processes of logic, reasoning, and analysis	A woman's husband is being transferred to a city far away from their hometown. She hides her anxiety by explaining to her parents the advantages associated with the move.	Rechanneling of drives or impulses that are personally or socially unacceptable into activities that are constructive	A mother whose son was killed by a drunk driver channels her anger and energy into being the president of the local chapter of Mothers Against Drunk Drivers.
INTROJECTION		**SUPPRESSION**	
Integrating the beliefs and values of another individual into one's own ego structure	Children integrate their parents' value system into the process of conscience formation. A child says to a friend, "Don't cheat. It's wrong."	The voluntary blocking of unpleasant feelings and experiences from one's awareness	"I don't want to think about that now. I'll think about that tomorrow."
ISOLATION		**UNDOING**	
Separating a thought or memory from the feeling, tone, or emotion associated with it	A young woman describes being attacked and raped without showing any emotion.	Symbolically negating or canceling out an experience that one finds intolerable	A man is nervous about his new job and yells at his wife. On his way home, he stops and buys her some flowers.
PROJECTION			
Attributing feelings or impulses unacceptable to oneself to another person	A man who is addicted to alcohol blames his wife for his excessive drinking.		

to impair a person's functioning. The following are common characteristics of people with neuroses:

- They are aware that they are experiencing distress.
- They are aware that their behaviors are maladaptive.
- They are unaware of any possible psychological causes of the distress.
- They feel helpless to change their situation.
- They experience no loss of contact with reality.

The following disorders are examples of psychoneurotic responses to severe anxiety as they appear in the *DSM-5-TR*:

- ***Anxiety disorders:*** Disorders in which the characteristic features are symptoms of anxiety and avoidance behavior (e.g., phobias, panic disorder, generalized anxiety disorder, and separation anxiety disorder)
- ***Somatic symptom and related disorders:*** Disorders in which the characteristic feature is a preoccupation with distressing somatic symptoms for which there is no demonstrable organic pathology; psychological factors are judged to play a significant role in the onset, severity, exacerbation, or maintenance of the symptoms (e.g., somatic symptom disorder, illness anxiety disorder, conversion disorder, and factitious disorder)
- ***Dissociative disorders:*** Disorders in which the characteristic feature is a disruption in the usually integrated functions of consciousness, memory, identity, or perception of the environment (e.g., dissociative amnesia, dissociative identity disorder, and depersonalization-derealization disorder)

Panic Anxiety

In this most intense state of anxiety, the individual is unable to focus on even one detail within the environment. Misperceptions are common, and a loss of contact with reality may occur. The individual may experience hallucinations or delusions. Behavior may be characterized by wild and desperate actions or extreme withdrawal. Human functioning and communication with others are ineffective. Panic anxiety is associated with a feeling of terror, and individuals may be convinced that they have a life-threatening illness or fear that they are "going crazy," are losing control, or are emotionally weak. Prolonged panic anxiety can lead to physical and emotional exhaustion and can be life threatening.

At this extreme level of anxiety, an individual is not capable of processing what is happening in the environment and may lose contact with reality.

Psychosis is defined as a significant thought disturbance in which reality testing is impaired, resulting in delusions, hallucinations, disorganized speech, or catatonic behavior. The following are common characteristics of people with psychoses:

- They exhibit minimal distress (emotional tone is flat, bland, or inappropriate).
- They are unaware that their behavior is mal-adaptive.
- They may be unaware of any psychological problems **(anosognosia)**.
- They are exhibiting a flight from reality into a less stressful world or into one in which they are attempting to adapt.

Examples of psychotic responses to anxiety include the schizophrenic, schizoaffective, and delusional disorders.

CORE CONCEPT

Grief

Grief is a subjective feeling of sorrow and sadness accompanied by emotional, physical, and social responses to the loss of a loved person or thing.

Grief

A loss is anything that is perceived as such by the individual. Losses may be real, in which case they can be substantiated by others (e.g., death of a loved one, loss of personal possessions), or they may be perceived by the individual alone and unable to be shared or identified by others (e.g., loss of the feeling of femininity following a mastectomy). Any situation that creates change for an individual can be identified as a loss. Failure (either real or perceived) can be viewed as a loss. Most individuals experience intense emotional anguish in response to a significant personal loss. Loss is typically a very stressful event and, like other stressors, an individual's response to loss may be adaptive or maladaptive.

The loss, or anticipated loss, of anything of value to an individual can trigger the grief response. This period of grief-related emotions and behaviors is called *mourning* and the duration of this process is individual and variable. The "normal" mourning process, which may include feelings of sadness, guilt, anger, helplessness, hopelessness, and despair, is adaptive. Indeed, an absence of mourning after a loss may be considered maladaptive. Grief is not considered a mental illness, but maladaptive responses to grief may culminate in clinical depression or other symptoms of mental illness, including risk for suicide. Careful assessment to differentiate normal grief responses from those that require additional treatment is critical to maintaining patient safety. An in-depth discussion of the usual stages of grief and maladaptive grief responses can be found in Chapter 27, "The Bereaved Individual."

Anxiety and grief have been described as two primary responses to stress. The severity of symptoms and the ability to adapt effectively are influential along a continuum of one's experience of mental health or mental illness.

Summary and Key Points

- Mental health is defined as "the successful adaptation to stressors from the internal or external environment evidenced by thoughts, feelings, and behaviors that are age appropriate and congruent with local and cultural norms" (Morgan & Townsend, 2021, p. 15).
- Mental illness is defined as "maladaptive responses to stressors from the internal or external environment, evidenced by thoughts, feelings, and behaviors that are incongruent with the local and cultural norms, and interfere with the individual's social, occupational, and/or physical functioning" (Morgan & Townsend, 2021, p. 16).
- From a sociocultural perspective, behavior may be labeled as mental illness on the basis of incomprehensibility and cultural relativity.
- When observers are unable to find meaning or comprehensibility in behavior, they are likely to label that behavior as mental illness. The meaning of behaviors is determined within individual cultures.
- Selye, who has become known as the founding father of stress research, defined stress as "the state manifested by a specific syndrome which consists of all the nonspecifically-induced changes within a biologic system" (Selye, 1976, p. 64).
- Selye determined that physical beings respond to stressful stimuli with a predictable set of physiological changes. He described the response in three stages of the general adaptation syndrome: (1) the alarm reaction stage, (2) the stage of resistance, and (3) the stage of exhaustion. Many illnesses, or diseases of adaptation, have their origin in this aroused state, which is the preparation for fight or flight.
- Anxiety and grief have been identified as the two primary responses to stress.
- Peplau (1963) defined anxiety by levels of symptom severity: mild, moderate, severe, and panic.
- Behaviors associated with levels of anxiety include coping mechanisms, ego defense mechanisms, psychophysiological responses, psychoneurotic responses, and psychotic responses.
- Grief is described as a response to loss of a valued entity. It can be an adaptive or a maladaptive experience.

Review Questions

Select the answer that is most appropriate for each of the following questions:

1. Which of the following is a true statement regarding Maslow's hierarchy of needs?
   a. Self-actualization cannot be effectively achieved if an individual is struggling with unmet safety and security needs.
   b. Self-actualized individuals have learned how to have no emotional reactions.
   c. Physiological health is the highest achievement in the hierarchy.
   d. All of the above.
2. A sociocultural perspective defines mental illness as:
   a. A disruption of brain chemicals in response to stress
   b. A *DSM-5-TR* diagnosis
   c. Behavior that is incomprehensible within one's culture
   d. Any illness that responds to psychotropic medication

Continued

3. When an individual remains under stress for a prolonged period, which of the following physiological effects occur? (Select all that apply.)
   a. Uncompensated inflammation
   b. Decreased immune response
   c. Fluid retention
   d. Hypotension
4. Which of the following are manifestations of mild anxiety?
   a. Less alertness to the environment and emotional numbness
   b. Sharp senses and motivation for productivity
   c. Ability to focus on only one detail
   d. Feeling out of control and exhibiting wild behavior
5. Extended periods of unmanaged or repressed severe anxiety may be associated with which of the following psychiatric symptoms?
   a. Panic disorder
   b. Phobias
   c. Somatic symptoms
   d. All of the above

Clinical Judgment Questions

6. A client with a history of substance use disorder is sent to the mental health clinic by their employer who expresses concern about their drinking alcohol on the job. The client denies having a problem and reports only drinking a little when the boss is "acting like a jerk". The nurse should document that the client is manifesting which defense mechanisms?
   a. Compensation and intellectualization
   b. Regression and reaction formation
   c. Denial and rationalization
   d. Undoing and projection
7. A client with a history of schizophrenia is brought to the emergency department by police who report that they were knocking down food displays at a grocery store and yelling that the food was all poisoned. The client reports to the nurse that they have no idea why they were brought to the emergency department because "there is nothing wrong with me." Which of these actions by the nurse demonstrates good clinical judgment?
   a. Instruct the police officer that this client should be incarcerated because there is nothing that can be done in an emergency department.
   b. Document that the client is manifesting psychotic symptoms and anosognosia.
   c. Ask the doctor to order gastric lavage because the client reports having been poisoned.
   d. Instruct the client that the food is not poisoned and there is something very wrong with them.
8. During a primary care physician appointment, a client who has been a widow for 7 years reports to the nurse not wanting to wake up in the morning and feeling like there is nothing left to live for. Which of these actions by the nurse is a priority?
   a. Listen empathically and encourage the client to find some activities to increase socialization.
   b. Encourage the client to discuss this with the physician.
   c. Assess the client for symptoms of depression and suicide risk.
   d. Instruct the client that grief takes a few months to resolve.

9. A client who has arrived at the health clinic for diabetic education is perspiring and states, "I'm so anxious about giving myself shots I can hardly breathe. I don't know what to do." Which of these actions by the nurse demonstrates good clinical judgment?
   a. Assist the client in relaxation exercises before commencing diabetes education.
   b. Instruct the client that it is not hard to give oneself a shot and commence teaching.
   c. Assess the client further for symptoms of anxiety.
   d. Cancel diabetic education and encourage the client to reschedule when they feel less anxious.
10. A client who was admitted to the psychiatric unit for major depressive disorder reports to the nurse, "Ever since my daughter died a year ago, I've been feeling depressed and thinking about suicide." Which of these actions by the nurse demonstrates good clinical judgment?
   a. Affirm that the client is not really depressed; but rather is simply experiencing grief.
   b. Assess the client's grief response and risk for suicide.
   c. Instruct the client that they just need time to heal from their grief.
   d. Assess what caused the daughter's death.

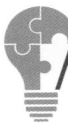

Go to **Davis Advantage** to complete your learning: strengthen understanding, apply your knowledge, and prepare for the Next Gen NCLEX®.

References

Abdullah, T., & Brown, T. L. (2011). Mental illness stigma and ethnocultural beliefs, values, and norms: An integrative review. *Clinical Psychology Review, 31*(6), 934–948.

American Psychiatric Association. (2022). *Diagnostic and statistical manual of mental disorders* (5th ed., text rev.).

Horwitz, A. V. (2010). *The social control of mental illness.* Percheron Press.

Morgan, K., & Townsend, M. C. (2021). *Psychiatric/mental health nursing: Concepts of care in evidence-based practice* (10th ed.). F.A. Davis.

Classical References

Freud, A. (1953). *The ego and mechanisms of defense.* International Universities Press.

Freud, S. (1961). *The ego and the id. In Standard edition of the complete psychological works of Freud (Vol. XIX).* Hogarth Press.

Maslow, A. (1970). *Motivation and personality* (2nd ed.). Harper & Row.

Menninger, K. (1963). *The vital balance.* Viking Press.

Peplau, H. (1963). A working definition of anxiety. In S. Burd & M. Marshall (Eds.), *Some clinical approaches to psychiatric nursing.* Macmillan.

Selye, H. (1956). *The stress of life.* McGraw-Hill.

Selye, H. (1974). *Stress without distress.* Signet Books.

Selye, H. (1976). *The stress of life* (Rev. ed.). McGraw-Hill.

2 Biological Implications

CORE CONCEPTS

Growth and Development: Genetics

Intracranial Regulation: Neuroendocrinology, Psychobiology, Nerve cells, Neurotransmitters

Immunity: Psychoneuroimmunology, Inflammation

Safety

CHAPTER OUTLINE

Objectives
Introduction
The Nervous System: An Anatomical Review
Neuroendocrinology
Genetics
Psychoneuroimmunology (PNI)
Psychopharmacology and the Brain
Implications for Nursing
Summary and Key Points
Review Questions

KEY TERMS

axon
cell body
circadian rhythms
dendrites
genotype
limbic system
neuron
neurotransmitters
phenotype
receptor sites
synapse

OBJECTIVES

After reading this chapter, the student will be able to:

1. Identify gross anatomical structures of the brain and describe their functions.
2. Discuss the physiology of neurotransmission in the central nervous system.
3. Describe the role of neurotransmitters in human behavior.
4. Discuss the association of endocrine functioning with the development of psychiatric disorders.
5. Describe the role of genetics in the development of psychiatric disorders.
6. Discuss the correlation of alteration in brain functioning to various psychiatric disorders.
7. Identify various diagnostic procedures used to detect alteration in biological functioning that may be contributing to psychiatric disorders.
8. Discuss the influence of psychological factors on the immune system.
9. Describe the biological mechanisms of psychoactive drugs at neural synapses.
10. Recognize various theorized influences in the development of psychiatric disorders, including brain physiology, genetics, endocrine function, immune system, and psychosocial and environmental factors.
11. Discuss the implications of psychobiological concepts for the practice of psychiatric mental health nursing.

Introduction

In recent years, a greater emphasis has been placed on the study of the organic basis for psychiatric illness. This "neuroscientific revolution," with its focus on the biological basis of behavior, has led to several mental illnesses now being considered neurodevelopmental disorders resulting from malfunctions and/or malformations of the brain.

That some behaviors and psychiatric illnesses can be traced to biological causes does not imply that psychosocial and sociocultural influences do not play a role in mental health disorders. For example, there is evidence that *psychological* interventions have an influence on brain activity that is similar to psychopharmacological intervention (Collerton, 2013; Flor, 2014; Mason et al., 2017), and evidence exists that lifestyle choices, such as marijuana use, can precipitate mental illness (psychosis) in individuals with genetic vulnerability (National Institutes of Health [NIH], 2020). Ongoing research will build a better understanding of the complex interplay of neural activities within the brain and in interaction with one's environment.

The systems of biology, psychology, and sociology are not mutually exclusive—they are interacting systems. This interaction is clearly indicated by the fact that individuals experience biological changes in response to various environmental events. Indeed, one or several of these systems may, at various times, explain behavioral phenomena.

This chapter focuses on the role of neurophysiological, neurochemical, genetic, and endocrine influences on psychiatric illness. An introduction to psychopharmacology is included (discussed in more detail in Chapter 4, "Psychopharmacology"), and various diagnostic procedures used to detect alteration in biological function that may contribute to psychiatric illness are identified. The implications for psychiatric mental health nursing are discussed.

CORE CONCEPT

Psychobiology

The study of the biological foundations of cognitive, emotional, and behavioral processes.

The Nervous System: An Anatomical Review

The Brain

The brain has three major divisions subdivided into five major parts:

1. Forebrain
   a. Cerebrum
   b. Diencephalon
2. Midbrain (Mesencephalon)
3. Hindbrain
   a. Pons
   b. Medulla
   c. Cerebellum

Each of these structures is discussed individually. A summary is presented in Table 2–1.

Cerebrum

The cerebrum consists of a right and left hemisphere and constitutes the largest part of the human brain. The right and left hemispheres are separated by a deep groove but remain connected to each other by a band of 200 million axons (nerve fibers) called the *corpus callosum.* Because each hemisphere controls different functions, information is processed through the corpus callosum so that each hemisphere is aware of the activity of the other.

The surface of the cerebrum consists of gray matter and is called the *cerebral cortex.* The gray matter is composed of neuron cell bodies that appear gray to the eye. These structures are thought to be the actual "thinking" structures of the brain. The *basal ganglia,* four subcortical nuclei of gray matter (the striatum, pallidum, substantia nigra, and subthalamic nuclei), are found deep within the cerebral hemispheres. They are responsible for certain subconscious aspects of voluntary movement, such as swinging the arms when walking and gesturing while speaking, and for regulating muscle tone (Scanlon & Sanders, 2018).

The cerebral cortex is identified by numerous folds, called *gyri,* and deep grooves between the folds, called *sulci.* This extensive folding extends the surface area of the cerebral cortex and thus permits the presence of millions more neurons than would be possible without it (as is the case in the brains of some animals, such as dogs and cats). Each hemisphere of the cerebral cortex is divided into the frontal lobe, parietal lobe, temporal lobe, and occipital

TABLE 2–1 Structure and Function of the Brain

STRUCTURE	PRIMARY FUNCTION
I. THE FOREBRAIN	
A. Cerebrum	Composed of two hemispheres connected by a band of nerve tissue that houses a band of 200 million axons called the *corpus callosum*. The outer layer is called the *cerebral cortex*. It is extensively folded and consists of billions of neurons. The left hemisphere appears to deal with logic and solving problems. The right hemisphere may be called the "creative" brain and is associated with affect, behavior, and spatial-perceptual functions. Each hemisphere is divided into four lobes:
1. Frontal lobes	Voluntary body movement, including movements that permit speaking, thinking and judgment formation, and expression of feelings.
2. Parietal lobes	Perception and interpretation of most sensory information (including touch, pain, taste, and body position).
3. Temporal lobes	Hearing, short-term memory, and sense of smell; expression of emotions through connection with limbic system.*
4. Occipital lobes	Visual reception and interpretation.
B. Diencephalon	Connects cerebrum with lower brain structures.
1. Thalamus	Integrates all sensory input (except smell) on way to cortex; some involvement with emotions and mood.
2. Hypothalamus	Regulates anterior and posterior lobes of pituitary gland; exerts control over actions of the autonomic nervous system; regulates appetite and temperature. Regulates visceral responses to emotional situations and body rhythms such as mood changes and sleep–wake cycles.
II. THE MIDBRAIN (mesencephalon)	Responsible for visual, auditory, and balance ("righting") reflexes.
III. THE HINDBRAIN	
A. Pons	Regulation of respiration and skeletal muscle tone; ascending and descending tracts connect brainstem with cerebellum and cortex.
B. Medulla	Pathway for all ascending and descending fiber tracts; contains vital centers that regulate heart rate, blood pressure, and respiration; reflex centers for swallowing, sneezing, coughing, and vomiting.
C. Cerebellum	Regulates muscle tone and coordination and maintains posture and equilibrium.

* The limbic system consists of medially placed cortical and subcortical structures and the fiber tracts connecting them with one another. Two of these structures are the thalamus and hypothalamus. It is sometimes called the "emotional brain"—associated with feelings of fear and anxiety; anger and aggression; and love, joy, and hope; and with sexuality and social behavior. As research has advanced our understanding of the connectivity in brain structures, it has become harder to define the boundaries of the limbic system.

lobe. These lobes, which are named for the overlying bones in the cranium, are identified in Figure 2–1.

The Frontal Lobes

Voluntary body movement is controlled by the impulses through the frontal lobes. The right frontal lobe controls motor activity on the left side of the body, and the left frontal lobe controls motor activity on the right side of the body. The frontal lobes may also play a role in emotional experience, as evidenced by changes in mood and character after damage to this area. Particularly, the prefrontal cortex (the front part of the frontal lobes) plays an essential role in the regulation and adaptation of our emotions to new situations. Morality, identified as one of the most sophisticated elements of human judgment, social cognition, decision making, and conflict resolution are impacted by the function of the prefrontal cortex (Lewis, 2017). Neuroimaging tests suggest that there may be some structural abnormalities in the frontal lobes (as well as temporal, parietal, and subcortical structures) in people with chronic schizophrenia (Lyall et al., 2017).

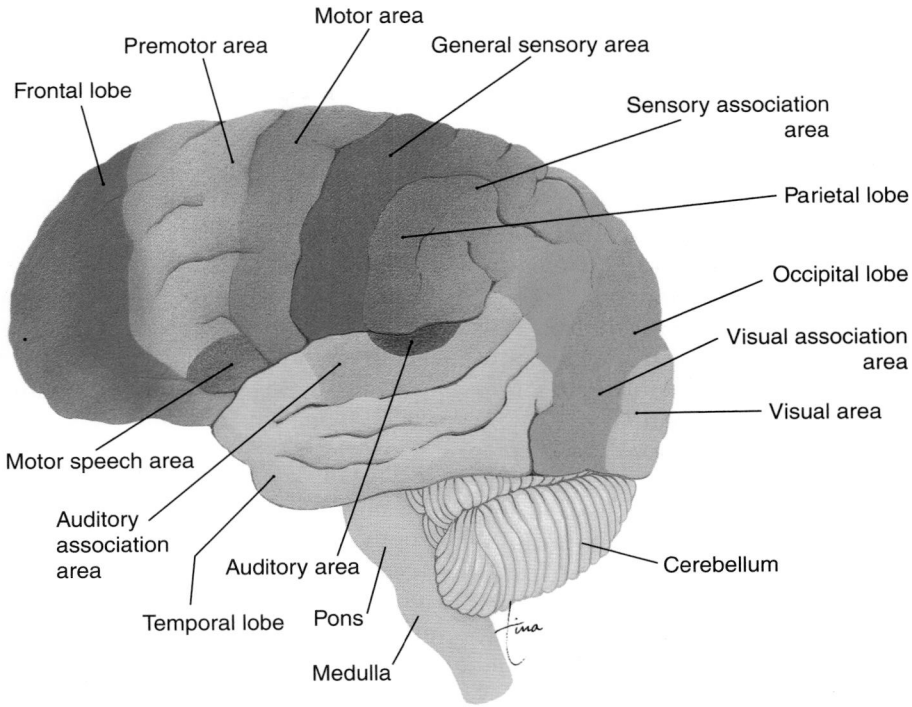

FIGURE 2–1 Left cerebral hemisphere showing some of the functional areas that have been mapped. (From *Essentials of Anatomy and Physiology* [8th ed.], by V. C. Scanlon and T. Sanders, 2018, F.A. Davis Company. Reprinted with permission.)

The Parietal Lobes

The parietal lobes manage somatosensory input, including touch, pain and pressure, taste, temperature, perception of joint and body position, and visceral sensations. The parietal lobes also contain association fibers linked to the primary sensory areas through which interpretation of sensory-perceptual information is made. Language interpretation is associated with the left hemisphere of the parietal lobe.

The Temporal Lobes

The upper anterior temporal lobe is concerned with auditory functions, and the lower part is dedicated to short-term memory. The sense of smell has a connection to the temporal lobes because the impulses carried by the olfactory nerves end in this area of the brain. The temporal lobes also play a role in the expression of emotions through an interconnection with the limbic system. The left temporal lobe, along with the left parietal lobe, is involved in language interpretation.

The Occipital Lobes

The occipital lobes are the primary area of visual reception and interpretation. Visual perception, which gives individuals the ability to judge spatial relationships such as distance and to see in three dimensions, is also processed in this area. Language interpretation is influenced by the occipital lobes through an association with the visual experience.

Diencephalon

The second part of the forebrain is the diencephalon, which connects the cerebrum with lower structures of the brain. The major components of the diencephalon include the thalamus and the hypothalamus, which are part of a neuroanatomical loop of structures known as the **limbic system.**

Thalamus

The thalamus integrates all sensory input (except smell) on its way to the cortex. This helps the cerebral cortex interpret the whole picture very rapidly rather than experiencing each sensation individually. The thalamus is also involved in temporarily blocking minor sensations so that an individual can concentrate on one important event when necessary. For example, an individual who is studying for an examination may be unaware of the clock ticking in the room, or even of another person walking into the room, because the thalamus has temporarily blocked these incoming sensations from the cortex. The impact of dopamine in the thalamus is associated with several neuropsychiatric disorders.

Hypothalamus

The hypothalamus is located just below the thalamus and just above the pituitary gland and has the following diverse functions:

1. ***Regulation of the pituitary gland:*** Many hormones are regulated by "releasing factors" from the hypothalamus. When the hormones are required by the body, the releasing factors stimulate the release of the hormone from the anterior pituitary, and the hormone in turn stimulates its target organ to carry out its specific functions.
2. ***Direct neural control over the actions of the autonomic nervous system:*** The hypothalamus regulates the appropriate visceral responses during various emotional states. The actions of the autonomic nervous system are described later in this chapter.
3. ***Regulation of appetite, temperature, blood pressure, thirst, and circadian rhythms (sleep and wakefulness):*** Appetite may be triggered or inhibited depending on which networks in the hypothalamus are stimulated. Temperature is regulated through the hypothalamus as it senses internal and external temperature changes on skin and in the blood. It then responds by triggering shivering or sweating to help maintain body temperature within the normal range. Thirst centers in the hypothalamus are stimulated by dry mouth or dehydration.
4. ***Regulation of blood pressure:*** Recent research has focused on the role of the hypothalamus in blood pressure regulation. The hypothalamus acts as an interface between the endocrine and nervous systems. It coordinates signal transduction from central and peripheral stimuli and has been identified as a key component in the development of hypertension when activated (Carmichael & Wainford, 2015). Inflammation in the hypothalamus has been found to disrupt signaling pathways affecting the control of blood pressure (Khor & Cai, 2017).

Limbic System

The limbic system is a group of structures including the amygdala, mammillary body, olfactory tract, hypothalamus, cingulate gyrus, septum pellucidum, thalamus, hippocampus, and fornix, that, through communication with the hypothalamus, controls several autonomic, endocrine, and somatic functions. This system has been called the "emotional brain" because of its association with feelings of fear and anxiety; anger, rage, and aggression; and love, joy, and hope and with sexuality and social behavior. However, as understanding of the complex connectivity within the brain has advanced, it has become increasingly difficult to define the boundaries of the limbic system, and recent research has demonstrated that some structures associated with the limbic system are involved in other complex brain processes such as memory (Melchitzky & Lewis, 2017). Nonetheless, the structures commonly associated with emotional regulation are identified in Figure 2–2. The amygdala seems to be a primary gateway for processing novel and ambiguous emotional stimuli, particularly related to fear, anxiety, and panic.

Mesencephalon (Midbrain)

The mesencephalon extends from the pons to the hypothalamus and is responsible for integration of various reflexes, including visual reflexes (e.g., automatically turning away from a dangerous object when it comes into view), auditory reflexes (e.g., automatically turning toward a sound that is heard), and righting reflexes (e.g., automatically keeping the head upright and maintaining balance).

Pons

The pons is part of the brainstem that acts as a relay station transmitting messages between various parts of the nervous system, including the cerebrum and cerebellum. It contains the central connections of cranial nerves V through VIII and centers for respiration and skeletal muscle tone. The pons is also associated with sleep and dreaming.

Medulla

The medulla is the connecting structure between the spinal cord and the pons, and all of the ascending and descending fiber tracts pass through it. The vital centers are contained in the medulla, and it is responsible for regulation of heart rate, blood pressure, and respiration. In the medulla are reflex centers for swallowing, sneezing, coughing, and vomiting. It also contains nuclei for cranial nerves IX through XII. The medulla, pons, and midbrain form the structure known as the *brainstem.*

Cerebellum

The cerebellum is separated from the brainstem by the fourth ventricle but has connections to the brainstem through bundles of fiber tracts (see Fig. 2–1). The functions of the cerebellum are concerned with involuntary aspects of movement, such as coordination, muscle tone, and the maintenance of posture and equilibrium.

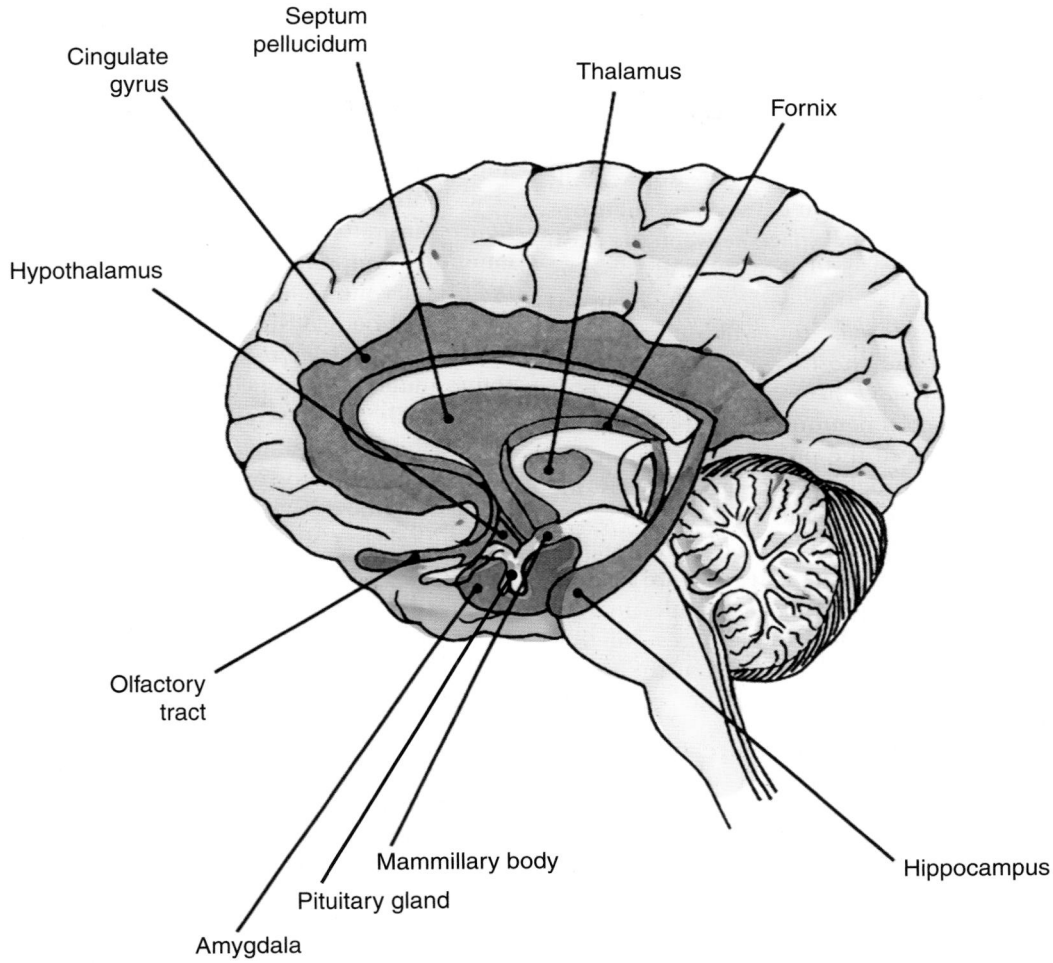

FIGURE 2–2 Structures of the limbic system. (Adapted from *Essentials of Anatomy and Physiology* [6th ed.], by V. C. Scanlon and T. Sanders, 2011, F.A. Davis Company. Reprinted with permission.)

Nerve Tissue

The tissue of the central nervous system (CNS) consists of nerve cells called *neurons* that generate and transmit electrochemical impulses. The **neuron** is composed of a cell body, an axon, and dendrites. The **cell body** contains the nucleus and is essential for the continued life of the neuron. The **dendrites** are processes that transmit impulses toward the cell body, and the **axon** transmits impulses away from the cell body. The axons and dendrites are covered by layers of cells called *neuroglia* that form a coating, or "sheath," of myelin. *Myelin* is a phospholipid that provides insulation against short-circuiting of the neurons during their electrical activity and increases the velocity of the impulse. The white matter of the brain and spinal cord is so called because of the whitish appearance of the myelin sheath over the axons and dendrites. The gray matter is composed of cell bodies that contain no myelin.

Classes of Neurons

The three classes of neurons include afferent (sensory), efferent (motor), and interneurons:

- ***Afferent neurons*** carry impulses from receptors in the internal and external periphery to the CNS, where they are then interpreted into various sensations.
- ***Efferent neurons*** carry impulses from the CNS to *effectors* in the periphery, such as muscles (that respond by contracting) and glands (that respond by secreting).
- ***Interneurons*** exist entirely within the CNS, and 99% of all nerve cells belong to this group. They may carry only sensory or motor impulses, or they may serve as integrators in the pathways between afferent and efferent neurons. They account in large part for thinking, feelings, learning, language, and memory.

Synapses

Information is transmitted through the body from one neuron to another. Some messages may be processed through only a few neurons, whereas others may require thousands of neuronal connections. The neurons that transmit the impulses do not actually touch each other. The junction between two neurons is called a **synapse.** The small space between the axon terminals of one neuron and the cell body or dendrites of another is called the *synaptic cleft.* Neurons conducting impulses toward the synapse are called *presynaptic neurons,* and those conducting impulses away are called *postsynaptic neurons.*

Chemicals that act as **neurotransmitters** are stored in the axon terminals of the presynaptic neuron. An electrical impulse through the neuron causes the release of this neurotransmitter into the synaptic cleft. The neurotransmitter then diffuses across the synaptic cleft and combines with **receptor sites** that are situated on the cell membrane of the postsynaptic neuron. The type of neurotransmitter determines whether another electrical impulse is generated at the receptor site. Excitatory neurotransmitters, when combined at the receptor site, generate an *excitatory response* and the electrical impulse moves on to the next synapse, where the same process recurs. Inhibitory neurotransmitters generate an *inhibitory response* at the receptor site, and synaptic transmission is terminated. Activity at the neural synapse is relevant in the study of psychiatric disorders because excessive or deficient activity of neurotransmitters influences a variety of cognitive and emotional symptoms, and the synapse is believed to be the primary site of activity for psychotropic drugs.

The cell body of the postsynaptic neuron also contains a chemical *inactivator* that is specific to the neurotransmitter that has been released by the presynaptic neuron. When the synaptic transmission has been completed, the chemical inactivator quickly inactivates the neurotransmitter to prevent unwanted, continuous impulses until a new impulse from the presynaptic neuron releases more neurotransmitter. Continuous impulses can result in excessive activity of neurotransmitters such as dopamine, which is believed to be responsible for symptoms such as hallucinations and delusions seen in people with schizophrenia. A schematic representation of a synapse is presented in Figure 2–3.

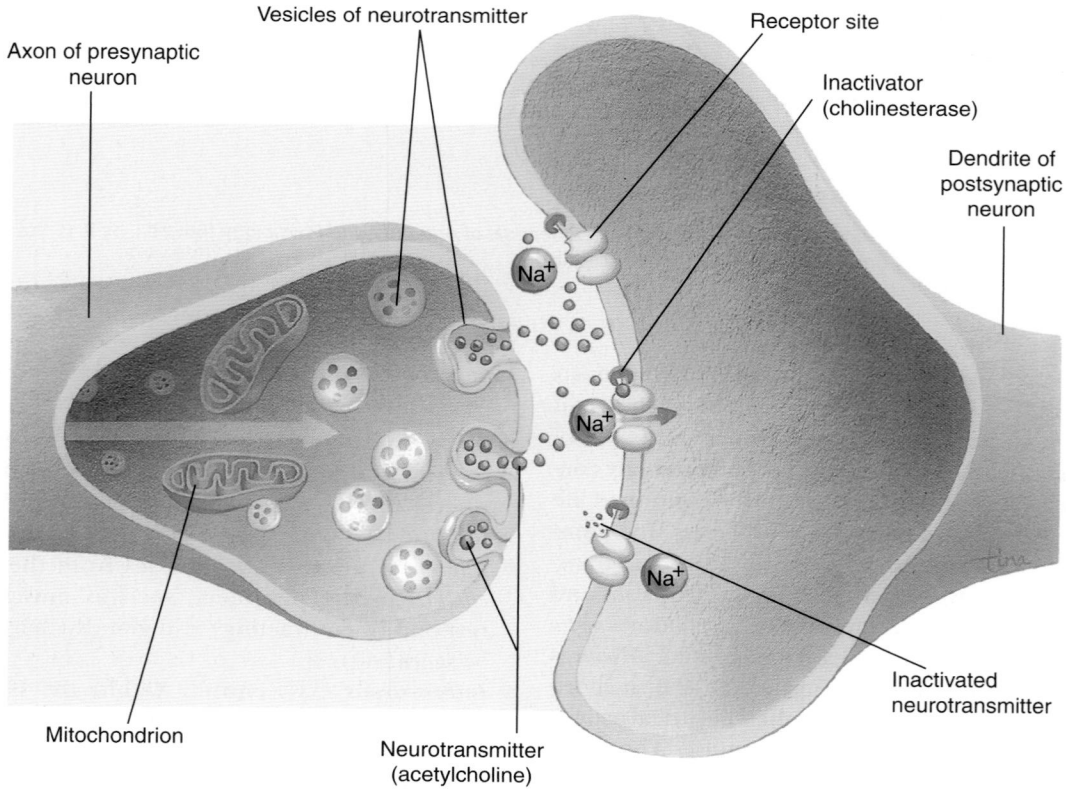

FIGURE 2–3 Impulse transmission at a synapse. The arrow indicates the direction of electrical impulses. (From *Essentials of Anatomy and Physiology* [8th ed.], by V. C. Scanlon and T. Sanders, 2018, F.A. Davis Company. Reprinted with permission.)

Autonomic Nervous System

The autonomic nervous system (ANS) is considered part of the peripheral nervous system. Its regulation is modulated by the hypothalamus, and emotions exert a great deal of influence over its functioning. For this reason, the ANS has been implicated in the etiology of a number of psychophysiological disorders.

The ANS has two divisions: the sympathetic and the parasympathetic. The sympathetic division is dominant in stressful situations and prepares the body for the fight-or-flight response (discussed in Chapter 1, "Mental Health and Mental Illness"). The fight-or-flight response causes an increase in heart rate and respirations and a decrease in digestive secretions and peristalsis. Blood is shunted to the vital organs and to skeletal muscles to ensure adequate oxygenation.

The parasympathetic division dominates when an individual is in a relaxed, nonstressful condition. The heart and respirations are maintained at a normal rate, and secretions and peristalsis increase for normal digestion. Elimination functions are promoted. A schematic representation of the ANS is presented in Figure 2–4.

Neurotransmitters

Although neurotransmitters were described during the explanation of synaptic activity, they are discussed here separately and in detail because of the essential role they have in human emotion and behavior. Neurotransmitters are also central to the therapeutic action of many psychotropic medications.

Neurotransmitters are chemicals that convey information across synaptic clefts to neighboring target cells. They are stored in small vesicles in the axon terminals of neurons. When the action potential, or electrical impulse, reaches this point, the neurotransmitters are released from the vesicles. They cross the synaptic cleft and bind with receptor sites on the cell body or dendrites of the adjacent neuron to allow the impulse to continue its course or to prevent the impulse from continuing. After the neurotransmitter has performed its function in the synapse, it returns to the vesicles to be stored and used again, or else it is inactivated and dissolved by enzymes. The process of being stored for reuse is called *reuptake*, a function that holds significance for understanding the mechanism of action of certain psychotropic medications.

Many neurotransmitters exist in the central and peripheral nervous systems, but only a limited number have implications for psychiatry. Major categories include cholinergic neurotransmitters, monoamines, amino acids, and neuropeptides. Each of these is discussed separately and summarized in Table 2–2.

Cholinergic Neurotransmitter

Acetylcholine

- ***Location:*** Acetylcholine was the first chemical to be identified and proven as a neurotransmitter. It is a major effector chemical in the ANS, producing activity at all sympathetic and parasympathetic presynaptic nerve terminals and all parasympathetic postsynaptic nerve terminals. It is highly significant in the neurotransmission that occurs at the junctions of nerve and muscles. Acetylcholinesterase is the enzyme that destroys acetylcholine or inhibits its activity. In the CNS, acetylcholine neurons innervate the cerebral cortex, hippocampus, and limbic structures. The pathways are especially dense through the area of the basal ganglia in the brain.
- ***Functions:*** Functions of acetylcholine are numerous and include sleep, arousal, pain perception, motor control, learning, and memory.
- ***Possible implications in mental illness:*** Cholinergic mechanisms may have some role in certain disorders of motor behavior and memory, such as Parkinson's disease, Huntington's disease, and Alzheimer's disease.

Monoamines

Norepinephrine

- ***Location:*** Norepinephrine is the neurotransmitter that produces activity at the sympathetic postsynaptic nerve terminals in the ANS, resulting in the fight-or-flight responses in the effector organs. In the CNS, norepinephrine pathways originate in the pons and medulla and innervate the thalamus, dorsal hypothalamus, limbic system, hippocampus, cerebellum, and cerebral cortex. When norepinephrine is not returned for storage in the vesicles of the axon terminals, it is metabolized and inactivated by the enzymes monoamine oxidase (MAO) and catechol-*O*-methyltransferase (COMT).
- ***Functions:*** The functions of norepinephrine include the regulation of mood, cognition, perception, attention, vigilance, memory, cardiovascular functioning, and sleep–wake cycles.
- ***Possible implications in mental illness:*** The activity of norepinephrine has been implicated in certain mood disorders such as depression and mania, in anxiety states, and in schizophrenia.

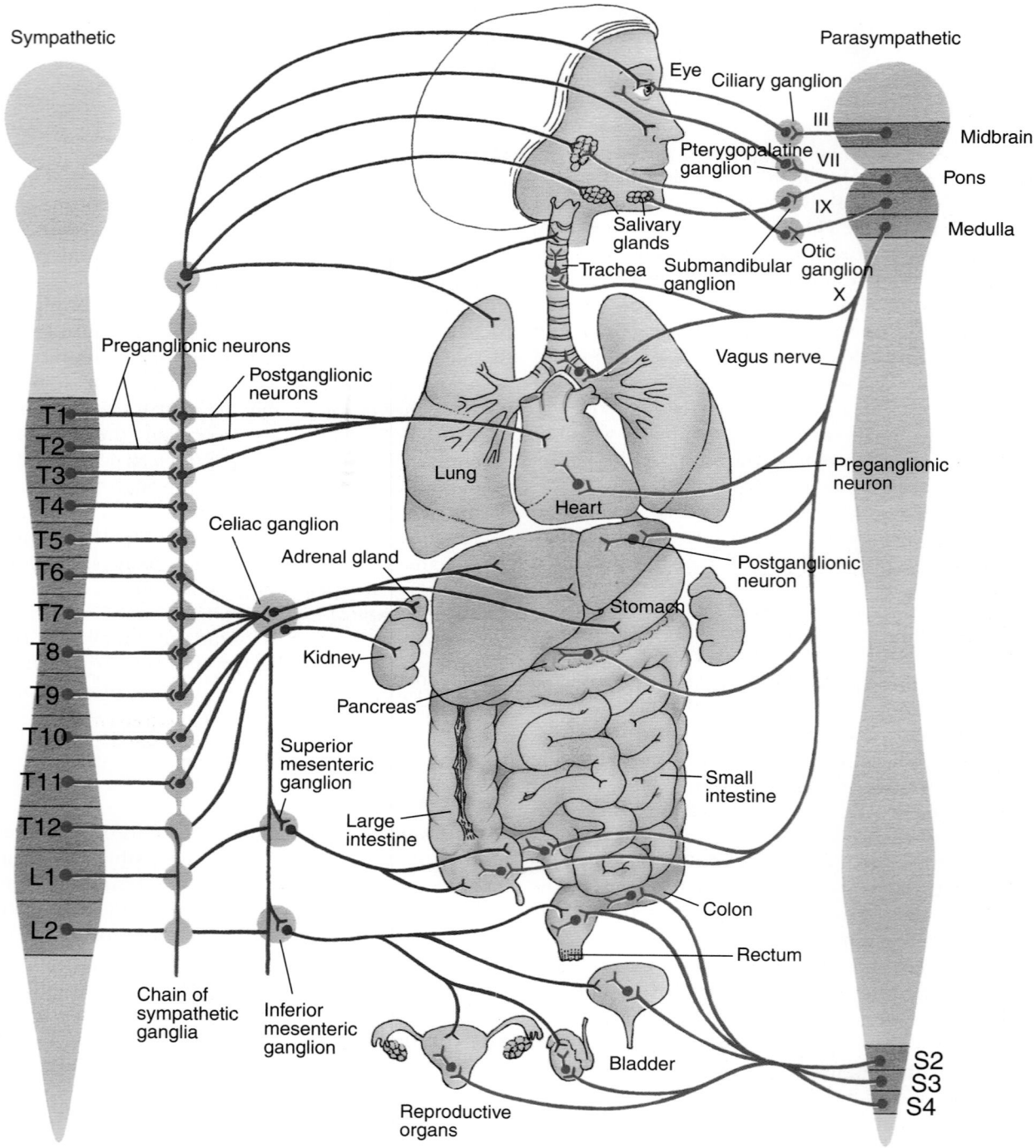

FIGURE 2–4 The autonomic nervous system. The sympathetic division is shown on the left, and the parasympathetic division is shown on the right (both divisions are bilateral). (From *Essentials of Anatomy and Physiology* [8th ed.], by V. C. Scanlon and T. Sanders, 2018, F.A. Davis Company. Reprinted with permission.)

TABLE 2–2 Neurotransmitters in the Central Nervous System

NEUROTRANSMITTER	LOCATION/FUNCTION	POSSIBLE IMPLICATIONS FOR MENTAL ILLNESS
I. CHOLINERGICS		
A. Acetylcholine	*ANS:* Sympathetic and parasympathetic presynaptic nerve terminals; parasympathetic postsynaptic nerve terminals. *CNS:* Cerebral cortex, hippocampus, limbic structures, and basal ganglia. *Functions:* Sleep, arousal, pain perception, movement, memory.	*Decreased levels:* Alzheimer's disease, Huntington's disease, Parkinson's disease *Increased levels:* Depression
II. MONOAMINES		
A. Norepinephrine	*ANS:* Sympathetic postsynaptic nerve terminals. *CNS:* Thalamus, hypothalamus, limbic system, hippocampus, cerebellum, cerebral cortex. *Functions:* Mood, cognition, perception, locomotion, cardiovascular functioning, and sleep and arousal.	*Decreased levels:* Depression *Increased levels:* Mania, anxiety states, schizophrenia
B. Dopamine	Frontal cortex, limbic system, basal ganglia, thalamus, posterior pituitary, and spinal cord. *Functions:* Movement and coordination, emotions, voluntary judgment, release of prolactin.	*Decreased levels:* Parkinson's disease, depression, Tourette syndrome, and ADHD *Increased levels:* Mania, schizophrenia, and addictions
C. Serotonin	Hypothalamus, thalamus, limbic system, cerebral cortex, cerebellum, spinal cord. *Functions:* Sleep and arousal, libido, appetite, mood, aggression, pain perception, coordination, judgment.	*Decreased levels:* Depression, anxiety *Increased levels:* Anxiety states (of the seven different types of serotonin receptors, increased levels of some [5HT1A] have an antianxiety effect, and increased levels of others [5HT3] may increase anxiety [Elsworth & Roth, 2017])
D. Histamine	Hypothalamus *Functions:* Wakefulness; pain sensation and inflammatory response.	*Decreased levels:* Depression *Increased levels:* Sleep disorders, anxiety, Alzheimer's disease, psychosis
III. AMINO ACIDS		
A. Gamma-aminobutyric acid (GABA)	Hypothalamus, hippocampus, cortex, cerebellum, basal ganglia, spinal cord, retina. *Functions:* Slowdown of body activity, reduces the activity of neurons to which it binds.	*Decreased levels:* Huntington's disease, anxiety disorders, schizophrenia, and various forms of epilepsy
B. Glycine	Spinal cord and brainstem. *Function:* Recurrent inhibition of motor neurons.	*Toxic levels:* "Glycine encephalopathy" *Decreased levels:* Correlated with spastic motor movements
C. Glutamate and aspartate	Pyramidal cells of the cortex, cerebellum, and the primary sensory afferent systems; hippocampus, thalamus, hypothalamus, spinal cord. *Functions:* Relay of sensory information and in the regulation of various motor and spinal reflexes.	*Increased levels:* Huntington's disease, temporal lobe epilepsy, spinal cerebellar degeneration, anxiety disorders, depressive disorders *Decreased levels:* Schizophrenia

Continued

TABLE 2–2 Neurotransmitters in the Central Nervous System—cont'd

NEUROTRANSMITTER	LOCATION/FUNCTION	POSSIBLE IMPLICATIONS FOR MENTAL ILLNESS
D. D-Serine	Cerebral cortex, forebrain, hippocampus, cerebellum, striatum, thalamus. *Functions:* Binds at NMDA receptors and with glutamate, is a co-agonist whose functions include mediating NMDA receptor transmission, synaptic plasticity, neurotoxicity.	*Decreased levels:* Schizophrenia
IV. NEUROPEPTIDES		
A. Endorphins and enkephalins	Hypothalamus, thalamus, limbic structures, midbrain, and brainstem; enkephalins are also found in the gastrointestinal tract *Functions:* Modulation of pain and reduced peristalsis (enkephalins).	Modulation of dopamine activity by opioid peptides may indicate some link to the symptoms of schizophrenia
B. Substance P	Hypothalamus, limbic structures, midbrain, brainstem, thalamus, basal ganglia, and spinal cord; also found in gastrointestinal tract and salivary glands. *Function:* Regulation of pain.	*Decreased levels:* Huntington's disease and Alzheimer's disease *Increased levels:* Depression
C. Somatostatin	Cerebral cortex, hippocampus, thalamus, basal ganglia, brainstem, and spinal cord *Functions:* Depending on part of the brain being affected, stimulates release of dopamine, serotonin, norepinephrine, and acetylcholine, and inhibits release of norepinephrine, histamine, and glutamate. Also acts as a neuromodulator for serotonin in the hypothalamus.	*Decreased levels:* Alzheimer's disease *Increased levels:* Huntington's disease

Dopamine

- ***Location:*** Dopamine pathways arise from the midbrain and hypothalamus and terminate in the frontal cortex, limbic system, basal ganglia, and thalamus. As with norepinephrine, the inactivating enzymes for dopamine are MAO and COMT.
- ***Functions:*** Dopamine functions include regulation of movements and coordination, emotions, reward signals, learning, memory, and voluntary decision-making ability; because of dopamine's influence on the pituitary gland, it inhibits the release of prolactin.
- ***Possible implications in mental illness:*** Increased levels of dopamine are associated with mania and schizophrenia. Decreased levels of dopamine have been associated with Parkinson's disease and depression. Dopamine may also have a role in addictions.

Serotonin

- ***Location:*** Serotonin pathways originate from cell bodies located in the pons and medulla and project to areas including the hypothalamus, thalamus, limbic system, cerebral cortex, cerebellum, and spinal cord. Serotonin that is not returned to be stored in the axon terminal vesicles is catabolized by the enzyme MAO.
- ***Functions:*** Serotonin may play a role in the sleep–wake cycle, sexual behavior, appetite, mood, anxiety, aggression, and pain perception. The fact that both too much and too little serotonin have been associated with anxiety has led to the hypothesis that serotonin may modulate intense emotional states rather than influencing one kind of mood disruption. Further, there are seven different subgroups of serotonin receptors, which, when activated, result in different effects (Elsworth & Roth, 2017).
- ***Possible implications in mental illness:*** The serotonergic system has been implicated in anxiety states, depression, and schizophrenia.

Histamine

- ***Location:*** The role of histamine in mediating allergic and inflammatory reactions has been well documented. Its role in the CNS as a neurotransmitter is the subject of ongoing research. The highest concentrations of histamine are found within various regions of the hypothalamus.

- ***Functions:*** Brain histamine regulates many physiological functions: neuroendocrine, circadian rhythms (the sleep–wake cycle), psychomotor activity, mood, learning, cognition, appetite, and eating behavior (Cacabelos et al., 2016). The enzyme that catabolizes histamine is MAO.
- ***Possible implications in mental illness:*** Alterations in brain histamine are associated with several pathological conditions, such as epilepsy, stroke, anxiety, depression, psychosis, neurodegeneration, and neuroinflammatory processes (Cacabelos et al., 2016).

Amino Acids

Inhibitory Amino Acids

Gamma-Aminobutyric Acid

- ***Location:*** Gamma-aminobutyric acid (GABA) has a widespread distribution in the CNS, with high concentrations in the hypothalamus, hippocampus, cortex, cerebellum, and basal ganglia of the brain; the gray matter of the dorsal horn of the spinal cord; and the retina. GABA is catabolized by the enzyme GABA transaminase.
- ***Functions:*** Inhibitory neurotransmitters, such as GABA, prevent postsynaptic excitation, interrupting the progression of the electrical impulse at the synaptic junction. This function is significant when slowdown of body activity is advantageous. Enhancement of the GABA system is the mechanism of action by which the benzodiazepines produce their calming effect.
- ***Possible implications in mental illness:*** Alterations in the GABA system have been implicated in anxiety disorders, depression, movement disorders (e.g., Huntington's disease), and various forms of epilepsy. GABA levels, in a complex interaction with other neurotransmitters such as dopamine, have also been implicated in substance use disorders and addiction.

Glycine

- ***Location:*** The highest concentrations of glycine in the CNS are found in the spinal cord and brainstem. Little is known about the possible enzymatic metabolism of glycine.
- ***Functions:*** Glycine appears to be the neurotransmitter of recurrent inhibition of motor neurons within the spinal cord and is possibly involved in the regulation of spinal and brainstem reflexes.
- ***Possible implications in mental illness:*** Glycine has been implicated in the pathogenesis of certain types of spastic disorders and in "glycine encephalopathy," which is known to occur with toxic accumulation of the neurotransmitter in the brain and cerebrospinal fluid (Van Hove et al., 2013).

Excitatory Amino Acids

Glutamate and Aspartate

- ***Location:*** Glutamate and aspartate appear to be primary excitatory neurotransmitters in the pyramidal cells of the cortex, the cerebellum, and the primary sensory afferent systems. They are also found in the hippocampus, thalamus, hypothalamus, and spinal cord. Glutamate and aspartate are inactivated by uptake into the tissues and through assimilation in various metabolic pathways.
- ***Functions:*** Glutamate and aspartate function in the relay of sensory information and in the regulation of various motor and spinal reflexes. Glutamate also plays a role in memory and learning.
- ***Possible implications in mental illness:*** Alterations in these systems have been implicated in the etiology of certain neurodegenerative disorders, such as Huntington's disease, temporal lobe epilepsy, and spinal cerebellar degeneration. Increases in glutamate have been associated with neuron degeneration in Alzheimer's disease (Coyle, 2017). Problems in making or using glutamate have been linked to many mental disorders, including autism spectrum disorder (ASD), obsessive-compulsive disorder (OCD), schizophrenia, and depression (National Institute of Mental Health [NIMH], n.d.).

Neuropeptides

Neuropeptides act as signaling molecules in the CNS. Their activities include regulating processes related to sex, sleep, stress, pain, emotion, and social cognition. They may contribute to symptoms and behaviors associated with psychosis, mood disorders, dementias, and ASD. Hormonal neuropeptides are discussed in the "Neuroendocrinology" section of this chapter.

Opioid Peptides

- ***Location:*** Opioid peptides, which include the endorphins and enkephalins, have been widely studied. Opioid peptides are found in various concentrations in the hypothalamus, thalamus, limbic structures, midbrain, and brainstem. Enkephalins are also found in the gastrointestinal tract.

- ***Functions:*** With their natural morphine-like properties, opioid peptides are thought to have a role in pain modulation. They are released in response to painful stimuli and may be responsible for producing the analgesic effect following acupuncture. Opioid peptides alter the release of dopamine and affect the spontaneous activity of the dopaminergic neurons.
- ***Possible implications in mental illness:*** Modulation of dopamine activity by opioid peptides may be associated with addiction and some symptoms of schizophrenia, and a growing body of research supports that opioid system dysregulation may contribute to depression (Peciña et al., 2019).

Substance P

- ***Location:*** Substance P was the first neuropeptide to be discovered. It is present in high concentrations in the hypothalamus, limbic structures, midbrain, and brainstem and is also found in the thalamus, basal ganglia, and spinal cord.
- ***Functions:*** Substance P plays a role in sensory transmission, particularly in the regulation of pain.
- ***Possible implications in mental illness:*** Substance P levels have been associated with depression and post-traumatic stress disorder (PTSD). Studies have demonstrated that people with depression and PTSD had elevated levels of substance P in their cerebral spinal fluid (Boland & Verduin, 2022). Recent research focused on PTSD identified more specifically an imbalance between serotonergic and substance P signaling systems (Frick et al., 2016).

Somatostatin

- ***Location:*** Somatostatin (also called *growth hormone-inhibiting hormone [GHIH]*) is found in the cerebral cortex, hippocampus, thalamus, basal ganglia, brainstem, and spinal cord.
- ***Functions:*** Somatostatin has been shown to stimulate dopamine, serotonin, norepinephrine, and acetylcholine and to inhibit norepinephrine, histamine, and glutamate. It also acts as a neuromodulator for serotonin in the hypothalamus, thereby regulating its release (i.e., controlling whether it is stimulated or inhibited). It is possible that somatostatin may serve this function for other neurotransmitters as well.
- ***Possible implications in mental illness:*** High concentrations of somatostatin have been reported in brain specimens of clients with Huntington's disease and low concentrations in those with Alzheimer's disease and depression.

CORE CONCEPT

Neuroendocrinology

Study of the interaction between the nervous system and the endocrine system and of the effects of various hormones on cognitive, emotional, and behavioral functioning.

Neuroendocrinology

Human endocrine functioning has a strong foundation in the CNS under the direction of the hypothalamus, which has direct control over the pituitary gland. The pituitary gland has two major lobes—the anterior lobe (also called the *adenohypophysis*) and the posterior lobe (also called the *neurohypophysis*). The pituitary gland is only about the size of a pea, but despite its size and because of the powerful control it exerts over endocrine functioning in humans, it is sometimes called the "master gland." (Figure 2–5 shows the hormones of the pituitary gland and their target organs.) Many of the hormones subject to hypothalamus-pituitary regulation may have implications for behavioral functioning. Discussion of these hormones is summarized in Table 2–3.

Pituitary Gland

The Posterior Pituitary (Neurohypophysis)

The hypothalamus has direct control over the posterior pituitary through efferent neural pathways. Two hormones are found in the posterior pituitary: vasopressin (antidiuretic hormone) and oxytocin. They are actually produced by the hypothalamus and stored in the posterior pituitary. Their release is mediated by neural impulses from the hypothalamus (Fig. 2–6).

Antidiuretic Hormone

The main function of antidiuretic hormone (ADH) is to conserve body water and maintain normal blood pressure. The release of ADH is stimulated by pain, emotional stress, dehydration, increased plasma concentration, and decreases in blood volume. An alteration in the secretion of this hormone is related to the polydipsia seen in patients with diabetes and may be one of many factors contributing to the polydipsia, or water intoxication, observed in about 10% to 20% of patients with severe mental illness, particularly those with schizophrenia. Other factors correlated with excessive thirst include adverse effects of psychotropic medications and features of the behavioral

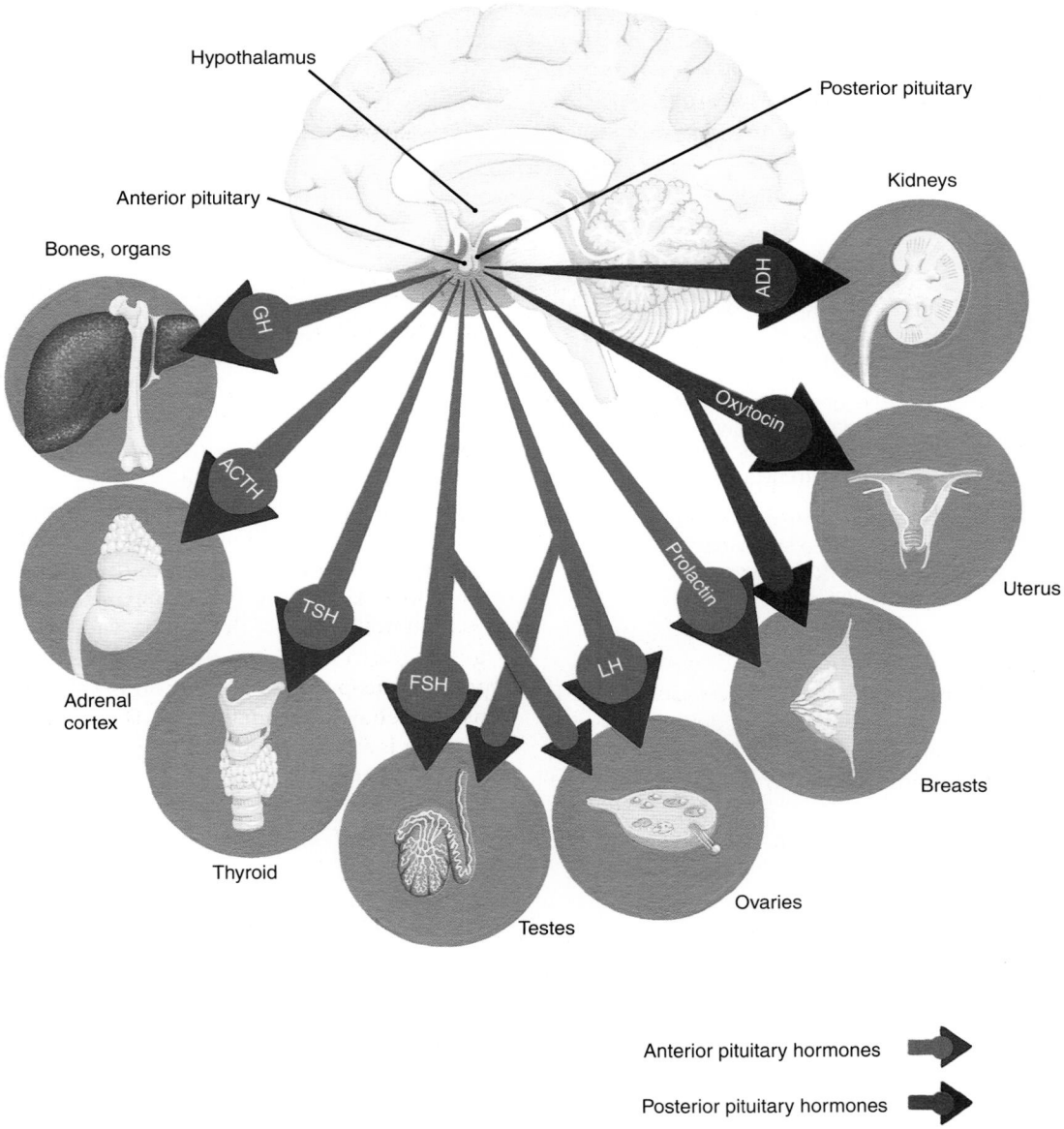

FIGURE 2–5 Hormones of the pituitary gland and their target organs. (From *Essentials of Anatomy and Physiology* [8th ed.], by V. C. Scanlon and T. Sanders, 2018, F.A. Davis Company. Reprinted with permission.)

disorder itself. It is important to note that severe polydipsia can result in electrolyte imbalance and death (Gill & McCauley, 2015). ADH also may play a role in learning and memory, in alteration of the pain response, and in the modification of sleep patterns.

Oxytocin

Oxytocin stimulates contraction of the uterus at the end of pregnancy and stimulates release of milk from the mammary glands (Scanlon & Sanders, 2018). It is also released in response to stress and during sexual arousal. Oxytocin functions to promote mother–infant bonding and bonding between sexes and has been used experimentally with children with ASD to increase socialization. Recent research found that oxytocin may be more beneficial in treating core symptoms of ASD when baseline levels of oxytocin were already low (Parker et al., 2017). Increases in oxytocin demonstrate anti-anxiety effects (in interaction with adrenocorticotropic hormone [ACTH]) and may facilitate development of

TABLE 2–3 Hormones of the Neuroendocrine System

HORMONE	LOCATION AND STIMULATION OF RELEASE	TARGET ORGAN	FUNCTION	POSSIBLE BEHAVIORAL CORRELATION TO ALTERED SECRETION
Antidiuretic hormone (ADH)	Posterior pituitary; release stimulated by dehydration, pain, stress	Kidney (causes increased reabsorption)	Conservation of body water and maintenance of blood pressure	Polydipsia; altered pain response; modified sleep pattern
Oxytocin	Posterior pituitary; release stimulated by end of pregnancy; stress; during sexual arousal	Uterus; breasts	Contraction of the uterus for labor; release of breast milk	May play role in stress response by stimulation of ACTH
Growth hormone (GH)	Anterior pituitary; release stimulated by growth hormone-releasing hormone from hypothalamus	Bones and tissues	Growth in children; protein synthesis in adults	Anorexia nervosa
Thyroid-stimulating hormone (TSH)	Anterior pituitary; release stimulated by thyrotropin-releasing hormone from hypothalamus	Thyroid gland	Stimulation of secretion of needed thyroid hormones for metabolism and regulation of temperature	*Increased levels of thyroid hormones (decreased secretion of TSH):* Insomnia, anxiety, emotional lability *Decreased levels of thyroid hormones (increased secretion of TSH):* Fatigue, depression
Adrenocorticotropic hormone (ACTH)	Anterior pituitary; release stimulated by corticotropin-releasing hormone from hypothalamus	Adrenal cortex	Stimulation of secretion of cortisol, which plays a role in response to stress	*Decreased levels:* Depression, apathy, fatigue *Increased levels:* Mood disorders, psychosis
Prolactin	Anterior pituitary; release stimulated by prolactin-releasing hormone from hypothalamus	Breasts	Stimulation of milk production	*Increased levels:* Depression, anxiety, decreased libido, irritability
Gonadotropic hormones	Anterior pituitary; release stimulated by gonadotropin-releasing hormone from hypothalamus	Ovaries and testes	Stimulation of secretion of estrogen, progesterone, and testosterone; role in ovulation and sperm production	*Decreased levels:* Depression and anorexia nervosa *Increased testosterone:* Increased sexual behavior and aggressiveness
Melanocyte-stimulating hormone	Anterior pituitary; release stimulated by onset of darkness	Pineal gland	Stimulation of secretion of melatonin	*Increased levels:* Depression

ADHD, attention deficit-hyperactivity disorder; NMDA, *N*-Methyl-D-aspartate

substance use disorders, especially with "party drugs" (MDMA [Ecstasy, Molly] and GHB [Liquid X, Goop]) often used to facilitate social interaction (Harris et al., 2017). Decreased levels of oxytocin have been reported in patients with ASD and anorexia.

The Anterior Pituitary (Adenohypophysis)

The hypothalamus produces *releasing hormones* that pass through capillaries and veins of the hypophyseal portal system to capillaries in the anterior pituitary, where they stimulate secretion of specialized hormones.

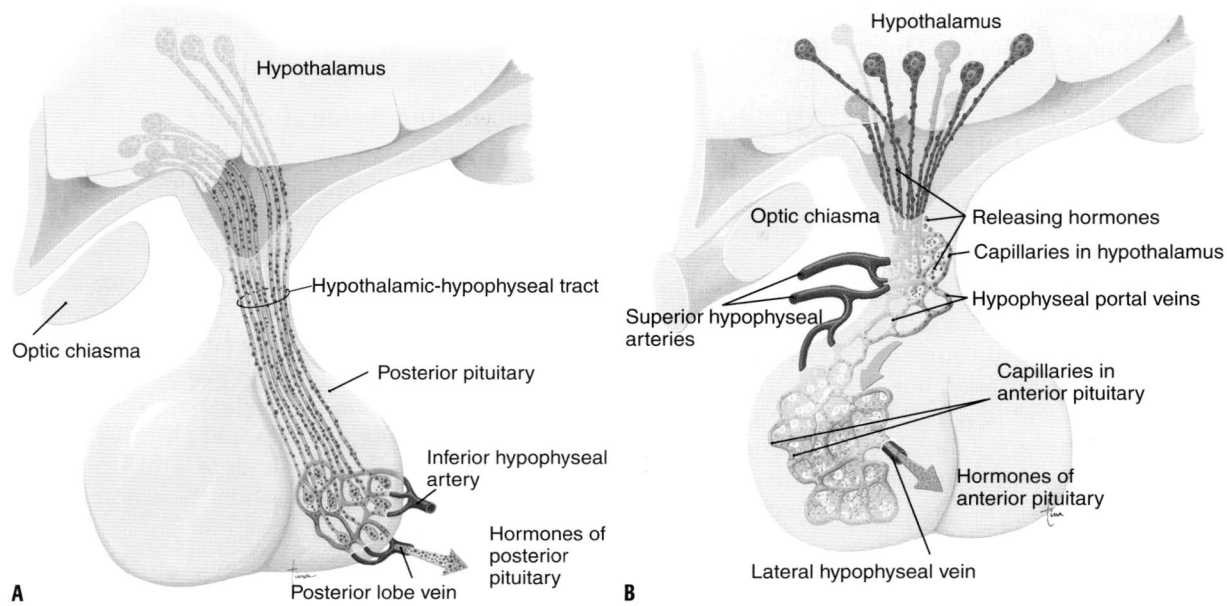

FIGURE 2–6 Structural relationships of hypothalamus and pituitary gland. (A) Posterior pituitary stores hormones produced in the hypothalamus. (B) Releasing hormones of the hypothalamus circulate directly to the anterior pituitary and influence its secretions. Notice the two networks of capillaries. (From *Essentials of Anatomy and Physiology* [8th ed.], by V. C. Scanlon and T. Sanders, 2018, F.A. Davis Company. Reprinted with permission.)

The hormones of the anterior pituitary gland regulate multiple body functions and include growth hormone, thyroid-stimulating hormone, ACTH, prolactin, gonadotropin-stimulating hormone, and melanocyte-stimulating hormone. Most of these hormones are regulated by a *negative feedback mechanism.* Once the hormone has exerted its effects, the information is "fed back" to the anterior pituitary, which inhibits the release, and ultimately decreases the effects, of the stimulating hormones.

Growth Hormone

The release of growth hormone (GH), also called somatotropin, is stimulated by growth hormone-releasing hormone (GHRH) from the hypothalamus. Its release is inhibited by GHIH (somatostatin), also from the hypothalamus. It is responsible for growth in children as well as for continued protein synthesis throughout life. During periods of fasting, it stimulates the release of fat from the adipose tissue to be used for increased energy. The release of GHIH is stimulated in response to periods of hyperglycemia. GHRH is stimulated in response to hypoglycemia and to stressful situations. During prolonged stress, GH has a direct effect on protein, carbohydrate, and lipid metabolism, resulting in increased serum glucose and free fatty acids to be used for increased energy. GH deficiency has been noted in many patients with major depressive disorder, and several GH abnormalities have been noted in patients with anorexia nervosa.

Thyroid-Stimulating Hormone

Thyrotropin-releasing hormone (TRH) from the hypothalamus stimulates the release of thyroid-stimulating hormone (TSH), or thyrotropin, from the anterior pituitary. TSH stimulates the thyroid gland to secrete triiodothyronine (T_3) and thyroxine (T_4). Thyroid hormones are integral to metabolism and the regulation of temperature.

A correlation between thyroid dysfunction and altered behavioral functioning has been well documented. Common symptoms of hyperthyroidism include irritability, insomnia, anxiety, restlessness, weight loss, emotional lability, and, in some instances, progression to delirium or psychosis. Symptoms of fatigue, decreased libido, memory impairment, depression, and suicidal ideations have been associated with chronic hypothyroidism. Studies have correlated various forms of thyroid dysfunction with mood disorders, anxiety, eating disorders, psychosis, and dementia.

Adrenocorticotropic Hormone (ACTH)

Corticotropin-releasing hormone (CRH) from the hypothalamus stimulates the release of ACTH from the anterior pituitary. ACTH stimulates the adrenal cortex to secrete cortisol. CRH, ACTH, and cortisol levels all rise in response to stress. Disorders of the adrenal cortex have been associated with mood disorders, PTSD, Alzheimer's dementia, and substance use disorders.

Addison's disease is the result of hyposecretion of the hormones of the adrenal cortex. Behavioral symptoms of hyposecretion include mood changes with apathy, social withdrawal, impaired sleep, decreased concentration, and fatigue. Hypersecretion of cortisol results in Cushing's disease and is associated with behaviors that include depression, mania, psychosis, and suicidal ideation. Cognitive impairments also have been commonly observed.

Prolactin

Prolactin is mainly involved in reproductive functions and milk production in the mammary glands during pregnancy. First generation antipsychotic medications (antipsychotic drugs that block dopamine receptors) increase prolactin levels and may be responsible for the undesired side effect of lactation. High prolactin levels are also associated with depression, decreased libido, anxiety, irritability, and the negative symptoms of schizophrenia.

Gonadotropic Hormones

The gonadotropic hormones are so called because they produce an effect on the gonads—the ovaries and the testes. The gonadotropins include follicle-stimulating hormone (FSH) and luteinizing hormone (LH). In women, FSH initiates maturation of ovarian follicles into the ova and stimulates their secretion of estrogen. LH is responsible for ovulation and the secretion of progesterone from the corpus luteum. In men, FSH initiates sperm production in the testes, and LH increases secretion of testosterone by the interstitial cells of the testes.

Limited evidence exists to correlate gonadotropins to behavioral functioning, although some observations have been made to warrant hypothetical consideration. Studies have indicated decreased levels of testosterone, LH, and FSH in men with depression (Bak et al., 2012; Jakka & Ramesh, 2017). Increased sexual behavior and aggressiveness have been linked to elevated testosterone levels in both men and women. Decreased plasma levels of LH and FSH commonly occur in patients with anorexia nervosa. Supplemental estrogen therapy has resulted in improved mentation and mood in some women with depression.

Melanocyte-Stimulating Hormone

Melanocyte-stimulating hormone from the hypothalamus stimulates the pineal gland to secrete melatonin. The release of melatonin appears to depend on the onset of darkness and is suppressed by light. Studies of this hormone have indicated that environmental light can affect neuronal activity and influence *circadian rhythms (Marcheva et al., 2013)*. Correlation between abnormal secretion of melatonin and symptoms of depression has led to the implication of melatonin in the etiology of seasonal affective disorder, in which individuals become depressed only during the fall and winter months when the amount of daylight decreases.

Circadian Rhythms

Human biological rhythms are largely determined by genetic coding with input from the external environment influencing the cyclic effects. **Circadian rhythms** in humans follow a near-24-hour cycle and may influence a variety of regulatory functions, including the sleep–wakefulness cycle, body temperature regulation, patterns of activity such as eating and drinking, and hormone secretion. The 24-hour rhythms in humans are affected to a large degree by the cycles of lightness and darkness.

Most of the biological rhythms of the body operate over a period of about 24 hours, but cycles of longer lengths have been studied. For example, women of menstruating age show monthly cycles of variable progesterone levels.

Some rhythms may last as long as a year. These circannual rhythms may influence the effectiveness of laboratory tests results and some medications. Clinical studies have shown that chemotherapy, when administered during the appropriate circadian phase, can significantly increase its efficacy and decrease the toxic effects of certain cytotoxic agents (Garlapow, 2016).

The Role of Circadian Rhythms in Psychopathology

Circadian rhythms may play a role in psychopathology. Abnormal circadian rhythms have been associated with a variety of mental illnesses including depression, bipolar disorder, and seasonal affective disorder. Because many hormones have been implicated in behavioral functioning, it is reasonable to believe that peak secretion times could be influential in predicting certain behaviors. The association of depression with increased secretion of melatonin during darkness hours has already been discussed. External manipulation of the light–dark cycle and removal of external time cues often have beneficial effects on mood disorders.

Symptoms that occur in the premenstrual cycle have been linked to disruptions in biological rhythms. A number of the symptoms associated with premenstrual dysphoric disorder (PMDD) strongly resemble those attributed to depression, and hormonal changes have been implicated in the etiology.

The sleep–wakefulness cycle is probably the most fundamental of biological rhythms, and sleep disturbances are common in both depression and PMDD. Neurochemicals such as serotonin and norepinephrine appear to be most active during non–rapid eye movement (REM) sleep, whereas the neurotransmitter acetylcholine is activated during REM sleep (Skudaev, 2019). Several studies have revealed information about the sleep-inducing characteristics of serotonin. L-tryptophan, the amino acid precursor to serotonin, has been used for many years as an effective sedative-hypnotic to induce sleep in individuals with sleep-onset disorder.

CORE CONCEPT

Genetics

Study of the biological transmission of certain characteristics (physical and/or behavioral) from parent to offspring.

Genetics

Human behavioral genetics seeks to understand both genetic and environmental contributions to individual variations in human behavior. This type of study is complicated by the fact that behaviors, like all complex traits, involve multiple genes.

The term **genotype** refers to the total set of genes present in an individual and coded in the DNA. The physical manifestations of a particular genotype are designated by characteristics that specify a specific **phenotype.** Examples of phenotypes include eye color, height, blood type, the characteristics of one's voice, and hair type. As evidenced by the examples presented, phenotypes are not *only* genetic but may also be acquired (i.e., influenced by the environment) or a combination of both. Many psychiatric disorders are likely the result of a combination of genetics and environmental influences.

Investigators who study the etiological implications for psychiatric illness may explore several risk factors. Studies to determine whether an illness is *familial* compare the percentages of family members with the illness to those in the general population or within a control group of unrelated individuals. These studies estimate the prevalence of psychopathology among relatives and make predictions about the predisposition to an illness based on familial risk factors. Schizophrenia, bipolar disorder, major depressive disorder, anorexia nervosa, panic disorder, somatic symptom disorder, antisocial personality disorder, and alcoholism are examples of psychiatric illnesses in which familial tendencies have been identified.

Studies that are purely genetic in nature search for a specific gene that is responsible for an individual having a particular illness. A number of disorders exist in which the mutation of a specific gene or change in the number or structure of a chromosome has been associated with the etiology. Examples include Huntington's disease, cystic fibrosis, phenylketonuria, Duchenne's muscular dystrophy, and Down's syndrome.

The search for pure genetic links to certain psychiatric disorders continues. Risk factors for early-onset Alzheimer's disease have been linked to mutations on chromosomes 21, 14, and 1 (National Institute on Aging, 2019). Other studies have linked a gene in the region of chromosome 19 that produces apolipoprotein E with late-onset Alzheimer's disease. One large study (Cross-Disorder Group of the Psychiatric Genomics Consortium, 2013) found similar genetic variations in five mental health disorders that were previously considered completely distinct. These disorders—ASD, attention deficit-hyperactivity disorder (ADHD), bipolar disorder, major depression, and schizophrenia—all showed some common gene variations, including differences in two genes that regulate the flow of calcium into cells. Although these findings are intriguing, they do not explain all the genetic risks for mental illness, the nongenetic risks, or the interaction between the two. Future research will continue to search for answers, with the ultimate goal of improving diagnosis and treatment and perhaps uncovering the keys to prevention of mental illness.

In addition to familial and purely genetic investigations, other types of studies have been conducted to estimate the existence and degree of genetic and environmental contributions to the etiology of certain psychiatric disorders. Twin studies and adoption studies have been successfully employed for this purpose.

Twin studies examine the frequency of a disorder in monozygotic (genetically identical) and dizygotic (fraternal; not genetically identical) twins. Twins are called *concordant* when both members have the same disorder in question. Concordance in monozygotic twins is considered stronger evidence of genetic involvement than it is in dizygotic twins. Twin studies have supported genetic vulnerability in the etiology of several mental illnesses including autism, PTSD, substance abuse (alcoholism), schizophrenia, bipolar disorder, major depression, OCD, risk for suicide, and others (Boland & Verduin, 2022). *Adoption studies* allow comparisons to be made between the influences of genetics and environment on the development of a psychiatric disorder. Adoption studies include the following four types:

1. The study of adopted children whose biological parent(s) had a psychiatric disorder but whose adoptive parent(s) did not.
2. The study of adopted children whose adoptive parent(s) had a psychiatric disorder but whose biological parent(s) did not.
3. The study of adoptive and biological relatives of adopted children who developed a psychiatric disorder.
4. The study of monozygotic twins reared apart by different adoptive parents.

Disorders in which adoption studies have suggested a possible genetic link include alcoholism, schizophrenia, major depression, bipolar disorder, ADHD, and antisocial personality disorder (Boland & Verduin, 2022).

A summary of various psychiatric disorders and the possible biological influences discussed in this chapter is presented in Table 2–4. Various diagnostic procedures used to detect alteration in biological functioning that may contribute to psychiatric disorders are presented in Table 2–5.

CORE CONCEPT

Psychoneuroimmunology

The study of the relationship between the immune system, the nervous system, and psychological processes such as thinking and behavior.

Psychoneuroimmunology (PNI)

Normal Immune Response

Cells responsible for *nonspecific* immune reactions include neutrophils, monocytes, and macrophages. They work to destroy the invasive organism and initiate and facilitate healing of damaged tissue. If these cells are not effective in accomplishing a satisfactory healing response, *specific* immune mechanisms take over.

Cytokines are one such mechanism. These molecules, which regulate immune and inflammatory responses, are active when an individual is fighting an infection or any other condition that creates inflammation in the body. Research has demonstrated that cytokines are part of an essential and complex system of responses that are crucial for reducing inflammation and bolstering the immune response, and they are active in mood disorders such as depression and bipolar disorder (Mao et al., 2018). Studies are also attempting to identify what happens when inflammation is not resolved and when cytokines remain active or cross the blood-brain barrier; there is evidence that these maladaptations may trigger a multitude of illnesses (Ratnayake et al., 2013).

Implications of the Immune System in Psychiatric Illness

Studies of the biological response to stress (Salleh, 2008) have shown that individuals become more susceptible to physical illness following exposure to a stressful stimulus or life event (see Chapter 1, "Mental Health and Mental Illness"). This response is thought to be due to the effect of increased glucocorticoid release from the adrenal cortex following stimulation from the hypothalamic-pituitary-adrenal axis during stressful situations ("axis" refers to the complex interactions among these three glands). The result is a suppression in lymphocyte proliferation and function.

Studies have shown that nerve endings exist in tissues of the immune system (Dantzer, 2018). The CNS has connections in both bone marrow and the thymus, where immune system cells are produced, and in the spleen and lymph nodes, where those cells are stored.

GH, which may be released in response to certain stressors, may enhance immune functioning, whereas testosterone is thought to inhibit immune functioning. Increased production of epinephrine and norepinephrine occurs in response to stress and may decrease immunity. Serotonin has been described as an immunomodulatory because it has demonstrated both enhancing and inhibitory effects on inflammation and immunity (Arreola et al., 2015).

Studies have correlated a decrease in lymphocyte functioning with periods of grief, bereavement, and depression, associating the degree of altered immunity

TABLE 2–4 Biological Implications in Psychiatric Disorders

ANATOMICAL BRAIN STRUCTURES INVOLVED	NEUROTRANSMITTER HYPOTHESIS	POSSIBLE ENDOCRINE CORRELATION	IMPLICATIONS OF CIRCADIAN RHYTHMS	POSSIBLE GENETIC LINK
SCHIZOPHRENIA				
Frontal cortex, temporal lobes, limbic system.	Dopamine hyperactivity; decreased glutamate.	Decreased prolactin levels.	May correlate antipsychotic medication administration to times of lowest level.	Twin, familial, and adoption studies suggest genetic link.
DEPRESSIVE DISORDERS				
Frontal lobes, limbic system, temporal lobes.	Decreased levels of norepinephrine, dopamine, and serotonin; increased glutamate.	Increased cortisol levels, thyroid hormone hyposecretion, increased melatonin.	DST* used to predict effectiveness of antidepressants; melatonin linked to depression during periods of darkness.	Twin, familial, and adoption studies suggest a genetic link.
BIPOLAR DISORDER				
Frontal lobes, limbic system, temporal lobes.	Increased levels of norepinephrine and dopamine in acute mania.	Elevated thyroid hormones may manifest as manic symptoms.	Abnormal circadian rhythms have been associated with bipolar disorder.	Twin, familial, and adoption studies suggest a genetic link.
PANIC DISORDER				
Limbic system, midbrain.	Increased levels of norepinephrine; decreased gamma amino butyric acid (GABA) activity.	Elevated levels of thyroid hormones.	May have some application for times of medication administration.	Twin and familial studies suggest a genetic link.
ANOREXIA NERVOSA				
Limbic system, particularly the hypothalamus.	Decreased levels of norepinephrine, serotonin, and dopamine.	Decreased levels of gonadotropins and growth hormone; increased cortisol levels.	DST* often shows same results as in depression.	Twin and familial studies suggest a genetic link.
OBSESSIVE-COMPULSIVE DISORDER				
Limbic system, basal ganglia (specifically caudate nucleus).	Decreased levels of serotonin.	Increased cortisol levels.	DST* often shows same results as in depression.	Twin studies suggest a possible genetic link.
ALZHEIMER'S DISEASE				
Temporal, parietal, and occipital regions of cerebral cortex; hippocampus.	Decreased levels of acetylcholine, norepinephrine, serotonin, and somatostatin.	Decreased corticotropin-releasing hormone.	Decreased levels of acetylcholine and serotonin may inhibit hypothalamic-pituitary-adrenal axis and interfere with hormonal releasing factors.	Familial studies suggest a genetic predisposition; late-onset disorder linked to marker on chromosome 19; early-onset to chromosomes 21, 14, and 1.

*DST, dexamethasone suppression test. Dexamethasone is a synthetic glucocorticoid that suppresses cortisol secretion via the feedback mechanism. In this test, 1 mg of dexamethasone is administered at 11:30 p.m., and blood samples are drawn at 8:00 a.m., 4:00 p.m., and 11:00 p.m. on the following day. A plasma value greater than 5 mcg/dL suggests that the individual is not suppressing cortisol in response to the dose of dexamethasone. This is a positive result for depression and may have implications for other disorders as well.

TABLE 2–5 Diagnostic Procedures Used to Detect Altered Brain Functioning

EXAM	TECHNIQUE USED	PURPOSE AND POSSIBLE FINDINGS
Electroencephalography (EEG)	Electrodes are placed on the scalp in a standardized position. Amplitude and frequency of beta, alpha, theta, and delta brain waves are graphically recorded on paper by ink markers for multiple areas of the brain surface.	Measures brain electrical activity; identifies dysrhythmias, asymmetries, or suppression of brain rhythms; used in the diagnosis of epilepsy, neoplasm, stroke, metabolic or degenerative disease.
Computerized EEG mapping	EEG tracings are summarized by computer-assisted systems in which various regions of the brain are identified and functioning is interpreted by color coding or gray shading.	Measures brain electrical activity; used largely in research to represent statistical relationships between individuals and groups or between two populations of subjects (e.g., patients with schizophrenia vs. control subjects).
Computed tomographic (CT) scan	CT scan may be used with or without contrast medium. X-rays are taken of various transverse planes of the brain while a computerized analysis produces a precise reconstructed image of each segment.	Measures accuracy of brain structure to detect possible lesions, abscesses, areas of infarction, or aneurysm. CT has also identified various anatomical differences in patients with schizophrenia, organic mental disorders, and bipolar disorder.
Magnetic resonance imaging (MRI)	Within a strong magnetic field, the nuclei of hydrogen atoms absorb and reemit electromagnetic energy that is computerized and transformed into image information. No radiation or contrast medium is used.	Measures anatomical and biochemical status of various segments of the brain; detects brain edema, ischemia, infection, neoplasm, trauma, and other changes such as demyelination. Morphological differences have been noted in brains of patients with schizophrenia as compared with control subjects.
Positron emission tomography (PET)	The patient receives an IV injection of a radioactive substance (type depends on brain activity to be visualized). The head is surrounded by detectors that relay data to a computer that interprets the signals and produces the image.	Measures specific brain functioning, such as glucose metabolism, oxygen utilization, blood flow, and, of particular interest in psychiatry, neurotransmitter-receptor interaction.
Single photon emission computed tomography (SPECT)	The technique is similar to PET, but longer-acting radioactive substance must be used to allow time for a gamma-camera to rotate about the head and gather the data, which are then computer assembled into a brain image.	Measures various aspects of brain functioning, as with PET; has also been used to image activity of cerebrospinal fluid circulation.

with severity of the depression (Buckley et al., 2012; Pasco et al., 2010). A number of research studies have been conducted attempting to correlate the onset of schizophrenia to abnormalities of the immune system. These studies have considered autoimmune responses, viral infections, and immunogenetics (Boland & Verduin, 2022). A link has been identified between toxoplasmosis and psychiatric disorders such as schizophrenia, bipolar disorder, and suicidal/aggressive behaviors (Del Grande et al., 2017). *Toxoplasma gondii*, the parasite responsible for toxoplasmosis, has an affinity for brain tissue where it causes brain inflammation and may affect neurotransmitters such as dopamine. Immunological abnormalities have also been investigated in a number of other psychiatric illnesses, including alcoholism, ASD, and neurocognitive disorder.

Evidence exists to support a correlation between psychosocial stress and the onset of illness. More research is needed to determine the specific processes involved in stress-induced modulation of the immune system.

Psychopharmacology and the Brain

Understanding the brain and the biological processes involved in thinking, feeling, and behaving has positive ramifications beyond better understanding of psychopharmacological treatment options. As mentioned earlier, future research may continue to demonstrate the impact of psychological interventions on brain activity and neurotransmitters, which would open opportunities to hone psychological treatments and avoid some of the troubling side effects that accompany many medications. Furthermore, continued research in areas such as psychoneuroimmunology may reveal causes of mental illness, which would provide the opportunity for primary prevention.

In spite of these potential opportunities, psychopharmacology remains a primary treatment modality for mental disorders, and current evidence suggests that early medication treatment of schizophrenia at the first signs of psychosis may prevent the damaging effects of multiple psychotic episodes on the brain (Nasrallah, 2018). Understanding, as best we can with current evidence, the biological mechanisms at work in psychoactive drugs is essential to nursing practice. See Chapter 4, "Psychopharmacology," for further discussion of the influence of psychoactive drugs on neurosynaptic transmission.

Implications for Nursing

Psychiatric mental health nurses must integrate knowledge of the biological sciences into their practices if they are to ensure safe and effective care for people with mental illness. Much progress has been made in understanding the biochemical, neuroanatomical, and genetic influences in mental illness, but much remains theoretical. Further, there is evidence that psychosocial influences, particularly a history of trauma such as abuse and neglect, interact significantly with an individual's biological vulnerabilities in the development of these illnesses.

To ensure a smooth transition from a strictly psychosocial focus to one of *bio*psychosocial emphasis, nurses must have a clear understanding of the following:

- ***Neuroanatomy and neurophysiology:*** The structure and functioning of the various parts of the brain and their correlation to human behavior and psychopathology.
- ***Neuronal processes:*** The various functions of the nerve cells, including the role of neurotransmitters, receptors, synaptic activity, and informational pathways.
- ***Neuroendocrinology:*** The interaction of the endocrine and nervous systems and the role that the endocrine glands and their respective hormones play in behavioral functioning.
- ***Circadian rhythms:*** The regulation of biochemical functioning over periods of rhythmic cycles and its influence in predicting certain behaviors.
- ***Genetic influences:*** The hereditary factors that predispose individuals to certain psychiatric disorders.
- ***Psychoneuroimmunology:*** The influence of stress on the immune system and its role in the susceptibility to illness.
- ***The impact of trauma:*** Both physical trauma (traumatic brain injury) and psychosocial trauma (especially early childhood trauma such as abuse, neglect, and abandonment) are influential in the development of several mental illnesses. (See Chapters 12, 19, and 28 for further discussion of trauma and trauma-informed care.)
- ***Psychopharmacology:*** The widespread use of psychotropic drugs in the treatment of mental illness demands knowledge of psychopharmacological principles and nursing interventions necessary for safe and effective management.
- ***Diagnostic technology:*** The importance of keeping informed about the latest in technological procedures for diagnosing alterations in brain structure and function.

Why are these concepts important to the practice of psychiatric mental health nursing? The interrelationship between psychosocial adaptation and physical functioning has been established. Integrating biological and behavioral concepts into psychiatric nursing practice is essential for nurses to meet the complex needs of patients with mental illness. Psychobiological perspectives must be incorporated into nursing practice, education, and research to attain evidence-based outcomes necessary for the delivery of competent care.

Summary and Key Points

- It is important for nurses to understand the interaction between biological and behavioral factors in the development and management of mental illness.
- Psychobiology is the study of the biological foundations of cognitive, emotional, and behavioral processes.

- The limbic system has been called the "emotional brain." It is associated with feelings of fear and anxiety; anger, rage, and aggression; love, joy, and hope; and sexuality and social behavior.
- The three classes of neurons include afferent (sensory), efferent (motor), and interneurons. The junction between two neurons is called a synapse.
- Neurotransmitters are chemicals that convey information across synaptic clefts to neighboring target cells. Many neurotransmitters have implications in the etiology of emotional disorders and in the pharmacological treatment of those disorders.
- Major categories of neurotransmitters include cholinergic neurotransmitters, monoamines, amino acids, and neuropeptides.
- The endocrine system plays an important role in human behavior through the hypothalamic-pituitary-adrenal axis.
- Hormones and their circadian rhythm of regulation significantly influence a number of physiological and psychological life-cycle phenomena, such as moods, sleep and arousal, stress response, appetite, libido, and fertility.
- Research continues to validate the role of genetics in mental illness.
- Familial, twin, and adoption studies suggest that genetics may be implicated in the etiology of schizophrenia, bipolar disorder, depressive disorder, panic disorder, anorexia nervosa, alcoholism, and OCD. Genetics studies, however, fail to entirely explain the complex factors involved in the development of mental disorders.
- Psychoneuroimmunology (PNI) examines the relationship between psychological factors, the immune system, and the nervous system.
- Evidence exists to support a link between psychosocial stressors and suppression of the immune response.
- Technologies such as magnetic resonance imaging (MRI), computed tomographic (CT) scan, positron emission tomography (PET), and electroencephalography (EEG) are used as diagnostic tools for detecting alterations in psychobiological functioning.
- Psychotropic medications act at the neural synapse to affect neurotransmitter activity and have been associated with improvement in symptoms of many mental disorders.
- Integrating knowledge of the expanding biological focus into psychiatric nursing is essential if nurses are to meet the changing needs of today's psychiatric clients.

Review Questions

Select the answer that is most appropriate for each of the following questions:

1. Which of the following parts of the brain is associated with multiple feelings and behaviors and is sometimes referred to as the "emotional brain"?
   a. Frontal lobe
   b. Thalamus
   c. Hypothalamus
   d. Limbic system
2. Which of the following parts of the brain is concerned with visual reception and interpretation?
   a. Frontal lobe
   b. Parietal lobe
   c. Temporal lobe
   d. Occipital lobe
3. Which of the following parts of the brain is associated with voluntary body movement, thinking and judgment, and expression of feeling?
   a. Frontal lobe
   b. Parietal lobe
   c. Temporal lobe
   d. Occipital lobe

4. Which of the following parts of the brain integrates all sensory input (except smell) on the way to the cortex?
   a. Temporal lobe
   b. Thalamus
   c. Limbic system
   d. Hypothalamus
5. Which of the following parts of the brain deals with sensory perception and interpretation?
   a. Hypothalamus
   b. Cerebellum
   c. Parietal lobe
   d. Hippocampus
6. Which of the following parts of the brain is concerned with hearing, short-term memory, and sense of smell?
   a. Temporal lobe
   b. Parietal lobe
   c. Cerebellum
   d. Hypothalamus
7. Which of the following parts of the brain has control over the pituitary gland and autonomic nervous system as well as regulation of appetite and temperature?
   a. Temporal lobe
   b. Parietal lobe
   c. Cerebellum
   d. Hypothalamus
8. At a synapse, the determination of further impulse transmission is accomplished by means of which of the following?
   a. Potassium ions
   b. Interneurons
   c. Neurotransmitters
   d. Myelin sheath
9. Inhibitory neurotransmitters such as GABA have which of the following actions?
   a. Initiate postsynaptic excitation
   b. Interrupt the progression of electrical impulses at the synapse
   c. Facilitate synaptic transmission
   d. All of the above
10. Which of the following hormones has been implicated in the etiology of mood disorder with seasonal pattern?
    a. Increased levels of melatonin
    b. Decreased levels of oxytocin
    c. Decreased levels of prolactin
    d. Increased levels of thyrotropin
11. Psychotropic medications may act at the neural synapse to accomplish which of the following? (Select all that apply.)
    a. Inhibit the reuptake of certain neurotransmitters, creating more availability
    b. Inhibit catabolic enzymes, promoting more availability of a neurotransmitter
    c. Block receptors, resulting in less neurotransmitter activity
    d. Add synthetic neurotransmitters found in the drug

Continued

12. Psychoneuroimmunology is a branch of science that involves which of the following? (Select all that apply.)
a. The impact of psychoactive medications at the neural synapse
b. The relationships among the immune system, the nervous system, and psychological processes, including mental illness
c. The correlation between psychosocial stress and the onset of illness
d. The potential role of viruses in the onset of schizophrenia
e. The genetic factors that influence prevention of mental illness

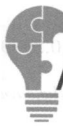

Go to **Davis Advantage** to complete your learning: strengthen understanding, apply your knowledge, and prepare for the Next Gen NCLEX®.

References

Arreola, R., Becerril-Villanueva, E., Cruz-Fuentes, C., Velasco-Velázquez, M. A., Garcés-Alvarez, M. E., Hurtado-Alvarado, G., Hurtado-Alvarado, G., Quintero-Fabian, S., & Pavón, L. (2015). Immunomodulatory effects mediated by serotonin. *Journal of Immunology Research.* http://doi.org/10.1155/2015/354957

Bak, C. W., Seok, H. H., Song, S. H., Kim, E. S., Her, Y. S., & Yoon, T. K. (2012). Hormonal infertile men. *Journal of Andrology, 33*(2), 181–189.

Boland, R., & Verduin, M. L. (2022). *Kaplan & Sadock's synopsis of psychiatry* (P. Ruiz, Ed.). (12th ed.). Wolters Kluwer.

Buckley, T., Sunari, D., Marshall, A., Bartrop, R., McKinley, S., & Tofler, G. (2012). Physiological correlates of bereavement and the impact of bereavement interventions. *Dialogues in Clinical Neuroscience, 14*(2), 129–139. https://doi.org/10.31887/DCNS.2012.14.2/tbuckley

Cacabelos, R., Torrellas, C., Fernandez-Novoa, L., & Lopez-Munoz, F. (2016). Histamine and immune biomarkers in CNS disorders. *Mediators of Inflammation, 2016,* 1924603. https://www.ncbi.nlm.nih.gov/pmc/articles/PMC4846752/

Carmichael, C. Y., & Wainford, R. D. (2015). Hypothalamic signaling mechanisms in hypertension. *Current Hypertension Reports, 17*(5), 39. https://doi.org/10.1007/s11906-015-0550-4

Collerton, D. (2013). Psychotherapy and brain plasticity. *Frontiers in Psychology,* 4, 548. https://doi.org/10.3389/fpsyg.2013.00548

Coyle, J. T. (2017). Amino acid neurotransmitters. In B. J. Sadock, V. A. Sadock, & P. Ruiz (Eds.), *Comprehensive textbook of psychiatry* (10th ed., pp. 76–84). Wolters Kluwer.

Cross-Disorder Group of the Psychiatric Genomics Consortium. (2013). Identification of risk loci with shared effects on five major psychiatric disorders: A genome-wide analysis. *Lancet, 381*(9875), 1371–1379. https://doi.org/10.1016/S0140-6736(12)62129-1

Dantzer, R. (2018). Neuroimmune interactions: From the brain to the immune system and vice versa. *Physiological Reviews, 98*(1), 477–504. https://doi.org/10.1152/physrev.00039.2016

Del Grande, C., Galli, L., Schiavi, E., Dell'Osso, L., & Bruschi, F. (2017). Is *Toxoplasma gondii* a trigger of bipolar disorder? *Pathogens, 6*(3), 1–20. https://doi.org/10.3390/pathogens6010003

Elsworth, J. D., & Roth, R. H. (2017). Biogenic amine transmitters. In B. J. Sadock, V. A. Sadock, & P. Ruiz (Eds.), *Comprehensive textbook of psychiatry* (10th ed., pp. 61–75). Wolters Kluwer.

Flor, H. (2014). Psychological pain interventions and neurophysiology: Implications for a mechanism-based approach. *American Psychologist, 69*(2), 188–196. https://doi.org/10.1037/a0035254

Frick, A., Åhs, F., Palmquist, Å., Pissiota, A., Wallenquist, U., Fernandez, M., Jonasson, M., Appel, L., Frans, O., Lubberink, M., Furmark, T., von Knorring, L., & Fredrikson, M. (2016). Alterations in the serotonergic and substance P systems in posttraumatic stress disorder. *Molecular Psychiatry, 21,* 1323. https://doi.org/10.1038/mp.2016.159

Garlapow, M. (2016). Timing chemotherapy administration to circadian rhythm improves drug effectiveness. *Oncology Nurse Advisor.* https://www.oncologynurseadvisor.com/side-effect-management/chemotherapy-more-effective-when-synced-with-circadian-rhythm/article/504455/

Gill, M., & McCauley, M. (2015). Psychogenic polydipsia: The result, or cause of, deteriorating psychotic symptoms? A case report of the consequences of water intoxication. *Case Reports in Psychiatry.* https://doi.org/10.1155/2015/846459

Harris, D. S., Wolkowitz, M. D., & Reus, V. I. (2017). Psychoneuroendocrinology. In B. J. Sadock, V. A. Sadock, & P. Ruiz (Eds.), *Comprehensive textbook of psychiatry* (10th ed., pp. 164–178). Wolters Kluwer.

Jakka, N. R., & Ramesh, J. (2017). Role of depression, anxiety, testosterone and luteinizing hormone levels in disorders of sexual function. *International Journal of Advances in Medicine, 4*(4). https://doi.org/10.18203/2349-3933.ijam20173241

Khor, S., & Cai, D. (2017). Hypothalamic and inflammatory basis of hypertension. *Clinical Science, 131*(3), 211–223. https://doi.org/10.1042/CS20160001

Lewis, D. O. (2017). Adult antisocial behavior, criminality, and violence. In B. J. Sadock, V. A. Sadock, & P. Ruiz (Eds.), *Comprehensive textbook of psychiatry* (10th ed., pp. 2413–2430). Wolters Kluwer.

Lyall, A. E., Kubicki, M., & Shenton, M. E. (2017). Structural brain imaging in schizophrenia. In B. J. Sadock, V. A. Sadock, & P. Ruiz (Eds.), *Comprehensive textbook of psychiatry* (10th ed., pp. 1463–1475). Wolters Kluwer.

Mao, R., Zhang, C., Chen, J., Zhao, G., Zhou, R., Wang, F., Xu, J., Yang, T., Su, Y., Huang, J., Wu, Z., Cao, L., Wang, Y., Hu, Y., Yuan, C., Yi, Z., Hong, W., Wang, Z., Peng, D., & Fang, Y. (2018). Different levels of pro- and anti-inflammatory cytokines in patients with unipolar and bipolar depression. *Journal of Affective Disorders, 237,* 65–72. https://doi.org/10.1016/j.jad.2018.04.115.

Marcheva, B., Ramsey, K. M., Peek, C. B., Affinati, A., Maury, E., & Bass, J. (2013). Circadian clocks and metabolism. *Handbook of Experimental Pharmacology, 217,* 127–155. https://doi.org/10.1007/978-3-642-25950-0_6

Mason, L., Peters, E., Williams, S. C., & Kumari, V. (2017). Brain connectivity changes occurring following cognitive behavioural therapy for psychosis predict long-term recovery. *Translational Psychiatry, 7*(1), e1001. https://doi.org/10.1038/tp.2016.263

Melchitzky, D. S., & Lewis, D. A. (2017). Functional neuroanatomy. In B. J. Sadock, V. A. Sadock, & P. Ruiz (Eds.), *Comprehensive textbook of psychiatry* (10th ed., pp. 3–39). Wolters Kluwer.

Nasrallah, H. A. (2018). Preventing brain damage in psychosis. *Current Psychiatry, 17*(10), 9–10. https://www.mdedge.com/psychiatry/article/175767/schizophreniaother-psychotic-disorders/page/0/1

National Institute of Mental Health. (n.d.) *Brain basics.* https://www.nimh.nih.gov/brainbasics/index.html

National Institute on Aging. (2019). *Alzheimer's disease genetics fact sheet.* https://www.nia.nih.gov/health/alzheimers-disease-genetics-fact-sheet

National Institutes of Health. (2020). *Is there a link between marijuana and psychiatric disorders?* https://www.drugabuse.gov/publications/research-reports/marijuana/there-link-between-marijuana-use-psychiatric-disorders

Parker, K. J., Oztan, O., Libove, R. A., Sumiyoshi, R. D., Jackson, L. P., Karhson, D. S., Summers, J. E., Hinman, K. E., Motonaga, K. S., Phillips, J. M., Carson, D. S., Garner, J. P., & Hardan, A. Y. (2017). Intranasal oxytocin treatment for social deficits and biomarkers of response in children with autism. *Proceedings of the National Academy of Sciences of the United States of America, 114*(30), 8119–8124.

Pasco, J. A., Nicholson, G. C., Williams, L. J., Jacka, F. N., Henry, M. J., Kotowicz, M. A., Schneider, H. G., Leonard, B. E., & Berk, M. (2010). Association of high-sensitivity C-reactive protein with de novo major depression. *British Journal of Psychiatry, 197,* 372–377.

Peciña, M., Karp, J. F., Mathew, S., Todtenkopf, M. S., Ehrich, E. W., & Zubieta, J. K. (2019). Endogenous opioid system dysregulation in depression: Implications for new therapeutic approaches. *Molecular Psychiatry, 24,* 576–587. https://doi.org/10.1038/s41380-018-0117-2

Ratnayake, U., Quinn, T., Walker, D. W., & Dickinson, H. (2013). Cytokines and the neurodevelopmental basis of mental illness. *Frontiers in Neuroscience, 7.* https://doi.org/10.3389/fnins.2013.00180

Salleh, M. R. (2008). Life event, stress and illness. *The Malaysian Journal of Medical Sciences, 15*(4), 9–18.

Scanlon, V. C., & Sanders, T. (2018). *Essentials of anatomy and physiology* (8th ed.). F.A. Davis.

Skudaev, S. (2019). *The neurophysiology and neurochemistry of sleep* [Review]. https://www.scribd.com/document/25882706/1022170-Neurophysiology-and-Neurochemistry-of-Sleep

Van Hove, J., Coughlin, C., & Sharer, G. (2013). Glycine encephalopathy. In R. A. Pagon, M. P. Adam, H. H. Ardinger, et al. (Eds.), *GeneReviews®*. National Library of Medicine. http://www.ncbi.nlm.nih.gov/books/NBK1357

3 Ethical and Legal Issues

CORE CONCEPTS

Professionalism: Ethics, Legal Aspects

Safety

Clinical Judgment

CHAPTER OUTLINE

Objectives
Introduction
Ethical Considerations
Legal Considerations
Summary and Key Points
Review Questions
Clinical Judgment Questions

KEY TERMS

advocacy
assault
autonomy
battery
beneficence
bioethics
Christian ethics
civil law
common law
criminal law
defamation of character
divine command ethics
ethical dilemma
ethical egoism
ethics
false imprisonment
informed consent
justice
Kantianism
libel
malpractice
morals
moral behavior
natural law theory
negligence
nonmaleficence
privileged communication
rights
slander
statutory law
tort
utilitarianism
values
values clarification
veracity

OBJECTIVES

After reading this chapter, the student will be able to:

1. Differentiate among *ethics, morals, values,* and *rights*.
2. Discuss ethical theories, including utilitarianism, Kantianism, Christian ethics, natural law theories, and ethical egoism.
3. Define *ethical dilemma*.
4. Discuss the ethical principles of autonomy, beneficence, nonmaleficence, justice, and veracity.
5. Use an ethical decision-making model to make an ethical decision.
6. Describe ethical issues relevant to psychiatric mental health nursing.
7. Define *statutory law* and *common law*.
8. Differentiate between *civil law* and *criminal law*.
9. Discuss legal issues relevant to psychiatric mental health nursing.
10. Differentiate between *malpractice* and *negligence*.
11. Identify behaviors relevant to the psychiatric mental health setting for which specific malpractice action could be taken.

Introduction

Nurses are constantly faced with the challenge of making difficult decisions regarding good and evil or life and death. Complex situations frequently arise in caring for individuals with mental illness, and nurses are held to the highest level of legal and ethical accountability in their professional practice. This chapter presents basic ethical and legal concepts and their relationship to psychiatric mental health nursing. A discussion of ethical theory is presented as a foundation upon which ethical decisions may be made. The American Nurses Association (ANA) has established a code of ethics for nurses to use as a framework within which to make ethical choices and decisions (ANA, 2015). These revised provisions and interpretive guidelines have been expanded to address some of the complexities of the current health-care environment and include ethical principles regarding nurses' duty not only to patients but also to themselves and to all persons with whom they interact. According to the code, the nurse's primary responsibility is to the patient (whether that is an individual, family, group, community, or population) and all relationships should be conducted within a culture of respect and civility.

The ANA Code of Ethics interpretive guidelines include a discussion of the importance of teamwork and collaboration, which is consistent with one of the recommendations of the Institute of Medicine (2003) [now renamed the National Academy of Medicine] for improving the future of health care and has become one of the Quality and Safety Education for Nurses competencies.

The American Psychiatric Nurses Association and the International Society of Psychiatric-Mental Health Nurses (2022) have published a scope and standards of practice manual specifically for psychiatric mental health nursing, which maintains consistency with the ANA code of ethics and applies those provisions to psychiatric mental health nursing issues. Knowledge about the ANA's *Code of Ethics for Nurses with Interpretive Statements* (ANA, 2015) and the *Psychiatric-Mental Health Nursing: Scope and Standards of Practice* (American Psychiatric Nurses Association & International Society of Psychiatric-Mental Health Nurses, 2022) is essential for guiding practice because these documents clarify the accepted expectations of the nurse in this field.

Because legislation determines what is *right* or *good* within a society, legal issues pertaining to psychiatric mental health nursing are also discussed in this chapter. Definitions are presented along with a description of the generally accepted and legal rights of psychiatric clients. Nursing competency and patient care accountability are compromised when the nurse has inadequate knowledge about the laws, rules, and guidelines that govern the practice of nursing.

Application of the legal and ethical concepts presented in this chapter promotes quality care in psychiatric mental health nursing practice and promotes legal accountability. The right to practice nursing carries with it the responsibility to maintain a specific level of competency and to practice in accordance with certain ethical and legal standards of care.

CORE CONCEPTS

Ethics is a branch of philosophy that deals with systematic approaches to distinguishing right from wrong behavior (Butts & Rich, 2019). **Bioethics** is the term applied to these principles when they refer to concepts within the scope of medicine, nursing, and allied health.

Morals are fundamental standards of right and wrong that are learned and internalized (Catalano, 2020). **Moral behavior** is conduct that results from serious critical thinking about how individuals ought to treat others. Moral behavior reflects the way a person interprets basic respect for other persons, such as the respect for autonomy, freedom, justice, honesty, and confidentiality.

Values are personal beliefs and ideals about what is important and desirable (Butts & Rich, 2019). **Values clarification** is a process of self-exploration through which individuals identify and rank their own personal values. This process increases awareness about why individuals behave in certain ways. Values clarification is important in nursing to increase understanding about why certain choices and decisions are made over others and how values affect nursing outcomes.

Rights are expectations to which an individual is entitled either by established laws, policies, or ethical principles. A right is *absolute* when there is no restriction whatsoever on the individual's entitlement. A *legal right* is one on which the society has agreed and formalized into law. Both the National League for Nursing (NLN) and the American Hospital Association (AHA) have established guidelines of patients' rights. Although these are not considered legal documents, nurses and hospitals are considered responsible for upholding these rights of patients.

Ethical Considerations

Theoretical Perspectives

An *ethical theory* is a set of philosophical principles that can be used to guide how an individual makes decisions on ethical questions and issues. Several ethical theories are described here.

Utilitarianism

The basis of **utilitarianism** is "the greatest-happiness principle." This principle holds that actions are right to the degree that they tend to promote happiness and wrong if they tend to produce the reverse of happiness. Thus, the good is happiness and the right is that which promotes the good. Conversely, the wrongness of an action is determined by its tendency to bring about unhappiness. An ethical decision based on the utilitarian view looks at the end results of the decision. Action is taken on the basis of the end results that produce the most good (happiness) for the most people.

Kantianism

Named for philosopher Immanuel Kant, **Kantianism** is directly opposed to utilitarianism. Kant argued that it is not the consequences or end results that make an action right or wrong; rather, it is the principle or motivation on which the action is based that is the morally decisive factor. Kantianism suggests that our actions are bound by a sense of duty. This theory is often called *deontology* (from the Greek word *deon*, which means "that which is binding; duty"). Kantian-directed ethical decisions are made out of respect for moral law. For example, "I make this choice because it is morally right and my duty to do so" (not because of consideration for a possible outcome).

Divine Command Ethics

The **divine command ethics** approach to decision making is focused on that which is commanded by God. Many contemporary religions, including Judaism, Islam, and Christianity and numerous polytheistic religions incorporate the importance of divine commands in ethical decision making (Rae, 2009). In **Christian ethics,** ethical decisions are based in the way of life and teachings of Jesus Christ. It advances the importance of virtues such as love, forgiveness, and honesty and is associated with the principle "Do unto others as you would have them do unto you." In Judaism, the Ten Commandments, which focus on loving God and loving others, are considered divine commands. In Islam, the focus is on the moral principles and virtues elaborated in Islamic religious texts, including good character, kindness, charity, and forgiveness.

Natural Law Theory

Natural law theory is based on the writings of St. Thomas Aquinas. It advances the idea that decisions about right versus wrong are self-evident and determined by human nature. The theory espouses that, as rational human beings, we inherently know the difference between good and evil (believed to be knowledge that is given to man from God), and this knowledge directs our decision making.

Ethical Egoism

Ethical egoism espouses that what is right and good is what is best for the individual making the decision. An individual's actions are determined by what is to their own advantage. The action may not be best for anyone else involved, but consideration is only for the individual making the decision.

Providing patient-centered care, an important health professions education competency identified in the IOM report (2013), speaks to some elements of ethical egoism. This competency promotes listening to and respecting the patient's values, preferences, and expressed needs in care management decisions.

Ethical Dilemmas

An **ethical dilemma** is a situation that requires an individual to make a choice between two equally balanced alternatives (Catalano, 2020). Evidence exists to support both moral "rightness" and moral "wrongness" related to a certain action. The individual who must make the choice experiences conscious conflict regarding the decision.

Not all ethical issues are dilemmas. An ethical dilemma arises when there is no clear reason to choose one action over another. Ethical dilemmas generally create a great deal of emotion. Often, the reasons supporting each side of the argument for action are logical and appropriate. The actions associated with both sides are desirable in some respects and undesirable in others. In most situations, taking no action is considered an action taken. For example, consider a patient who refuses to take a prescribed cardiac medication, claiming that they do not believe it is necessary. Although each patient has the right to refuse medication under ordinary circumstances, if the same patient is known to be depressed and suicidal, might they be intending self-harm by their refusal to take such a medication? And, if so, what is the best course of action? Many health-care settings have established guidelines for how to proceed should an ethical question or dilemma arise. Hospitals typically have a formal committee to explore and analyze ethical issues from several vantage points. Nurses can improve their critical thinking and clinical judgment skills by identifying such issues and seeking clarification through collaborative exploration with others and through ethics committee involvement.

Ethical Principles

Ethical principles are fundamental guidelines that influence decision making. The ethical principles of autonomy, beneficence, nonmaleficence, veracity, and justice are helpful and used frequently by health-care workers to assist with ethical decision making.

Autonomy

The principle of **autonomy** arises from the Kantian view of persons as independent moral agents whose right to determine their own destinies should always be respected. Autonomy presumes that individuals are always capable of making independent choices for themselves. Health-care workers know that this is not always the case. Children, comatose individuals, and some people with serious mental illness are incapable of making informed choices. In these instances, a representative for the individual is usually asked to intervene and give consent. However, health-care workers must ensure that respect for an individual's autonomy is not disregarded in favor of what another person may view as best for the client.

Beneficence

Beneficence refers to one's duty to benefit or promote the good of others. Health-care workers who act in their patients' interests are beneficent, provided their actions really do serve the patient's best interest. In fact, some duties seem to take preference over other duties. For example, the duty to respect the autonomy of an individual may be overridden when that individual has been deemed harmful to self or others. "Doing good" for the patient should not be confused with "doing whatever the patient wants" ("What Do I Do Now?" 2013). Good care must include a holistic focus that considers the patient's beliefs, feelings, and wishes; the wishes of the family and significant others; and considerations about competent nursing care (Catalano, 2020). Despite these guidelines, it is not always clear which action *is* in the best interest of the patient. When such dilemmas occur, nurses should reach out to available resources such as supervisors and ethics committees to build confidence that decisions about patient care have explored various vantage points.

Peplau (1991), a noted nursing theorist, recognized client **advocacy** as an essential role for the psychiatric nurse. The term *advocacy* means acting in another's behalf—being a supporter or defender. Being a patient advocate in psychiatric nursing means helping patients fulfill needs that, without assistance and because of their illness, may go unfulfilled. Individuals with mental illness are not always able to speak for themselves. Nurses serve in this manner to protect the patients' rights and interests. Strategies include educating patients and their families about their legal rights, ensuring that patients have sufficient information to make informed decisions or to give informed consent, and assisting patients to consider alternatives and supporting them in the decisions they make. Additionally, nurses may act as advocates by speaking on behalf of individuals with mental illness to secure essential mental health services.

Nonmaleficence

Nonmaleficence is the requirement that health-care providers do no harm to their patients, either intentionally or unintentionally. Some philosophers suggest that this principle is more important than beneficence; that is, they support the notion that it is more important to avoid doing harm than it is to do good. In any event, ethical dilemmas arise when a conflict exists between an individual's rights and what is thought to best represent the welfare of the individual. An example of this conflict might occur when a psychiatric patient refuses antipsychotic medication (consistent with their rights), and the nurse must then decide how to maintain patient safety while psychotic symptoms continue.

Justice

The principle of **justice** has been referred to as the "justice as fairness" principle. It is sometimes called *distributive justice*, and its basic premise lies with the right of individuals to be treated equally and fairly regardless of race, gender, sexual orientation, marital status, medical diagnosis, social standing, economic level, or religious beliefs (Catalano, 2020). When applied to health care, this principle suggests that all resources within the society (including health-care services) ought to be distributed equally to all people.

Thus, according to this principle, the vast disparity in the quality of care dispensed to the various socioeconomic classes within our society would be considered unjust. *Retribution* or *restorative justice* refers to the rules for responding when expectations for fairness are violated. *Social justice* assumes that rules for both distribution and rules for retribution should be fair and people should play by the rules (Maiese, 2017). It is important for nurses to recognize that in the latest revision of the Code of Ethics for Nurses (ANA, 2015), a new focus in one of the provisions states that nursing should integrate principles of social justice both in practice and in developing health policy.

Veracity

The principle of **veracity** refers to one's duty to always be truthful. Catalano (2020) states that veracity "requires the health care provider to tell the truth and not to intentionally deceive or mislead clients" (p. 128). There are times when limitations must be placed on this principle, such as when the truth would knowingly produce harm or interfere with the recovery process. Being honest is not always easy, but lying rarely is justified. Clients have the right to know about their diagnosis, treatment, and prognosis.

A Model for Making Ethical Decisions

The following is a set of steps that may be used in making an ethical decision. These steps are consistent with the steps of the nursing process:

1. ***Assessment:*** Gather the subjective and objective data about a situation. Consider personal values as well as values of others involved in the ethical dilemma.
2. ***Problem identification:*** Identify the conflict between two or more alternative actions.
3. ***Planning:***
   a. Explore the benefits and consequences of each alternative.
   b. Consider principles of ethical theories.
   c. Select an alternative.
4. ***Implementation:*** Act on the decision made and communicate the decision to others.
5. ***Evaluation:*** Evaluate outcomes.

A schematic of this model is presented in Figure 3–1. A case study using this decision-making model is presented in Box 3–1. If the outcome is acceptable, action continues in the manner selected. If the outcome is unacceptable, benefits and consequences of the remaining alternatives are reexamined, and steps three through seven in Box 3–1 are repeated.

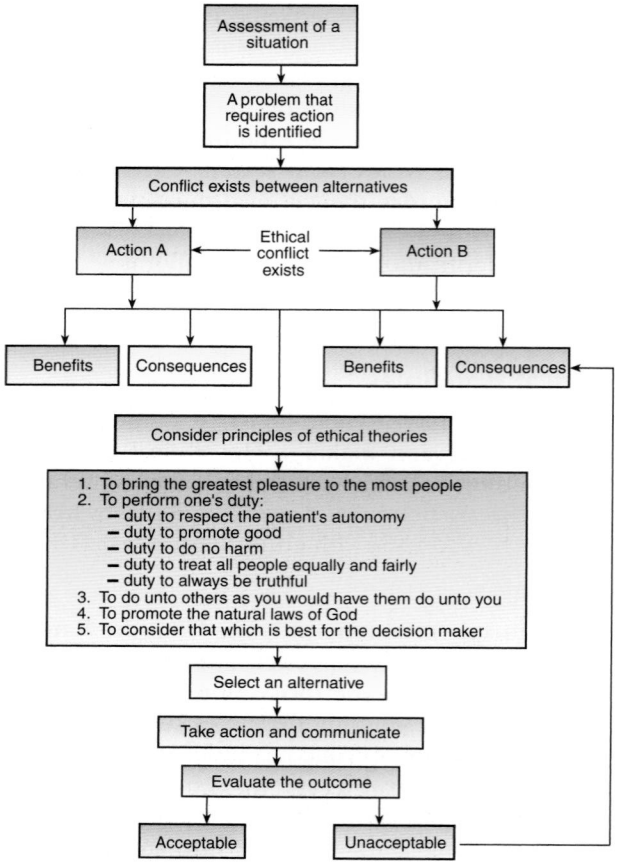

FIGURE 3–1 Ethical decision-making model.

Ethical and Legal Issues in Psychiatric Mental Health Nursing

The Right to Treatment

Anyone who is admitted to a hospital has the right to treatment. For example, a psychiatric patient cannot legally be hospitalized and then denied appropriate treatment. The AHA, although not having the authority of law, has also identified the rights of any hospitalized patient. The AHA patient Bill of Rights was historically written with an emphasis on protecting the patient from a breach of reasonable standards while hospitalized. These rights were revised in 2003 to create an emphasis on the importance of the collaborative relationship between the client and the hospital health-care team. Titled *The Patient Care Partnership*, this brochure informs patients that they have a right to high-quality care while hospitalized, to a clean and safe environment, to be involved in their care, to have their privacy protected, to get help when leaving the hospital, and to get help with their billing claims (AHA, 2003).

BOX 3–1 Ethical Decision Making—A Case Study

STEP 1. ASSESSMENT

Tonja is a 17-year-old girl who is currently on the psychiatric unit with a diagnosis of conduct disorder. Tonja reports that she has been sexually active since she was 14. She had an abortion when she was 15 and a second one just 6 weeks ago. She states that her mother told her she has "had her last abortion" and that she has to start taking birth control pills. She asks her nurse, Kimberly, to give her some information about the pills and to tell her how to go about getting some. Kimberly believes Tonja desperately needs information about birth control pills, as well as other types of contraceptives, but the psychiatric unit is part of a Catholic hospital, and hospital policy prohibits distributing this type of information.

STEP 2. PROBLEM IDENTIFICATION

A conflict exists between the patient's need for information, the nurse's desire to provide that information, and the institution's policy prohibiting the provision of that information.

STEP 3. ALTERNATIVES—BENEFITS AND CONSEQUENCES

Alternative 1: Give the patient information and risk losing job.

Alternative 2: Do not give patient information and compromise own values of holistic nursing.

Alternative 3: Refer the patient to another source outside the hospital and risk reprimand from supervisor.

STEP 4. CONSIDER PRINCIPLES OF ETHICAL THEORIES

Alternative 1: Giving the patient information would certainly respect the patient's autonomy and would benefit the patient by decreasing her chances of becoming pregnant again. It would not be to Kimberly's best advantage, because she would likely lose her job. And according to the beliefs of the Catholic hospital, the natural laws of God would be violated.

Alternative 2: Withholding information restricts the patient's autonomy. It has the potential for doing harm, because without the use of contraceptives, the patient may become pregnant again (and she implies that this is not what she wants). Kimberly's Christian ethic is violated in that this action is not what she would want "done unto her."

Alternative 3: A referral would respect the patient's autonomy, would promote good, and would do no harm (except perhaps to Kimberly's ego from the possible reprimand), and this decision would comply with Kimberly's Christian ethic.

STEP 5. SELECT AN ALTERNATIVE

Alternative 3 is selected on the basis of the ethical theories of utilitarianism (does the most good for the greatest number), Christian ethics (Kimberly's belief of "Do unto others as you would have others do unto you"), Kantianism (to perform one's duty), and the ethical principles of autonomy, beneficence, and nonmaleficence. The success of this decision depends on the patient's follow-through with the referral and compliance with use of the contraceptives.

STEP 6. TAKE ACTION AND COMMUNICATE

Taking action involves providing information in writing for Tonja, perhaps making a phone call and setting up an appointment for her with Planned Parenthood. Communicating involves sharing the information with Tonja's mother. Communication also includes documentation of the referral in the patient's chart.

STEP 7. EVALUATE THE OUTCOME

An acceptable outcome might indicate that Tonja did indeed keep her appointment at Planned Parenthood and is complying with the prescribed contraceptive regimen. It might also include Kimberly's input into the change process in her institution to implement these types of referrals to other patients who request them.

An unacceptable outcome might be indicated by Tonja's lack of follow-through with the appointment at Planned Parenthood or lack of compliance in using the contraceptives, resulting in another pregnancy. Kimberly may also view a reprimand from her supervisor as an unacceptable outcome, particularly if she is told that she must select other alternatives should this situation arise in the future. This may motivate Kimberly to make another decision—that of seeking employment in an institution that supports a philosophy more consistent with her own.

In 2010, federal law expanded patient rights to include insurability in spite of pre-existing conditions. However, federal health-care law continues to be a debated issue and will no doubt continue to see changes depending on the prevailing political climate. Nurses practicing in hospital settings need to be aware of and adhere to legal statutes, accepted standards of practice, and organizational policies with regard to a patient's rights during hospital treatment.

The Right to Refuse Treatment (Including Medication)

Legally, patients have the right to refuse treatment unless the treatment requires immediate intervention to prevent death or serious harm to the patient or another person or to prevent deterioration of the patient's clinical state (Boland & Verduin, 2022). The U.S. Constitution and several of its amendments affirm this right (e.g., the First Amendment, which addresses the rights of speech, thought, and expression; the Eighth Amendment, which grants the right to freedom from cruel and unusual punishment; and the Fifth and Fourteenth Amendments, which grant due process of law and equal protection for all). In psychiatry, however, there are both ethical and legal issues that must be considered. Sometimes patients are involuntarily hospitalized because they are at risk of harming themselves or others and do not recognize the dangerousness of their symptoms. To protect the client's rights, specific legal criteria must be met to assure that the involuntary hospitalization is justified. However, Saya and associates (2019) note the strictness of criteria for involuntarily hospitalization in the United States has led to a criminalization of mental illness and consequently this population is detained in prisons in the United States more so than in any other country.

In emergency cases, sedative medication may be administered without the patient's consent in order to protect patients from harming themselves or others. Unlike some other countries (such as Italy) where involuntary medication is automatically allowed for a hospitalized patient, in the United States there are, typically, specific criteria that must be met to justify medicating a patient without their consent (Saya et al., 2019). Because laws vary from state to state, it is important for nurses to know the laws that pertain to their local jurisdiction. Organizational policies in the nurse's practice setting should also guide decision making.

Although many courts support a client's right to refuse medications in psychiatric treatment, exceptions do exist. When making a decision about forced medication, Weiss-Kaffie and Purtell (2001) state:

> The treatment team must determine that three criteria be met to force medication without client consent. The client must exhibit behavior that is dangerous to self or others; the medication ordered by the physician must have a reasonable chance of providing help to the client; and clients who refuse medication must be judged incompetent to evaluate the benefits of the treatment in question. (p. 361)

Evidence supports the long-term benefits of involuntary medication, particularly for patients with schizophrenia and bipolar disorders (Mental Illness Policy Org., 2017). Current research (Dixon et al., 2018) demonstrating the particular benefits of treating a first episode of psychosis as important in decreasing long-term negative consequences may increase acceptability of involuntary medication as an early intervention when needed.

More recently, some states have adopted laws that allow a court to mandate outpatient treatment for people with mental illness who have a history of violent behavior. In New York City, this law (known as *Kendra's Law*; see discussion later in this chapter) also includes a provision for ordering an individual to take medication as part of the treatment plan.

The Right to the Least Restrictive Treatment Alternative

The right to the least restrictive treatment alternative means that clients who can be adequately treated in an outpatient setting should not be hospitalized, and if they are hospitalized, they should not be sedated, restrained, or secluded unless other less restrictive measures were found to be unsuccessful. In other words, clients have a right to whatever level of treatment is effective and least restricts their freedom. The "restrictiveness" of psychiatric therapy can be described in the context of a continuum based on severity of illness. Clients may be treated on an outpatient basis, in day hospitals, or through voluntary or involuntary hospitalization. Symptoms may be treated with verbal rehabilitative techniques and move successively to behavioral techniques, chemical interventions, mechanical restraints, or electroconvulsive therapy. However, ethical issues arise in selecting the least restrictive means among involuntary chemical intervention, seclusion, and mechanical restraints. Boland and Verduin (2022) state that

> distinguishing among these interventions on the basis of restrictiveness proves to be a purely subjective exercise fraught with personal bias. Moreover, each of these three interventions is both more and less restrictive than each of the other two. Nevertheless, the effort should be made to think in terms of restrictiveness when deciding how to treat patients. (p. 841)

Although these rights may seem reasonable and expected, it is important to recognize that clients with mental illness have historically been hospitalized against their will simply because they had a mental illness. In the case of *O'Connor* v. *Donaldson* (1976), the Supreme Court ruled that harmless mentally ill individuals cannot be confined against their will if they are able to remain safe outside of a hospital setting. Only if they are considered dangerous to themselves or others or are so unable to care for themselves that their safety and survival are at risk may they be confined involuntarily. In 1981, the case of *Roger* v. *Oken* culminated in the ruling that all patients, even those involuntarily hospitalized, are competent to refuse treatment, but a legal guardian may authorize treatment (Boland & Verduin, 2022). These laws and policies have attempted to better protect the rights of clients with mental illness while still recognizing that, at times, individuals with acute mental illness may be unable to make decisions in the interest of their safety and survival.

Ideally, it is hoped that the person with mental illness recognizes their need for treatment and agrees voluntarily to be hospitalized if this measure is recommended by the health-care provider. The client who is voluntarily hospitalized typically signs a consent to treatment upon admission, but it remains the client's right, as a voluntary patient, to revoke that consent and to be discharged from the hospital if they so choose.

Legal Considerations

Patient Rights

The Patient Self-Determination Act, as part of the Omnibus Budget Reconciliation Act of 1990, went into effect on December 1, 1991. Cady (2010) states:

> The Patient Self-determination Act requires healthcare facilities to provide clear written information for every patient concerning his/her legal rights to make healthcare decisions, including the right to accept or refuse treatment. (p. 118)

Box 3–2 lists the rights of patients affirmed by this law.

Nurse Practice Acts

The legal parameters of professional and practical nursing are defined within each state by the state's

BOX 3–2 Patient Self-Determination Act—Patient Rights

A person admitted to a program or facility for the purpose of receiving mental health services should be accorded the following:

1. The right to appropriate treatment and related services in a setting and under conditions that are the most supportive of such person's personal liability and that restrict such liberty only to the extent necessary consistent with such person's treatment needs, applicable requirements of law, and applicable judicial orders.
2. The right to an individualized, written treatment or service plan (such plan to be developed promptly after admission of such person), the right to treatment based on such plan, the right to periodic review and reassessment of treatment and related service needs, and the right to appropriate revision of such plan, including any revision necessary to provide a description of mental health services that may be needed after such person is discharged from such program or facility.
3. The right to ongoing participation, in a manner appropriate to a person's capabilities, in the planning of mental health services to be provided (including the right to participate in the development and periodic revision of the plan).
4. The right to be provided, in terms and language appropriate to a person's condition and ability to understand, a reasonable explanation of the person's general mental and physical (if appropriate) condition, the objectives of treatment, the nature and significant possible adverse effects of recommended treatment, the reasons a particular treatment is considered appropriate, the reasons access to certain visitors may not be appropriate, and any appropriate and available alternative treatments, services, and types of providers of mental health services.
5. The right not to receive a mode or course of treatment in the absence of informed, voluntary, written consent to treatment except during an emergency situation or as permitted by law when the person is being treated as a result of a court order.
6. The right not to participate in experimentation in the absence of informed, voluntary, written consent (includes human subject protection).
7. The right to freedom from restraint or seclusion, other than as a mode or course of treatment or restraint or seclusion during an emergency situation with a written order by a responsible mental health professional.
8. The right to a humane treatment environment that affords reasonable protection from harm and appropriate privacy with regard to personal needs.
9. The right to access, on request, to such person's mental health-care records.
10. The right, in the case of a person admitted on a residential or inpatient care basis, to converse with others privately, to have convenient and reasonable access to the telephone and mail, and to see visitors during regularly scheduled hours. (For treatment purposes, specific individuals may be excluded.)
11. The right to be informed promptly and in writing at the time of admission of these rights.
12. The right to assert grievances with respect to infringement of these rights.
13. The right to exercise these rights without reprisal.
14. The right of referral to other providers upon discharge.

Source: Adapted from the U.S. Code, Title 42, Section 10841, The Public Health and Welfare, 1991.

nurse practice act. These documents are passed by the state legislature and in general are concerned with such provisions as the following:

- The definition of important terms, including the definition of *nursing* and the various types of nurses recognized
- A statement of the education and other training or requirements for licensure and reciprocity
- Broad statements that describe the scope of practice for various levels of nursing (APRN, RN, LPN)
- Conditions under which a nurse's license may be suspended or revoked, and instructions for appeal
- The general authority and powers of the state board of nursing

Most nurse practice acts are general in their terminology and do not provide specific guidelines for practice. Nurses must understand the scope of practice that is protected by their license and should seek assistance from legal counsel if they are unsure about the proper interpretation of a nurse practice act.

Types of Law

There are two general categories of law that are of most concern to nurses: statutory law and common law. These laws are identified by their source or origin.

Statutory Law

A **statutory law** is a law that has been enacted by a legislative body, such as a county or city council, state legislature, or the U.S. Congress. An example of statutory law is a nurse practice act.

Common Law

Common laws are derived from decisions made in previous cases. These laws apply to a body of principles that evolve from court decisions resolving various controversies. Because common law in the United States has been developed on a state basis, the law on specific subjects may differ from state to state. An example of a common law might be how different states deal with a nurse's refusal to provide care for a specific client.

Classifications Within Statutory and Common Law

Broadly speaking, there are two kinds of unlawful acts: civil and criminal. Both statutory law and common law have civil and criminal components.

Civil Law

Civil law protects the private and property rights of individuals and businesses. Private individuals or groups may bring a legal action to court for breach of civil law. These legal actions are of two basic types: torts and contracts.

Torts

A **tort** is a violation of a civil law in which an individual has been wronged. In a tort action, one party asserts that wrongful conduct on the part of the other has caused harm, and the first party seeks compensation for harm suffered. A tort may be *intentional* or *unintentional*. Examples of unintentional torts are malpractice and negligence actions. An example of an intentional tort is the touching of another person without that person's consent. Intentional touching (e.g., a medical treatment) without the client's consent can result in a charge of battery, an intentional tort.

Contracts

In a contract action, one party asserts that the other party, in failing to fulfill an obligation, has breached the contract, and either compensation or performance of the obligation is sought as remedy. An example is an action by a mental health professional whose clinical privileges have been reduced or terminated in violation of an implied contract between the professional and a hospital.

Criminal Law

Criminal law provides protection from conduct deemed injurious to the public welfare. It provides for punishment of those found to have engaged in such conduct, which can range from community service and fines to imprisonment and death depending on the scope of the crime (Aiken, 2020). An example of a violation of criminal law is the theft of supplies or drugs by a hospital employee. Catalano (2020) notes, "The most common violation by nurses of the criminal law is failure to renew nursing licenses. In this situation, the nurse is practicing nursing without a license, which is a crime in all states" (p. 184). He adds that recent cases of intentional or unintentional death of clients and assisted suicide have also led to criminal charges against nurses.

Legal Issues in Psychiatric Mental Health Nursing

Confidentiality and Right to Privacy

The Fourth, Fifth, and Fourteenth Amendments to the U.S. Constitution protect an individual's privacy. Most states have statutes protecting the confidentiality of client records and communications. Nurses must recognize that the only individuals who have a right to observe a client or have access to medical information are those involved in their medical care. The patient must provide written consent for health-care information to be shared with anyone outside the current treatment team.

HIPAA

Until 1996, client confidentiality in medical records was not protected by federal law. In August 1996, President Clinton signed the Health Insurance Portability and Accountability Act (HIPAA) into law. This federal privacy rule pertains to data called *protected health information* (PHI) and applies to most individuals and institutions involved in health care. PHI is defined as individually identifiable health information indicators that "relate to past, present, or future physical or mental health or condition of the individual, or the past, present, or future payment for the provision of health care to an individual; and (1) that identifies the individual; or (2) with respect to which there is a reasonable basis to believe the information can be used to identify the individual" (U.S. Department of Health & Human Services, 2003). These specific identifiers are listed in Box 3–3.

Under HIPAA, individuals have the right to access their medical records, to have corrections made to their medical records, and to decide with whom their medical information may be shared. The actual document belongs to the facility or the therapist, but the information contained therein belongs to the client. The passage of HIPAA increased the level of control clients have over the information maintained in their medical records. Notice of privacy policies must be provided to clients upon entry into the health-care system.

In 2013, HIPAA privacy and security rules were expanded to afford more rights to patients with regard to their medical information and to ensure greater security of a person's health information. For example, when patients are paying out of pocket for care, they can tell a provider that they do not want treatment information shared with their health insurance provider (U.S. Department of Health & Human Services, 2013). Nurses in any practice setting need to be aware of these HIPAA laws and of any new provisions in law that will impact the conduct of their practice.

Pertinent medical information may be released without consent in a life-threatening situation. If information is released in an emergency, the following information must be recorded in the client's record: date of disclosure, person to whom information was disclosed, reason for disclosure, reason written consent could not be obtained, and the specific information disclosed.

BOX 3–3 Protected Health Information (PHI): Individually Identifiable Indicators

1. Names
2. Postal address information (except state), including street address, city, county, precinct, and zip code
3. All elements of dates (except year) for dates directly related to an individual, including birth date, admission date, discharge date, date of death; and all ages over 89 and all elements of dates (including year) indicative of such age, except that such ages and elements may be aggregated into a single category of age 90 or older
4. Telephone numbers
5. Fax numbers
6. Electronic mail addresses
7. Social Security numbers
8. Medical record numbers
9. Health plan beneficiary numbers
10. Account numbers
11. Certificate/license numbers
12. Vehicle identifiers and serial numbers, including license plate numbers
13. Device identifiers and serial numbers
14. Web Universal Resource Locators (URLs)
15. Internet protocol (IP) address numbers
16. Biometric identifiers, including finger and voice prints
17. Full face photographic images and any comparable images
18. Any other unique identifying number, characteristic, or code

Source: U.S. Department of Health and Human Services *(2003). Standards for privacy of individually identifiable health information.*

Most states have statutes that pertain to the doctrine of **privileged communication.** Although the codes differ markedly from state to state, most grant certain professionals privileges under which they may refuse to reveal information about and communications with clients. In most states, the doctrine of privileged communication applies to psychiatrists and attorneys; in some instances, psychologists, clergy, and nurses are also included.

In certain instances, nurses may be called on to testify in cases in which the medical record is used as evidence. In most states, the right to privacy of these records is exempted in civil or criminal proceedings. Therefore, it is important that nurses document with these possibilities in mind. Careful record-keeping using statements that are objective and nonjudgmental, care plans that are specific in their prescriptive interventions, and documentation that describes those interventions and their subsequent evaluation all serve the best interests of the client, the nurse, and the institution should questions regarding care arise. Documentation very often weighs heavily in malpractice case decisions.

The right to confidentiality is a basic one, and especially so in psychiatry. Although societal attitudes are improving, individuals have experienced discrimination in the past for no other reason than that they have a history of mental illness. Nurses working in psychiatric mental health nursing must guard the privacy of their patients with great diligence.

Exception: A Duty to Warn (Protection of a Third Party)

There are exceptions to the laws of privacy and confidentiality. One of these exceptions stems from the 1974 case of *Tarasoff* v. *Regents of the University of California.* The incident from which this case evolved came about in the late 1960s. Mr. P., a young man from Bengal, India, who was a graduate student at the University of California (UC), Berkeley, fell in love with another university student (Ms. Tarasoff). Because she was not interested in an exclusive relationship with Mr. P., he became very resentful and angry. He began to stalk her and to record some of their conversations in an effort to determine why she did not love him. He soon became very depressed and neglected his health, appearance, and studies.

Ms. Tarasoff spent the summer of 1969 in South America. During this time, Mr. P. entered therapy with a psychologist at UC. He confided in the psychologist that he intended to kill his former girlfriend (identifying her by name) when she returned from vacation. The psychologist recommended civil commitment for Mr. P., claiming that he was suffering from acute and severe paranoid schizophrenia. Mr. P. was picked up by the campus police but released a short time later because he appeared rational and promised to stay away from Ms. Tarasoff. Neither Ms. Tarasoff nor her parents received any warning of the threat of Mr. P.'s intention to kill her.

When Ms. Tarasoff returned to campus in October 1969, Mr. P. resumed his stalking behavior and eventually stabbed her to death. Ms. Tarasoff's parents sued the psychologist, several psychiatrists, and the university for failure to warn the family of the danger. The case was referred to the California Supreme Court, which ruled that a mental health professional has a duty not only to a client but also to individuals who are being threatened by that client. The Court stated:

> Once a therapist does in fact determine, or under applicable professional standards should have determined, that a patient poses a serious danger of violence to others, he bears a duty to exercise reasonable care to protect the foreseeable victim of that danger. While the discharge of this duty of due care will necessarily vary with the facts of each case, in each instance the adequacy of the therapist's conduct must be measured against the traditional negligence standard of reasonable care under the circumstances. (*Tarasoff* v. *Regents of University of California*, 1974a)

The defendants argued that warning the woman or her family would have breached professional ethics and violated the client's right to privacy. But the court ruled that "the confidential character of patient-psychotherapist communications must yield to the extent that disclosure is essential to avert danger to others. The protective privilege ends where the public peril begins" (*Tarasoff* v. *Regents of University of California*, 1974b).

In 1976, the California Supreme Court expanded the original case ruling (now referred to as *Tarasoff I*). The second ruling (known as *Tarasoff II*) broadened the ruling of "duty to warn" to include "duty to protect." They stated that, under certain circumstances, a therapist might be required to warn an individual, notify police, or take whatever steps are necessary to protect the intended victim from harm. This duty to protect can also occur in instances when patients must be protected by health-care providers because they are vulnerable as a result of their inability to identify harmful situations (Guido, 2014).

The *Tarasoff* rulings created a great deal of controversy in the psychiatric community regarding breach of confidentiality and the subsequent negative impact on the client-therapist relationship. However, most states now recognize that therapists have ethical and legal obligations to prevent their clients from harming themselves or others. Many states have passed their own variations on the original "protect and warn" legislation, but in most cases, courts have outlined the following guidelines for therapists to follow in determining their obligation to take protective measures:

1. Assessment of a threat of violence by a client toward another individual
2. Identification of the intended victim
3. Ability to intervene in a feasible, meaningful way to protect the intended victim

When these guidelines apply to a specific situation, it is reasonable for the therapist to notify the victim, law enforcement authorities, and/or relatives of the intended victim. The therapist may also consider initiating voluntary or involuntary commitment of the client in an effort to prevent potential violence.

Implications for Nursing Although the original decision in the *Tarasoff* ruling was directed toward psychotherapists, it has become more broadly applied since that time. Not all states identify registered nurses as having a duty to warn, but other statutes include a duty to warn for anyone from a licensed practical nurse to licensed certified advanced practice nurses. As of 2018, there are three states (Maine, Nevada, and North Dakota) that have not yet addressed the issue of duty to warn and one state (North Carolina) that does not recognize the duty to warn (National Conference of State Legislatures, 2018). In 2018, New Jersey expanded its "duty to warn" law to require mental health professionals (including nurses) to notify local authorities whenever patients threaten to harm *themselves* or others (Sitrin, 2018). Although intended to promote greater gun safety by removing guns from people who are at risk of harming themselves or others with firearms, the law has far broader implications both professionally and politically.

Even in states that do not address a duty to warn, practitioners still need to make an ethical decision about warning a potential victim. Every nurse, not just those practicing in psychiatric nursing, should be informed about the laws in their state regarding duty to warn. As Henderson (2015) notes, emergency nurses are often the frontline health-care workers and thus are in a position to first identify persons at risk for violence and to protect the safety of the patient and others.

In psychiatric mental health nursing practice, if a client confides in the nurse the potential for harm to an intended victim, it is the duty of the nurse to report this information to the psychiatrist and to other team members. Reporting this information is not a breach of confidentiality, and the nurse may be considered negligent for failure to report. All members of the treatment team must be made aware of the potential danger that the client poses to self or others. Detailed written documentation of the situation is essential.

Exception: Suspected Child or Elder Abuse

The Federal Child Abuse Prevention and Treatment Act (CAPTA) requires each state to have provisions or procedures for requiring certain individuals to report known or suspected instances of child abuse and neglect (Child Welfare Information Gateway, 2019a). Many jurisdictions also have statutes requiring that suspected elder abuse or neglect be reported. At times, health-care professionals are worried that they may be liable for false allegations and therefore may be reluctant to report, but reporting statutes generally grant immunity to anyone making a good faith report about a reasonable suspicion. In fact, nearly every state and U.S. territory imposes penalties, from imposing fines or possible imprisonment for mandatory reporters who *fail* to report suspected child abuse or neglect as required by law; in some jurisdictions, failure to report is identified as a felony (Child Welfare Information Gateway, 2019b).

Implications for Nursing There is often an element of clinical judgment about whether a patient's communication raises a reasonable suspicion of abuse. For example, when a person is experiencing hallucinations or delusions, their perception about events may be distorted. The nurse has a responsibility to explore all of the patient's perceptions of abuse or mistreatment and discuss them with other health-care team members to identify the most appropriate decision considering legal, ethical, and clinical factors.

Informed Consent

According to law, all individuals have the right to decide whether to accept or reject treatment. A health-care provider can be charged with assault and battery for providing treatment to a client when the client has not agreed to it. The rationale for the doctrine of **informed consent** is the preservation and protection of individual autonomy in determining what will and will not happen to the person's body (Guido, 2014).

Informed consent is a client's permission granted to a health-care provider to perform a therapeutic procedure after information about the procedure has been presented to the client with adequate time given for consideration about the pros and cons. The client should receive information such as what treatment alternatives are available; why the health-care provider believes this treatment is most appropriate; the possible outcomes, risks, and adverse effects; the possible outcome should the client select another treatment alternative; and the possible outcome should the client choose to have no treatment. An example of a treatment in the psychiatric area that requires informed consent is electroconvulsive therapy.

Under some conditions, treatment may be performed without obtaining informed consent from the client. A client's refusal to accept treatment may be challenged under the following circumstances (Guido, 2014):

1. When a client is mentally incompetent to make a decision and treatment is necessary to preserve life or avoid serious harm
2. When refusing treatment endangers the life or health of another
3. During an emergency in which a client is in no condition to exercise judgment
4. When the client is a child (consent is obtained from parent or surrogate)
5. In the case of therapeutic privilege (a situation where it is acceptable for the physician to withhold some information from the patient): Information about a treatment may be withheld if the physician can show that full disclosure would:
   a. Hinder or complicate necessary treatment,
   b. Cause severe psychological harm, or
   c. Be so upsetting as to render a rational decision by the client impossible.

Although most clients in psychiatric and mental health facilities are competent and capable of giving informed consent, those with severe psychiatric illness may not possess the cognitive ability to do so. If an individual has been legally determined to be mentally incompetent, consent is obtained from the legal guardian. Difficulty arises when no legal determination has been made, but the individual's current mental state prohibits informed decision making (e.g., the person who is psychotic, unconscious, or inebriated). In these instances, informed consent is usually obtained from the individual's nearest relative, or if none exists and time permits, the health-care provider may ask the court to appoint a conservator or guardian. When time does not permit court intervention, permission may be sought from the hospital administrator.

A client or guardian always has the right to withdraw consent after it has been given. When this occurs, the health-care provider should inform (or re-inform) the client about the consequences of refusing treatment. If treatment has already been initiated, the health-care provider should terminate treatment in a way least likely to cause injury to the client and inform the client or guardian of the risks associated with interrupted treatment (Guido, 2014).

The staff nurse's role in obtaining informed consent is usually defined by agency policy. A nurse may sign the consent form as witness for the client's signature. However, legal liability for informed consent lies with the physician. The nurse acts as client advocate, ensuring that the following three major elements of informed consent have been addressed:

1. ***Knowledge:*** The client has received adequate information on which to base their decision.
2. ***Competency:*** The individual's cognition is not impaired to an extent that would interfere with decision making, but if cognition is so impaired, the individual has a legal representative.
3. ***Free will:*** The individual has given consent voluntarily without pressure or coercion from others.

Restraints and Seclusion

An individual's privacy and personal security are protected by the Patient Self-Determination Act of 1991. This legislation includes a set of patient rights, one of which is an individual's right to freedom from restraint and from seclusion except in an emergency situation. The use of seclusion and restraint as a therapeutic intervention for psychiatric patients has been controversial, and many efforts have been made through federal and state regulations and through standards set forth by accrediting bodies to minimize or eliminate its use. In addition, an element of moral decision making is involved when any kind of treatment is coerced, as is often the case with seclusion and restraint. Landeweer et al. (2011) point out that although coercion may sometimes be necessary, it can be detrimental to the patient because it may produce trauma and mistrust. Most hospitals have a forum, such as an ethics committee, to discuss these ethical issues. One advantage of using such forums to guide moral decision making is that, by exploring issues (such as the use of seclusion and restraint) with a diverse group of people who have different vantage points, alternative treatments can be identified and explored.

Because injuries and deaths have been associated with restraint and seclusion, this treatment requires careful attention whenever it is used. Further, the laws, regulations, accreditation standards, and hospital policies are frequently revised, so it is important for anyone practicing in inpatient psychiatric settings to be well informed in each of these areas.

In psychiatry, the term *restraints* generally refers to a set of leather straps that is used to restrain the extremities of an individual whose behavior is out of control and who poses an immediate risk to the physical safety and psychological well-being of the individual and others. It is important to note, however, that the current generally accepted definition of restraint refers not only to leather restraints but also to any manual method or medication used to restrict a person's freedom of movement. Restraints are never to be used as punishment or for the convenience of staff. Other measures to decrease agitation, such as "talking down" (verbal intervention) and chemical restraints (tranquilizing medication) are the preferred first-line interventions. If these interventions are ineffective, mechanical restraints may be instituted (although some controversy exists as to whether chemical restraints are indeed less restrictive than mechanical restraints). *Seclusion* is another type of physical restraint in which the client is confined alone in a room from which they are unable to leave. The room is usually minimally furnished to promote the client's comfort and safety.

Since seclusion and restraint are both considered high-risk interventions, institutions, health-care accrediting bodies (such as The Joint Commission), and state mental health departments define specific expectations for their use. These standards typically include requirements for staff training and competency in the use of seclusion or restraint; expectations that these interventions will be used only as a last resort and for the shortest amount of time necessary; and what kinds of assessment and intervention are required before, during, and after the individual is secluded or restrained.

The laws, regulations, accreditation standards, and hospital policies pertaining to restraint and seclusion share a common priority of maintaining patient safety for a procedure that has the potential to incur injury or death. The importance of close and careful monitoring, following institutional policies, and accurate documentation cannot be overstated.

False imprisonment is the deliberate and unauthorized confinement of a competent person with the intent to prevent them from leaving the hospital; this includes use of threats or medications that interfere with the client's ability to leave the facility (Aiken, 2020). Health-care workers may be charged with false imprisonment for restraining or secluding—against the wishes of the client—anyone having been admitted to the hospital voluntarily. Should a voluntarily admitted client decompensate to a point that restraint or seclusion for protection of self or others is necessary, court intervention to determine competency and involuntary commitment is required to preserve the client's rights to privacy and freedom.

Hospitalization

Voluntary Admissions

Although the vast majority of mental health services are provided on a voluntary basis (Substance Abuse and Mental Health Services Administration [SAMHSA], 2019), much of voluntary treatment occurs in settings other than inpatient hospitalization. This has been influenced by the availability of a greater number of outpatient treatment options including partial hospitalization, intensive outpatient programs, and other specialized treatment programs. To be admitted voluntarily to a hospital setting, an individual signs a voluntary admission consent and may stay as long as treatment is deemed necessary. They may sign out of the hospital at any time unless, following a mental status examination, the health-care professional determines that the client may be harmful to self or others and recommends that the admission status be changed from voluntary to involuntary (in which case legal criteria must be met). Even when an admission is voluntary, it is still important to ensure that the individual comprehends the meaning of their actions, has not been coerced in any manner, and is willing to proceed with admission.

Involuntary Commitment

Although the term *involuntary hospitalization* is preferred by some rather than the term *involuntary commitment* or *civil commitment*, it must be understood that this process needs to be conducted with respect to state and federal law. Because involuntary hospitalization results in substantial restrictions of the rights of an individual, the admission process is subject to the guarantee of the Fourteenth Amendment to the U.S. Constitution that provides citizens protection against loss of liberty and ensures due process rights. Involuntary hospitalizations are made for various reasons. Most states commonly cite the following criteria:

- The person is imminently dangerous to himself or herself (i.e., suicidal intent).
- The person is a danger to others (i.e., aggressive, violent, or homicidal).
- The person is unable to take care of basic personal needs (the "gravely disabled").

Under the Fourth Amendment, individuals are protected from unlawful searches and seizures without probable cause. Therefore, the individual recommending involuntary hospitalization must show probable cause for hospitalizing the client against their wishes; that is, the person must show that there is cause to believe that the client would be dangerous to self or others, is mentally ill and in need of treatment, or is gravely disabled.

Emergency Commitments

Emergency commitments are sought when an individual manifests behavior that is clearly and imminently dangerous to self or others. These admissions are usually instigated by relatives or friends of the individual, police officers, the court, or health-care professionals. Emergency commitments are time-limited, and a court hearing for the individual is scheduled, usually within 72 hours. At that time, the court may decide that the client may be discharged; or, if deemed necessary, and voluntary admission is refused by the client, an additional period of involuntary hospitalization may be ordered. In most instances, another hearing is scheduled for a specified time (usually in 7 to 21 days).

The Mentally Ill Person in Need of Treatment

A second type of involuntary commitment is for the observation and treatment of mentally ill persons in need of treatment. These are typically longer than emergency commitments. Most states have established definitions of what constitutes "mentally ill" for purposes of state involuntary admission statutes. Some examples include individuals who, because of severe mental illness, are

- Unable to make informed decisions concerning treatment
- Likely to cause harm to self or others
- Unable to fulfill basic personal needs necessary for health and safety

In determining whether commitment is required, the court looks for substantial evidence of abnormal conduct—evidence that cannot be explained as the result of a physical cause. There must be "clear and convincing evidence" as well as "probable cause" to substantiate the need for involuntary hospitalization to ensure that an individual's rights under the Constitution are protected. As mentioned earlier, the U.S. Supreme Court, in *O'Connor* v. *Donaldson*, held that the existence of mental illness alone does not justify involuntary hospitalization. State standards require a specific impact or consequence to flow from the mental illness that involves danger or an inability to care for one's own needs. These clients are entitled to court hearings with representation, at which time determination of commitment and length of stay are considered. Legislative statutes governing involuntary commitments vary from state to state.

Involuntary Outpatient Commitment

Involuntary outpatient commitment (IOC) is a court-ordered mechanism used to compel a person with mental illness to submit to treatment on an outpatient basis. As these laws have evolved, they have taken a more "preventive approach." In this scenario a person with mental illness who is not currently dangerous, and therefore not legally committable to a hospital, could be ordered to community treatment on the basis of a complex clinical assessment and prediction about the future. Examples of eligibility criteria (SAMHSA, 2019) include those outlined in North Carolina's state statutes:

- The person must have a mental illness.
- The person is capable of surviving safely in the community with available supervision from family, friends, or others.
- Based on the person's psychiatric history, the person is in need of treatment in order to prevent further disability or deterioration that would predictably result in dangerousness.
- The person's current mental status or the nature of their illness limits or negates their ability to make an informed decision to seek voluntary admission or comply with recommended treatment.

Most states have already enacted IOC legislation or currently have resolutions that speak to this topic on their agendas. Most commonly, clients who are committed into the IOC programs are those with severe and persistent mental illness, such as schizophrenia. The rationale behind the legislation is to improve preventive care and reduce the number of readmissions and lengths of hospital stays of these clients. The need for this kind of legislation arose after it was recognized that individuals with schizophrenia who did not meet criteria for involuntary hospital treatment were, in some cases, ultimately dangerous to themselves or others.

Public attention to this need arose in New York after a man with schizophrenia who had stopped taking his medication pushed a young woman into the path of a subway train. He would not have met criteria for involuntary hospitalization until he was deemed dangerous to others, but advocates for this legislation argued that there should be provisions to prevent violence rather than waiting until it happens. The subsequent law governing IOC in New York became known as Kendra's Law in reference to the woman who was pushed to her death. Opponents of this legislation fear that it may violate the individual rights of psychiatric clients without significant improvement in outcomes. While many states have enacted similar laws, New York's Kendra's Law adds a stricter stipulation that the person must have been hospitalized at least twice within the prior three years as a result of noncompliance with treatment, or have committed, attempted, or threatened an act of violence or self-harm within the prior two years and they would benefit from this type of treatment.

Research studies have attempted to evaluate whether IOC improves care, reduces lengths of stay in the hospital, and/or reduces episodes of violence. Some studies have shown positive outcomes with IOC, including a decrease in hospital readmissions (Ridgely et al., 2001; Swartz et al., 2001; Swartz & Swanson, 2008). But a Cochran literature review (Kisely et al., 2017) concluded that compulsory community treatment resulted in no significant differences in service use, social functioning, mental state, or quality of life, although those in mandated outpatient treatment were less likely to be victims of crimes. The issues around whether IOC will improve treatment compliance and enhance quality of life in the community for individuals with severe and persistent mental illness will continue to be a focus of study and debate.

The Gravely Disabled Client

A number of states have statutes that specifically define the "gravely disabled" client. For those that do not use this label, the description of the individual who, because of mental illness, is unable to take care of basic personal needs is very similar.

Gravely disabled is generally defined as a condition in which an individual, as a result of mental illness, is in danger of serious physical harm resulting from an inability to provide for basic needs such as food, clothing, shelter, medical care, and personal safety. Inability to care for oneself cannot be established by showing that an individual lacks the resources to provide the necessities of life. Rather, it is established by showing the individual's inability to make use of available resources.

Should it be determined that an individual is gravely disabled, a guardian, conservator, or committee is appointed by the court to ensure the management of the person and their estate. To legally restore competency requires another court hearing to reverse the previous ruling. The individual whose competency is being determined has the right to be represented by an attorney.

It is an ethical and legal duty to ensure that whenever coercive treatments are used, including involuntary hospitalizations, seclusion and restraint, involuntary outpatient commitments, mandated medication, and even prison commitments, the least restrictive intervention must first be considered. Sashadahran and Saraceno (2017) identified a concern that there is a current shift globally toward more coercive care similar to that which existed prior to the community mental health movement. They cite increasing numbers of involuntary hospitalizations. They also note that in the United States there are currently three times as many individuals with mental illness in prisons as there are in hospitals, and that sexual predator laws in the United States allow indefinite hospital stays for serious sex offenders beyond their prison sentence completion. The authors posit that when risk management supersedes the most appropriate level of care for treatment, stigmatization of this population may increase (Sashadahran & Saraceno, 2017).

Nursing Liability

Mental health practitioners—psychiatrists, psychologists, psychiatric nurses, and social workers—have a duty to provide appropriate care based on the standards of their professions and the standards set by law. The standards of practice for psychiatric mental health nursing are presented in Chapter 6, "The Nursing Process in Psychiatric Mental Health Nursing."

Malpractice and Negligence

The terms *malpractice* and *negligence* are often used interchangeably. **Negligence** has been defined as failure to exercise the care toward others that a reasonable or prudent person would do in the circumstances, or taking action that such a reasonable person would not. Negligence is accidental as distinguished from "intentional torts" (assault or trespass, for example) or from crimes, but a crime can also constitute negligence, such as reckless driving (Hill & Hill, 2018).

Any person may be negligent. In contrast, malpractice is a specialized form of negligence applicable only to professionals. **Malpractice** may be defined as an act or continuing conduct of a professional that does not meet the standard of professional competence and results in provable damages to their client or patient. Such an error or omission may be through negligence, ignorance (when the professional should have known), or intentional wrongdoing (Hill & Hill, 2018).

In the absence of any state statutes, common law is the basis of liability for injuries to clients caused by acts of malpractice and negligence of individual practitioners. In other words, most decisions of negligence in the professional setting are based on legal precedent (decisions that have previously been made about similar cases) rather than any specific action taken by the legislature.

To summarize, when the breach of duty is characterized as malpractice, the action is weighed against the professional standard. When it is brought forth as negligence, action is contrasted with what a reasonably prudent professional would have done in the same or similar circumstances.

Austin (2011) cites the following basic elements of a nursing malpractice lawsuit:

1. A duty to the patient existed based on the recognized standard of care.
2. A breach of duty occurred, meaning that the care rendered was not consistent with the recognized standard of care.
3. The client was injured.
4. The injury was directly caused by the breach of a standard of care.

For the client to prevail in a malpractice claim, each of these elements must be proved. Juries' decisions are generally based on the testimony of expert witnesses because members of the jury are laypeople and cannot be expected to know what nursing interventions should have been carried out. Without the testimony of expert witnesses, a favorable verdict usually goes to the defendant nurse.

Types of Lawsuits That Occur in Psychiatric Nursing

Most malpractice suits against nurses are civil actions; that is, they are considered breach of conduct actions on the part of the professional, for which compensation is being sought. The nurse in the psychiatric setting should be aware of the types of behaviors that may result in charges of malpractice.

The hospitalized psychiatric client has a basic right to confidentiality and privacy. A nurse may be charged with *breach of confidentiality* for revealing aspects about a client's case, or even for revealing that an individual has been hospitalized, if that person can show that making this information known resulted in harm.

When shared information is detrimental to the client's reputation, the person sharing the information may be liable for **defamation of character.** When the information is in writing, the action is called **libel.** Oral defamation is called **slander.** Defamation of character involves communication that is malicious and false (Aiken, 2020). Occasionally, libel arises out of critical, judgmental statements written in the client's medical record. Nurses need to be very objective in their charting, backing up all statements with factual evidence.

Invasion of privacy is a charge that may result when a client is searched without probable cause. Many institutions conduct body searches on clients with mental illness as a routine intervention. In these cases, there should be a physician's order and written rationale showing probable cause for the intervention. Many institutions are reexamining their policies regarding this procedure.

Assault is an act that results in a person's genuine fear and apprehension that they will be touched without consent. **Battery** is the unconsented touching of another person. These charges can result when a treatment is administered to a client against their wishes and outside of an emergency situation. Harm or injury need not have occurred for these charges to be legitimate.

For confining a client against their wishes, and outside of an emergency situation, the nurse may be charged with false imprisonment. Examples of actions that may invoke these charges include locking an individual in a room; taking a client's clothes for purposes of detainment against their will; and retaining in mechanical restraints a competent, voluntary client who demands to be released.

Avoiding Liability

Aiken (2020) suggests the following proactive nursing actions in an effort to avoid nursing malpractice and the risk of lawsuits:

1. ***Effective communication*** with patients and other caregivers. The SBAR model of reporting information, which stands for Situation, Background, Assessment, and Recommendations, has been identified as a useful tool for effective communication with caregivers. Establishing rapport with clients encourages open and honest communication.
2. ***Accurate and complete documentation in the medical record***

The electronic health record (EHR) has been identified as the best way to document and share this information. The use of best informatics sources is identified as an essential nursing competency (Institute of Medicine, 2003) and an important standard for quality and safety education in nursing (QSEN Institute, 2013).

3. ***Complying with standards of care,*** including those established within the profession (such as ANA standards) and those identified by specific hospital policies
4. ***Rapport with and knowledge of clients,*** which includes helping the client become involved in their care as well as understanding and responding to aspects of care in which the client is dissatisfied
5. ***Practicing within the nurse's level of competence and scope of practice,*** which includes not only adhering to professional standards (those of the ANA and state boards of nursing) but also keeping knowledge and nursing skills current through evidence-based literature, in-services, and continuing education

Some clients appear to be more "suit prone" than others. Suit-prone clients are often very critical, complaining, uncooperative, and even hostile. A natural staff response to these clients is to become defensive or withdrawn. Aiken (2020) recommends instead that it is important to be direct and engage the client in problem-solving. No matter how high the nurse's technical competence and skill, their insensitivity to a patient's complaints and failure to meet the patient's emotional needs often influence whether or not a lawsuit is generated. A great deal depends on the psychosocial skills of the health-care professional.

CLINICAL PEARL
- **Always put the patient's rights and welfare first.**
- **Develop and maintain a good interpersonal relationship with each patient and their family.**

Summary and Key Points

- *Ethics* is a branch of philosophy that addresses methods for determining the rightness or wrongness of one's actions.
- *Bioethics* is the term applied to these principles when they refer to concepts within the scope of medicine, nursing, and allied health.
- *Morals* are fundamental standards of right and wrong that are learned and internalized.
- *Moral behavior* is conduct that results from serious critical thinking about how individuals ought to treat others.
- *Values* are personal beliefs about what is important or desirable.
- *Rights* are expectations to which an individual is entitled either by established laws, policies, or ethical principles.
- The ethical theory of utilitarianism is based on the premise that what is right and good is that which produces the most happiness for the most people.
- The ethical theory of Kantianism suggests that actions are bound by a sense of duty and that ethical decisions are made out of respect for moral law.
- Divine command ethics identifies ethical decisions as those that follow the divine commands of God.
- The moral precept of the natural law theory is "do good and avoid evil." Good is viewed as that which is inscribed by God into the nature of things. Evil acts are never condoned, even if they are intended to advance the noblest of ends.
- Ethical egoism espouses that what is right and good is what is best for the individual making the decision.
- Ethical principles include autonomy, beneficence, nonmaleficence, veracity, and justice.
- An ethical dilemma is a situation that requires an individual to make a choice between two equally unfavorable alternatives.
- Ethical issues may arise in psychiatric mental health nursing around the client's right to refuse medication and the right to the least restrictive treatment alternative.
- Statutory laws are those that have been enacted by legislative bodies, and common laws are derived from decisions made in previous cases. Both types of laws have civil and criminal components.
- Civil law protects the private and property rights of individuals and businesses, and criminal law provides protection from conduct deemed injurious to the public welfare.
- Legal issues in psychiatric mental health nursing center on confidentiality and the right to privacy, informed consent, restraints and seclusion, and commitment issues.
- Nurses are accountable for their own actions in relation to legal issues, and violation can result in malpractice lawsuits against the physician, the hospital, and the nurse.
- Developing and maintaining a good interpersonal relationship with the patient and their family is a positive factor when the question of malpractice is being considered.

Review Questions

Select the answer that is most appropriate for each of the following questions:

1. The nurse decides to go against family wishes and tell the client of their terminal status because that is what they would want if the nurse were the patient. Which of the following ethical theories is considered in this decision?
   a. Kantianism
   b. Christian ethics
   c. Natural law theories
   d. Ethical egoism
2. The nurse decides to respect family wishes and not tell the client of their terminal status because that would bring the most happiness to the most people. Which of the following ethical theories is considered in this decision?
   a. Utilitarianism
   b. Kantianism
   c. Divine command ethics
   d. Ethical egoism
3. The nurse decides to tell the client of their terminal status because the nurse believes it is their duty to do so. Which of the following ethical theories is considered in this decision?
   a. Natural law theories
   b. Ethical egoism
   c. Kantianism
   d. Utilitarianism
4. The nurse assists the physician with electroconvulsive therapy on their client who has refused to give consent. With which of the following legal actions might the nurse be charged because of this nursing action?
   a. Assault
   b. Battery
   c. False imprisonment
   d. Breach of confidentiality
5. A competent, voluntary client has stated that they want to leave the hospital. The nurse hides the client's clothes in an effort to keep them from leaving. With which of the following legal actions might the nurse be charged because of this nursing action?
   a. Assault
   b. Battery
   c. False imprisonment
   d. Breach of confidentiality
6. A hospitalized client is very restless and is pacing a lot. The nurse says, "If you don't sit down in the chair and be still, I'm going to put you in restraints!" With which of the following legal actions might the nurse be charged because of this nursing action?
   a. Defamation of character
   b. Battery
   c. Breach of confidentiality
   d. Assault

Clinical Judgment Questions

7. A nurse reports to the supervisor that a depressed client is refusing medication to treat their heart condition and states they "would rather just die." The nurse is not sure how to intervene because, although clients have a right to refuse medication, this client may be so depressed that the client's behavior represents risk for suicide. Which of these actions by the supervisor is a priority?
   a. Tell the nurse that medication will have to be given forcibly if the client continues to refuse medication.
   b. Instruct the nurse that, because the client is elderly, they are unable to make this decision and medication will need to be secretly mixed in their food.
   c. Educate the nurse that the physician has the final say, so the nurse should ask the physician what to do.
   d. Activate appropriate hospital resources, such as an ethics committee, so this issue can be explored further.
8. A client on the psychiatric unit begins yelling loudly that no one is listening to them and that they are going to "blow up" soon. The orderly asks the nurse if they should go ahead and put the client in restraints for the safety of others. Which of these responses by the nurse is most appropriate?
   a. Educate the orderly that restraints may never be initiated without a physician's order.
   b. Instruct the orderly that it would be best to see if the client can be assisted to calm down by listening to their concerns.
   c. Instruct the orderly to put the client in restraints but make sure to assess the client every 15 minutes for issues regarding circulation, nutrition, respiration, hydration, and elimination.
   d. Instruct the orderly to get others to assist them in restraining the client, but be aware restraints should be discontinued at the earliest possible time regardless of when a physician's order is scheduled to expire.
9. The nurse collects the following information during the admission assessment. For which of these data should the nurse take additional action to ensure that "duty to warn" laws are followed?
   a. The client threatens violence toward another individual.
   b. The client states they want to kill everyone who has demons.
   c. The client is having command hallucinations.
   d. The client reveals paranoid delusions about another individual.
10. Which of these actions by the nurse demonstrates an application of the QSEN competency related to informatics?
   a. Learns how to effectively communicate information using electronic health records.
   b. Provides a verbal report of client behavioral issues at shift change.
   c. Asks the supervisor for guidelines on how to prevent lawsuits.
   d. Reads journals to learn information about new treatments and approaches to nursing care.

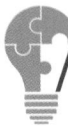

Go to **Davis Advantage** to complete your learning: strengthen understanding, apply your knowledge, and prepare for the Next Gen NCLEX®.

References

Aiken, M. E. T. (2020). Nursing law and liability. In J. T. Catalano (Ed.), *Nursing now! Today's issues, tomorrow's trends* (8th ed., pp. 183–212). F.A. Davis.

American Hospital Association. (2003). *The patient care partnership: Understanding expectations, rights, and responsibilities.* https://www.aha.org/system/files/2018-01/aha-patient-care-partnership.pdf

American Nurses Association. (2015). *Code of ethics for nurses with interpretive statements.*

American Psychiatric Nurses Association & International Society of Psychiatric-Mental Health Nurses. (2022). *Psychiatric-mental health nursing: Scope and standards of practice* (3rd ed.). American Nurses Association.

Austin, S. (2011). Stay out of court with proper documentation. *Nursing, 41*(4), 25–29.

Boland, R., & Verduin, M. L. (2022). *Kaplan & Sadock's synopsis of psychiatry* (P. Ruiz, Ed.). (12th ed.). Wolters Kluwer.

Butts, J., & Rich, K. (2019). *Nursing ethics: Across the curriculum and into practice* (5th ed.). Jones & Bartlett.

Cady, R. F. (2010). A review of basic patient rights in psychiatric care. *JONA's Healthcare Law, Ethics, and Regulation, 12*(4), 117–125.

Catalano, J. T. (2020). *Nursing now! Today's issues, tomorrow's trends* (8th ed.). F.A. Davis.

Child Welfare Information Gateway. (2019a). *Mandatory reporters of child abuse and neglect.* https://www.childwelfare.gov/pubPDFs/manda.pdf

Child Welfare Information Gateway. (2019b). *Penalties for failure to report and false reporting of child abuse and neglect.* https://www.childwelfare.gov/pubPDFs/report.pdf

Dixon, L. B., Goldman, H. H., Srihari, V. H., & Kane, J. M. (2018). Transforming the treatment of schizophrenia in the United States: The RAISE initiative. *Annual Review of Clinical Psychology, 7*(14), 237–258. https://doi.org/10.1146/annurev-clinpsy-050817-084934

Guido, G. W. (2014). *Legal and ethical issues in nursing* (6th ed.). Pearson.

Henderson, E. (2015). Potentially dangerous patients: A review of the duty to warn. *Journal of Emergency Nursing, 41*(3), 193–200.

Hill, G., & Hill, K. (2018). *The people's law dictionary.* https://dictionary.law.com

Institute of Medicine. (2003). *Health professions education: A bridge to quality.*

Kisely, S. R., Campbell, L. A., & O'Reilly, R. (2017). *Compulsory community and involuntary outpatient treatment for people with severe mental disorders. Cochrane Database of Systematic Reviews.* http://www.cochrane.org/CD004408/SCHIZ_compulsory-community-and-involuntary-outpatient-treatment-people-severe-mental-disorders

Landeweer, E., Abma, T. A., & Widdershoven, G. (2011). Moral margins concerning the use of coercion in psychiatry. *Nursing Ethics, 18*(3), 304–316.

Maiese, M. (2017 [originally posted July 2003]). Principles of justice and fairness. In C. Burgess & H. Burgess (Eds.), *Beyond intractability.* Conflict Information Consortium, University of Colorado, Boulder. http://www.beyondintractability.org/essay/principles-of-justice

Mental Illness Policy Org. (2017). *The effects of involuntary medication on individuals with schizophrenia and manic-depressive disorder.* https://mentalillnesspolicy.org/medical/involuntary-medication.html

National Conference of State Legislatures. (2018). *Mental health professionals' duty to warn.* http://www.ncsl.org/research/health/mental-health-professionals-duty-to-warn.aspx

QSEN Institute. (2013). *Competencies.* http://qsen.org/competencies/

Rae, S. (2009). *Moral choices: An introduction to ethics.* Zondervan.

Ridgely, M. S., Borum, R., & Petrila, J. (2001). *The effectiveness of involuntary outpatient treatment: Empirical evidence and the experience of eight states.* Rand Publications.

Sashadahran, S. P., & Saraceno, B. (2017). Is psychiatry becoming more coercive? *The British Medical Journal, 357.* https://doi.org/10.1136/bmj.j2904

Saya, A., Brugnoli, C., Piazzi, G., Liberato, D., Di Ciaccia, G., Niolu, C., & Siracusano, A. (2019). Criteria, procedures, and future prospects of involuntary treatment in psychiatry around the world: A narrative review. *Frontiers in Psychiatry, 10,* 271. https://doi.org/10.3389/fpsyt.2019.00271

Sitrin, C. (2018). Gov. Murphy signs New Jersey into new era of gun safety. *NJ Spotlight News.* https://www.njspotlight.com/stories/18/06/13/gov-murphy-signs-new-jersey-into-new-era-of-gun-safety/

Substance Abuse and Mental Health Services Administration. (2019). *Civil commitment and the mental health care continuum: Historical trends and principles for law and practice.*

Swartz, M. S., & Swanson, J. W. (2008). Outpatient commitment: When it improves patient outcomes. *Current Psychiatry, 7*(4), 25–35. https://doi.org/10.1176/appi.ps.52.3.325

Tarasoff v. Regents of University of California et al. (1974a), 551 P.d 345.

Tarasoff v. Regents of University of California et al. (1974b), 554 P.d 347.

U.S. Department of Health & Human Services. (2003). *Standards for privacy of individually identifiable health information.*

U.S. Department of Health & Human Services. (2013, January 17). *New rule protects patient privacy, secures health information* [Press release].

What do I do now? Ethical dilemmas in nursing and health care. (2013). *ISNA Bulletin, 13*(2), 5–12.

Classical References

Patient Self-Determination Act – Restatement of Bill of Rights for Mental Health Patients. (1991). U.S. Code, Title 42, Section 10841, The Public Health and Welfare.

Peplau, H. E. (1991). *Interpersonal relations in nursing: A conceptual frame of reference for psychodynamic nursing.* Springer.

Swartz, M., Swanson, J., Hiday, V., Wagner, H. R., Burns, B., & Borum, R. (2001). A randomized controlled trial of outpatient commitment in North Carolina. *Psychiatric Services, 52*(3), 325–329.

Weiss-Kaffie, C. J., & Purtell, N. E. (2001). Psychiatric nursing. In M. E. O'Keefe (Ed.), *Nursing practice and the law: Avoiding malpractice and other legal risks* (pp. 352–371). F.A. Davis.

4 Psychopharmacology

CHAPTER OUTLINE

Objectives
Introduction
Historical Perspectives
Role of the Nurse in Psychopharmacology
How Do Psychotropics Work?
Applying the Nursing Process in Psychopharmacological Therapy
Summary and Key Points
Review Questions
Clinical Judgment Questions

CORE CONCEPTS

Intracranial Regulation: Neurotransmitters
Safety: Psychotropic medication
Clinical Judgment

KEY TERMS

agonist
agranulocytosis
akathisia
akinesia
amenorrhea
antagonist
antianxiety agents
antidepressants
antiparkinsonian agents
antipsychotic agents
attention deficit-hyperactivity disorder (ADHD) agents
black box warning
dystonia
extrapyramidal symptoms (EPS)
gynecomastia
hypertensive crisis
mood-stabilizing agents
neuroleptic malignant syndrome
neurotransmitter
oculogyric crisis
priapism
receptor sites
retrograde ejaculation
reuptake
sedative-hypnotics
serotonin syndrome
tardive dyskinesia

OBJECTIVES

After reading this chapter, the student will be able to:

1. Discuss historical perspectives related to psychopharmacology.
2. Describe indications, actions, contraindications, precautions, side effects, and nursing implications for the following classifications of drugs:
   a. Antianxiety agents
   b. Antidepressants
   c. Mood-stabilizing agents
   d. Antipsychotics and agents for the treatment of tardive dyskinesia
   e. Antiparkinsonian agents
   f. Sedative-hypnotics
   g. Agents for attention deficit-hyperactivity disorder
3. Apply the steps of the nursing process to the administration of psychotropic medications.

Introduction

The middle of the 20th century represents a pivotal period in the treatment of individuals with mental illness. It was during this time that the phenothiazine class of antipsychotics was introduced in the United States. Before that time, phenothiazines had been used in France as preoperative medications. As Dr. Henri Laborit of the Hospital Boucicaut in Paris stated:

> It was our aim to decrease the anxiety of the patients to prepare them in advance for their postoperative recovery. With these new drugs, the phenothiazines, we were seeing a profound psychic and physical relaxation . . . a real indifference to the environment and to the upcoming operation. It seemed to me these drugs must have an application in psychiatry. (Sage, 1984)

Indeed, they have had a significant application in psychiatry. Not only have they helped many individuals to function effectively, but they have also provided researchers and clinicians with information to study the origins and etiologies of mental illness. Knowledge gained from learning how these drugs work has promoted advancement in understanding how behavioral disorders develop. Dr. Arnold Scheibel, director of the UCLA Brain Research Institute, stated:

> [When these drugs came out] there was a sense of disbelief that we could actually do something substantive for the patients . . . see them for the first time as sick individuals and not as something bizarre that we could literally not talk to. (Sage, 1984)

This chapter explores historical perspectives in the use of psychotropic medications in the treatment of mental illness. Seven classifications of medications are discussed, and their implications for psychiatric nursing are presented in the context of the steps of the nursing process.

CORE CONCEPT

Psychotropic Medication

Medication that affects psychic function, behavior, or experience.

Historical Perspectives

Historically, reaction to and treatment of individuals with mental illness ranged from benign involvement to intervention some would consider inhumane. Individuals with mental illness were feared because of common beliefs associating them with demons or the supernatural. They were looked upon as loathsome and often were mistreated.

Beginning in the late 18th century, a type of "moral reform" in the treatment of persons with mental illness began to occur. Community and state hospitals concerned with the needs of persons with mental illness were established. Considered a breakthrough in the humanization of care, these institutions, however well intentioned, fostered the concept of custodial care. Clients were ensured food and shelter but received little or no hope of change for the future. As they became increasingly dependent on the institution to fulfill their needs, the likelihood of their return to the family or community diminished.

The early part of the 20th century saw the advent of the somatic therapies in psychiatry. Individuals with mental illness were treated with insulin shock therapy, wet sheet packs, ice baths, electroconvulsive therapy, and psychosurgery. Before 1950, sedatives and amphetamines were the only significant psychotropic medications available. Even these drugs had limited use because of their potential for toxicity and physical dependence. Since the 1950s, the development of psychopharmacology has expanded to include widespread use of antipsychotic, antidepressant, antianxiety, and mood stabilizer medications. Research into how these drugs work has provided an understanding of the biochemical influences in many psychiatric disorders.

Psychotropic medications are not a "cure" for mental illness. Most mental health practitioners who prescribe these medications for their clients use them as an adjunct to individual or group psychotherapy. Although their contribution to psychiatric care cannot be minimized, it must be emphasized that psychotropic medications relieve some physical and behavioral symptoms. They do not eliminate mental disorders.

The Role of the Nurse in Psychopharmacology

Ethical and Legal Implications

Nurses must understand the ethical and legal implications associated with the administration of psychotropic medications. Laws differ from state to state, but most adhere to the client's right to refuse treatment. Exceptions exist in emergency situations when it has been determined that clients are likely to harm themselves or others. Many states have adopted laws that allow courts to order outpatient treatment, which may include medication, in circumstances in which an individual is not seeking treatment and has a history of violent, aggressive behavior. The original law, called Kendra's law, was enacted after a young woman, Kendra Webdale, was pushed in front of a New York City subway by a man who was living in the community but was not seeking treatment for his mental illness (New York State Office of Mental Health, 2012). This law is perhaps more developed in New York state than are similar laws in other states. It includes a medication grant clause that provides uninterrupted medication for those transitioning from hospitals or correctional facilities. Some states do not have similar laws at all. It is important, then, for nurses to be informed about local, state, and federal laws when they are working in any health-care setting or correctional facility and providing care to clients with a psychiatric disorder.

Assessment

A thorough baseline assessment must be conducted before a client is placed on a regimen of psychopharmacological therapy. A history and physical examination (see Chapter 6, "The Nursing Process in Psychiatric Mental Health Nursing"), an ethnocultural assessment, and a comprehensive medication assessment (see Box 4–1) are all essential components of this assessment. The ethnocultural assessment is necessary because genetic variations in selected populations and cultural factors, including dietary preferences, may influence response to some medications; Cytochrome P450 isoenzyme variations, for example, influence metabolism of some medications and pharmacogenetic testing may be ordered to identify individuals at risk for being poor metabolizers (see Table 4–1 for degrees of risk for poor

BOX 4–1 Medication Assessment Tool

Date _____

Patient's Name _____ Age _____

Marital Status _____ Children _____

Occupation _____

Presenting Symptoms (subjective & objective) _____

_____

_____

Diagnosis (*DSM-5-TR*) _____

Current Vital Signs: Blood Pressure: Sitting _____/_____ Standing _____/_____

Pulse _____

Respirations _____

Height _____ Weight _____

CURRENT/PAST USE OF PRESCRIPTION DRUGS (Indicate with "c" or "p" beside name of drug whether current or past use):

Name	Dosage	How Long Used	Why Prescribed	By Whom	Side Effects/Results
_____	_____	_____	_____	_____	_____
_____	_____	_____	_____	_____	_____
_____	_____	_____	_____	_____	_____

CURRENT/PAST USE OF OVER-THE-COUNTER DRUGS (Indicate with "c" or "p" beside name of drug whether current or past use):

Name	Dosage	How Long Used	Why Prescribed	By Whom	Side Effects/Results
_____	_____	_____	_____	_____	_____
_____	_____	_____	_____	_____	_____
_____	_____	_____	_____	_____	_____

Continued

BOX 4–1 Medication Assessment Tool—cont'd

CURRENT/PAST USE OF STREET DRUGS, ALCOHOL, NICOTINE, AND/OR CAFFEINE (Indicate with "c" or "p" beside name of drug):

Name	Amount Used	How Often Used	When Last Used	Effects Produced
_____	_____	_____	_____	_____
_____	_____	_____	_____	_____
_____	_____	_____	_____	_____

Any allergies to food or drugs?

_____

Any special diet considerations?

_____

Do you have (or have you ever had) any of the following? If yes, provide explanation on the back of this sheet.

Yes No	Yes No	Yes No
Difficulty swallowing _____	Chest pain _____	Lumps in your breasts _____
Delayed wound healing _____	Blood clots/pain in legs _____	Blurred or double vision _____
Constipation problems _____	Fainting spells _____	Ringing in the ears _____
Urination problems _____	Swollen ankles/legs/hands _____	Insomnia _____
Recent change in elimination patterns _____	Asthma _____	Skin Rashes _____
	Varicose veins _____	Diabetes _____
Weakness or tremors _____	Numbness/tingling (location?) _____	Hepatitis (or other liver disease) _____
Seizures _____	Ulcers _____	Kidney disease _____
Headaches _____	Nausea/vomiting _____	Glaucoma _____
Dizziness _____	Problems with diarrhea _____	
High blood pressure _____	Shortness of breath _____	
Palpitations _____	Sexual dysfunction _____	

Are you pregnant or breast feeding? _____ Date of last menses_____ Type of contraception used _____

Describe any restrictions/limitations that might interfere with your use of medication for your current problem: _____

_____

_____

Prescription orders:

Patient teaching related to medications prescribed:

Lab work or referrals prescribed:

Nurse's signature _____

Patient's signature _____

TABLE 4–1 Variations in CYP450 Enzymes and Response to Selected Psychotropic Medications*

CYP450 ISOENZYME	RISK FOR BEING POOR METABOLIZERS BY ETHNIC GROUP (%)	SELECTED PSYCHOTROPIC MEDICATIONS AFFECTED	SELECTED POTENTIAL OUTCOMES
2C19	Asian 12%–23% African, African American 18% Caucasian 3%–7%	Diazepam, tricyclics, citalopram	1. Higher blood levels and faster therapeutic response to tricyclic antidepressants. Experience more toxic side effects and more risk for tricyclic antidepressant delirium. 2. Increased sensitivity to effects of alcohol.
2D6	East Asian 0%–2% African, African American 0%–19% Caucasian 3%–9%	Tricyclics, fluoxetine, paroxetine venlafaxine, sertraline, chlorpromazine, haloperidol, clozapine, risperidone	1. Higher incidence of extrapyramidal side effects with haloperidol. 2. More sensitive to the effects of many psychotropic medications.
3A4	Although results are inconsistent, poor metabolizers are rare (<1%) but drug-drug and drug-food interactions, such as interactions with grapefruit juice, may inhibit metabolism	Mirtazapine, sertraline, haloperidol, clozapine, quetiapine, risperidone, ziprasidone, gabapentin, lamotrigine, clonazepam, diazepam, zolpidem, buspirone, lurasidone, pimozide, ketamine, fentanyl, oxycodone, alfentanil dextromethorphan triazolam	1. Higher risk for respiratory depression with alfentanil, fentanyl, ketamine, and oxycodone. 2. Higher risk for torsade de pointes with lurasidone, pimozide, and ziprasidone. 3. Risk for hallucinations and somnolence with dextromethorphan. 4. Increased sedation with buspirone and triazolam.

*CYP450 enzymes are responsible for metabolizing many medications. Variations can occur due to genetic vulnerability or through drug-drug or drug-food interactions. CYP450 induction increases the metabolism of selected drugs thereby decreasing their effectiveness. Inhibition of CYP450 enzymes decreases the metabolism of selected drugs which can result in severe toxicity and several adverse effects.
Sources: Compiled from Anderson (2018); Horn and Hansten (2008); Jones (2006); Lynch and Price (2007).

metabolism of selected medications). Individuals who metabolize drugs poorly are more vulnerable to adverse drug reactions including toxicity.

Medication Administration and Evaluation

The nurse is the key health-care professional in direct contact with patients receiving psychotropic medication in inpatient settings, partial hospitalization programs, day treatment centers, home health care, and other settings. Medication administration is followed by continuous monitoring for side effects and adverse reactions. The nurse also evaluates the therapeutic effectiveness of the medication. It is essential for the nurse to have a thorough knowledge of psychotropic medications to be able to anticipate potential problems and outcomes associated with their administration.

Patient Education

The information associated with psychotropic medications is copious and complex. An important role of the nurse is to translate that complex information into terms that can be easily understood by the patient. Patients must understand why the medication has been prescribed, when it should be taken, and what they may expect in terms of side effects and possible adverse reactions. They must know whom to contact when they have a question and when it is important to report to their physician. Medication education encourages patient cooperation and promotes accurate and effective management of the treatment regimen.

For women of childbearing age, pregnancy risk information is an essential aspect of patient education. In 2015, a new U.S. Food and Drug Administration (FDA) rule went into effect that requires drug labeling to include specific narrative information on pregnancy-associated risks, lactation considerations, and reproductive potential (Drugs.com, 2020). This new system replaces the lettered risk categories that were criticized for being overly simplistic. Nurses should use the latest informatics resources to provide current and relevant education on this and other medication-related topics.

How Do Psychotropics Work?

Neurotransmitters are chemicals stored in the axon terminals of the presynaptic neuron. An electrical impulse through the neuron stimulates the release of the neurotransmitter into the synaptic cleft, which in turn determines whether another electrical impulse is generated. **Receptor sites** are molecules on the cell membrane that are binding sites for neurotransmitters. Most of the psychotropic medications have their effects at the neuronal synapse, producing changes in neurotransmitter release and the receptor sites to which they bind (see Fig. 4–1). **Antagonist** drugs exert their effect by blocking a receptor and dampening the biological reaction. Conversely, **agonist** drugs activate receptors. Researchers hypothesize that most antidepressants work by blocking the reuptake of neurotransmitters (acting as antagonists), particularly serotonin and norepinephrine. **Reuptake** is the process of neurotransmitter inactivation by which the neurotransmitter is reabsorbed into the presynaptic neuron from which it had been released. Blocking the reuptake process allows more of the neurotransmitter to be available for neuronal transmission. This mechanism of action may also result in undesirable side effects (see Table 4–2). Some antidepressants also block receptor sites that are unrelated to their mechanisms of action on mood and emotions. These include α-adrenergic, histaminergic, and muscarinic cholinergic receptors. Blocking these receptors is associated with the development of certain side effects. Individuals being treated with tricyclic antidepressants, for example, are at risk for developing postural hypotension. The specific type of receptor that a medication binds to is also relevant to the medication's level of antianxiety, antidepressant, and sedative properties (see Table 4–2).

Antipsychotic medications block dopamine receptors, and some affect muscarinic cholinergic,

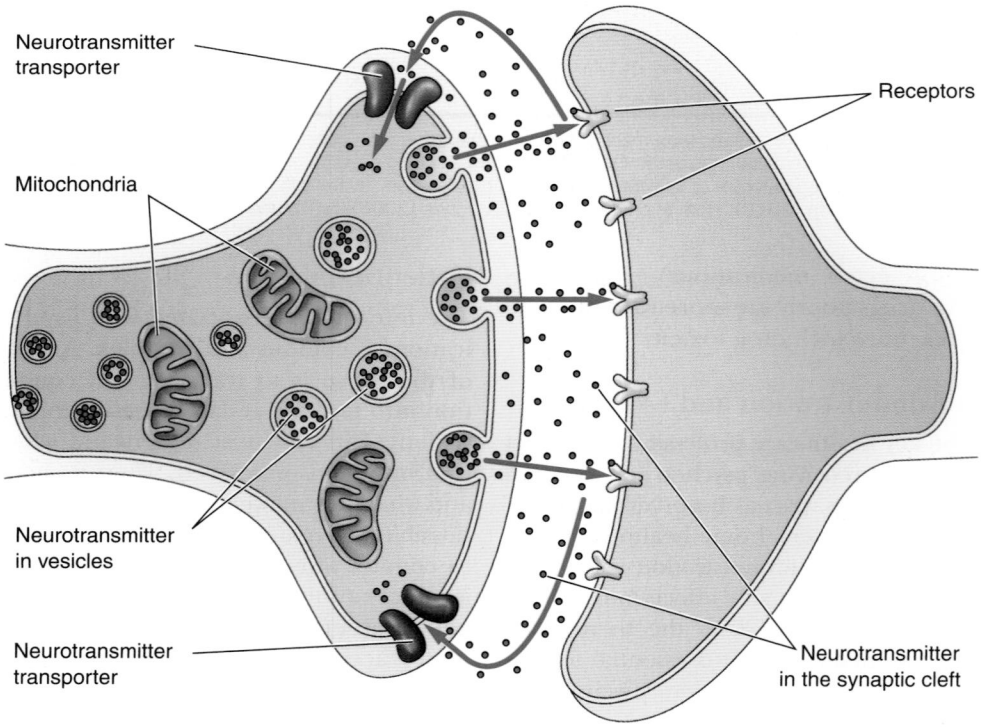

FIGURE 4–1 Area of synaptic transmission that is altered by drugs.

TABLE 4–2 Effects of Psychotropic Influence on Neurotransmitters

EXAMPLE OF MEDICATION	ACTION ON NEUROTRANSMITTER AND/OR RECEPTOR	PHYSIOLOGICAL EFFECTS	SIDE EFFECTS
SSRIs	Inhibit reuptake of serotonin (5-HT)	Reduce depression Control anxiety Control obsessions	Nausea, agitation, headache, sexual dysfunction
Tricyclic antidepressants	Inhibit reuptake of serotonin (5-HT) Inhibit reuptake of norepinephrine (NE) Block NE (α_1) receptor Block ACh receptor Block histamine (H_1) receptor	Reduce depression Relief of severe pain Prevent panic attacks	Sexual dysfunction (NE & 5-HT) Sedation, weight gain (H_1) Dry mouth, constipation, blurred vision, urinary retention (ACh) Postural hypotension and tachycardia (α_1)
MAO inhibitors	Increase NE and 5-HT by inhibiting the enzyme that degrades them (MAO-A)	Reduce depression Control anxiety	Sedation, dizziness Sexual dysfunction Hypertensive crisis (interaction with tyramine)
Trazodone and nefazodone	5-HT reuptake block 5-HT_2 receptor antagonism Adrenergic receptor blockade	Reduce depression Reduce anxiety Promote sleep	Nausea (5-HT) Sedation (5-HT_2) Orthostasis (α_1) Priapism (α_2)
SNRIs: venlafaxine, desvenlafaxine, duloxetine, and levomilnacipran	Potent inhibitors of serotonin and norepinephrine reuptake Weak inhibitors of dopamine reuptake	Reduce depression Relieve pain of neuropathy (duloxetine) Relieve anxiety (venlafaxine)	Nausea (5-HT) Increased sweating (NE) Insomnia (NE) Tremors (NE) Sexual dysfunction (5-HT)
Bupropion	Inhibits reuptake of NE and dopamine (D)	Reduces depression Aids in smoking cessation Decreases symptoms of ADHD	Insomnia, dry mouth, tremor, seizures
Esketamine (nasal spray)	Nonselective, noncompetitive antagonist of the NMDA receptor (an ionotropic glutamate receptor)	Reduce depression in treatment-resistant depression (in conjunction with an oral antidepressant)	Dissociation, dizziness, hypoesthesia (decreased sensation; numbness), anxiety, lethargy, increased blood pressure, and vomiting
Antipsychotics: phenothiazines and haloperidol	Strong D_2 receptor blockade Weaker blockade of ACh, H_1, α_1-adrenergic, and 5-HT_2 receptors	Relief of psychosis Relief of anxiety (Some) provide relief from nausea and vomiting and intractable hiccoughs	Blurred vision, dry mouth, decreased sweating, constipation, urinary retention, tachycardia (ACh) EPS (D_2) Increases plasma prolactin (D_2) Sedation; weight gain (H_1) Ejaculatory difficulty (5-HT_2) Postural hypotension (α; H_1)

Continued

TABLE 4–2 Effects of Psychotropic Influence on Neurotransmitters—cont'd

EXAMPLE OF MEDICATION	ACTION ON NEUROTRANSMITTER AND/OR RECEPTOR	PHYSIOLOGICAL EFFECTS	SIDE EFFECTS
Antipsychotics (second generation, atypical): aripiprazole, asenapine, brexpiprazole, clozapine, iloperidone, lurasidone, olanzapine, paliperidone, quetiapine, risperidone, ziprasidone	Receptor antagonism of 5-HT_1 and 5-HT_2, D_1–D_5 (varies with drug), H_1, α_1-adrenergic, muscarinic (ACh)	Relief of psychosis (with minimal or no EPS) Relief of anxiety Relief of acute mania	Potential with some of the drugs for mild EPS (D_2) Sedation, weight gain (H_1) Orthostasis and dizziness (α-adrenergic) Blurred vision, dry mouth, decreased sweating, constipation, urinary retention, tachycardia (ACh)
Antianxiety: benzodiazepines	Bind to BZ receptor sites on the $GABA_A$ receptor complex; increase receptor affinity for GABA	Relief of anxiety Sedation	Dependence (with long-term use) Confusion; memory impairment; motor incoordination
Antianxiety: buspirone	5-HT_{1A} agonist D_2 agonist D_2 antagonist	Relief of anxiety	Nausea, headache, dizziness, restlessness

ACh, acetylcholine; ADHD, attention deficit-hyperactivity disorder; BZ, benzodiazepine; D, dopamine; EPS, extrapyramidal symptoms; GABA, gamma-aminobutyric acid; H, histamine; 5-HT, 5-hydroxytryptamine (serotonin); MAO, monoamine oxidase; NE, norepinephrine; NMDA, *N*-methyl-D-aspartate; SNRI, serotonin-norepinephrine reuptake inhibitor; SSRI, selective serotonin reuptake inhibitor.

histaminergic, and α-adrenergic receptors. The "atypical" (or second generation) antipsychotics focus primarily on blocking specific serotonin receptors. Benzodiazepines facilitate the transmission of the inhibitory neurotransmitter gamma-aminobutyric acid (GABA). The psychostimulants work by increasing norepinephrine, serotonin, and dopamine release.

Although each psychotropic medication affects neurotransmission, the specific drugs within each class have varying neuronal effects. Their exact mechanisms of action are unknown. Many of the neuronal effects occur rapidly; however, the therapeutic effects of some medications, such as antidepressants and atypical antipsychotics, may take weeks to become apparent. Acute alterations in neuronal function do not fully explain how these medications work. Boland and Verduin (2022) note that

> if merely raising or lowering levels of neurotransmitter activity is associated with the clinical effects of a drug, then all drugs that cause these changes should produce equivalent benefits [and] this predictability is not the case. (p. 592)

Long-term neuropharmacological reactions to increased norepinephrine and serotonin levels may better explain their mechanisms of action. Recent research suggests that the therapeutic effects are related to the nervous system's adaptation to increased levels of neurotransmitters. These adaptive changes result from a homeostatic mechanism, much like a thermostat, that regulates the cell and maintains equilibrium.

Applying the Nursing Process in Psychopharmacological Therapy

An assessment tool for obtaining a drug history is provided in Box 4–1. This tool may be adapted for use by staff nurses admitting patients to the hospital or by nurse practitioners with prescriptive privileges. Some psychotropic medications (such as benzodiazepines, ketamine, and many sedative-hypnotic medications) are controlled substances because of their potential for abuse Box 4–2 describes the different levels of controlled substance schedules.

BOX 4–2 Controlled Substance Schedules

Schedule I: Substances in this schedule have no currently accepted medical use in the United States, a lack of accepted safety for use under medical supervision, and a high potential for abuse.
Schedule II: Substances in this schedule have a high potential for abuse which may lead to severe psychological or physical dependence.
Schedule III: Substances in this schedule have a potential for abuse less than substances in schedules I or II and abuse may lead to moderate or low physical dependence or high psychological dependence.
Schedule IV: Substances in this schedule have a low potential for abuse relative to substances in Schedule III.
Schedule V: Substances in this schedule have a low potential for abuse relative to substances listed in Schedule IV and consist primarily of preparations containing limited quantities of certain narcotics.

Source: U.S. Department of Justice (n.d.).

One of the Quality and Safety in Nursing Education (QSEN) criteria culminating from the Institute of Medicine (2003) report on essential competencies for health-care professionals stresses that the patient must be at the center of decisions about treatment (patient-centered care) and this type of assessment tool provides an opportunity to actively engage the patient in describing what medications have been effective or ineffective and identifying side effects that may impact their willingness to adhere to a medication regimen.

Antianxiety Agents

Antianxiety agents are also called *anxiolytics* and historically were referred to as *minor tranquilizers*. Other medications that have been used off-label to treat anxiety disorders include anticonvulsants (such as divalproex, gabapentin, and pregabalin), beta blockers (such as atenolol, propranolol, and nadolol), antihistamines (hydroxyzine), and the antipsychotic medication quetiapine.

Background Assessment Data

Indications

Antianxiety agents are used in the treatment of anxiety disorders, anxiety symptoms, acute alcohol withdrawal, skeletal muscle spasms, convulsive disorders, status epilepticus, and preoperative sedation. They are most appropriate for the treatment of acute anxiety states rather than for long-term treatment. Their use and efficacy for periods greater than 4 months have not been evaluated. For longer-term management of anxiety disorders, antidepressants are often used as the first line of treatment because they are not addictive. (A table of current FDA-approved antianxiety agents, controlled substance schedules, and daily dosage ranges can be found in Chapter 18, "Anxiety, Obsessive-Compulsive, and Related Disorders.")

Action

Antianxiety drugs depress subcortical levels of the central nervous system (CNS), particularly the limbic system and reticular formation. They may potentiate the effects of the powerful inhibitory neurotransmitter GABA in the brain (inhibiting excitation) and thereby produce a calmative effect. All levels of CNS depression can be affected, from mild sedation to hypnosis to coma. The most commonly prescribed antianxiety agents are benzodiazepines (which are schedule IV controlled substances), including clonazepam (Klonopin), diazepam (Valium), lorazepam (Ativan), and alprazolam (Xanax). Benzodiazepines are much like alcohol in their effects on GABA receptors, which explains why benzodiazepines may be used for the management of alcohol withdrawal.

The antianxiety agent buspirone is not a benzodiazepine and does not depress the CNS. Although its action is unknown, the drug is believed to produce the desired effects through interactions with serotonin, dopamine, and other neurotransmitter receptors. Patients should be instructed that this drug has a lag period of 7 to 10 days before full therapeutic benefits are achieved. It does not have the physical dependence potential that some of the other antianxiety agents have and, therefore, may be a better option for patients with anxiety disorders who also have substance use disorders.

One trend noted by Olfson and colleagues (2015) is the increased use of benzodiazepines in the older adult population despite known safety concerns, including psychomotor impairment, impaired cognitive function, and paradoxical increase in anxiety. The researchers add that 33% of benzodiazepine prescriptions are for *long-term use* in older adults, a practice that has not been supported by scientific evidence and one that increases risks for side effects and dependence. Further, Maust and associates (2016) found that most older adults who were prescribed benzodiazepines did not receive a clinical mental health diagnosis and almost none were referred for psychotherapy. Nurses are in a position to assess safety risks and, in collaboration with the patient, physician, and other health-care team members, explore other options for treatment of anxiety and insomnia.

Despite the concerns about long-term use, side effects, and potential for dependence, benzodiazepines remain a mainstream treatment choice. In 2020 a new vehicle for diazepam administration came with the approval of diazepam nasal spray, but it should be noted that this is approved only for the rescue treatment of seizure clusters in patients with epilepsy age 6 years and older (Remaly, 2020).

Interactions

- Increased effects of antianxiety agents can occur when they are taken concomitantly with alcohol, barbiturates, narcotics, antipsychotics, antidepressants, antihistamines, neuromuscular blocking agents, cimetidine, or disulfiram.
- The FDA (2016a) added a boxed warning (its strongest warning, commonly called a **black box warning**) related to the serious risks and possible death associated with combining benzodiazepines with opioid pain or cough medicines.
- Increased effects can also occur with herbal depressants (e.g., kava, valerian, lemon verbena, L-tryptophan, melatonin, and chamomile).
- Decreased effects can be noted with cigarette smoking and caffeine consumption.

Diagnosis

The following nursing diagnoses may be considered for patients receiving therapy with antianxiety agents:

- Risk for injury related to seizures, panic anxiety, acute agitation from alcohol withdrawal (indications), abrupt withdrawal from the medication after long-term use, effects of medication intoxication or overdose.
- Anxiety related to threat to physical integrity or self-concept.
- Risk for activity intolerance related to side effects of sedation, confusion, and/or lethargy.
- Disturbed sleep pattern related to situational crises, physical condition, or severe level of anxiety.

Safety Issues in Planning and Implementing Care

The Institute of Medicine (IOM) (2003) identified *ensuring safety* as a core competency for health-care professionals. With that goal in mind, the following are some of the significant safety issues to be considered for clients taking antianxiety agents. Nursing interventions related to each side effect are noted to the right of each safety issue in Table 4–3.

Outcome Criteria and Evaluation

The following criteria may be used for evaluating the effectiveness of therapy with antianxiety agents. The patient:

- Demonstrates a reduction in anxiety, tension, and restless activity.
- Experiences no seizure activity.
- Experiences no physical injury.
- Is able to tolerate usual activities without excessive sedation.
- Exhibits no evidence of confusion.
- Tolerates the medication without gastrointestinal distress.
- Verbalizes understanding of the need for, side effects of, and regimen for self-administration.
- Verbalizes possible consequences of abrupt withdrawal from the medication.

Antidepressants

There are several types of **antidepressants,** some of which are also prescribed in the treatment of anxiety disorders. The first "antidepressant" drug was a *monoamine oxidase inhibitor (MAOI),* isoniazid, which was used to treat tuberculosis. When patients began describing their increased feelings of well-being while taking these drugs, MAOIs were developed specifically for the treatment of depression. Unfortunately, they were also potentially deadly for anyone who ate foods high in tyramine while taking these drugs, and several serious interactions occurred with other drugs. Because MAOIs increase the availability of norepinephrine, researchers focused on developing drugs that impacted norepinephrine without the need for food restrictions, leading to the introduction of *tricyclic antidepressants (TCAs).*

Tricyclics, for many years, were the first-line treatment for depression, but not everyone responded to them (it was generally identified that about 70% of people with depression improved with treatment). In addition, because all neurotransmitters bind to various receptor sites, increasing the availability of norepinephrine also has anticholinergic effects and increases the potential for postural hypotension. These side effects limit their usefulness in the elderly and those with cardiovascular problems.

In the late 1980s, serotonin, an antianxiety hormone and neurotransmitter, became the latest biochemical believed to promote improvement in depression and anxiety without significant anticholinergic side effects. Consequently, a new group of

TABLE 4–3 Safety Issues and Nursing Interventions for Patients Taking Antianxiety Agents

SAFETY ISSUES	NURSING INTERVENTIONS
Tolerance and physical dependence **Abrupt withdrawal can be life threatening** (except buspirone) Signs include sweating, agitation, tremors, nausea and vomiting, delirium, seizures	Instruct the patient not to stop taking the drug abruptly Assess the patient for signs of developing tolerance (requiring higher doses of medication to achieve effects) Educate the patient about symptoms of withdrawal Contact the doctor immediately if symptoms of withdrawal are assessed
Drowsiness, confusion, lethargy (most common side effects)	Instruct the patient not to drive or operate dangerous machinery while until response to medication is known
Increases the effect of other CNS depressants	Instruct the patient not to drink alcohol or take other CNS depressants, as well as antihistamines, cimetidine, antidepressants, neuromuscular blocking agents, and disulfiram, while taking antianxiety agents
May aggravate symptoms of depression	Assess the patient's mood and assess for suicide risk
Orthostatic hypotension	Instruct the patient to rise slowly from a sitting to standing position to minimize risks for falls Monitor lying and standing blood pressures each shift to assess for orthostatic hypotension
Paradoxical excitement (opposite from the desired effect) Especially the elderly may be at higher risk for agitation and increased anxiety	Hold the medication and notify the doctor
Blood dyscrasias, although rare, can be serious or life threatening	Assess for sore throat, fever, bruising, or unusual bleeding Hold medication and report these symptoms immediately to the doctor
Congenital malformations have been associated with use of these drugs during the first trimester of pregnancy	Instruct the female patient to discuss with her physician if she is pregnant or anticipating pregnancy while on these drugs to explore alternative treatment options

drugs, the *selective serotonin reuptake inhibitors (SSRIs)* and *serotonin/norepinephrine reuptake inhibitors (SNRIs)*, became the preferred first-line treatment.

Atypical antidepressants are a group of drugs that work differently and do not fit into the previously mentioned classes. These include the following drugs:

- Bupropion (Wellbutrin)—decreases reuptake of dopamine and, to a lesser extent, serotonin and norepinephrine
- Mirtazapine (Remeron)—potentiates the effects of norepinephrine and serotonin
- Nefazodone—inhibits reuptake of serotonin and norepinephrine by acting as an antagonist at the central 5-HT_2 receptor
- Vortioxetine (Trintellix)—action not well understood
- Vilazodone (Viibryd)—partial agonist at serotonergic 5-HT_{1A} receptors
- Trazodone (Desyrel)—unknown but alters the effect of serotonin

One of the more recent additions to the pharmacological treatments for depression and anxiety are atypical antipsychotics that increase the availability of serotonin and dopamine. These medications are being promoted as adjunctive to antidepressant therapy. The most popular example is aripiprazole (Abilify). In a recent large study sponsored by the National Institute of Mental Health, 44% of elderly adults who were not responding to venlafaxine showed improvement when aripiprazole was added to treatment with venlafaxine. This finding has important implications for the treatment of elderly clients because over half of older adults with clinical depression do not respond to antidepressants alone (Lenze et al., 2015).

Despite all of these developments and client subjective reports of improvement with these medications, our understanding of the exact mechanism of action remains theoretical. Currently, the levels of neurotransmitters in the brain cannot be directly measured. Further, in the STAR*D study (a large study funded by the National Institute of Mental Health), it was found that two-thirds of patients on antidepressant medication do not experience full recovery (Tartakovsky, 2016).

Research continues with the goal of identifying antidepressant therapies that are more effective and more rapid in achieving therapeutic benefits. All antidepressant therapies (TCA, SSRI, SNRI, and MAOI) may take up to 2 weeks before signs of improvement are noted and up to 4 weeks to achieve full therapeutic benefits. Several of the newest drugs on the market for treatment of depression are not significantly different from existing products. For example, a "new" antidepressant approved by the FDA in 2016, Oleptro, is a reformulation of trazodone. But new mechanisms are being explored in clinical trials. Glutamate receptors (*N*-methyl-D-aspartate [NMDA]) and a novel GABA modulator (Gunduz-Bruce et al., 2019) are being studied for potential antidepressant effects; ketamine and midazolam (a benzodiazepine with transient effects similar to those of ketamine) are being explored as potentially faster acting than traditional antidepressants.

In 2019, the FDA approved nasal spray esketamine (Spravato) in conjunction with an oral antidepressant for individuals with treatment-resistant depression and in 2020 approved acute suicidal ideation as an additional indication. In one of three short-term studies used to evaluate the drug's efficacy, Spravato demonstrated statistically significant benefit in reducing depressive symptoms, and some effect was seen within 2 days (FDA, 2019). Research into esketamine's mechanism of action, applications, and risks is ongoing. Because there are risks for serious adverse outcomes related to sedation, dissociation (difficulty with attention, judgment, and thinking), and the potential for substance abuse and misuse, this drug is classified as a schedule III controlled drug and is only available through a restricted distribution system. It must be administered in a certified medical office where the patient is under observation, and it requires a Risk Evaluation and Mitigation Strategy (REMS) (FDA, 2019).

Drugs that act on melatonin receptors are currently in clinical trials for use in depression (one is already approved for use in Europe). One study found a synergistic antidepressant effect when melatonin was combined with fluoxetine (Li et al., 2018), but more research is needed. There is concern that melatonin, although it may improve sleep disturbances in people with depression, may also worsen other symptoms of depression in some individuals (WebMD, 2019). A new group of antidepressants called *triple reuptake inhibitors* that simultaneously block reuptake of serotonin, norepinephrine, and dopamine has been studied but has demonstrated mixed results with regard to any superior benefits over highly selective serotonergic agents alone (Kose & Cetin, 2018).

The most current research is exploring the potential benefits of the psychedelic drugs ayahuasca, psilocybin, and lysergic acid diethylamide (LSD), for treatment-resistant depression. Studies thus far have found that when administered in a supportive setting, antidepressant and anxiolytic effects were immediate, consistent, and enduring for several months (Muttoni et al., 2019). The researchers caution, though, that at present the studies have been limited and small.

Pharmacogenetic research is ongoing to identify factors that may influence whether an individual is more likely to respond to one kind of antidepressant than to another. This type of research may provide a valuable resource for making decisions about which antidepressant to prescribe first.

The myriad searches for different treatment options speaks to the enormity of depression and suicide as public health concerns and the need for a more effective response. Nurses need to be informed of current, evidence-based pharmacological *and* nonpharmacological treatments to provide education and counseling to patients in and outside of psychiatric settings.

Background Assessment Data

Indications

In addition to the obvious indications for antidepressant medications in the treatment of major depressive and dysthymic disorders, some SSRIs, SNRIs, and atypical antidepressants have received FDA approval for the treatment of some anxiety disorders, bulimia nervosa and other eating disorders, premenstrual dysphoric disorder, borderline personality disorder, obesity, and smoking cessation.

A landmark review of the research on antidepressants (Fournier et al., 2010) found that the benefits of antidepressant therapy for clients with mild to moderate symptoms of depression may be minimal or nonexistent but that for clients with severe depression, the benefits, when compared to placebo effects, are substantial. Therefore, these medications are particularly indicated when an individual is identified as having severe levels of depression. (A table of current FDA-approved antidepressants, and daily dosage ranges can be found in Chapter 16, "Depressive Disorders.")

Action

Most antidepressants work to increase the concentration of norepinephrine, serotonin, and/or dopamine through a complex series of interactions in the body. For TCAs, SSRIs, SNRIs, and some atypical antidepressants, this is believed to be accomplished in the brain by blocking the reuptake of these neurotransmitters. MAOI antidepressants act by inhibiting the enzyme monoamine oxidase (MAO), which is known to inactivate norepinephrine, serotonin, and dopamine.

CLINICAL PEARL All antidepressants carry an FDA black box warning for increased risk of suicidality in children, adolescents, and young adults up to 25 years of age.

CLINICAL PEARL As antidepressants take effect and mood begins to lift, the individual may have increased energy with which to implement a suicide plan. The nurse should be particularly alert to sudden lifts or other dramatic changes in mood.

Interactions

Tables 4–4, 4–5, 4–6, and 4–7 identify some of the significant, dangerous drug interactions with antidepressant medications. It is important to recognize

TABLE 4–4 Drug Interactions With SSRIs

INTERACTING DRUGS	ADVERSE EFFECTS
Buspirone (Buspar), tricyclic antidepressants (especially clomipramine), selegiline (Eldepryl), St. John's wort	Serotonin syndrome[a]
Monoamine oxidase inhibitors	Hypertensive crisis
Warfarin, NSAIDs	Increased risk of bleeding
Alcohol, benzodiazepines	Increased sedation
Antiepileptics	Lowered seizure threshold

[a] Serotonin syndrome is a potentially fatal syndrome of serotonin overstimulation with rapid onset that progresses from diarrhea, restlessness, agitation, hyperreflexia, and fluctuations in vital signs to later symptoms of myoclonus, seizures, hyperthermia, uncontrolled shivering, and muscle rigidity, and ultimately it can lead to delirium, coma, status epilepticus, cardiovascular collapse, and death. Immediate cessation of offending drugs and comprehensive supportive intervention are essential (Boland & Verduin, 2022).

TABLE 4–5 Drug Interactions With Tricyclic Antidepressants (TCAs)

INTERACTING DRUGS	ADVERSE EFFECTS
Monoamine oxidase inhibitors	High fever, convulsions, death
St. John's wort, tramadol (Ultram)	Seizures, serotonin syndrome
Clonidine (Catapres), epinephrine	Severe hypertension
Acetylcholine blockers	Paralytic ileus
Alcohol and carbamazepine (Tegretol)	Blocks antidepressant action, increases sedation
Cimetidine (Tagamet), bupropion (Buspar)	Increased TCA blood levels and increased side effects

TABLE 4–6 Drug Interactions With Monoamine Oxidase Inhibitors (MAOIs)

INTERACTING DRUGS	ADVERSE EFFECTS
SSRIs, TCAs, atomoxetine (Strattera), duloxetine (Cymbalta), dextromethorphan (an ingredient in many cough syrups), venlafaxine (Effexor), St. John's wort, ginkgo	Serotonin syndrome
Morphine and other narcotic pain relievers, antihypertensives	Hypotension
All other antidepressants, pseudoephedrine, amphetamines, cocaine cyclobenzaprine (Flexeril), dopamine, methyldopa, levodopa, epinephrine, buspirone (Buspar)	Hypertensive crisis (these side effects can occur even if taken within 2 weeks of stopping MAOIs)
Buspirone (Buspar)	Psychosis, agitation, seizures
Antidiabetics	Hypoglycemia
Tegretol	Fever, hypertension, seizures

TABLE 4–7 Diet Restrictions for Clients on Monoamine Oxidase Inhibitor (MAOI) Therapy

FOODS CONTAINING TYRAMINE		
HIGH TYRAMINE CONTENT (AVOID WHILE ON MAOI THERAPY)	MODERATE TYRAMINE CONTENT (MAY EAT OCCASIONALLY WHILE ON MAOI THERAPY)	LOW TYRAMINE CONTENT (LIMITED QUANTITIES PERMISSIBLE WHILE ON MAOI THERAPY)
Aged cheeses (cheddar, Swiss, Camembert, blue cheese, Parmesan, provolone, Romano, brie) Raisins, fava beans, flat Italian beans, Chinese pea pods Red wines (Chianti, burgundy, cabernet sauvignon) Liqueurs Smoked and processed meats (salami, bologna, pepperoni, summer sausage) Caviar, pickled herring, corned beef, chicken or beef liver Soy sauce, brewer's yeast, meat tenderizer (MSG) Sauerkraut (Krakus)	Gouda cheese, processed American cheese, mozzarella Yogurt, sour cream Avocados, bananas Beer, white wine, coffee, colas, tea, hot chocolate Meat extracts, such as bouillon Chocolate	Pasteurized cheeses (cream cheese, cottage cheese, ricotta) Figs Distilled spirits (in moderation)

Sources: Complied from Boland and Verduin (2022); Vallerand and Sanoski (2021).

that new information about drug interactions is being discovered and published frequently. To fully understand safety issues related to medication administration, nurses need to access the most current, evidence-based informatics on drug interaction information.

Drug interactions vary widely within these groups. The following are several examples:

- Concomitant use with MAOIs results in serious, sometimes fatal, effects resembling **neuroleptic malignant syndrome.** Coadministration is contraindicated.
- **Serotonin syndrome** may occur when any of the following are used together: St. John's wort, sumatriptan, sibutramine, trazodone, nefazodone, venlafaxine, duloxetine, levomilnacipran, SSRIs, 5-HT receptor agonists (triptans).
- Increased effects of haloperidol, clozapine, and desipramine occur with concomitant use of venlafaxine.
- Increased effects of levomilnacipran occur with concomitant use of CYP3A4 inhibitors.
- Increased effects of venlafaxine occur with concomitant use of cimetidine.
- Increased effects of duloxetine occur with concomitant use of CYP1A2 inhibitors (e.g., fluvoxamine, quinolone antibiotics) or CYP2D6 inhibitors (e.g., fluoxetine, quinidine, paroxetine).

- Risk of liver injury is increased with concomitant use of alcohol and duloxetine.
- Risk of toxicity or adverse effects is increased when drugs extensively metabolized by CYP2D6 (e.g., flecainide, phenothiazines, propafenone, TCAs, thioridazine) are used concomitantly with duloxetine or bupropion.
- Decreased effects of bupropion and trazodone occur with concomitant use of carbamazepine.
- The anticoagulant effect of warfarin may be altered with concomitant use of bupropion, venlafaxine, desvenlafaxine, duloxetine, levomilnacipran, or trazodone.
- Risk of seizures is increased when bupropion is coadministered with drugs that lower the seizure threshold (e.g., antidepressants, antipsychotics, systemic steroids, theophylline, tramadol).
- Effects of midazolam are decreased with concomitant use of desvenlafaxine.
- Effects of desvenlafaxine and levomilnacipran are increased with concomitant use of potent CYP3A4 inhibitors (e.g., ketoconazole).

Diagnosis

The following nursing diagnoses may be considered for patients receiving therapy with antidepressant medications:

- Risk for suicide related to depressed mood
- Risk for injury related to side effects of sedation, lowered seizure threshold, orthostatic hypotension, **priapism,** photosensitivity, arrhythmias, **hypertensive crisis,** or serotonin syndrome
- Social isolation related to depressed mood
- Risk for constipation related to side effects of the medication
- Insomnia related to depressed mood and elevated level of anxiety

Safety Issues in Planning and Implementing Care

Some of the common but manageable side effects of antidepressant medications include dry mouth, sedation, and nausea. General nursing interventions such as offering hard candies, ice, and frequent sips of water are helpful in alleviating dry mouth. Clients may find that sedation is less bothersome if they take the daily dose of antidepressant at bedtime. They should be encouraged to discuss this side effect with the prescribing physician or nurse practitioner. Taking antidepressant medication with food may be helpful in minimizing the common side effect of nausea.

Some patients taking SSRIs or SNRIs complain of sexual dysfunction while on these medications. Men may report abnormal ejaculation or impotence, and women may report loss of orgasm. Because of these side effects, clients sometimes stop the medication abruptly, which may put them at risk for discontinuation syndrome and worsen their symptoms of depression. Nurses must develop an open attitude regarding discussion and assessment of client sexual concerns, and clients who are particularly troubled by this side effect can be encouraged to discuss their concerns with their physician or nurse practitioner to explore an alternative medication.

Other side effects or adverse reactions may be dangerous or even fatal. Many are related to drug-drug or drug-food interactions, as discussed previously.

Because there is so much new information and new drug development is ongoing, practicing nurses should assure that they are accessing evidence-based informatics to keep up to date on side effects and significant drug or food interactions. Many health-care organizations provide online medication resources to employees, and mobile device applications may also provide a readily available resource for up-to-date drug information. Some important safety issues and nursing interventions are listed in Table 4–8.

Outcome Criteria and Evaluation

The following criteria may be used for evaluating the effectiveness of therapy with antidepressant medications. The patient:

- Has not harmed self.
- Has not experienced injury caused by side effects.
- Exhibits vital signs within normal limits.
- Manifests symptoms of improvement in mood (brighter affect, interacts with others, demonstrates improved hygiene, expresses clear thoughts, expresses hopefulness, shows improved ability to make decisions).
- Willingly participates in activities and interacts appropriately with others.

Mood-Stabilizing Agents

For many years, the drug of choice for treatment and management of bipolar mania was lithium carbonate. However, in recent years, several other **mood-stabilizing agents** have demonstrated effectiveness either alone or in combination with lithium. Most notable are many drugs in the class of anticonvulsant medications, which are now FDA approved as indicated for mood stabilization. Some second generation, atypical antipsychotics have also demonstrated benefits for management of this disorder.

TABLE 4–8 Safety Issues and Nursing Interventions for Patients Taking Antidepressants

Drug interactions (multiple, as discussed in the text)	Instruct patients to inform their physician or nurse practitioner of *all* medications they are taking, including herbal preparations, over-the-counter (OTC) drugs, and any medications they have stopped taking within the previous 2 weeks. Notify the physician immediately when any symptoms of serotonin syndrome are assessed. Do not administer the offending agent. ■ Monitor vital signs ■ Protect from injury secondary to muscle rigidity or change in mental status ■ Cooling blankets for temperature regulation ■ Monitor intake and output The condition usually resolves when the offending agent is promptly discontinued but can be fatal without intervention (Cooper & Sejnowski, 2013).
Increased risk for suicide	Assess frequently for presence or worsening of suicide ideation Initiate suicide precautions as needed Monitor patient's use of medication as prescribed, since these medications can be lethal in overdose
Sedation	Instruct patient not to drive or operate dangerous machinery when experiencing sedation
Discontinuation syndrome: SSRIs—dizziness, lethargy, headache, nausea TCAs—hypomania, akathisia, cardiac arrhythmias, GI upset, panic attacks MAOIs—flu-like symptoms, confusion, hypomania	Instruct patients that all antidepressants have some potential for discontinuation syndrome and should not be stopped abruptly but rather should be tapered off. Paroxetine is associated with the highest risk for discontinuation syndrome (Janicak & Hussain, 2017).
Photosensitivity	Instruct patients of vulnerability to severe sunburn, and recommend sunscreen
Orthostatic hypotension (TCAs)	Instruct patients to rise slowly from sitting to standing Monitor blood pressure to assess for symptoms
Tachycardia, arrhythmias (TCAs)	Monitor vital signs, especially in elderly patients with preexisting cardiovascular disorders
Hyponatremia (SSRIs), especially among the elderly	Instruct patients to report any symptoms of nausea, malaise, lethargy, muscle cramps Assess for disorientation or restlessness ■ Monitor sodium levels ■ <120 mEq/L risk for seizure, coma, respiratory arrest Withhold medication, contact physician, restrict water intake Take a detailed history of antidepressant therapy particularly the duration of new antidepressant use (Lien, 2018).
Blurred vision (TCAs and atypicals)	Instruct patients to avoid driving, and reassure patients that this side effect usually resolves within 3 weeks Monitor blood pressure to rule out symptoms of hypertension
Constipation	Recommend a high-fiber diet and regular exercise, and instruct patients to report any symptoms of ongoing difficulty with bowel movements

MAOIs, monoamine oxidase inhibitors; SSRIs, selective serotonin reuptake inhibitors; TCAs, tricyclic antidepressants

Background Assessment Data

Indications

Bipolar disorder is characterized by cycles of depression and manic episodes that may manifest as grandiose thinking and behavior, rapid thoughts, hyperactivity, and/or impulsive agitation. The effective medication treatment for this disorder is one that reduces the rollercoaster of "ups and downs" often described by clients; thus, the name "mood stabilizer" is an apt description of their purpose. Lithium was first identified as an antimanic but was later recognized as useful for stabilizing the mood swings of bipolar disorder as well.

Action

Lithium is a salt that is present in mineral springs and added to spa baths. Although it also was also used for other medicinal purposes, in 1949, John Cade, a physician in Australia, reported that he was using lithium to treat manic excitement and found that it was so successful for some that they became symptom free and were able to be discharged after years of institutionalization (Shorter, 2009). It remains true today that people who respond to lithium and remain on the medication may show no evidence of bipolar moods swings. Although lithium is not a cure for bipolar disorder, it is often described as "like insulin to a diabetic" in that proper use and response can reduce or eliminate symptoms. Unfortunately, not everyone responds to lithium with the same degree of success, and too much lithium can be fatal. Today, we are able to measure specifically the blood levels of lithium and can be confident of its safety when maintained within the specified therapeutic range (0.6–1.2 mEq/L). The exact mechanism of action remains unknown, but it is believed to have an impact on the same neurotransmitters (serotonin, norepinephrine, glutamate, GABA, and dopamine), as previously discussed.

In 1995, the FDA approved valproate (Depakote) as a mood stabilizer, and since then, a great shift toward this group of anticonvulsant/mood stabilizers (including carbamazepine, clonazepam, topiramate, and lamotrigine) and away from lithium has occurred (Shorter, 2009). The mechanism of action for these drugs, as with lithium, is also unclear. Impact on cellular sodium transport, GABA modulation, and raising the seizure threshold have all been advanced as possible explanations for their effectiveness.

Both first generation and second generation antipsychotics have been used alone or as adjuncts to other medication treatment for bipolar mania. Because lithium has a lag period of 7 to 10 days, first generation antipsychotics such as haloperidol may be helpful in initial treatment because of their immediate sedative effects. They also increase the effects of lithium, so monitoring blood serum levels is especially important in the initial phase of treatment when these two drugs are used in combination. (A table of current FDA-approved mood stabilizer medication agents, half-life, and daily dosage ranges can be found online in Chapter 17, "Bipolar and Related Disorders.").

Several studies have explored dietary supplements and anti-inflammatory agents for their benefits as adjunct treatments in bipolar disorder (Aiken, 2020). While studies have demonstrated benefits of *N*-acetylcysteine as an adjunctive treatment of subsyndromal depressive symptoms, the results for treatment of bipolar disorder have been mixed. Two anti-inflammatory agents, celecoxib and aspirin, have shown more promising results as adjunct treatments in major depressive disorder and depressive symptoms associated with bipolar disorder (Köhler-Forsberg et al., 2019). A recent systematic review and meta-analysis also supported that skill-based psychosocial interventions, like cognitive behavior therapy (in combination with pharmacotherapy), reduced the recurrence of illness episodes better than medication treatment alone (Miklowitz et al., 2020).

Interactions

One of the interesting things about drug interactions with mood stabilizers is that many drugs either increase or decrease their effectiveness, as shown in Table 4–9. Understanding that lithium is a salt is relevant in explaining some of these interactions. Because lithium is an imperfect substitute for sodium, anything that depletes sodium will make more receptor sites available to lithium and increase the risk for lithium toxicity. This effect is why individuals taking lithium must maintain regular dietary sodium and fluid intake to avoid major fluctuations in their lithium levels and the resulting effects. For example, significant increases in dietary sodium intake may reduce the effectiveness of lithium because sodium will bind at more receptor sites and decrease the amount of lithium that can bind to these receptors. Other drugs that increase or decrease serum sodium levels will also have an impact on lithium levels.

TABLE 4–9 **Drug Interactions With Mood-Stabilizing Agents**

THE EFFECTS OF	ARE INCREASED BY	ARE DECREASED BY	CONCOMITANT USE MAY RESULT IN
Antimanic: Lithium	Carbamazepine, fluoxetine, haloperidol, loop diuretics, methyldopa, NSAIDs, and thiazide diuretics	Acetazolamide, osmotic diuretics, theophylline, and urinary alkalinizers	Increased effects of neuromuscular blocking agents and TCAs; decreased pressor sensitivity of sympathomimetics; neurotoxicity may occur with phenothiazines or calcium channel blockers
Anticonvulsants: Clonazepam	CNS depressants, cimetidine, hormonal contraceptives, disulfiram, fluoxetine, isoniazid, ketoconazole, metoprolol, propranolol, valproic acid, probenecid	Rifampin, theophylline (↓ sedative effects), phenytoin	Increased phenytoin levels; decreased efficacy of levodopa
Carbamazepine	Verapamil, diltiazem, propoxyphene, erythromycin, clarithromycin, SSRIs, TCAs, cimetidine, isoniazid, danazol, lamotrigine, niacin, acetazolamide, dalfopristin, valproate, nefazodone	Cisplatin, doxorubicin, felbamate, rifampin, barbiturates, hydantoins, primidone, theophylline	Decreased levels of corticosteroids, doxycycline, quinidine, warfarin, estrogen-containing contraceptives, cyclosporine, benzodiazepines, theophylline, lamotrigine, valproic acid, bupropion, haloperidol, olanzapine, tiagabine, topiramate, voriconazole, ziprasidone, felbamate, levothyroxine, or antidepressants; increased levels of lithium; life-threatening hypertensive reaction with MAOIs
Valproic Acid	Chlorpromazine, cimetidine, erythromycin, felbamate, salicylates	Rifampin, carbamazepine, cholestyramine, lamotrigine, phenobarbital, ethosuximide, hydantoins	Increased effects of TCAs, carbamazepine, CNS depressants, ethosuximide, lamotrigine, phenobarbital, warfarin, zidovudine, hydantoins
Lamotrigine	Valproic acid	Primidone, phenobarbital, phenytoin, rifamycin, succinimides, oral contraceptives, oxcarbazepine, carbamazepine, acetaminophen	Decreased levels of valproic acid; increased levels of carbamazepine and topiramate
Topiramate	Metformin, hydrochlorothiazide	Phenytoin, carbamazepine, valproic acid, lamotrigine	Increased risk of CNS depression with alcohol or other CNS depressants; increased risk of kidney stones with carbonic anhydrase inhibitors; increased effects of phenytoin, metformin, amitriptyline; decreased effects of oral contraceptives, digoxin, lithium, risperidone, and valproic acid
Oxcarbazepine		Carbamazepine, phenobarbital, phenytoin, valproic acid, verapamil	Increased concentrations of phenobarbital and phenytoin; decreased effects of oral contraceptives, felodipine, and lamotrigine
Calcium Channel Blocker: Verapamil	Amiodarone, beta blockers, cimetidine, ranitidine, and grapefruit juice	Barbiturates, calcium salts, hydantoins, rifampin, and antineoplastics	Increased effects of beta blockers, disopyramide, flecainide, doxorubicin, benzodiazepines, buspirone, carbamazepine, digoxin, dofetilide, ethanol, imipramine, nondepolarizing muscle relaxants, prazosin, quinidine, sirolimus, tacrolimus, and theophylline; altered serum lithium levels

Antipsychotics: Olanzapine	Fluvoxamine and other CYP1A2 inhibitors, fluoxetine	Carbamazepine and other CYP1A2 inducers, omeprazole, rifampin	Decreased effects of levodopa and dopamine agonists; increased hypotension with antihypertensives; increased CNS depression with alcohol or other CNS depressants
Aripiprazole	Ketoconazole and other CYP3A4 inhibitors; quinidine, fluoxetine, paroxetine, or other potential CYP2D6 inhibitors	Carbamazepine, famotidine, valproate	Increased CNS depression with alcohol or other CNS depressants; increased hypotension with antihypertensives
Chlorpromazine	Beta blockers, paroxetine	Centrally acting anticholinergics	Increased effects of beta blockers; excessive sedation and hypotension with meperidine; decreased hypotensive effect of guanethidine; decreased effect of oral anticoagulants; decreased or increased phenytoin levels; increased orthostatic hypotension with thiazide diuretics; increased CNS depression with alcohol or other CNS depressants; increased hypotension with antihypertensives; increased anticholinergic effects with anticholinergic agents.
Quetiapine	Cimetidine; ketoconazole, itraconazole, fluconazole, erythromycin, or other CYP3A4 inhibitors	Phenytoin, thioridazine	Decreased effects of levodopa and dopamine agonists; increased CNS depression with alcohol or other CNS depressants; increased hypotension with antihypertensives
Risperidone	Clozapine, fluoxetine, paroxetine, or ritonavir	Carbamazepine	Decreased effects of levodopa and dopamine agonists; increased effects of clozapine and valproate; increased CNS depression with alcohol or other CNS depressants; increased hypotension with antihypertensives
Ziprasidone	Ketoconazole and other CYP3A4 inhibitors	Carbamazepine	Life-threatening prolongation of QT interval with quinidine, dofetilide, other class Ia and III antiarrhythmics, pimozide, sotalol, thioridazine, chlorpromazine, pentamidine, arsenic trioxide, mefloquine, dolasetron, tacrolimus, droperidol, gatifloxacin, or moxifloxacin; decreased effects of levodopa and dopamine agonists; increased CNS depression with alcohol or other CNS depressants; increased hypotension with antihypertensives
Asenapine	Fluvoxamine, imipramine, valproate	Carbamazepine, cimetidine, paroxetine	Increased effects of paroxetine and dextromethorphan; increased CNS depression with alcohol or other CNS depressants; increased hypotension with antihypertensives; additive effects of QT interval prolongation with quinidine, dofetilide, other class Ia and III antiarrhythmics, pimozide, sotalol, thioridazine, chlorpromazine, pentamidine, arsenic trioxide, mefloquine, dolasetron, tacrolimus, droperidol, gatifloxacin, or moxifloxacin

Diagnosis

The following nursing diagnoses may be considered for patients receiving therapy with mood-stabilizing agents:

- Risk for injury related to manic hyperactivity
- Risk for self-directed or other-directed violence related to unresolved anger turned inward on the self or outward on the environment
- Risk for injury related to lithium toxicity
- Risk for injury related to adverse effects of mood-stabilizing drugs
- Risk for activity intolerance related to side effects of drowsiness and dizziness

Safety Issues in Planning and Implementing Care

One of the primary safety issues with lithium has to do with its narrow therapeutic range. A description of lithium toxicity, selected other safety concerns with mood-stabilizing agents, and relevant nursing interventions are discussed in Table 4–10.

TABLE 4–10 Safety Issues and Nursing Interventions for Patients Taking Mood Stabilizers

SAFETY ISSUES	NURSING INTERVENTIONS
Lithium toxicity: ■ Blood levels >0.8 mmol (or mEq)/L are associated with increased risk for renal toxicity (*N*-acetylcysteine may prevent lithium-induced renal damage [Rege, 2020]) ■ At blood levels >1.2 mEq/L early signs of toxicity include vomiting and diarrhea ■ At blood levels >1.5 mEq/L gastrointestinal (increasing nausea, anorexia, diarrhea) and CNS effects (muscle weakness, drowsiness, ataxia, coarse tremor and muscle twitching) occur (Rege, 2020) ■ At blood levels >2 mEq/L: increasing disorientation and seizures can occur ■ Blood levels ≥3.5 mEq/L are associated with coma, cardiovascular collapse, and death. Chlorpromazine and Thorazine may mask early signs of lithium toxicity (Vallerand & Sanoski, 2021)	Instruct patient to report all medications, herbals, and caffeine use to physician or nurse practitioner to evaluate for drug interactions Encourage patient to maintain fluid intake at 2,000–3,000 mL/day and to avoid activities that cause excessive sweating or fluid loss because inadequate fluid intake can impact lithium levels Instruct patient about the importance of regular monitoring of serum lithium levels Blood levels should be drawn 12 hours after the last dose
Increased risk of suicide for all antiepileptics (black box warning, FDA, 2008)	Assess for suicide risk regularly, and inform patients of risks associated with anticonvulsants
Hyponatremia (lithium, carbamazepine)	Instruct patients to maintain usual dietary intake of sodium Assess for and educate patients to report any episodes of nausea, vomiting, headache, muscle weakness, confusion, seizures; these may be signs of hyponatremia
Stevens-Johnson syndrome (especially with lamotrigine and carbamazepine) This toxic skin necrolysis can be life threatening	Assess for and educate patients to report any signs of rash or unusual skin breakdown
Hypotension, arrhythmias (lithium)	Monitor vital signs and instruct patient to report any symptoms of dizziness or palpitations
Blood dyscrasias (valproic acid, carbamazepine)	Educate patients to report infections or other illness while on these medications Ensure that platelet counts and bleeding time are determined before initiation of therapy. Monitor for spontaneous bleeding or bruising.
Increased risk of birth defects (anticonvulsant/mood stabilizers)	Instruct female patients on the risks of birth defects, and provide education about contraception as desired
Drowsiness (lithium and all anticonvulsants)	Instruct patients to avoid driving or operating dangerous machinery when experiencing this side effect Assess patient's mental status for level of alertness

Clients who respond to lithium will typically remain on the medication indefinitely. To assure safe maintenance and prevent lithium toxicity, patient education and regular monitoring are essential. An important component of monitoring is evaluation of serum lithium levels to assure that they remain within the therapeutic range.

While a typical therapeutic range for lithium is from 0.6 to 1.2 mEq/L, current American Psychiatric Association clinical practice guidelines recommend that when initiating treatment, the levels should be closer to 1.2 (the higher end of the range) and that in maintenance treatment the optimum levels should be closer to 0.6 (the lower end of the range) (Rege, 2020). An international study group recently completed a systematic review and came to a consensus on a more conservative optimal range of 0.4 to 0.6 mEq/L if the patient is responding well to lithium therapy (Nolen et al., 2019). While higher levels (closer to 1.0) may be more efficacious for patients that are prone to more manic episodes (rather than more depressive episodes), higher levels are also associated with more adverse effects. At levels over 1.5 mEq/L, increasing nausea, anorexia, and diarrhea are common as well as CNS symptoms such as muscle weakness, drowsiness, ataxia, tremors, and muscle twitching. Even higher levels can lead to delirium, seizures, cardiovascular collapse, or death.

Serum lithium levels should be monitored once or twice a week after initial treatment until dosage and serum levels are stable, then monthly during maintenance therapy. Blood samples should be drawn 12 hours after the last dose.

Some clients complain that they miss the "high" feeling of being in a manic or hypomanic state once they begin mood-stabilizing medications. They may be at risk for self-adjusting medication or discontinuing it all together.

Open discussion and exploring the benefits versus disadvantages of medication treatment promote patient-centered care and enable the nurse to troubleshoot with the patient ways to minimize risks.

One generally undesirable side effect of lithium is weight gain. Patients should be educated about this potential, and weight should be monitored at regular intervals. It may be helpful to discuss low-calorie diets while stressing the importance of not making large changes in sodium intake because of its impact on serum blood levels of lithium.

CLINICAL PEARL The U.S. Food and Drug Administration requires that all antiepileptic (anticonvulsant) drugs carry a warning label indicating that use of the drug increases risk for suicidal thoughts and behaviors. Patients being treated with these medications should be monitored for the emergence or worsening of depression, suicidal thoughts or behavior, or any unusual changes in mood or behavior.

Outcome Criteria and Evaluation

The following criteria may be used for evaluating the effectiveness of therapy with mood-stabilizing agents. The patient:

- Is maintaining stability of mood.
- Has not harmed self or others.
- Has experienced no injury from hyperactivity.
- Is able to participate in activities without excessive sedation or dizziness.
- Is maintaining appropriate weight.
- Exhibits no signs of lithium toxicity.
- Verbalizes importance of taking medication regularly and reporting for regular laboratory blood tests.

Antipsychotic Agents

Antipsychotic medications are also called *neuroleptics*. Historically, they have been referred to as *major tranquilizers*, and have clear sedative effects. The term *antipsychotic* is most descriptive because the primary benefit over time is the alleviation of psychotic symptoms such as hallucinations and delusions.

Background Assessment Data

Antipsychotic medications were introduced in the United States in the 1950s with the phenothiazines. Other drugs in this classification soon followed, and they are now called typical, or first generation, antipsychotics. Unfortunately, this group of medications has the potential for extrapyramidal side effects, also called **extrapyramidal symptoms (EPS)** that interfere with normal movements, including acute **dystonias** (muscle spasms), which can be life threatening; Parkinsonian-like symptoms; and **tardive dyskinesias** (later onset involuntary movement disorders primarily in the tongue, lips, and jaw but may also involve other movement disturbances). Some of these side effects can be permanent even after the drug is discontinued. The first generation, typical antipsychotics include the phenothiazines, haloperidol, loxapine, pimozide, and thiothixene.

Second generation antipsychotic medications have since been developed with less potential for

EPS. They have become the preferred first-line treatment. These are most often referred to as atypical antipsychotics and they include aripiprazole, asenapine and asenapine transdermal (Secuado), clozapine, olanzapine, quetiapine, risperidone, paliperidone, iloperidone, lurasidone, ziprasidone, brexpiprazole (Rexulti), cariprazine (Vraylar), pimavanserin (Nuplazid), and lumateperone (Caplyta). Pimavanserin is indicated for hallucinations and delusions associated with Parkinson's disease psychosis. This group of drugs is used to alleviate positive symptoms: hallucinations, delusions, and agitation and may be beneficial in treating some of the negative symptoms as well.

The atypical antipsychotic aripiprazole (Abilify) has sometimes been described as a third generation antipsychotic because of its unique functional profile with dopamine receptors, and it has been identified as having minimal risk for EPS (Brust et al., 2015). In 2017 the FDA approved a novel (and controversial) formulation of aripiprazole (called Abilify MyCite) that includes a sensor device embedded in the pill that enables the patient (and others) to track whether they are taking the medication. In 2020 the FDA approved a novel antipsychotic medication, lumateperone (Caplyta), which, although the action is unknown, reportedly demonstrates benefit in treating both positive and negative symptoms of schizophrenia.

Indications

Antipsychotics are used in the treatment of schizophrenia and other psychotic disorders. Selected agents are used in the treatment of bipolar mania (see previous section, "Mood-Stabilizing Agents"). Others are used as antiemetics (chlorpromazine, perphenazine, prochlorperazine) in the treatment of intractable hiccoughs (chlorpromazine), and for the control of tics and vocal utterances in Tourette's disorder (haloperidol, pimozide). Selected second generation, atypical, antipsychotics, including aripiprazole, are being identified as adjuncts to the treatment of major depressive disorders. (A table of current FDA-approved antipsychotics, and daily dosage ranges and medications used to treat EPS of antipsychotic medications can be found in Chapter 15, "Schizophrenia Spectrum and Other Psychotic Disorders.")

Action

First generation, typical antipsychotics are antagonists that work by blocking postsynaptic dopamine receptors in the basal ganglia, hypothalamus, limbic system, brainstem, and medulla. They also demonstrate varying affinity for cholinergic, alpha$_1$-adrenergic, and histaminic receptors.

Second generation, atypical antipsychotics are weaker dopamine receptor antagonists than the first generation antipsychotics, but they are more potent antagonists of the serotonin type 2A (5-HT$_{2A}$) receptors. They also exhibit antagonism for cholinergic, histaminic, and adrenergic receptors. As mentioned previously, aripiprazole (Abilify) is a dopamine receptor antagonist that seems to have a unique way of accomplishing its action and thus has a minimal risk of EPS.

Contraindications and Precautions

Certain individuals may be at greater risk for experiencing side effects associated with antipsychotic agents. The elderly have been identified as an at-risk population related to reports of stroke and sudden death while taking antipsychotic medication. Studies have indicated that elderly patients with psychosis related to neurocognitive disorder (NCD) who are treated with antipsychotic drugs are at increased risk of death compared with those taking a placebo (Gareri et al., 2014). Causes of death are most commonly related to infections or cardiovascular problems. All antipsychotic drugs now carry black box warnings to this effect. They are not approved for treatment of elderly patients with neurocognitive-related psychosis.

Both first and second generation antipsychotics are contraindicated in clients with known hypersensitivity. They should not be used in patients in comatose states or when CNS depression is evident; when blood dyscrasias exist; in clients with Parkinson's disease or narrow-angle glaucoma (first generation); in those with liver, renal, or cardiac insufficiency; in individuals with poorly controlled seizure disorders; or in elderly clients with dementia-related psychosis.

Ziprasidone, risperidone, paliperidone, asenapine, and iloperidone are contraindicated in patients with a history of QT prolongation or cardiac arrhythmias, recent myocardial infarction (MI), or uncompensated heart failure, and concomitant use with other drugs that prolong the QT interval is also contraindicated. Clozapine is contraindicated in patients with myeloproliferative disorders, with a history of clozapine-induced **agranulocytosis** (an acute condition involving a severe and dangerous lowered white blood cell count) or severe granulocytopenia, and in uncontrolled epilepsy. Lurasidone is contraindicated in concomitant use with strong inhibitors of cytochrome P450 isozyme 3A4 (CYP3A4) (e.g., ketoconazole, an antifungal) and strong CYP3A4 inducers (e.g., rifampin, an antitubercular).

Caution should be taken in administering these drugs to elderly or debilitated patients; to patients with cardiac, hepatic, or renal insufficiency; to those with a history of seizures; to patients with diabetes or risk factors for diabetes; to clients exposed to temperature extremes; under conditions that cause hypotension (dehydration, hypovolemia, treatment with antihypertensive medication); and to pregnant clients (several atypical antipsychotic medications, such as olanzapine, risperidone, and quetiapine, have been associated with congenital malformations [Babu et al., 2015]). Six atypical antipsychotic medications (aripiprazole, asenapine, olanzapine, paliperidone, quetiapine, and risperidone) have FDA approval for use in children and adolescents. Both aripiprazole and quetiapine (also approved for adjunctive treatment in depression) carry black box warnings about increased risk for suicidal thinking in children, adolescents, and young adults.

Interactions

Table 4–11 highlights some drug interactions that warrant monitoring and assessment by nurses.

Diagnosis

The following nursing diagnoses may be considered for patients receiving antipsychotic therapy:

- Risk for other-directed violence related to panic anxiety and mistrust of others
- Risk for injury related to medication side effects of sedation, photosensitivity, reduction of seizure threshold, agranulocytosis, EPS, tardive dyskinesia, neuroleptic malignant syndrome, and/or QT prolongation
- Risk for activity intolerance related to medication side effects of sedation, blurred vision, and/or weakness
- Nonadherence with medication regimen related to suspiciousness and mistrust of others

Safety Issues in Planning and Implementing Care

Table 4–12 discusses some significant safety issues to consider and relevant nursing interventions for patients taking antipsychotic medication.

Additional Issues for Patient Education

- Smoking increases the metabolism of antipsychotics, requiring an adjustment in dosage to achieve a therapeutic effect. Encourage the patient to discuss this issue with the prescribing physician or nurse practitioner.

TABLE 4–11 Drug interactions With Antipsychotic Medications

DRUG INTERACTION	ADVERSE EFFECT
Antihypertensives, CNS depressants Epinephrine or dopamine in combination with haloperidol or phenothiazines	Additive and potentially severe hypotension
Oral anticoagulants with phenothiazines	Less effective anticoagulant effects
Drugs that prolong QT intervals	Additive effects
Drugs that trigger orthostatic hypotension	Additive hypotension
Drugs with anticholinergic effects, prescription, and OTC drugs	Additive anticholinergic effects, including anticholinergic toxicity, which includes: ■ Flushing ■ Dry mouth ■ Mydriasis ■ Altered mental status ■ Tachycardia ■ Urinary retention ■ Tremulousness ■ Hypertension

Source: Compiled from Ramnarine (2020).

TABLE 4–12 Safety Issues in Planning and Implementing Care for Patients Taking Antipsychotic Medication

Extrapyramidal side effects[a]	Instruct the patient to report any signs of muscle stiffness or spasms; hold the medication if signs occur Administer antiparkinsonian agents as ordered and immediately when signs of acute dystonia are present Assess the patient for abnormal involuntary movements (see Box 4–2) (See the section "Additional Issues for Patient Education" for additional discussion)
Hyperglycemia, weight gain, and diabetes (More common with atypical antipsychotic agents)	Assess for history of diabetes Evaluate blood sugars Instruct the patient in these risks and the importance of diet and exercise Assess for signs of hyperglycemia, including polydipsia, polyphagia, polyuria, and weakness
Hypotension	Educate the patient about risk for hypotension Monitor blood pressure
Orthostatic hypotension	Instruct the patient to rise slowly from sitting to standing Monitor blood pressure lying and then standing to assess for postural changes
Lower seizure threshold (especially with clozapine)	Assess the patient for history of seizure disorder Monitor the patient for evidence of seizure activity, and report to prescribing physician or nurse practitioner
Prolonged QT interval[b] Especially ziprasidone, thioridazine, pimozide, haloperidol, paliperidone, iloperidone, asenapine, and clozapine	Assess the patient for history of arrhythmias, recent myocardial infarction, or heart failure, and report to prescribing physician or nurse practitioner because these events are contraindications Assess for other medications the patient is taking that prolong QT interval (there are many; online resources such as www.crediblemeds.org provide a composite list for comparison), but note that erythromycin and clarithromycin are two that are commonly prescribed Instruct the patient to report any rapid heartbeat, dizziness, or fainting Check baseline ECG before beginning treatment
Anticholinergic effects	Instruct the patient about additive effects of other anticholinergic drugs in combination with antipsychotics and to report any other medications being taken, including over-the-counter and herbal remedies For minor symptoms such as dry mouth, recommend hard candies and sips of water Instruct the patient regarding the importance of good oral hygiene Instruct the patient to report and assess for any evidence of urinary retention, tachycardia, tremulousness, or hypertension, since these may be signs of anticholinergic toxicity
Sedation	Educate the patient about this side effect, and instruct the patient not to drive or operate dangerous machinery if experiencing sedation
Photosensitivity	Instruct the patient to use sunblock and sunglasses and to wear protective clothing when in the sun because of the increased risk for severe sunburn while on these medications
Agranulocytosis (more common with typical antipsychotics but especially with the atypical antipsychotic agent clozapine)	Instruct the patient receiving clozapine that regular monitoring of white blood cell and absolute neutrophil blood levels is essential Instruct the patient to report any signs of sore throat, fever, or malaise (See additional guidelines below)

TABLE 4–12 Safety Issues in Planning and Implementing Care for Patients Taking Antipsychotic Medication—cont'd

Neuroleptic malignant syndrome (NMS)[c]	Instruct the patient to report immediately any fever, muscle rigidity, diaphoresis, tachycardia Assess vital signs regularly, including temperature Assess for deteriorating mental status or any other sign of NMS; presence of any of these signs requires holding the medication and contacting the prescribing physician or nurse practitioner immediately and monitoring vital signs and intake and output
Drug reaction with eosinophilia and systemic symptoms (DRESS) (olanzapine)[d] (FDA, 2016b)	Assess for symptoms of DRESS including fever, rash, swollen lymph glands, swelling in the face. Hold medication and contact physician immediately.
New impulse control problems such as compulsive or uncontrollable urges to gamble, binge eat, shop, and have sex (aripiprazole) (FDA, 2016c)	Assess for newly developing impulse control problems for patients taking aripiprazole. Closely monitor patients who may be at increased risk for impulse control problems such as those with personal or family history of obsessive-compulsive disorder, bipolar disorder, impulsive personality, alcohol, drug, or other addictive behaviors.

[a] Acute dystonias can be life threatening (more common with typical (first generation) antipsychotic medications).
[b] Potentially life threatening.
[c] Rare but potentially life-threatening side effect characterized by muscle rigidity, severe hyperthermia, and cardiac effects, which can be rapidly progressive over 24–72 hours and is potentially fatal.
[d] Rare but serious; can lead to organ injury and even death.

- Body temperature is harder to maintain with antipsychotic medication, so patients should be encouraged to dress warmly in cold weather and avoid extended exposure to very high or low temperatures.
- Alcohol and antipsychotic drugs potentiate each other's effects, so patients should be advised to avoid drinking alcohol while on antipsychotic therapy.
- Many medications contain substances that interact with antipsychotics in a way that may be harmful, so patients should be advised to avoid taking other medications (including over-the-counter products) without first consulting the physician.
- A significant number of patients on clozapine report excessive salivation. Sugar-free gum and medications (anticholinergic or alpha$_2$-adrenoceptor agonists) may alleviate symptoms. Patients should be encouraged to discuss these options with the prescribing physician or nurse practitioner.
- Advise patients of possible risks of taking antipsychotics during pregnancy. Antipsychotics are thought to readily cross the placental barrier; if so, a fetus could experience adverse effects of the drug. Patients should inform the physician immediately if pregnancy occurs, is suspected, or is planned.
- Clozapine carries a particular risk for agranulocytosis, which increases risk for severe infection. Patients should be instructed that regular measurement of neutrophils is essential (this is discussed in more detail below).
- Clozapine also carries a risk for ileus (intestinal blockage) with a 15% to 28% fatality rate. Eighty percent of clozapine-treated patients have some hypomotility in their bowels, and in 2020 the FDA strengthened its warning on the risks of ileus (FDA, 2020). Instruct patients to report any change in bowel habits to their physician and to explore dietary and medications to reduce constipation.

Issues in Antipsychotic Maintenance Therapy

The nurse must understand the management of side effects associated with antipsychotic medication in order to conduct a thorough assessment and minimize risks. In addition, some of these side effects can be difficult for patients to manage or to understand, particularly when they are struggling with impaired mental status including psychosis and cognitive deficits. Three of these side effects are discussed next.

Clozaril and the Risk for Agranulocytosis

The FDA requires close monitoring for patients on medications that increase the risk for life-threatening side effects. Clozapine (Clozaril) is one such drug. Due to the risk of agranulocytosis, the FDA requires that clozapine be part of a Risk Evaluation and Mitigation Strategy (REMS) program to ensure that risk for agranulocytosis is monitored, managed, and reported. Agranulocytosis is a potentially fatal blood disorder in which the patient's absolute neutrophil count (ANC) drops to extremely low levels (less than or equal to 500 μL). This condition is called neutropenia. An ANC must be assessed before initiation of treatment with clozapine and weekly for the first 6 months of treatment. Initially, only a 1-week supply of medication is dispensed at a time. If the ANC remains within acceptable levels (i.e., ANC of at least 1,500 μL) during the first 6 months, blood counts may be monitored biweekly for another 6 months and monthly thereafter. Some individuals with dark skin, particularly those of African and Middle Eastern descent, have normally lower ANC (benign ethnic neutropenia); in such cases the parameters for identifying clinically significant neutropenia are altered (Clozapine REMS, 2015).

Although the benefits of clozapine can be profound, this medication is typically used when patients fail to respond to other antipsychotics because of the strict protocols for adherence. If the patient agrees to this option, the nurse can be a vital link in assuring that support services, both professional and personal (such as family members or peers), are engaged to assist the patient with follow-through as needed.

Extrapyramidal Symptoms (EPS)

To conduct a thorough assessment the nurse must be familiar with several distinct types of EPS:

- **Akathisia:** Continuous restlessness and fidgeting; occurs most frequently in women and may manifest 50 to 60 days following initiation of therapy. Combining atypical antipsychotics has demonstrated a threefold risk for developing akathisia compared with monotherapy with a single second generation antipsychotic (Berna et al., 2015).
- **Akinesia:** Absence or impairment in voluntary movement.
- **Dystonia:** Involuntary muscle spasms in the face, arms, legs, and neck; occurs most often in men and in people younger than 25 years of age. Dystonia should be treated as an emergency because laryngospasm follows in untreated symptoms and can be fatal. The physician should be contacted, and intravenous or intramuscular benztropine mesylate (Cogentin) is commonly administered (see Chapter 15, "Schizophrenia Spectrum and Other Psychotic Disorders," for a list of **antiparkinsonian agents** used to treat EPS). Nurses should stay with the patient and offer reassurance.
- **Oculogyric crisis:** Uncontrolled rolling back of the eyes is a symptom of acute dystonias and can be mistaken for seizure activity. As with other symptoms of acute dystonias, oculogyric crisis should be treated as a medical emergency.
- **Pseudoparkinsonism** (tremor, shuffling gait, drooling, rigidity): Symptoms may appear 1 to 5 days following initiation of antipsychotic medication; occurs most often in women, the elderly, and dehydrated clients.
- **Tardive dyskinesia:** Bizarre facial and tongue movements, stiff neck, and difficulty swallowing may occur with all antipsychotics but is more common with first generation antipsychotics.

Some EPS can be life threatening and those that are not can sometimes be permanent. The abnormal movements of the tongue and lips are sometimes very visible and even severe enough to interfere with a person's ability to speak or swallow.

All clients receiving long-term (months or years) antipsychotic therapy are at risk for tardive dyskinesia, and the symptoms are potentially irreversible. Early signs of tardive dyskinesia (usually vermiform movements of the tongue) should be reported immediately to the prescribing physician or nurse practitioner. Often, the drug is discontinued, the dosage is altered, or a different antipsychotic is prescribed. In 2017 the FDA approved the first drugs for treating tardive dyskinesia, valbenazine (Ingrezza) and deutetrabenazine (Austedo). It is hoped that these novel drugs will effectively reduce this troubling condition and its sometimes stigmatizing effects. The involuntary movements associated with tardive dyskinesia can be measured by the Abnormal Involuntary Movement Scale (AIMS), developed in the 1970s by the National Institute of Mental Health. AIMS aids in early detection of movement disorders and provides means for ongoing surveillance. AIMS is featured in Box 4–3.

The nurse's empathic approach in listening to the patient's wishes with regard to medication and advocating for exploring other options for management of symptoms is one way to promote patient-centered care, an essential nursing competency (IOM, 2003) and to promote a recovery model that empowers patients to make decisions about management of their illness. There is evidence (Haddad et al., 2014) that remaining on antipsychotic medication can reduce the frequency of hospitalizations and early treatment at the first psychotic episode may reduce some long-term consequences of illness. Educating patients about these risks and benefits is important in assisting them to make an informed decisions about medication treatment.

BOX 4–3 Abnormal Involuntary Movement Scale (AIMS)

Name _____ Rater Name _____ Date _____

Instructions: Complete the examination procedure before making ratings. For movement ratings, circle the highest severity observed. Rate movements that occur upon activation one *less* than those observed spontaneously. Circle movement as well as code number that applies.

Code: 0 = None
1 = Minimal, may be normal
2 = Mild
3 = Moderate
4 = Severe

Facial and Oral Movements	**Muscles of Facial Expression** (e.g., movements of forehead, eyebrows, periorbital area, cheeks, including frowning, blinking, smiling, grimacing)	**0 1 2 3 4**
	Lips and Perioral Area (e.g., puckering, pouting, smacking)	**0 1 2 3 4**
	Jaw (e.g., biting, clenching, chewing, mouth opening, lateral movement)	**0 1 2 3 4**
	Tongue (Rate only increases in movement both in and out of mouth. NOT inability to sustain movement. Darting in and out of mouth.)	**0 1 2 3 4**
Extremity Movements	**Upper (arms, wrists, hands, fingers)** Include choreic movements (i.e., rapid, objectively purposeless, irregular, spontaneous) and athetoid movements (i.e., slow, irregular, complex serpentine). *Do not include tremor* (i.e., repetitive, regular, rhythmic)	**0 1 2 3 4**
	Lower (legs, knees, ankles, toes) (e.g., lateral knee movement, foot tapping, heel dropping, foot squirming, inversion and eversion of foot)	**0 1 2 3 4**
Trunk Movements	**Neck, shoulders, hips** (e.g., rocking, twisting, squirming, pelvic gyrations)	**0 1 2 3 4**
Global Judgments	**Severity of abnormal movements overall**	**0 1 2 3 4**
	Incapacitation due to abnormal movements	**0 1 2 3 4**
	Patient's awareness of abnormal movements (Rate only the patient's report)	
	No awareness	**0**
	Aware, no distress	**1**
	Aware, mild distress	**2**
	Aware, moderate distress	**3**
	Aware, severe distress	**4**
Dental Status	**Current problems with teeth and/or dentures?**	**No Yes**
	Are dentures usually worn?	**No Yes**
	Edentia?	**No Yes**
	Do movements disappear in sleep?	**No Yes**

Continued

BOX 4–3 Abnormal Involuntary Movement Scale (AIMS)—cont'd

Either before or after completing the examination procedure, observe the patient unobtrusively, at rest (e.g., in waiting room). The chair to be used in this examination should be a hard, firm one without arms.

1. Ask patient to remove shoes and socks.
2. Ask patient whether there is anything in their mouth (e.g., gum, candy), and if so, to remove it.
3. Ask patient about the current condition of their teeth. Ask patient if they wear dentures. Do teeth or dentures bother patient now?
4. Ask patient whether they notice any movements in mouth, face, hands, or feet. If yes, ask to describe and to what extent movements currently bother patient or interfere with his/her activities.
5. Have patient sit in chair with both hands on knees, legs slightly apart, and feet flat on floor. (Look at entire body for movements while in this position.)
6. Ask patient to sit with hands hanging unsupported. If male, between legs, if female and wearing a dress, hanging over knees. (Observe hands and other body areas.)
7. Ask patient to open mouth. (Observe tongue at rest within mouth.) Do this twice.
8. Ask patient to protrude tongue. (Observe abnormalities of tongue movement.) Do this twice.
9. Ask patient to tap thumb with each finger as rapidly as possible for 10 to 15 seconds; separately with right hand, then with left hand. (Observe facial and leg movements.)
10. Flex and extend patient's left and right arms (one at a time). (Note any rigidity.)
11. Ask patient to stand up. (Observe in profile. Observe all body areas again, hips included.)
12. Ask patient to extend both arms outstretched in front with palms down. (Observe trunk, legs, and mouth.)
13. Have patient walk a few paces, turn, and walk back to chair. (Observe hands and gait.) Do this twice.

INTERPRETATION OF AIMS SCORE

Add patient scores and note areas of difficulty.

Score of:

0 to 1 = Low risk

2 in only ONE of the areas assessed = borderline/observe closely

2 in TWO or more of the areas assessed **or** 3 to 4 in ONLY ONE area = indicative of TD

Source: U.S. Department of Health and Human Services. Available for use in the public domain from Guy W. ECDEU Assessment Manual for Psychopharmacology: Revised (DHEW publication number ADM 76-338). Rockville, MD, US Department of Health, Education and Welfare, Public Health Service, Alcohol, Drug Abuse and Mental Health Administration, NIMH Psychopharmacology Research Branch, Division of Extramural Research Programs, 1976: 534–537.

Hormonal Side Effects

Following are hormonal side effects that may accompany these medications:

- ***Male side effects:*** Decreased libido, **retrograde ejaculation** (the discharge of seminal fluid into the bladder rather than through the urethra); **gynecomastia** (breast enlargement)
- ***Female side effects:*** **Amenorrhea** (absence of menses); galactorrhea (milky discharge from breasts of non-breastfeeding woman)

These side effects can be very troubling for anyone, and for a patient struggling with thought disturbances, they can become the foundation for delusions. A male patient with gynecomastia, for example, might begin to believe that external forces are taking over his body and turning him into a woman. An amenorrheic woman may begin to believe that she has been divinely impregnated. It is important for the nurse to be clear that these are side effects of the medication and to offer reassurance that they are reversible. Women with amenorrhea should be instructed that this side effect does not indicate cessation of ovulation, so use of contraception should continue as usual. Patients should be encouraged to explore alternative treatment if these side effects are deemed intolerable.

Current Developments in Psychopharmacological Treatment of Schizophrenia

One of the identified limitations of medication treatments available for schizophrenia is the cognitive deficits that are core symptoms of this illness, including deficits in working memory, long-term memory, reduced processing speed, verbal fluency, and impaired executive functions. Some atypical antipsychotics have demonstrated efficacy in lessening cognitive deficits but not eliminating residual effects.

Cariprazine (Vraylar) has demonstrated efficacy in treating some negative symptoms of schizophrenia, including flat affect, social withdrawal, and apathy (Harrison, 2015). Although cariprazine is similar to other atypical antipsychotics, its particular affinity for certain dopamine receptors (D3) is believed to be associated with its superior impact on negative symptoms, particularly improving social behavior and self-care. In addition, cariprazine has demonstrated effectiveness in reducing substance use, a common comorbidity in patients with schizophrenia, and its long half-life enables maintenance of therapeutic levels even when a few doses are missed (Scarff, 2017). Negative symptoms can complicate the prognosis in treatment of schizophrenia, and as Scarff (2017) points out, the evidence supports "cautious optimism" that cariprazine may become the first-line treatment for patients with "disabling negative symptoms or impairment in self-care and interpersonal relationships" (p. 237). As mentioned previously, an even newer medication, lumateperone (Caplyta) is also being advanced as effective for treating both positive and negative symptoms of schizophrenia, although its action is unknown.

Outcome Criteria and Evaluation

The following criteria may be used for evaluating the effectiveness of therapy with antipsychotic medications. The patient:

- Has not harmed self or others.
- Has not experienced injury caused by side effects of lowered seizure threshold or photosensitivity.
- Maintains an ANC within normal limits.
- Exhibits no symptoms of EPS, neuroleptic malignant syndrome, or hyperglycemia.
- Maintains weight within normal limits.
- Tolerates activity unaltered by the effects of sedation or weakness.
- Takes medication willingly.
- Verbalizes understanding of medication regimen and the importance of regular administration.
- Demonstrates improvement in self-care and prosocial behavior

Sedative-Hypnotics

Background Assessment Data

Indications

Sedative-hypnotics are used in the short-term management of various anxiety states and to treat insomnia. Selected agents are used as anticonvulsants (pentobarbital, phenobarbital) and preoperative sedatives (pentobarbital, secobarbital) and in the management of alcohol withdrawal.

Clinical guidelines typically recommend cognitive behavior therapy (CBT) as the first choice of treatment for insomnia, but there are currently four categories of medications approved by the FDA for this purpose (Neubauer, 2020):

- ***Benzodiazepines*** (estazolam, flurazepam, quazepam, temazepam, and triazolam) and alternative structured medications (eszopiclone, zaleplon, and zolpidem) with benzodiazepine-like properties
- ***Melatonin receptor agonists*** (ramelteon)
- ***Histamine receptor antagonist*** (low-dose doxepin)
- ***Orexin receptor antagonists*** (suvorexant and lemborexant)

Action

Sedative-hypnotics cause generalized CNS depression. They may produce tolerance with chronic use and have the potential for psychological or physical dependence. Consequently, most are schedule IV controlled substances. **EXCEPTION:** Ramelteon (Rozerem) is not a controlled substance. It does not produce tolerance or physical dependence. Sleep-promoting properties are the result of ramelteon's agonist activity on selective melatonin receptors.

Contraindications and Precautions

Sedative-hypnotics are contraindicated in individuals with hypersensitivity to the drug or to any drug within the chemical class; during pregnancy (exceptions based on benefit-to-risk ratio may be made in certain cases) and lactation; with severe hepatic, cardiac, respiratory, or renal disease; in children younger than age 15 for flurazepam and children younger than age 18 estazolam, quazepam, temazepam, triazolam. Triazolam is contraindicated with concomitant use of medications that impair the metabolism of triazolam by cytochrome P4503A (CYP3A) such as ketoconazole, itraconazole, or nefazodone. Ramelteon is contraindicated in concomitant use with fluvoxamine. Zolpidem, zaleplon, eszopiclone, and ramelteon are contraindicated in children.

Caution should be used in administering sedative-hypnotics to patients with cardiac, hepatic, renal, or respiratory insufficiency. They should be used with caution in patients who may be suicidal or who may previously have been addicted to drugs. Hypnotic

TABLE 4–13 Sedative-Hypnotic Agents

CHEMICAL CLASS	GENERIC (TRADE) NAME	CATEGORIES	DAILY DOSAGE RANGE (mg)
Barbiturates	Amobarbital	CII	60–200
	Butabarbital (Butisol)	CIII	45–120
	Pentobarbital (Nembutal)	CII	150–200
	Phenobarbital (Luminal; Solfoton)	CIV	30–200
	Secobarbital (Seconal)	CII	100 (hypnotic) 200–300 (pre-op sedation)
Benzodiazepines	Estazolam	CIV	1–2
	Flurazepam	CIV	15–30
	Quazepam (Doral)	CIV	7.5–15
	Temazepam (Restoril)	CIV	15–30
	Triazolam (Halcion)	CIV	0.125–0.5
Miscellaneous	Eszopiclone (Lunesta)	CIV	1–3
	Ramelteon (Rozerem)	N/A	8
	Zaleplon (Sonata)	CIV	5–20
	Zolpidem (Ambien)	CIV	5–10 (immediate release), 12.5 (extended release)
	Suvorexant (Belsomra)	CIV	5–20
	Lemborexant (Dayvigo)	CIV	5–10

use should be short term. Elderly clients may be more sensitive to CNS depressant effects, and dosage reduction may be required.

Interactions

- ***Barbiturates.*** The effects of barbiturates are increased with concomitant use of alcohol, other CNS depressants, MAOIs, or valproic acid. The effects of barbiturates may be decreased with rifampin. Possible decreased effects of the following drugs may occur when used concomitantly with barbiturates: anticoagulants, beta blockers, carbamazepine, clonazepam, oral contraceptives, corticosteroids, digitoxin, doxorubicin, doxycycline, felodipine, fenoprofen, griseofulvin, metronidazole, phenylbutazone, quinidine, theophylline, and verapamil. Concomitant use with methoxyflurane may enhance renal toxicity.
- ***Benzodiazepines:*** The effects of the benzodiazepine hypnotics are increased with concomitant use of alcohol or other CNS depressants, cimetidine, oral contraceptives, disulfiram, isoniazid, or probenecid. Concomitant use with opioids increases the risk of respiratory depression, coma, and death. The effects of the benzodiazepine hypnotics are decreased with concomitant use of rifampin, theophylline, carbamazepine, fluoxetine, and St. John's wort and with cigarette smoking. The effects of digoxin or phenytoin are increased when used concomitantly with benzodiazepines. There is increased bioavailability of triazolam with concomitant use of macrolides.
- ***Eszopiclone:*** Additive effects of eszopiclone occur with alcohol or other CNS depressants. Decreased effects of eszopiclone occur with CYP3A4 inducers (e.g., rifampin, phenytoin, carbamazepine, phenobarbital), with lorazepam, or following a high-fat or heavy meal. Increased effects of eszopiclone occur with CYP3A4 inhibitors (e.g., ketoconazole, clarithromycin, nefazodone, ritonavir). There are decreased effects of lorazepam with concomitant use.
- ***Zaleplon:*** Additive effects of zaleplon occur with alcohol or other CNS depressants. Decreased effects of zaleplon occur with CYP3A4 inducers (e.g., rifampin, phenytoin, carbamazepine, phenobarbital) or following a high-fat or heavy meal. There are increased effects of zaleplon with cimetidine.
- ***Zolpidem:*** Increased effects of zolpidem occur with alcohol or other CNS depressants, azole antifungals, ritonavir, or SSRIs. Decreased effects of zolpidem occur with flumazenil, rifampin, and with food. There is a risk of life-threatening cardiac arrhythmias with concomitant use of amiodarone.
- ***Ramelteon:*** Increased effects of ramelteon occur with alcohol, ketoconazole (and other CYP3A4

inhibitors), or fluvoxamine (and other CYP1A2 inhibitors). Decreased effects of ramelteon occur with rifampin (and other CYP3A4 inducers) and following a heavy or high-fat meal.

Diagnosis

The following nursing diagnoses may be considered for patients receiving therapy with sedative hypnotics:

- Risk for injury related to abrupt withdrawal from long-term use or decreased mental alertness caused by residual sedation
- Disturbed sleep pattern/insomnia related to situational crises, physical condition, or severe level of anxiety
- Risk for activity intolerance related to side effects of lethargy, drowsiness, and dizziness
- Risk for acute confusion related to action of the medication on the central nervous system

Safety Issues in Planning and Implementing Care

Refer to the earlier discussion of safety issues in the section "Antianxiety Agents." In addition to the side effects listed in that section, abnormal thinking and behavioral changes, including aggressiveness, hallucinations, and suicidal ideation, have been reported in some individuals taking sedative-hypnotics. Certain complex behaviors, such as sleep-driving, preparing and eating food, and making phone calls, with no memory of the behavior, have occurred. Although a direct correlation to the behavior with the use of sedative-hypnotics cannot be made, the emergence of any new behavioral sign or symptom of concern requires careful and immediate evaluation.

Outcome Criteria and Evaluation

The following criteria may be used for evaluating the effectiveness of therapy with sedative-hypnotic medications. The patient:

- Demonstrates a reduction in anxiety, tension, and restless activity.
- Falls asleep within 30 minutes of taking the medication and remains asleep for 6 to 8 hours without interruption.
- Is able to participate in usual activities without residual sedation.
- Experiences no physical injury.
- Exhibits no evidence of confusion.
- Verbalizes understanding of taking the medication on a short-term basis.
- Verbalizes understanding of potential for development of tolerance and dependence with long-term use.

Agents for Attention Deficit-Hyperactivity Disorder (ADHD)

Background Assessment Data

Attention deficit-hyperactivity disorder (ADHD) agents are used for treating ADHD in children and adults. They include some medications that are classified as stimulants and some that are nonstimulants.

Indications

CNS stimulants (amphetamines) are also used in the treatment of narcolepsy and exogenous obesity. Amphetamines are schedule II controlled substances indicating their high potential for abuse and dependence. Nonstimulant medications include atomoxetine and bupropion (also used in the treatment of major depression and for smoking cessation [Zyban only]) and clonidine and guanfacine (also used to treat hypertension). (A table of current FDA approved agents for ADHD, and daily dosage ranges can be found in Chapter 23, "Children and Adolescents.")

Action

CNS stimulants increase levels of neurotransmitters (probably norepinephrine, dopamine, and serotonin) in the CNS. They produce CNS and respiratory stimulation, dilated pupils, increased motor activity and mental alertness, diminished sense of fatigue, and brighter spirits. The CNS stimulants discussed in this section include dextroamphetamine sulfate, methamphetamine, lisdexamfetamine, amphetamine mixtures, methylphenidate, and dexmethylphenidate. Action in the treatment of ADHD is unclear. However, research indicates that their effectiveness in the treatment of hyperactivity disorders is based on the activation of dopamine D_4 receptors in the basal ganglia and thalamus, which depress, rather than enhance, motor activity (Erlij et al., 2012).

Atomoxetine is a nonstimulant that inhibits the reuptake of norepinephrine, and bupropion blocks the neuronal uptake of serotonin, norepinephrine, and dopamine. Clonidine and guanfacine stimulate central alpha-adrenergic receptors in the brain, resulting in reduced sympathetic outflow from the CNS. The exact mechanism by which these nonstimulant drugs produce the therapeutic effect in ADHD is unclear.

One of the most recent FDA approvals (2020) for the treatment of ADHD was not a drug but instead a novel interactive video game, EndeavorRx. Its developers identify that it directly targets neurological function and that studies support its effectiveness in improving attention (Tumolo, 2020). It requires a prescription and is currently advanced as a nondrug adjunctive treatment option.

Contraindications and Precautions

CNS stimulants are contraindicated in individuals with hypersensitivity to sympathomimetic amines. They should not be used in clients with advanced arteriosclerosis, cardiovascular disease, hypertension, hyperthyroidism, glaucoma, agitated or hyperexcitability states; or in clients with a history of drug abuse, during or within 14 days of receiving therapy with MAOIs, in children younger than 3 years of age, and in pregnancy and lactation. Atomoxetine and bupropion are contraindicated in clients with hypersensitivity to the drugs or their components, in lactation, and in concomitant use with or within 2 weeks of using MAOIs. Atomoxetine is contraindicated in clients with narrow-angle glaucoma. Bupropion is contraindicated in individuals with known or suspected seizure disorder, in the acute phase of myocardial infarction, and in clients with bulimia or anorexia nervosa. Because bupropion reduces the seizure threshold, doses should be given in equally spaced time increments during the day to minimize the risk of seizures. Risk of seizures increases fourfold in doses greater than 450 mg per day (Vallerand & Sanoski, 2021). Alpha-adrenergic agonists are contraindicated in clients with known hypersensitivity to the drugs.

Caution is advised in using CNS stimulants in children with psychosis; in clients with Tourette's disorder anorexia, or insomnia; in elderly, debilitated, or asthenic clients; and in clients with a history of suicidal or homicidal tendencies. Prolonged use may result in tolerance and physical or psychological dependence. Use atomoxetine and bupropion cautiously in clients with urinary retention; hypertension; hepatic, renal, or cardiovascular disease; in suicidal clients; in clients who are pregnant; and in elderly and debilitated clients. Alpha-adrenergic agonists should be used with caution in clients with coronary insufficiency, recent myocardial infarction, or cerebrovascular disease; in clients with chronic renal or hepatic failure; in the elderly; and during pregnancy and lactation.

Interactions

- ***CNS stimulants (amphetamines):*** Effects of amphetamines are increased with furazolidone or urinary alkalinizers. Hypertensive crisis may occur with concomitant use of (and up to several weeks after discontinuing) MAOIs. Increased risk of serotonin syndrome occurs with coadministration of SSRIs. Decreased effects of amphetamines occur with urinary acidifiers, and decreased hypotensive effects of guanethidine occur with amphetamines.
- ***Dexmethylphenidate and methylphenidate:*** Effects of antihypertensive agents and pressor agents (e.g., dopamine, epinephrine, phenylephrine) are decreased with concomitant use of the methylphenidates. Effects of coumarin anticoagulants, anticonvulsants (e.g., phenobarbital, phenytoin, primidone), TCAs, and SSRIs are increased with the methylphenidates. Hypertensive crisis may occur with coadministration of MAOIs.
- ***Atomoxetine:*** Effects of atomoxetine are increased with concomitant use of CYP2D6 inhibitors (e.g., paroxetine, fluoxetine, quinidine). Potentially fatal reactions may occur with concomitant use of (or within 2 weeks of discontinuation of) MAOIs. Risk of cardiovascular effects is increased with concomitant use of albuterol or vasopressors.
- ***Bupropion:*** Effects of bupropion are increased with amantadine, levodopa, or ritonavir. Effects of bupropion are decreased with carbamazepine. There is increased risk of acute toxicity with MAOIs. Increased risk of hypertension may occur with nicotine replacement agents, and adverse neuropsychiatric events may occur with alcohol. Increased anticoagulant effects of warfarin, as well as increased effects of drugs metabolized by CYP2D6 (e.g., nortriptyline, imipramine, desipramine, paroxetine, fluoxetine, sertraline, haloperidol, risperidone, thioridazine, metoprolol, propafenone, and flecainide), occur with concomitant use.
- ***Alpha-adrenergic agonists:*** Synergistic pharmacologic and toxic effects, possibly causing atrioventricular block, bradycardia, and severe hypotension, may occur with concomitant use of calcium channel blockers or beta blockers. Additive sedation occurs with CNS depressants, including alcohol, antihistamines, opioid analgesics, and sedative-hypnotics. Effects of clonidine may be decreased with concomitant use of tricyclic antidepressants and prazosin. Decreased effects of levodopa may occur with clonidine, and effects of guanfacine are decreased with barbiturates or phenytoin.

Diagnosis

The following nursing diagnoses may be considered for patients receiving therapy with agents for ADHD:

- Risk for injury related to overstimulation and hyperactivity (CNS stimulants) or seizures (possible side effect of bupropion)
- Risk for suicide secondary to major depression related to abrupt withdrawal after extended use (CNS stimulants)
- Risk for suicide (children and adolescents) as a side effect of atomoxetine and bupropion (black box warning)
- Imbalanced nutrition, less than body requirements, related to side effects of anorexia and weight loss (CNS stimulants)
- Insomnia related to side effects of overstimulation
- Nausea related to side effects of atomoxetine or bupropion
- Pain related to side effect of abdominal pain (atomoxetine, bupropion) or headache (all agents)
- Risk for activity intolerance related to side effects of sedation and dizziness with atomoxetine or bupropion

Safety Issues in Planning and Implementing Care

The plan of care should include monitoring for the following side effects from agents for ADHD. Relevant nursing interventions related to each side effect are designated by an asterisk (*).

- ***Overstimulation, restlessness, insomnia*** (CNS stimulants)
  - Assess mental status for changes in mood, level of activity, degree of stimulation, and aggressiveness.
  - Ensure that the patient is protected from injury.
  - Keep stimuli low and environment as quiet as possible to discourage overstimulation.
  - To prevent insomnia, administer the last dose at least 6 hours before bedtime. Administer sustained-release forms in the morning.
- ***Palpitations, tachycardia*** (CNS stimulants, atomoxetine, bupropion, clonidine), or bradycardia (clonidine, guanfacine)
  - Monitor and record vital signs at regular intervals (two or three times a day) throughout therapy. Report significant changes to the physician immediately.

  NOTE: The FDA has issued warnings associated with CNS stimulants and atomoxetine of the risk for sudden death in patients who have cardiovascular disease. A careful personal and family history of heart disease, heart defects, or hypertension should be obtained before these medications are prescribed. Careful monitoring of cardiovascular function during administration must be ongoing.
- ***Anorexia, weight loss*** (CNS stimulants, atomoxetine, bupropion)
  - To reduce anorexia, the medication may be administered immediately after meals. The patient should be weighed regularly (at least weekly) when receiving therapy with CNS stimulants, atomoxetine, or bupropion because of the potential for anorexia and weight loss and temporary interruption of growth and development.
- ***Tolerance, physical and psychological dependence*** (CNS stimulants)
  - In children with ADHD, a drug "holiday" should be attempted periodically under direction of the physician to determine the effectiveness of the medication and the need for continuation.
  - The drug should not be withdrawn abruptly. To do so could initiate the following syndrome of symptoms: nausea, vomiting, abdominal cramping, headache, fatigue, weakness, mental depression, suicidal ideation, increased dreaming, and psychotic behavior.
- ***Nausea and vomiting*** (atomoxetine and bupropion)
  - Recommend taking with food to minimize gastrointestinal (GI) upset.
- ***Constipation*** (atomoxetine, bupropion, clonidine, guanfacine)
  - Recommend increasing fiber and fluid in diet if not contraindicated.
- ***Dry mouth*** (clonidine and guanfacine)
  - Offer sugarless candy, ice, frequent sips of water.
  - Instruct about the importance of strict oral hygiene.
- ***Sedation*** (clonidine and guanfacine)
  - Warn the patient that this effect is increased by concomitant use of alcohol and other CNS drugs.
  - Warn the patient to refrain from driving or performing hazardous tasks until response has been established.
- ***Potential for seizures*** (bupropion)
  - Protect the patient from injury if seizure should occur. Instruct family and significant others of patients on bupropion therapy how to protect the patient during a seizure if one should occur.
  - Ensure that doses of the immediate-release medication are administered at least 4 to 6 hours apart and doses of the sustained-release medication are administered at least 8 hours apart.

- ***Severe liver damage*** (with atomoxetine)
  - Monitor for the following side effects and report to physician immediately: itching, dark urine, right upper quadrant pain, yellow skin or eyes, sore throat, fever, malaise.
- ***New or worsened psychiatric symptoms*** (with CNS stimulants and atomoxetine)
  - Monitor for psychotic symptoms (e.g., hearing voices, paranoid behaviors, delusions).
  - Monitor for manic symptoms, including aggressive and hostile behaviors.
- ***Rebound syndrome*** (with clonidine and guanfacine)
  - The patient should be instructed not to discontinue therapy abruptly. To do so may result in symptoms of nervousness, agitation, headache, and tremor, and a rapid rise in blood pressure. Dosage should be tapered gradually under the supervision of the physician.
  - Assess the patient for signs of depression and risk for suicide since abrupt withdrawal increases these risks.

Patient and Family Education

Instruct the patient and family that the patient should:

- Use caution while driving or operating dangerous machinery. Drowsiness, dizziness, and blurred vision can occur.
- Not stop taking CNS stimulants abruptly. To do so could produce serious withdrawal symptoms.
- Avoid taking CNS stimulants late in the day to prevent insomnia. Take no later than 6 hours before bedtime.
- Not take other medications (including over-the-counter drugs) without physician's approval. Many medications contain substances that, in combination with agents for ADHD, can be harmful.
- Monitor blood sugar two or three times a day or as instructed by the physician if the patient is diabetic. Be aware of the need for possible alteration in insulin requirements because of changes in food intake, weight, and activity.
- Avoid consumption of large amounts of caffeinated products (coffee, tea, colas, chocolate), as they may enhance the CNS stimulant effect.
- Notify the physician if restlessness, insomnia, anorexia, or dry mouth becomes severe or if rapid, pounding heartbeat becomes evident.
- Report any of the following side effects to the physician immediately: shortness of breath, chest pain, jaw/left arm pain, fainting, seizures, sudden vision changes, weakness on one side of the body, slurred speech, confusion, itching, dark urine, right upper quadrant pain, yellow skin or eyes, sore throat, fever, malaise, increased hyperactivity, believing things that are not true, or hearing voices.
- Be aware of possible risks of taking agents for ADHD during pregnancy. Safe use during pregnancy and lactation has not been established. Inform the physician immediately if pregnancy is suspected or planned.
- Be aware of potential side effects of agents for ADHD. Refer to written materials furnished by health-care providers for safe self-administration.
- Carry a card or other identification at all times describing medications being taken.

Outcome Criteria and Evaluation

The following criteria may be used for evaluating the effectiveness of therapy with agents for ADHD. The patient:

- Does not exhibit excessive hyperactivity.
- Has not experienced injury.
- Is maintaining expected parameters of growth and development.
- Verbalizes understanding of safe self- administration and the importance of not withdrawing medication abruptly.

Summary and Key Points

- Psychotropic medications are intended to be used as adjunctive therapy to individual or group psychotherapy.
- *Antianxiety agents* are used in the treatment of anxiety disorders and to alleviate acute anxiety symptoms. The benzodiazepines are the most commonly used group. They are central nervous system (CNS) depressants and have a potential for physical and psychological dependence. They should not be discontinued abruptly following long-term use because they can produce a life-threatening withdrawal syndrome. The most common side effects are drowsiness, confusion, and lethargy.
- *Antidepressants* elevate mood and alleviate other symptoms associated with moderate-to-severe depression. These drugs are believed to work by increasing the concentration of norepinephrine and serotonin in the body.
- The tricyclics and related drugs accomplish this action by blocking the reuptake of these chemicals by the neurons.

- Another group of antidepressants inhibits monoamine oxidase (MAO), an enzyme that is known to inactivate norepinephrine and serotonin. They are called MAO inhibitors (MAOIs).
- A third category of drugs blocks neuronal reuptake of serotonin and has minimal or no effect on reuptake of norepinephrine or dopamine. They are called selective serotonin reuptake inhibitors (SSRIs).
- SNRIs are antidepressant medications that block reuptake of serotonin and norepinephrine.
- Antidepressant medications may take up to 2 weeks before desired effects are noticed and up to 4 weeks to achieve full therapeutic benefits. The most common side effects are anticholinergic effects, sedation, and orthostatic hypotension. They can also reduce the seizure threshold.
- MAOIs can cause hypertensive crisis if products containing tyramine are consumed while taking these medications.
- Lithium carbonate is widely used as a *mood-stabilizing agent.* Its mechanism of action is not fully understood, but it is thought to enhance the reuptake of norepinephrine and serotonin in the brain, thereby lowering the levels in the body, resulting in decreased hyperactivity. The most common side effects are dry mouth, gastrointestinal (GI) upset, polyuria, and weight gain. There is a very narrow margin between the therapeutic and toxic levels of lithium. Serum levels must be drawn regularly to monitor for toxicity. An accepted therapeutic range is 0.6 to 1.2 mEq/L.
- Symptoms of lithium toxicity are most noticeable at or above 1.5 mEq/L. If left untreated, lithium toxicity can be life threatening.
- Several other medications are used as mood-stabilizing agents. Two groups, anticonvulsants (carbamazepine, clonazepam, valproic acid, lamotrigine, oxcarbazepine, and topiramate) and the calcium channel blocker verapamil, have been used with some effectiveness. Their action in the treatment of bipolar mania is unknown.
- More recently, a number of atypical antipsychotic medications have been used with success in the treatment of bipolar mania. These include olanzapine, aripiprazole, quetiapine, risperidone, asenapine, and ziprasidone. The phenothiazine chlorpromazine has also been used effectively. The action of antipsychotics in the treatment of bipolar mania is not understood.
- *Antipsychotic drugs* are primarliy used in the treatment of acute and chronic psychoses. The action of first generation (or typical) medications, such as the phenothiazines, is caused by blocking postsynaptic dopamine receptors in the basal ganglia. Their most common side effects include anticholinergic effects, sedation, weight gain, reduction in seizure threshold, photosensitivity, and extrapyramidal symptoms.
- Atypical antipsychotic medications, which include clozapine, risperidone, paliperidone, olanzapine, quetiapine, aripiprazole, asenapine, iloperidone, lurasidone, and ziprasidone, may have an effect on dopamine, serotonin, and other neurotransmitters. They show evidence of greater efficacy with fewer extrapyramidal symptoms (EPS) but have been associated with increased risk for metabolic disturbances and weight gain.
- *Antiparkinsonian agents* are used to counteract the EPS associated with antipsychotic medications. Antiparkinsonian drugs work to restore the natural balance of acetylcholine and dopamine in the brain. The most common side effects of these drugs are the anticholinergic effects. They may also cause sedation and orthostatic hypotension.
- Agents for the treatment of tardive dyskinesia are used to reduce movement disturbances associated with antipsychotic medications. Their action is unknown but believed to be associated with inhibition of monoamine transport. Valbenazine (Ingrezza) and deutetrabenazine (Austedo) were both approved by the FDA for this indication in 2017.
- *Sedative-hypnotics* are used in the management of anxiety states and to treat insomnia. These CNS depressants have the potential for physical and psychological dependence (with the exception of ramelteon). They are indicated for short-term use only. Side effects and nursing implications are similar to those described for antianxiety medications.
- Several medications have been designated as *agents for treatment of attention deficit-hyperactivity disorder (ADHD).* These include CNS stimulants, which have the potential for physical and psychological dependence. Tolerance develops quickly with CNS stimulants, and they should not be withdrawn abruptly because they can produce serious withdrawal symptoms. The most common side effects are restlessness, anorexia, and insomnia. Other medications that have shown to be effective with ADHD include atomoxetine, bupropion, and the alpha-adrenergic agonists clonidine and guanfacine. Their mechanism of action in the treatment of ADHD is not clear.

Review Questions

Select the answer that is most appropriate for each of the following questions:

1. How do antianxiety medications, such as benzodiazepines, produce a calming effect?
   a. Depressing the CNS
   b. Decreasing levels of norepinephrine and serotonin in the brain
   c. Decreasing levels of dopamine in the brain
   d. Inhibiting production of the enzyme MAO
2. There is a narrow margin between the therapeutic and toxic levels of lithium carbonate. Symptoms of toxicity are most likely to appear when the serum levels exceed:
   a. 0.15 mEq/L
   b. 1.5 mEq/L
   c. 15.0 mEq/L
   d. 150 mEq/L
3. Initial symptoms of lithium toxicity include:
   a. Constipation, dry mouth
   b. Dizziness, thirst
   c. Vomiting, diarrhea
   d. Anuria, arrhythmias
4. Antipsychotic medications are thought to decrease psychotic symptoms by:
   a. Blocking reuptake of norepinephrine and serotonin
   b. Blocking the action of dopamine in the brain
   c. Inhibiting production of the enzyme MAO
   d. Depressing the CNS
5. Part of the nurse's ongoing assessment of the client taking antipsychotic medications is to observe for extrapyramidal symptoms. Which of the following are examples of extrapyramidal symptoms?
   a. Muscular weakness, rigidity, tremors, facial spasms
   b. Dry mouth, blurred vision, urinary retention, orthostatic hypotension
   c. Amenorrhea, gynecomastia, retrograde ejaculation
   d. Elevated blood pressure, severe occipital headache, stiff neck

Clinical Judgment Questions

6. A client who is prescribed haloperidol is observed to be staring at the ceiling and says they cannot move their eyes. The nurse notices that the client also appears to have muscle spasms in their legs and hands. What is the most appropriate action for the nurse to take at this point?
   a. Conduct an AIMS test.
   b. Administer prn benztropine (Cogentin).
   c. Withhold the next dose of antipsychotic medication.
   d. Contact the physician.
7. A client reports to the nurse that, after having been on their antidepressant medication (fluoxetine) for almost 2 weeks, they don't feel much better. Which of these actions by the nurse demonstrates the best clinical judgment?
   a. Educate the client that this medication may not be fully effective for up to 4 weeks.
   b. Hold the next dose and contact the physician to recommend an alternative antidepressant.
   c. Check the client's vital signs and check labs for therapeutic blood levels.
   d. Assess whether the client is aware of mood swings or history of bipolar disorder in their family.

8. A client who was recently prescribed an MAOI tells the nurse that they drink 3 to 4 cups of coffee with each meal. Which of these actions by the nurse demonstrates the best clinical judgment?
   a. Instruct the client that they only need to avoid foods high in tyramine; coffee consumption is not an issue with this medication.
   b. Inform the client that foods or beverages with high caffeine content increase the risk for serious hypertension and arrhythmias.
   c. Inform the client that caffeine interferes with the effectiveness of this medication.
   d. Instruct the client that red wines are a better beverage choice because they do not contain tyramine.
9. A young adult client has been prescribed an SSRI antidepressant, which they have been taking for 1 week. The client reports that they feel that they are getting worse and that nothing is going to help. Which of these actions by the nurse is a priority?
   a. Educate the client that SSRIs have a lag period before full therapeutic effectiveness is apparent.
   b. Ask the client to describe why they think they are depressed.
   c. Contact the physician to recommend a different medication.
   d. Conduct a suicide risk assessment.
10. A licensed practical nurse who is administering medications reports to the RN in charge that he forgot to give the last scheduled dose of bupropion to a client. He asks the RN if he should give the client two doses at the next scheduled time. Which of these responses by the nurse demonstrates the best clinical judgment?
   a. "Yes, that would be fine. Just make sure the client stays in bed since this is a sedating medication."
   b. "No. Doses of this medication should not be doubled since that poses an increased risk for seizures."
   c. "Yes, as long as the client has not changed their sodium intake recently."
   d. "No, doses should not be doubled because there is an increased risk of tolerance and addiction."

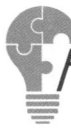

Go to **Davis Advantage** to complete your learning: strengthen understanding, apply your knowledge, and prepare for the Next Gen NCLEX®.

References

Anderson, L. (2018). *Drug interactions with grapefruit juice.* https://www.drugs.com/article/grapefruitdrug-interactions.html

Aiken, C. (2020). Novel approaches to bipolar: What worked, and what did not, in 2019. *Psychiatric Times.* https://www.psychiatrictimes.com/view/novel-approaches-bipolar-what-worked-and-what-did-not-2019

Babu, G. N., Desai, G., & Chandra, P. S. (2015). Antipsychotics in pregnancy and lactation. *Indian Journal of Psychiatry, 57*(Suppl 2), S303–S307. https://doi.org/10.4103/0019-5545.161497

Berna, F., Misdrahi, D., Boyer, L., Aouizerate, B., Brunel, L., Capdevielle, D., & Liorca, P. M. (2015). Prevalence and risk factors in a community dwelling sample of patients with schizophrenia. Results from the FACE-SZ dataset. *Schizophrenia Research, 169*(1-3), 255–261.

Boland, R., & Verduin, M. L. (2022). *Kaplan & Sadock's synopsis of psychiatry* (P. Ruiz, Ed.). (12th ed.). Wolters Kluwer.

Brust, T. F., Hayes, M. P., Roman, D. L., & Watts, V. J. (2015). New functional activity of aripiprazole revealed: Robust antagonism of D2 dopamine receptor-stimulated Gβγ signaling. *Biochemical Pharmacology, 93*(1), 85–91. https://doi.org/10.1016/j.bcp.2014 10.014

Clozapine REMS. (2015). *Clozapine and the risk of neutropenia: A guide for healthcare providers.* https://www.clozapinerems.com/CpmgClozapineUI/rems/pdf/resources/Clozapine_REMS_HCP_Guide.pdf

Cooper, B. E., & Sejnowski, C. A. (2013). Serotonin syndrome: Recognition and treatment. *AACN Advanced Critical Care, 24*(1), 15–20.

Drugs.com. (2020). *FDA pregnancy categories: FDA pregnancy risk information: An update.* https://www.drugs.com/pregnancy-categories.html

Erlij, D., Acosta-Garcia, J., Rojas-Marquez, M., Gonzalez-Hernandez, B., Escartin-Perez, E., Aceves, J., & Floran, B.

(2012). Dopamine D_4 receptor stimulation in GABAergic projections of the globus pallidus to the reticular thalamic nucleus and the substantia nigra reticulate of the rat decreases locomotor activity. *Neuropharmacology, 62*(2), 1111–1118.

Fournier, J. C., DeRubeis, R. J., Hollon, S. D., Dimidjian, S., Amsterdam, J. D., Shelton, R. C., & Fawcett, J. (2010). Antidepressant drug effects and depression severity: A patient-level meta-analysis. *Journal of the American Medical Association, 303*(1), 47–53. https://doi.org/10.1001/jama.2009.1943

Gareri, P., Segura-García, C., Manfredi, V. G., Bruni, A., Ciambrone, P., Cerminara, G., De Sarro, G., & De Fazio, P. (2014). Use of atypical antipsychotics in the elderly: A clinical review. *Clinical Interventions in Aging, 9*, 1363–1373. https://doi.org/10.2147/CIA.S63942

Gunduz-Bruce, H., Silber, C., Kaul, I., Rothschild. A. J., Riesenberg, R., Sankoh, A. J., Li, H., Lasser, R., Zorumski, C. F., Rubinow, D. R., Paul, S. M., Jonas, J., Doherty, J. J., & Kanes, S. J. (2019). Trial of SAGE-217 in patients with major depressive disorder. *New England Journal of Medicine, 381*(10), 903–911. https://doi.org/10.1056/NEJMoa1815981

Haddad, P. M., Brain, C., & Scott, J. (2014). Nonadherence with antipsychotic medication in schizophrenia: Challenges and management strategies. *Patient Related Outcome Measures*, 5, 43–62. http://www.ncbi.nlm.nih.gov/pmc/articles/PMC4085309/

Harrison, P. (2015). Novel drug first to treat negative symptoms in schizophrenia. *Medscape.* www.medscape.com/viewarticle/850701

Horn, J. R., & Hansten, P. D. (2008). Get to know an enzyme: CYP2C19. *Pharmacy Times.* https://www.pharmacytimes.com/publications/issue/2008/2008-05/2008-05-8538

Institute of Medicine. (2003). *Health professions education: A bridge to quality.*

Janicak, P. G., & Hussain, K. (2017). Medication induced movement disorders. In B. J. Sadock, V. A. Sadock, & P. Ruiz (Eds.), *Comprehensive textbook of psychiatry* (10th ed., pp. 2936–2944). Wolters Kluwer.

Jones, D. S. (2006). Racial profiling in psychiatry: Does it help patients? *Psychiatric Times, 23*(4).

Köhler-Forsberg, O., N. Lydholm, C., Hjorthøj, C., Nordentoft, M., Mors, O., Benros, M.E. (2019). Efficacy of anti-inflammatory treatment on major depressive disorder or depressive symptoms: meta-analysis of clinical trials. *Acta Psychiatrica Scandinavica, 139*(5), 404–419. https://doi.org/10.1111/acps.13016.

Kose, S., & Cetin, M. (2018). Triple reuptake inhibitors (TRIs): Do they promise us a rose garden? *Psychiatry and Clinical Pharmacology, 28*(2), 119—122. https://doi.org/10.1080/24750573. 2018.1443386

Lenze, E. J., Mulsant, B. H., Blumberger, D. M., Karp, J. F., Newcomer, J. W., Anderson, S. J., & Reynolds, C. F. (2015). Efficacy, safety, and tolerability of augmentation pharmacotherapy with aripiprazole for treatment resistant depression in late life: A randomized placebo-controlled study. *Lancet, 386*(10011), 2404–2412.

Li, K., Shen, S., Ji, Y. T., Li, X. Y., Zhang, L., & Wang, X. D. (2018). Melatonin BDNF-TrkB signaling. *Neuroscience Bulletin, 34*(2), 303–311. https://doi.org/10.1007/s12264-017-019-z

Lien, Y. H. H. (2018). Antidepressants and hyponatremia. *American Journal of Medicine, 131*(1), 7–8. https://doi.org/10.1016/j.amjmed.2017.09.002

Lynch, T., & Price, A. (2007). The effect of cytochrome P450 metabolism on drug response, interactions, and adverse effects. *American Family Physician, 76*(3), 391–396.

Maust, D. T., Kales, H. C., Weichers, I. R., Blow, F. C., & Olfson, M. (2016). No end in sight: Benzodiazepine use among older adults in the United States. *Journal of the American Geriatric Society, 64*(12), 2546–2553. https://doi.org/10.1111/jgs.14379

Miklowitz, D. J., Efthimiou, O., Furukawa, T. A., Scott, J., McLaren, R., Geddes, J. R., & Cipriani, A. (2020). Adjunctive psychotherapy for bipolar disorder: A systematic review and component network meta-analysis. *JAMA Psychiatry, 78*(2), 141–150. https://doi.org/10.1001/jamapsychiatry.2020.2993

Muttoni, S., Ardissino, M., & John, C. (2019). Classical psychedelics for the treatment of depression and anxiety: A systematic review. *Journal of Affective Disorders*, 258, 11–24. https://doi.org/10.1016/j.jad.2019.07.076

Neubauer, D. N. (2020). Lemborexant for insomnia. *Current Psychiatry, 19*(11), 43–49.

New York State Office of Mental Health. (2012). An explanation of Kendra's law. www.omh.ny.gov/omhweb/Kendra_web/Ksummary.htm

Nolen, W. A., Licht, R. W., Young, A. H., Malhi, G. S., Tohen, M., Vieta, E., Kupka, R. W., Zarate, C., Nielsen, R. E., Baldessarini, R. J., Severus, E., & ISBD/IGSLI Task Force on the Treatment with Lithium. (2019). What is the optimal serum level for lithium in the maintenance treatment of bipolar disorder? A systematic review and recommendations from the ISBD/IGSLI Task Force on treatment with lithium. *Bipolar Disorders, 21*(5), 394–409. https://doi.org/10.1111/bdi.12805

Olfson, M., King, M., & Schoenbaum, M. (2015). Benzodiazepine use in the United States. *JAMA Psychiatry, 72*(2), 136–142. https://doi.org/10.1001/jamapsychiatry.2014.1763

Ramnarine, M. (2020). Anticholinergic toxicity. *Medscape.* emedicine.medscape.com/article/812644-overview

Rege, S. (2020). Lithium prescribing and monitoring in clinical practice – A practical guide. *Psychscenehub.* https://psychscenehub.com/psychinsights/lithium-prescribing-monitoring-clinical-practice/#:~:text=CLINICAL

Remaly, J. (2020). FDA approves diazepam nasal spray for seizure clusters. *Neurology Reviews.* https://www.mdedge.com/neurology/article/215442/epilepsy-seizures/fda-approves-diazepam-nasal-spray-seizure-clusters

Sage, D. L. (Producer). (1984). *The brain: Madness.* Public Broadcasting Company.

Scarff, J. R. (2017). The prospects of cariprazine in the treatment of schizophrenia. *Therapeutic Advances in Psychopharmacology, 7*(11), 237–239. doi:10.1177/2045125317727260

Shorter, E. (2009). The history of lithium therapy. *Bipolar Disorders, 11*(2), 4–9. https://doi.org/10.1111/j.1399-5618.2009.00706.x

Tartakovsky, M. (2016). *Depression: New medications on the horizon.* https://psychcentral.com/lib/depressionnew-medications-on-the-horizon/

Tumolo, J. (2020). FDA clears video game as treatment for ADHD. *Psych Congress Network.* https://www.psychcongress.com/article/fda-clears-video-game-treatment-adhd?hmpid=

U.S. Department of Justice. (n.d.). *Controlled substance schedules.* https://www.deadiversion.usdoj.gov/schedules/#:~:text=Definition%

U.S. Food and Drug Administration. (2008). *FDA requires warnings about risk of suicidal thoughts and behavior for antiepileptic medications.* http://www.fda.gov/Drugs/DrugSafety/PostmarketDrugSafetyInformationforPatientsandProviders/ucm100197.htm

U.S. Food and Drug Administration. (2016a). *FDA Drug Safety Communication: FDA warns about serious risks and death when combining opioid pain or cough medicines with benzodiazepines; requires its strongest warning.* http://www.fda.gov/Drugs/DrugSafety/ucm518473.htm

U.S. Food and Drug Administration. (2016b). *FDA Drug Safety Communication: FDA warns about rare but serious skin reactions with mental health drug olanzapine (Zyprexa, Zyprexa Zydis, Zyprexa Relprevv, and Symbyax).* https://www.fda.gov/Drugs/DrugSafety/ucm499441.htm

U.S. Food and Drug Administration. (2016c). *FDA Drug Safety Communication: FDA warns about new impulse-control problems associated with mental health drug aripiprazole (Abilify, Abilify Maintena, Aristada).* https://www.fda.gov/Drugs/DrugSafety/ucm498662.htm

U.S. Food and Drug Administration. (2017). *FDA approves first drug to treat tardive dyskinesia.* https://www.fda.gov/NewsEvents/Newsroom/PressAnnouncements/ucm552418.htm

U.S. Food and Drug Administration. (2019). *FDA approves new nasal spray medication for treatment-resistant depression; available only at a certified doctor's office or clinic [Press Release].* https://www.fda.gov/news-events/pressannouncements/fda-approves-new-nasal-spray-medicationtreatment-resistant-depression-available-only-certified

U.S. Food and Drug Administration. (2020). *FDA strengthens warning that untreated constipation caused by schizophrenia medicine clozapine (Clozaril) can lead to serious bowel problems.* https://www.fda.gov/drugs/fda-drug-safety-podcasts/fda-strengthens-warning-untreated-constipation-caused-schizophrenia-medicine-clozapine-clozaril-can#:~:text=

Vallerand, A. H., & Sanoski, C. A. (2021). *Davis drug guide for nurses* (17th ed.). F.A. Davis.

WebMD. (2019). *Melatonin.* https://www.webmd.com/vitamins/ai/ingredientmono-940/melatonin

UNIT 2

Psychiatric Mental Health Nursing Interventions

5 Relationship Development and Therapeutic Communication

CORE CONCEPTS

Communication: Therapeutic communication

Caring: Therapeutic relationship

Clinical Judgment

CHAPTER OUTLINE

Objectives
Introduction
The Therapeutic Nurse-Patient Relationship
Conditions Essential to Development of a Therapeutic Relationship
Phases of a Therapeutic Nurse-Patient Relationship
Boundaries in the Nurse-Patient Relationship
Interpersonal Communication
Therapeutic Communication Techniques
Nontherapeutic Communication Techniques
Active Listening
Process Recordings
Feedback
Summary and Key Points
Review Questions
Clinical Judgment Questions

KEY TERMS

concrete thinking
confidentiality
countertransference
density
empathy
genuineness
intimate distance
material boundaries
motivational interviewing
paralanguage
personal boundaries
personal distance
professional boundaries
public distance
rapport
social boundaries
social distance
sympathy
territoriality
transference
unconditional positive regard

OBJECTIVES

After reading this chapter, the student will be able to:

1. Describe the relevance and dynamics of a therapeutic nurse-patient relationship.
2. Identify types of pre-existing conditions that influence the outcome of the communication process.
3. Define *territoriality, density*, and *distance* as components of the environment.
4. Identify components of nonverbal expression.
5. Describe therapeutic and nontherapeutic verbal communication techniques.
6. Describe motivational interviewing as a communication strategy.
7. Describe active listening.
8. Discuss therapeutic feedback.
9. Identify and discuss essential conditions for a therapeutic relationship to occur.
10. Describe the phases of relationship development and the tasks associated with each phase.

Introduction

The nurse-patient relationship is the foundation on which psychiatric nursing is established. It is a relationship in which both participants must recognize each other as unique and important human beings. It is also a relationship in which mutual learning occurs. In today's health-care environment, patient-centered care is being promoted as central to quality and safety, and the therapeutic relationship remains at the foundation. Concepts that were developed over 50 years ago (Peplau, 1952) and have been the core of nursing practice to the present day are now being recognized by the larger medical community as not only still relevant but also critical to improving quality and safety in the future of health care. Peplau (1991) describes the foundation for therapeutic relationship development (and the accomplishment of nursing care) as follows:

> Shall a nurse do things *for* a patient or can participant relationships be emphasized so that a nurse comes to do things *with* a patient as her share of an agenda of work to be accomplished in reaching a goal—health. *It is likely that the nursing process is educative and therapeutic when nurse and patient can come to know and to respect each other, as persons who are alike, and yet, different, as persons who share in the solution of problems.* (p. 9)

Hays and Larson (1963) add that a therapeutic relationship requires the nurse's understanding of their role and its relationship to the patient's illness. They describe the role of the nurse as providing the patient with the opportunity to

- Identify and explore problems in relating to others.
- Discover healthy ways of meeting emotional needs.
- Experience a satisfying interpersonal relationship.

The *therapeutic interpersonal relationship* is the process by which nurses provide care for patients in need of psychosocial intervention. *Therapeutic use of self* is the instrument for delivery of that care. *Interpersonal communication techniques* (both verbal and nonverbal) are the "tools" of psychosocial intervention.

This chapter describes the phases of development of a therapeutic nurse-patient relationship. Therapeutic use of self and techniques of interpersonal communication are discussed.

CORE CONCEPT

Therapeutic relationship

An interaction between two people (usually a caregiver and a care receiver) in which input from both participants contributes to a climate of healing, growth promotion, and/or illness prevention.

The Therapeutic Nurse-Patient Relationship

Travelbee (1971), who expanded on Peplau's theory of interpersonal relations in nursing, stated that it is only when each individual in the interaction perceives the other as a human being that a relationship is possible. She refers not to a nurse-patient relationship but to a human-to-human relationship, which she describes as a "mutually significant experience." That is, both the nurse and the recipient of care have needs met when each views the other as a unique human being, not as "an illness," "a room number," or "all nurses" in general.

Therapeutic relationships are goal oriented. Ideally, the nurse and patient decide together what the goal of the relationship will be. Most often, the goal is directed at learning and growth promotion in an effort to bring about some type of change in the patient's life. In general, the goal of a therapeutic relationship may be based on a problem-solving model.

EXAMPLE

Goal

The patient will demonstrate more adaptive coping strategies for dealing with (specific life situation).

Intervention

- Identify what is troubling the patient at this time.
- Encourage the patient to discuss changes the patient would like to make.
- Discuss with the patient which changes are possible and which are not possible.
- Have the patient explore feelings about aspects that cannot be changed and alternative ways of coping more adaptively.
- Discuss alternative strategies for creating changes the patient desires to make.
- Weigh the benefits and consequences of each alternative.
- Assist the patient to select an alternative.
- Encourage the patient to implement the change.
- Provide positive feedback for the patient's attempts to create change.
- Assist the patient to evaluate outcomes of the change and make modifications as required.

Therapeutic Use of Self

Travelbee (1971) described the instrument for delivery of the process of interpersonal nursing as the *therapeutic use of self*, which she defined as "the ability to use one's personality consciously and in full awareness in an attempt to establish relatedness and to structure nursing interventions" (p. 19).

Use of the self in a therapeutic manner requires that the nurse have a great deal of self-awareness and self-understanding, having arrived at a philosophical belief about life, death, and the overall human condition. The nurse must understand that the ability to, and the extent to which one can, effectively help others in time of need is strongly influenced by this internal value system—a combination of intellect and emotions.

Conditions Essential to Development of a Therapeutic Relationship

Several characteristics that enhance the achievement of a therapeutic relationship have been identified. These concepts are highly significant to the use of self as the therapeutic tool in interpersonal relationship development.

Rapport

Getting acquainted and establishing rapport are the primary tasks in relationship development. **Rapport** implies special feelings on the part of both the patient and the nurse based on acceptance, warmth, friendliness, common interest, a sense of trust, and a nonjudgmental attitude. Establishing rapport may be accomplished by discussing non–health-related topics. Travelbee (1971) states,

> [To establish rapport] is to create a sense of harmony based on knowledge and appreciation of each individual's uniqueness. It is the ability to be still and experience the other as a human being—to appreciate the unfolding of each personality one to the other. The ability to truly care for and about others is the core of rapport. (pp. 152, 155)

Trust

To trust another, one must feel confidence in that person's presence, reliability, integrity, veracity, and sincere desire to provide assistance when requested. As discussed in Chapter 29, "Concepts of Personality Development," available online at fadavis.com, trust is the initial developmental task described by Erikson. If the task has not been achieved, this component of relationship development becomes more difficult. That is not to say that trust cannot be established but only that additional time and patience may be required on the part of the nurse.

Trust cannot be presumed; it must be earned. Trustworthiness is demonstrated through nursing interventions that convey a sense of warmth and caring to the patient. These interventions are initiated simply and concretely and are directed toward activities that address the patient's basic needs for physiological and psychological safety and security. Psychiatric patients with thought disorders, such as schizophrenia, may also have difficulty thinking abstractly (a symptom called **concrete thinking**) so it becomes even more important that the nurse communicate and behave in a simple, concrete manner to promote the development of trust. Examples of nursing interventions that would promote trust in an individual who is thinking concretely include the following:

- Providing a blanket when the patient is cold
- Providing food when the patient is hungry
- Keeping promises
- Being honest (e.g., saying, "I don't know the answer to your question, but I'll try to find out") and then following through
- Simply and clearly providing reasons for certain policies, procedures, and rules
- Providing a written, structured schedule of activities
- Attending activities with the patient who is reluctant to go alone
- Being consistent in adhering to unit guidelines
- Listening to the patient's preferences, requests, and opinions and making collaborative decisions concerning care
- Ensuring **confidentiality;** providing reassurance that what is discussed will not be repeated outside the boundaries of the health-care team

Trust is the basis of a therapeutic relationship. The nurse working in psychiatry must perfect the skills that foster the development of trust. Trust must be established in order for the nurse-patient relationship to progress beyond the superficial level of tending to the patient's immediate needs.

Real Nurses, Real Advice

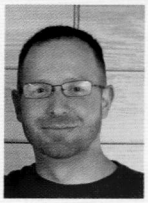

"Many patients admitted to inpatient psychiatric settings are there involuntarily so establishing trust can sometimes be a challenge. Truthfulness, honesty, and genuineness are the best ways to earn a patient's trust. Trust is essential for earning the patient's respect and growing your nurse-patient relationship."

—**Matt Mangus,** RN, BSN

Respect

To show respect is to believe in the dignity and worth of an individual regardless of unacceptable behavior. The psychologist Carl Rogers called this **unconditional positive regard** (Raskin et al., 2014). The attitude is nonjudgmental, and the respect is unconditional in that it does not depend on the behavior of the patient to meet certain standards. The nurse, in fact, may not approve of the patient's lifestyle or pattern of behaving. However, with unconditional positive regard, patients are accepted and respected for no other reason than that they are considered to be worthwhile and unique human beings.

Many psychiatric patients have very little self-respect. Lack of self-respect may be related to the low self-esteem that accompanies illnesses such as clinical depression or it may be related to rejection and stigmatization by others. Recognition that patients are being accepted and respected as unique individuals on an unconditional basis can serve to elevate feelings of self-worth and self-respect. The nurse can convey an attitude of respect in the following ways:

- Calling the patient by their preferred name, pronouns, and title
- Spending time with the patient
- Allowing for sufficient time to answer the patient's questions and concerns
- Promoting an atmosphere of privacy during therapeutic interactions with the patient or when the patient may be undergoing physical examination or therapy
- Always being open and honest with the patient, even when the truth may be difficult to discuss
- Listening to the patient's ideas, preferences, and requests, and making collaborative decisions concerning his or her care whenever possible
- Striving to understand the motivation behind the patient's behavior, regardless of how unacceptable it may seem

Genuineness

The concept of **genuineness** refers to the nurse's ability to be open, honest, and "real" in interactions with the patient. To be real is to be aware of what one is experiencing internally and to allow the quality of this inner experiencing to be apparent in the therapeutic relationship. When one is genuine, there is congruence between what is felt and what is being expressed (Raskin et al., 2014). The nurse who possesses the quality of genuineness responds to the patient with truth and honesty rather than with responses that may be considered more "professional" or that merely reflect the "nursing role."

Genuineness may call for a degree of self-disclosure on the part of the nurse. This is not to say that the nurse must disclose to the patient *every* feeling or *all* personal experiences that may relate to what the patient is going through. Indeed, care must be taken when using self-disclosure to avoid reversing the roles of the nurse and patient.

For example, when a patient tells the nurse "I just get so upset when someone disrespects me, sometimes you just have to smack someone to teach them a lesson," the nurse might respond, "I get upset by that, too. Let's talk about some different ways to respond to this anger rather than hitting someone." In this example the nurse acknowledges a common feeling while maintaining a focus on the patient's need for problem-solving. When the nurse uses self-disclosure, a quality of "humanness" is revealed to the patient, creating a role for the patient to model in similar situations. The patient may then feel more comfortable revealing personal information to the nurse.

Most individuals have an uncanny ability to detect other people's artificiality. When the nurse does not bring the quality of genuineness to the relationship, a reality base for trust cannot be established. These qualities are essential to helping the patient actualize their potential within the nurse-patient relationship and for change and growth to occur (Raskin et al., 2014).

Empathy

Empathy is the ability to see beyond outward behavior and to understand the situation from the patient's point of view. With empathy, the nurse can accurately perceive and understand the meaning and relevance of the patient's thoughts and feelings. The nurse must also be able to communicate this perception to the patient by attempting to translate words and behaviors into feelings.

It is not uncommon for the concept of empathy to be confused with that of **sympathy.** The major difference is that with empathy the nurse "accurately perceives or understands" what the patient is feeling and encourages the patient to explore these feelings. With sympathy the nurse actually becomes emotionally involved in what the patient is feeling and experiences a need to alleviate distress.

Empathy is considered to be one of the most important characteristics of a therapeutic relationship. Accurate empathetic perceptions on the part of the nurse assist the patient to identify feelings that may have been suppressed or denied. Positive emotions are generated as the patient realizes the feeling of being understood by another. As the feelings surface and are explored, the patient learns aspects of self about which they may have been unaware. This exploration contributes to the process of self-awareness and the promotion of positive self-concept.

With empathy, while understanding the patient's thoughts and feelings, the nurse is able to maintain sufficient objectivity to allow the patient to achieve problem resolution with minimal assistance. With sympathy, the nurse actually feels what the patient is feeling, objectivity is lost, and the nurse may become focused on relief of personal distress rather than on helping the patient resolve the problem at hand. The following example describes an empathetic and sympathetic response to the same situation.

EXAMPLE

Situation: BJ is a patient on the psychiatric unit with a diagnosis of dysthymic disorder. She is 5 ft 5 inches tall and weighs 295 lb. BJ has been overweight all of her life. She is single, has no close friends, and has never had an intimate relationship with another person. It is her first day on the unit, and she is refusing to come out of her room. When she appeared for lunch in the dining room following admission, she expressed feeling embarrassed when one of the other patients laughed out loud and call her "fatso."

Sympathetic response: Nurse: "I can certainly identify with what you are feeling. I've been overweight most of my life, too. I just get so angry when people act like that. It's so insensitive and so typical of skinny people to act that way! You have a right to want to stay away from them. I'd stay away from them, too."

Empathetic response: Nurse: "I can understand your feeling upset about what happened at lunch today." As tears fill BJ's eyes, the nurse encourages her to cry if she feels like it and to express her anger at the situation. She stays with BJ but does not dwell on her own feelings about what happened. Instead, she focuses on BJ and what the patient perceives are her most immediate needs.

Rapport, trust, respect, genuineness, and empathy all are essential to forming therapeutic relationships, and they can certainly be assets in social relationships, too. The primary differences between social and therapeutic relationships are that therapeutic relationships always remain focused on the health-care needs of the patient, they are never for the purpose of addressing the nurse's personal needs, and they progress through identified phases of development for the purpose of helping the patient to solve health-related problems.

Phases of a Therapeutic Nurse-Patient Relationship

Psychiatric nurses use interpersonal relationship development as the primary intervention with patients in various psychiatric mental health settings. Developing an interpersonal relationship with the patient is congruent with Peplau's (1962) identification of *counseling* as the major subrole of nursing in psychiatry. Sullivan (1953), after whom Peplau patterned her own interpersonal theory of nursing, strongly believed that many emotional problems were closely related to difficulties with interpersonal relationships. With this concept in mind, this role of the nurse in psychiatry becomes especially meaningful and purposeful—an integral part of the total therapeutic regimen.

The therapeutic interpersonal relationship is the means by which the nursing process is implemented. Through the relationship, problems are identified and resolution is sought. Tasks of the relationship have been categorized into four phases:

1. Preinteraction phase
2. Orientation (introductory) phase
3. Working phase
4. Termination phase

Although each phase is presented as specific and distinct from the others, some tasks may overlap, particularly when the interaction is limited. The major goals during each phase of the nurse-patient relationship are listed in Table 5–1.

The Preinteraction Phase

The preinteraction phase involves preparation for the first encounter with the patient. Tasks include the following:

- Obtaining available information about the patient from their chart, significant others, or other health team members. From this information, the initial

TABLE 5–1 Phases of Relationship Development and Major Nursing Goals

PHASE	GOALS
1. Preinteraction	Explore self-perceptions
2. Orientation (introductory)	Establish trust and formulate contract for intervention
3. Working	Promote patient change
4. Termination	Evaluate goal attainment and ensure therapeutic closure

assessment is begun. This initial information may also allow the nurse to become aware of personal responses to knowledge about the patient.
- Examining one's feelings, fears, and anxieties about working with a particular patient. For example, the nurse may have been reared in an alcoholic family and have ambivalent feelings about caring for a patient who is alcohol dependent. All individuals bring attitudes and feelings from prior experiences to the clinical setting. The nurse needs to be aware of how these preconceptions may affect their ability to care for individual patients.

The Orientation (Introductory) Phase

During the orientation phase, the nurse and patient become acquainted. Tasks include the following:

- Creating an environment for the establishment of trust and rapport
- Establishing a contract for intervention that details the expectations and responsibilities of both the nurse and patient
- Gathering assessment information to build a strong patient database
- Identifying the patient's strengths and limitations
- Formulating nursing diagnoses
- Setting goals that are mutually agreeable to the nurse and patient
- Developing a plan of action that is realistic for meeting the established goals
- Exploring feelings of both the patient and nurse in terms of the introductory phase

Introductions often are uncomfortable, and the participants may experience some anxiety until a degree of rapport has been established. Interactions may remain on a superficial level until anxiety subsides. Several interactions may be required to fulfill the tasks associated with this phase.

The Working Phase

The therapeutic work of the relationship is accomplished during this phase. Tasks include the following:

- Maintaining the trust and rapport that was established during the orientation phase
- Promoting insight and perception of reality
- Problem-solving using the model presented earlier in this chapter
- Overcoming resistance behaviors as the level of anxiety rises in response to discussion of painful issues
- Continuously evaluating progress toward goal attainment

Transference and Countertransference

Transference and countertransference are common phenomena that often arise during the course of a therapeutic relationship.

Transference

Transference occurs when the patient unconsciously displaces (or "transfers") to the nurse feelings formed toward a person from their past. These feelings toward the nurse may be triggered by something about the nurse's appearance or personality that reminds the patient of the person. Transference can interfere with the therapeutic interaction when the feelings being expressed include anger and hostility. Anger toward the nurse can be manifested by uncooperativeness and resistance to the therapy.

Transference can also take the form of overwhelming affection for the nurse or excessive dependency on the nurse. The nurse is overvalued, and the patient forms unrealistic expectations of the nurse. When the nurse is unable to fulfill those expectations or meet the excessive dependency needs, the patient may become angry and hostile.

Interventions for Transference

Hilz (2013) stated:

> In cases of transference, the relationship does not usually need to be terminated, except when the transference poses a serious barrier to therapy or safety. The nurse should work with the patient in sorting out the past from the present, assist the patient into identifying the transference, and reassign a new and more appropriate meaning to the current nurse-patient relationship. The goal is to guide the patient to independence by teaching them to assume responsibility for their own behaviors, feelings, and thoughts, and to assign the correct meanings to the relationships based on present circumstances instead of the past.

Countertransference

Countertransference refers to the nurse's behavioral and emotional response to the patient. These responses may be related to unresolved feelings toward significant others from the nurse's past, or they may be generated in response to transference feelings on the part of the patient. It is not easy to refrain from becoming angry when the patient is consistently antagonistic, to feel flattered when showered with affection and attention by the patient, or even to feel quite powerful when the patient exhibits excessive dependency on the nurse. These feelings can interfere with the therapeutic relationship when they initiate the following types of behaviors:

- The nurse overidentifies with the patient's feelings because they remind him or her of problems from the nurse's past or present.
- The nurse and patient develop a social or personal relationship.
- The nurse begins to give advice or attempts to "rescue" the patient.
- The nurse encourages and promotes the patient's dependence.
- The nurse's anger engenders feelings of disgust toward the patient.
- The nurse feels anxious and uneasy in the presence of the patient.
- The nurse is bored and apathetic in sessions with the patient.
- The nurse has difficulty setting limits on the patient's behavior.
- The nurse defends the patient's behavior to other staff members.

The nurse may be completely unaware or only minimally aware of the countertransference as it is occurring (Hilz, 2013).

Interventions for Countertransference

Hilz (2013) states:

> The relationship usually should not be terminated in the presence of countertransference. Rather, the nurse or staff member experiencing the countertransference should be supportively assisted by other staff members to identify his or her feelings and behaviors and recognize the occurrence of the phenomenon. It may be helpful to have evaluative sessions with the nurse after his or her encounter with the patient, in which both the nurse and other staff members (who are observing the interactions) discuss and compare the exhibited behaviors in the relationship.

The Termination Phase

Termination of the relationship may occur for a variety of reasons: the mutually agreed-on goals may have been reached; the patient may be discharged from the hospital; or, in the case of a student nurse, it may be the end of a clinical rotation. Termination can be a difficult phase for both the patient and nurse. The main task involves bringing a therapeutic conclusion to the relationship. The relationship concludes when the following occur:

- Progress has been made toward attainment of mutually set goals.
- A plan for continuing care or for assistance during stressful life experiences is mutually established by the nurse and patient.
- Feelings about termination of the relationship are recognized and explored. Both the nurse and patient may experience feelings of sadness and loss. The nurse should share feelings with the patient. Through these interactions, the patient learns that it is acceptable to have these feelings at a time of separation. Through this knowledge, the patient experiences growth during the process of termination. This is also a time when both nurse and patient may evaluate and summarize the learning that occurred as an outgrowth of their relationship.

CLINICAL PEARL When the patient feels sadness and loss, behaviors to delay termination may become evident. If the nurse experiences the same feelings, the nurse may allow the patient's behaviors to delay termination. For therapeutic closure, the nurse must establish the reality of the separation and resist being manipulated into repeated delays by the patient.

Boundaries in the Nurse-Patient Relationship

A boundary indicates a border or a limit. It determines the extent of acceptable limits. Many types of boundaries exist. Examples include the following:

- ***Material boundaries:*** These are physical boundaries that can be seen, such as fences that border land.
- ***Social boundaries:*** These boundaries are established within a culture and define how individuals are expected to behave in social situations.
- ***Personal boundaries:*** These are boundaries that individuals define for themselves. These include *physical distance boundaries*, or just how close individuals will allow others to invade their physical space; and *emotional boundaries*, or how much individuals choose to disclose of their most private and intimate selves to others.
- ***Professional boundaries:*** These boundaries limit and outline expectations for appropriate professional relationships with patients. "Professional boundaries are the spaces between a nurse's power and the patient's vulnerability" (National Council of State Boards of Nursing [NCSBN], 2018). Nurses must recognize that they have an imbalance of power with their patients by virtue of their role and the patient information to which they have access. They must be consistently conscientious

in avoiding any circumstance in which they might achieve personal gain within that relationship.

Concerns regarding professional boundaries are commonly related to the following issues:

1. ***Self-disclosure:*** Self-disclosure on the part of the nurse may be appropriate when it is judged that the information may therapeutically benefit the patient. It should never be undertaken for the purpose of meeting the nurse's needs.
2. ***Gift giving:*** Individuals who are receiving care often feel indebted toward health-care providers. The British Columbia College of Professional Nurses (BCCPN, 2019) clarifies in their practice standards that, although nurses do not generally exchange gifts with patients, when it is deemed to have therapeutic intent, groups of nurses may accept a token gift, but significant gifts should be returned or redirected. There is always a degree of clinical judgment necessary in deciding to accept or refuse a gift, including the appropriateness, the value, and the reason the gift is being offered. Cultural belief and values may also enter into the decision of whether to accept a gift from a patient. In some cultures, failure to do so would be interpreted as an insult (Pie, 2012). Accepting financial gifts is never appropriate, but in some instances, nurses may be permitted to suggest instead a donation to a charity of the patient's choice. If acceptance of a small gift of gratitude is deemed appropriate, the nurse may choose to share it with other staff members who have been involved in the patient's care. Refusal to accept a gift should be done with sensitivity for the patient's feelings. Attention should be given not only to what the gift giving means to the patient but also to institutional policy, the American Nurses Association's (ANA) *Code of Ethics for Nurses*, and the ANA's *Scope and Standards of Practice*.
3. ***Touch:*** Nursing by its very nature involves touching patients. Touching is required to perform the many therapeutic procedures involved in the physical care of patients. Caring touch is the touching of patients when there is no physical need to do so. Touching or hugging can be beneficial when it is implemented with therapeutic intent *and* patient consent. When using caring touch, make sure it is appropriate, supportive, and welcomed (BCCPN, 2019). Caring touch may provide comfort or encouragement, but some vulnerable patients may misinterpret the meaning of touch. In some cultures, touch is not considered acceptable unless the parties know each other very well. The nurse must be sensitive to these cultural nuances and aware when touch is crossing a personal boundary. Additionally, patients who are experiencing high levels of anxiety, suspiciousness, or psychosis may interpret touch as aggressiveness. These are times when touch should be avoided or considered with extreme caution.
4. ***Friendship or romantic association:*** When a nurse is already acquainted with a patient, the relationship must move from personal to professional. If the nurse is unable to accomplish this separation, the nurse should withdraw from the professional relationship. Likewise, nurses must guard against personal relationships developing as a result of the nurse-patient relationship. Romantic, sexual, or similar personal relationships are never appropriate between nurse and patient.

Certain warning signs exist that indicate that professional boundaries of the nurse-patient relationship may be in jeopardy. Some of these include the following (Coltrane & Pugh, 1978):

- Favoring one patient's care over that of another
- Keeping secrets with a patient
- Changing dress style for working with a particular patient
- Swapping patient assignments to care for a particular patient
- Giving special attention or treatment to one patient over others
- Spending free time with a patient
- Frequently thinking about the patient when away from work
- Sharing personal information or work concerns with the patient
- Receiving gifts from or continuing communication with the patient after discharge

Boundary crossing can threaten the integrity of the nurse-patient relationship. Nurses must gain self-awareness and insight to be able to recognize when professional integrity is being compromised. Although some variables such as the care setting, community influences, patient needs, and the nature of therapy affect how boundaries are delineated, "any action that oversteps the established boundaries to meet the needs of the nurse are boundary violations" (NCSBN, 2018).

CORE CONCEPT

Communication

An interactive process of transmitting information between two or more entities.

Interpersonal Communication

It has been said that individuals "cannot *not* communicate." Every word that is spoken, every movement that is made, and every action that is taken or is not taken gives a message to someone. Interpersonal communication is a *transaction* between the sender and the receiver. In the transactional model of communication, both participants simultaneously perceive each other, listen to each other, and mutually are involved in creating meaning in a relationship.

The Impact of Pre-existing Conditions

In all interpersonal transactions, both the sender and receiver bring certain pre-existing conditions to the exchange that influence both the intended message and the way in which it is interpreted. Examples of these conditions include one's value system, internalized attitudes and beliefs, culture or religion, social status, gender, background knowledge and experience, and age or developmental level. The type of environment in which the communication takes place also may influence the outcome of the transaction.

Values, Attitudes, and Beliefs

Values, attitudes, and beliefs are learned ways of thinking. Children generally adopt the value systems and internalize the attitudes and beliefs of their parents. Children may retain this way of thinking into adulthood or develop a different set of attitudes and values as they mature.

Values, attitudes, and beliefs can influence communication in numerous ways. For example, prejudice is expressed verbally through negative stereotyping.

One's value system may be communicated with behaviors that are more symbolic in nature. For example, an individual who values youth may dress and behave in a manner that is characteristic of one who is much younger. Persons who value socioeconomic status may choose large homes, luxury cars, and other expensive personal possessions. In each of these situations, a message is being communicated.

Culture and Religion

Communication has its roots in culture. Cultural mores, norms, ideas, and customs provide the basis for our way of thinking. Cultural values are learned and differ from society to society. For example, in some European countries (e.g., Italy, Spain, and France), men may greet each other with hugs and kisses; in the United States or England, shaking hands is a more culturally accepted style of greeting among men.

Religion also can influence communication. Priests and ministers who wear clerical collars publicly communicate their mission in life. The collar also may influence the way in which others relate to them, either positively or negatively. Other symbolic gestures, such as wearing a cross around the neck or wearing a hijab (a religious veil worn by some Muslim women in public), also communicate an individual's religious beliefs.

Social Status

Studies of nonverbal indicators of social status or power have suggested that high-status persons are associated with gestures that communicate their higher-power position (Hall et al., 2005; Ridgeway et al., 1985). For example, they use more eye contact, have a more erect and open posture, use louder voice pitch, and talk more, dress more formally, and interact at closer interpersonal distance.

Gender

Gender influences the manner in which individuals communicate. Most cultures have *gender signals* that are recognized as either masculine or feminine and provide a basis for distinguishing between members of each gender. Examples include differences in posture, both standing and sitting, between many men and women. In the United States, generally, men tend to expand in their physical space, whereas women are more likely to cross legs and arms and reduce their physical space. Men tend to lean away from a speaker, whereas women are more likely to lean toward a speaker and use more eye contact (Valamis, 2021). It should be reinforced, though, that these are generalizations rather than absolute differences.

Roles have historically been identified as either male or female. For example, in the United States, masculinity typically was communicated through such roles as husband, father, breadwinner, doctor, lawyer, and engineer. Traditional female roles included wife, mother, homemaker, nurse, teacher, and secretary.

Gender signals are changing in U.S. society as gender roles become less distinct. Behaviors that once were considered typically masculine or feminine may now be generally accepted in members of both genders. Words such as *nonbinary* communicate a desire by some individuals to diminish the distinction between the genders and minimize the discrimination of either. Gender roles are changing as both women and men enter professions that once were dominated by members of the opposite gender.

Age or Developmental Level

Age influences communication, and it is especially evident during adolescence. In their struggle to separate from parental confines and establish their own identity, adolescents generate a unique pattern of communication that changes from generation to generation. Words such as *dude, dope, lit,* and *wasted* have had special meaning for different generations of adolescents. The technological age has produced a whole new language for today's adolescents. Communication by text messaging includes such acronyms as BRB ("be right back"), BFF ("best friends forever"), and YOLO ("you only live once").

Developmental physiological alterations may also influence communication. For people who are deaf or hearing impaired, American Sign Language may be their preferred method of communication. Individuals who are blind at birth never learn the subtle nonverbal gestures that typically accompany language and can totally change the meaning of the spoken word.

Environment in Which the Transaction Takes Place

The place where the communication occurs influences the outcome of the interaction. Some individuals who feel uncomfortable and refuse to speak during a group therapy session may be open and willing to discuss problems privately with the nurse.

Territoriality, density, and distance are aspects of environment that communicate messages. **Territoriality** is the innate tendency to own space. Individuals lay claim to areas around them as their own. This influences communication when an interaction takes place in the territory "owned" by one or the other. Interpersonal communication can be more successful if the interaction takes place in a "neutral" area. For example, with the concept of territoriality in mind, the nurse may choose to conduct the psychosocial assessment in an interview room rather than in an office or in the patient's room.

Density refers to the number of people within a given environmental space, and it has been shown to influence interpersonal interaction. Some studies indicate that a correlation exists between prolonged high-density situations and certain behaviors, such as aggression and withdrawal, but Regoeczi (2002) identifies support for the notion that this relationship is nonlinear based on variation in individual self-selected behaviors.

Distance is the means by which various cultures use space to communicate. Hall (1966) identified four kinds of spatial interaction, or distances, that people maintain from each other in their interpersonal interactions and the kinds of activities in which people engage at these various distances.

1. ***Intimate distance*** is the closest distance that individuals will allow between themselves and others. In the United States, this distance, which is restricted to interactions of an intimate nature, is 0 to 18 inches.
2. ***Personal distance*** is approximately 18 to 40 inches and is reserved for interactions that are personal in nature, such as close conversations with friends or colleagues.
3. ***Social distance*** is about 4 to 12 feet away from the body. Interactions at this distance include conversations with strangers or acquaintances, such as at a cocktail party or in a public building.
4. ***Public distance*** is one that exceeds 12 feet. Examples include speaking in public or yelling to someone some distance away. This distance is considered public space, and communicants are free to move about in it during the interaction.

Nonverbal Communication

Various studies have identified nonverbal communication as more reliable than verbal communication in expressing one's attitudes and feelings, and some describe it as the single most powerful way in which communication occurs (Heathfield, 2019). Some aspects of nonverbal expression were discussed in the previous section on pre-existing conditions that influence communication. Other components of nonverbal communication include physical appearance and dress, body movement and posture, touch, facial expressions, eye behavior, and vocal cues or *paralanguage* (such as intonation, pitch, and speed; a more detailed description follows). These nonverbal messages vary from culture to culture.

Physical Appearance and Dress

Physical appearance and dress are part of the total nonverbal stimuli that influence interpersonal responses, and, under some conditions, they are the primary determinants of such responses. Body coverings—both dress and hair—are manipulated by the wearer in a manner that conveys a distinct message to the receiver. Dress can be formal or casual, stylish or unkempt. Hair can be long or short, and even the presence or absence of hair conveys a message about the person. Other body adornments that are considered potential communicative stimuli include tattoos, masks, cosmetics, badges, jewelry, and eyeglasses. Some jewelry worn in specific ways can give special messages (e.g., a gold band or diamond ring worn on the fourth finger of the left hand, a pin bearing Greek letters worn on the lapel, or the wearing of a ring that is inscribed with the insignia of a college or university). Some individuals convey a specific message with the total absence of any type of body adornment.

Body Movement and Posture

The way in which an individual positions his or her body communicates messages regarding self-esteem, gender identity, status, and interpersonal warmth or coldness. The individual whose posture is slumped, with head and eyes pointed downward, conveys a message of low self-esteem. Specific ways of standing or sitting are considered to be either feminine or masculine within a defined culture. To stand straight and tall with head high and hands on hips indicates a superior status over the person being addressed.

Reece and Whitman (1962) identified response behaviors that were used to designate individuals as either "warm" or "cold" persons. Individuals who were perceived as warm responded to others with a shift of posture toward the other person, a smile, direct eye contact, and hands that remained still. Individuals who responded to others with a slumped posture, by looking around the room, drumming fingers on the desk, and not smiling were perceived as cold.

Touch

Touch is a powerful communication tool. It can elicit both negative and positive reactions, depending on the people involved and the circumstances of the interaction. It is a very basic and primitive form of communication, and the appropriateness of its use is culturally determined.

Touch can be categorized according to the message communicated (Knapp & Hall, 2014):

- ***Functional-professional:*** This type of touch is impersonal and businesslike. It is used to accomplish a task.

EXAMPLE

A tailor measuring a customer for a suit or a physician examining a patient

- ***Social-polite:*** This type of touch is still rather impersonal, but it conveys an affirmation or acceptance of the other person.

EXAMPLE

A handshake

- ***Friendship-warmth:*** Touch at this level indicates a strong liking for the other person—a feeling of friendship.

EXAMPLE

Laying one's hand on the shoulder of another

- ***Love-intimacy:*** This type of touch conveys an emotional attachment or attraction to another person.

EXAMPLE

Engaging in a strong, mutual embrace

- ***Sexual arousal:*** Touch at this level is an expression of physical attraction only.

EXAMPLE

Caressing or touching another with intent to create sexual arousal

Some cultures encourage more touching of various types than do others. The nurse should understand the cultural meaning of touch before using this method of communication in specific situations. The best practice is to ask the patient's permission before using touch as an intervention.

Facial Expressions

Next to human speech, facial expression is the primary source of communication. Facial expressions primarily reveal an individual's emotional states, such as happiness, sadness, anger, surprise, and fear. The face is a complex multi-message system. Facial expressions serve to complement and qualify other communication behaviors and at times even take the place of verbal messages. A summary of feelings associated with various facial expressions is presented in Table 5–2.

Eye Behavior

Eyes have been called the "windows of the soul." It is through eye contact that individuals view and are viewed by others in a revealing way, creating an interpersonal connection. In American culture, eye contact conveys a personal interest in the other person. Eye contact indicates that the communication channel is open, and it is often the initiating factor in verbal interaction between two people.

Eye behavior is regulated by social rules. These rules dictate where, when, for how long, and at whom we can look. Staring is often used to register disapproval of the behavior of another. People are extremely sensitive to being looked at, and if the gazing or staring behavior violates social rules, they often assign meaning to it, such as the following statement implies: "He kept staring at me, and I began to

TABLE 5–2 Summary of Facial Expressions

FACIAL EXPRESSION	ASSOCIATED FEELINGS
NOSE	
Nostril flare	Anger; arousal
Wrinkling up	Dislike; disgust
LIPS	
Grin; smile	Happiness; contentment
Grimace	Fear; pain
Compressed	Anger; frustration
Canine-type snarl	Disgust
Pouted; frown	Unhappiness; discontented; disapproval
Pursing	Disagreement
Sneer	Contempt; disdain
BROWS	
Frown	Anger; unhappiness; concentration
Raised	Surprise; enthusiasm
TONGUE	
Stick out	Dislike; disagree
EYES	
Widened	Surprise; excitement
Narrowed; lids squeezed shut	Threat; fear
Stare	Threat
Stare, blink, then look away	Dislike; uninterest
Eyes downcast; lack of eye contact	Submission; low self-esteem
Eye contact (generally intermittent as opposed to a stare)	Self-confidence; interest

Sources: Compiled from Cherry (2019) and Simon (2005).

wonder if I was dressed inappropriately or had mustard on my face!"

Vocal Cues or Paralanguage

Paralanguage is the vocal component of the spoken word. It consists of pitch, tone, and loudness of spoken messages, the rate of speaking, expressively placed pauses, and emphasis assigned to certain words. These vocal cues greatly influence the way individuals interpret verbal messages. A normally soft-spoken individual whose pitch and rate of speaking increases may be perceived as being anxious or tense.

Different vocal emphases can alter interpretation of the message. For example,

- "I felt SURE you would notice the change."
  Interpretation: I was SURE you would, but you didn't.
- "I felt sure YOU would notice the change."
  Interpretation: I thought YOU would, even if nobody else did.
- "I felt sure you would notice the CHANGE."
  Interpretation: Even if you didn't notice anything else, I thought you would notice the CHANGE.

Verbal cues play a major role in determining responses in human communication situations. *How* a message is verbalized can be as important as *what* is verbalized.

CORE CONCEPT

Therapeutic Communication

Caregiver verbal and nonverbal techniques that focus on the care receiver's needs and advance the promotion of healing and change. Therapeutic communication encourages exploration of feelings and fosters understanding of behavioral motivation. It is nonjudgmental, discourages defensiveness, and promotes trust.

Therapeutic Communication Techniques

Hays and Larson (1963) identified a number of techniques to assist the nurse in interacting more therapeutically with patients. These are important "technical procedures" carried out by the nurse working in psychiatry, and they should serve to enhance development of a therapeutic nurse-patient relationship. Table 5–3 includes a list of these techniques, a short explanation of their usefulness, and examples of each.

Nontherapeutic Communication Techniques

Several approaches are considered to be barriers to open communication between the nurse and patient. Hays and Larson (1963) identified a number of these techniques, which are presented in Table 5–4. Nurses should recognize and eliminate the use of these patterns in their relationships with patients. Avoiding these communication barriers will maximize the effectiveness of communication and enhance the nurse-patient relationship.

Active Listening

To listen actively is to be attentive and to really desire to hear and understand what the patient is saying, both verbally and nonverbally. Attentive listening

Text continued on page 116

TABLE 5–3 Therapeutic Communication Techniques

TECHNIQUE	EXPLANATION/RATIONALE	EXAMPLES
Using silence	Silence encourages the patient to organize thoughts and put them into words and allows the patient time to think about the significance of events, thoughts, and feelings. Allowing the patient to break the silence often provides the nurse with important information about the patient's foremost concerns.	Patient: "My husband divorced me so I must be undesirable." Nurse: (silence) Patient: "You know, when I think about it, no matter what my husband does I always assume it's my fault or it's something wrong with me."
Accepting	Acceptance conveys an attitude of understanding and willingness to interact.	"Yes, I understand what you said." Eye contact; nodding
Giving recognition	Acknowledging and indicating awareness is better than complimenting, which reflects the nurse's judgment.	"Hello, Mr. J. I notice that you made a ceramic ash tray in OT." "I see you made your bed."
Offering self	Willingness to spend time with the patient and show interest on an unconditional basis promotes the patient's feelings of self-worth.	"I'll stay with you awhile." "How are you feeling today?" "I'm interested in hearing your thoughts about the group you just attended."
Giving broad openings	Broad openings allow the patient to direct the focus of the interaction and emphasize the importance of the patient's role in the communication process.	"What would you like to talk about today?" "Is there anything you want to discuss?"
Offering general leads	General leads offer the patient encouragement to continue with minimal input from the nurse.	"Yes, I see." "Go on." "And after that?"
Placing the event in time or sequence	Encouraging the patient to identify the sequence of events and when they occurred in time facilitates organizing one's thoughts about their experiences.	"What happened first?" "What happened next?" "Was this before or after . . . ?" "When did this happen?"
Making observations	Verbalizing observations about a patient's behavior or appearance encourages the patient to develop awareness of how they are perceived by others and promotes exploration of issues that may be problematic.	"You appear sad today." "I notice you are pacing a lot." "I notice that when I ask you about whether you have thoughts of suicide you change the subject."
Encouraging description of perceptions	Asking the patient to verbalize his or her perceptions facilitates the patient's ability to develop awareness and understanding. For the patient experiencing hallucinations, it can facilitate both nurse's and patient's clarification about what the patient's perceptual experiences are communicating.	"Tell me more about the voices you said you are hearing." "What was it that increased your agitation during the group activity?" "Are these voices you hear directing you to take some action?"
Encouraging comparison	Asking the patient to compare similarities and differences in ideas, experiences, or interpersonal relationships helps the patient recognize life experiences that tend to recur and those aspects of life that are changeable.	"Was this episode similar to . . . ?" "How does this compare with the time when . . . ?" "What was your response the last time this situation occurred?"

TABLE 5–3 Therapeutic Communication Techniques—cont'd

TECHNIQUE	EXPLANATION/RATIONALE	EXAMPLES
Restating	Repeating the main idea of what the patient has said lets the patient know whether an expressed statement has been understood and gives him or her the chance to continue, or to clarify if necessary.	Patient: "I can't study. My mind keeps wandering." Nurse: "You have trouble concentrating." Patient: "I can't take that new job. What if I can't do it?" Nurse: "You're afraid you will fail in this new position."
Reflecting	Questions and feelings are referred back to the patient so that the patient is empowered to actively engage in problem-solving rather than simply asking the nurse for advice.	Patient: "Don't you think I should tell my boss I'm not putting up with that?" Nurse: "What do *you* think you should do?" Patient: "She makes me so upset!" Nurse: "So you're feeling angry at your boss?"
Focusing	Taking notice of a single idea or even a single word encourages specific discussion about a relevant issue and is especially helpful with patients who are moving rapidly from one thought to another. However, focusing is very difficult for a patient with severe anxiety so in this case the nurse should not pursue focusing until the anxiety level lessens.	"Tell me more about this specific point."
Exploring	When the nurse hears the patient mention an issue or theme that seems relevant, the nurse asks the patient to explore this further. Exploring facilitates the patient's development of awareness and understanding about events, thoughts, and feelings. However, if the patient chooses not to disclose further information, the nurse should refrain from pushing or probing in an area that obviously creates discomfort.	"Please explain that situation in more detail." "Tell me more about that particular situation." "You mentioned feeling like no one cares about you. Tell me more about those feelings."
Seeking clarification and validation	Striving to explain vague or incomprehensible statements and searching for mutual understanding facilitates and increases understanding for both patient and nurse.	"I'm not sure that I understand. Would you please explain?" "Tell me if my understanding agrees with yours." "Do I understand correctly that you said . . . ?"
Presenting reality	When the patient has a misperception of the environment, the nurse defines reality by expressing his or her perception of the situation without challenging the patient's perceptions.	"I understand that the voices seem real to you, but I do not hear any voices." "I don't see anyone else in the room but you and me."
Voicing doubt	Expressing uncertainty about the validity of the patient's perceptions is a technique often used with patients experiencing delusional thinking.	"It's difficult to believe that the president of the United States would be listening to all of your phone calls." "I find that hard to believe [or accept]." "That seems rather doubtful to me."

Continued

TABLE 5–3 Therapeutic Communication Techniques—cont'd

TECHNIQUE	EXPLANATION/RATIONALE	EXAMPLES
Verbalizing the implied	Putting into words what the patient has only implied or said indirectly is a technique that can be helpful with patients experiencing impaired verbal communication.	Patient: "I can't talk about this. . . . You haven't been where I've been." Nurse: "Does it seem like no one could understand your thoughts and feelings unless they've had the same experiences you've had?" Patient: "I . . . I don't know where to begin." Nurse: "So it feels overwhelming to think about sharing the details of this experience."
Attempting to translate words into feelings	When the patient has difficulty identifying feelings or feelings are expressed indirectly, the nurse tries to "desymbolize" what has been said and to find clues to the underlying true feelings.	Patient: "I'm just an empty pit." Nurse: "It sounds like you are feeling hopeless, is that right?"
Formulating a plan of action	Encouraging the patient to identify a plan for behavior change promotes developing better coping skills.	"What could you do differently if you are faced with this situation in the future?" "What are some steps you could take to manage your anger without punching someone?" "What is one thing you might be willing to try to decrease your anxiety instead of using alcohol?"

Sources: Compiled from Engard (2018), Hays and Larson (1963), and Sullivan (1954).

TABLE 5–4 Nontherapeutic Communication Techniques

TECHNIQUE	EXPLANATION/RATIONALE	EXAMPLES
Giving false reassurance	False reassurance conveys that the nurse already knows the outcome of a situation and minimizes the patient's expressed concerns. It may discourage the patient from further expression of feelings if the patient believes the feelings will be downplayed or ridiculed.	Patient: "My husband doesn't love me anymore. I think he wants a divorce." Nurse: "I'm sure he must still love you. Everything will be fine." ***Better alternative:*** "Tell me more about what's been happening in your relationship with your husband."
Rejecting	Refusing to consider or showing contempt for the patient's ideas or behavior may cause the patient to discontinue interaction with the nurse for fear of further rejection.	Patient: "Since I started taking this medication I can't be intimate with my girlfriend." Nurse: "Let's not talk about that right now." ***Better alternative:*** "Tell me more about what you mean by not being able 'to be intimate' with your girlfriend."
Approving or disapproving	Sanctioning or denouncing the patient's ideas or behavior implies that the nurse's role is to pass judgment on whether the patient's ideas or behaviors are "good" or "bad" and that the patient is expected to please the nurse. The nurse's acceptance of the patient is then seen as conditional depending on the patient's behavior.	"It's good that you confronted your wife about her behavior." "You shouldn't yell at your wife." ***Better alternative:*** "What happened after you confronted your wife in a loud voice?"

TABLE 5–4 Nontherapeutic Communication Techniques—cont'd

TECHNIQUE	EXPLANATION/RATIONALE	EXAMPLES
Agreeing or disagreeing	Indicating accord with or opposition to the patient's ideas or opinions implies that the nurse has the right to pass judgment on whether the patient's ideas or opinions are "right" or "wrong." Agreement prevents the patient from later modifying his or her point of view without the risk of displeasing the nurse. Disagreement may provoke defensiveness on the part of the patient.	Patient: "I think my doctor doesn't care about me." Nurse: "I disagree. You shouldn't think that way." or "I can't believe that's true." ***Better alternative:*** "Tell me more about why you think your doctor doesn't care."
Giving advice	Telling the patient what to do or how to behave implies that the nurse knows what is best and nurtures the patient in the dependent role by discouraging independent thinking.	"You need to do deep breathing exercises when you become anxious." "You should stop drinking alcohol and start going to Alcoholics Anonymous meetings." ***Better alternative:*** "What do *you* think you should do?" or "Let's explore some options for solving this problem."
Probing	Persistent questioning of the patient and pushing for answers to issues the patient does not wish to discuss or does not know the answers to may contribute to the patient feeling used only for what information the nurse is seeking and may place the patient on the defensive.	"Why was your family angry with you?" "How many times did you receive poor evaluations before you got fired?" "How many girlfriends were you lying to?" ***Better alternative:*** The nurse should actively listen to the patient's response and discontinue the interaction at the first sign of discomfort.
Defending	Defending someone or something the patient has criticized minimizes or completely ignores the patient's concerns. Defending may cause the patient to think the nurse is taking sides against him or her.	"None of the nurses here would lie to you." "You have a very capable physician." "Your children want only what's best for you." ***Better alternative:*** "Tell me more about these concerns you've expressed."
Requesting an explanation	This technique involves asking why the patient has certain thoughts, feelings, and behaviors. Asking "why" a patient did something or feels a certain way can be very intimidating and implies that the patient must defend his or her behavior or feelings.	"Why do you think people are out to get you?" "Why do you feel depressed?" "Why were you taking drugs?" ***Better alternative:*** "Describe what you were feeling just before that happened."
Indicating the existence of an external source of power	Attributing the source of thoughts, feelings, and behavior to something or someone other than the patient encourages the patient to project blame for his or her thoughts or behaviors on others rather than accepting the responsibility personally.	"What *made* you go on a drinking binge?" "What *made* you say that you are a worthless person?" ***Better alternative:*** "What was happening just before you started binge drinking?" "What do you mean when you say you are 'a worthless person'?"
Belittling feelings expressed	When the nurse minimizes the degree of the patient's discomfort, a lack of empathy and understanding may be conveyed. When the nurse tells the patient to "cheer up" or "everybody feels that way," the patient may feel that his or her concerns are insignificant or unimportant.	Patient: "I don't even have the energy to go to work." Nurse: "We've all felt like that at times. You've just got to perk up and get moving." ***Better alternative:*** "Tell me more about what you are feeling right now."

Continued

TABLE 5–4 Nontherapeutic Communication Techniques—cont'd

TECHNIQUE	EXPLANATION/RATIONALE	EXAMPLES
Making stereotyped comments	Trite expressions are meaningless in a nurse-patient relationship. When the nurse uses meaningless expressions, it encourages a similar response from the patient.	"How are you?" "Hang in there." "It'll all work out." ***Better alternative:*** Choose words, sentences, and nonverbal language that convey a sincere interest in encouraging the patient to share more about the patient's thoughts, feelings, and behaviors.
Using denial	Denying that a problem exists blocks discussion with the patient and avoids helping the patient identify and explore areas of difficulty.	Patient: "I have a problem interacting with people." Nurse: "You're doing fine." ***Better alternative:*** "Tell me more about that."
Interpreting	Interpreting attempts to tell the patient the meaning of his or her experience. Erroneous interpretations may leave the patient feeling that the nurse doesn't understand him or her, or that the nurse is being smug.	"What you really mean is . . ." "You're angry because . . ." ***Better alternative:*** The nurse must leave interpretation of the patient's behavior to a therapist who is trained to use interpretation in the context of specialized therapy.
Introducing an unrelated topic	When the nurse prematurely changes the subject, it conveys to the patient that the nurse does not want to discuss the original topic any further. This may occur in order to get to something that the nurse wants to discuss with the patient or to get away from a topic that the patient would prefer not to discuss.	Patient: "I don't have anything to live for." Nurse: "How well did you sleep last night?" ***Better alternative:*** "Tell me more." Sometimes silence may be appropriate to convey that the nurse is willing to hear all of what the patient wants to say before moving on to a different topic.

Sources: Compiled from Hays and Larson (1963) and Sullivan (1954).

creates a climate in which the patient can communicate; the nurse communicates acceptance and respect for the patient, and trust is enhanced. A climate is established in the relationship that promotes openness and honest expression.

Several nonverbal behaviors have been designated as facilitative skills for attentive listening. Those listed here can be identified by the acronym SOLER:

Sit **S**quarely facing the patient. This gives the message that the nurse is there to listen and is interested in what the patient has to say.

Open posture. Posture is considered "open" when arms and legs remain uncrossed. This posture suggests that the nurse is "open" to what the patient has to say. With a "closed" posture, the nurse can convey a somewhat defensive stance, possibly invoking a similar response in the patient.

Lean forward toward the patient. This nonverbal behavior conveys to the patient that you are involved in the interaction, interested in what is being said, and making a sincere effort to be attentive.

Eyecontact. Direct eye contact is another behavior that conveys the nurse's involvement and willingness to listen to what the patient has to say. The absence of eye contact, or the constant shifting of eye contact, gives the message that the nurse is not really interested in what is being said.

Relax. Whether sitting or standing during the interaction, the nurse should communicate a sense of being relaxed and comfortable with the patient. Restlessness and fidgetiness communicate a lack of interest and may convey a feeling of discomfort that is likely to be transferred to the patient.

CLINICAL PEARL Ensure that eye contact conveys warmth, is accompanied by smiling and intermittent nodding of the head, and does not come across as staring or glaring, which can create intense discomfort in the patient. Active observation and listening to discern an individual's comfort level with eye contact facilitates adapting one's level of eye contact if it appears to increase the patient's anxiety. For example, patient's experiencing paranoia and some individuals with autism spectrum disorder may be very sensitive to levels of eye contact that in other situations would seem appropriate.

MOTIVATIONAL INTERVIEWING

Patient-centered care has been identified as an important focus in the quest to improve the quality of communication and therapeutic relationships with patients (Institute of Medicine, Board on Health Care Services and Committee on the Health Professions Education Summit, 2003). **Motivational interviewing** is an evidence-based, patient-centered style of communication that promotes behavior change by guiding patients to explore their own motivation for change and the advantages and disadvantages of their decisions (Rubak et al., 2005).

This style of communication incorporates active listening and therapeutic communication techniques, but it is focused on what the patient wants to do rather than what the nurse thinks *should* be the next steps in behavior change. Motivational interviewing was originally developed for use with patients who have substance use disorders, primarily because this style of communication may decrease defensive responses. It has since gained widespread acceptance as a patient-centered communication strategy that promotes behavior change for patients with many different health-care issues. See the "Real People, Real Stories" feature for an example of motivational interviewing described in a process recording format.

Real People, Real Stories: A Sample of Motivational Interviewing in a Process Recording Format

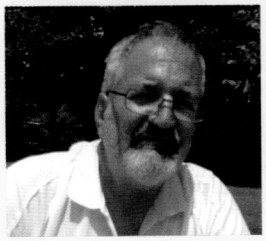

The following is part of an interaction with Alan, incorporating motivational interviewing communication strategies in a process recording format. Learn more about Alan's story in the chapter on substance use disorders.

Interaction	Nurse's Thoughts and Feelings	Communication Technique/ Evaluation
Karyn: You mentioned that you were at an event and you commented that you "needed a drink." Tell me more about what was happening. (SOLER)	I wasn't sure if Alan was willing to talk about this, but I thought it was important to facilitate his looking at his behavior in response to this experience.	***Technique:*** *Exploring* ***Evaluation:*** This approach was effective. Alan talked more about the event and was able to articulate some thoughts and feelings as well.
Alan: (nodding) I was perturbed. I felt like I was stuck at this event. There was supposed to be entertainment, but it got cancelled due to rain, and suddenly I noticed people were drinking and smoking. It brought back a lot of memories. (looks down)	I was glad that Alan was open to discussing this experience, but he said so many things in this short statement that I had to be thoughtful about what to follow up on.	
Karyn: So you felt perturbed and stuck. . . . (looking up, not making direct eye contact)	I was thinking that I don't usually explore feelings right off the bat because I believe it's better to help someone fully describe events and thoughts first (or at least it's less threatening), but I've interacted with Alan many times, he's been through rehab, sober for seven years, and he's pretty comfortable talking about feelings.	***Technique:*** *Reflecting* ***Evaluation:*** This technique was effective. Alan began to process his thoughts about why he might be feeling perturbed and stuck. I think I may have been not making direct eye contact because of my perception that feelings can be a little more threatening for some people to talk about.

Continued

Real People, Real Stories: A Sample of Motivational Interviewing in a Process Recording Format—cont'd

Interaction	Nurse's Thoughts and Feelings	Communication Technique/ Evaluation
Alan: Yeah, but it didn't last long. Maybe it had something to do with the fact that there was nothing else going on and it seemed like the whole thing became about drinking. But then I just blacked it out.	My immediate thought was that I want to tell him to go to an AA meeting or call his sponsor, but I was trying to incorporate a motivational interviewing strategy, and that meant it would be better to help him explore his motivation for how to respond to this experience. I didn't know what he meant by "blacked it out," but I felt uncomfortable when he said that.	
Karyn: What do you mean when you say you blacked it out? (SOLER)	I thought this was an important statement to clarify, since it might help him explore how he behaved in response to this event.	***Technique:*** *Clarifying* ***Evaluation:*** Asking this question was effective. Alan talked at length about his thoughts and feelings.
Alan: (silent for several seconds) I do need to go back to an AA meeting. I mean, am I different than other people? I know there are other people out there that have to be struggling with the same kind of things. When I was in rehab, my mom and her boyfriend were always there taking me to meetings. My sister went, too. . . . (silent for several more seconds) I know it's important (silence) . . . about 75% of the people I went to rehab with are back out there using again.	Alan seemed to be thinking a lot about this and was responding with several different thoughts, so I felt like it was important to just use silence and facilitate his reflection. I thought Alan seemed to be genuinely considering a behavior change.	
Karyn: You said that you need to go back to a meeting and that they are important. Is it more helpful to go to meetings when you just start thinking about needing a drink, or do you think that meetings are only necessary after you actually take a drink?	I knew that Alan had not been going to meetings regularly for the last couple of years, even though he acknowledges their importance, so I wanted to know more about whether he thought behavior change (such as going to AA meetings) was necessary at this point.	***Techniques:*** *Restating, focusing* ***Evaluation:*** Restatement was effective. The way I chose to focus was probably leading Alan to choose the "right" answer, and that makes it harder to evaluate whether he is just telling me what I want to hear or is really motivated. It might have been better to use the technique of formulating a plan of action.
Alan: Oh no, you've got to go long before you take that first drink. (silence) People told me when I was in rehab that they could tell I was really listening in meetings . . . the meetings were helpful (silence), and I just reconnected with my sponsor on Facebook, so I need to get back to a meeting to see him.	Alan seemed like he was thinking about what is important to him, so I continued to remain silent to facilitate that process.	

Real People, Real Stories: A Sample of Motivational Interviewing in a Process Recording Format—cont'd

Interaction	Nurse's Thoughts and Feelings	Communication Technique/ Evaluation
Karyn: You've identified three reasons why you believe you need to go to a meeting: because they are helpful to you, because you want to find out if others are struggling with the same kinds of thoughts that you are, and because you need to reconnect with your sponsor. Do you have a plan in mind for how to follow through with that?	I was thinking that he talks about needing to go to AA, and *I* was feeling anxious about wanting him to commit to that, but at the same time, I recognized that the motivation for change and commitment to a plan of action has to come from him.	***Techniques:*** *Summarizing, formulating a plan of action* ***Evaluation:*** I think the techniques were effective, although Alan may not be ready to formulate an action plan at present.
Alan: Well, I haven't done it yet. I guess I'm still just thinking about it.	I was appreciating his honesty and thinking that this is the challenge of motivational interviewing: accepting where the patient is while continuing to explore and facilitate his or her motivations for behavior change.	

Process Recordings

Process recordings are written reports of verbal interactions with patients. They are verbatim (to the extent that this is possible) accounts written by the nurse or student as a tool for improving interpersonal communication techniques. Process recordings can take many forms but usually includes the verbal and nonverbal communication of both nurse and patient. The exercise provides a means for the nurse to analyze the content and pattern of the interaction. The process recording, which is not considered documentation, is intended to be used as a learning tool for professional development. An example of one type of process recording is presented in Table 5–5.

Feedback

Feedback is a method of communication that helps the patient consider a modification of behavior by providing information about how the patient is perceived by others. Feedback can be useful to the patient if presented with objectivity by a trusted individual in a manner that discourages defensiveness. Characteristics of useful feedback and examples of each include the following:

- ***Feedback should be descriptive rather than evaluative and focused on the behavior rather than on the person.*** Avoiding evaluative language reduces the need for the patient to react defensively. Objective descriptions allow patients to take the information and use it in whatever way they choose. When the focus is on the person, rather than the behavior, the patient may perceive that they are being judged as "good" or "bad."

  Descriptive and focused on behavior: "Jane was very upset in group today when you called her 'fatty' and laughed at her in front of the others."
  Evaluative: "You were very rude and inconsiderate to Jane in group today."
  Focused on patient: "You are a very insensitive person."

- ***Feedback should be specific rather than general.*** Information that gives details about the patient's behavior can be used more easily than a generalized description for modifying the behavior.

  Specific: "You were talking to Joe when we were deciding on the issue. Now you want to argue about the outcome."
  General: "You just don't pay attention."

- ***Feedback should be directed toward behavior that the patient has the capacity to modify.*** To provide feedback about a characteristic or situation that the patient cannot change will only provoke frustration.

  Can modify: "I noticed that you did not want to hold your baby when the nurse brought her to you."
  Cannot modify: "Your baby daughter is mentally retarded because you took drugs when you were pregnant."

TABLE 5–5 Sample Process Recording

NURSE VERBAL (NONVERBAL)	PATIENT VERBAL (NONVERBAL)	NURSE'S THOUGHTS AND FEELINGS CONCERNING THE INTERACTION	ANALYSIS OF THE INTERACTION
"Do you still have thoughts about harming yourself?" (Sitting facing patient; looking directly at patient.)	"Not really. I still feel sad, but I don't want to die." (Looking at hands in lap.)	Felt a little uncomfortable. Always a hard question to ask.	***Therapeutic:*** *Asking a direct, closed-ended question* about suicidal intent to elicit specific information
"Tell me what you were feeling before you took all the pills the other night." (Using SOLER techniques of active listening.)	"I was just so angry! To think that my husband wants a divorce now that he has a good job. I worked hard to put him through college." (Fists clenched. Face and neck reddened.)	Beginning to feel more comfortable. She seems willing to talk, and I think she trusts me.	***Therapeutic:*** *Exploring.* Delving further into patient's feelings to help patient better understand her experience
"You wanted to hurt him because you felt betrayed." (SOLER)	"Yes! If I died, maybe he'd realize that he loved me more than that other woman." (Tears starting to well up in her eyes.)	Starting to feel sorry for her.	***Therapeutic:*** *Attempting to translate words into feelings* to convey active listening
"Seems like a pretty drastic way to get your point across." (Small frown.)	"I know. It was a stupid thing to do." (Wiping eyes.)	Trying hard to remain objective.	***Nontherapeutic:*** Sounds disapproving. Better to have focused on the patient's feelings such as "How are you feeling about that now?"
"How are you feeling about the situation now?" (SOLER)	"I don't know. I still love him. I want him to come home. I don't want him to marry her." (Starting to cry again.)	Wishing there was an easy way to help relieve some of her pain.	***Therapeutic:*** *Focusing* on her current feelings to assess current mental status
"Yes, I can understand that you would like things to be the way they were before." (Offer patient a tissue.)	(Silence. Continues to cry softly.)	I'm starting to feel some anger toward her husband. Sometimes it's so hard to remain objective!	***Therapeutic:*** *Conveying empathy* to support caring and connectedness
"What do you think are the chances of your getting back together?" (SOLER)	"None. He's refused marriage counseling. He's already moved in with her. He says it's over." (Wipes tears. Looks directly at nurse.)	Relieved to know that she isn't using denial about the reality of the situation.	***Therapeutic:*** *Reflecting* on the patient's expressed desires to encourage her to recognize and clarify her perceptions
"So how are you preparing to deal with this inevitable outcome?" (SOLER)	"I'm going to do the things we talked about: join a divorced women's support group; increase my job hours to full-time; do some volunteer work; and call the suicide hotline if I feel like taking pills again." (Looks directly at nurse. Smiles.)	Positive feeling to know that she remembers what we discussed earlier and plans to follow through.	***Therapeutic:*** *Formulating a plan of action* to set the foundation for problem-solving
"It won't be easy. But you have come a long way, and you've gained strength in your ability to cope." (Standing. Looking at patient. Smiling.)	"Yes, I know I will have hard times. But I also know I have support, and I want to go on with my life and be happy again." (Standing, smiling at nurse.)	Feeling confident that the session has gone well; hopeful that she will succeed in what she wants to do with her life.	***Therapeutic:*** *Presenting reality, making observations, and giving recognition* to support her progress in problem-solving

- ***Feedback should impart information rather than offer advice.*** Giving advice fosters dependence and may convey the patient a message of not being capable of making decisions and solving problems independently. It is the patient's right and privilege to be as self-sufficient as possible.

> *Imparting information:* "There are various methods of assistance for people who want to lose weight, such as Overeaters Anonymous, Weight Watchers, regular visits to a dietitian, and the Physician's Weight Loss Program. You can decide what is best for you."
>
> *Giving advice:* "You obviously need to lose a great deal of weight. I think the Physician's Weight Loss Program would be best for you."

- ***Feedback should be well timed.*** Feedback is most useful when given at the earliest appropriate opportunity following the specific behavior.

> *Prompt response:* "I saw you hit the wall with your fist just now when you hung up the phone from talking to your mother."
>
> *Delayed response:* "You need to learn some more appropriate ways of dealing with your anger. Last week after group I saw you pounding your fist against the wall."

Summary and Key Points

- Nurses who work in the psychiatric mental health field use special skills of relationship development and therapeutic communication to assist patients in adapting to difficulties or changes in life experiences.
- Therapeutic nurse-patient relationships are goal oriented. Ideally, the goal is mutually agreed on by the nurse and patient and is directed at learning and growth promotion.
- The instrument of delivery for the process of interpersonal nursing is the therapeutic use of self, which requires that the nurse possess a strong sense of self-awareness and self-understanding.
- Several characteristics that enhance the achievement of a therapeutic relationship have been identified. They include rapport, trust, respect, genuineness, and empathy.
- The tasks associated with the development of a therapeutic interpersonal relationship have been categorized into four phases: pre-interaction phase, orientation (introductory) phase, working phase, and termination phase.
- Interpersonal communication is a transaction between the sender and the receiver.
- In all interpersonal transactions, both the sender and receiver bring certain pre-existing conditions to the exchange that influence both the intended message and the way in which it is interpreted. Examples of these conditions include one's value system, internalized attitudes and beliefs, culture or religion, social status, gender, background knowledge and experience, age or developmental level, and the type of environment in which the communication takes place.
- Nonverbal expression is a primary component of communication in which meaning is assigned to various gestures and patterns of behavior.
- Some components of nonverbal communication include physical appearance and dress, body movement and posture, touch, facial expressions, eye behavior, and vocal cues or paralanguage. The meaning of each of these nonverbal components is culturally determined.
- Active listening is described as attentiveness to what the patient is saying through both verbal and nonverbal cues. Skills associated with active listening include **SOLER**: **S**itting **S**quarely facing the patient, maintaining an **O**pen posture, **L**eaning forward toward the patient, establishing **E**ye contact, and being **R**elaxed. The nurse must be aware of and avoid techniques that are barriers to effective communication.
- Motivational interviewing is an evidence-based, patient-centered style of communication that facilitates patients' exploration of their own motivations for behavior change and guides the patient to explore the advantages and disadvantages of their decisions.
- Process recordings are written analyses of the interaction between nurse and patient. They are used as tools for critical thinking and professional development.
- The nurse must be aware of the therapeutic or nontherapeutic value of the communication techniques used with the patient because they are the primary tools of psychosocial intervention.
- Feedback is a method of communication for helping the patient to develop self-awareness and consider modification of his or her behavior.

Review Questions

Select the answer that is most appropriate for each of the following questions:

1. Which of the following behaviors suggest a possible breach of professional boundaries? (Select all that apply.)
   a. The nurse repeatedly requests to be assigned to a specific client.
   b. The nurse shares the details of their divorce with the client.
   c. The nurse makes arrangements to meet the patient outside of the therapeutic environment.
   d. The nurse shares how they dealt with a similar difficult situation.
2. The nurse, who is an adult child of an alcoholic, is working with a client who abuses alcohol. The client has experienced a successful detoxification process and is beginning a rehabilitation program. The client says to the nurse, "I'm not going to go to those stupid AA meetings. They don't help anything." The nurse, whose father died of complications from alcoholism, responds with anger: "Don't you even care what happens to your children?" The nurse's response is an example of which of the following?
   a. Transference
   b. Countertransference
   c. Self-disclosure
   d. A breach of professional boundaries
3. When there is congruence between what is felt and what is expressed, the nurse is exhibiting which of the following characteristics?
   a. Trust
   b. Respect
   c. Genuineness
   d. Empathy
4. A client says to the nurse, "I've been offered a promotion, but I don't know if I can handle it." The nurse replies, "The thought of this promotion seems overwhelming." This is an example of which therapeutic technique?
   a. Restating
   b. Making observations
   c. Focusing
   d. Verbalizing the implied
5. A client who has been in rehabilitation for alcohol dependence returns from a visit to their home and tells the nurse, "We were having a celebration and I did have one drink, but it really wasn't a problem." The nurse notices that his breath smells of alcohol. Which of the following responses by the nurse demonstrates a motivational interviewing style of communication?
   a. "You are obviously not motivated to change, so perhaps we should discuss your discharge from the treatment program."
   b. "You need to abstain from alcohol in order to recover, so let me talk to the doctor about the consequences of your behavior."
   c. "Why would you destroy everything you've worked so hard to achieve?"
   d. "What do you mean when you say, 'It really wasn't a problem'?"

Clinical Judgment Questions

6. A client with schizophrenia appears very watchful of others and tells the nurse, "There are infiltrators everywhere and I think they are trying to kill me." Which of these actions by the nurse would best promote development of trust with this client?
   a. Touch the client's shoulder and state, "I want you to feel safe here."
   b. State to the client, "I'm interested in hearing your thoughts. Would you like to talk more about this?"
   c. Ask the client, "Why would you think such a thing?"
   d. Tell the client, "It is an expectation that we will not talk about things that aren't real."
7. A client is being discharged from the inpatient psychiatric unit and states to their primary nurse, "Everyone abandons me and now you're probably going to abandon me, too." Which of these actions by the nurse best accomplishes termination of the therapeutic relationship?
   a. Discuss the boundaries of this relationship and assist the client to explore their feelings.
   b. Terminate the therapeutic relationship while exploring ways to remain connected as friends.
   c. Provide discharge medication instructions and encourage the client to follow up with their physician.
   d. Assure the client that they are not being abandoned and remind the client that they can return to the unit in the future.
8. A client who is being discharged from an inpatient hospital stay has their wife bring a box of chocolates and a bouquet of flowers for the client's primary nurse. The client presents these gifts to the nurse, saying, "Thank you for taking care of me." What is the most appropriate response by the nurse?
   a. "I don't accept gifts from patients."
   b. "Thank you so much! It is so nice to be appreciated."
   c. "Thank you. I will share these with the rest of the staff."
   d. "Hospital policy forbids me to accept any positive feedback from patients."
9. A client was involved in an automobile accident while under the influence of alcohol. The client swerved their car into a tree and narrowly missed hitting a child on a bicycle. The client is in the hospital with multiple abrasions and contusions. They are talking about the accident with the nurse. Which of the following statements by the nurse is most appropriate?
   a. "Now that you know what can happen when you drink and drive, I'm sure you won't let it happen again."
   b. "You know that was a terrible thing you did. That child could have been killed."
   c. "I'm sure everything is going to be okay now that you understand the possible consequences of such behavior."
   d. "How are you feeling about what happened?"
10. A client, who has been in the hospital for 3 weeks, has used Valium "to settle their nerves" for the past 15 years. The client was admitted by their psychiatrist for safe withdrawal from the drug. They have passed the physical symptoms of withdrawal at this time but states to the nurse, "I don't know if I will be able to make it without Valium after I go home. I'm already starting to feel nervous. I have so many personal problems." Which is the most appropriate response by the nurse?
    a. "Why do you think you need drugs to deal with your problems?"
    b. "Everybody has problems, but not everybody uses drugs to deal with them. You'll just have to do the best that you can."
    c. "Let's explore some things you can do to decrease your anxiety without resorting to drugs."
    d. "Just hang in there. I'm sure everything is going to be okay."

Continued

11. A client asks the nurse, "Do you think I should tell my husband about my affair with my boss?" Which is the most appropriate response by the nurse?
    a. "What do you think would be best for you to do?"
    b. "Of course you should. Marriage has to be based on truth."
    c. "Of course not. That would only make things worse."
    d. "I can't tell you what to do. You have to decide for yourself."
12. An adolescent who has just returned from group therapy is crying. The client says to the nurse, "All the other kids laughed at me! I try to fit in, but I always seem to say the wrong thing. I've never had a close friend and I guess I never will." Which is the most therapeutic response by the nurse?
    a. "What makes you think you will never have any friends?"
    b. "You're feeling pretty down on yourself right now."
    c. "I'm sure they didn't mean to hurt your feelings."
    d. "Why do you feel this way about yourself?"

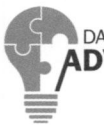

Go to **Davis Advantage** to complete your learning: strengthen understanding, apply your knowledge, and prepare for the Next Gen NCLEX®.

References

British Columbia College of Professional Nurses. (2019). *Boundaries in the nurse-client relationship practice standard.* https://www.bccnp.ca/Glossary/Pages/boundaries.aspx

Cherry, K. (2019). Understanding body language and facial expressions. https://www.verywellmind.com/understand-body-language-and-facial-expressions-4147228

Engard, B. (2018). *17 therapeutic communication techniques.* https://online.rivier.edu/therapeutic-communication-techniques/

Hall, J. A., Coats, E. J., & Smith LeBeau, L. (2005). Nonverbal behavior and the vertical dimension of social relations: A meta-analysis. *Psychological Bulletin, 131,* 898–924.

Heathfield, S. M. (2019). *How to understand your coworkers' nonverbal communication.* https://www.thebalancecareers.com/tips-for-understanding-nonverbalcommunication-1918459

Hilz, L. M. (2013). Transference and countertransference. *Kathi's Mental Health Review.* http://www.toddlertime.com/mh/terms/countertransference-transference-3.htm

Institute of Medicine, Board on Health Care Services and Committee on the Health Professions Education Summit. (2003). *Health professions education: A bridge to quality.* National Academies Press.

Knapp, M. L., & Hall, J. A. (2014). *Nonverbal communication in human interaction* (8th ed.). Wadsworth.

National Council of State Boards of Nursing. (2018). *A nurse's guide to professional boundaries.* https://www.ncsbn.org/Professional Boundaries_Complete.pdf

Pie, R. W. (2012). The patient gift conundrum. *Medscape Psychiatric and Mental Health.* http://www.medscape.com/viewarticle/775575

Raskin, N. J., Rogers, C. R., & Witty, M. C. (2014). Client-centered therapy. In D. Wedding & R. J. Corsini (Eds.), *Current psychotherapies* (10th ed., pp. 95–145). Brooks/Cole.

Regoeczi, W. C. (2002). The impact of density: The importance of nonlinearity and selection on flight and fight responses. *Social Forces, 81*(2), 505–530.

Rubak, S., Sandbaek, A., Lauritzen, T., & Christensen, B. (2005). Motivational interviewing: A systematic review and meta-analysis. *The British Journal of General Practice: The Journal of the Royal College of General Practitioners, 55*(513), 305–312.

Simon, M. (2005). *Facial expressions: A visual reference for artists.* Watson-Guptill.

Valamis. (2021). *Gender differences in communication.* https://www.valamis.com/hub/gender-differences-in-communication

Classical References

Coltrane, F., & Pugh, C. (1978). Danger signals in staff/patient relationships. *Journal of Psychiatric Nursing & Mental Health Services, 16*(6), 34–36.

Hall, E. T. (1966). *The hidden dimension.* Doubleday.

Hays, J. S., & Larson, K. H. (1963). *Interacting with patients.* Macmillan.

Peplau, H. E. (1952). *Interpersonal relations in nursing.* G.P. Putnam.

Peplau, H. E. (1962). Interpersonal techniques: The crux of psychiatric nursing. *American Journal of Nursing, 62*(6), 50–54.

Peplau, H. (1991). *Interpersonal relations in nursing: A conceptual frame of reference for psychodynamic nursing.* Springer.

Reece, M., & Whitman, R. (1962). Expressive movements, warmth, and verbal reinforcement. *Journal of Abnormal and Social Psychology, 64*(3), 234–236.

Ridgeway, C. L., Berger, J., & Smith, L. (1985). Nonverbal cues and status: An expectation states approach. *American Journal of Sociology, 90,* 955–978.

Sullivan, H. S. (1953). *The interpersonal theory of psychiatry.* Norton.

Sullivan, H. S. (1954). *The psychiatric interview.* Norton.

Travelbee, J. (1971). *Interpersonal aspects of nursing* (2nd ed.). F.A. Davis.

The Nursing Process in Psychiatric Mental Health Nursing 6

CHAPTER OUTLINE

Objectives
Introduction
The Nursing Process
Why Nursing Diagnosis?
Nursing Case Management
Applying the Nursing Process in the Psychiatric Setting
Concept Mapping
Documentation of the Nursing Process
Summary and Key Points
Review Questions
Clinical Judgment Questions

CORE CONCEPTS

Professionalism: The nursing process
Assessment
Nursing Diagnosis
Outcomes
Planning
Implementation
Evaluation
Clinical Judgment

KEY TERMS

assessment
case management
case manager
concept mapping
critical pathways of care (CPCs)
evaluation
Focus Charting
implementation
interdisciplinary
managed care
nursing diagnosis
Nursing Interventions Classification (NIC)
Nursing Outcomes Classification (NOC)
nursing process
outcomes
planning
PIE charting
problem-oriented recording

OBJECTIVES

After reading this chapter, the student will be able to:

1. Define the nursing process.
2. Identify six steps of the nursing process and describe nursing actions associated with each.
3. Describe the benefits of using nursing diagnoses.
4. Discuss the list of nursing diagnoses approved by NANDA International for clinical use and testing.
5. Define and discuss the use of case management and critical pathways of care in the clinical setting.
6. Apply the six steps of the nursing process in the care of a patient in the psychiatric setting.
7. Document patient care that validates use of the nursing process.

Introduction

For many years, the **nursing process** has provided a systematic framework for the delivery of nursing care. It is nursing's means of fulfilling the requirement for a *scientific methodology* in order to be considered a profession.

This chapter examines the steps of the nursing process as they are set forth by the American Nurses Association (ANA) in *Nursing: Scope and Standards of Practice* (ANA, 2021). The landmark Institute of Medicine report (2003) identifies six critical areas of focus (patient-centered care, safety, teamwork and collaboration, evidence-based practice, informatics, and quality improvement) that are needed to shape the future and improve quality of health care. The six critical areas are incorporated as an important model for implementing nursing care. These have become known as Quality and Safety Education for Nurses (QSEN) competencies (Cronenwett et al., 2007). An explanation is provided for the implementation of case management and the critical pathways tool used in the delivery of care with this methodology. A description of concept mapping is included, and documentation that validates the use of the nursing process is discussed.

The Nursing Process

Definition

The **nursing process** consists of six steps (Fig. 6–1) and uses a problem-solving approach that has come to be accepted as nursing's scientific methodology.

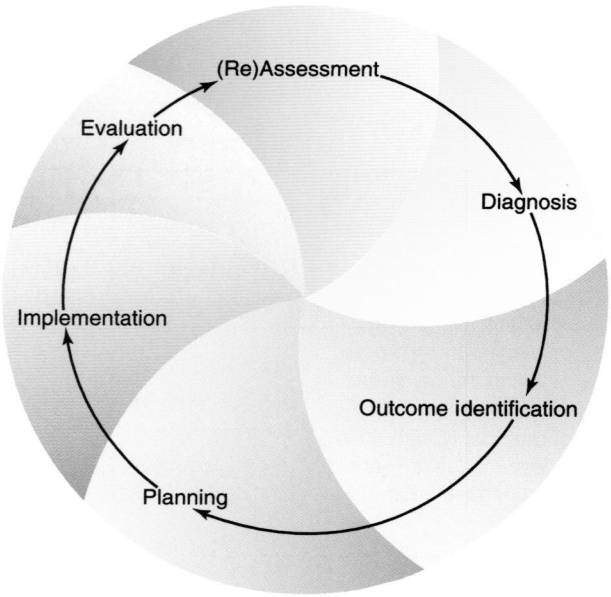

FIGURE 6–1 The ongoing nursing process.

It is goal directed with the objective being delivery of quality patient care.

The nursing process is dynamic, not static. It is an ongoing process that continues for as long as the nurse and patient have interactions directed toward change in the patient's physical or behavioral responses. Figure 6–1 presents a schematic of the ongoing nursing process.

Standards of Practice

The American Psychiatric Nurses Association (APNA) and the International Society of Psychiatric-Mental Health Nurses (ISPN) have delineated a set of standards that psychiatric nurses are expected to follow as they provide care for their patients (APNA & ISPN, 2021). The ANA (2021) describes a *standard of practice* as an authoritative statement that is defined and promoted by the profession and that provides the foundation for evaluating quality of nursing practice. The nursing process is a critical-thinking model that integrates professional standards of practice to assess, diagnose, identify outcomes, plan, implement, and evaluate nursing care.

Following are the standards of practice for psychiatric mental health nurses as set forth by the APNA and ISPN related to the steps of the nursing process (2014).

Counseling interventions (performed by the psychiatric mental health registered nurse) are differentiated from psychotherapy (performed by the psychiatric mental health *advanced practice* registered nurse) and are used to assist patients in their "individual recovery journeys" (ANA, APNA, & ISPN, 2014). This language supports the recovery model of intervention, which is a current trend toward focusing intervention on a collaborative recovery process rather than on health-care provider–prescribed treatment alone. (See Chapter 10, "The Recovery Model," for more information.)

Standard 1. Assessment

The Psychiatric–Mental Health Registered Nurse collects and synthesizes comprehensive health data that are pertinent to the healthcare consumer's health and/or situation (ANA, APNA, & ISPN, 2014, p. 44).

In this first step, information is gathered from which to establish a database for determining the best possible care for patients. Information for this database is gathered from a variety of sources, including interviews with patients and/or family, observation of patients and their environments, consultation with other health team members, review of patient records, and a nursing physical examination. A biopsychosocial assessment tool based on the stress-adaptation framework is included in Box 6–1.

CORE CONCEPT

Assessment

Assessment is a systematic, dynamic process by which the registered nurse, through interaction with the patient, family, groups, communities, populations, and health-care providers, collects and analyzes data. Assessment may include the following dimensions: physical, psychological, sociocultural, spiritual, cognitive, functional abilities, developmental, economic, and lifestyle (ANA, APNA, & ISPN, 2014, p. 87).

An example of a simple and quick mental status evaluation is presented in Table 6–1. Sometimes the term *mental status assessment* is used to describe an assessment strictly of the cognitive aspects of functioning. This is the case with tools such as Folstein's Mini-Mental status evaluation (Folstein et al., 1975). Likewise, the tool in Table 6–1 focuses solely on a brief assessment of cognitive aspects of mental functioning. In psychiatry and psychiatric mental health nursing, mental status assessment assumes a much broader definition and includes assessment of mood,

Text continued on page 133

BOX 6–1 Nursing History and Assessment Tool

I. General Information

Patient name: _____ Allergies: _____

Room number: _____ Diet: _____

Doctor: _____ Height/weight: _____

Age: _____ Vital signs: TPR/BP _____

Sex: _____ Name and phone no. of significant other: _____

Race: _____

Dominant language: _____ City of residence: _____

Marital status: _____ Diagnosis (admitting & current): _____

Chief complaint: _____

_____

Conditions of admission: _____

Date: _____ Time: _____

Accompanied by: _____

Route of admission (wheelchair; ambulatory; cart): _____

Admitted from: _____

II. Predisposing Factors

A. *Genetic Influences*

1. Family configuration (use genograms):

   Family of origin: Present family:

   Family dynamics (describe significant relationships between family members): _____

   _____

   _____

2. Medical/psychiatric history:

   a. Patient: _____

   _____

   _____

   b. Family members: _____

   _____

   _____

3. Other genetic influences affecting present adaptation. This might include effects specific to gender, race, appearance, such as genetic physical defects, or any other factor related to genetics that is affecting the patient's adaptation that has not been mentioned elsewhere in this assessment.

   _____

   _____

Continued

BOX 6–1 Nursing History and Assessment Tool—cont'd

B. *Past Experiences*
1. Cultural and social history:
   a. Environmental factors (family living arrangements, type of neighborhood, special working conditions): _____
   b. Health beliefs and practices (personal responsibility for health; special self-care practices): _____
   c. Religious beliefs and practices: _____
   d. Educational background: _____
   e. Significant losses/changes (include dates): _____
   f. Peer/friendship relationships: _____
   g. Occupational history: _____
   h. Previous pattern of coping with stress: _____
   i. Other lifestyle factors contributing to present adaptation: _____

C. *Existing Conditions*
1. Stage of development (Erikson):
   a. Theoretically: _____
   b. Behaviorally: _____
   c. Rationale: _____
2. Support systems: _____
3. Economic security: _____
4. Avenues of productivity/contribution:
   a. Current job status: _____
   b. Role contributions and responsibility for others: _____

III. Precipitating Event
Describe the situation or events that precipitated this illness/hospitalization: _____

BOX 6–1 Nursing History and Assessment Tool—cont'd

IV. Patient's Perception of the Stressor
Patient's or family member's understanding or description of stressor/illness and expectations of hospitalization:
_____
_____
_____
_____

V. Adaptation Responses
A. *Psychosocial*
1. Anxiety level (circle one of the 4 levels and check the behaviors that apply):
Mild Moderate Severe Panic
calm _____ friendly _____ passive _____ alert _____ perceives environment correctly _____
cooperative _____ impaired attention _____ "jittery" _____ unable to concentrate _____
hypervigilant _____ tremors _____ rapid speech _____ withdrawn _____ confused _____
disoriented _____ fearful _____ hyperventilating _____ misinterpreting the environment
(hallucinations or delusions) _____ depersonalization _____ obsessions _____ compulsions _____
somatic complaints _____ excessive hyperactivity _____ other _____

Judgment: Intact _____ Impaired _____
Associated behaviors: _____
Insight: Intact: _____ Impaired _____
Associated patient statements: _____

2. Mood/affect (circle as many as apply):
happiness sadness dejection despair elation euphoria suspiciousness apathy (little emotional tone)
anger/hostility

3. Level of self-esteem (circle one): low moderate high
Things patient likes about self _____
_____
Things patient would like to change about self _____
_____
Objective assessment of self-esteem:
Eye contact _____
General appearance _____
_____
Personal hygiene _____
_____
Participation in group activities and interactions with others _____
_____

4. Stage and manifestations of grief (circle one):
Denial Anger Bargaining Depression Acceptance
Describe the patient's behaviors and communication that are associated with this stage of grieving in response to loss or change.
_____
_____
_____

5. Thought processes (circle as many as apply): clear logical easy to follow relevant confused blocking delusional rapid flow of thoughts slowness in thought suspicious

6. Memory
Recent memory (circle one): loss intact
Remote memory (circle one): loss intact
Other: _____
_____

Continued

BOX 6–1 Nursing History and Assessment Tool—cont'd

7. Communication patterns (circle as many as apply):
   clear coherent slurred speech incoherent
   neologisms loose associations flight of ideas aphasic perseveration rumination
   tangential speech loquaciousness slow, impoverished speech,
   speech impediment (describe) _____
   Other _____
   _____

8. Interaction patterns (describe patient's pattern of interpersonal interactions with staff and peers on the unit, e.g., manipulative, withdrawn, isolated, verbally or physically hostile, argumentative, passive, assertive, aggressive, passive-aggressive, other): _____
   _____
   _____
   _____

9. Reality orientation (check those that apply):
   Oriented to: Time _____ Person _____
   Place _____ Situation _____

10. Ideas of destruction to self/others? Yes No
    If yes, consider plan; available means _____
    _____

11. Nonsuicidal intent to self-injury? Yes No

12. Intent to die? Yes No
    If yes, consider plan; available means: _____
    _____
    _____
    _____

13. Previous history of ideation and/or attempts (describe) _____

14. Intensity of current ideation (if present) _____

15. Other risk factors _____

16. Other warning signs _____

B. *Physiological*

1. Psychosomatic manifestations (describe any somatic complaints that may be stress-related):
   _____
   _____
   _____

2. Drug history and assessment:
   Use of prescribed drugs:

Name	Dosage	Prescribed for	Results

   Use of over-the-counter drugs:

Name	Dosage	Used for	Results

BOX 6–1 Nursing History and Assessment Tool—cont'd

Medication Side Effects:
What symptoms is the client experiencing that may be attributed to current medication usage? _____

Use of street drugs or alcohol:

Name	Amount Used	How Often Used	When Last Used	Effects Produced

3. Pertinent physical assessments:
   a. Respirations: normal _____ labored _____
      Rate _____ Rhythm _____
   b. Skin: warm _____ dry _____ moist _____ cool _____ clammy _____ pink _____
      cyanotic _____ poor turgor _____ edematous _____
      Evidence of: rash _____ bruising _____ needle tracks _____ hirsutism _____
      loss of hair _____ other _____
   c. Musculoskeletal status: weakness _____ tremors _____
      Degree of range of motion (describe limitations) _____
      Pain (describe) _____
      Skeletal deformities (describe) _____
      Coordination (describe limitations) _____
   d. Neurological status:
      History of (check all that apply): seizures _____ (describe method of control) _____
      headaches (describe location and frequency) _____
      fainting spells _____ dizziness _____
      tingling/numbness (describe location) _____
   e. Cardiovascular: B/P _____ Pulse _____
      History of (check all that apply):
      hypertension _____ palpitations _____
      heart murmur _____ chest pain _____
      shortness of breath _____ pain in legs _____
      phlebitis _____ ankle/leg edema _____
      numbness/tingling in extremities _____
      varicose veins _____
   f. Gastrointestinal:
      Usual diet pattern: _____
      Food allergies: _____
      Dentures? Upper _____ Lower _____
      Any problems with chewing or swallowing? _____
      Any recent change in weight? _____
      Any problems with: _____
      Indigestion/heartburn? _____
         Relieved by _____
      Nausea/vomiting? _____
         Relieved by _____
      History of ulcers? _____

Continued

BOX 6–1 Nursing History and Assessment Tool—cont'd

Usual bowel pattern _____

Constipation? _____ Diarrhea? _____

Type of self-care assistance provided for either of the above problems _____

_____

g. Genitourinary/Reproductive:

Usual voiding pattern _____

Urinary hesitancy? _____ Frequency? _____

Nocturia? _____ Pain/burning? _____

Incontinence? _____

Any genital lesions? _____

Discharge? _____ Odor? _____

History of sexually transmitted disease? _____

If yes, please explain: _____

_____

Any concerns about sexuality/sexual activity? _____

_____

Method of birth control used _____

Females:

Date of last menstrual cycle _____

Length of cycle _____

Problems associated with menstruation? _____

_____

Breasts: Pain/tenderness?

Swelling? _____ Discharge? _____

Lumps? _____ Dimpling? _____

Practice breast self-examination? _____

Frequency? _____

Males:

Penile discharge? _____

Prostate problems? _____

h. Eyes:

	Yes	No	Explain
Glasses?	_____	_____	_____
Contacts?	_____	_____	_____
Swelling?	_____	_____	_____
Discharge?	_____	_____	_____
Itching?	_____	_____	_____
Blurring?	_____	_____	_____
Double vision?	_____	_____	_____

i. Ears

	Yes	No	Explain
Pain?	_____	_____	_____
Drainage?	_____	_____	_____
Difficulty hearing?	_____	_____	_____
Hearing aid?	_____	_____	_____
Tinnitus?	_____	_____	_____

j. Altered lab values and possible significance:

_____

_____

BOX 6–1 Nursing History and Assessment Tool—cont'd

k. Activity/rest patterns:
Exercise (amount, type, frequency) _____
_____
Leisure time activities: _____
_____
Patterns of sleep: Number of hours per night _____
Use of sleep aids? _____
Pattern of awakening during the night? _____
_____
Feel rested upon awakening? _____

l. Personal hygiene/activities of daily living:
Patterns of self-care: independent _____
Requires assistance with:
mobility _____
hygiene _____
toileting _____
feeding _____
dressing _____
other _____
Statement describing personal hygiene and general appearance _____
_____
_____

m. Other pertinent physical assessments: _____
_____
_____

VI. Summary of Initial Psychosocial/Physical Assessment:

Knowledge Deficits Identified:

Nursing Diagnoses Indicated:

affect, behavior, relationships, speech, perceptual disturbances, insight, and judgment in addition to an assessment of cognitive functioning. A comprehensive mental status assessment guide, with explanations and selected sample interview questions, is provided in Appendix A, "Mental Status Assessment."

CORE CONCEPT

Nursing Diagnosis

A **nursing diagnosis** involves clinical judgments concerning human responses to health conditions and life processes, or susceptibility to responses, that are recognized in an individual, caregiver, family, group, or community. It also provides the basis for selection of nursing interventions to achieve outcomes for which the nurse has accountability (Herdman et al., 2021).

Standard 2. Diagnosis

The Psychiatric–Mental Health Registered Nurse analyzes the assessment data to determine diagnoses, problems, and areas of focus for care and treatment, including level of risk (ANA, APNA, & ISPN, 2014, p. 46).

In the second step, data gathered during the assessment are analyzed. Diagnoses and potential problem statements are formulated and prioritized. Diagnoses are congruent with available and accepted classification systems.

Standard 3. Outcomes Identification

The Psychiatric–Mental Health Registered Nurse identifies expected outcomes and the healthcare consumer's goals and develops a plan individualized to the healthcare consumer or to the situation (ANA, APNA, & ISPN, 2014, p. 48).

TABLE 6–1 Brief Mental Status Evaluation

AREA OF MENTAL FUNCTION EVALUATED	EVALUATION ACTIVITY
Orientation to time	"What year is it? What month is it? What day is it?" (3 points)
Orientation to place	"Where are you now?" (1 point)
Attention and immediate recall	"Repeat these words now: bell, book, and candle." (3 points) "Remember these words, and I will ask you to repeat them in a few minutes."
Abstract thinking	"What does this mean: No use crying over spilled milk." (3 points)
Recent memory	"Say the three words I asked you to remember earlier." (3 points)
Naming objects	Point to eyeglasses and ask, "What is this?" Repeat with one other item (e.g., calendar, watch, pencil). (2 points possible)
Ability to follow simple verbal command	"Tear this piece of paper in half and put it in the trash container." (2 points)
Ability to follow simple written command	Write a command on a piece of paper (e.g., TOUCH YOUR NOSE), give the paper to the patient, and say, "Do what it says on this paper." (1 point for correct action)
Ability to use language correctly	Ask the patient to write a sentence. (3 points if sentence has a subject, a verb, and valid meaning)
Ability to concentrate	"Say the months of the year in reverse, starting with December." (1 point each for correct answers from November through August; 4 points possible)
Understanding spatial relationships	Instruct patient to draw a clock; put in all the numbers; and set the hands on 3 o'clock. (clock circle = 1 point; numbers in correct sequence = 1 point; numbers placed on clock correctly = 1 point; two hands on the clock = 1 point; hands set at correct time = 1 point) (5 points possible)

Scoring: 30–21 = normal; 20–11 = mild cognitive impairment; 10–0 = severe cognitive impairment. (Scores are not absolute and must be considered within the comprehensive diagnostic assessment.)
Source: Compiled from Folstein, M. F., Folstein, S. E., & McHugh, P. R. (1975). Mini-mental state: A practical method for grading the cognitive state of patients for the clinician. *Journal of Psychiatric Research, 12*(3), 189–198; Kaufman, D. M., & Zun, L. (1995). A quantifiable, brief mental status examination for emergency patients. *Journal of Emergency Medicine, 13*(4), 440–456; Kokman, E., Smith, G. E., Petersen, R. C., Tangalos, E., & Ivnik, R. C. (1991). The short test of mental status: Correlations with standardized psychometric testing. *Archives of Neurology, 48*(7), 725–728; Pfeiffer, E. (1975). A short portable mental status questionnaire for the assessment of organic brain deficit in elderly patients. *Journal of the American Geriatric Society, 23*(10), 433–441.

CORE CONCEPT

Outcomes

Outcomes are patient behaviors and responses that are collaboratively agreed upon, measurable, desired results of nursing interventions.

Expected outcomes are derived from the diagnosis. They must be measurable and include a time estimate for attainment. They must be realistic for the patient's capabilities and are most effective when formulated cooperatively by the interdisciplinary team members, the patient, and significant others.

Nursing Outcomes Classification (NOC)

The **Nursing Outcomes Classification (NOC)** is a comprehensive, standardized classification of patient outcomes developed to evaluate the effects of nursing interventions (Moorhead et al., 2018). The outcomes have been linked to NANDA International (NANDA-I) nursing diagnoses and to the **Nursing Interventions Classification (NIC).** NANDA-I, NIC, and NOC represent all domains of nursing and can be used together or separately (Moorhead & Dochterman, 2012). Each of the NOC outcomes has a label name, a definition, a list of indicators to evaluate patient status in relation to the outcome, and a five-point Likert scale to measure patient status (Moorhead et al., 2018).

CORE CONCEPT

Planning

Planning involves selection of nursing interventions directed toward helping the patient achieve identified outcomes.

Standard 4. Planning

The Psychiatric–Mental Health Registered Nurse develops a plan that prescribes strategies and alternatives to assist the healthcare consumer in attainment of expected outcomes (ANA, APNA, & ISPN, 2014, p. 50).

The care plan is individualized to address the mental health problems, condition, or needs of the patient and is developed in collaboration with the patient, significant others, and interdisciplinary team members if possible. For each diagnosis identified, the most appropriate interventions, based on current psychiatric mental health nursing practice, standards, relevant statutes, and research evidence, are selected. Patient education and necessary referrals are included. Thorough and ongoing assessment is an important intervention to ensure that referrals are appropriate and timely. Priorities for delivery of nursing care are determined on the basis of physiological safety needs and risk for harm to self or others.

Nursing Interventions Classification (NIC)

NIC is a comprehensive, standardized language describing treatments that nurses perform in all settings and in all specialties (Butcher et al., 2019). NIC includes both physiological and psychosocial interventions as well as interventions for illness treatment, illness prevention, and health promotion. NIC interventions are comprehensive, based on research, and reflect current clinical practice. They were developed inductively on the basis of existing practice.

Each NIC intervention has a definition and a detailed set of activities that describe what a nurse does to implement the intervention. The use of a standardized language is thought to enhance continuity of care and facilitate communication among nurses and between nurses and other providers.

CORE CONCEPT

Implementation

Implementation is the execution of identified nursing interventions.

Standard 5. Implementation

The Psychiatric–Mental Health Registered Nurse implements the identified plan (ANA, APNA, & ISPN, 2014, p. 52).

Interventions selected during the planning stage are executed, taking into consideration the nurse's level of practice, education, and certification. The care plan serves as a blueprint for delivery of safe, ethical, and appropriate interventions. Documentation of interventions also occurs at this step in the nursing process.

Several specific interventions, described in standards 5A through 5H, are included in the standards of psychiatric mental health clinical nursing practice (APNA & ISPN, 2021).

Standard 5A. Coordination of Care

The Psychiatric–Mental Health Registered Nurse coordinates care delivery (ANA, APNA, & ISPN, 2014, p. 54).

One of the QSEN competencies, teamwork and collaboration, is related to this ANA standard of practice. In order for the nurse to coordinate care, it is critical that they understand the roles of other healthcare team members and develop strategies for effectively collaborating to meet the patient's needs.

Standard 5B. Health Teaching and Health Promotion

The Psychiatric–Mental Health Registered Nurse employs strategies to promote health and a safe environment (ANA, APNA, & ISPN, 2014, p. 55).

For the psychiatric patient, this often includes education about medications and strategies to manage side effects. It may also include teaching and health promotion from a recovery-oriented approach so that the patient has information about various treatment options and available community resources.

Standard 5C. Consultation

The Psychiatric–Mental Health Advanced Practice Registered Nurse provides consultation to influence the identified plan, enhance the abilities of other clinicians to provide services for healthcare consumers, and effect change (APNA & ISPN, 2021, p. 57).

Standard 5D. Prescriptive Authority and Treatment

The Psychiatric–Mental Health Advanced Practice Registered Nurse uses prescriptive authority, procedures, referrals, treatments, and therapies in accordance with state and federal laws and regulations (ANA, APNA, & ISPN, 2014, p. 58).

Standard 5E. Pharmacological, Biological, and Integrative Therapies

The Psychiatric–Mental Health Registered Nurse incorporates knowledge of pharmacological, biological, and complementary interventions with applied clinical skills to restore the healthcare consumer's health and prevent further disability (ANA, APNA, & ISPN, 2014, p. 59).

Standard 5F. Milieu Therapy

The Psychiatric–Mental Health Registered Nurse provides, structures, and maintains a safe, therapeutic, recovery-oriented environment in collaboration with healthcare consumers, families, and other healthcare clinicians (ANA, APNA, & ISPN, 2014, p. 60).

Several models have been developed to identify what constitutes a therapeutic environment, and these are discussed further in Chapter 7, "Psychosocial Interventions and Spiritual Care." Incorporation of the health-care environment (including the community of patients, their families, and health-care providers) is a unique aspect of treatment for the patient with a psychiatric mental health disorder.

Standard 5G. Therapeutic Relationship and Counseling

The Psychiatric–Mental Health Registered Nurse uses the therapeutic relationship and counseling interventions to assist healthcare consumers in their individual recovery journeys by improving and regaining their previous coping abilities, fostering mental health and preventing mental disorder and disability (ANA, APNA, & ISPN, 2014, p. 62).

As mentioned previously, therapeutic relationship and counseling interventions are part of the role of registered nurses practicing in psychiatric mental health settings. These are basic psychoeducational and problem discussion interventions and are differentiated from psychotherapy that requires advanced practice education and competency.

Standard 5H. Psychotherapy

The Psychiatric–Mental Health Advanced Practice Registered Nurse conducts individual, couples, group, and family psychotherapy using evidence-based psychotherapeutic frameworks and the nurse-client therapeutic relationship (ANA, APNA, & ISPN, 2014, p. 63).

CORE CONCEPT

Evaluation

Evaluation is the process of determining the patient's progress toward attainment of expected outcomes and the effectiveness of the registered nurse's interventions.

Standard 6. Evaluation

The Psychiatric–Mental Health Registered Nurse evaluates progress toward attainment of expected outcomes (ANA, APNA, & ISPN, 2014, p. 65).

During the evaluation step, the nurse measures the success of the interventions in meeting the outcome criteria. The patient's response to treatment is documented, validating use of the nursing process in the delivery of care. The diagnoses, outcomes, and plan of care are reviewed and revised as determined by the evaluation.

Why Nursing Diagnosis?

The concept of nursing diagnosis is not new. For centuries, nurses have identified specific unhealthy responses to health-care problems for which nursing interventions were used in an effort to improve the patient's quality of life. Historically, because of the limitations imposed by their licensure, nurses have lacked autonomy in the provision of care. Nurses assisted physicians as required and performed a group of specific tasks that were considered within their scope of responsibility. Formal identification of nursing diagnoses, however, affirms those aspects of nursing practice that are within their scope of practice *and* independently directed or implemented.

The term *diagnosis* in relation to nursing first began to appear in the literature in the early 1950s. The formalized organization of the concept was initiated in 1973 with the convening of the First Task Force to Name and Classify Nursing Diagnoses. The Task Force of the National Conference Group on the Classification of Nursing Diagnoses was developed during this conference. These individuals were charged with the task of identifying and classifying nursing diagnoses.

Also in the 1970s, the ANA began to write standards of practice around the steps of the nursing process, of which nursing diagnosis is an inherent part. This format encompassed both the general and specialty standards outlined by the ANA.

From this progression a statement of policy was published in 1980 and included a definition of nursing. The ANA defined *nursing* as "the diagnosis and treatment of human responses to actual or potential health problems" (ANA, 2010). This definition has been expanded to describe more appropriately nursing's commitment to society and to the profession itself. The ANA (n.d.) currently defines *nursing* as follows:

> Beyond the time-honored reputation for compassion and dedication lies a highly specialized profession, which is constantly evolving to address the

> needs of society. From ensuring the most accurate diagnoses to the ongoing education of the public about critical health issues; nurses are indispensable in safeguarding public health. . . . Through the critical thinking exemplified in the nursing process, nurses use their judgment to integrate objective data with subjective experience of a patient's biological, physical, and behavioral needs. This ensures that every patient, from city hospital to community health center; state prison to summer camp, receives the best possible care regardless of who they are, or where they may be.

A number of states have incorporated the steps of the nursing process, including nursing diagnosis, into the scope of nursing practice described in their nursing practice acts. Decisions regarding professional negligence are made on the basis of standards of practice defined by the ANA and the individual state nursing practice acts. When this is the case, it is the legal duty of the nurse to show that nursing process and nursing diagnosis were accurately implemented in the delivery of nursing care.

NANDA-I evolved from the original task force that was convened in 1973 to name and classify nursing diagnoses. The major purpose of NANDA-I is "to develop, refine and promote terminology that accurately reflects nurses' clinical judgments. . . . NANDA-I will be a global force for the development and use of nursing's standardized terminology to ensure patient safety through evidence-based care, thereby improving the health care of all people" (NANDA-I, 2021b). The list of NANDA-I-approved nursing diagnoses is by no means all-inclusive. In an effort to maintain a common language within nursing and to encourage clinical testing of what is available, most of the nursing diagnoses used in this text come from the 2021–2023 list approved by NANDA-I (Herdman et al., 2021). However, in some instances, nursing diagnoses that have been retired by NANDA-I will continue to be used because of their appropriateness and suitability in describing specific behaviors. New diagnoses continue to be researched and developed as the scope of practice and nursing care evolve.

The use of nursing diagnoses affords a degree of autonomy that historically has been lacking in the practice of nursing. A nursing diagnosis describes the patient's unhealthy or potentially unhealthy responses, facilitating the prescription of interventions and establishment of parameters for outcome criteria based on aspects of practice that are unique to nursing. The ultimate benefit is to patients who receive effective and consistent nursing care based on knowledge of the problems they are experiencing and of the most beneficial nursing interventions to resolve them.

Nursing Case Management

The concept of **case management** evolved with the advent of diagnosis-related groups (DRGs) and shorter hospital stays. Case management is a model of care delivery that can result in improved patient care. In this model, patients are assigned a manager who negotiates with multiple providers to obtain diverse services. This type of health-care delivery process serves to decrease fragmentation of care while striving to contain cost of services.

Case management in the acute care setting strives to organize patient care through an episode of illness or injury so that specific clinical and financial outcomes are achieved within an allotted time frame. Commonly, the allotted time frame is determined by the established protocols for length of stay as defined by the DRGs.

Case management has been shown to be an effective method of treatment for individuals with a severe and persistent mental illness. This type of care strives to improve functioning by assisting the individual to solve problems, improve work and socialization skills, promote leisure-time activities, and enhance overall independence.

Ideally, case management incorporates concepts of care at the primary, secondary, and tertiary levels of prevention (see Chapter 26, "Community Mental Health Nursing," for further discussion of the different levels of prevention). Various definitions have emerged and should be clarified, as follows.

Managed care refers to a strategy employed by purchasers of health services who make determinations about various types of services in order to maintain quality and control costs. In a managed care program, individuals receive health care based on need, as assessed by coordinators of the providership. Managed care exists in many settings, including (but not limited to) the following:

- Insurance-based programs
- Employer-based medical providerships
- Social service programs
- The public health sector

Managed care may exist in virtually any setting in which medical providership is a part of the service—that is, in any setting in which an organization (whether private or government based) is responsible for payment of health-care services for a group of people. Examples of managed care are health maintenance organizations (HMOs) and preferred provider organizations (PPOs).

Case management is the method used to achieve managed care. It is the actual coordination of services required to meet the needs of a patient within the fragmented health-care system. Case management strives to help at-risk patients prevent avoidable episodes of illness. Its goal is to provide these services while attempting to control health-care costs to the consumer and third-party payers.

Types of patients who benefit from case management include (but are not limited to) the following:

- The frail elderly
- Individuals with developmental disabilities
- Individuals with physical disabilities
- Individuals with severe mental disabilities
- Individuals with long-term medically complex problems that require multifaceted, costly care (e.g., high-risk infants, individuals with HIV or AIDS, and patients with transplanted organs)
- Individuals who are severely compromised by an acute episode of illness or an acute exacerbation of a severe and persistent illness (e.g., schizophrenia)

The **case manager** is responsible for negotiating with multiple health-care providers to obtain a variety of services for the patient. Nurses are exceptionally qualified to serve as case managers. The very nature of nursing, which incorporates knowledge about the biological, psychological, and sociocultural aspects related to human functioning, makes nurses highly appropriate case managers. Several years of experience as a registered nurse are usually required for employment as a case manager. Some case management programs prefer advanced practice registered nurses who have experience working with the specific populations for whom the case management service will be rendered. The American Nurses Credentialing Center (ANCC) offers an examination for nurses to become board certified in nursing case management.

Critical Pathways of Care

Critical pathways of care (CPCs) may be used as the tools for provision of care in a case management system. A critical pathway is a type of abbreviated plan of care that provides outcome-based guidelines for goal achievement within a designated length of stay. A sample CPC is presented in Table 6–2. Only one nursing diagnosis is used in this sample, but a comprehensive CPC may have nursing diagnoses for several problems and incorporates the responsibilities of other team members as well.

CPCs are intended to be used by the entire interdisciplinary team, which may include a nurse, case manager, clinical nurse specialist, social worker, psychiatrist, psychologist, dietitian, occupational therapist, recreational therapist, chaplain, and others. The team decides what categories of care are to be performed, by what date, and by whom. Each member of the team is then expected to carry out assigned functions according to the timeline designated on the CPC.

Unlike a nursing care plan, CPCs have the benefit of describing what an episode of care will look like when implemented by team members working collaboratively. Clarity about how *team members collaborate* is important not only for providing efficient patient care but also for improving *quality* and *safety*.

As a case manager, the nurse is ultimately responsible for ensuring that each of the assignments is carried out. If variations occur at any time in any of the categories of care, rationale must be documented in the progress notes. For example, with the sample CPC presented in Table 6–2, the nurse case manager may admit the patient into the detoxification center. The nurse informs the psychiatrist about the admission. The psychiatrist performs additional assessments to determine whether other consultations are required and writes the orders for the initial diagnostic work-up and medication regimen. Within 24 hours, the interdisciplinary team meets to decide on other categories of care, to complete the CPC, and to make individual care assignments from the CPC. This particular sample CPC relies heavily on nursing care of the patient through the critical withdrawal period. However, other problems for the same patient, such as imbalanced nutrition, impaired physical mobility, or spiritual distress, may involve other members of the team to a greater degree. Each member of the team stays in contact with the case manager regarding individual assignments. Ideally, team meetings are held daily or every other day to review progress and modify the plan as required.

CPCs can be standardized, as they are intended to be used with uncomplicated cases. A CPC can be viewed as protocol for patients who have specific problems for which a designated outcome can be predicted.

Applying the Nursing Process in the Psychiatric Setting

Based on the definition of *mental health* set forth in Chapter 1, "Mental Health and Mental Illness," the role of the nurse in psychiatry focuses on helping the patient successfully adapt to stressors in the

TABLE 6–2 Sample Critical Pathway of Care for Patient in Alcohol Withdrawal

Estimated Length of Stay: 7 days—variations from designated pathway should be documented in progress notes.

NURSING DIAGNOSES AND CATEGORIES OF CARE	TIME DIMENSION	GOALS AND/OR ACTIONS	TIME DIMENSION	GOALS AND/OR ACTIONS	TIME DIMENSION	DISCHARGE OUTCOME
Risk for injury related to CNS agitation					Day 7	Patient shows no evidence of injury sustained during ETOH withdrawal
Referrals	Day 1	Psychiatrist Assess need for neurologist, cardiologist, internist			Day 7	Discharge with follow-up appointments as required
Diagnostic studies	Day 1	Blood alcohol level Drug screen (urine and blood) Complete blood count with MCV Clotting screen Liver function test (with albumin and GGT) Urea/electrolytes Blood glucose Folate/B_{12}, magnesium, and phosphate levels	Day 4	Repeat of selected diagnostic studies as necessary		
Additional assessments	Day 1 Day 1–5 Ongoing	VS q4h I&O Assess withdrawal symptoms: tremors, nausea/vomiting, tachycardia, sweating, high blood pressure, seizures, insomnia, hallucinations	Day 2–3 Day 6 Day 4	VS q8h if stable DC I&O Marked decrease in objective withdrawal symptoms	Day 4–7 Day 7	VS bid; remain stable Discharge; absence of objective withdrawal symptoms
Medications	Day 1 Day 2 Day 1–6 Day 1–7	Chlordiazepoxide* 200 mg in divided doses Chlordiazepoxide 160 mg in divided doses Chlordiazepoxide prn (maximum of 250 mg total daily dose including regular and prn doses) Maalox pc & hs	Day 3 Day 4	Chlordiazepoxide 120 mg in divided doses Chlordiazepoxide 80 mg in divided doses	Day 5 Day 6 Day 7	Chlordiazepoxide 40 mg DC chlordiazepoxide Discharge; no withdrawal symptoms
Patient education			Day 5	Discuss goals of AA and need for outpatient therapy	Day 7	Discharge with information regarding AA attendance or outpatient treatment

*Some physicians may elect to use oxazepam (Serax) or carbamazepine (Tegretol) in the detoxification process.
AA, Alcoholics Anonymous; bid, twice a day; DC, discontinue; ECT, electrocardiogram; ETOH, alcohol; hs, bedtime; GGT, gamma-glutamyl transferase; I&O, intake and output; MCV, mean corpuscular volume; pc, after meals; prn, as needed; q4h, every 4 hours; q8h, every 8 hours; VS, vital signs.

environment. Goals are directed toward changes in thoughts, feelings, and behaviors that are age appropriate and congruent with local and cultural norms.

Treatment within the psychiatric setting is very often team oriented, or **interdisciplinary.** Therefore, it is important to delineate nursing's involvement in the interdisciplinary care plan. Nurses are valuable members of the team, providing services that are defined within the scope of nursing practice. Nursing diagnosis helps to define these nursing boundaries and provides a degree of autonomy and professionalism.

For example, a newly admitted patient with the medical diagnosis of schizophrenia may be demonstrating the following behaviors:

- Inability to trust others
- Verbalizing hearing voices
- Refusing to interact with staff and peers
- Expressing a fear of failure
- Poor personal hygiene

From these assessments, the treatment team may determine that the patient has the following problems:

- Paranoid delusions
- Auditory hallucinations
- Social withdrawal
- Developmental regression

Team goals would be directed toward the following:

- Reducing suspiciousness
- Minimizing or eliminating auditory hallucinations
- Increasing feelings of self-worth

From this team treatment plan, nursing may identify the following nursing diagnoses:

- Disturbed sensory perception, auditory (evidenced by hearing voices)[1]
- Disturbed thought processes (evidenced by delusions)
- Low self-esteem (evidenced by fear of failure and social withdrawal)
- Self-care deficit (evidenced by poor personal hygiene)
- Social isolation (evidenced by suspiciousness and social withdrawal)

Nursing diagnoses are prioritized according to life-threatening potential. Maslow's hierarchy of needs is a good model to follow in prioritizing nursing diagnoses. In this instance, disturbed sensory perception (auditory) is identified as the priority nursing diagnosis because the patient may be hearing voices commanding harm to self or others. Psychiatric nursing, regardless of the setting—hospital (inpatient or outpatient), office, home, community—is goal-directed care. The goals (or expected outcomes) are patient-oriented, measurable, and focused on problem resolution (if this is realistic) or on a more short-term outcome (if resolution is unrealistic). For example, in the previous situation, expected outcomes for the identified nursing diagnoses might be as follows:

The patient:

1. Demonstrates trust in one staff member within 3 days.
2. Verbalizes understanding that the voices are not real (not heard by others) within 5 days.
3. Completes one simple craft project within 5 days.
4. Takes responsibility for self-care and performs activities of daily living independently by time of discharge.

Nursing's contribution to the interdisciplinary treatment regimen will focus on establishing trust on a one-to-one basis (thus reducing the level of anxiety that may be promoting hallucinations), giving positive feedback for small day-to-day accomplishments in an effort to promote self-esteem, and assisting with and encouraging independent self-care. These interventions describe *independent nursing* actions and goals that are evaluated apart from, while also being directed toward achievement of, the *team's* treatment goals.

In this manner of collaboration with other team members, nursing provides a unique service based on sound knowledge of psychopathology, scope of practice, and legal implications of the role. Although implementing the physician's orders is acknowledged as an important aspect of nursing care, nursing interventions that enhance achievement of the overall goals of treatment are important as well. The nurse who administers a medication prescribed by the physician to decrease anxiety may also choose to stay with the anxious patient and offer reassurance of safety and security, thereby providing an independent nursing action that is distinct from, yet complementary to, the medical treatment.

Concept Mapping[2]

Concept mapping is a diagrammatic teaching and learning strategy that allows students and faculty to

[1] Disturbed sensory perception and Disturbed thought processes (see next list item) were removed from the NANDA-I list of approved nursing diagnoses in 2012. "Disturbed thought processes" has been reintroduced in the latest (2021) edition. "Disturbed sensory perception" will continue to be used in this textbook because of its appropriateness to certain symptoms.

[2] Content in this section is adapted from Doenges et al. (2019) and Schuster (2016).

visualize interrelationships between medical diagnoses, nursing diagnoses, assessment data, and treatments. The concept map is a diagram of patient problems and interventions. Compared with the commonly used care plans in a column format, concept map care plans are more visual. They primarily serve to enhance critical-thinking skills and clinical reasoning ability by creating a holistic picture of various problems and their interconnectedness to one another.

The nursing process is foundational to developing and using the concept map care plan, just as it is with all types of nursing care plans. Patient data are collected and analyzed, nursing diagnoses are formulated, outcome criteria are identified, nursing actions are planned and implemented, and the success of the interventions in meeting the outcome criteria is evaluated.

The concept map care plan may be presented in its entirety on one page, or the assessment data and nursing diagnoses may appear in diagram format on one page, with outcomes, interventions, and evaluations written on a second page. Alternatively, the diagram may appear in circular format, with nursing diagnoses and interventions branching off the "patient" in the center of the diagram. Or, it may begin with the "patient" at the top of the diagram, with branches emanating in a linear fashion downward.

Whatever format is chosen to visualize the concept map, the diagram should reflect the nursing process in a stepwise fashion, beginning with the patient and their reason for needing care, nursing diagnoses with subjective and objective clinical evidence for each, nursing interventions, and outcome criteria for evaluation.

Figure 6–2 presents one example of a concept map care plan. It is assembled for the hypothetical patient with schizophrenia discussed in the previous section, "Applying the Nursing Process in the Psychiatric Setting." Different colors may be used in the diagram to designate various components of the care plan. Connecting lines are drawn between components to indicate any relationships that exist. For example, there may be a relationship between two nursing diagnoses (e.g., between the nursing diagnoses of pain or anxiety and disturbed sleep pattern). A line between these nursing diagnoses should be drawn to show that relationship.

Concept map care plans permit viewing the "whole picture" without generating a great deal of paperwork. Because they reflect the steps of the nursing process, concept map care plans also are valuable guides for documentation of patient care. Doenges et al. (2019) note that traditional care plans fail to clarify how all of the patient's identified needs are related so the user may not develop a holistic view. The concept map clarifies those linkages. Whether these care-planning strategies are used for learning or in actual practice, both the concept map and traditional care plan are useful tools for developing and visualizing the critical-thinking process that goes into planning patient care.

The concept map can be expanded to visualize an episode of care that not only includes various patient needs and associated nursing care but also visualizes how other disciplines within the treatment team are collaborating to address those needs. In this format, the concept map informs about *teamwork and collaboration*, one of the six QSEN competencies.

Documentation of the Nursing Process

Equally important as using the nursing process in the delivery of care is documenting its use in writing. Some contemporary nursing leaders are advocating that with solid standards of practice and procedures in place within the institution, nurses need only chart when there has been a deviation in the care as outlined by that standard. This method of documentation, known as *charting by exception*, is not widely accepted because many legal decisions are still based on the precept that "if it was not charted, it was not done."

Because nursing process and nursing diagnosis are mandated by nursing practice acts in some states, documentation of their use is being considered in those states as evidence in determining certain cases of negligence by nurses. Some health-care organization accrediting agencies also require that nursing process be reflected in the delivery of care.

Types of Documentation Methods

A variety of documentation methods can be used to reflect use of the nursing process in the delivery of nursing care. Three examples are presented here: problem-oriented recording (POR); Focus Charting; and the problem, intervention, evaluation (PIE) system of documentation.

Electronic health records (EHRs) have become a primary vehicle for documentation of patient care, and many rely heavily on preset menus and checklists. However, the various methods of documentation described below remain an important model for critical thinking about the essential aspects to be included in communicating and documenting patient care. These methods can be incorporated in electronic nurses' notes when there is an opportunity or need to provide additional documentation in the EHR.

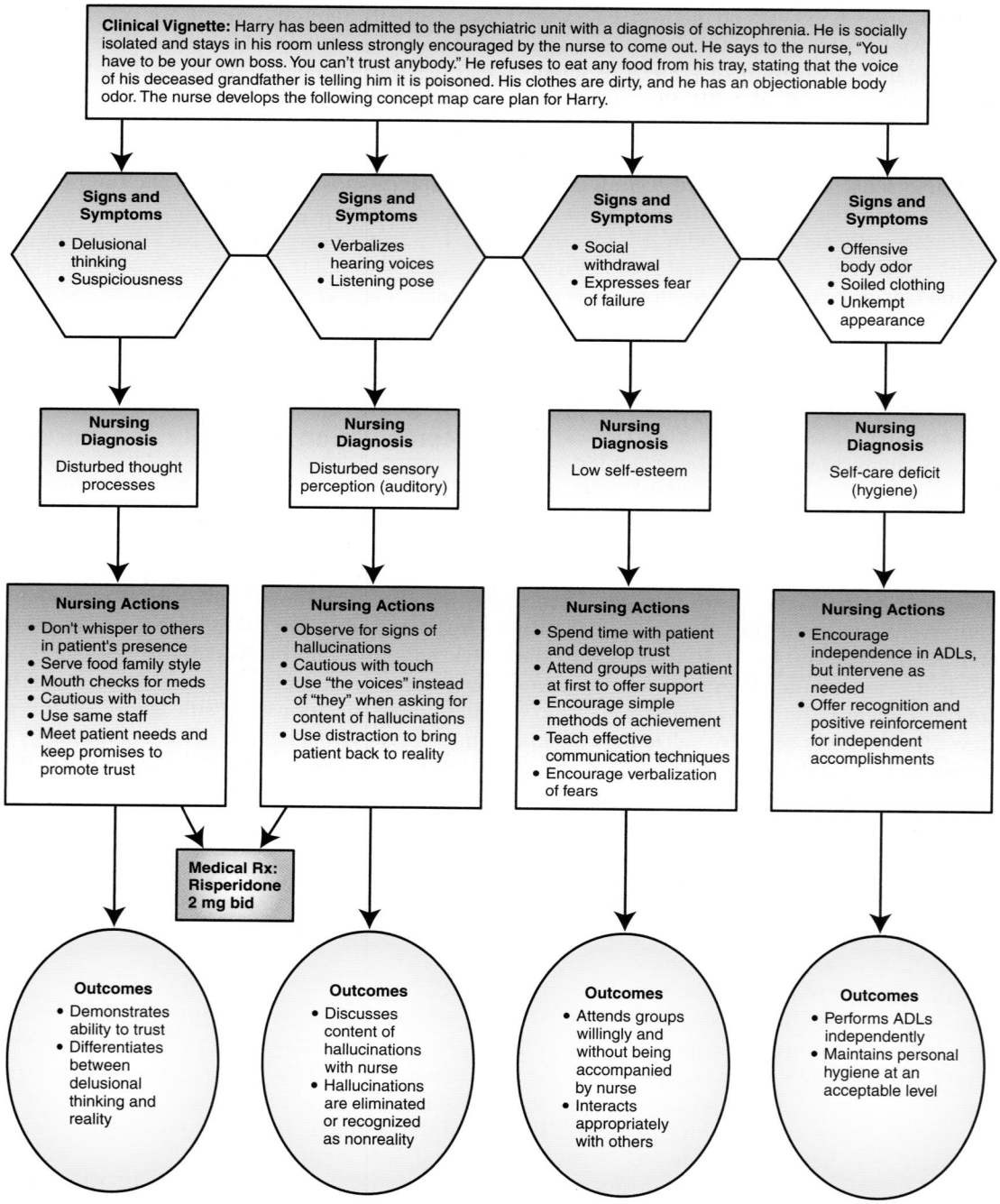

FIGURE 6–2 Example: Concept map care plan for a patient with schizophrenia.

Problem-Oriented Recording

Problem-oriented recording follows the subjective, objective, assessment, plan, implementation, and evaluation (SOAPIE) format. It has as its basis a list of problems. When it is used in nursing, the problems (nursing diagnoses) are identified on a written plan of care, with appropriate nursing interventions described for each. Documentation written in the SOAPIE format includes the following:

S = Subjective data: Information gathered from what the patient, family, or other source has said or reported.

O = Objective data: Information gathered through direct observation by the person performing the assessment; may include a physiological measurement such as blood pressure or a behavioral response such as affect.

A = Assessment: The nurse's interpretation of the subjective and objective data.

P = Plan: The actions or treatments to be carried out (may be omitted in daily charting if the plan is clearly explained in the written nursing care plan and no changes are expected).

I = Intervention: Those nursing actions that were actually carried out.

E = Evaluation: An appraisal of the problem following nursing intervention (some nursing interventions cannot be evaluated immediately, so this section may be optional).

Table 6–3 shows how problem-oriented recording corresponds to the steps of the nursing process.

The following is an example of a three-column documentation in the problem-oriented recording format.

EXAMPLE

Date/Time	Problem	Progress Notes
9-12-21 1000	Social isolation	**S:** States he does not want to sit with or talk to others; "They frighten me." **O:** Stays in room alone unless strongly encouraged to come out; no group involvement; at times listens to group conversations from a distance but does not interact; some hypervigilance and scanning noted. **A:** Inability to trust; panic level of anxiety; delusional thinking. **I:** Initiated trusting relationship by spending time alone with patient; discussed his feelings regarding interactions with others; accompanied patient to group activities; provided positive feedback for voluntarily participating in assertiveness training.

Focus Charting

Another type of documentation that reflects use of the nursing process is **Focus Charting®**. Focus Charting® differs from problem-oriented recording in that the main perspective is "focus" instead of "problem," and a data, action, and response (DAR) format replaces SOAPIE.

Lampe (1985) suggested that a focus for documentation can be any of the following:

- Nursing diagnosis
- Current patient concern or behavior
- Significant change in the patient's status or behavior
- Significant event in the patient's therapy

TABLE 6–3 Validation of the Nursing Process With Problem-Oriented Recording

PROBLEM-ORIENTED RECORDING	WHAT IS RECORDED	NURSING PROCESS
S and O (Subjective and Objective data)	Verbal reports to, and direct observation and examination by, the nurse	Assessment
A (Assessment)	Nurse's interpretation of S and O	Diagnosis and outcome identification
P (Plan) (Omitted in charting if written plan describes care to be given)	Description of appropriate nursing actions to resolve the identified problem	Planning
I (Intervention)	Description of nursing actions actually carried out	Implementation
E (Evaluation)	A reassessment of the situation to determine results of nursing actions implemented	Evaluation

TABLE 6–4 Validation of the Nursing Process With Focus Charting

FOCUS CHARTING	WHAT IS RECORDED	NURSING PROCESS
D (Data)	Information that supports the stated focus or describes pertinent observations about the patient	Assessment
Focus	A nursing diagnosis; current patient concern or behavior; significant change in patient status; significant event in the patient's therapy (*Note:* If outcome appears on written care plan, does not need to be repeated in daily documentation unless a change occurs.)	Diagnosis and outcome identification
A (Action)	Immediate or future nursing actions that address the focus; appraisal of the care plan along with any changes required	Plan and implementation
R (Response)	Description of patient responses to any part of the medical or nursing care	Evaluation

The focus cannot be a medical diagnosis. The documentation is organized in the format of DAR. These categories are defined as follows:

D = Data: Information that supports the stated focus or describes pertinent observations about the patient.

A = Action: Immediate or future nursing actions that address the focus and evaluation of the present care plan along with any changes required.

R = Response: Description of the patient's responses to any part of the medical or nursing care.

Table 6–4 shows how Focus Charting® corresponds to the steps of the nursing process.

The following is an example of a three-column documentation in the DAR format.

EXAMPLE

Date/Time	Focus	Progress Notes
9-12-21 1000	Social isolation related to mistrust, panic anxiety, delusions	**D:** States he does not want to sit with or talk to others; they "frighten" him; stays in room alone unless strongly encouraged to come out; no group involvement; at times listens to group conversations from a distance but does not interact; some hypervigilance and scanning noted. **A:** Initiated trusting relationship by spending time alone with patient; discussed his feelings regarding interactions with others; accompanied patient to group activities; provided positive feedback for voluntarily participating in assertiveness training. **R:** Cooperative with therapy; still acts uncomfortable in the presence of a group of people; accepted positive feedback from nurse.

The PIE Method

The PIE method, sometimes referred to as "APIE" (assessment, problem, intervention, evaluation), is a systematic approach to documenting the nursing process and nursing diagnosis. A problem-oriented system, **PIE charting** uses accompanying flow sheets that are individualized by each institution. Criteria for documentation are organized in the following manner:

A = Assessment: A complete patient assessment is conducted at the beginning of each shift. Results are documented under this section in the progress notes. Some institutions elect instead to use a daily patient assessment sheet designed to address specific assessment needs within particular units. Explanation of any deviation from the norm is included in the progress notes.

P = Problem: A problem list, or list of nursing diagnoses, is an important part of the APIE method of charting. The name or number of the problem being addressed is documented in this section.

I = Intervention: Nursing actions are performed, directed at resolution of the problem.

E = Evaluation: Outcomes of the implemented interventions are documented, including an evaluation of patient responses to determine the effectiveness of nursing interventions and the presence or absence of progress toward resolution of a problem.

Table 6–5 shows how APIE charting corresponds to the steps of the nursing process.

The following is an example of a three-column documentation in the APIE format.

EXAMPLE

Date/Time	Focus	Progress Notes
9-12-21 1000	Social isolation	**A:** States he does not want to sit with or talk to others; they "frighten" him; stays in room alone unless strongly encouraged to come out; no group involvement; at times listens to group conversations from a distance but does not interact; some hypervigilance and scanning noted. **P:** Social isolation related to inability to trust, panic level of anxiety, and delusional thinking. **I:** Initiated trusting relationship by spending time alone with patient; discussed his feelings regarding interactions with others; accompanied patient to group activities; provided positive feedback for voluntarily participating in assertiveness training. **E:** Cooperative with therapy; still uncomfortable in the presence of a group of people; accepted positive feedback from nurse.

Electronic Documentation

Most health-care facilities have implemented—or are in the process of implementing—some type of EHRs or electronic documentation system. Federal regulations and programs have incentivized the move to EHR systems by requiring health-care organizations to use them in order to receive Medicare and Medicaid reimbursement; in 2015, progressive reductions in reimbursement were initiated for health-care providers not demonstrating meaningful use of EHRs.

The rationale for this move is that EHRs have been shown to improve both the quality of patient care and the efficiency of the health-care system (U.S. Government Accountability Office, 2010). *Quality improvement* and *informatics* are both QSEN competencies.

In 2003, the U.S. Department of Health and Human Services commissioned the Institute of Medicine (IOM) to study the capabilities of EHR systems. The IOM identified a set of eight core functions that EHR systems should perform in the delivery of

TABLE 6–5 Validation of the Nursing Process With APIE Method

APIE CHARTING	WHAT IS RECORDED	NURSING PROCESS
A (Assessment)	Subjective and objective data about the patient that are gathered at the beginning of each shift	Assessment
P (Problem)	Name (or number) of nursing diagnosis being addressed from written problem list, and identified outcome for that problem (*Note:* If outcome appears on written care plan, it does not need to be repeated in daily documentation unless a change occurs.)	Diagnosis and outcome identification
I (Intervention)	Nursing actions performed, directed at problem resolution	Plan and implementation
E (Evaluation)	Appraisal of patient responses to determine effectiveness of nursing interventions	Evaluation

safer, higher quality, and more efficient health care (Institute of Medicine, 2003):

1. ***Health information and data:*** EHRs provide more rapid access to important patient information (e.g., allergies, laboratory test results, a medication list, demographic information, and clinical narratives), thereby improving care providers' ability to make sound clinical decisions in a timely manner.
2. ***Results management:*** Computerized results of all types (e.g., laboratory test results, radiology procedure result reports) can be accessed more easily by the provider at the time and place they are needed.
3. ***Order entry/order management:*** Computer-based order entries improve workflow processes by eliminating lost orders and ambiguities caused by illegible handwriting, generating related orders automatically, monitoring for duplicate orders, and improving the speed with which orders are executed.
4. ***Decision support:*** Computerized decision support systems enhance clinical performance for many aspects of health care. Using reminders and prompts, improvement in regular screenings and other preventive practices can be accomplished. Other aspects of health-care support include identifying possible drug interactions and facilitating diagnosis and treatment.
5. ***Electronic communication and connectivity:*** Improved communication among care associates, such as medicine, nursing, laboratory, pharmacy, and radiology, can enhance patient safety and quality of care. Efficient communication among providers improves continuity of care, allows for more timely interventions, and reduces the risk of adverse events.
6. ***Patient support:*** Computer-based interactive patient education, self-testing, and self-monitoring have been shown to improve control of chronic illnesses.
7. ***Administrative processes:*** Electronic scheduling systems (e.g., for hospital admissions and outpatient procedures) increase the efficiency of health-care organizations and provide more timely service to patients.
8. ***Reporting and population health management:*** Health-care organizations are required to report health-care data to government and private sectors for patient safety and public health. Uniform electronic data standards facilitate this process at the provider level, reduce the associated costs, and increase the speed and accuracy of the data reported.

Summary and Key Points

- The nursing process provides a methodology by which nurses may deliver care using a systematic, scientific approach.
- The focus of nursing process is goal directed and based on a decision-making or problem-solving model consisting of six steps: assessment, diagnosis, outcome identification, planning, implementation, and evaluation.
- Assessment is a systematic, dynamic process by which the nurse, through interaction with the patient, significant others, and health-care providers, collects and analyzes data about the patient.
- Nursing diagnoses are clinical judgments about individual, family, or community responses to actual or potential health problems and life processes.
- Outcomes are measurable, expected, patient-focused goals that translate into observable behaviors.
- Evaluation is the process of determining both the patient's progress toward the attainment of expected outcomes and the effectiveness of nursing care.
- The psychiatric nurse uses the nursing process to assist patients to adapt successfully to stressors within the environment.
- Standards of practice for psychiatric-mental health nurses, set forth by the ANA, APNA, and ISPN, outline the nurse's role in each step of the nursing process when caring for the patient within psychiatric services.
- The nurse serves as a valuable member of the interdisciplinary treatment team, working both independently and cooperatively with other team members.
- Case management is a model of care delivery that serves to provide quality patient care while controlling health-care costs. CPCs serve as the tools for provision of care in a case management system.
- Nurses may serve as case managers, who are responsible for negotiating with multiple health-care providers to obtain a variety of services for the patient.
- Concept mapping is a diagrammatic teaching and learning strategy that allows students and faculty to visualize interrelationships among medical diagnoses, nursing diagnoses, assessment data, and treatments. It can be expanded to include a visual picture of how other disciplines are collaborating with nursing to meet specific patient needs. Nurses must document that the nursing process has been used in the delivery of care. Three methods of documentation that reflect use of the nursing process include problem-oriented recording, Focus Charting®, and the PIE method.
- Many health-care facilities have implemented the use of EHRs, or electronic documentation systems. EHRs have been shown to improve both the quality of patient care and the efficiency of the health-care system.

Review Questions

Select the answer that is most appropriate for each of the following questions:

1. The nurse is using nursing process to care for a client who is suicidal. Which of the following nursing actions is a part of the assessment step of the nursing process?
   a. Identifies the nursing diagnosis: Risk for suicide
   b. Notes that client's family reports recent suicide attempt
   c. Prioritizes the necessity for maintaining a safe environment for the client
   d. Obtains a commitment from the client to work collaboratively to identify adaptive coping
2. The nurse is using nursing process to care for a client who is suicidal. Which of the following nursing actions is a part of the diagnosis step of the nursing process?
   a. Identifies client as "At risk for suicide"
   b. Notes that client's family reports recent suicide attempt
   c. Prioritizes the necessity for maintaining a safe environment for the client
   d. Obtains a commitment from the client to work collaboratively to identify adaptive coping skills
3. The nurse is using nursing process to care for a client who is suicidal. Which of the following nursing actions is a part of the outcome identification step of the nursing process?
   a. Prioritizes the necessity for maintaining a safe environment for the client
   b. Determines whether nursing interventions have been appropriate to achieve desired results
   c. Obtains a commitment from the client to work collaboratively to identify adaptive coping skills
   d. Identifies that the "Client will not harm self during hospitalization"
4. The nurse is using nursing process to care for a client who is suicidal. Which of the following nursing actions is a part of the planning step of the nursing process?
   a. Prioritizes the necessity for maintaining a safe environment for the client
   b. Determines whether nursing interventions have been appropriate to achieve desired results
   c. Obtains a commitment from the client to work collaboratively to identify adaptive coping skills
   d. Identifies that the "Client will not harm self during hospitalization"
5. The nurse is using nursing process to care for a client who is suicidal. Which of the following nursing actions is a part of the implementation step of the nursing process?
   a. Prioritizes the necessity for maintaining a safe environment for the client
   b. Determines whether nursing interventions have been appropriate to achieve desired results
   c. Collaborates with the client to develop a plan for ongoing safety and suicide prevention
   d. Identifies that "Client will not harm self during hospitalization"
6. The nurse is using nursing process to care for a client who is suicidal. Which of the following nursing actions is a part of the evaluation step of the nursing process?
   a. Prioritizes the necessity for maintaining a safe environment for the client
   b. Determines whether nursing interventions have been appropriate to achieve desired results
   c. Obtains a commitment from the client to collaboratively work to identify adaptive coping skills
   d. Identifies that the "Client will not harm self during hospitalization"

Clinical Judgment Questions

7. A 15-year-old female client has just been admitted to the adolescent psychiatric unit with a diagnosis of anorexia nervosa. She is 5 ft 5 inches tall and weighs 82 lb. She was elected to the cheerleading squad for the fall but states that she is not as good as the others on the squad. The treatment team has identified the following problems: refusal to eat, occasional purging, refusing to interact with staff and peers, and fear of failure. Which of the following nursing diagnoses would be appropriate for this client? (Select all that apply.)
   a. Social isolation
   b. Disturbed body image
   c. Low self-esteem
   d. Imbalanced nutrition: Less than body requirements

Continued

8. Which of the following nursing diagnoses would be the highest **priority** diagnosis for the client described in question 7?
   a. Social isolation
   b. Disturbed body image
   c. Low self-esteem
   d. Imbalanced nutrition: Less than body requirements
9. The nurse is transferring a client to a different unit and is providing a transfer report to the nurse who will be receiving this client. The receiving nurse asks what medications this client received within the past 2 hours. Which action should the nurse take to convey this information?
   a. Read the handwritten notes from a shift change report
   b. Try to recall from memory what was given to the client earlier
   c. Read the information recorded in the electronic health record
   d. Ask the unit secretary to read the record and then convey that information to the receiving nurse
10. A client is admitted to the psychiatric unit with depression. Which of these nursing activities is a priority?
   a. Assess the client's risk for suicide
   b. Establish a care plan that includes suicide precautions
   c. Contact the physician for orders
   d. Orient the client to unit activities

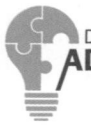

Go to **Davis Advantage** to complete your learning: strengthen understanding, apply your knowledge, and prepare for the Next Gen NCLEX®.

References

American Nurses Association. (n.d.). *What is nursing?* https://www.nursingworld.org/practice-policy/workforce/what-is-nursing/

American Nurses Association. (2010). *Nursing's social policy statement: The essence of the profession* (3rd ed.). Nursesbooks.org.

American Nurses Association. (2021). *Nursing: Scope and standards of practice* (4th ed.). Nursesbooks.org.

American Nurses Association, American Psychiatric Nurses Association, & International Society of Psychiatric-Mental Health Nurses. (2014). *Psychiatric-mental health nursing: Scope and standards of practice* (2nd ed.). Nursebooks.org.

Butcher, H., Bulechek, G., Dochterman, J., & Wagner, C. (Eds.). (2019). *Nursing interventions classification (NIC)* (7th ed.). Elsevier.

Cronenwett, L., Sherwood, G., Barnsteiner, J., Disch, J., Johnson, J., Mitchell, P., Sullivan, D. T., & Warren, D. J. (2007). Quality and safety education for nurses. *Nursing Outlook, 55*(3), 122–131. https://doi.org/10.1016/j.outlook.2007.02.006

Doenges, M. E., Moorhouse, M. F., & Murr, A. C. (2019). *Nursing diagnosis manual: Planning, individualizing, and documenting client care* (6th ed.). F.A. Davis.

Herdman, T. H., Kamitsuru, S., & Lopes, C. T. (Eds.). (2021). *NANDA-International Nursing diagnoses: Definitions and classification, 2021–2023* (12th ed.). Thieme.

Institute of Medicine. (2003). *Key capabilities of an electronic health record system: Letter report.* The National Academies Press. https://doi.org/10.17226/10781

Kaufman, D. M., & Zun, L. (1995). A quantifiable, brief mental status examination for emergency patients. *Journal of Emergency Medicine, 13*(4), 440–456.

Kokman, E., Smith, G. E., Petersen, R. C., Tangalos, E., & Ivnik, R. C. (1991). The short test of mental status: Correlations with standardized psychometric testing. *Archives of Neurology, 48*(7), 725–728.

Lampe, S. S. (1985). Focus charting: Streamlining documentation. *Nursing Management, 16*(7), 43–46.

Moorhead, S., & Dochterman, J. M. (2012). Languages and development of the linkages. In M. Johnson, S. Moorhead, G. Bulechek, M. Butcher, M. Maas, & E. Swanson, *NOC and NIC linkages to NANDA-I and clinical conditions: Supporting critical reasoning and quality care* (3rd ed., pp. 1–10). Mosby.

Moorhead, S., Swanson, E., Johnson, M., & Maas, M. (2018). *Nursing Outcomes Classification (NOC): Measurement of health outcomes* (6th ed.). Elsevier.

NANDA International. (2021b). *About NANDA International.* https://nanda.org/who-we-are/our-story/

Pfeiffer, E. (1975). A short portable mental status questionnaire for the assessment of organic brain deficit in elderly patients. *Journal of the American Geriatric Society, 23*(10), 433–441.

Schuster, P. M. (2016). *Concept mapping: A critical-thinking approach to care planning* (4th ed.). F.A. Davis.

U.S. Government Accountability Office. (2010). *Features of integrated systems support patient care strategies and access to care, but systems face challenges.*

Classical Reference

Folstein, M. F., Folstein, S. E., & McHugh, P. R. (1975). Mini-mental state: A practical method for grading the cognitive state of patients for the clinician. *Journal of Psychiatric Research, 12*(3), 189–198.

Psychosocial Interventions and Spiritual Care

7

CHAPTER OUTLINE

Objectives
Introduction
Individual Psychosocial Therapies
Psychosocial Interventions in Nursing Practice
Spiritual Care
Addressing Spiritual and Religious Needs Through the Nursing Process
Summary and Key Points
Review Questions
Clinical Judgment Questions

CORE CONCEPTS

Health Promotion: Psychosocial therapies
Stress and Coping: Psychosocial interventions
Teaching & Learning: Assertiveness training
Caring, Comfort: Spiritual care
Clinical Judgment

KEY TERMS

aggressive
assertive
automatic thoughts
cognitive behavior therapy (CBT)
dialectical behavior therapy (DBT)
interpersonal psychotherapy (IPT)
milieu therapy
nonassertive
passive-aggressive
psychoanalysis
reality therapy
relaxation therapy
religion
spirituality
therapeutic community

OBJECTIVES

After reading this chapter, the student will be able to:

1. Discuss objectives and therapeutic strategies of various psychosocial therapies, including individual psychotherapy, dialectical behavior therapy, and cognitive behavior therapy.
2. Discuss objectives and therapeutic strategies for various psychosocial interventions including, assertiveness training, relaxation therapy, and milieu therapy.
3. Differentiate formal therapy from psychosocial interventions that are conducted by generalist and psychiatric nurses.
4. Define and differentiate between spirituality and religion.
5. Conduct an assessment of a patient's spiritual needs.
6. Apply the six steps of the nursing process to individuals with spiritual and religious needs.

Introduction

Conventional interventions for patients with a mental illness include psychopharmacological, psychosocial, spiritual, and physical interventions such as electroconvulsive therapy, transcranial magnetic stimulation, and light therapy. Complementary care comprises a variety of adjunctive interventions that may include over-the-counter supplements, exercise and diet interventions, acupuncture, and chiropractic services among others. The term *integrative health* has been used to describe a holistic approach that incorporates complementary and conventional interventions in a coordinated, comprehensive treatment plan.

Psychopharmacological interventions (see Chapter 4, "Psychopharmacology"), selected physical interventions (see Chapter 16, "Depressive Disorders"), and complementary care (see Chapter 30, "Complementary Therapies and Integrative Care") are covered elsewhere in the textbook.

The focus of this chapter is on selected psychosocial therapies, psychosocial interventions, and spiritual care. Psychosocial therapy, in the formal sense, refers to a variety of specialized treatment strategies that require advanced education, licensure, or certification. Other psychosocial interventions, such as milieu therapy, relaxation therapy, and assertiveness training, are not therapies in a formal sense but rather a series of interventions that are well within the scope of practice for generalist and psychiatric nurses with basic education.

Individual Psychosocial Therapies

Individual psychotherapy takes place on a one-to-one basis between a client and a therapist. Mental health professionals who usually perform individual psychotherapy include advanced practice registered nurses, psychiatric social workers, psychiatrists, psychologists, and licensed mental health counselors. An agreement is established, and, within a therapeutic environment, the therapist assists the client to overcome behavioral symptoms or resolve interpersonal problems. Several models of individual psychotherapy are discussed in this section.

Psychoanalysis and Psychoanalytic Psychotherapy

Psychoanalysis is considered by many to be the historical foundation for individual psychotherapy. It was originated by Freud in the early 20th century. In **psychoanalysis,** a major goal is for the client to gain insight and understanding about current relationships and behavior patterns by confronting unconscious conflicts that surface in therapy with the analyst. Psychoanalysis is a lengthy and costly treatment. Psychoanalytic *psychotherapy* is typically briefer and may be focused on specific conflicts. Some of the techniques used in psychoanalysis are described in the following subsections.

Free Association

Free association is a technique in which the therapist is largely nonverbal, perhaps simply introducing words or phrases. The client then verbalizes whatever thoughts come to mind. Proponents of this form of therapy believe that through freely associating, a conflict or issue may surface. Psychoanalytic psychotherapy rarely uses free association because it is more focused on already-identified conflicts.

Dream Analysis

In psychoanalysis, dreams are considered a symbolic window to unconscious conflict, so interpreting dreams is an important tool in this type of therapy. Freud even believed that some symbols that occur in dreams are universal symbols. Analyzing dreams may include free association as well as exploring the meaning of symbols expressed in dream content.

Hypnosis

Hypnotherapy is sometimes used in psychoanalysis as a tool for unlocking the unconscious. Hypnosis is very deep relaxation during which the therapist, who has been trained in techniques of trance formation, asks certain questions of the client. Guided imagery also may be used to help the client envision a specific situation to explore aspects of a problem that were not available in the client's conscious memory. At the close of the session, while the individual is still in the trance state, the therapist may offer some posthypnotic suggestions.

Catharsis

Catharsis is defined as a releasing of unconscious conflicts into conscious awareness, generally through individual or group psychotherapy, accompanied by emotional release. Psychoanalysis proposes that maladaptive symptoms may be resolved by bringing unconscious thoughts and feelings into consciousness. Sometimes the individual not only may recall the painful experience but also may actually relive it, experiencing the feelings and emotions associated with the event. This process is called *abreaction.*

Interpersonal Psychotherapy

Interpersonal psychotherapy (IPT) is a time-limited therapy that was originally developed for the treatment of major depression. Time-limited psychotherapies (also called *brief psychotherapy*) have a specific focus, identified goals, and a limited number of sessions. Theoretical approaches include psychoanalytic, psychodynamic, interpersonal, and integrative. IPT is based on the concepts of Harry Stack Sullivan (1953) and assumes that the symptoms and social dysfunction associated with depression (and other psychiatric disorders) are correlated with difficulties in interpersonal relations. The overall goal of IPT is improvement in current interpersonal skills. Sessions generally occur weekly for about 12 to 16 weeks.

In the initial sessions, the therapist gathers information by taking a psychiatric history, identifying the major problem, establishing a diagnosis, and, together with the client, outlining the goals of therapy. A plan of action for the remaining therapy sessions defines specific interventions targeted at resolving the identified problem. The therapist's role is to guide the patient to meet specifically identified treatment goals that are focused on change in interpersonal behaviors and responses. Guynn (2017, p. 2779) identifies phrases such as "moving forward on your goals" and "making important changes" are used to encourage patients to be responsible for their treatment while reminding them that altering interpersonal patterns requires attention and persistence.

Outcome studies have demonstrated IPT's efficacy in treating various types of depression, including nonpsychotic major depression, recurrent depression, bipolar disorder, postpartum depression, and dysthymic disorder as well as bulimia nervosa and binge eating disorder (Guynn, 2017). Some evidence suggests that IPT may also be effective for treating substance use disorders with dual diagnoses (a co-occurring mental disorder, such as depression, with an addiction) (Crane, 2018). In this context, motivational interviewing is often incorporated, and the focus is on interpersonal patterns that are detrimental to recovery.

Reality Therapy

Reality therapy was developed in the mid-1960s by the American psychiatrist William Glasser (1965). **Reality therapy** suggests that all individuals are responsible for what they choose to do.

Personality development is viewed as an attempt to fulfill five basic needs: power, belonging, freedom, fun, and survival. Individuals choose behaviors that will either be effective or ineffective in satisfying those needs. The therapist helps the client identify needs that are not being met, correlate the unmet needs to current ineffective behaviors, and make conscious choices to change to more effective patterns of behavior in an effort to satisfy basic needs. In reality therapy, emphasis is on the present: the here and now. The past is addressed only as it affects present choices or future behavior. A primary function of the therapist is to assist the client in dealing with getting needs met in the present.

In reality therapy, psychopathology is viewed in terms of ineffective behaviors rather mental illnesses. Diagnoses and labels (e.g., neurotic or dysfunctional) are perceived as not particularly useful. As such, it is not entirely compatible in a medical model of psychiatric treatment. The concept of responsibility is emphasized. Accepting responsibility for one's own behavior is equated with mental health. An individual who behaves responsibly is able to fulfill his or her basic needs without interfering with others' attempts at need fulfillment. An important part of the therapist's role is serving as a positive role model for responsible behavior.

Cognitive Behavior Therapy

Cognitive behavior therapy (CBT), developed by Aaron Beck (1976) and originally identified as simply cognitive therapy, was originally developed for the treatment of mood disorders, but evidence supports its benefits in the treatment of many other disorders including schizophrenia, eating disorders, posttraumatic stress disorders, substance use disorders, and personality disorders. In the cognitive model, irrational thoughts (also referred to as *thought distortions*) are considered a factor in the development and maintenance of mental and emotional disorders. Teaching and guiding the client to challenge and reframe dysfunctional patterns of thinking is believed to contribute to more positive mood and behavior and relief of symptoms. Developing skill in mindfulness is considered foundational to achieving these outcomes.

The general goals in cognitive behavior therapy are to obtain symptom relief as quickly as possible. Therapy focuses on changing *automatic* thought patterns that contribute to mood and thought disturbances. Examples of **automatic thoughts** common in depression include:

- ***Personalizing:*** "I'm the only one who failed."
- ***All or nothing:*** "I'm a failure at everything I do."
- ***Mind reading:*** "He thinks I'm foolish."
- ***Discounting positives:*** "Even though I got the promotion, it was probably because no one else wanted the job."

One technique in CBT involves asking the client to describe evidence that both supports and disputes an automatic troubling thought. The logic underlying their inferences is then reviewed with the client. Another technique involves evaluating what the client thinks would most likely happen if their automatic thoughts were true. Implications of consequences are then discussed. In general, CBT involves a critical thinking process of analyzing one's thoughts, exploring how the way one thinks affects the way one feels and behaves, and finding what might be alternative, more rational approaches to thinking about a given situation.

Dialectical Behavior Therapy

Dialectical behavior therapy (DBT) was originally developed by Marsha Linehan (1993) as a treatment approach for patients with borderline personality disorder (BPD) and suicidal ideation. Originally conceptualized as a cognitive behavior therapy, it shares several features with CBT including mindfulness as a foundational skill. Like CBT, DBT focuses on the therapist working with the client to develop a series of skills. Where the central focus in CBT is learning how to reframe troubling thoughts, DBT focuses more on learning how to regulate troubling emotions. Some of the skills that are unique to DBT include learning nonjudgmental self-acceptance, structuring the environment to positively reinforce progress, developing skills in distress tolerance, and interpersonal effectiveness. Evidence supports the effectiveness of DBT for patients with several psychiatric disorders including BPD, eating disorders, substance use disorders, mood disorders, and substance use disorders.

Psychosocial Interventions in Nursing Practice

Psychiatric nurses, while not prepared to conduct formal therapy, are often involved in education and counseling on psychosocial issues. Three psychosocial interventions within the scope of nursing practice include milieu therapy, relaxation therapy, and assertiveness training.

Milieu Therapy: The Therapeutic Community

Standard 5F of the *Psychiatric–Mental Health Nursing: Scope and Standards of Practice* (American Nurses Association [ANA], American Psychiatric Nurses Association, & International Society of Psychiatric Nurses, 2014) states, "The psychiatric-mental health nurse provides, structures, and maintains a safe, therapeutic, and recovery-oriented environment in collaboration with healthcare consumers, families, and other healthcare clinicians" (p. 60).

Milieu, Defined

The word *milieu*, French for "middle," is translated in English as "surroundings, or environment." In psychiatry, therapy involving the milieu, or environment, may be called **milieu therapy,** the **therapeutic community,** the therapeutic environment, or the therapeutic milieu. The goal of milieu therapy is to manipulate the environment so that all aspects of the patient's hospital experience are considered therapeutic. Within this therapeutic community setting, the patient is expected to learn adaptive coping, interaction, and relationship skills that can be adapted to other aspects of his or her life.

CORE CONCEPT

Milieu Therapy

A scientific structuring of the environment in order to effect behavioral changes and improve the psychological health and functioning of the individual (Skinner, 1979).

Milieu therapy came into its own from the 1960s through the early 1980s. The milieu was the inpatient hospital setting. During this period, psychiatric inpatient treatment provided sufficient time to implement programs of therapy aimed at social rehabilitation. Lengths of stay averaged from 28 to 30 days for acute care hospitalizations and several months or years for long-term hospitalizations. Nursing's focus on establishing interpersonal relationships with patients fit well within this concept of therapy. Patients were encouraged to be active participants in their therapy, and individual autonomy was emphasized. Since acute care hospital lengths of stay now average 2 to 3 days, the focus of inpatient psychiatric care has changed to primarily biologically based stabilization of acute symptoms, but patients still interact within a community environment that can be used to promote their recovery.

Although some of the original strategies for milieu therapy are still used, they have been modified to conform to the short-term approach to care or to outpatient treatment programs. Some programs (e.g., those for children and adolescents, clients with substance use disorders, and geriatric clients) have successfully adapted the concepts of milieu treatment to their specialty needs (Menninger Clinic, 2020; O-School, 2018; Valley View, 2020).

Evidence supports the benefits of therapeutic communities in prison settings for individuals with substance use disorders (National Institutes of Health [NIH], 2015). In this context, work assignments, peer support, formal treatment, and accepting responsibility for one's actions are key elements, and the therapeutic community treatment may last 12 months or more. Evidence also supports milieu therapy for longer-term treatment of patients with schizophrenia. For these patients, milieu therapy has demonstrated positive benefits at lower doses of antipsychotic medications, leading researchers to conclude that the positive emotional experience of milieu therapy is not only an important aspect of treatment but also one that may enable lower doses of medication (Ciompi & Hoffman, 2004; Kvarnstrom, 2017).

Whether the inpatient treatment setting is short term or longer term, some basic principles of milieu therapy are applicable. In a therapeutic community, the setting is the foundation, and everything that happens to the patient or within the patient's environment is considered part of the treatment program. Unlike a medical or surgical hospital setting, patients in an inpatient psychiatric setting are exposed to a tremendous amount of interaction and activity with one another. Community factors—such as social interactions, the physical structure of the treatment setting, and schedule of activities—may generate negative responses from some patients. These stressful experiences are used as opportunities to help the patient learn how to manage stress more adaptively in real-life situations.

Under what conditions, then, is a hospital environment considered therapeutic? Gunderson (1978) identified five elements of a community environment that are necessary for therapeutic outcomes:

1. ***Containment:*** The environment is contained to create a sense of safety and security. Patients who are struggling with strong suicidal intentions, for example, often find that locked doors and lack of access to easy methods of self-harm provide the containment they need to resist self-destructive impulses.
2. ***Structure:*** The environment needs to have a structure that promotes the goals of treatment. This includes a schedule of activities so that patients know what, when, and where activities are taking place. Group therapies, for example, are scheduled at specific times so patients can structure their day to attend. Knowing to whom they should go (perhaps a primary nurse or team leader) to express concerns, ask for medication, or contact other team members is another aspect of unit structure that promotes therapeutic outcomes.
3. ***Involvement:*** The environment must encourage involvement so that patients develop a sense of social community. Common dining areas, small group seating arrangements, and community meetings to discuss aspects of community living are examples of elements that promote involvement.
4. ***Support:*** The environment must be supportive and affirming rather than rigid or punitive. The nurse plays an active role in offering emotional support, reinforcing the expectations within the community environment by promoting supportive interaction, and redirecting patients who are struggling to accomplish therapeutic interaction with others. Support also includes creating a sense that patients are not only involved in treatment but empowered in decision making and direction about their care.
5. ***Validation:*** The environment must support and affirm the needs of the individual both within and separate from the community. Active, empathic listening to the patient's perceptions and concerns and promoting autonomy are examples of validation.

The Role of the Nurse in Milieu Therapy

Several professional health-care disciplines contribute to the function of the therapeutic milieu and collaborate with one another through interdisciplinary team treatment planning and intervention. Table 7–1 describes some of the roles and functions of these team members. Nursing, however, is the only discipline that provides in-person care for patients 24 hours a day and, as such, plays a crucial role in establishing and maintaining the therapeutic milieu.

One of the most important initial nursing interventions in establishing a therapeutic milieu and a foundation for trust is orienting the new patient to the environment, including his or her rights and responsibilities within the unit milieu, the structured activities designed for personal growth, and any limits or restrictions necessary to maintain safety. Availability to provide support and validation to patients throughout their treatment is also an essential nursing competency in milieu therapy (ANA et al., 2014), and this, too, is rooted in a trusting relationship. Active listening and inquiring about the patient's expectations for treatment are key communication skills in providing support and validation and in establishing a foundation for patient-centered care.

In acute care hospitalizations, the ability to establish trust quickly and to assess and collaborate with patients about their post-discharge needs has become an essential role for nurses because many aspects of the recovery treatment plan will occur in treatment settings other than inpatient hospitalization. Do not underestimate the importance

TABLE 7–1 The Interdisciplinary Treatment Team in Psychiatry

TEAM MEMBER	RESPONSIBILITIES	CREDENTIALS
Psychiatrist	Serves as the leader of the team. Responsible for diagnosis and treatment of mental disorders. Prescribes medication and other somatic therapies. May perform psychotherapy.	Medical degree with residency in psychiatry and license to practice medicine.
Clinical Psychologist	Conducts individual, group, and family therapy. Administers, interprets, and evaluates psychological tests that assist in the diagnostic process.	Doctorate in clinical psychology with 2- to 3-year internship supervised by a licensed clinical psychologist. State license is required to practice.
Psychiatric Clinical Nurse Specialist or Psychiatric Nurse Practitioner	Conducts individual, group, and family therapy. Presents educational programs for nursing staff. Provides consultation services to nurses who require assistance in the planning and implementation of care for individual patients. May also prescribe and manage the medication regimen.	Registered nurse with a minimum of a master's degree in psychiatric nursing. Some institutions require certification by national credentialing association.
Psychiatric Nurse	Provides ongoing mental and physical assessment of the patient's condition. Manages the therapeutic milieu on a 24-hour basis. Administers medications. Assists patients with all therapeutic activities as required. Focus is on one-to-one relationship development.	Registered nurse with hospital diploma, associate degree, or baccalaureate degree. Some psychiatric nurses have national certification.
Mental Health Technician (also called psychiatric aide or assistant or psychiatric technician)	Functions under the supervision of the psychiatric nurse. Provides assistance to patients in the fulfillment of their activities of daily living. Assists activity therapists as required in conducting their groups. May also participate in one-to-one relationship development.	Varies by state. Requirements include high school education, with additional vocational education or on-the-job training. Some hospitals hire individuals with a baccalaureate degree in psychology in this capacity. Some states require a licensure examination to practice.
Psychiatric Social Worker	Conducts individual, group, and family therapy. Is concerned with patient's social needs, such as placement, financial support, and community requirements. Conducts in-depth psychosocial history on which the needs assessment is based. Works with patient and family to ensure that requirements for discharge are fulfilled and needs can be met by appropriate community resources.	Minimum of a master's degree in social work. Some states require additional supervision and subsequent licensure by examination.
Occupational Therapist	Works with patients to help develop (or redevelop) independence in performance of activities of daily living. Focus is on rehabilitation and vocational training in which clients learn to be productive, thereby enhancing self-esteem. Creative activities and therapeutic relationship skills are used.	Baccalaureate or master's degree in occupational therapy.
Recreation Therapist	Uses recreational activities to promote patients to redirect their thinking or to rechannel destructive energy in an appropriate manner. Patients learn skills (e.g., bowling, volleyball, exercises, jogging) that can be used during leisure time and during times of stress following discharge from treatment. Some longer-term settings include activities such as picnics, swimming, and group attendance at certain events (e.g., the state fair).	Baccalaureate or master's degree in recreational therapy.

TABLE 7–1 The Interdisciplinary Treatment Team in Psychiatry—cont'd

TEAM MEMBER	RESPONSIBILITIES	CREDENTIALS
Music Therapist	Encourages patients in self-expression through music. Patients listen to music, play instruments, sing, dance, and compose songs that help them get in touch with feelings and emotions that they may not be able to experience in any other way.	Graduate degree with a specialty in music therapy.
Art Therapist	Uses the patient's creative abilities to encourage the expression of emotions and feelings through artwork. Helps patients to analyze their own work in an effort to recognize and resolve underlying conflict.	Graduate degree with a specialty in art therapy.
Dietician	Plans nutritious meals for all patients. Consults with patients with specific eating disorders, such as anorexia nervosa, bulimia nervosa, obesity, and pica.	Baccalaureate or master's degree with a specialty in dietetics.
Chaplain	Assesses, identifies, and attends to the spiritual needs of patients and their family members. Provides spiritual support and comfort as requested by the patient or family. May provide counseling if educational background includes this type of preparation.	College degree with advanced education in theology, seminary, or rabbinical studies.

of these short-term relationships. Patients in outpatient treatment often identify that something a nurse said or something they learned within the hospital milieu planted the seeds for their ongoing recovery plan.

CLINICAL PEARL Developing trust entails being reliable and transparent. It requires acceptance of the individual as a person, separate from behaviors that are unacceptable. It means responding to the patient with concrete actions that are easy to understand (e.g., "If you are frightened, I will stay with you"; "If you are cold, I will bring you a blanket"; "If you are thirsty, I will bring you a drink of water").

Reorienting patients who are confused, redirecting and setting limits when patient behavior is disruptive within the community, patient education, and role-modeling communication and social skills are all activities in which nurses contribute to promoting a therapeutic milieu.

In the therapeutic milieu, nurses are also responsible for ensuring that patients' physiological needs are met. Patients must be encouraged to perform as independently as possible in fulfilling activities of daily living. However, the nurse must make ongoing assessments and provide assistance for those who require it. Assessing physical status is an important nursing responsibility that must not be overlooked in a psychiatric setting.

Therapeutic Milieu as a Professional Nursing Practice Model

Meehan (2019) reimagines the idea of therapeutic milieu as a model for professional practice that involves six principles and can be adopted in any practice setting. Some of these principles are patient centered; others pertain to the nurses; and some are the responsibility of the health-care team. These principles are listed as follows:

1. ***Contagious calmness:*** This principle refers to the nurse's ability to maintain composure, even during stressful events. Nurses encounter patients' anxiety on a daily basis, and the nurse's ability to respond with calm composure creates the foundation for a healing environment for the patient.
2. ***Respect for inherent human dignity:*** Widely recognized as a core value in nursing, this principle can be overlooked in practice if not given careful thought. Patients with mental illness have been victims of stigmatizing attitudes and behaviors. Referring to patients with derogatory language such as "those crazies" or "nuts," even when doing so with other health-care professionals, devalues the inherent dignity of the patient.
3. ***Nurse's care for self and one another:*** Caring for self implies attending to one's own needs to achieve inner and outer wellness. Caring for

others implies attending to relational wellness. Nurses sometimes express that their relationships with patients and their relationships with other team members are two mutually exclusive entities. However, patients who see inconsistencies in how health-care professionals relate to one another and their patients may have more difficulty trusting that the milieu is safe and therapeutic.

4. ***Intellectual engagement:*** The therapeutic milieu is developed and enhanced by the nurse's active engagement in critical thinking, creativity, and problem-solving around relevant practice issues. Examples may include exploring the best ways to maintain a safe environment or studying a patient care intervention to improve its effectiveness. Intellectual engagement is the essence of quality improvement, which has been identified as an essential Quality and Safety Education for Nurses (QSEN) competency.
5. ***Caritas:*** Caritas refers to the nurse's ability to experience and express benevolent affection for patients regardless of their characteristics. Patients with mental illness may say things that are reflections of disrupted thought processes; they may be anxious and angry; they may behave in ways that are not socially acceptable. The ability to relate to patients with caritas, or what Carl Rogers (1951; the founder of client-centered psychology) described as "unconditional positive regard," is foundational to establishing a healing, therapeutic environment.
6. ***Safe and restorative physical surroundings:*** In the inpatient psychiatric unit, safety of the physical environment is paramount. Many adjustments are made to doors, windows, and furniture to minimize risks for suicide or violence toward others. Standards and unit policies dictate the manner and frequency with which patients are observed and assessed to ensure their safety. All of these efforts communicate to the patient a concern for a safe, therapeutic milieu and begin to lay the foundation for establishing trust. Whether the therapeutic milieu is adopted as a treatment strategy within psychiatric treatment settings or broadened in scope to be viewed as a professional practice model for nurses in any setting, evidence supports that establishing a therapeutic environment of care is essential to the development of trust, relationship building, and therapeutic outcomes in patient care.

Relaxation Therapy

Stress is a part of our everyday lives. It can be positive or negative, but it cannot be eliminated. Keeping stress at a manageable level is a lifelong process. Individuals under stress respond with a physiological arousal that can be dangerous over long periods. Indeed, the stress response has been shown to be a major contributor, either directly or indirectly, to coronary heart disease, cancer, lung ailments, accidental injuries, cirrhosis of the liver, and suicide—six of the leading causes of death in the United States.

Relaxation therapy is an effective means of reducing the stress response in some individuals. The degree of anxiety that an individual experiences in response to stress is related to certain predisposing factors, such as innate temperament, past experiences resulting in learned patterns of responding, and existing conditions, such as health status, coping strategies, and adequacy of support systems. Nurses can play an active role in educating patients about the stress response and various methods to achieve relaxation. Deep relaxation can counteract the physiological and behavioral manifestations of stress. Various methods of relaxation are described in the following subsections.

Deep-Breathing Exercises

Tension is released when the lungs are allowed to breathe in as much oxygen as possible. Deep-breathing exercises involve inhaling slowly and deeply through the nose, holding the breath for a few seconds, and then exhaling slowly through the mouth, pursing the lips as if trying to whistle.

Progressive Relaxation

Progressive relaxation is a method of deep-muscle relaxation that is based on the premise that the body responds to anxiety-provoking thoughts and events with muscle tension. Each muscle group is tensed for 5 to 7 seconds and then relaxed for 20 to 30 seconds, during which time the individual concentrates on the difference in sensations between the two conditions. Soft, slow background music may facilitate relaxation. A modified version of this technique, called *passive progressive relaxation*, involves relaxation of the muscles by concentrating on the feeling of relaxation within the muscle, rather than on the actual tensing and relaxing of the muscle.

Meditation

The goal of meditation is to gain mastery over attention. It brings on a special state of consciousness as attention is concentrated solely on one thought or object. During meditation, as the individual becomes completely preoccupied with the selected focus, respiration rate, heart rate, and blood pressure decrease.

Mindfulness meditation, a practice rooted in Buddhist traditions, has gained popularity as a foundational skill in several psychological therapies. The practice of mindfulness is a form of meditation focused on nonjudgmental awareness of the present moment. Developing the skill of "being present in the moment" is believed to facilitate focus on problem-solving and behavior change.

Mental Imagery

Mental imagery uses the imagination of a relaxing environment to reduce the body's response to stress. The frame of reference is very personal, based on what each individual considers to be a relaxing environment. The relaxing scenario is most useful when taped and played back at a time when the individual wishes to achieve relaxation.

Biofeedback

Biofeedback is the use of instrumentation to become aware of processes in the body that usually go unnoticed and to help bring them under voluntary control. Biological conditions, such as muscle tension, skin surface temperature, blood pressure, and heart rate, are monitored by the biofeedback equipment. As biofeedback training progresses, the individual learns to use relaxation and voluntary control to modify the biological condition, in turn indicating a modification of the autonomic function it represents. Biofeedback is often used together with other relaxation techniques such as deep breathing, progressive relaxation, and mental imagery. Nurses may be involved in providing biofeedback services after completing specialized training and/or certification.

Assertiveness Training

Assertive behavior and communication promote positive self-esteem by encouraging open and honest expression of one's needs and respecting one's basic human rights as well as the rights of others. Assertive communication is an important skill for nurses to develop in professional relationships with peers and supervisors in any practice setting. In psychiatric nursing, assertive communication and behavior are important tools that can be taught and role-modeled in interaction with patients to promote their development of effective communication skills in interpersonal relationships.

Individuals develop patterns of responding in various ways, such as through role-modeling, receiving positive or negative reinforcement, or making conscious choices. These patterns can take the form of nonassertiveness, assertiveness, aggressiveness, or passive-aggressiveness. **Nonassertive** patterns of communication have the effect of pleasing others at the expense of denying one's own basic human rights. Assertive patterns of communication have the effect of expressing one's needs or rights while protecting the rights of others. Those who respond with an **aggressive** approach defend their rights by violating the basic rights of others. Individuals who respond in a **passive-aggressive** manner defend their rights by resisting social and occupational demands without open, direct communication.

Some important behavioral considerations of assertive behavior include eye contact, body posture, personal distance, physical contact, gestures, facial expression, voice, fluency, timing, listening, thoughts, and content. Various techniques have been developed to assist individuals in the process of becoming more assertive. Some of these are described in Table 7–2.

The basic goal in assertive communication training is to teach clients to express what they feel and need without becoming defensive and without violating the rights of others. Some clients who are beginning to learn these skills wrongly believe that assertive communication will get people to respond in certain ways or will allow clients to get what they want from another person. Manipulation is not the goal of assertive communication. Further, no one can control another person's behaviors or responses, and if clients do not understand these limitations at the outset, they may be setting themselves up for failure. It is important to educate clients that assertive communication skills are designed to empower them to express themselves and their needs more effectively.

Spiritual Care

Assessing a patient's spiritual needs is recognized as an important aspect of holistic nursing care, but definitions and activities to accomplish this have not always been well understood. Historically,

TABLE 7–2 Techniques for Becoming More Assertive

TECHNIQUE	DEFINITION	EXAMPLE
Standing up for one's basic human rights	Expressing and asserting one's rights in relationship with others.	"I have the right to express my opinion."
Assuming responsibility for one's own statements	Acknowledging one's feelings accurately.	"I don't want to go out with you tonight," instead of "I can't go out with you tonight." The latter implies a lack of power or ability.
Responding as a "broken record"	Persistently repeating in a calm voice what is wanted.	TELEPHONE SALESPERSON: "I want to help you save money by changing long-distance services." ASSERTIVE RESPONSE: "I don't want to change my long-distance service." TELEPHONE SALESPERSON: "I can't believe you don't want to save money!" ASSERTIVE RESPONSE: "I don't want to change my long-distance service."
Agreeing assertively	Assertively accepting negative aspects about oneself. Admitting when an error has been made.	MS. JONES: "You sure let that meeting get out of hand. What a waste of time." MS. SMITH: "Yes, I didn't do a very good job of conducting the meeting today."
Inquiring assertively	Seeking additional information about critical statements.	MALE BOARD MEMBER: "You made a real fool of yourself at the board meeting last night." FEMALE BOARD MEMBER: "Oh, really? Just what about my behavior offended you?" MALE BOARD MEMBER: "You were so damned pushy!" FEMALE BOARD MEMBER: "Were you offended that I spoke up for my beliefs, or was it because my beliefs are in direct opposition to yours?"
Shifting from content to process	Changing the focus of the communication from discussing the topic at hand to analyzing what is actually going on in the interaction.	WIFE: "Would you please call me if you will be late for dinner?" HUSBAND: "Why don't you just get off my back! I always have to account for every minute of my time with you!" WIFE: "Sounds to me like we need to discuss some other things here. What are you really angry about?"
Clouding/fogging	Concurring with the critic's argument without becoming defensive and without agreeing to change.	NURSE 1: "You make so many mistakes. I don't know how you ever got this job!" NURSE 2: "You're right. I have made some mistakes since I started this job."
Defusing	Putting off further discussion with an angry individual until they are calmer.	"You are very angry right now. I don't want to discuss this matter with you while you are so upset. I will discuss it with you in my office at 3 o'clock this afternoon."
Delaying assertively	Putting off further discussion with another individual until one is calmer.	"That's a very challenging position you have taken, Mr. Brown. I'll need time to give it some thought. I'll call you later this afternoon."

spiritual care has had distinctly religious connections, with a spiritual person being described as "someone with whom the Spirit of God dwelt." Koenig (2012) describes **spirituality** as distinguished by its connection to that which is considered sacred and transcendent. He identifies spirituality as connected to the supernatural, the mystical, and organized religion but extending beyond and beginning before organized religion. In other words, spirituality may be considered a quest for the transcendent that might lead to staunch belief or nonbelief.

CORE CONCEPT

Spirituality

The human quality that gives meaning and sense of purpose to an individual's existence. Spirituality exists within each individual regardless of belief system and serves as a force for interconnectedness between the self and others, the environment, and a higher power.

Contemporary research (more than 60 studies) supports the value of addressing spirituality for both medical and psychiatric patients (Lichter, 2013; Liefbroer et al., 2019; Reeves & Reynolds, 2009). Within nursing, focus on spirituality is identified as a nursing responsibility in the International Council of Nurses *Code of Ethics* (2012) and the American Holistic Nurses Association (in collaboration with the American Nurses Association) *Holistic Nursing: Scope and Standards of Practice* (2019). Spiritual care is recognized as an important aspect of care in two *NANDA International* nursing diagnoses: Spiritual distress and spiritual well-being (Herdman et al., 2021). Although spiritual care has been identified as an important aspect of recovery, a recent study (Neathery et al., 2020) found that nurses who had a spiritual perspective with a religious affiliation and more years of experience as a psychiatric mental health nurse were more likely to provide spiritual care. The authors suggest that more development for nurses in their understanding of spiritual care is necessary to enhance the frequency with which this aspect of nursing care is provided.

Specifically in psychiatric nursing, issues related to spiritual distress and spiritual well-being are common. The sense of hopelessness that is symptomatic in major depressive disorders raises spiritual questions for many patients with this condition. The thought disruptions that are characteristic in schizophrenia lead some to misinterpret their experience as induced by evil forces. Patients with grandiose delusions may falsely believe they are a prophet, the messiah, or other person of great religious or spiritual significance. How should the nurse respond to these issues and questions around spirituality with respect for the patient's needs, values, and beliefs? A prerequisite to conducting a meaningful spiritual assessment is exploration of concepts related to meaning and purpose in life, faith, hope, love, and forgiveness.

Spiritual Needs

Meaning and Purpose in Life

Humans by nature strive for order and structure in their lives. Having a purpose in life gives one a sense of control and the feeling that life is worth living. Each individual's exploration of what is most important in their lives is foundational to one's awareness of their spirituality and provides a platform for spiritual growth. Further, each nurse's exploration of their own spirituality and efforts to grow spiritually are foundational to being responsive to those needs in others. Walsh (1999) describes seven perennial practices that he believes promote enlightenment, aid in transformation, and encourage spiritual growth:

1. ***Transform your motivation:*** Reduce craving and find your soul's desire.
2. ***Cultivate emotional wisdom:*** Heal your heart and learn to love.
3. ***Live ethically:*** Feel good by doing good.
4. ***Concentrate and calm your mind:*** Accept the challenge of mastering attention and mindfulness.
5. ***Awaken your spiritual vision:*** See clearly and recognize the sacred in all things.
6. ***Cultivate spiritual intelligence:*** Develop wisdom and understand the purpose of life.
7. ***Express spirit in action:*** Embrace generosity and the joy of service. (p. 14)

In the final analysis, individuals must determine their own perception of what is important and what gives meaning to life. Throughout one's existence, the meaning of life will undoubtedly be challenged many times. A solid spiritual foundation may help an individual confront the challenges that result from life's experiences.

Erik Erikson, who elaborated a classic model of developmental tasks throughout the life span (1950), recognized that as people continue to live into older adulthood, his identified tasks did not address what he referred to as the older, older adult (those adults age 80 years and older). His widow compiled his notes and subsequently published his work on an additional developmental stage. This stage is *transcendence*, in which adults 80 years and older focus more on clarifying meaning in their life as well as those things that transcend beyond themselves. Erikson suggests that as individuals continue to grow older, spirituality becomes a more important part of their development.

Faith

Faith is often thought of as the acceptance of a belief in the absence of physical or empirical evidence. Smucker (2001) stated:

> For all people, faith is an important concept. From childhood on, our psychological health depends on having faith or trust in something or someone to help meet our needs. (p. 7)

Having faith requires that individuals rise above that which they can experience only through the five senses. Faith transcends the appearance of the physical world. An increasing amount of medical and scientific research is showing that what individuals believe exists can have as powerful an impact as what actually exists (Bogousslavski & Inglin, 2007; Harvard Health, 2019; Sathyanarayana Rao et al., 2009; Tétreault et al., 2016). Karren and associates (2010) add that there is a growing appreciation of the healing power of faith among members of the medical community.

Hope

Hope is defined as a positive, optimistic outlook. With hope, individuals look at a situation, and no matter how negative, find something positive on which to focus. Hope functions as an energizing force. In addition, research indicates that hope may promote healing, facilitate coping, and enhance the quality of life (Enayati, 2013; Nekolaichuk et al., 1999).

Kübler-Ross (1969), in her classic study of dying patients, stressed the importance of hope. She suggested that even though these patients could not hope for a cure, they could hope for additional time to live, to be with loved ones, for freedom from pain, or for a peaceful death with dignity. She found hope to be a satisfaction unto itself, whether or not it was fulfilled. She stated, "If a patient stops expressing hope, it is usually a sign of imminent death" (p. 140).

Researchers in the field of psychoneuroimmunology have found that the attitudes we have and the emotions we experience have a definite effect on inflammation in the body (Jones, 2019; Jones & Graham-Engeland, 2021). An optimistic feeling of hope is not just a mental state. Hope and optimism produce positive physical changes in the body that can influence the immune system and the functioning of specific body organs. The medical literature abounds with countless examples of individuals with terminal conditions who suddenly improve when they find hope. Conversely, there are many accounts of patients whose conditions deteriorate when they lose hope.

Love

Love may be identified as a projection of one's own good feelings onto others. To love others, one must first experience love of self and then be able and willing to project that warmth and affectionate concern for others (Karren et al., 2013). Smucker (2001) states:

> Love, in its purest unconditional form, is probably life's most powerful force and our greatest spiritual need. Not only is it important to receive love, but equally important to give love to others. Thinking about and caring for the needs of others keeps us from being too absorbed with ourselves and our needs to the exclusion of others. We all have experienced the good feelings that come from caring for and loving others. (p. 10)

Love may be an important component of the healing process. Thaik, a cardiologist, states that love, as one of many strong human emotions, releases a cascade of hundreds or thousands of neuropeptides and hormones that can affect physical and mental health (2013). Among the beneficial effects, Thaik reports that:

1. Love counteracts the fight-or-flight syndrome and decreases production of the stress hormone cortisol.
2. Love encourages the production of oxytocin, the "feel-good" hormone, which can reduce cardiovascular stress and improve the immune system.
3. Love increases the production of norepinephrine and dopamine and may stave off depression.
4. Love decreases inflammation, which affects immune function and pain relief.

Some researchers present evidence that love has a positive effect on the immune system in adults, children, and animals (Murray et al., 2019; Ornish, 1998; Pace et al., 2009). The giving and receiving of love may also result in higher levels of endorphins, thereby contributing to a sense of euphoria and helping to reduce pain.

In a classic long-term study, researchers Werner and Smith (1992) studied children who were reared in impoverished environments. Their homes were troubled by discord, desertion, or divorce or were marred by parental alcoholism or mental illness. The participants were studied at birth, childhood, adolescence, and adulthood. Two out of three of these high-risk children had developed serious learning and/or behavioral problems by age 10 or had a record of delinquencies, mental health problems, or pregnancies by age 18. One-fourth of them had developed "very serious" physical and psychosocial problems. By the time they reached adulthood, more than three-fourths had profound psychological and behavioral problems, and even more were in poor physical health. But of particular interest to the researchers were the 15% to 20% who remained resilient and well despite their impoverished and difficult existence. These children had experienced a warm and loving relationship with another person during their first year of life, whereas the children who developed serious psychological and physical problems did not. This research indicates that the earlier people have the benefit of a strong, loving relationship, the better they seem able to resist the effects of a deleterious lifestyle.

Forgiveness

Forgiveness has been defined as the letting go of resentments and thoughts of revenge (Mayo Clinic, 2020). Feelings of bitterness and resentment take a physical toll on an individual by generating stress hormones. When maintained for long periods, these feelings can have a detrimental effect on health. Forgiveness enables a person to cast off resentment and begin the pathway to healing. Owen, as cited by Harrison (2011), conducted research with patients who were HIV positive to study the effects of forgiveness on the immune system and found that forgiveness was correlated with improvements in immune function.

Forgiveness is not easy. Individuals often have great difficulty when called upon to forgive others, and even greater difficulty in attempting to forgive themselves. To forgive is not necessarily to condone or excuse one's own or someone else's inappropriate behavior. Karren and associates (2013) suggest that forgiveness is an attitude of owning responsibility for one's own perceptions and moving beyond the perception of being a helpless victim to the perception of being empowered in choosing one's own responses to hurts and offenses.

It is important for nurses to be able to assess the spiritual needs of their patients. The aforementioned aspects are relevant to one's spiritual well-being as well as their physical well-being. Nurses need not serve the role of a professional counselor or spiritual guide, but because of the ongoing contact with patients and the trust that is developed within a therapeutic nurse-patient relationship, nurses may be the part of the health-care team to whom patients reveal the most intimate details of their lives. Smucker (2001) stated:

> Just as answering a patient's question honestly and with accurate information and responding to his needs in a timely and sensitive manner communicates caring, so also does high-quality professional nursing care reach beyond the physical body or the illness to that part of the person where identity, self-worth, and spirit lie. In this sense, good nursing care is also good spiritual care. (pp. 11–12)

Religion

CORE CONCEPT

Religion

Religion is a set of beliefs, values, rites, and rituals adopted by a group of people. The practices are usually grounded in the teachings of a spiritual leader.

Religion is one way an individual's spirituality may be expressed. There are more than 6,500 religions in the world (Bronson, 2005). Globally, Christianity remains the largest religious group (31.2%), followed by Islam (24.1%), and unaffiliated individuals (16%) (Pew Research Center, 2017). Some individuals seek out various religions in an attempt to find answers to fundamental questions that they have about life and, indeed, about their very existence. Others, although they may regard themselves as spiritual, choose not to affiliate with an organized religious group. In either situation, however, it is inevitable that questions related to life and the human condition arise during the progression of spiritual maturation.

Evidence supports that affiliation with a religious group is a health-enhancing endeavor (Karren et al., 2013). Several studies indicate a correlation between religious faith, church attendance, increased chance of survival following serious illness, fewer instances of depression and mental illness, longer life, and overall better physical and mental health. In an extensive review of the literature, Levin (2010) concludes that the weight of the evidence across studies suggests that religious involvement is a general protective factor for mental illness and psychological distress.

Despite these findings, confidence in organized religion and church attendance have been declining in American society. Over the past four decades, there has been a steady decline in Americans' confidence in religion. In 2018, church membership reached an all-time low, with 50% of Americans reporting belonging to a church, synagogue, or mosque (Jones, 2019). The trend toward declining membership has been particularly pronounced over the past two decades. Church attendance has shown similar declines.

Despite declining church membership, a recent Gallup poll (Jones, 2019) identified that 77% of Americans report identifying with some organized religion. Although the majority of Americans still identify as affiliated with some branch of Christianity, the number of Americans identifying as having no religious affiliation has more than doubled (from 8% to 19%) since the turn of the century (Jones, 2019). These findings suggest that although a majority of Americans may still value faith and worship, their mechanisms for expressing those values are undergoing cultural change.

Addressing Spiritual and Religious Needs Through the Nursing Process

Assessment

It is important for nurses to consider spiritual and religious needs when planning care for their patients. The Joint Commission, as part of its accreditation standards, identifies that nurses should address the psychosocial, spiritual, and cultural variables that influence their perception of illness. Dossey (1998) developed a spiritual assessment tool about which she stated:

> The Spiritual Assessment Tool provides reflective questions for assessing, evaluating, and increasing awareness of spirituality in patients and their significant others. The tool's reflective questions can facilitate healing because they stimulate spontaneous, independent, meaningful initiatives to improve the patient's capacity for recovery and healing. (p. 45)

An adapted version of this spiritual assessment tool can be found in Box 7–1.

Assessing the spiritual needs of a patient with a psychotic disorder can pose some additional challenges. Approximately 25% of people with schizophrenia and 15% to 22% of people with bipolar disorder have religious delusions (Koenig, 2012). Sometimes these delusions can be difficult to differentiate from general religious or cultural beliefs, but nonpsychotic religious activity may actually improve long-term prognosis in patients with psychotic disorders (Koenig, 2012). Engaging family members and significant others in the assessment process can be a great help in determining which religious beliefs and activities have been beneficial to the patient and which have been detrimental to their progress.

Diagnoses/Outcome Identification

Nursing diagnoses that may be used when addressing spiritual and religious needs of patients include the following:

- Risk for spiritual distress
- Spiritual distress
- Readiness for enhanced spiritual well-being
- Risk for impaired religiosity
- Impaired religiosity
- Readiness for enhanced religiosity

The following outcomes may be used as guidelines for care and to evaluate effectiveness of the nursing interventions. The patient:

- Identifies meaning and purpose in life that reinforce hope, peace, and contentment.
- Verbalizes acceptance of self as a worthwhile human being.
- Accepts and incorporates change into life in a healthy manner.
- Expresses understanding of the relationship between difficulties in current life situation and Interruption in previous religious beliefs and activities.
- Discusses beliefs and values about spiritual and religious issues.
- Expresses desire and ability to participate in beliefs and activities of desired religion.

Planning and Implementation

Sample care plans using NANDA-I nursing diagnoses for spiritual distress and impaired religiosity are presented in Table 7–3.

Evaluation

Evaluation of nursing actions is directed at achievement of the established outcomes. Part of the evaluation process is continuous reassessment to ensure that the selected actions are appropriate and the goals and outcomes are realistic. Including the family and extended support systems in the evaluation process is essential if spiritual and religious implications of nursing care are to be measured. Modifications to the plan of care are made as the need is determined.

BOX 7–1 Spiritual Assessment Tool

The following reflective questions may assist you in assessing, evaluating, and increasing awareness of spirituality in yourself and others.

MEANING AND PURPOSE

These questions assess a person's ability to seek meaning and fulfillment in life, manifest hope, and accept ambiguity and uncertainty.

- What gives your life meaning?
- Describe your sense of purpose in life.
- How does your illness affect your life goals?
- How hopeful are you about obtaining a better degree of health?
- How would you describe your role in maintaining your health?
- What kind of changes will you be able to make in your life to maintain your health?
- Describe your level of motivation to get well.
- What is the most important or powerful thing your life?

INNER STRENGTHS

These questions assess a person's ability to manifest joy and recognize strengths, choices, goals, and faith.

- What brings you joy and peace in your life?
- What can you do to feel alive and full of spirit?
- What traits do you like about yourself?
- What are your personal strengths?
- What choices are available to you to enhance your healing?
- What life goals have you set for yourself?
- What do you think is the role of stress, if any, in your illness?
- How aware were you of your body before you became sick?
- What do you believe in?
- How has your illness influenced your faith?
- How important is faith in your overall health and sense of well-being?

INTERCONNECTIONS

These questions assess a person's positive self-concept, self-esteem, and sense of self; sense of belonging in the world with others; capacity to pursue personal interests; and ability to demonstrate love of self and self-forgiveness.

- How do you feel about yourself right now?
- How do you feel when you have a true sense of yourself?
- Describe any activities of personal interest that you pursue.
- What do you do to show love for yourself?
- Can you forgive yourself?
- What do you do to heal your spirit?

RELATIONSHIPS

These questions assess a person's ability to connect in life-giving ways with family, friends, and social groups and to engage in the forgiveness of others.

- Who are the significant people in your life?
- Who are your readily available, nearby, support people?
- Who are the people to whom you are closest?
- Describe any groups in which you are an active participant.
- How comfortable are you with asking people for help when you need it?
- How comfortable are you with sharing your feelings with others?
- What are some of the most loving things that others have done for you?
- What are the loving things that you do for other people?
- What are your thoughts about forgiving others?

BEHAVIOR AND ACTIVITIES

These questions assess a person's capacity for finding meaning in worship or religious activities and a connectedness with a divinity.

- How important is worship to you?
- What do you consider the most significant act of worship in your life?
- Describe any religious activities in which you are an active participant.
- Describe any spiritual activities, if any, that you find meaningful.
- Do you find prayer meaningful?
- To whom do you turn for support?
- Describe any activities in which you engage for coping and support.
- Describe any activities in which you have previously engaged and have not found helpful.

ENVIRONMENT

These questions assess a person's ability to experience a sense of connection with life and nature, an awareness of the effects of the environment on life and well-being, and a capacity or concern for the health of the environment.

- How does your environment have an impact on your state of well-being?
- What are your environmental stressors at work and at home?
- What strategies reduce your environmental stressors?
- Do you have any concerns for the state of your immediate environment?
- Are you involved with environmental issues such as recycling environmental resources at home, work, or in your community?
- Are you concerned about the survival of the planet?

Source: Compiled from Burkhardt (1989); Dossey & American Holistic Nurses' Association (1995); and Dossey (1998).

Table 7–3 | CARE PLAN FOR THE PATIENT WITH SPIRITUAL AND RELIGIOUS NEEDS

NURSING DIAGNOSIS: RISK FOR SPIRITUAL DISTRESS

RELATED TO: Life changes; environmental changes; stress; anxiety; depression

OUTCOME CRITERIA	NURSING INTERVENTIONS	RATIONALE
Patient identifies meaning and purpose in life that reinforce hope, peace, contentment, and self-satisfaction.	1. Assess current situation.	1–8. Thorough assessment is necessary to develop an accurate care plan.
	2. Listen to the patient's expressions of anger, concern, self-blame.	
	3. Note the patient's perceptions about reason for living and whether it is directly related to situation.	
	4. Determine the patient's religious and/or spiritual orientation, current involvement, and presence of conflicts, especially in current circumstances.	
	5. Assess sense of self-concept, worth, ability to enter into loving relationships.	
	6. Observe behavior indicative of poor relationships with others.	
	7. Determine support systems available to and used by the patient and significant others.	
	8. Assess substance use/abuse.	
	9. Establish an environment that promotes free expression of feelings and concerns.	9. Trust is the basis of a therapeutic nurse-patient relationship.
	10. Have the patient identify and prioritize current/immediate spiritual needs.	10. Helps patients focus on what needs to be done and identify manageable steps to take.
	11. Discuss philosophical issues related to impact of current situation on spiritual beliefs and values.	11. Helps patients to understand that certain life experiences can cause individuals to question personal values and that this response is not uncommon.
	12. Use therapeutic communication skills of reflection and active listening.	12. Helps patients explore and identify solutions to concerns.
	13. Review coping skills used and their effectiveness in current situation.	13. Identifies strengths to incorporate into plan and techniques that need revision.
	14. Provide a role model for open discussion of spiritual concerns.	14. Sharing of experiences and hope assists patients to deal with reality.
	15. Suggest use of journaling.	15. Journaling can assist in clarifying beliefs and values and in recognizing and resolving feelings about current life situation.
	16. Discuss the patient's interest in the arts, music, and literature.	16. Provides insight into meaning of these issues and how they are integrated into an individual's life.

Table 7–3 | CARE PLAN FOR THE PATIENT WITH SPIRITUAL AND RELIGIOUS NEEDS—cont'd

OUTCOME CRITERIA	NURSING INTERVENTIONS	RATIONALE
	17. Role-play new coping techniques. Discuss possibilities of taking classes, becoming involved in discussion groups, cultural activities of the patient's choice.	17. These activities will help to enhance integration of new skills and necessary changes in the patient's lifestyle.
	18. Refer the patient to appropriate resources for spiritual support and guidance.	18. Patients may require additional assistance with an individual who specializes in these types of concerns.

NURSING DIAGNOSIS: RISK FOR IMPAIRED RELIGIOSITY

RELATED TO: Suffering; depression; illness; life transitions

OUTCOME CRITERIA	NURSING INTERVENTIONS	RATIONALE
Patient expresses achievement of support and personal satisfaction from spiritual and/or religious practices.	1. Assess current situation (e.g., illness, hospitalization, prognosis of death, presence of support systems, financial concerns).	1. This information identifies problems the patient is dealing with in the moment that is affecting desire to be involved with religious activities.
	2. Listen nonjudgmentally to the patient's expressions of anger and possible belief that illness or condition may be a result of lack of faith.	2. Individuals often blame themselves for what has happened and reject previous religious beliefs and/or God.
	3. Determine the patient's usual religious and/or spiritual beliefs, current involvement in specific church activities.	3. This information is important background for establishing a database about the patient's impaired religiosity.
	4. Note quality of relationships with significant others and friends.	4. Individuals may withdraw from others in relation to the stress of illness, pain, and suffering.
	5. Assess substance use/abuse.	5. When in distress, individuals may turn to use of various substances, which can affect the ability to deal with problems in a positive manner.
	6. Develop nurse-patient relationship in which the individual can express feelings and concerns freely.	6. Trust is the basis for a therapeutic nurse-patient relationship.
	7. Use therapeutic communication skills of active listening, reflection, and "I" messages.	7. Helps patients explore and identify solutions to problems and concerns and promotes sense of control.
	8. Be accepting and nonjudgmental when the patient expresses anger and bitterness toward God. Stay with the patient.	8. The nurse's presence and nonjudgmental attitude increase the patient's feelings of self-worth and promote trust in the relationship.
	9. Encourage the patient to discuss previous religious practices and how these practices provided support in the past.	9. A nonjudgmental discussion of previous sources of support may help the patient work through current rejection of them as potential sources of support.

Continued

Table 7–3 | CARE PLAN FOR THE PATIENT WITH SPIRITUAL AND RELIGIOUS NEEDS—cont'd

OUTCOME CRITERIA	NURSING INTERVENTIONS	RATIONALE
	10. Allow the patient to take the lead in initiating participation in religious activities, such as prayer.	10. Patients may be vulnerable in current situation and needs to be allowed to decide own resumption of these actions.
	11. Contact spiritual leader of patient's choice, if they request one.	11. These individuals serve to provide relief from spiritual distress and often can do so when other support persons cannot.

Source: The interventions for this care plan were adapted from Doenges et al. (2019).

Summary and Key Points

- Selected psychosocial therapies include psychoanalysis, interpersonal psychotherapy, reality therapy, cognitive behavior therapy, and dialectical behavior therapy. Advanced practice psychiatric nurses may use some of these therapies in their practices.
- Generalist psychiatric nurses play active roles in milieu therapy and educating patients about relaxation and assertiveness skills.
- In psychiatry, milieu therapy (or the therapeutic community) constitutes a manipulation of the environment to create behavioral changes and to improve the psychological health and functioning of the individual.
- The goal of a therapeutic community is for the patient to learn adaptive coping, interaction, and relationship skills that can be generalized to other aspects of his or her life.
- Six principles for establishing therapeutic milieu as a practice model for nurses in any healthcare setting are contagious calmness, respect for inherent human dignity, nurse's care for self and others, intellectual engagement, caritas, and maintaining safe and restorative physical surroundings (Meehan, 2019).
- Spirituality is the human quality that gives meaning and sense of purpose to an individual's existence.
- Individuals possess a number of spiritual needs that include meaning and purpose in life; faith or trust in someone or something beyond themselves; hope; love; and forgiveness.
- Religion is a set of beliefs, values, rites, and rituals adopted by a group of people.
- Religion is one way in which an individual's spirituality may be expressed.
- Affiliation with a religious group has been shown to be a health-enhancing endeavor.

Review Questions

Select the answer that is most appropriate for each of the following questions:

1. Interpersonal psychotherapy assumes that a client's psychiatric disorder is related to:
   a. Irrational, automatic thought patterns
   b. Emotional dysregulation
   c. Difficulties in relationships
   d. Negative reinforcement
2. Which of the following are basic assumptions of milieu therapy? (Select all that apply.)
   a. Individuals own their own environment.
   b. Individuals own their own behavior.
   c. Peer pressure is a useful and powerful tool.
   d. Inappropriate behaviors are punished immediately.

3. Within the therapeutic milieu of an inpatient psychiatric unit, duties of the staff psychiatric nurse include which of the following? (Select all that apply.)
   a. Medication administration
   b. Client teaching
   c. Medical diagnosis
   d. Reality orientation
   e. Relationship development
   f. Group therapy
4. Relaxation therapy is composed of a variety of interventions designed to:
   a. Educate the client to reframe automatic thought distortions
   b. Reduce the stress response
   c. Decrease oxygen intake
   d. Treat epilepsy

Clinical Judgment Questions

5. In a medication education group, which of the following actions is most important for reinforcing the therapeutic milieu?
   a. Allowing each person a specific and equal amount of time to talk.
   b. Reviewing group rules and behavioral limits that apply to all clients.
   c. Reading the medication information.
   d. Restricting the group to only those clients who are currently adhering to medication schedules.
6. One of the goals of therapeutic milieu is for clients to become more independent and accept self-responsibility. Which of the following approaches by staff best encourages the fulfillment of this goal?
   a. Including client input and decisions into the treatment plan
   b. Insisting that each client take a turn leading a group activity
   c. Making decisions for the client regarding plans for treatment
   d. Requiring that the client bathe, dress, and attend breakfast on time each morning
7. A client admitted to the inpatient psychiatric unit appears anxious and states, "I've never been on a unit like this before." Which action by the nurse is a priority for beginning to establish a therapeutic milieu?
   a. Instruct the client to remain in their room until they feel less anxious.
   b. Orient the client to the physical surroundings, milieu rules, and activities.
   c. Offer to medicate the client with antianxiety medication.
   d. Instruct the client not to worry because they will only be on the unit for a few days.
8. A client approaches the nurse and says, "I'm sick of the rules on this unit about not touching each other. I'm an adult and if I want to give one of the ladies a massage, it's my own business." Which of these responses best incorporates milieu therapy principles?
   a. "If you don't follow the established rules, you will be put in seclusion."
   b. "You don't make the rules, so just do as you're told."
   c. "Why are you on this unit?"
   d. "Let me try to explain why these rules are important for everyone's safety."

Continued

9. A client reports feeling "anxious all the time" but doesn't want to take the benzodiazepine medication prescribed by their family physician. Which of these is the most appropriate action for the nurse to take next?
   a. Instruct the client to continue to take the prescribed medication for several weeks in order to begin to feel relaxed.
   b. Recommend that the client begin using melatonin nightly.
   c. Assess whether the client has tried relaxation exercises or meditation.
   d. Provide medical massage therapy.
10. A fellow nurse approaches you and states, "Since you knew I was swamped you could have offered to pass my medications. You are so lazy!" Which response by the nurse is most assertive?
   a. "I'm sorry you're feeling overwhelmed. I'll try to be more sensitive next time."
   b. "You're the lazy one. I've got my own work to do."
   c. "I will go ahead and pass your medications this time, but in the future, you need to stop talking to me that way."
   d. "I deserve to be treated with respect and I will not be bullied into doing your work."
11. A client who has come to the mental health clinic with symptoms of depression says to the nurse, "My father is dying. I have always hated my father. He physically abused me when I was a child. We haven't spoken for many years. He wants to see me now, but I don't know if I want to see him." Which nursing diagnoses is a priority?
   a. Spiritual distress
   b. Risk for physical injury
   c. Altered mental status
   d. Risk for self-harm
12. As a child, a client was physically abused by their father. The father is now dying and has expressed a desire to see his child before he dies. The client is depressed and says to the mental health nurse, "I'm so angry! Why did God have to give me a father like this? I feel cheated of a father! I've always been a good person. I deserved better. I hate God!" Which nursing intervention is a priority?
   a. Ask the client why they think God gave them such an abusive father.
   b. Instruct the client to set aside their feelings temporarily to meet the needs of their dying father.
   c. Ask the client to describe in detail how they were physically abused.
   d. Ask the client if they would be willing to talk with a chaplain.

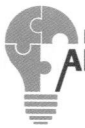

Go to **Davis Advantage** to complete your learning: strengthen understanding, apply your knowledge, and prepare for the Next Gen NCLEX®.

References

American Holistic Nurses Association & American Nurses Association. (2019). *Holistic nursing: Scope and standards of practice.* (3rd ed.).

American Nurses Association, American Psychiatric Nurses Association, & International Society of Psychiatric Nurses. (2014). *Psychiatric-mental health nursing: Scope and standards of practice.*

Bogousslavsky, J., & Inglin, M. (2007). Beliefs and the brain. *European Neurology, 58,* 129–132.

Bronson, M. (2005). *Why are there so many religions?* http://www.biblehelp.org/relig.htm

Ciompi, L., & Hoffman, H. (2004). Soteria Berne: An innovative milieu therapeutic approach to acute schizophrenia based on the concept of affect-logic. *World Psychiatry, 3*(3), 140–146.

Crane, M. (2018). Interpersonal therapy for mood disorders and substance abuse. https://www.recovery.org/topics/interpersonal-therapy-for-mood-disorders-and-substance-abuse/

Doenges, M. E., Moorhouse, M. F., & Murr, A. C. (2019). *Nursing diagnosis manual: Planning, individualizing, and documenting client care* (6th ed.). F.A. Davis.

Enayati, A. (2013). *How hope can help you heal.* http://www.cnn.com/2013/04/11/health/hope-healingenayati

Graham-Engeland, J., Sin, N., Smyth, M., Jones, D. R., Knight, E. L., Sliwinski, M. J., Almeida, D. M., Katz, M. J., Lipton. R. B., & Engeland, C. (2018). Negative and positive affect as predictors of inflammation: Timing matters. *Brain, Behavior, and Immunity 74,* 222–230. https://doi.org/10.1016/j.bbi.2018.09.011

Guynn, R. W. (2017). Interpersonal psychotherapy. In B. J. Sadock, V. A. Sadock, & P. Ruiz (Eds.), *Comprehensive textbook of psychiatry* (10th ed., pp. 2775–2784). Wolters Kluwer.

Harrison, P. (2011). *Forgiveness can improve immune function.* http://www.medscape.com/viewarticle/742198

Harvard Health. (2019). *The power of the placebo effect.* https://www.health.harvard.edu/mental-health/the-power-of-the-placebo-effect

Herdman, T. H., Kamitsuru, S., & Lopes, C. T. (Eds.). (2021). *NANDA-I nursing diagnoses: Definitions and classification, 2021–2023* (12th ed.). Thieme.

International Council of Nurses. (2012). *The ICN code of ethics for nurses.* https://www.icn.ch/sites/default/files/inlinefiles/2012_ICN_Codeofethicsfornurses_%20eng.pdf

Jones, J. (2019). U.S. church membership down sharply in past two decades. Gallup. https://news.gallup.com/poll/248837/church-membership-down-sharply-past-two- decades.aspx?g

Jones, D. R., & Graham-Engeland, J. E. (2021). Positive affect and peripheral inflammatory markers among adults: A narrative review. *Psychoneuroendocrinology, 123.* https//doi.org/10.1016/j.psyneuen.2020.104892

Karren, K. J., Hafen, B. Q., Smith, N. L., & Jenkins, K. J. (2010). *Mind/body health: The effects of attitudes, emotions, and relationships* (4th ed.). Benjamin Cummings.

Karren, K. J., Smith, N. L., Gordon, K., & Frandsen, K. J. (2013). *Mind/body health: The effects of attitudes, emotions, and relationships* (5th ed.). Pearson.

Kvarnstrom, E. (2017). *A social treatment: Mental health benefits of milieu therapy for people living with schizophrenia.* https://www.hanbleceya.com/blog/a-social-treatmentmental-health-benefits-of-milieu-therapy-for-people-living-withschizophrenia/

Koenig, H. G. (2012). Religion, spirituality, and health: The research and clinical implications. *International Scholarly Research Notices, 2012.* https://doi.org/10.5402/2012/278730

Levin, J. (2010). Religion and mental health: Theory and research. *International Journal of Applied Psychoanalytic Studies, 7*(2), 102–115. https://doi.org/10.1002/aps.240

Lichter, D. A. (2013, March-April). Studies show spiritual care linked to better health outcomes. *Health Progress.* https://www.chausa.org/publications/health-progress/article/march-april-2013/studies-show-spiritual-care-linked-to-better-health-outcomes

Liefbroer, A. I., Ganzevoort, R. R., & Olsman, E. (2019). Addressing the spiritual domain in a plural society: What is the best mode of integrating spiritual care into healthcare? *Mental Health, Religion & Culture, 22*(3), 244–260. https://doi.org/10.1080/13674676.2019.1590806

Mayo Clinic. (2020). *Forgiveness: Letting go of grudges and bitterness.* http://www.mayoclinic.org/healthy-lifestyle/adult-health/in-depth/forgiveness/art-20047692

Meehan, T. C. (2019). *The therapeutic milieu.* https://www.carefulnursing.ie/go/overview/professional_practice_model/therapeutic_milieu

Menninger Clinic. (2020). *Professionals program.* https://www.menningerclinic.com/patients/professionals-in-crisis-program/milieu-therapy

Murray, D. R., Haselton, M. G., Fales, M., & Cole, S. W. (2019). Falling in love is associated with immune system gene regulation. *Psychoneuroendocrinology 100,* 120–126. https://doi.org/10.1016/j.psyneuen.2018.09.043

National Institutes of Health. (2015). *How are therapeutic communities integrated into the criminal justice system?* https://www.drugabuse.gov/publications/research-reports/therapeutic-communities/how-are-therapeutic-communities-integrated-criminal-justice-system

Neathery, M., He, Z., Johnston Taylor, E., & Deal, B. (2020). Spiritual perspectives, spiritual care, and knowledge of recovery among psychiatric mental health nurses. *Journal of the American Psychiatric Nurses Association 26*(1), 364–372. https://doi.org/10.1177/1078390319846548

O-School. (2018). *The six components of modern milieu therapy.* http://oschool.org/the-six-components-of-modern-milieu-therapy/

Pace, T. W., Negi, T. L., Adame, D. D., Cole, S. P., Sivilli, T. I., Brown, T. D., Issa, M. J., & Raison, C. L. (2009). Effect of compassion meditation on neuroendocrine, innate immune and behavioral responses to psychosocial stress. *Psychoneuroendocrinology, 34*(1), 87–98. https://doi.org/10.1016/j.psyneuen.2008.08.011

Pew Research Center. (2017). *The changing global religious landscape.* http://assets.pewresearch.org/wpcontent/uploads/sites/11/2017/04/07092755/FULLREPORT-WITH-APPENDIXES-A-AND-B-APRIL-3.pdf

Reeves, R., & Reynolds, M. (2009). What is the role of spirituality in mental health treatment? *Journal of Psychosocial Nursing, 54*(5), 8–9. https://doi.org/10.3928/02793695-20090301-05

Sathyanarayana Rao, T. S., Asha, M. R., Jagannatha Rao, K. S., & Vasudevaraju, P. (2009). The biochemistry of belief. *Indian Journal of Psychiatry, 51*(4), 239–241. https://doi.org/10.4103/0019-5545.58285

Tétreault, P., Mansour, A., Vachon-Presseau, E., Schnitzer, T. J., Apkarian, A. V., & Baliki, M. N. (2016). Brain connectivity predicts placebo response across chronic pain clinical trials. *PLoS Biology 14*(10), e1002570. https://doi.org/10.1371/journal.pbio.1002570

Thaik, C. (2013). *Love heals!* http://www.huffingtonpost.com/dr-cynthia-thaik/love-health-benefits_b_3131370.html

Valley View. (2020). *Therapeutic milieu.* https://www.valleyviewschool.org/Therapeutic-Milieu

Classical References

Beck, A. (1976). *Cognitive therapy and the emotional disorders.* Penguin Books.

Dossey, B. M. (1998). Holistic modalities and healing moments. *American Journal of Nursing, 98*(6), 44–47.

Dossey, B. M., & American Holistic Nurses' Association. (1995). *Holistic nursing: A handbook for practice* (2nd ed.). Aspen.

Erikson, E. H. (1950). *Childhood and society.* Norton.

Glasser, W. (1965). *Reality therapy: A new approach to psychiatry.* Harper & Row.

Gunderson, J. G. (1978). Defining the therapeutic processes in psychiatric milieus. *Psychiatry: Interpersonal and Biological Processes, 41*(4), 327–335.

Kübler-Ross, E. (1969). *On death and dying.* Macmillan.

Linehan, M. M. (1993). *Cognitive-behavioral treatment of borderline personality disorder.* Guilford Press.

Nekolaichuk, C. L., Jevne, R. F., & Maguire, T. O. (1999). Structuring the meaning of hope in health and illness. *Social Science and Medicine, 48*(5), 591–605. http://doi.org/10.1016/S0277-9536(98)00348-7

Ornish, D. (1998). *Love and survival: Eight pathways to intimacy and health.* Harper Perennial.

Rogers, C. (1951). *Client-centered therapy: Its current practice, implications and theory.* Constable.

Skinner, B. F. (1979). *Beyond freedom and dignity.* Knopf.

Smucker, C. J. (2001). Overview of nursing the spirit. In D. L. Wilt & C. J. Smucker (Eds.), *Nursing the spirit: The art and science of applying spiritual care* (pp. 1–18). American Nurses.

Sullivan, H. S. (1953). *The interpersonal theory of psychiatry.* W.W. Norton and Company.

Walsh, R. (1999). *Essential spirituality.* Wiley.

Werner, E. E., & Smith, R. S. (1992). *Overcoming the odds: High risk children from birth to adulthood.* Cornell University Press.

8 Intervention in Groups

CORE CONCEPTS

Professional Behavior: Intervention in groups

Family: Family therapy

Clinical Judgment

CHAPTER OUTLINE

Objectives
Introduction
Functions of a Group
Types of Groups
Physical Conditions That Influence Group Dynamics
Therapeutic Factors
Phases of Group Development
Leadership Styles
Member Roles
Psychodrama
The Family as a Group
The Role of the Nurse in Therapeutic Groups
Summary and Key Points
Review Questions
Clinical Judgment Questions

KEY TERMS

altruism
autocratic leaders
catharsis
democratic leaders
genogram
group
laissez-faire leader
psychodrama
universality

OBJECTIVES

After reading this chapter, the student will be able to:

1. Define a group.
2. Discuss eight functions of a group.
3. Identify various types of groups.
4. Describe physical conditions that influence groups.
5. Discuss "therapeutic factors" that occur in groups.
6. Describe the phases of group development.
7. Identify various leadership styles in groups.
8. Identify various roles that members assume within a group.
9. Discuss psychodrama and family therapy as specialized forms of group therapy.
10. Describe the role of the nurse in group therapy.

Introduction

Human beings are complex creatures who share their activities of daily living (ADLs) with various groups of people. As Forsyth (2019) stated, "The tendency to join with others in groups is perhaps the single most important characteristic of humans and the processes that unfold within these groups leave an indelible imprint on their members and on society" (p. 1). Groups provide a sense of belonging, establish norms for accepted behavior, and facilitate problem-solving.

Health-care professionals encounter multiple group situations in their professional activities. Team conferences, committee meetings, grand rounds, and in-service sessions are but a few instances in which this occurs. In psychiatry, work with patients and families is often conducted within groups. With group work, not only does the nurse have the opportunity to reach out to a greater number of people at one time, but the group members also assist each other by sharing feelings, opinions, ideas, and behaviors within the group. Patients learn from each other in a group setting.

This chapter explores various types of therapeutic groups that can be used in psychiatric settings and the role of the nurse in group intervention.

CORE CONCEPT

Group

A **group** is a collection of individuals whose association is founded on shared interests, values, norms, or purpose. Membership in a group is generally by chance (born into the group), by choice (voluntary affiliation), or by circumstance (the result of life-cycle events over which an individual may or may not have control).

Functions of a Group

In their classic work, Sampson and Marthas (1990) outlined the following eight functions that groups serve for their members. They contend that groups may serve more than one function and usually serve different functions for different members of the group.

1. ***Socialization:*** The cultural group into which we are born begins the process of teaching social norms. This process continues throughout our lives as we interact with members of other groups with which we become affiliated.
2. ***Support:*** One's fellow group members are available in time of need. Individuals derive a feeling of security from group involvement.
3. ***Task completion:*** Group members provide assistance in endeavors that are beyond the capacity of one individual alone or when results can be achieved more effectively as a team.
4. ***Camaraderie:*** Members of a group provide the joy and pleasure that individuals seek from interactions with significant others.
5. ***Information sharing:*** Learning takes place within groups. Knowledge is gained when individual members learn how others in the group have resolved situations similar to those with which they are currently struggling.
6. ***Normative influence:*** This function relates to the ways in which groups enforce the established norms. As group members interact, they begin to influence each other regarding the expected norms for communication and behavior.
7. ***Empowerment:*** Groups help to bring about improvement in existing conditions by providing support to individual members who seek to bring about change. Groups have power that individuals alone do not.
8. ***Governance:*** Groups may provide oversight functions and direction of activities (such as strategic planning or quality improvement) often within the context of a larger organization.

Types of Groups

The functions of a group vary depending on the reason the group was formed. Clark (2009) identified three types of groups in which nurses most often participate: task, teaching, and supportive/therapeutic groups.

Task Groups

The function of a task group is to accomplish a specific outcome or task. The focus is on solving problems and making decisions to achieve this outcome. Often a deadline is placed on completion of the task, and such importance is placed on a satisfactory outcome that conflict in the group may be smoothed over or ignored in order to focus on the priority at hand.

Teaching Groups

Teaching, or educational, groups exist to convey knowledge and information to a number of individuals. Nurses can be involved in many types of teaching groups, such as medication education, childbirth education, and effective parenting classes. These groups usually have a set time frame or a specific number of meetings. Members learn from each other as well as from the designated instructor. The objective of teaching groups is for the learner to verbalize or demonstrate mastery of the material presented by the end of the designated period.

Supportive/Therapeutic Groups

Supportive or therapeutic groups are primarily concerned with participants sharing thoughts, feelings, events, and coping strategies to help them learn effective ways to deal with emotional stress arising from situational or developmental crises.

CORE CONCEPT

Group therapy

Group therapy is a form of psychosocial treatment in which a number of clients meet together with a therapist for purposes of sharing, gaining personal insight, and improving interpersonal coping strategies.

For the purposes of this text, it is important to differentiate between *therapeutic groups* and *group therapy*. Leaders of group therapy generally have advanced degrees in psychology, social work, nursing, or medicine. They often have additional training or experience under the supervision of an accomplished professional in conducting group psychotherapy based on various theoretical frameworks such as cognitive behavioral, psychodynamic, interpersonal, and family dynamics. Approaches based on these theories are used by the group therapy leaders to encourage improvement in the ability of group members to function on an interpersonal level.

Supportive/therapeutic groups, on the other hand, are not designed to conduct psychotherapy. They focus instead on group relations, interactions among group members, and the consideration of a selected issue. Like group therapists, individuals who lead therapeutic groups must be knowledgeable in *group process*—that is, the *way* in which group members interact with each other. Interruptions, silences, judgments, glares, and scapegoating are examples of group processes. These interactions may occur whether or not there is a designated group leader, but nurses who are acting as group leaders can guide the way in which members interact with one another to facilitate accomplishing the goals or tasks of the group. This is one reason that group leaders are often referred to as *group facilitators*. They must also have a thorough knowledge of *group content* (the topic or issue being discussed among the group), and the ability to present the topic in language that can be understood by all group members. Many nurses who work in psychiatry lead supportive/therapeutic groups.

Self-Help Groups

Nurses may also be involved in self-help groups. This type of group that has grown in number and credibility in recent years. Self-help groups allow clients to talk about their fears and relieve feelings of isolation while receiving comfort and advice from others undergoing similar experiences. Examples of self-help groups are those for dealing with disorders such as Alzheimer's disease or anorexia nervosa, Weight Watchers, Alcoholics Anonymous, Reach to Recovery, Parents Without Partners, Overeaters Anonymous, Adult Children of Alcoholics, and many others related to specific needs or illnesses. These groups may or may not have a professional leader or consultant. They are run by the members, and leadership often rotates from member to member.

Nurses may become involved with self-help groups either voluntarily or because members have requested their advice or participation. The nurse may function as a referral agent, resource person, member of an advisory board, or leader of the group. Self-help groups are a valuable source of referral for clients with specific problems. However, nurses must be knowledgeable about the purposes of the group, membership, leadership, benefits, and problems that might threaten the success of the group before referring their clients to a specific self-help group. The nurse may find it necessary to attend several meetings of a particular group, if possible, to assess its effectiveness of purpose and appropriateness for client referral.

Physical Conditions That Influence Group Dynamics

The physical aspects, including arrangement of seating, the number of group members, and whether the membership is consistent or variable, has an impact on the dynamics of interaction within the group.

Seating

When preparing the seating for a group, there should be no barrier between the members. For example, a circle of chairs is better than chairs set around a table. Members should be encouraged to sit in different chairs at each meeting. The openness and change of seating create a feeling of discomfort that encourages anxious and unsettled behaviors that can then be explored within the group.

Size

Various authors have suggested different ranges of size as ideal for group interaction: 5 to 10 (Yalom & Leszcz, 2005), 2 to 15 (Sampson & Marthas, 1990), and 4 to 12 (Clark, 2009). Group size does make a difference in the interaction among members. The larger the group, the less time there is available to devote to individual members. In larger groups, aggressive individuals are most likely to be heard, whereas quiet members may be left out of the discussions altogether. Understanding this dynamic alerts nurse group leaders to this possibility and allows them to facilitate interaction in ways that promote greater involvement for all members. However, larger groups provide more opportunities for individuals to learn from other members. The wider range of life experiences and knowledge provides a greater potential for effective group problem-solving. Ultimately, there is no single right answer in identifying optimal group size because it is influenced by several variables including the group's purpose, group members' functional abilities, and expected outcomes.

Membership

Whether the group is open-ended or closed-ended is another condition that influences the dynamics of group process. Open-ended groups are those in which members leave and others join at any time while the group is active. The continuous movement of members in and out of the group creates discomfort that encourages individual members to explore their feelings about their own progress. These are the most common types of groups held on short-term inpatient units, although they are used in outpatient and long-term care facilities as well. Closed-ended groups usually have a predetermined, fixed time frame. All members join at the time the group is organized and terminate at the end of the designated time period. Closed-ended groups are often composed of individuals with common issues or problems they wish to address.

Therapeutic Factors

Why are therapeutic groups helpful? Yalom and Leszcz (2005) described 11 therapeutic factors that individuals can achieve through interpersonal interactions within the group, some of which are present in most groups in varying degrees:

1. ***Instillation of hope:*** By observing the progress of others in the group with similar problems, a group member garners hope that his or her problems can also be resolved.
2. ***Universality:*** Through **universality,** individuals come to realize that they are not alone in the problems, thoughts, and feelings they are experiencing. Anxiety is relieved by the support and understanding of others in the group who share similar (universal) experiences.
3. ***Imparting of information:*** Knowledge is gained through formal instruction as well as the sharing of advice and suggestions among group members.
4. ***Altruism:*** **Altruism** is mutual sharing and concern for each other. Providing assistance and support to others creates a positive self-image and promotes self-growth.
5. ***Corrective recapitulation of the primary family group:*** Group members are able to reexperience early family conflicts that remain unresolved. Attempts at resolution are promoted through feedback and exploration.
6. ***Development of socializing techniques:*** Through interaction with and feedback from other members of the group, individuals are able to correct maladaptive social behaviors and learn and develop new social skills.
7. ***Imitative behavior:*** In a group setting, members who have mastered particular psychosocial skills or developmental tasks can be valuable role models for others. Individuals may imitate selected behaviors that they wish to develop in themselves.
8. ***Interpersonal learning:*** The group offers many and varied opportunities for interacting with other people. Insight is gained regarding how one perceives and is being perceived by others.
9. ***Group cohesiveness:*** Members develop a sense of belonging that separates the individual ("I am") from the group ("we are"). Out of this alliance emerges a common feeling that individual members and the total group are of value to each other.
10. ***Catharsis:*** Within the group, members are able to express both positive and negative feelings—perhaps feelings that have never been expressed before—in a nonthreatening atmosphere. This **catharsis,** or open expression of feelings, is beneficial for the individual within the group.
11. ***Existential factors:*** The group is able to help individual members take direction of their own lives and to accept responsibility for the quality of their existence.

It may be helpful for a group leader to explain these therapeutic factors to members of the group. Positive responses are experienced by individuals who understand and are able to recognize therapeutic factors as they occur within the group.

Phases of Group Development

Groups, like individuals, move through phases of life-cycle development. Ideally, groups progress from the phase of infancy to advanced maturity in an effort to fulfill the objectives set forth by the membership.

As with individuals, some groups become fixed in early developmental levels and never progress, or they experience periods of regression in the developmental process. Three phases of group development are discussed here.

Phase I. Initial or Orientation Phase

Group Activities

The leader and members work together to establish the rules that govern the group (e.g., when and where meetings will occur, the importance of confidentiality, how meetings will be structured). Goals of the group are established. Members are introduced to each other.

Leader Expectations

The leader is expected to orient members to specific group processes, encourage members to participate without disclosing too much too soon, promote an environment of trust, and ensure that rules established by the group do not interfere with fulfillment of the goals.

Member Behaviors

In phase I, members have not yet established trust and will respond to this lack of trust by being overly polite. There is a fear of not being accepted by the group. They may try to "get on the good side" of the leader with compliments and conforming behaviors. A power struggle may ensue as members compete for their position in the "pecking order" of the group.

Phase II. Middle or Working Phase

Group Activities

Ideally, during the working phase, cohesiveness has been established within the group. This is when the productive work toward completion of the task is undertaken. Problem-solving and decision making occur within the group. In the mature group, cooperation prevails, and differences and disagreements are confronted and resolved.

Leader Expectations

The leader becomes less of a leader and more of a facilitator during the working phase. Some leadership functions are shared by certain members of the group as they progress toward resolution. The leader helps to resolve conflict and continues to foster cohesiveness among the members while ensuring that they do not deviate from the intended task or purpose for which the group was organized.

Member Behaviors

At this point, trust has been established among the members. They turn more often to each other and less often to the leader for guidance. They accept criticism from each other, using it in a constructive manner to create change. Occasionally, subgroups will form in which two or more members conspire with each other to the exclusion of the rest of the group. These subgroups must be confronted and discussed by the entire membership to maintain group cohesion. Conflict is managed by the group with minimal assistance from the leader.

Phase III. Final or Termination Phase

Group Activities

The longer a group has been in existence, the more difficult termination is likely to be for the members. Termination should be mentioned from the outset of group formation. It should be discussed in depth for several meetings prior to the final session. A sense of loss that precipitates the grief process may be in evidence, particularly in groups that have been successful in their stated purpose.

Leader Expectations

In the termination phase, the leader encourages the group members to reminisce about what has occurred within the group, to review the goals and discuss the actual outcomes, and provide feedback to each other about individual progress within the group. The leader encourages members to discuss feelings of loss associated with termination of the group.

Member Behaviors

Members may express surprise when the group actually ends. This expression represents the grief response of denial, which may then progress to anger. Anger toward other group members or toward the leader may reflect feelings of abandonment (Sampson & Marthas, 1990). These feelings may lead to individual members' discussions of previous losses for which similar emotions were experienced. Successful termination of the group may help members develop the skills needed when losses occur in other dimensions of their lives.

Leadership Styles

Lippitt and White's classic work (1958) identified three of the most common group leadership styles: autocratic, democratic, and laissez-faire. Table 8–1 outlines various similarities and differences among the three leadership styles.

TABLE 8–1 **Leadership Styles—Similarities and Differences**

CHARACTERISTICS	AUTOCRATIC	DEMOCRATIC	LAISSEZ-FAIRE
1. Focus	Leader	Members	Undetermined
2. Task strategy	Members are persuaded to adopt leader ideas	Members engage in group problem-solving	No defined strategy exists
3. Member participation	Limited	Unlimited	Inconsistent
4. Individual creativity	Stifled	Encouraged	Not addressed
5. Member enthusiasm and morale	Low	High	Low
6. Group cohesiveness	Low	High	Low
7. Productivity	High	High (may not be as high as autocratic)	Low
8. Individual motivation and commitment	Low (tend to work only when leader is present to urge them to do so)	High (satisfaction derived from personal input and participation)	Low (feelings of frustration from lack of direction or guidance)

Autocratic

Autocratic leaders have personal goals for the group. They withhold information from group members, particularly issues that may interfere with achievement of their own objectives. The message that is conveyed to the group is: "We will do it my way. My way is best." The focus in this style of leadership is on the leader. Members are dependent on the leader for problem-solving, decision making, and permission to perform. The approach of autocratic leaders is one of persuasion, striving to persuade others in the group that their ideas and methods are superior. Productivity is high with this type of leadership, but often morale within the group is low because of lack of member input and creativity.

Democratic

Democratic leaders focus on the members of the group. Information is shared with members in an effort to allow them to make decisions regarding achieving the goals for the group. Members are encouraged to participate fully in solving problems that relate to the group, including taking action to effect change. The message conveyed to the group is: "Decide what must be done, consider the alternatives, make a selection, and proceed with the actions required to complete the task." The leader provides guidance and expertise as needed. Productivity is lower than it is with autocratic leadership, but morale is much higher because of the extent of input allowed all members of the group and the potential for individual creativity.

Laissez-Faire

This leadership style allows people to do as they please. There is no direction from the leader. In fact, the approach of the **laissez-faire leader** is noninvolvement. Goals for the group are undefined. No decisions are made, no problems are solved, and no action is taken. Members become frustrated and confused, and productivity and morale are low.

Member Roles

Benne and Sheat's classic work (1948) identified three major types of roles that individuals play within the membership of the group. These are roles that serve to

1. Complete the task of the group.
2. Maintain or enhance group processes.
3. Fulfill personal or individual needs.

Task roles and maintenance roles contribute to the success or effectiveness of the group. Personal roles satisfy needs of the individual members, sometimes to the extent of interfering with the effectiveness of the group.

Table 8–2 outlines specific roles within these three major types and the behaviors associated with each.

Psychodrama

A specialized type of therapeutic group, called **psychodrama,** was introduced in 1921 by J. L. Moreno, a Viennese psychiatrist. Moreno's method employs a

TABLE 8–2 Member Roles Within Groups

ROLE	BEHAVIORS
TASK ROLES	
Coordinator	Clarifies ideas and suggestions that have been made within the group; brings relationships together to pursue common goals.
Evaluator	Examines group plans and performance, measuring against group standards and goals.
Elaborator	Explains and expands upon group plans and ideas.
Energizer	Encourages and motivates group to perform at its maximum potential.
Initiator	Outlines the task at hand for the group and proposes methods for solution.
Orienter	Maintains direction within the group.
MAINTENANCE ROLES	
Compromiser	Relieves conflict within the group by assisting members to reach a compromise agreeable to all.
Encourager	Offers recognition and acceptance of others' ideas and contributions.
Follower	Listens attentively to group interaction; is a passive participant.
Gatekeeper	Encourages acceptance of and participation by all members of the group.
Harmonizer	Minimizes tension within the group by intervening when disagreements produce conflict.
INDIVIDUAL (PERSONAL) ROLES	
Aggressor	Expresses negativism and hostility toward other members; may use sarcasm in effort to degrade the status of others.
Blocker	Resists group efforts; demonstrates rigid and sometimes irrational behaviors that impede group progress.
Dominator	Manipulates others to gain control; behaves in authoritarian manner.
Help-seeker	Uses the group to gain sympathy from others; seeks to increase self-confidence from group feedback; lacks concern for others or for the group as a whole.
Monopolizer	Maintains control of the group by dominating the conversation.
Mute or silent member	Does not participate verbally; remains silent for a variety of reasons—may feel uncomfortable with self-disclosure or may be seeking attention through silence.
Recognition seeker	Talks about personal accomplishments in an effort to gain attention for self.
Seducer	Shares intimate details about self with group; is the least reluctant of the group to do so; may frighten others in the group and inhibit group progress with excessive premature self-disclosure.

Source: Compiled from Benne and Sheats (1948, Spring) and Hobbs and Powers (1981).

dramatic approach in which clients become "actors" in life-situation scenarios. Cruz and associates (2018), in a systematic review of the literature, identified and defined 11 distinct techniques that are core techniques of Morenian psychodrama, all of which are directed toward offering the client, in a group format, an opportunity to "act out" roles and situations in which the client has unresolved conflicts.

The group leader is called the *director*, group members are the *audience*, and the *set*, or *stage*, may be specially designed or may just be any room or part of a room selected for this purpose. Group members agree to take part in the "drama" by role-playing a situation about which they have been informed by the director. Usually, the situation is an issue with which one individual client has been struggling.

That individual plays themself and is called the *protagonist.* The psychodrama setting provides the client with a safer and less threatening atmosphere than the real situation in which to express true feelings. Resolution of interpersonal conflicts is facilitated.

When the drama has been completed, group members from the audience discuss the situation they have observed, offer feedback, express their feelings, and relate their own similar experiences. In this way, all group members benefit from the session, either directly or indirectly.

Nurses often serve as actors, or role players, in psychodrama sessions. Leaders of psychodrama typically have graduate degrees in psychology, social work, nursing, or medicine with additional training in group therapy and specialty preparation to become a psychodramatist.

CORE CONCEPTS

Family

Two or more individuals who depend on one another for emotional, physical, and economical support. The members of the family are self-defined.

A treatment modality that identifies the family, rather than any one individual, as the client. The family is assisted to solve identified problems within the context of the family group.

The Family as a Group

In family therapy, the family is viewed as a system in which the members are interdependent; a change in one part (member) within the system affects or creates change in all other parts (members). Thus, the major goal is to facilitate system change rather than focus on any one individual as the one in need of treatment.

Because the primary goal of family therapy is to facilitate change within the family as a group, it is important for the family therapist to identify who the family perceives to be family members and, ideally, to conduct an assessment with the entire family. One assessment tool often used by family therapists is a **genogram.** The genogram is a visual presentation of the members, their relationships, and sometimes their health issues, across several generations. It provides a convenient way to visualize and summarize a great deal of information in a concise format. A sample genogram is presented in Figure 8–1.

Nurses who conduct family therapy are expected to possess a graduate degree and have considerable knowledge of family theories. However, it is within the realm of the generalist registered nurse in psychiatric settings to contribute to the assessment, planning, and interventions with families for the purpose of counseling and education. All nurses should have a basic understanding of family dynamics and the ability to distinguish between functional and dysfunctional behaviors within a family system.

The Role of the Nurse in Therapeutic Groups

Nurses participate in group situations on a daily basis. In health-care settings, nurses serve on or lead task groups that create policy, describe procedures, and plan patient care. They are also involved in a variety of other groups aimed at the institutional effort of serving the health-care consumer. Nurses are encouraged to use the steps of the nursing process as a framework for task group leadership.

In psychiatry, nurses may lead various types of therapeutic groups, such as patient education, assertiveness training, grief support, parenting, and transition to discharge groups, among others. To function effectively in the leadership capacity for these groups, nurses need to be able to recognize various processes that occur in groups, such as the phases of group development, the various roles that people play within group situations, and the motivation behind these behaviors. They also need to be able to select the most appropriate leadership style for the type of group. Generalist nurses may develop these skills as part of their undergraduate education, or they may pursue additional study while serving and learning as the co-leader of a group with a more experienced nurse leader.

Generalist nurses in psychiatry should not serve as leaders of psychotherapy groups. The *Psychiatric–Mental Health Nursing Scope and Standards of Practice* (American Nurses Association, American Psychiatric Nurses Association, & International Society of Psychiatric Nurses, 2022) specifies that nurses who serve as group psychotherapists should have a minimum of a master's degree in psychiatric nursing. Educational preparation in group theory, extended practice as a group co-leader or leader under the supervision of an experienced psychotherapist, and participation in group therapy on an experiential level are also recommended. Additional specialist training is required beyond the master's level to prepare nurses to become family therapists or psychodramatists.

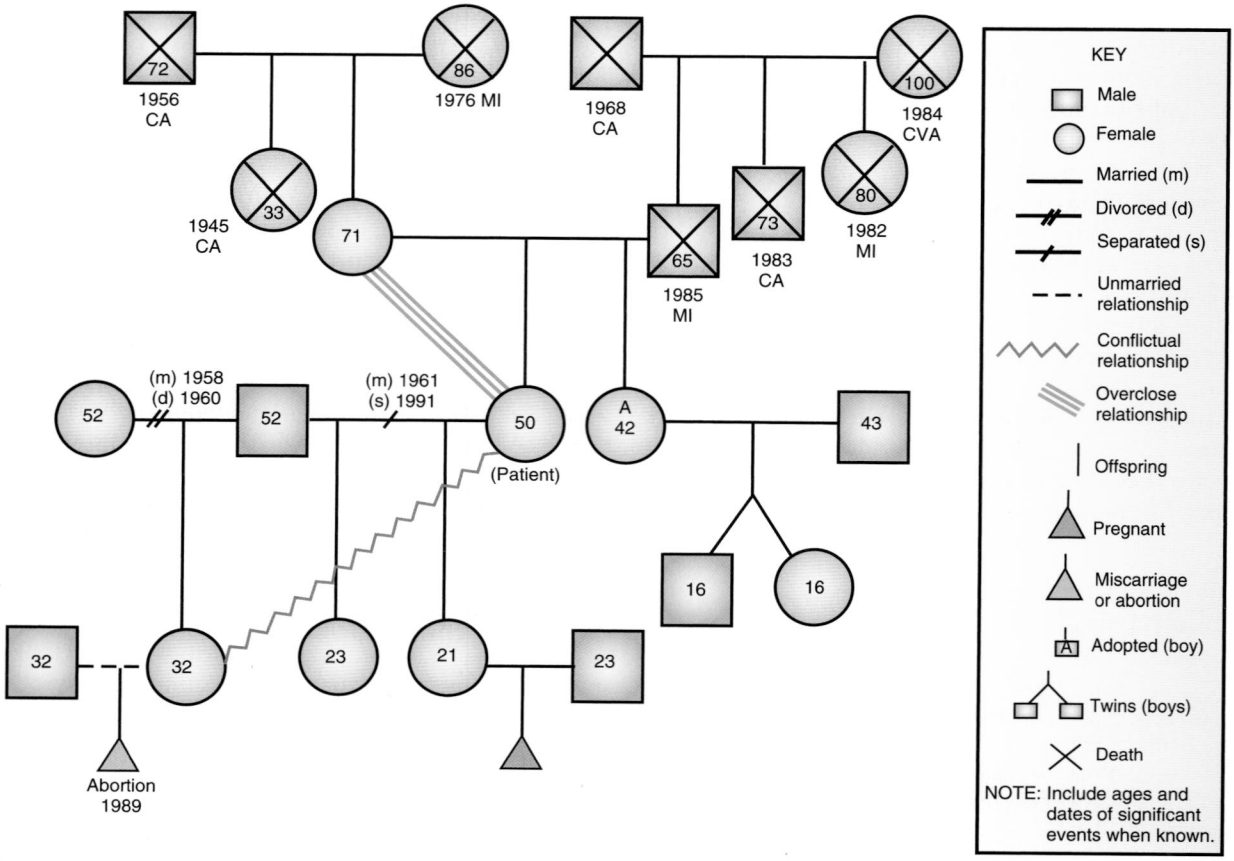

FIGURE 8–1 Sample genogram.

Leading therapeutic groups is within the realm of nursing practice. Because group work is such a common therapeutic approach in the discipline of psychiatry, nurses working in this field must continually strive to expand their knowledge and use of group process as a significant psychiatric nursing intervention.

CLINICAL PEARL Knowledge of human behavior in general and the group process in particular is essential to effective group leadership.

Summary and Key Points

- A *group* is defined as a collection of individuals whose association is founded on shared interests, values, norms, or purpose.
- Eight group functions identified by Sampson and Marthas (1990) are socialization, support, task completion, camaraderie, information sharing, normative influence, empowerment, and governance.
- The three major types of groups are task groups, teaching groups, and supportive/therapeutic groups.
- The function of task groups is to solve problems, make decisions, and achieve a specific outcome.
- In teaching groups, knowledge and information are conveyed to a number of individuals.
- The function of supportive/therapeutic groups is to facilitate members' learning how to deal effectively with emotional stress in their lives.
- In self-help groups, members share the same type of problem and help each other to prevent decompensation related to that problem.
- Therapeutic groups differ from group therapy in that the focus is not on psychotherapy but on interaction and relationships among group members with regard to a selected issue. Group therapy is more focused on specific models of psychotherapy, and the leaders generally have advanced degrees in psychology, social work, nursing, or medicine.

- Placement of the seating and size of the group can influence group interaction.
- Groups can be open-ended (when members leave and others join at any time while the group is active) or closed-ended (when groups have a predetermined, fixed time frame and all members join at the same time and leave when the group disbands).
- Yalom and Leszcz (2005) describe the following therapeutic factors that individuals derive from participation in therapeutic groups: the instillation of hope, universality, the imparting of information, altruism, the corrective recapitulation of the primary family group, the development of socializing techniques, imitative behavior, interpersonal learning, group cohesiveness, catharsis, and existential factors.
- Groups progress through three phases: the initial (orientation) phase, the working phase, and the termination phase.
- Group leadership styles include autocratic, democratic, and laissez-faire.
- Members play various roles within groups. These roles are categorized according to task roles, maintenance roles, and personal roles.
- Psychodrama is a specialized type of group therapy that uses a dramatic approach in which clients become "actors" in life-situation scenarios.
- The psychodrama setting provides the client with a safer and less threatening atmosphere than the real situation in which to express and work through unresolved conflicts.
- Family therapy is a specialized form of group intervention in which the client is the whole family rather than any one individual and the goal is to facilitate change in the family system.
- Nurses lead various types of therapeutic groups in the psychiatric setting. Knowledge of human behavior in general and the group process in particular is essential to effective group leadership.
- Specialized training, in addition to a master's degree, is required for nurses to serve as group psychotherapists or psychodramatists.

Review Questions

Select the answer that is most appropriate for each of the following questions:

1. A nurse leader of a childbirth preparation group shows various films each week and sets out reading materials. Participants are expected to utilize their time on a topic of their choice or practice skills they have observed on the films. Two couples have dropped out of the group, stating, "This is a big waste of time." Which type of group and style of leadership is described in this situation?
   a. Task; democratic
   b. Teaching; laissez-faire
   c. Self-help; democratic
   d. Supportive/therapeutic; autocratic
2. A psychiatric nurse is leading a group for women who desire to lose weight. The criterion for membership is that they must be at least 20 pounds overweight. All have tried to lose weight on their own many times in the past without success. At their first meeting, the nurse provides suggestions as the members determine what their goals will be and how they plan to achieve those goals. They decide how often they want to meet and what they plan to do at each meeting. Which type of group and style of leadership is described in this situation?
   a. Task; autocratic
   b. Teaching; democratic
   c. Self-help; laissez-faire
   d. Supportive/therapeutic; democratic

Continued

3. A staff nurse on a surgical unit has been selected to lead a group of staff nurses organized to determine ways to decrease the number of medication errors occurring on the unit. The group leader has definite ideas about how to bring this about and believes that if they are successful in leading the group toward achievement of its goals, it will facilitate their chances for promotion. At each meeting, the nurse addresses the group in an effort to convince the members to adopt their ideas. Which type of group and style of leadership is described in this situation?
   a. Task; autocratic
   b. Teaching; autocratic
   c. Self-help; democratic
   d. Supportive/therapeutic; laissez-faire
4. The nurse leader, who is explaining about group "therapeutic factors" to members of the group, tells the members that group situations are beneficial because members can see that they are not alone in their experiences. This is an example of which therapeutic factor?
   a. Altruism
   b. Imitative behavior
   c. Universality
   d. Imparting of information
5. Nancy is a new member of a bereavement group for widows. She listens to the group and learns that Jane has been a widow for 5 years. Jane has adjusted well, and Nancy thinks maybe she can too. This is an example of which therapeutic factor?
   a. Universality
   b. Imitative behavior
   c. Installation of hope
   d. Imparting of information
6. A client is a member of an anger management group. The client knows that people do not want to be their friend because of their violent temper. In the group, the client has learned to control their temper and form satisfactory interpersonal relationships with others. This is an example of which therapeutic factor?
   a. Catharsis
   b. Altruism
   c. Imparting of information
   d. Development of socializing techniques
7. In a supportive/therapeutic group for individuals with anxiety disorders, one of the members, Helen, talks incessantly. When other members try to make a comment, Helen refuses to allow them to speak. What type of member role is Helen assuming in this group?
   a. Aggressor
   b. Monopolizer
   c. Blocker
   d. Seducer

Clinical Judgment Questions

8. A nurse who is a diabetic educator is offering a support group for clients who are having difficulty adhering to the recommended diet. Thirty people have signed up for the group. Which next action by the nurse is most appropriate?
   a. Change the focus of the group from a support group to an education group.
   b. Defer starting the group until at least 50 people have signed up.
   c. Limit the group size to a maximum of 15 people and consider having two separate groups.
   d. In lieu of meeting as a group, provide written materials with suggestions for how to adhere to dietary recommendations.
9. A newly admitted client asks the psychiatric unit staff nurse to describe what's going to happen in the support group that is scheduled on the unit. Which of these actions by the nurse is most appropriate?
   a. Instruct the client that support groups are an opportunity for participants to share thoughts and feelings and learn ways to effectively manage stress.
   b. Instruct the client that this is something that only the physician is permitted to describe to the client.
   c. Instruct the client not to attend since the other participants have been on the unit longer.
   d. Instruct the client that they will just have to go and see for themselves.
10. A staff nurse on the psychiatric unit is approached by a psychologist who requests that the staff nurse conduct a therapy group for trauma clients. Which of these actions by the nurse is most appropriate?
   a. Ask the psychologist to recommend what activities should be completed.
   b. Offer to lead the group as long as there is a co-leader assigned.
   c. Instruct the psychologist that leading a therapy group is not within the scope of practice for a generalist staff nurse.
   d. Agree to lead the group but limit the focus to art therapy activities.

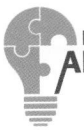

Go to **Davis Advantage** to complete your learning: strengthen understanding, apply your knowledge, and prepare for the Next Gen NCLEX®.

References

American Nurses Association, American Psychiatric Nurses Association, & International Society of Psychiatric Nurses. (2022). *Psychiatric–mental health nursing: Scope and standards of practice* (3rd ed.). Nursesbooks.org.

Clark, C. C. (2009). *Group leadership skills for nurses and health professionals* (5th ed.). Springer.

Cruz, A., Sales, C., Alves, P., & Moita, G. (2018). The core techniques of Morenian psychodrama: A systematic review of literature. *Frontiers in Psychology, 9*, 1263. https://doi.org/10.3389/fpsyg.2018.01263

Forsyth, D. R. (2019). *Group dynamics* (7th ed.). Cengage Learning.

Yalom, I. D., & Leszcz, M. (2005). *The theory and practice of group psychotherapy* (5th ed.). Basic Books.

Classical References

Benne, K. D., & Sheats, P. (1948, Spring). Functional roles of group members. *Journal of Social Issues, 4*(2), 41–49.

Hobbs, D. J., & Powers, R. C. (1981). *Group member roles: For group effectiveness.* Iowa State University, Cooperative Extension Service.

Lippitt, R., & White, R. K. (1958). An experimental study of leadership and group life. In E. E. Maccoby, T. M. Newcomb, & E. L. Hartley (Eds.), *Readings in social psychology* (3rd ed.). Holt, Rinehart & Winston.

Sampson, E. E., & Marthas, M. (1990). *Group process for the health professions* (3rd ed.). Delmar.

9 Crisis Intervention

CORE CONCEPTS
Stress and Coping: Crisis
Safety: Crisis intervention
Clinical Judgment

CHAPTER OUTLINE

Objectives
Introduction
Characteristics of a Crisis
Phases in the Development of a Crisis
Types of Crises
Crisis on the Inpatient Unit: Anger and Aggression Management
Crisis Intervention
Phases of Crisis Intervention: The Role of the Nurse
Disaster Nursing
Application of the Nursing Process to Disaster Nursing
Summary and Key Points
Review Questions
Clinical Judgment Questions
Communication Exercises

KEY TERMS

aggression
anger
crisis
crisis intervention
disaster
prodromal syndrome

OBJECTIVES

After reading this chapter, the student will be able to:

1. Define *crisis*.
2. Describe four phases in the development of a crisis.
3. Identify types of crises that occur in people's lives.
4. Discuss the goal of crisis intervention.
5. Describe the steps in crisis intervention.
6. Identify the role of the nurse in crisis intervention.
7. Apply the nursing process to care of victims of disasters.
8. Define and differentiate between *anger* and *aggression*.
9. Discuss predisposing factors to the maladaptive expression of anger.

Introduction

Stressful situations are a part of everyday life. Any stressful situation can precipitate a crisis. Crises result in a disequilibrium from which many individuals require assistance to recover. Crisis resolution requires problem-solving skills that are often diminished by the level of anxiety accompanying disequilibrium. Assistance with problem-solving during the crisis period preserves self-esteem and promotes growth with resolution.

In recent years, individuals in the United States have been faced with a number of catastrophic events, including a worldwide pandemic and natural disasters such as tornados, earthquakes, hurricanes, and floods. Man-made disasters, such as the Oklahoma City and

Boston Marathon bombings, the attacks on the World Trade Center and the Pentagon, and mass shootings, have created psychological stress of enormous proportions in populations around the world.

This chapter examines the phases in the development of a crisis and the types of crises that commonly occur in people's lives. The methodology of crisis intervention, including the role of the nurse, is explored. A discussion of disaster nursing is also presented.

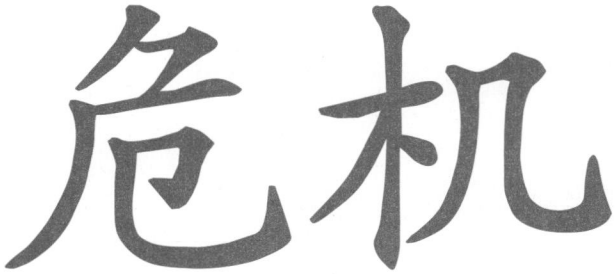

FIGURE 9–1 Chinese symbol for crisis.

CORE CONCEPT

Crisis

A **crisis** is an acute event perceived by the individual as distressing and in which coping mechanisms and support systems are inadequate to manage associated anxiety.

Characteristics of a Crisis

The concept of crisis has several defining characteristics (Aguilera, 1998; Caplan, 1964). They include the following:

1. Crisis occurs in all individuals at one time or another and is not necessarily equated with psychopathology.
2. Crises are precipitated by specific identifiable events.
3. Crises are personal by nature. What may be considered a crisis situation by one individual may not be so for another.
4. Crises are acute, not chronic, and will be resolved in one way or another within a brief period.
5. A crisis situation contains the potential for psychological growth or deterioration.

Individuals who are in crisis feel helpless to change. They do not believe they have the resources to deal with the precipitating stressor. Levels of anxiety rise to the point that the individual becomes nonfunctional, thoughts become obsessional, and all behavior is aimed at relief of the anxiety being experienced. The feeling is overwhelming and may affect the individual physically as well as psychologically.

Bateman and Peternelj-Taylor (1998) stated:

> Outside Western culture, a crisis is often viewed as a time for movement and growth. The Chinese symbol for crisis consists of the characters for *danger* and *opportunity* [Fig. 9–1]. When a crisis is viewed as an opportunity for growth, those involved are much more capable of resolving related issues and more able to move toward positive changes. When the crisis experience is overwhelming because of its scope and nature or when there has not been adequate preparation for the necessary changes, the dangers seem paramount and overshadow any potential growth. The results are maladaptive coping and dysfunctional behavior. (pp. 144–145)

Phases in the Development of a Crisis

The development of a crisis situation follows a relatively predictable course. Caplan (1964) outlined four specific phases through which individuals progress in response to a precipitating stressor and that culminate in the state of acute crisis:

- ***Phase 1:*** *The individual is exposed to a precipitating stressor.* Anxiety increases; previous problem-solving techniques are employed.
- ***Phase 2:*** *When previous problem-solving techniques do not relieve the stressor, anxiety increases further.* The individual begins to feel a great deal of discomfort at this point. Coping techniques that have worked in the past are attempted, only to create feelings of helplessness when they are not successful. Feelings of confusion and disorganization prevail.
- ***Phase 3:*** *All possible resources, both internal and external, are called on to resolve the problem and relieve the discomfort.* The individual may try to view the problem from a different perspective or even to overlook certain aspects of it. New problem-solving techniques may be used and, if effective, resolution may occur at this phase, with the individual returning to a higher, a lower, or previous level of precrisis functioning.
- ***Phase 4:*** *If resolution does not occur in previous phases, "the tension mounts beyond a further threshold or its burden increases over time to a breaking point. Major disorganization of the individual with drastic results often occurs"* (Caplan, 1998, p. 41). Anxiety may reach panic levels. Cognitive functions are disordered, emotions are labile, and behavior may reflect the presence of psychotic thinking.

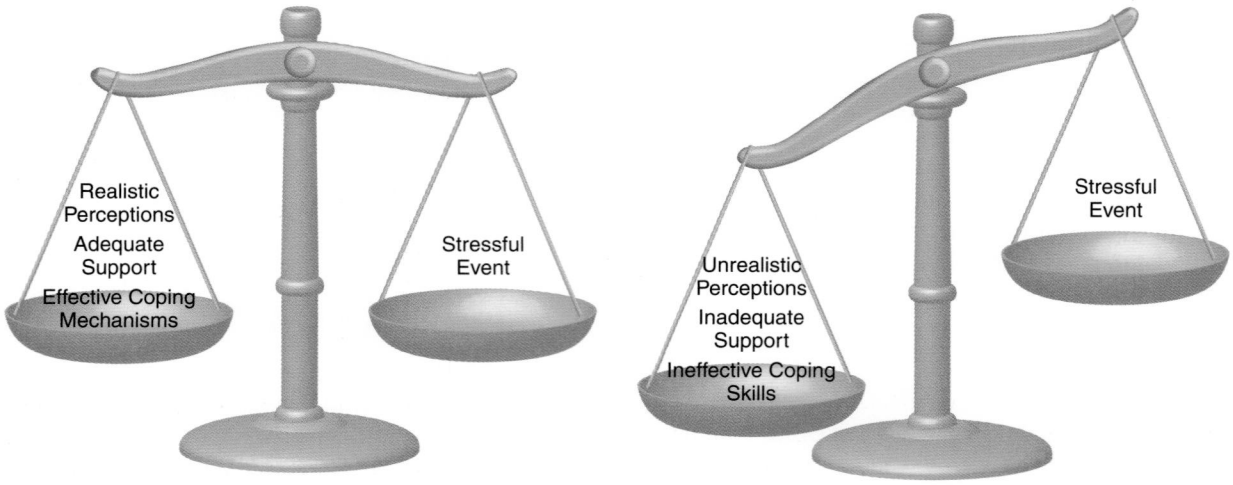

FIGURE 9–2 The effect of balancing factors in a stressful event.

These phases are congruent with the concept of "balancing factors" as described by Aguilera (1998). When individuals perceive a stressor as a threat to their well-being and they lack adaptive coping strategies or employ maladaptive strategies, crisis ensues. Similarly, Aguilera (1998) spoke of "balancing factors" that affect the way in which individuals perceive and respond to a precipitating stressor. A schematic of these balancing factors is illustrated in Figure 9–2.

The paradigm set forth by Aguilera suggests that whether an individual experiences a crisis in response to a stressful situation depends on the following three factors:

1. ***The individual's perception of the event:*** If the event is perceived realistically, the individual is more likely to draw upon adequate resources to restore equilibrium. If the perception of the event is distorted, attempts at problem-solving are likely to be ineffective, and equilibrium is not restored.
2. ***The availability of situational supports:*** Aguilera stated, "Situational supports are those persons who are available in the environment and who can be depended on to help solve the problem" (p. 37). Without adequate situational supports during a stressful situation, an individual is most likely to feel overwhelmed and alone.
3. ***The availability of adequate coping mechanisms:*** When a stressful situation occurs, individuals draw upon behavioral strategies that have been successful for them in the past. If these coping strategies work, a crisis may be diverted. If not, disequilibrium may continue, and tension and anxiety increase.

As previously stated, it is assumed that crises are acute, not chronic, situations that will be resolved one way or another within 1 to 3 months. Crises can become growth opportunities when individuals learn new methods of coping that can be preserved and used when similar stressors recur. However, when new coping mechanisms or balancing factors are not identified and incorporated, the crisis can evolve into longer-term problems, sometimes including symptoms of mental illness such as depression, anxiety, and trauma/stressor-related disorders.

Types of Crises

Baldwin (1978) identified six classes of emotional crises, which progress by degree of severity. As the measure of psychopathology increases, the source of the stressor changes from external to internal. The type of crisis determines the method of intervention selected.

Class 1: Dispositional Crises

Definition

An acute response to an external situational stressor.

EXAMPLE

Brittany and Ethan have been married for 3 years and have a 1-year-old daughter. Ethan has been having difficulty with his boss at work. Twice during the past 6 months he exploded in anger at home and became abusive with Brittany. When Ethan discovered that Brittany had purchased clothing for the baby that he felt was overpriced, he grabbed the baby from Brittany and tossed her, screaming, into her crib. He hit and punched Brittany until she feared for her life. The next morning when Ethan left for work, Brittany took the baby and went to the emergency department of the city hospital, not knowing what else to do.

Intervention

Physical care of wounds and screening for domestic violence issues should be conducted in the emergency department. The mental health counselor can provide support and guidance in terms of presenting alternatives for managing the health and safety of herself and her child. The emergency nurse should encourage and empower Brittany to clarify her needs and issues so that referrals for agency assistance can be made.

Class 2: Crises of Anticipated Life Transitions

Definition

Normal life-cycle transitions may be anticipated but the individual may feel a lack of control over them.

EXAMPLE

College student J.T. lost his scholarship when he had to reduce his course load to pick up more hours at work. His wife had a baby and had to quit her job. He increased his working hours from part-time to full-time to compensate and therefore had little time for studies. He presents himself to the student-health nurse practitioner and describes numerous vague physical complaints.

Intervention

Physical examination should be performed (physical symptoms could be caused by depression), and ventilation of feelings encouraged. Reassurance and support should be provided as needed. J.T. should be referred to services that can provide financial and other types of needed assistance. Problematic areas should be identified and approaches to change discussed.

Class 3: Crises Resulting From Traumatic Stress

Definition

Crisis precipitated by an unexpected external stressor over which the individual has little or no control, resulting in feelings of being emotionally overwhelmed and defeated.

EXAMPLE

Ava is a doctor whose last shift ended at midnight two weeks ago. At that point, while walking to her car, she was abducted by two men with guns, taken to an abandoned building, and raped and beaten. Since that time, her physical wounds have nearly healed. However, Ava cannot be alone, is constantly fearful, relives the experience in flashbacks and dreams, and is unable to eat, sleep, or return to work at the hospital. A friend offers to accompany her to the mental health clinic.

Intervention

The nurse should offer Ava the opportunity to talk about the experience and to express her feelings about the trauma when she demonstrates readiness. The nurse should offer reassurance and support; discuss stages of grief and how rape may precipitate feelings of loss, including loss of control, loss of power, and loss of a sense of self-worth, that trigger the grief response. After a discussion of the stages of grief, the nurse should identify resources and explore new coping mechanisms and support systems that can help Ava to resume her normal activities. These interventions should be conducted in an environment that is sensitive to the impact of trauma on a person's sense of self and all interventions should convey dignity, respect, and hopefulness and promote the patient's empowerment to make choices in their care (Substance Abuse and Mental Health Services Administration, 2014). See Chapter 19, "Trauma- and Stressor-Related Disorders," for more information on trauma-informed care.

Class 4: Maturational and Developmental Crises

Definition

Crises that occur in response to failed attempts to master developmental tasks associated with transitions in the life cycle.

EXAMPLE

Jada and Caleb have been married for 2 years, and their firstborn child is 4 months old. Jada's mother was recently diagnosed with cancer, and the prognosis is unclear. Over the past 3 weeks Jada has become increasingly anxious and disorganized. She has been calling the nurse practitioner 10 to 15 times each day with new fears that she is not addressing her child's health needs. Jada has been screaming at Caleb that he is never there when she needs help with the baby and states she is thinking of dropping their child off at the children's services agency because she believes they are both unable to be effective parents. She agrees to see a counselor at Caleb's insistence.

Intervention

The primary intervention is to help Jada with anxiety reduction. When individuals have intense anxiety, their ability to gain insight about contributing factors and explore options for behavior change is impaired. The safety of their child should also be carefully assessed. Referrals and guidance in parenting skills may also lessen the anxiety associated with this new developmental phase. Anxiety and grief related to Jada's mother's illness could also be explored as a possible contributing factor to the current crisis.

Class 5: Crises Reflecting Psychopathology

Definition

A crisis that is influenced or triggered by pre-existing psychopathology. Examples of psychopathology that may precipitate crises include personality disorders, anxiety disorders, bipolar disorder, and schizophrenia.

EXAMPLE

Sonja, age 29, was diagnosed with borderline personality disorder at age 18. This disorder is believed to be rooted in deep fear of abandonment. She has been in therapy on a weekly basis for 10 years with several hospitalizations for suicide attempts during that time. She has had the same therapist for the past 6 years. This therapist told Sonja today that she is moving across the country to accept an administrative position. Sonja is distraught, stating that no one cares about her and that she would be better off dead. She is found wandering in and out of traffic on a busy expressway, oblivious to her surroundings. Police bring her to the emergency department of the hospital.

Intervention

The initial goal is aimed at helping Sonja to reduce her anxiety. She requires that someone stay with her and reassure her of her safety and security. After the feelings of panic and anxiety have subsided, she should be encouraged to verbalize her feelings of abandonment. Regressive behaviors should be discouraged. Positive reinforcement should be given for independent activities and accomplishments. The primary therapist will need to pursue this issue of termination with Sonja and facilitate transfer of services to another therapist or treatment program. Hospitalization may be necessary to maintain patient safety.

Class 6: Psychiatric Emergencies

Definition

Crisis situations in which general functioning has been severely impaired and the individual rendered incompetent or unable to assume personal responsibility for their behavior. Examples include acutely suicidal individuals, drug overdoses, reactions to hallucinogenic drugs, acute psychoses, uncontrollable anger, and alcohol intoxication.

EXAMPLE

Olivia, age 14, had been dating Liam, a high school football player, for 6 months. After the game on Friday night, Olivia and Liam went to Alexandra's house, where a number of high school students had gathered for an after-game party. No adults were present. At about midnight, Liam told Olivia that he did not want to date her anymore. Olivia became hysterical, and Alexandra was frightened by her behavior. She took Olivia to her parent's bedroom and gave her a Valium from a bottle in her mother's medicine cabinet. She left Olivia lying on her parent's bed and returned to the party downstairs. About an hour later, she returned to her parent's bedroom and found that Olivia had removed the bottle of Valium from the cabinet and swallowed all of the tablets. Olivia was unconscious, and Alexandra could not awaken her. An ambulance was called, and Olivia was transported to the local hospital.

Intervention

Emergency medical care, including monitoring vital signs, ensuring maintenance of adequate airway, and initiating gastric lavage and/or activated charcoal, is the priority in this case. Olivia is a minor, so notifying the parents is essential as well. Inpatient hospitalization is justifiable to ensure patient safety. Discussing feelings about self-esteem, rejection, and loss will help Olivia explore more adaptive methods of dealing with stressful situations.

Crisis on the Inpatient Unit: Anger and Aggression Management

Assessment

Sometimes crises occur for hospitalized psychiatric patients when they become unable to manage personal responsibility for their behaviors in response to anger. Nurses must be aware of the symptoms associated with anger and aggression in order to make an accurate assessment. Because the best intervention is prevention, risk factors for assessing violence potential are also presented.

Symptoms Associated With Anger and Aggression

Anger

Anger is often described as a secondary emotion. For example, it may be a response to unresolved grief, depression, fear, anxiety, or unresolved post-traumatic stress. Anger is often manifested in the following ways:

- Anxious, tense, frowning, or angry facial expression (affect)
- Clenched fists
- Low-pitched verbalizations forced through clenched teeth
- Yelling and shouting
- Intense eye contact or avoidance of eye contact
- Hypersensitivity, easily offended
- Defensive response to criticism
- Passive-aggressive behaviors
- Lack of control or overcontrolled emotions
- Intense discomfort; continuous state of tension
- Flushed face

Anger is one of the stages of the normal grief process and thus is an expected emotion. Because of the negative connotation to the word *anger*, some clients will not acknowledge that they are angry. These individuals need assistance to recognize their true feelings and to understand that anger is a perfectly acceptable emotion when it is expressed appropriately; it is one's *behavior* in response to anger that may be unacceptable, such as when it results in aggression.

Aggression

Aggression can arise from a number of feeling states, including anger, anxiety, guilt, frustration, or suspiciousness. Kassinove (2021) states that **aggression** includes verbal and physical attacks that intend harm to another and often reflect a desire for dominance and control. Aggressive behaviors can be classified as mild (e.g., sarcasm), moderate (e.g., slamming doors), severe (e.g., threats of physical violence against others), or extreme (e.g., physical acts of violence against others). Aggression may be evidenced in many behaviors, including (but not limited to) the following defining characteristics:

- Pacing, restlessness
- Threatening body language
- Verbal or physical threats
- Loud voice, shouting, use of obscenities, argumentativeness
- Threats of homicide or suicide
- Increase in agitation, with overreaction to environmental stimuli
- Panic anxiety, leading to misinterpretation of the environment
- Suspiciousness and defensive posturing
- Angry mood, often disproportionate to the situation
- Destruction of property
- Acts of physical harm toward another person

Aggression may be differentiated as reactive versus proactive. Reactive aggression is defined as fear-based and impulsive; proactive aggression is described as predatory and calculated. In both cases there is intent to harm another, but the motives differ. *Intent* is a requisite in the definition of aggression. It refers to behavior that is *intended* to inflict harm or destruction. Accidents that lead to *unintentional* harm or destruction are not considered aggression.

Assessing Risk Factors

Prevention is the key issue in the management of aggressive or violent behavior. The individual who becomes violent usually feels an underlying helplessness. Three factors have been identified as important considerations in assessing for potential violence:

1. Past history of violence
2. Client diagnosis
3. Current behavior

Past history of violence is widely recognized as a major risk factor for violence in a treatment setting (Iozzino et al., 2015). Assaultive behavior is also highly correlated with diagnosis. Substance abuse (alone or in combination with a mental illness) is the single largest risk factor for violence; the lifetime prevalence is 35% in individuals with substance abuse or dependence compared to 16% for those with schizophrenia or a bipolar disorder and a notable 43.6% in those with a comorbid mental illness and substance abuse (Victoroff, 2017).

Novitsky et al. (2009) stated:

> The successful management of violence is predicated on an understanding of the dynamics of violence. A patient's threatening behavior is commonly an overreaction to feelings of impotence, helplessness, and perceived or actual humiliation. Aggression rarely occurs suddenly and unexpectedly. (p. 50)

Novitsky and associates describe a **prodromal syndrome** that is characterized by anxiety and tension, verbal abuse and profanity, and increasing hyperactivity. These escalating behaviors usually do not occur in stages but most often overlap and sometimes occur simultaneously. Behaviors associated with this prodromal stage include rigid posture; clenched fists and jaws; grim, defiant affect; talking in a rapid, raised voice; arguing and demanding; using profanity and threatening verbalizations; agitation and pacing; and pounding and slamming.

Most assaultive behavior is preceded by a period of increasing hyperactivity. Behaviors associated with the prodromal syndrome should be considered emergent and demand immediate attention. Keen observation skills and background knowledge for accurate assessment are critical factors in predicting potential for violent behavior. The Brøset Violence Checklist (BVC), presented in Box 9–1, is a quick, simple, and reliable checklist that can be used as a risk assessment for potential violence. Testing has shown 63% accuracy for prediction of violence at a score of 2 or above (Almvik et al., 2000). De-escalation techniques are also included.

Diagnosis and Outcome Identification

NANDA International does not include a separate nursing diagnosis for anger, and in and of itself, anger is not an unhealthy response. Anger is one of a broad range of normal emotional responses, but becomes an unhealthy response only when the behaviors that accompany anger are harmful to self or others. The nursing diagnosis of maladaptive grieving may be used when anger is related to a loss and is being expressed inappropriately.

The following nursing diagnoses may be considered for patients demonstrating inappropriate behaviors in response to anger:

- Ineffective coping
- Risk for self-directed or other-directed violence

BOX 9–1 The Brøset Violence Checklist

BEHAVIORS	SCORE (Score 1 point for each behavior observed. At a score of ≥2, begin de-escalation techniques.)
Confusion	_____
Irritability	_____
Boisterousness	_____
Physical threats	_____
Verbal threats	_____
Attacks on objects	_____
Total Score	_____
DE-ESCALATION TECHNIQUES:	
Calm voice	Walk outdoors or fresh air
Helpful attitude	Reduction in demands
Identify consequences	Group participation
Open hands and nonthreatening posture	Relaxation techniques
Allow phone call	Express concern
Offer food or drink	Reduce stimulation and loud noise
Decrease waiting times and request refusals	Verbal redirection and limit setting
Distract with a more positive activity (e.g., soft music or a quiet room)	Time out, quiet time, open seclusion
	Offer prn medication
IF DE-ESCALATION TECHNIQUES FAIL:	
Suggest prn medications	
Time out or unlocked seclusion, which can progress to locked seclusion if all other de-escalation strategies and less restrictive measures have been unsuccessful	

Source: Almvik, R., Woods, P., & Rasmussen, K. (2000). The Brøset violence checklist: Sensitivity, specificity, and interrater reliability. Journal of Interpersonal Violence, 15*(12), 1284–1296. With permission. De-escalation techniques reprinted with permission from Barbara Barnes, Milwaukee County Behavioral Health Division.*

Outcome Criteria

Outcome criteria include short- and long-term goals. Timelines are individually determined. The following criteria may be used for measurement of outcomes in the care of the patient needing assistance with management of anger and aggression.

The patient:

1. Recognizes their anger and seeks out staff/support person to talk about their feelings.
2. Takes responsibility for feelings of anger.
3. Demonstrates the ability to exert self-control over feelings of anger.
4. Demonstrates ability to diffuse anger before losing control.
5. Uses the tension generated by the anger in a constructive manner.
6. Causes no harm to self or others.
7. Uses steps of the problem-solving process rather than becoming violent as a means of seeking solutions.

Planning and Implementation

In Table 9–1, a plan of care is presented for the patient who expresses anger inappropriately. Outcome criteria and appropriate nursing interventions with rationales are included for each diagnosis.

Table 9–1 | CARE PLAN FOR THE INDIVIDUAL WHO EXPRESSES ANGER INAPPROPRIATELY

NURSING DIAGNOSIS: INEFFECTIVE COPING
RELATED TO: (Possible) negative role modeling, feelings of helplessness
EVIDENCED BY: Yelling, name calling, hitting others, and temper tantrums as expressions of anger

OUTCOME CRITERIA	NURSING INTERVENTION	RATIONALE
Patient recognizes anger in self and takes responsibility before losing control.	1. Remain calm when dealing with an angry patient.	1. Anger expressed by the nurse will most likely incite increased anger in the patient.
	2. Set verbal limits on behavior. Clearly delineate the consequences of inappropriate expression of anger, and always follow through.	2. Consistency in enforcing the consequences is essential if positive outcomes are to be achieved. Inconsistency creates confusion and encourages testing of limits.
	3. Have the patient keep a diary of angry feelings, what triggered them, and how they were handled.	3. Journaling provides a more objective measure of the problem.
	4. Avoid touching the patient when they become angry.	4. Patients may view touch as threatening and could become violent.
	5. Help the patient determine the true source of the anger.	5. Often, anger is being displaced onto a safer object or person. If resolution is to occur, the first step is to identify the source of the problem.
	6. Help the patient find alternative ways to release tension, such as physical outlets, and more appropriate ways to express anger, such as seeking out staff when feelings emerge.	6. Patients will likely need assistance to problem solve more appropriate ways of behaving.
	7. Role model appropriate ways to express anger assertively, such as, "I dislike being called names. I get angry when I hear you saying those things about me."	7. Role modeling is one of the strongest methods of learning.

Continued

Table 9–1 | CARE PLAN FOR THE INDIVIDUAL WHO EXPRESSES ANGER INAPPROPRIATELY—cont'd

NURSING DIAGNOSIS: RISK FOR SELF-DIRECTED OR OTHER-DIRECTED VIOLENCE

RELATED TO: History of violence, inadequate management of anger, post-trauma stress

OUTCOME CRITERIA	NURSING INTERVENTION	RATIONALE
Patient does not harm self or others. Patient verbalizes anger rather than hit others.	1. Observe for escalation of anger (called the *prodromal syndrome*): increased motor activity, pounding, slamming, tense posture, defiant affect, clenched teeth and fists, arguing, demanding, and challenging or threatening staff.	1. Violence may be prevented if risks are identified in time.
	2. When these behaviors are observed, first ensure that sufficient staff are available to help with a potentially violent situation. Attempt to defuse the anger beginning with the least restrictive means.	2. The initial consideration must be having enough help to diffuse a potentially violent situation. Patient rights must be honored while preventing harm to patient and others.
	3. Techniques for dealing with aggression include: a. *Talking down*. For example, say, "John, you seem very angry. Let's sit down and talk about it." (Maintain safe distance and opportunity to leave the immediate area if needed.)	3. Aggression control techniques promote safety and reduce risk of harm to the patient and others: a. Promote a trusting relationship and may prevent patient's anxiety from escalating.
	b. *Physical outlets*. For example, say, "Maybe it would help if you did some walking or other exercise for a while to help you safely release this energy" or "I'll stay here with you if you want."	b. Provide effective way for the patient to release tension associated with high levels of anger.
	c. *Medication*. If agitation continues to escalate, offer the patient a choice of taking medication voluntarily. If they refuse, reassess the situation to determine whether harm to self or others is imminent.	c. Tranquilizing medication may calm the patient and prevent violence from escalating.
	d. *Call for assistance*. Remove self and other patients from the immediate area. Call violence code, push "panic" button, call for assault team, or institute measures established by the institution. Sufficient staff to indicate a show of strength may be enough to de-escalate the situation, and patient may agree to take the medication.	d. Patient and staff safety are of primary concern. Many states, accrediting bodies, and/or facilities require that staff members working with hospitalized psychiatric patients be trained and/or certified in psychiatric emergency interventions to ensure that the strategies used are in the best interest of staff and patient safety.
	e. *Seclusion or restraints*. If the patient is not calmed by talking down or by medication, use of mechanical restraints and/or seclusion may be necessary. Be sure to have sufficient staff available to assist and appropriately deal with an out-of-control patient. Follow protocol for restraints/seclusion established by the institution. Restraints should be used as a last resort after all other interventions have been unsuccessful and the patient is clearly at risk of harm to self or others.	e. Patients who do not have internal control over their own behavior may require external controls, such as mechanical restraints, in order to prevent harm to self or others.

Table 9–1 | CARE PLAN FOR THE INDIVIDUAL WHO EXPRESSES ANGER INAPPROPRIATELY—cont'd

OUTCOME CRITERIA	NURSING INTERVENTION	RATIONALE
	f. *Observation and documentation*. Hospital policy typically dictates the requirements for observation of patient in restraints. Basic safety principles include that patient in restraints should be observed throughout the period of restraint. Every 15 minutes, the patient should be monitored to ensure that circulation to extremities is not compromised (check temperature, color, pulses). Assist the patient with needs related to nutrition, hydration, and elimination. Position patient so that comfort is facilitated and aspiration can be prevented. (Patients should never be restrained in a prone position.) Document all observations.	f. Patient and staff safety are of primary concern. Many state regulations, accrediting bodies (such as The Joint Commission), and/or facility policies require that staff members working with hospitalized psychiatric patients be trained and/or certified in psychiatric emergency interventions to ensure that the strategies used are in the best interest of staff and patient safety. Patient well-being is a nursing priority.
	g. *Ongoing assessment*. As agitation decreases, assess the patient's readiness for restraint removal or reduction. With assistance from other staff members, remove one restraint at a time while assessing the patient's response. This measure minimizes the risk of injury to patient and staff.	g. Gradual removal of the restraints allows for testing of the patient's self-control. Patient and staff safety are of primary concern, as is ensuring that the patient is offered the least restrictive treatment option effective in maintaining safety.
	h. *Debriefing*. It is important when a patient loses control for staff to follow up with a discussion about the situation. This discussion should occur with the patient and among other staff. The staff should discuss factors that necessitated the crisis intervention, factors that contributed to the failure of less restrictive interventions, and staff's thoughts about the safety and effectiveness of the intervention. When the patient has regained control, a debriefing should occur in which the patient is encouraged to discuss thoughts about what contributed to the crisis situation and about staff interventions and to explore strategies to avert a crisis situation in the future. It is also important to discuss the situation with other patients who witnessed the episode so they understand and process what happened. Some patients may fear that they could be at risk for experiencing a crisis or that they might be in danger when someone else's behavior becomes aggressive.	h. Debriefing helps to process the impact of the intervention. Mutual feedback is shared; staff and patient have an opportunity to process and learn from the event.

Cognitive behavior therapy (CBT) is an evidence-based strategy for anger management and aggression that, especially in treatment of children and adolescents, has demonstrated effectiveness in reducing aggression (Smeets et al., 2015). Although CBT is typically conducted by advanced practice nurses and other trained specialists, the generalist psychiatric nurse can incorporate principles of this modality in psychoeducation, which provides a foundation for referral to formal CBT treatment.

Evaluation

Evaluation consists of reassessment to determine whether the nursing interventions have been successful in achieving the objectives of care. The following type of information may be gathered to determine the success of working with a patient exhibiting inappropriate expression of anger:

- Is the patient now able to recognize their anger?
- Can the patient take responsibility for these feelings and keep them in check without losing control?
- Does the patient seek out staff to talk about feelings when they occur?
- Is the patient able to transfer tension generated by the anger into constructive activities?
- Has harm to the patient and others been avoided?
- Is the patient able to solve problems adaptively without undue frustration and without becoming violent?

Crisis Intervention

Individuals experiencing crises have an urgent need for assistance. In **crisis intervention,** therapists, or other interveners, become a part of the individuals' life situations. Because of the individuals' emotional states, they are unable to problem solve and, therefore, require guidance and support from others to help mobilize the resources needed to resolve the crisis.

Lengthy psychological interpretations are not appropriate for crisis intervention. It is a time for doing what is needed to help an individual get relief and for calling into action all of the people and other resources required to do so. Aguilera (1998) stated:

> The goal of crisis intervention is the resolution of an immediate crisis. Its focus is on the supportive, with the restoration of the individual to his precrisis level of functioning or possibly to a higher level of functioning. The therapist's role is direct, supportive, and that of an active participant. (p. 24)

Crisis intervention takes place in inpatient settings, outpatient settings, and in the community. In the past few decades, people with mental illness have been increasingly involved with criminal justice personnel as first responders to manage mental health crisis situations. In 1988, the fatal shooting by police officers of a man with mental illness prompted the development of the *crisis intervention team (CIT) model* to ensure that select police officers are trained to identify mental illness and substance abuse, use de-escalation techniques, and divert individuals from criminal justice systems to mental health professionals (Watson & Fulambarker, 2012). Not all states have developed CIT training programs, but several studies have demonstrated improved safety outcomes for patients with mental illness and officers where CIT-trained officers are available (National Alliance on Mental Illness, 2021). Other resources that may be available for patients with mental illness who are experiencing an acute crisis include 24-hour crisis phone lines, walk-in crisis centers, mobile crisis teams, respite and residential services, and hospital services, including 23-hour observation beds. Nurses have a responsibility to know what resources exist in their community of practice. They can then become an important advocate for crisis intervention training in communities and can also be a support to families by encouraging them to ask for CIT-trained officers (where available) when they are faced with a family member's psychiatric crisis.

A more recent development in some states, counties, and mental health facilities is to utilize *peer support specialists.* These are individuals who have personal experience with mental illness and who are trained and/or credentialed to help clients navigate everyday challenges of living with a mental illness. Evidence has demonstrated their effectiveness in diffusing psychiatric crises (Bouchery et al., 2018).

The basic methodology for crisis intervention work by health-care professionals relies heavily on orderly problem-solving techniques and structured activities that are focused on change. Through adaptive change, crises are resolved and growth occurs. Because of the time limitation of crisis intervention, the individual must experience some degree of relief almost from the first interaction. Crisis intervention, then, is not aimed at major personality change or reconstruction (as may be the case in long-term psychotherapy) but rather at using a given crisis situation, at the very least, to restore functioning and, at most, to enhance personal growth.

Phases of Crisis Intervention: The Role of the Nurse

Nurses respond to crisis situations on a daily basis. Crises can occur on every unit in the general hospital, in the home setting, in the community health-care setting, in schools and offices, and in private practice. Nurses may be called on to function as crisis helpers in virtually any setting committed to the practice of nursing.

Aguilera (1998) described four specific phases in the technique of crisis intervention that are clearly comparable to the steps of the nursing process. These phases are discussed in the following sections.

Phase 1. Assessment

In this phase, the nurse gathers information regarding the precipitating stressor and the resulting crisis that prompted the individual to seek professional help. A nurse in crisis intervention might perform some of the following assessments:

- Ask the individual to describe the event that precipitated this crisis.
- Determine when it occurred.
- Assess the individual's mental *and* physical status.
- Determine if the individual has experienced this stressor before. If so, what method of coping was used? Have these methods been tried this time?
- If previous coping methods were tried, what was the result?
- If new coping methods were tried, what was the result?
- Assess suicide or homicide potential, plan, and means.
- Assess the adequacy of support systems.
- Determine level of precrisis functioning. Assess the usual coping methods, available support systems, and ability to problem solve.
- Assess the individual's perception of personal strengths and limitations.
- Assess the individual's use of substances.

Next, information from the comprehensive assessment is analyzed, and appropriate nursing diagnoses reflecting the immediacy of the crisis situation are identified. Some nursing diagnoses that may be relevant include the following:

- Ineffective coping
- Anxiety (severe to panic)
- Disturbed thought processes
- Risk for self- or other-directed violence
- Rape-trauma syndrome
- Post-trauma syndrome
- Fear

Phase 2. Planning of Therapeutic Intervention

In the planning phase of crisis intervention, the nurse selects the appropriate nursing actions for the identified nursing diagnoses. In planning the interventions, the type of crisis, as well as the individual's strengths, desired choices, and available resources for support, are taken into consideration. Goals are established for crisis resolution and a return to, or increase in, the precrisis level of functioning.

Phase 3. Intervention

During phase 3, the actions that were identified in phase 2 are implemented. The following interventions are the focus of nursing in crisis intervention:

- Use a reality-oriented approach. The focus of the problem is on the here and now.
- Remain with the individual who is experiencing panic anxiety.
- Establish a rapid working relationship by showing unconditional acceptance, by active listening, and by attending to immediate needs.
- Discourage lengthy explanations or rationalizations of the situation; promote an atmosphere for verbalization of true feelings.
- Set firm limits on aggressive, destructive behaviors. At high levels of anxiety, behavior is likely to be impulsive and regressive. Establish at the outset what is acceptable and what is not and maintain consistency.
- Clarify the problem that the individual is facing. The nurse does this by describing their perception of the problem and comparing it with the individual's perception of the problem.

- Help the individual determine what they believe precipitated the crisis.
- Acknowledge feelings of anger, guilt, helplessness, and powerlessness without judgment.
- Guide the individual through a problem-solving process by which they may move in the direction of positive life change:
  - Help the individual confront the factors that are contributing to the experience of crisis.
  - Encourage the individual to discuss changes they would like to make. Jointly determine whether or not desired changes are realistic.
  - Encourage exploration of feelings about aspects that cannot be changed and explore alternative ways of coping more adaptively in these situations.
  - Discuss alternative strategies for creating changes that are realistically possible.
  - Weigh benefits and consequences of each alternative.
- Assist the individual to select alternative coping strategies that will help alleviate future crisis situations.
- Identify external support systems and new social networks from which the individual may seek assistance in times of stress.

CLINICAL PEARL Coping mechanisms are highly individual and the choice ultimately must be made by the patient. The nurse may offer suggestions and provide guidance to help the patient identify coping mechanisms that are realistic for them, and that can promote positive outcomes in a crisis situation.

Phase 4. Evaluation of Crisis Resolution and Anticipatory Planning

To evaluate the outcome of crisis intervention, a reassessment is made to determine whether the stated objective was achieved:

- Have positive behavioral changes occurred?
- Has the individual developed more adaptive coping strategies? Have they been effective?
- Has the individual grown from the experience by gaining insight into their responses to crisis situations?
- Does the individual believe that they could respond with healthy adaptation in future stressful situations to prevent crisis development?
- Can the individual describe a plan of action for dealing with stressors similar to the one that precipitated this crisis?

During the evaluation period, the nurse and client summarize what has occurred during the intervention. They review what the individual has learned and "anticipate" how they will respond in the future. A determination is made regarding follow-up therapy; if needed, the nurse provides referral information.

Disaster Nursing

Although there are many definitions of **disaster,** a common feature is that the event overwhelms local resources and threatens the function and safety of the community. A violent disaster, whether natural or man-made, may leave devastation to property or life. Such tragedies leave victims with a damaged sense of safety and well-being and varying degrees of emotional trauma. Often, spiritual distress is an issue as victims ask, "How could this have happened?" and "What is most important in life?" A care plan for responding to spiritual distress is included in Table 9–2. Children, who lack life experiences and coping skills, are particularly vulnerable. Their sense of order and security has been seriously disrupted, and they are unable to understand that the disruption is time limited and that their world will eventually return to normal.

Application of the Nursing Process to Disaster Nursing

Background Assessment Data

Individuals respond to traumatic events in many ways. Grieving is a natural response following any loss, and it may be more extreme if the disaster is directly experienced or witnessed. The emotional effects of loss and disruption may show up immediately or may appear weeks or months later.

Psychological and behavioral responses common in adults following trauma and disaster include anger; disbelief; sadness; anxiety; fear; irritability; arousal; numbing; sleep disturbance; and increases in alcohol, caffeine, and tobacco use. Preschool children commonly experience separation anxiety, regressive behaviors, nightmares, and hyperactive or withdrawn behaviors.

Older children may have difficulty concentrating, somatic complaints, sleep disturbances, and concerns about safety. Adolescents' responses are often similar to those of adults.

Traumatic bereavement is a term used to describe the grief process that accompanies sudden, unexpected losses resulting from traumatic events such as disasters (but may also be applicable to other sudden losses such as the loss of a family member to suicide). In such circumstances the survivor must come to grips not only with the loss but also the manner in which the loss occurred, and this can include powerful emotions ranging from guilt (at having survived when others lost their lives) to overwhelming fear of additional traumas (catastrophic thinking) and anger. Barlé et al. (2017) report that, most often, the symptoms associated with traumatic loss are more intense and more prolonged than those following a natural death. These authors propose that three critical elements for intervention include building resources, processing trauma, and facilitating mourning. Ongoing assessment includes looking for signs of post-traumatic stress disorder (PTSD) and major depression or anxiety disorders that require additional intervention and treatment.

Nursing Diagnoses and Outcome Identification

Information from the assessment is analyzed, and appropriate nursing diagnoses reflecting the immediacy of the situation are identified. Some nursing diagnoses that may be relevant include the following:

- Risk for injury (trauma, suffocation, poisoning)
- Risk for infection
- Anxiety (panic)
- Fear
- Spiritual distress
- Risk for post-trauma syndrome
- Ineffective community coping

The following criteria may be used for measurement of outcomes in the care of the patient having experienced a traumatic event. Timelines are individually determined.

The patient:

- Demonstrates behaviors necessary to protect self from further injury.
- Identifies interventions to prevent/reduce risk of infection.
- Maintains anxiety at a manageable level.
- Expresses beliefs and values about spiritual issues.
- Demonstrates ability to deal with emotional reactions in an individually appropriate manner.
- Demonstrates an increase in activities to improve community functioning.

Planning and Implementation

Table 9–2 provides a plan of care for the patient who has experienced a traumatic event. Selected nursing diagnoses are presented, along with outcome criteria, appropriate nursing interventions, and rationales for each.

Evaluation

In the final step of the nursing process, a reassessment is conducted to determine whether the nursing actions have been successful in achieving the objectives of care. Evaluation of the nursing actions for the patient who has experienced a traumatic event may be facilitated by gathering information utilizing the following types of questions.

Has the patient:

- Been assessed and treated for serious injury or infections or have they been resolved?
- Been able to maintain anxiety at a manageable level?
- Demonstrated appropriate problem-solving skills?
- Discussed their beliefs about spiritual issues?
- Demonstrated the ability to deal with emotional reactions in an individually appropriate manner?
- Verbalized a subsiding of the physical symptoms (e.g., pain, nightmares, flashbacks, fatigue) associated with the traumatic event?
- Recognized factors affecting the community's ability to meet its own demands or needs?
- Demonstrated increased activities to improve community functioning?
- Established and put in place a plan to deal with future contingencies?

When acute crises are not resolved, an individual may be vulnerable to acute stress disorders and trauma-related disorders. See Chapter 19 ("Trauma and Stressor-Related Disorders") for more information on these topics.

Text continued on page 201

Table 9–2 | CARE PLAN FOR THE PATIENT WHO HAS EXPERIENCED A TRAUMATIC EVENT

NURSING DIAGNOSIS: ANXIETY (PANIC)/FEAR

RELATED TO: Real or perceived threat to physical well-being; threat of death; situational crisis; exposure to toxins; unmet needs

EVIDENCED BY: Persistent feelings of apprehension and uneasiness; sense of impending doom; impaired functioning; verbal expressions of having no control or influence over situation, outcome, or self-care; sympathetic stimulation; extraneous physical movements

OUTCOME CRITERIA	NURSING INTERVENTIONS	RATIONALE
Patient demonstrates that anxiety is at a manageable level. Patient demonstrates use of positive coping mechanisms to manage anxiety.	1. Determine degree of anxiety/fear present, associated behaviors (e.g., laughter, crying, calm or agitation, excited/hysterical behavior, expressions of disbelief and/or self-blame), and reality of perceived threat.	1. Clearly understanding the patient's perception is pivotal to providing appropriate assistance in overcoming the fear. Individual may be agitated or totally overwhelmed. Panic state increases risk for harm to self or others in the environment.
	2. Note degree of disorganization.	2. The patient may be unable to handle ADLs or work requirements and may need more intensive intervention.
	3. Create as quiet an area as possible. Maintain a calm, confident manner. Speak in even tone using short, simple sentences.	3. Decreases sense of confusion or overstimulation; enhances sense of safety. Helps the patient focus on what is said and reduces transmission of anxiety.
	4. Develop trusting relationship.	4. Trust is the basis of a therapeutic nurse-patient relationship and enables them to work effectively together.
	5. Identify whether incident has reactivated pre-existing or coexisting situations (physical or psychological).	5. Concerns and psychological issues are recycled every time trauma is re-experienced and affect how the individual views the current situation.
	6. Determine presence of physical symptoms (e.g., numbness, headache, tightness in chest, nausea, and pounding heart).	6. Physical problems need to be differentiated from anxiety symptoms so appropriate treatment can be given.
	7. Identify psychological responses (e.g., anger, shock, acute anxiety, panic, confusion, denial). Record emotional changes.	7. Although these are normal responses at the time of the trauma, they will recycle repeatedly until they are dealt with adequately.
	8. Discuss the patient's perception of what is causing the anxiety.	8. Increases the patient's ability to connect symptoms to subjective feeling of anxiety, providing opportunity to gain insight/control and make desired changes.
	9. Assist the patient to correct any distortions being experienced. Share perceptions with patient.	9. Perceptions based on reality help to decrease fearfulness. How the nurse views the situation may help the patient to see it differently.

Table 9–2 | CARE PLAN FOR THE PATIENT WHO HAS EXPERIENCED A TRAUMATIC EVENT—cont'd

OUTCOME CRITERIA	NURSING INTERVENTIONS	RATIONALE
	10. Explore with the patient or significant other the manner in which the patient has previously coped with anxiety-producing events.	10. May help the patient regain sense of control and recognize significance of trauma.
	11. Engage the patient in learning new coping behaviors (e.g., progressive muscle relaxation, thought-stopping).	11. Replacing maladaptive behaviors can enhance ability to manage and deal with stress. Interrupting obsessive thinking allows the patient to use energy to address underlying anxiety, whereas continued rumination about the incident can retard recovery.
	12. Encourage use of techniques to manage stress and vent emotions such as anger and hostility.	12. Reduces the likelihood of eruptions that can result in abusive behavior.
	13. Give positive feedback when the patient demonstrates better ways to manage anxiety and is able to calmly and realistically appraise the situation.	13. Provides acknowledgment and reinforcement, encouraging use of new coping strategies. Enhances the patient's ability to deal with fearful feelings and gain control over situation, promoting future successes.
	14. Administer medications as indicated: Antianxiety—diazepam, alprazolam, oxazepam. Antidepressants—fluoxetine, paroxetine, bupropion.	14. Antianxiety medication provides temporary relief of anxiety symptoms, enhancing ability to cope with situation. Antidepressants lift mood and help suppress intrusive thoughts and explosive anger.

NURSING DIAGNOSIS: SPIRITUAL DISTRESS

RELATED TO: Physical or psychological stress; energy-consuming anxiety; loss(es), intense suffering; separation from religious or cultural ties; challenged belief and value system

EVIDENCED BY: Expressions of concern about disaster and the meaning of life and death or belief systems; inner conflict about current loss of normality and effects of the disaster; anger directed at deity; engaging in self-blame; seeking spiritual assistance

OUTCOME CRITERIA	NURSING INTERVENTIONS	RATIONALE
Patient expresses beliefs and values about spiritual issues.	1. Determine the patient's religious/spiritual orientation, current involvement, and presence of conflicts.	1. Provides baseline for planning care and accessing appropriate resources.
	2. Establish environment that promotes free expression of feelings and concerns. Provide calm, peaceful setting when possible.	2. Promotes awareness and identification of feelings so they can be dealt with.
	3. Listen to the patient's and significant other's expressions of anger, concern, alienation from God, belief that situation is a punishment for wrongdoing, and similar concerns.	3. It is helpful to understand the patient's and significant other's points of view and how they are questioning their faith in the face of tragedy.

Continued

Table 9–2 | CARE PLAN FOR THE PATIENT WHO HAS EXPERIENCED A TRAUMATIC EVENT—cont'd

OUTCOME CRITERIA	NURSING INTERVENTIONS	RATIONALE
	4. Note sense of futility, feelings of hopelessness and helplessness, lack of motivation to help self.	4. These thoughts and feelings can result in patients feeling paralyzed and unable to move forward to resolve the situation.
	5. Listen to expressions of inability to find meaning in life and reason for living. Evaluate for suicidal ideation.	5. May indicate need for further intervention to prevent suicide attempt.
	6. Determine support systems available to the patient.	6. Presence or lack of support systems can affect the patient's recovery.
	7. Ask how you can be most helpful. Convey acceptance of the patient's spiritual beliefs and concerns.	7. Promotes trust and comfort, encouraging the patient to be open about sensitive matters.
	8. Make time for nonjudgmental discussion of philosophic issues and questions about spiritual impact of current situation.	8. Helps the patient begin to look at basis for spiritual confusion. *Note:* There is a potential for care provider's belief system to interfere with the patient finding their own way. Therefore, it is most beneficial to remain neutral and not espouse own beliefs.
	9. Discuss difference between grief and guilt, and help the patient to identify and deal with each, assuming responsibility for own actions, expressing awareness of the consequences of acting out of false guilt.	9. Blaming self for what has happened impedes dealing with the grief process and needs to be discussed and dealt with.
	10. Use therapeutic communication skills of reflection and active listening.	10. Helps the patient find own solutions to concerns.
	11. Facilitate the patient's expressed interest in practicing meditation, prayer, and forgiveness. Provide information that anger with God is a normal part of the grieving process.	11. This can help to heal past and present pain.
	12. Assist the patient to develop goals for dealing with life situation.	12. Enhances commitment to goal, optimizing outcomes and promoting sense of hope.
	13. Identify and refer to resources that can be helpful, such as pastoral/parish nurse or religious counselor, crisis counselor, psychotherapy, Alcoholics Anonymous and/or Narcotics Anonymous.	13. Specific assistance may be helpful to recovery (e.g., relationship problems, substance abuse, suicidal ideation).
	14. Encourage participation in support groups.	14. Discussing concerns and questions with others can help the patient resolve feelings.

Table 9–2 | CARE PLAN FOR THE PATIENT WHO HAS EXPERIENCED A TRAUMATIC EVENT—cont'd

NURSING DIAGNOSIS: RISK FOR POST-TRAUMA SYNDROME

RELATED TO: Events outside the range of usual human experience; serious threat or injury to self or loved ones; witnessing horrors or tragic events; exaggerated sense of responsibility; survivor's guilt or role in the event; inadequate social support

OUTCOME CRITERIA	NURSING INTERVENTIONS	RATIONALE
Patient demonstrates ability to deal with emotional reactions in an individually appropriate manner.	1. Determine involvement in event (e.g., survivor, significant other, rescue/aid worker, health-care provider, family member).	1. All those concerned with a traumatic event are at risk for emotional trauma and have needs related to their involvement in the event.
	2. Evaluate current factors associated with the event, such as displacement from home due to illness/injury, natural disaster, or terrorist attack. Identify how the patient's past experiences may affect current situation.	2. Affects the patient's reaction to current event and is basis for planning care and identifying appropriate support systems and resources.
	3. Listen for comments of taking on responsibility (e.g., "I should have been more careful or gone back to get her").	3. Statements such as these are indicators of "survivor's guilt" and blaming self for actions.
	4. Identify the patient's current coping mechanisms.	4. Noting positive or negative coping skills provides direction for care.
	5. Determine availability and usefulness of the patient's support systems, family, social contacts, and community resources.	5. Family and others close to the patient may also be at risk and require assistance to cope with the trauma.
	6. Provide information about signs and symptoms of post-trauma response, especially if the patient is involved in a high-risk occupation.	6. Awareness of these factors helps the patient identify need for assistance when signs and symptoms occur.
	7. Identify and discuss the patient's strengths as well as vulnerabilities.	7. Provides information to build on for coping with traumatic experience.
	8. Evaluate the patient's perceptions of events and personal significance (e.g., rescue worker trained to provide lifesaving assistance but recovering only dead bodies).	8. Events that trigger feelings of despair and hopelessness may be more difficult to deal with and require long-term interventions.
	9. Provide emotional and physical presence by sitting with the patient/significant other and offering solace.	9. Strengthens coping abilities.
	10. Encourage expression of feelings. Note whether feelings expressed appear congruent with events experienced.	10. It is important to talk about the incident repeatedly. Incongruencies may indicate deeper conflict and can impede resolution.
	11. Note presence of nightmares, reliving the incident, loss of appetite, irritability, numbness and crying, and family or relationship disruption.	11. These responses are normal in the early, post-incident time frame. If prolonged and persistent, they may indicate need for more intensive therapy.

Continued

Table 9–2 | CARE PLAN FOR THE PATIENT WHO HAS EXPERIENCED A TRAUMATIC EVENT—cont'd

OUTCOME CRITERIA	NURSING INTERVENTIONS	RATIONALE
	12. Provide a calm, safe environment.	12. Helps the patient deal with the disruption in their life.
	13. Encourage and assist the patient in learning stress-management techniques.	13. Promotes relaxation and helps the patient exercise control over self and what has happened.
	14. Recommend participation in debriefing sessions that may be provided following major disaster events.	14. Dealing with the stresses promptly may facilitate recovery from the event or prevent exacerbation.
	15. Identify employment, community resource groups.	15. Provides opportunity for ongoing support to deal with recurrent feelings related to the trauma.
	16. Administer medications as indicated, such as antipsychotics (e.g., chlorpromazine, haloperidol, olanzapine, or quetiapine) or carbamazepine (Tegretol).	16. Low doses of antipsychotics may be used for reduction of psychotic symptoms when loss of contact with reality occurs, usually for patients with especially disturbing flashbacks. Carbamazepine may be used to alleviate intrusive recollections or flashbacks, impulsivity, and violent behavior.

NURSING DIAGNOSIS: INEFFECTIVE COMMUNITY COPING

RELATED TO: Natural or man-made disasters (earthquakes, tornados, floods, reemerging infectious agents, terrorist activity); ineffective or nonexistent community systems (e.g., lack of or inadequate emergency medical system, transportation system, or disaster planning systems)

EVIDENCED BY: Deficits of community participation; community does not meet its own expectations; expressed vulnerability; community powerlessness; stressors perceived as excessive; excessive community conflicts; high illness rates

OUTCOME CRITERIA	NURSING INTERVENTIONS	RATIONALE
Patient demonstrates an increase in activities to improve community functioning.	1. Evaluate community activities related to meeting collective needs within the community and between the community and the larger society. Note immediate needs, such as health care, food, shelter, funds.	1. Provides a baseline to determine community needs in relation to current concerns or threats.
	2. Note community reports of functioning, including areas of weakness or conflict.	2. Provides a view of how the community sees these areas.
	3. Identify effects of related factors on community activities.	3. In the face of a current threat, local or national, community resources need to be evaluated, updated, and given priority to meet the identified need.
	4. Determine availability and use of resources. Identify unmet demands or needs of the community.	4. Information is necessary to identify what else is needed to meet the current situation.
	5. Determine community strengths.	5. Promotes understanding of the ways in which the community is already meeting the identified needs.

Table 9–2 | CARE PLAN FOR THE PATIENT WHO HAS EXPERIENCED A TRAUMATIC EVENT—cont'd

OUTCOME CRITERIA	NURSING INTERVENTIONS	RATIONALE
	6. Encourage community members and groups to engage in problem-solving activities.	6. Promotes a sense of working together to meet community needs.
	7. Develop a plan jointly with the members of the community to address immediate needs.	7. Deals with deficits in support of identified goals.
	8. Create plans managing interactions within the community and between the community and the larger society.	8. Meets collective needs when the concerns or threats are shared beyond a local community.
	9. Make information accessible to the public. Provide channels for dissemination of information to the community as a whole (e.g., print media, radio and television reports and community bulletin boards, Internet sites, speaker's bureau, reports to committees, councils, advisory boards).	9. Readily available, accurate information can help citizens deal with the situation.
	10. Make information available in different modalities and geared to differing educational levels and cultures of the community.	10. Using languages other than English and making written materials accessible to all members of the community promotes understanding.
	11. Seek out and evaluate needs of underserved populations.	11. Homeless and those residing in lower income areas may have special requirements that need to be addressed with additional resources.

Source: Doenges, M. E., Moorhouse, M. F., & Murr, A. C. (2019). *Nurse's pocket guide: Diagnoses, prioritized interventions, and rationales* (15th ed.). F.A. Davis. With permission.

Summary and Key Points

- A *crisis* is defined as an acute event in one's life, perceived by the individual as distressing and in which usual coping mechanisms and support systems are inadequate to manage associated anxiety.
- All individuals experience crises at one time or another. A crisis does not necessarily indicate psychopathology. However, individuals with psychopathology are also vulnerable to crisis and may experience an exacerbation of psychiatric symptoms when in crisis.
- Crises are precipitated by specific identifiable events and are determined by an individual's personal perception of the situation.
- Crises are acute rather than chronic and generally last no more than a few weeks to a few months.
- Crises occur when an individual is exposed to a stressor and previous problem-solving techniques are ineffective. This causes the level of anxiety to rise. Panic may ensue when new techniques are tried and resolution fails to occur.
- Six types of crises have been identified: dispositional crises, crises of anticipated life transitions, crises resulting from traumatic stress, maturational and developmental crises, crises reflecting psychopathology, and psychiatric emergencies. The type of crisis determines the method of intervention selected.
- Crisis intervention is designed to provide rapid assistance for individuals who have an urgent need.
- The minimum therapeutic goal of crisis intervention is psychological resolution of the individual's immediate crisis and restoration to at least the level of functioning that existed before the crisis period. The ideal goal is improvement in functioning above the precrisis level.
- Nurses regularly respond to individuals in crisis in all types of settings. Nursing process is the vehicle by which nurses assist individuals in crisis with a short-term problem-solving approach to change.

- A four-phase technique of crisis intervention includes assessment, planning of therapeutic intervention, intervention, and evaluation of crisis resolution and anticipatory planning.
- Through this structured method of assistance, nurses help individuals in crisis to develop more adaptive coping strategies for dealing with stressful situations in the future.
- Nurses have many important skills that can assist individuals and communities in the wake of traumatic events. Nursing interventions presented in this chapter were developed for the nursing diagnoses of panic anxiety/fear, spiritual distress, risk for post-trauma syndrome, and ineffective community coping.

Review Questions

Select the answer that is most appropriate for each of the following questions:

1. Which of the following is a correct assumption regarding the concept of crisis?
   a. Crises occur only in individuals with psychopathology.
   b. The stressful event that precipitates crisis is seldom identifiable.
   c. A crisis situation contains the potential for psychological growth or deterioration.
   d. Crises are chronic situations that recur many times during an individual's life.
2. Crises occur when an individual:
   a. Is exposed to a precipitating stressor
   b. Perceives a stressor to be threatening
   c. Has no support systems
   d. Experiences a stressor and perceives coping strategies to be ineffective
3. Which of the following is a desired outcome of working with an individual who has witnessed a traumatic event and is now experiencing panic anxiety?
   a. The individual will experience no anxiety.
   b. The individual will demonstrate hope for the future.
   c. The individual will identify that anxiety is at a manageable level.
   d. The individual will verbalize the acceptance of self as worthy.
4. The client, a firefighter who responded to an industrial explosion, lost a coworker and close friend when they entered a building that collapsed. The client reports that since this event, they have had frequent nightmares and anxiety attacks. The client says to the mental health worker, "I should have died, but instead I lost my best friend!" This statement suggests that the client is experiencing:
   a. Spiritual distress
   b. Night terrors
   c. Survivor's guilt
   d. Suicidal ideation
5. Which assessment data should the nurse consider as risk factors for possible violence in a client? (Select all that apply.)
   a. A diagnosis of somatization disorder
   b. A diagnosis of schizophrenia or bipolar disorder
   c. Substance intoxication
   d. Argumentative and demanding behavior
   e. Past history of violence
6. Which statement is true regarding traumatic bereavement?
   a. The bereavement period is more prolonged but symptoms are less intense.
   b. Traumatic bereavement is characterized by the presence of survivor guilt.
   c. Traumatic bereavement only occurs following a natural disaster.
   d. Symptoms are most often more intense and prolonged than those associated with a natural death.

Clinical Judgment Questions

7. A client whose home was destroyed during a tornado expresses to the nurse that they have been having disabling anxiety and nightmares for the past 2 weeks following this disaster. The most appropriate crisis intervention would be to:
   a. Encourage the client to recognize how lucky they are to be alive
   b. Discuss stages of grief and feelings associated with each
   c. Identify community resources that can help the client
   d. Suggest that the client find a place to live that provides a storm shelter
8. A client with a history of violence is yelling in the dayroom and knocking over chairs. The nurse observes their increased agitation, clenched fists, and loud, demanding voice. The client is challenging and threatening staff and the other clients. The nurse's priority intervention would be to:
   a. Call for assistance
   b. Draw up a syringe of prn haloperidol
   c. Ask the client if they would like to talk about their anger
   d. Tell the client if they do not calm down, they will have to be restrained
9. A client who has been in restraints is now calm. The client apologizes to the nurse and says, "I hope I didn't hurt anyone." Which action by the nurse demonstrates the best clinical judgment?
   a. Ignore the patient's comment to extinguish their aggressive behavior.
   b. Affirm to the patient that everyone loses control sometimes and tell them not to worry about it.
   c. Reinforce that it is fortunate that no one was hurt and assist the client to explore alternative behaviors when they become angry.
   d. Set firm limits with the client, instructing them that if they become angry again they will be secluded and restrained.
10. A client is noted to be pacing with clenched fists and saying, "I'm not putting up with this anymore. They've been trying to trick me all along." Which action by the nurse is most appropriate at this point?
    a. Gently touch the client's shoulder and reassure them that no one is trying to trick them.
    b. Ask the client to describe what's upsetting them.
    c. Offer the client medication.
    d. Don't intervene but continue to watch the client from a distance.
11. A client is brought to the emergency room by her roommate, who reports that she was raped at a party earlier that evening. The client appears emotionless. Which action by the nurse is a priority?
    a. Ask the client if she would like to shower before she is examined.
    b. Confront the client about her apparent lack of emotion and ask if this was consensual sex.
    c. Affirm the client for seeking help and ask her to describe what happened.
    d. Ask the roommate if the client is typically so emotionless.
12. A client is admitted to the inpatient psychiatric unit after a suicide attempt. The client reports that they have a history of depression, but they became acutely suicidal after they recently lost their job. Which nursing action is a priority in response to this client's psychiatric crisis?
    a. Assess why the client lost their job.
    b. Ensure that the client remains safe and free from further self-injury.
    c. Explore career interests and other job opportunities.
    d. Assess for substance use disorder.

Communication Exercises

1. A patient you have been working with for several days approaches you with apparent signs of agitation and yells in a loud voice, "I want out of this hospital right now! You don't listen to a thing I say, and my doctor just wants my money!"
   How will you respond?
2. Shelley enters the emergency department accompanied by a friend who reports that Shelley was raped after leaving a college campus party the night before. Shelley is staring off into space, exhibits a closed posture, and is mumbling inaudibly.
   How will you introduce yourself and begin to intervene in this crisis situation?
3. Thomas was secluded and restrained after punching another patient on the inpatient psychiatric unit. The next day he asks you what happened last night, stating he doesn't remember, and says he wants to know why he was arrested and tied up like an animal.
   What will you communicate to Thomas about the prior events and the crisis intervention process?

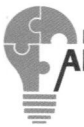

Go to **Davis Advantage** to complete your learning: strengthen understanding, apply your knowledge, and prepare for the Next Gen NCLEX®.

References

Almvik, R., Woods, P., & Rasmussen, K. (2000). The Brøset violence checklist: Sensitivity, specificity, and interrater reliability. *Journal of Interpersonal Violence, 15*(12), 1284–1296.

Barlé, N., Wortman, C. B., & Latack, J. A. (2017). Traumatic bereavement: Basic research and clinical implications. *Journal of Psychotherapy Integration, 27*(2), 127–139. https://doi.org/10.1037/int0000013

Bouchery, E. E., Barna, M., Babalola, E., Friend, D., Brown, J. D., Blyler, C., & Ireys, H. T. (2018). The effectiveness of a peer-staffed crisis respite program as an alternative to hospitalization. *Psychiatric Services, 69*(10), 1069–1074. https://doi.org/10.1176/appi.ps.201700451

Doenges, M. E., Moorhouse, M. F., & Murr, A. C. (2019). *Nurse's pocket guide: Diagnoses, prioritized interventions, and rationales* (15th ed.). F.A. Davis.

Iozzino, L., Ferrari, C., Large, M., Nielssen, O., & de Girolamo, G. (2015). Prevalence and risk factors of violence by psychiatric acute inpatients: A systematic review and meta-analysis. *PloS one, 10*(6), e0128536. https://doi.org/10.1371/journal.pone.0128536

Kassinove, H. (2021). *How to recognize and deal with anger.* http://www.apa.org/helpcenter/recognize-anger.aspx

National Alliance on Mental Illness. (2021). *Crisis intervention team (CIT) programs.* https://www.nami.org/Advocacy/Crisis-Intervention/Crisis-Intervention-Team-(CIT)-Programs

Novitsky, M. A., Julius, R. J., & Dubin, W. R. (2009). Nonpharmacologic management of violence in psychiatric emergencies. *Primary Psychiatry, 16*(9), 49–53.

Smeets, K. C., Leeijen, A. A. M., van der Molen, M. J., Scheepers, F. E., Buitelaar, J. K., & Rommelse, N. N. J. (2015). Treatment moderators of cognitive behavior therapy to reduce aggressive behavior: A meta-analysis. *European Child & Adolescent Psychiatry, 24,* 255–264. https://doi.org/10.1007/s00787-014-0592-1

Substance Abuse and Mental Health Services Administration. (2014). *SAMHSA's concept of trauma and guidance for a trauma-informed approach.* https://store.samhsa.gov/shin/content//SMA14-4884/SMA14-4884.pdf

Victoroff, J. (2017). The neuropsychiatry of human aggression. In B. A. Sadock, V. A. Sadock, & P. Ruiz (Eds.), *Comprehensive textbook of psychiatry* (10th ed.). Wolters Kluwer.

Watson, A. C., & Fulambarker, A. J. (2012). The crisis intervention team model of police response to mental health crisis: A primer for mental health practitioners. *Best Practices in Mental Health, 8*(2), 71.

Classical References

Aguilera, D. C. (1998). *Crisis intervention: Theory and methodology* (8th ed.). C.V. Mosby.

Baldwin, B. A. (1978, July). A paradigm for the classification of emotional crises: Implications for crisis intervention. *American Journal of Orthopsychiatry, 48*(3), 538–551.

Bateman, A., & Peternelj-Taylor, C. (1998). Crisis intervention. In C. A. Glod (Ed.), *Contemporary psychiatric-mental health nursing: The brain-behavior connection.* F.A. Davis.

Caplan, G. (1964). *Principles of preventive psychiatry.* Basic Books.

10 The Recovery Model

CHAPTER OUTLINE

Objectives
Introduction
What Is Recovery?
Guiding Principles of Recovery
Models of Recovery
Nursing Interventions That Assist With Recovery
Summary and Key Points
Review Questions
Clinical Judgment Questions
Communication Exercises

CORE CONCEPTS

Health Promotion: Recovery
Clinical Judgment

KEY TERMS

hope
Psychological Recovery Model
purpose
recovery
Tidal Model
WRAP Model

OBJECTIVES

After reading this chapter, the student will be able to:

1. Define *recovery*.
2. Discuss the 10 guiding principles of recovery as delineated by the Substance Abuse and Mental Health Services Administration.
3. Describe three models of recovery: the Tidal Model, the WRAP Model, and the Psychological Recovery Model.
4. Identify nursing interventions to assist individuals with mental illness in the process of recovery.

Introduction

For many years, the belief was that individuals with mental illnesses do not recover. Optimistically, the course of the illness was viewed in terms of maintenance, and pessimistically, it was viewed with the expectation for deterioration. The medical model has focused primarily on the treatment of symptoms, largely with psychotropic medications. However, as Jacobs (2015) notes, despite these available treatments, people with severe mental illness "continue to have residual positive symptoms, negative symptoms, and marked cognitive deficits" and, as a result, have difficulty "getting their lives back on track." Current research suggests that striving for and achieving recovery is, in fact, realistic for many individuals. Although critics of the recovery model argue that it contradicts the scientific model, other sources highlight the complementary and integrative potential of both models working collaboratively (Duckworth, 2015; Jacobs 2015).

The concept of recovery is not new. It originally began in the addictions field, referring to the process of recovering from a substance-related disorder. The term has been adopted by mental health professionals who believe that recovery from mental illness is also possible.

CORE CONCEPT

Recovery

Recovery is an ongoing process of movement toward improvement in health and quality of life.

What Is Recovery?

A number of definitions of recovery as it applies to mental illness have been proposed. The Substance Abuse and Mental Health Services Administration (SAMHSA, 2017) suggests the following:

> Recovery [from mental health disorders and substance use disorders] is a process of change through which individuals improve their health and wellness, live a self-directed life, and strive to reach their full potential. Recovery is built on access to evidence-based clinical treatment and recovery support services for all populations.

Essential to understanding recovery definitions and models is the focus on recovery as an ongoing process rather than a set of interventions with a distinct endpoint.

SAMHSA suggests that a life in recovery is supported by four major dimensions:

1. ***Health:*** Overcoming or managing one's disease as well as living in a physically and emotionally healthy way
2. ***Home:*** A stable and safe place to live
3. ***Purpose:*** Meaningful daily activities, such as a job, school, volunteerism, family caretaking, or creative endeavors, and the independence, income, and resources to participate in society
4. ***Community:*** Relationships and social networks that provide support, friendship, love, and hope

SAMHSA (2017) adds that the process of recovery from mental illness and substance use disorders is highly personal and occurs via many pathways. It may include clinical treatment medications, faith-based approaches, peer support, family support, self-care, and other approaches. Recovery is characterized by continual growth and improvement in one's health and wellness that may involve setbacks. Because setbacks are a natural part of life, resilience becomes a key component of recovery.

The focus on recovery as a model for treatment is widely supported. The President's New Freedom Commission on Mental Health (2003) proposed to transform the mental health system by shifting the paradigm of care of persons with serious mental illness (SMI) from traditional medical psychiatric treatment toward the concept of recovery. The American Psychiatric Association has endorsed a recovery model from a psychiatric services perspective (Sharfstein, 2005) and the American Psychological Association (2009) endorsed the recovery model as a person-centered treatment for SMI that is sensitive to consumer-defined goals and one that is only effective when efforts to reduce stigmatization are employed as well.

In a systematic review and synthesis of the various approaches to what has become known as the recovery model, Leamy and associates (2011) identified six recovery processes that form a common foundation for this model: connectedness, hope, optimism about the future, identity, meaning in life, and empowerment. Empowerment means that individuals take primary control over decisions about their own care whenever possible. The National Association of Social Workers (2006) adds, "Consumers need to be as fully informed as possible about the potential benefits and consequences of each decision. They also need to know the possible results if they become a danger to themselves or others."

Guiding Principles of Recovery

As part of its Recovery Support Strategic Initiative, a year-long effort by SAMHSA and a wide range of partners in the behavioral health-care community and other fields, a working definition of recovery from mental health and substance use disorders (previously stated) was developed. In addition, a set of guiding principles that support the recovery definition were delineated. These guiding principles include the following (SAMHSA, 2012):

- ***Recovery emerges from hope:*** The belief that recovery is real provides the essential and motivating message of a better future—that people can and do overcome the internal and external challenges, barriers, and obstacles that confront them. **Hope** is internalized and can be fostered by peers, families, providers, allies, and others. Hope is the catalyst of the recovery process.
- ***Recovery is person-driven:*** Self-determination and self-direction are the foundations for recovery as individuals define their own life goals and design their unique paths toward those goals. Individuals optimize their autonomy and independence to the greatest extent possible by leading, controlling, and exercising choice over the services and supports that assist their recovery and resilience.

In so doing, they are empowered and provided the resources to make informed decisions, initiate recovery, build on their strengths, and gain or regain control over their lives.

- ***Recovery occurs via many pathways:*** Individuals are unique with distinct needs, strengths, preferences, goals, culture, and backgrounds (including traumatic experiences) that affect and determine their pathways to recovery. Recovery is built on the multiple capacities, strengths, talents, coping abilities, resources, and inherent value of each individual. Recovery pathways are highly personalized. They may include professional clinical treatment, use of medications, support from families and in schools, faith-based approaches, peer support, and other approaches. Recovery is nonlinear, characterized by continual growth and improved functioning that may involve setbacks. Because setbacks are a natural, though not inevitable, part of the recovery process, it is essential to foster resilience for all individuals and families. Abstinence is the safest approach for those with substance use disorders. Use of tobacco and nonprescribed or illicit drugs is not safe for anyone. In some cases, recovery pathways can be enabled by creating a supportive environment. This is especially true for children, who may not have the legal or developmental capacity to set their own course.
- ***Recovery is holistic:*** Recovery encompasses an individual's whole life, including mind, body, spirit, and community. A holistic approach to recovery addresses self-care practices, family, housing, employment, education, clinical treatment for mental disorders and substance use disorders, services and supports, primary health care, dental care, complementary and alternative services, faith, spirituality, creativity, social networks, transportation, and community participation. The array of services and supports available should be integrated and coordinated.
- ***Recovery is supported by peers and allies:*** Mutual support and mutual aid groups, including the sharing of experiential knowledge and skills, as well as social learning, play an invaluable role in recovery. Peers encourage and engage other peers and provide each other with a vital sense of belonging, supportive relationships, valued roles, and community. Through helping others and giving back to the community, individuals also help themselves. Peer-operated supports and services provide important resources to assist people along their journeys of recovery and wellness. In addictions recovery, peer support has long been recognized as foundational, especially in 12-step programs such as Alcoholics Anonymous. In mental health treatment, although formal peer support is a newer approach, the premises are similar. Sometimes called peer support specialists, individuals who facilitate peer-operated supports and services may be trained and/or certified in supportive skills; all participants share the experience of lived experience with mental illness and, as such, can provide a unique perspective for support and trust in ongoing relationships. In a fully implemented recovery model, peer support specialists should be considered equal members of the treatment team (Getty, 2015). Professionals can also play an important role in the recovery process by providing clinical treatment and other services that support individuals in their chosen recovery paths. Although peers and allies play an important role for many in recovery, their role for children and youth may be slightly different. Peer supports for families are very important for children with behavioral health problems and can also play a supportive role for youth in recovery.
- ***Recovery is supported through relationship and social networks:*** An important factor in the recovery process is the presence and involvement of people who believe in the person's ability to recover; who offer hope, support, and encouragement; and who also suggest strategies and resources for change. Family members, peers, providers, faith groups, community members, and other allies form vital support networks. Through these relationships, people leave unhealthy and/or unfulfilling life roles behind and engage in new roles (e.g., partner, caregiver, friend, student, employee) that lead to a greater sense of belonging, personhood, empowerment, autonomy, social inclusion, and community participation.
- ***Recovery is culturally based and influenced:*** Culture and cultural background in all of its diverse representations (including values, traditions, and beliefs) are keys in determining a person's journey and unique pathway to recovery. Services should be culturally grounded, attuned, sensitive, congruent, and competent as well as personalized to meet each individual's unique needs. SAMHSA (2017) stresses that mental health and substance addiction services must not only respect and actively address the cultural and linguistic needs of diverse populations but should also reduce disparities in access to care.

- ***Recovery is supported by addressing trauma:*** The experience of trauma (such as physical or sexual abuse, domestic violence, war, disaster, and others) is often a precursor to or associated with alcohol and drug use, mental health problems, and related issues. Services and supports should be trauma-informed to foster safety (physical and emotional) and trust as well as promote choice, empowerment, and collaboration.
- ***Recovery involves individual, family, and community strengths and responsibilities:*** Individuals, families, and communities have strengths and resources that serve as a foundation for recovery. In addition, individuals have a personal responsibility for their own self-care and journeys of recovery. Individuals should be supported in speaking for themselves. Families and significant others have responsibilities to support their loved ones, especially for children and youth in recovery. Communities have responsibilities to provide opportunities and resources to address discrimination and to foster social inclusion and recovery. Individuals in recovery also have a social responsibility and should have the ability to join with peers to speak collectively about their strengths, needs, desires, and aspirations.
- ***Recovery is based on respect:*** Community systems, social acceptance, and appreciation of people's lived experience with mental illness and substance use problems—including protecting their rights and eliminating discrimination—are crucial in supporting recovery. There is a need to acknowledge that taking steps toward recovery may require great courage. Self-acceptance, developing a positive and meaningful sense of identity, and regaining belief in oneself are particularly important.

The recovery model integrates services provided by professionals (e.g., medication, therapy, case management), services provided by consumers (e.g., advocacy, peer support programs, hotlines, mentoring), and services provided in collaboration (e.g., recovery education, crisis planning, community integration, consumer rights education) (Jacobson & Greenley, 2001). Jacobson and Greenley state,

> Although many of these services may sound similar to services currently being offered in many mental health systems, it is important to recognize that no service is recovery-oriented unless it incorporates the attitude that recovery is possible and has the goal of promoting hope, healing, empowerment, and connection. (p. 485)

The concepts of consumer-driven care and empowerment are closely related to the concept of patient-centered care that has been advanced by the Institute of Medicine (2003) as one of the key elements necessary to improve the quality of health care in the future. As this cultural shift evolves, nurses need to be thoughtful about language and attitudes that support patient-centered recovery models. For example, a traditional goal for a patient has been described as "Patient will comply with prescribed medication regime." In a patient-centered recovery model, a more appropriate goal might be stated as, "Patient will discuss preferences, advantages, and disadvantages of psychotropic medication in the management of his or her illness."

Models of Recovery

There are many different evidence-based models of recovery. SAMHSA lists these models in a database at the National Registry for Evidence-Based Programs and Practices (www.nrepp.samhsa.gov). Three of these models—the Tidal Model, the Wellness Action Recovery Plan (WRAP), and the Psychological Recovery Model—are discussed in the following sections.

The Tidal Model

The **Tidal Model** was developed in the late 1990s by Phil Barker and Poppy Buchanan-Barker of Newcastle, United Kingdom. It is a mental health nursing recovery model that may be used as the basis for interdisciplinary mental health care (Barker & Buchanan-Barker, 2012). The authors use the power of metaphor to engage with the person in distress. The metaphor of *water* is used to describe how individuals in distress can become emotionally, physically, and spiritually *shipwrecked* (Barker & Buchanan-Barker, 2005). The Tidal Model was the first recovery model to be developed by nurses in practice, drawing largely on nursing research and in collaboration with users and consumers of mental health services (Barker & Buchanan-Barker, 2005; Brookes, 2006).

The Tidal Model uses a person-centered approach to help people deal with their problems of human living. Focus is on the individual's personal story, which is where their problems first appeared and where any growth, benefit, or recovery will be found (Barker & Buchanan-Barker, 2015).

Barker and Buchanan-Barker (2005) developed a set of essential values upon which the model is based. These values, which they call the *10 Tidal Commitments*, provide practitioners with a philosophical focus for empowering people to make their own life changes rather than health-care professionals trying to manage or control "patient symptoms" (Buchanan-Barker & Barker, 2008). From these commitments, the authors developed Tidal Competencies, which reflect the way the commitments are practiced in the clinical setting. These commitments and competencies include the following:

1. ***Value the voice:*** People are encouraged to tell their stories. "The person's story represents the beginning and endpoint of the helping encounter, embracing not only an account of the person's distress, but also the hope for its resolution" (p. 95). Practitioner competencies include a capacity to actively listen to the person's story and to help the person record the story in their own words.
2. ***Respect the language:*** Individuals are encouraged to speak their own words in their own unique way. "The language of the story—complete with its unusual grammar and personal metaphors—is the ideal medium for illuminating the way to recovery. We encourage people to speak their own words in their distinctive voice" (pp. 95–96). Practitioner competencies include helping individuals express in their own language their understanding of personal experiences through use of stories, anecdotes, and metaphors.
3. ***Develop genuine curiosity:*** Nurses and other caregivers "need to express genuine interest in the story so that they can better understand the storyteller and the story. Genuine curiosity reflects an interest in the person and the person's unique experience" (p. 96). Practitioner competencies include showing interest in the person's story, asking for clarification of certain points, and assisting the person to unfold the story at their own pace.
4. ***Become the apprentice:*** Individual are the experts on their life stories, and they must be the leader in deciding what needs to be done. "Professionals may learn something of the power of that story, but only if they apply themselves diligently and respectfully to the task by becoming apprentice-minded" (p. 96). Practitioner competencies include developing a plan of care for the individual, based on expressed needs or wishes, and helping the individual identify specific problems and ways to address them.
5. ***Use the available toolkit:*** Concentration is given to the individual's strengths, which are the major tools in the recovery process. "The story contains examples of 'what has worked' for the person in the past or beliefs about 'what might work' for this person in the future. These represent the main tools that need to be used to unlock or build the story of recovery" (p. 96). Practitioner competencies include helping individuals identify what efforts may be successful in relation to solving identified problems and which persons in the individual's life may be able to provide assistance.
6. ***Craft the step beyond:*** The individual and the practitioner decide together what needs to be done immediately. "Any 'first step' is a crucial step, revealing the power of change and potentially pointing towards the ultimate goal of recovery" (p. 96). Practitioner competencies include helping individuals determine what kind of change would represent a step toward recovery and what they need to do to take that first step toward that goal.
7. ***Give the gift of time:*** Change happens when the individual and practitioner spend quality time in a therapeutic relationship. "The challenge is using time for things that are important" (Young, 2010, p. 573). Practitioner competencies include acknowledging (and helping the individual understand) the importance of time dedicated to addressing the needs of the individual and the planning and implementing of care.
8. ***Reveal personal wisdom:*** People often do not realize their own personal wisdom, strengths, and abilities. "A key task for the professional is to help the person reveal and come to value that wisdom, so that it might be used to sustain the person throughout the voyage of recovery" (Buchanan-Barker & Barker, 2008, p. 97). Practitioner competencies include helping individuals to identify personal strengths and weaknesses and to develop self-confidence in their ability to help themselves.
9. ***Know that change is constant:*** Because change is a constant in everyone's life, important decisions and choices must be made along the path to recovery in order for growth to occur. Professional competencies include helping individuals develop awareness of the changes that are occurring and how they have influenced these changes. "The task of the professional helper is to develop awareness of how change is happening and to support the person in making decisions regarding the course of the recovery voyage" (Buchanan-Barker & Barker, 2008, p. 97).

10. ***Be transparent:*** Transparency is important in the teambuilding process between the individual and the professional helper. "Professionals are in a privileged position and should model confidence by being transparent at all times, helping the person understand exactly what is being done and why" (Buchanan-Barker & Barker, 2008, p. 97). Professional competencies include ensuring that individuals are aware of the significance of all interventions and that they receive copies of all documents related to the plan of care.

Young (2010) states,

> The Tidal Model is not a typical boxes-and-arrows diagram to use and follow. Instead, it is a way of thinking, a paradigm for giving person-centered care that is strength-based, empowering, and relational. (p. 574)

The Wellness Recovery Action Plan (WRAP)

The **WRAP Model** was developed in 1997 by a group of 30 individuals who were attending a mental health recovery skills seminar conducted by Mary Ellen Copeland in Vermont. This group (which included persons with psychiatric symptoms, family members, and care providers) determined the need for a system to incorporate into their everyday lives the skills and strategies they were learning during the seminar. Copeland (2001) states,

> [WRAP] is a structured system for monitoring uncomfortable and distressing symptoms and, through planned responses, reducing, modifying or eliminating those symptoms. It also includes plans for responses from others when a person's symptoms have made it impossible to continue to make decisions, take care of him/herself and keep him/herself safe. (p. 129)

Copeland suggests that all a person needs to begin the program is a system for storing information (e.g., a notebook, computer, or tape recorder) and possibly a friend, health-care provider, or other supporter to give assistance and feedback. The program is a stepwise process through which an individual is able to monitor and manage distressing symptoms that occur in daily life. Individuals may be assisted in the process by others (e.g., health-care professionals, significant others, friends), "but to be effective and empowering, the person experiencing the symptoms must develop the plan for himself/herself" (2001, p. 129). The WRAP process involves six steps:

Step 1. Developing a wellness toolbox: The individual creates a list of tools, strategies, and skills that have been used in the past (or has heard of in the past and would like to try) to assist in relieving disturbing symptoms. Copeland (2001) offers a number of examples:

- Talking to a friend or health-care professional
- Peer counseling or exchange listening
- Relaxation and stress reduction exercises
- Guided imagery
- Journaling
- Physical exercise
- Attending a support group
- Doing something special for someone else
- Listening to music

Step 2. Daily maintenance list: This list is divided into three parts. In part 1, individuals write a description of how they feel (or would like to feel) when experiencing wellness (e.g., bright, cheerful, talkative, happy, optimistic, capable). This information is used as a reference point. In part 2, using the wellness toolbox as a reference, individuals make a list of things they need to do every day to maintain wellness. This is an important part of the plan and must be realistic so as not to set individuals up for failure or create additional frustration. Example items for part 2 may include the following (Copeland, 2001):

- Eat three healthy meals and three healthy snacks.
- Drink at least six 8-ounce glasses of water.
- Avoid caffeine, sugar, junk foods, and alcohol.
- Exercise for at least 30 minutes.
- Have 20 minutes of relaxation or meditation time.
- Write in my journal for at least 15 minutes.
- Take medications and vitamin supplements.
- Spend at least 30 minutes enjoying a fun, affirming, and/or creative activity.

In part 3 of this step, individuals keep a list of things that need to be done. Individuals read this list daily as a reminder, and items may be considered for accomplishment on any given day at the individual's discretion. For part 3, Copeland (2001) suggests items such as the following:

- Spend time with my counselor or case manager.
- Make an appointment with my health-care professional.
- Spend time with my friend or partner.
- Be in touch with my family.
- Spend time with children or pets.
- Buy groceries.

- Do the laundry.
- Write some letters.
- Remember someone's birthday or anniversary.

Step 3. Triggers: This step is divided into two parts. In part 1, individuals list events or circumstances that, should they occur, would cause distress or discomfort. These triggers are situations to which the individuals are susceptible or that have triggered or increased symptoms in the past. Copeland (2001) lists the following examples:

- The anniversary dates of losses or trauma
- Being overtired or exhausted
- Work stress
- Family friction
- A relationship ending
- Being judged, criticized, or teased
- Financial problems
- Physical illness
- Sexual harassment or inappropriate sexual behavior
- Substance abuse

In part 2, individuals use items from the wellness toolbox to develop a plan for what to do if triggers interfere with wellness.

Step 4. Early warning signs: This step is divided into two parts. Part 1 involves identification of subtle signs that indicate a possible worsening of the situation. Copeland (2001) states, "Recognizing early warning signs and reviewing them regularly will help the person to become more aware of these early warning signs, allowing the person to take action before the signs worsen" (p. 136). Some types of early warning signs include anxiety, forgetfulness, lack of motivation, avoiding others or isolating, increased irritability, increase in smoking, using substances, or feeling worthless and inadequate. In part 2, individuals develop a plan for responding to the early warning signs that result in relief or in preventing them from escalating. The plan may include items such as consulting a supporter or counselor, increasing focus on peer counseling, increasing time spent in relaxation exercises, or utilizing other interventions from the wellness toolbox until warning signs diminish.

Step 5. Things are breaking down or getting worse: This step is divided into two parts. In part 1, individuals list symptoms that are occurring that indicate that the situation has worsened. In this stage, the symptoms are producing great discomfort, but individuals are still able to take some action on their own behalf. Immediate action is required to prevent a crisis from developing. Symptoms at this stage differ greatly from person to person, and Copeland (2001) states, "What may mean 'things are breaking down' to one person may mean 'crisis' to another" (p. 137). She lists a number of examples of symptoms, which may include the following:

- Irrational responses to events and the actions of others
- Inability to sleep or sleeping all the time
- Headaches
- Not eating or overeating
- Social isolation
- Thoughts of self-harm
- Substance abuse or chain smoking
- Bizarre behaviors
- Seeing things that are not there
- Paranoia

In part 2, individuals make a plan that they think will help when the symptoms have worsened to this degree. Plans must be very specific and direct, with clear instructions. Some examples include the following (Copeland, 2001):

- Call my health-care professional; ask for and follow directions.
- Arrange for someone to stay with me around the clock until my symptoms subside.
- Take action so that I cannot hurt myself if my symptoms get worse, such as give my medication, checkbook, credit cards, and car keys to a previously designated friend for safe keeping.
- Make sure I do everything on my daily checklist.
- Have at least two peer counseling sessions daily.
- Increase use of items from wellness toolbox (e.g., relaxation exercises, physical exercises, creative activities).

Step 6. Crisis planning: This stage identifies symptoms indicating that individuals can no longer care for themselves, make independent decisions, or keep themselves safe. This stage is multifaceted and is meant for use by caregivers on behalf of the individual who developed the plan. It is composed of the following parts (Copeland, 2001, p. 130):

- *Part 1.* Gathers information that describes what the person is like when well.
- *Part 2.* Identifies the symptoms that indicate when others need to take responsibility for the person's care.
- *Part 3.* Provides names of supporters previously identified by the individual to speak on their behalf.

- *Part 4.* Includes the name of health-care providers and phone numbers, medications currently being used, allergies to medications, medications the individual would prefer to take if additional medication is necessary, and medications that the individual refuses to take.
- *Part 5.* Includes the individual's preferred treatments and treatments to be avoided.
- *Part 6.* Identifies the individual's preferences in treatment facilities (e.g., home, community care, respite center).
- *Part 7.* Identifies acceptable facilities if previous preferences cannot be executed. Facilities to be avoided are also indicated.
- *Part 8.* Includes an extensive description of what the individual expects from identified supporters who are acting on their behalf during a crisis situation.
- *Part 9.* Consists of a list of indicators, developed by individuals, that communicates to supporters when their services are no longer required. Individuals should update this plan periodically when they learn new information or change their mind about certain situations. Assurance of the use of the crisis plan may be increased if it is notarized and signed in the presence of two witnesses. To further increase its potential for use, people may appoint a durable power of attorney, although because of the variability of the legality of these documents from state to state, there is no guarantee that the plan will be followed.

Copeland (2001) states,

> WRAP is a systematic method for developing skills in self-management and empowerment. It provides a means for individuals with a mental illness to work more collaboratively with healthcare providers. It is highly individualized and addresses the unique needs of the person and his/her situation. It is applicable to most any long-term illness/disability or problem situation. These benefits suggest that it can be used more widely and should be introduced as an option for individuals in need of a self-management system. (p. 149)

The Copeland Center for Wellness and Recovery (2020) offers resources for training in the WRAP model and has established certification programs for peer support specialists and for programs that provide structured WRAP services.

The Psychological Recovery Model

Andresen and associates (2011) define *psychological recovery* as "the establishment of a fulfilling, meaningful life and a positive sense of identity founded on hopefulness and self-determination. Psychological recovery is necessary whether mental illness is biologically based or the result of the exacerbation of emotional problems caused by stress" (p. 40). The **Psychological Recovery Model** does not emphasize the absence of symptoms but focuses on individuals' self-determination in the course of their recovery process.

In examining a number of studies, Andresen and associates (2011) identified four components that were consistently evident in the recovery process:

- ***Hope:*** Finding and maintaining hope that recovery can occur
- ***Responsibility:*** Taking responsibility for one's life and well-being
- ***Self and identity:*** Renewing the sense of self and building a positive identity
- ***Meaning and purpose:*** Finding **purpose** and meaning in life

Andresen and associates (2011) conceptualized a five-stage model of recovery, which they define by integrating into each stage the four components of the recovery process:

Stage 1. Moratorium: This stage is identified by dark despair and confusion. "It is called moratorium, because it seems 'life is on hold'" (p. 47).

- *Hope:* In the moratorium stage, hopelessness prevails. Clients may even perceive feelings of hopelessness from practitioners when treatment plans emphasize stabilization and maintenance, thereby conveying messages of no hope for recovery.
- *Responsibility:* In the moratorium stage, the individual feels out of control and powerless to change.
- *Self and identity:* In the moratorium stage, individuals feel "as though they no longer know who they are as a person" (p. 59). An individual's sense of identity as a valuable and functional member of society can be lost with a diagnosis of mental illness.
- *Meaning and purpose:* The diagnosis of severe mental illness is a traumatic event that can challenge an individual's fundamental beliefs, creating a loss of meaning and purpose in life.

Stage 2. Awareness: In this stage, the individual comes to a realization that a possibility for recovery exists. Andresen and associates state, "It involves an awareness of a possible self other than that of 'sick person': a self that is capable of recovery" (p. 47).

- *Hope:* In the awareness stage, there is a dawn of hope that "life is not over." This feeling of hope may emanate from significant others, professionals, or family members. Individuals may also be inspired by others who have recovered. Hope may also be derived from strong inner determination and from personal faith and spirituality.

- *Responsibility:* In this stage, the individual develops an awareness of the need to take control of their life. Feelings of control and responsibility lead to a sense of personal empowerment that paves the way for recovery.
- *Self and identity:* In the awareness stage, individuals come to realize they are people independent of the illness. "The person realizes that there still exists an 'intact self' capable of taking action on one's own behalf" (p. 72).
- *Meaning and purpose:* In the awareness stage, the individual strives for a personal comprehension of the illness, why it occurred, and what the implications of the illness are for their future. "Seeking a meaning of the illness can be explained by theories of cognitive control, in which one tries to understand unexplainable negative events by finding a reason for them" (p. 74).

Stage 3. Preparation: This stage begins with the individual's resolve to begin the work of recovery.

- *Hope:* In the preparation stage, hope is manifested in the mobilization of personal and external resources to foster self-care and find pathways to goals. The individual identifies strengths and weaknesses, gathers knowledge and information, and seeks out available support systems.
- *Responsibility:* Taking responsibility in the preparation stage involves learning about the effects of the illness and how to recognize, monitor, and manage symptoms. Taking charge of one's life also includes the ability to be independent and take care of basic needs.
- *Self and identity:* Andresen and associates state, "During the preparation stage, the person takes stock of his or her skills and strengths in order to build on them to rediscover a positive sense of identity" (p. 81). The person is willing to take risks and try new activities to re-establish a sense of self. Lost aspects of self are rediscovered, new aspects are identified, and both are incorporated into a new self-identity.
- *Meaning and purpose:* The basis for a meaningful life lies in solid core values. "Living according to one's valued directions gives meaning to the work of recovery, and for this reason, some people hold on tenaciously to their goals" (p. 83). Each individual must live by certain tenets that make life personally valuable and enriching. Individuals living with a severe mental illness may require a reordering of priorities and setting of new goals as part of their recovery.

Stage 4. Rebuilding: The hard work of recovery takes place in the rebuilding stage. The individual "takes the necessary steps to work towards his or her goals in rebuilding a meaningful life" (p. 87).

- *Hope:* In the rebuilding stage, the individual has hope for and looks forward to a more fulfilling life. Realistic goals are set, and the individual is encouraged to pursue the recovery process at their own pace. With each success, hope is renewed.
- *Responsibility:* "Through setting and working towards goals, the person begins to actively take control of his or her life; not only management of symptoms, but also enlisting social support, improvement of self-image, handling social pressures, and building social competence" (p. 90). Assuming control of treatment decisions and illness management is an essential part of the recovery process.
- *Self and identity:* The individual elaborates and enhances their sense of identity by having succeeded in previous stages in developing a positive self-identity separate from the illness and a new sense of self-confidence by succeeding at new activities. In the rebuilding stage, the work of examining core values and working toward value-congruent goals reinforce a positive sense of identity and a commitment to recovery.
- *Meaning and purpose:* Having realistic goals and a positive sense of identity provides a sense of purpose in life. Individuals need a reason to start each day. Andresen and associates state, "Finding meaning [in life] is more than finding a valued occupation, but rather is more akin to finding a way to live. This may include, but is not limited to, vocational goals. It includes examining one's spirituality or philosophy of life. The journey is, in itself, a source of meaning for many" (p. 99).

Stage 5. Growth: The outcome of the psychological recovery process is growth. Although it is called the *final* stage of the psychological recovery model, it is important to remember that this is a dynamic stage and that personal growth is a continuing life process.

- *Hope:* In the growth stage, the individual feels a sense of optimism and hope of a rewarding future. Skills that have been nurtured in the previous stages are applied with confidence, and the individual strives for higher levels of well-being.

- *Responsibility:* "Achieving control requires sustained commitment in the face of set-backs" (p. 106). In the growth phase, individuals exhibit confidence in managing their illnesses and are resilient when relapses occur. They are empowered by personal input and decision making regarding their treatment.
- *Self and identity:* The individual in the growth stage has developed a strong, positive sense of self and identity. Andresen and associates state, "Many consumers have reported feeling that they are a better person as a result of their struggle with the illness. [In one research study] participants reported developing personal qualities, including strength and courage; more confidence in the self; resourcefulness and responsibility; a new philosophy of life; compassion and empathy; a sense of self-worth; and being happier and more carefree" (pp. 108–109).
- *Meaning and purpose:* Individuals who have reached the growth stage often report a more profound sense of meaning. Some describe having achieved a sense of serenity and peace, and for others it takes the form of a spiritual awakening. Some individuals find reward in educating others about the experience of mental illness and recovery.

Andresen and associates (2011) state,

> Recovery from serious mental illness is more than staying out of the hospital or a return to some arbitrary level of functioning. It is more than merely coping with the illness. In [the growth] stage, the notion of wellbeing replaces that of wellness. While wellness implies the absence of illness, wellbeing refers to a more holistic psychological experience of fulfilling life. Although we may not expect everyone (including those who do not have a mental illness) to reach the highest levels of self-actualization, we can expect that all people have the opportunity to develop a positive sense of self and identity and to live a meaningful life filled with purpose and hope for the future. (p. 113)

Nursing Interventions That Assist With Recovery

It is within the scope of nursing to assist individuals in many aspects of the mental health recovery process. Caldwell and colleagues (2010) state,

> Professional nurses must play an active role in client recovery because they are employed in all aspects of service delivery systems, and most times professional nurses are responsible for the delivery and coordination of care. The professional nurse must be center stage in the development and implementation of any action plan involving client recovery. (p. 44)

Nurses have historically held the promotion of wellness within a collaborative nurse-patient relationship as a primary goal. Peplau (1991) described nursing as "a human relationship between an individual who is sick, or in need of health services, and a nurse especially educated to recognize and to respond to the need for help" (pp. 5–6). As previously noted, recovery models are inherently collaborative in that services are provided by professionals, by consumers, and cooperatively by both. Examples of interventions and activities in which nurses and patients may collaborate in the individual's journey to recovery are outlined in Table 10–1.

Advocates for the recovery model stress its positive, hopeful, and empowering aspects that have been lacking in traditional medical models of treatment. Critics argue that an individual's subjective perception of recovery does not necessarily validate the quality of health-care interventions, particularly in cases where individuals (as in schizophrenia) may experience the symptom of anosognosia (in which they do not see themselves as having an illness despite apparent, significant symptoms). Duckworth (2015) promotes integrating recovery and medical models of treatment to ensure that scientific processes are used to validate outcomes associated with recovery models of intervention. He cites several examples of recovery-focused treatments that have been supported by research, such as the WRAP model (previously discussed); dialectical behavioral therapy (DBT) for borderline personality disorders; cognitive enhancement therapy (CET) for improving cognition problems in patients with early-stage psychosis; and the National Alliance on Mental Health's (NAMI) Family-to Family Program, an education and peer support program for families experiencing mental illness.

Many nurse leaders see the current period of health-care reform as an opportunity for nurses to expand their roles and assume key positions in education, prevention, assessment, and referral. Nurses are, and will continue to be, in key positions to assist individuals with mental illness to remain as independent as possible, to manage their illness within the community setting, and to strive to minimize the number of hospitalizations required. A vision of recovery from mental illness exists, and hope, trust, and self-determination should be incorporated into all treatment models.

TABLE 10–1 Nurse-Patient Collaboration in the Mental Health Recovery Process

	TIDAL MODEL	WRAP MODEL	PSYCHOLOGICAL RECOVERY MODEL
Assessment	■ The patient tells their personal story ■ Nurse actively listens and expresses interest in the story ■ Nurse helps the patient record their story in the patient's own language ■ The patient identifies specific problems to be addressed ■ Nurse and patient identify the patient's strengths and weaknesses	■ The patient develops a wellness toolbox by creating a list of tools, strategies, and skills that have been helpful in the past ■ The patient identifies strengths and weaknesses ■ Nurse provides assistance and feedback	■ The patient is feeling hopeless and powerless ■ The patient seeks meaning of the illness ■ Nurse helps by offering hope ■ The patient begins to develop an awareness of the need to take control of and responsibility for their life
Interventions	■ Nurse and patient determine what has worked in the past ■ The patient suggests new tools to try ■ The patient decides what changes to make and sets realistic goals ■ Nurse and patient decide what must be done as the first step ■ Nurse gives positive feedback for the patient's efforts to make life changes and for successes achieved ■ Nurse encourages the patient to be as independent as possible but offers assistance when required ■ Nurse gives the "gift of time"	■ The patient creates a daily maintenance list: - How the patient is feeling at best - What must be done daily to maintain wellness - Reminder list of other things that need to be accomplished ■ The patient identifies triggers that cause distress or discomfort and identifies what to do if triggers interfere with wellness ■ The patient identifies signs of worsening of symptoms and develops a plan to prevent escalation ■ The patient identifies when symptoms have worsened and help is needed ■ The patient identifies when unable to care for self and makes decisions (in writing) about treatment issues (what type, who will provide, who will represent the patient's interests) ■ Nurse offers support and provides feedback and assistance when needed	■ The patient resolves to begin work of recovery ■ The patient and nurse identify strengths and weaknesses ■ Nurse assists the patient to learn about effects of the illness and how to recognize, monitor, and manage symptoms ■ The patient identifies desired changes and sets realistic goals to rebuild a meaningful life ■ The patient examines personal spirituality and philosophy of life in search of a meaning and purpose—one that gives them a "reason to start each day"
Outcomes	■ The patient acknowledges that change has occurred and is ongoing ■ The patient feels empowered to manage own self-care ■ Nurse is available for support	■ The patient develops skills in self-management ■ The patient develops self-confidence and hope for a brighter future	■ The patient develops a positive self-identity separate from the illness ■ The patient maintains commitment to recovery in the face of setbacks ■ The patient feels a sense of optimism and hope of a rewarding future

Summary and Key Points

- Recovery is characterized by continual growth and improvement in one's health and wellness that may involve setbacks.
- SAMHSA identifies four major dimensions that support a life in recovery: health, home, purpose, and community.
- The President's New Freedom Commission on Mental Health (2003) proposed to transform the mental health system by shifting the paradigm of care of persons with serious mental illness from traditional medical psychiatric treatment toward the concept of recovery.
- SAMHSA outlines 10 guiding principles that support recovery:
  - Recovery emerges from hope.
  - Recovery is person-driven.
  - Recovery occurs via many pathways.
  - Recovery is holistic.
  - Recovery is supported by peers and allies.
  - Recovery is supported through relationship and social networks.
  - Recovery is culturally based and influenced.
  - Recovery is supported by addressing trauma.
  - Recovery involves individual, family, and community strengths and responsibilities.
  - Recovery is based on respect.
- Many models of recovery exist. Three models that are discussed in this chapter are the Tidal Model, the Wellness Action Recovery Plan (WRAP), and the Psychological Recovery Model.
- Nurses work in key positions to assist individuals with mental illness in the recovery process. Interventions based on the three previously mentioned recovery models are included in this chapter.

Review Questions

Select the answer that is most appropriate for each of the following questions:

1. Which is a true statement about mental health recovery? (Select all that apply.)
a. Mental health recovery applies only to severe and persistent mental illnesses.
b. Mental health recovery serves to provide empowerment to the consumer.
c. Mental health recovery is based on the medical model.
d. Mental health recovery is a collaborative process.

2. A nurse is assisting an individual with mental illness recovery using the Tidal Model. Which is a component of this model?
a. The wellness toolbox
b. The daily maintenance list
c. The individual's personal story
d. Triggers

Clinical Judgment Questions

3. A nurse is assisting an individual with mental illness recovery using the Psychological Recovery Model. The client states to the nurse, "I have schizophrenia. Nothing can be done. I might as well die." In which stage of the Psychological Recovery Model should the nurse assess this individual to be?
a. Awareness
b. Preparation
c. Rebuilding
d. Moratorium

4. A nurse who is helping a client in the preparation stage of the Psychological Recovery Model should include which intervention?
a. Teach about effects of the illness and how to recognize, monitor, and manage symptoms.
b. Help the client identify "triggers" that cause distress or discomfort.
c. Help the client establish a daily maintenance list.
d. Listen actively while the client composes their personal story.

5. A client approaches the nurse and states, "I don't want to go to outpatient group therapy. I don't like groups." Which response by the nurse supports a recovery model focus?
   a. "You need to attend weekly groups to support your ongoing recovery."
   b. "If you don't comply with treatment you will need to be hospitalized again."
   c. "Let's discuss some options for follow-up care and explore the advantages and disadvantages."
   d. "Your psychiatrist recommended this, but we can't force you to comply with treatment."
6. A client with bipolar disorder tells the nurse at the community mental health center that they stopped taking their medication and they are getting so much more done. The client's speech is rapid and they admit that they haven't gotten much sleep but states they are not tired. The client doesn't want to be hospitalized because they are "about to save the world" with their new invention. Which intervention by the nurse is a priority?
   a. Administer an IM dose of the client's previously ordered medication.
   b. Make arrangements for the client to be admitted to the psychiatric hospital.
   c. Explore the advantages and disadvantages of medication adherence.
   d. Assess the client for risk of harm to self and others.
7. A client is voluntarily admitted to the hospital with suicide ideation. The client tells the nurse, "I thought I was recovered from this depression, but this is my sixth episode. I guess I can't do anything right so I may as well just end it all." Which action by the nurse is a priority?
   a. Educate the client that depression is not an illness that one can recover from; they must instead learn how to manage it with a comprehensive treatment strategy.
   b. Educate the client that recovery is a process that sometimes has setbacks and reinforce their decision to seek hospitalization.
   c. Assess the client's perception of what they've been doing that "is not right."
   d. Assess why the client believes they are depressed.

Communication Exercises

1. Joshua comes to his appointment at the mental health clinic and states, "I can't sit still when I take those medications, so I don't want to take them anymore."
   Using principles of the recovery model, what are some options for responding to this patient?
2. Kelly is a war veteran who was admitted to inpatient hospitalization with depression, alcohol addiction, and complaints of troubling nightmares. She states, at the admission assessment, "I don't trust any 'mental health gurus.' You can't possibly understand what I've been through."
   How will you respond, and what principles of the recovery model will guide your response?

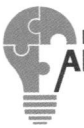

Go to **Davis Advantage** to complete your learning: strengthen understanding, apply your knowledge, and prepare for the Next Gen NCLEX®.

References

American Psychological Association. (2009). *Resolution on APA endorsement of the concept of recovery for people with serious mental illness.* https://web.archive.org/web/20121222063240/http://www.apa.org/practice/leadership/smi/recovery-resolution.pdf

Andresen, R., Oades, L. G., & Caputi, P. (2011). *Psychological recovery: Beyond mental illness.* John Wiley & Sons.

Barker, P. J., & Buchanan-Barker, P. (2005). *The Tidal Model: A guide for mental health professionals.* Brunner-Routledge.

Barker, P. J., & Buchanan-Barker, P. (2012). Tidal Model of mental health nursing. *Current Nursing.* http://www.currentnursing.com/nursing_theory/Tidal_Model.html

Barker, P. J., & Buchanan-Barker, P. (2015). *The Tidal Model: Reclaiming stories, recovering lives.* http://www.tidal-model.com

Brookes, N. (2006). Phil Barker: The Tidal Model of mental health recovery. In A. M. Tomey & M. R. Alligood (Eds.), *Nursing theorists and their work* (6th ed., pp. 696–725). Elsevier.

Buchanan-Barker, P., & Barker, P. J. (2008). The Tidal commitments: Extending the value base of mental health recovery. *Journal of Psychiatric and Mental Health Nursing, 15*(2), 93–100.

Caldwell, B. A., Sclafani, M., Swarbrick, M., & Piren, K. (2010). Psychiatric nursing practice and the recovery model of care. *Journal of Psychosocial Nursing, 48*(7), 42–48.

Copeland, M. E. (2001). Wellness recovery action plan: A system for monitoring, reducing and eliminating uncomfortable or dangerous physical symptoms and emotional feelings. In C. Brown (Ed.), *Recovery and wellness: Models of hope and empowerment for people with mental illness* (pp. 127–150). Haworth Press.

Copeland Center for Wellness and Recovery. (2020). *Certified peer specialist training.* https://copelandcenter.com/our-services/certified-peer-specialist-training-cps

Duckworth, K. (2015). Science meets the human experience: Integrating the medical and recovery models. *NAMI.* https://www.nami.org/blogs/nami-blog/april-2015/science-meets-the-human-experience-integrating-th

Getty, S. M. (2015). Implementing a mental health program using the recovery model. *OT Practice, 20*(3), 1–8.

Institute of Medicine. (2003). *Health professions education: A bridge to quality.*

Jacobs, K. S. (2015). Recovery model of mental illness: A complementary approach to psychiatric care. *Indian Journal of Psychological Medicine, 37*(2), 117–119. https://doi.org/10.4103/0253-7176.155605

Jacobson, N., & Greenley, D. (2001). What is recovery? A conceptual model and explication. *Psychiatric Services, 52*(4), 482–485.

Leamy, M., Bird, V., LeBoutillier, C., Williams, J., & Slade, M. (2011). Conceptual framework for personal recovery in mental health: Systematic review and narrative synthesis. *British Journal of Psychiatry, 199,* 445–452. https://doi.org/10.1192/bjp.bp.110.083733

National Association of Social Workers. (2006). *NASW Practice snapshot: The mental health recovery model.* http://www.socialworkers.org/practice/behavioral_health/0206snapshot.asp?

President's New Freedom Commission on Mental Health. (2003). *Achieving the promise: Transforming mental health care in America.* http://govinfo.library.unt.edu/mentalhealthcommission/index.htm

Sharfstein, S. (2005). Recovery model will strengthen psychiatrist-patient relationship. *Psychiatric News, 40*(20), 3.

Substance Abuse and Mental Health Services Administration. (2012). *SAMHSA's working definition of recovery: 10 guiding principles of recovery* [Brochure].

Substance Abuse and Mental Health Services Administration. (2017). *Recovery and recovery support.* https://www.samhsa.gov/recovery

Young, B. B. (2010). Using the Tidal Model of mental health recovery to plan primary health care for women in residential substance abuse recovery. *Issues in Mental Health Nursing, 31*(9), 569–575.

Classical Reference

Peplau, H. E. (1991). *Interpersonal relations in nursing: A conceptual frame of reference for psychodynamic nursing.* Springer.

11 Suicide Prevention

CHAPTER OUTLINE

Objectives
Introduction
Historical Perspectives
Epidemiology
Risk Factors
Predisposing Factors: Theories of Suicide
Application of the Nursing Process With the Suicidal Patient
Summary and Key Points
Review Questions
Clinical Judgment Questions
Communication Exercises

KEY TERMS

collaborative safety plan
suicide
suicide risk factors
suicide warning signs

OBJECTIVES

After reading this chapter, the student will be able to:

1. Discuss epidemiological statistics and risk factors related to suicide.
2. Describe predisposing factors implicated in the etiology of suicide.
3. Differentiate between facts and myths regarding suicide.
4. Apply the nursing process to individuals exhibiting suicidal behavior.

CORE CONCEPTS

Behaviors: Suicide
Caring: Therapeutic relationship
Safety: Suicide risk assessment, Suicide prevention
Evidence-Based Practice: Suicide prevention
Health Promotion: Suicide risk assessment
Professional Behavior: Nursing process in the care of patients with suicidal ideation or behaviors
Clinical Judgment

Introduction

Suicide is not a diagnosis or a disorder; it is a behavior. Specifically, it is the act of taking one's own life, and it derives from the Latin words for "one's own killing." Many religions hold that suicide is a sin, and it is strictly forbidden. Cultural norms and attitudes also influence an individual's beliefs about suicide. Although some populations are considered at higher risk for suicide (such as American Indians and Alaska Natives; active and veteran military members; lesbian, gay, bisexual, or transgender individuals; and people in justice or child welfare settings), suicide touches the lives of all age-, ethnic, and racial groups in all parts of the country. A complex interaction of factors, such as mental illness, substance abuse, painful losses, exposure to violence, and social isolation, are all influential in increasing these risks (Substance Abuse and Mental Health Services Administration [SAMHSA], 2020).

In the past decade, many state legislatures have debated the acceptability of physician-assisted suicide. Although it is legal in all parts of the United States for an individual or the individual's power of attorney to refuse life-preserving medical treatment, the majority of states have not legalized physician-assisted suicide. As of 2020, nine states (California, Colorado, Hawaii, Maine, Montana, New Jersey, Oregon, Washington, and Vermont) and Washington, DC, have legalized physician-assisted suicide. New Mexico also adopted a similar law, but it was overturned on appeal in August 2015. Can suicide be a rational act? Most people in our society do not yet believe that it can.

In the field of psychiatry, suicide is considered an irrational act associated with mental illness and most commonly, but not exclusively, with depression. However, not everyone who dies by suicide has a mental illness. Individuals in non-psychiatric health-care settings and in the community may also be at risk. This chapter explores suicide from an epidemiological and etiological perspective. Care of the suicidal patient is presented in the context of the nursing process.

Historical Perspectives

In ancient Greece, individuals were said to have "committed" suicide because it was an offense against the state, and individuals who did so were denied burial in community sites (Minois, 2001). In the culture of ancient Rome, individuals sometimes resorted to suicide to escape humiliation or abuse.

In the Middle Ages, suicide was viewed as a selfish or criminal act (Minois, 2001). Individuals who "committed suicide" were often denied cemetery burial and their property was confiscated and shared by the crown and the courts (MacDonald & Murphy, 1991). The issue of suicide changed during the Renaissance period. Although condemnation was still expected, the view became more philosophical, and intellectuals could discuss the issue more freely.

Most philosophers of the 17th and 18th centuries condemned suicide, but some writers recognized a connection between suicide and melancholy or other severe mental disturbances (Minois, 2001). Suicide was illegal in England until 1961, and only in 1993 was it decriminalized in Ireland. With the decriminalization of suicide, many have advanced the idea that the term *committed suicide* should be removed from our vocabulary because it is inaccurate and potentially maintains a stigmatizing attitude toward this population.

Most religions consider suicide as a sin: Judaism, Christianity, Islam, Hinduism, and Buddhism all condemn suicide. The Catholic Church still teaches that suicide is wrong, that it is in opposition to proper love of self and love of God, and that it wrongs others through the experience of loss and grief (Byron, 2016). But as Byron points out, some of the church's condemnation may have been rooted in a "denial of the responsibility to understand the pain" that produces such an act, and he stresses the importance of encouraging those who "are hurting to open up," which, it is hoped, will remove some of the taboos of discussing suicide within the church. Likewise, replacing the term *committed suicide* (which has persisted long since its decriminalization) may also help to reduce the stigma and taboo that has historically been associated with discussing suicide.

Epidemiology

In 2019, the most recent year for which statistics have been recorded, 47,511 people died by suicide in the United States (Centers for Disease Control and Prevention [CDC], 2021a). Most of those deaths were firearm suicides. These statistics have established suicide as the second-leading cause of death (behind unintentional injuries) among young Americans ages 10 to 24 (19.2% of deaths) and 25 to 44 (10.9%), the eighth-leading cause for those ages 45 to 64 (3.1% of deaths), and the 10th-leading cause of death overall (CDC, 2019a). (While suicide has been the 10th-leading cause of death for several years, provisional statistics for 2020 indicate suicide as the 11th-leading cause of death for a year where COVID-19 deaths became the third-leading cause of death overall in the United States [Ahmad et al., 2021].) Many more people attempt suicide than succeed (about 12:1), and countless others seriously contemplate the act without carrying it out. With a steady incline in rates of suicide over the period from 2000 to 2018, suicide has become a major health-care problem in the United States today.

Not only have the number of suicides been on the incline but the demographics have changed. Historically, the highest rates of suicide were among the elderly. However, the current highest rates of suicide are among individuals ages 45 to 54 and the second-highest are those over 85 years of age (American Foundation for Suicide Prevention [AFSP], 2021). Historically, the suicide rate has been lower among military personnel than among the general population. However, in some time periods since the Iraq War began—including in 2010 and 2011—more soldiers died by suicide than died in combat (Nock et al., 2013). The Department of Defense reports that among all military populations, the 2018 rate of suicide was consistent over the last two years but rates from the active military component were statistically higher than the last five years (Lopez, 2019). See Chapter 28, "Military Families," for further discussion.

Research is being conducted to better understand the best methods for assessment of suicide risk, what differentiates those with suicidal ideation from those who attempt, and evidence-based treatments and interventions. The federal government, through the Substance Abuse and Mental Health Services Administration (SAMHSA), has endorsed the "Zero Suicide" movement; a partnership of several national organizations dedicated to identifying evidence-based strategies for suicide prevention. Within the next several years, we may discover that our understanding of and approaches to treatment will dramatically change. We are certainly beginning to recognize that, with the rise in suicide rates, our conventional interventions have not adequately addressed the complex needs of this population.

Confusion exists over the reality of various notions regarding suicide. Some currently accepted facts and some myths relating to suicide are presented in Table 11–1.

TABLE 11–1 Facts and Myths About Suicide

MYTHS	FACTS
People who talk about suicide do not act on their ideas. Suicide happens without warning.	Eight out of 10 people who kill themselves have given definite clues and warnings about their suicidal intentions. Very subtle clues may be ignored or disregarded by others.
You cannot stop suicidal people. They are fully intent on dying.	Most suicidal people are very ambivalent about their feelings regarding living or dying. Most are "gambling with death" and see it as a cry for someone to save them.
Once people are suicidal, they are suicidal forever.	Suicidal ideation and risk fluctuate over time and may be time limited. If provided adequate support and resources, a suicidal person can go on to lead a normal life. However, multiple suicide attempts may reflect greater chronicity of suicidal ideation. Reassessment over time is important to identify current risks.
Improvement after severe depression means that the suicidal risk is over.	Most suicides occur within about 3 months after the beginning of "improvement," when the individual has the energy to carry out suicidal intentions.
Suicide is inherited, or "runs in families."	Suicide is not inherited. Many mental illnesses like depression, bipolar disorder, and substance abuse run in families and confer an increased risk, but suicidal behavior is not inevitable in these populations. However, suicide by a close family member does increase the risk of similar behavior in other family members.
All suicidal individuals are mentally ill, and suicide is the act of a psychotic person.	Although a majority of people who attempt suicide are extremely unhappy, or clinically depressed, they are not necessarily psychotic. They are merely unable at that point in time to see an alternative solution to what they consider an unbearable problem.
Suicidal thoughts and attempts should be considered manipulative or attention-seeking behavior and should not be taken seriously.	All suicidal behavior must be approached with the gravity of the potential act in mind. Attention should be given to the possibility that the individual is issuing a cry for help.
People usually take their own lives by taking an overdose of drugs.	Gunshot wounds are the leading cause of death among suicide victims.
If individuals have attempted suicide, they will not do it again.	Between 50% and 80% of all people who ultimately kill themselves have a history of at least one previous attempt.
Suicide always happens in an impulsive moment.	People who are suicidal often contemplate, imagine, plan strategies, write notes, post things on the Web. The importance of in-depth exploration and assessment cannot be overstated.
Young children (ages 5–12) cannot be suicidal.	Each year, 30 to 35 children younger than age 12 take their own lives and not all are clinically depressed.

Sources: Compiled from Fuller (2020); National Alliance on Mental Illness (NAMI) (2021); and The Samaritans (2021).

Risk Factors

Suicide risk factors are identified as factors that have statistically been correlated with a higher incidence of suicide. They should be differentiated from **suicide warning signs,** which are identified as factors suggesting a more immediate concern. Both are included as part of a comprehensive assessment of overall risk for suicide.

Marital Status

Widows and widowers, in some studies, have been identified as high risk, but a longitudinal study found that being single or widowed had no effect on suicide rates (Kposowa, 2000). However, the Kposowa study did find that divorced men were twice as likely as married men to die by suicide.

For those who are divorced or widowed, the stresses associated with major life changes and loss are influential. Evidence has demonstrated that change in marital status increases risk for suicidal behavior, particularly in the first year after the change and particularly among older people (Roškar et al., 2011; Yamauchi et al., 2013). Again, it should be noted that demographics such as marital status, age, and sex may inform about populations that are statistically at higher risk, but none of these factors is predictive of immediate risk. A thorough assessment of variables, including risk factors, warning signs, and a host of other data, is essential to identifying individuals at acute risk for attempting suicide.

Sex

More women than men attempt suicide, but men succeed more often (about 70% of men who attempt suicide succeed, and 30% of women who attempt it succeed). This rate reflects the lethality of the means. Women tend to overdose on drugs; men use more lethal means, such as firearms. These differences between men and women may also reflect differing societal expectations; women are more likely than men to seek and accept help from friends or professionals.

Age

Suicide risk and age are, in general, positively correlated, particularly with men. Although rates among women remain fairly constant throughout life, rates among men increase with age. The most recent statistics, according to the AFSP (2021), revealed that in 2018, the highest rate of suicide occurred in the 45-to-64-year-old age-group (with the highest rates among those 52 to 59 years of age, and men 3.56 times more often than women), and the second-highest rate was for those 85 or older.

Although adolescents may statistically have a lower rate of suicide than some other age-groups, it is still important to note that it has been, over several years, the third-leading cause of death in this population, and in 2013 it jumped to the second-leading cause of death where it remained in 2019 (CDC, 2021b). Several factors put adolescents at risk for suicide, including impulsive and high-risk behaviors, untreated mood disorders (e.g., major depression and bipolar disorder), access to lethal means (e.g., firearms), and substance abuse. One study (Reyes et al., 2015) found a link between some modes of anger expression in adolescents and suicide risk; in particular, hopelessness and hostility modes of anger expression were associated with an increase in suicidal tendency.

Among children younger than 10 years of age, the statistics demonstrate a low number of suicides, and some have argued that younger children do not have the capacity to intentionally consider and follow through with a suicide attempt. Anecdotal evidence has shown that this is not always the case, with some therapists identifying 5- to 9-year-olds actively talking about suicide (Jobes, 2015). Research is beginning to emerge that supports real risk in young children (Duran & McGuinness, 2016). Bridge and associates (2015) studied a large sample of children ages 5 to 11 and found that an average of 33 children per year die by suicide within this age-group in the United States, predominately from suffocation and hanging. These researchers also noted that suicide was never coded as a cause of death for children under 5 years of age. When Whalen and associates (2015) studied children in the 3-to-7-year-old age-group, they found about 11% with suicidal ideation. Increased risk was correlated with male gender, psychiatric illness in their mothers, and psychiatric illness in the child. In young girls ages 10 to 14 years, the incidence of self-inflicted injury has risen 18.8% every year between 2008 and 2015, and self-inflicted injury is one of the strongest risk factors for suicide (Mercado et al., 2017). Duran and McGuinness (2016, p. 29) stress that the implications for nursing are clear; direct inquiry about suicide ideas is a "necessary component in healthcare encounters with children," including those in primary care, emergency departments, and with the school nurse.

The American Association of Suicidology (2021) reports that although the overall number of suicides for 2019 (47,511) was less than it was in 2018 (48,344), rates for some demographic groups increased. For example, the rate of suicide for those over 85 years of age increased by 5.2%. It cannot be overstated, however, that although statistics reveal degrees of risk in certain age-groups, screening for risk of suicide should be conducted for all individuals regardless of demographic characteristics.

Religion

Assessing religion's role in risk for suicide is complicated by variables such as degree of affiliation, participation, religious doctrine, and others. Further, some studies have found it to be protective while others have found it to be a risk factor (Lawrence et al., 2016). A systematic review of the research on religion and suicide risk (Lawrence et al., 2016) found that although religious affiliation is not protective against suicide *ideation*, it is protective against suicide attempts, and that religious service attendance is possibly protective against suicide. The authors of another study (Rasic et al., 2009) found that religious affiliation is associated with a decreased risk of suicide attempts in both the general population and in those with a mental illness, independent of the availability of social support systems.

Socioeconomic Influences

Financial strain and unemployment have often been identified as risk factors for suicide. To what extent these factors act alone (as opposed to a complex interaction of several variables) requires further study. The CDC (2019b) discusses loss (including loss of employment) as one risk factor for suicide.

Suicide rates are higher in rural areas and with a twofold greater use of firearms as the means (Ivey-Stephenson et al., 2017). Kim and associates (2016) studied the factors influencing a move from suicide ideation to suicide attempts and found that low education and unemployment significantly increased the prevalence of attempts among young adult men and women with suicide ideation. Because previous attempts are a leading risk factor for eventual suicide, assessing for suicide ideation and previous attempts along with demographic risk factors are important aspects of risk assessment.

Ethnicity

In 2019 the highest U.S. age-adjusted suicide rate (per 100,000 individuals) was among white populations (15.67), and the second-highest rate was among American Indians and Alaska Natives (13.64). Much lower rates were found among black populations (7.04) and Asians and Pacific Islanders (7.04) (AFSP, 2021). In 2019, although the overall suicide rate was lower, there were increases in rates for black men (1.7% increase) and Asian/Pacific Islanders (2.8% increase). It is difficult to pinpoint the associated variables and whether these changes will become trends, but the statistics focus attention on the changing face of suicide in the United States and can contribute to early identification of problems.

Research has highlighted two trends that illuminate issues of concern within specific ethnic groups. First, although national suicide rates among white populations are higher in adults and the elderly, within the American Indian community, young adults are the highest-risk age-group, and the rate of suicide is 2.5 times higher than the national average (National Indian Council on Aging, 2019). Almendrala (2015) relays the story of a psychiatrist called to a reservation where there had been 17 suicides in the previous 8 months, and the community members described themselves as "grieved out." The second trend of concern, as Almendrala reports, is that the rates of suicide may be underestimated in this population because death certificates do not always report accurately regarding ethnicity.

Another study examined suicide trends among school-age children younger than age 12 (Bridge et al., 2015) and found that suicide rates for black children 5 to 11 years of age nearly doubled over the period from 1993 to 2012, while the overall suicide rate in this age-group remained relatively stable during the same period. As of 2018, suicide became the second-leading cause of death in black children ages 10 to 14, and the third-leading cause of death in black adolescents ages 15 to 19 (Gordon, 2020). It is hard to imagine what causes children so young to take their own lives. The contributing factors to these recent trends are not well understood and will require further research, including a review of the impact of health-care disparities for select communities or populations.

Other Risk Factors

The majority of people who die by suicide have a diagnosable mental illness, most commonly depression, bipolar disorder, or substance use disorder. Studies support that individuals who have been hospitalized for a psychiatric illness have a higher risk of suicide than those with psychiatric illness in the general population and particularly in the first week and first month following hospitalization

(Chung et al., 2019). This higher risk may be a reflection of the severity of their mental illness. Other recent research supports that the increased risk of suicide in the period following discharge from psychiatric hospitalization is especially higher for those not connected to a system of care (Forte et al., 2019; Olfson et al., 2016). Suicide risk may increase during early treatment with antidepressants. One possible reason is that as energy returns to those taking antidepressants, they may have an increased ability to act out self-destructive wishes. Although suicide is often thought of as strictly related to depression, there is also a recognized risk of suicide among people with schizophrenia, bipolar disorders, personality disorders, eating disorders, anxiety disorders, and substance use disorders. A thorough suicide risk assessment should be conducted for anyone seeking mental health services.

Other major physical conditions have also been identified as contributing to increased risk for suicide (Ahmedani et al., 2017), with three conditions (traumatic brain injury, sleep disorders, and HIV/AIDS) conferring a twofold increase in risk. Severe insomnia is associated with increased suicide risk even in the absence of depression. Use of alcohol, and particularly a combination of alcohol and barbiturates, increases the risk of suicide. Withdrawal from stimulants increases suicide risk as the person begins to "crash." Psychosis, especially with command hallucinations (hearing voices telling one to harm or kill oneself), poses a higher risk as does having a chronic painful or disabling illness.

Several studies have indicated a higher risk for suicide among lesbian, gay, bisexual, and transgender (LGBT) individuals (Cassels, 2011; Eisenberg & Resnick, 2006; King et al., 2008; Plöderl et al., 2013). The Trevor Project (2021), a national organization providing crisis intervention and suicide prevention services for young adults in the LGBTQ community, cites studies that found an 8.4% increase in suicide attempts among LGBTQ youth who come from families who reject them, and an average of a 2.5 times greater risk of self-harming behavior for each episode of LGBTQ victimization, such as physical or verbal harassment or abuse. A report from the CDC (2016) identified that in a study of youths in grades 7 to 12, lesbian, gay, and bisexual youth were twice as likely to attempt suicide than their heterosexual peers (this study did not address the risk for transgender individuals). Another study, however, found that transgender individuals are also a high-risk population for suicide, with an alarming 41% lifetime prevalence (Stroumsa, 2014).

Higher risk is also associated with a family history of suicide, especially in a same-gender parent and with individuals who have made previous suicide attempts. About one-half of individuals who kill themselves have previously attempted suicide. Because roughly equal numbers die by suicide on their first attempt, all individuals with suicide ideation should be assessed carefully for risk factors and warning signs. Significant losses, including relational, social, work, or financial losses, have also been identified as risk factors (CDC, 2019b).

In recent years, a number of suicides have been reported in the media among young people who are the victims of bullying. Zweig and Dank (2013) reported that 41% of youth are victims of physical bullying (most often boys), 17% are victims of cyberbullying, and girls are more likely to be victims of psychological bullying. Clearly, bullying is a prevalent concern among youth.

Cyberbullying has also been associated with increased risk of depression and suicidal behavior among young people. Researchers found that both perpetrators and victims of cyberbullying had more suicidal ideation, more incidents of self-harm, and more suicide behaviors than those who had not experienced such forms of peer aggression (Bauman et al., 2013; John et al., 2018). Edgerton and Limber (2013), in a research brief on suicide and bullying, caution that although research does show that those who are bullied have high levels of suicidal thoughts and attempts, there is not enough research to identify a cause-and-effect relationship. Other risk factors such as mental health problems appear to play a larger role.

Predisposing Factors: Theories of Suicide

Psychological Theories

Psychological theories focus primarily on cognitive, emotional, and behavioral factors that are associated with risk for suicide. While suicidal behavior is most commonly associated with depression, several other emotions and behaviors have been identified as influential. Following is a description of several of these psychological factors.

Anger Turned Inward

Freud (1957) believed that suicide was a response to intense self-hatred. The anger is first directed toward a love object but is ultimately turned inward against the self.

Hopelessness and Other Symptoms of Depression

Hopelessness has long been identified as both a symptom of depression and an underlying factor in the predisposition to suicide. Although many of the symptoms that are identified in suicide risk assessment tools attempt to assess for seriousness of suicide ideation, current research is attempting to glean which symptoms might be more predictive of the move from ideation to attempts, and although hopelessness is identified as a contributing factor, the strength of the person's intention to die may be more significant in triggering an attempt (Jobes, 2015).

History of Aggression and Violence

Outwardly directed aggression has been found to be associated with suicide attempts but not with suicide ideation, and among psychiatric patients outwardly directed aggression was associated with planned rather than unplanned attempts (Swogger et al., 2014). Some evidence suggests that impulsive traits are higher in individuals with suicide ideation but not necessarily associated with more attempts (Klonsky & May, 2015b).

Shame and Humiliation

Some individuals view suicide as a "face-saving" mechanism—a way to prevent public humiliation following a social defeat, such as a sudden loss of status or income. Both shame and humiliation may also interrupt one's sense of connectedness with others, and sense of belonging and connectedness are considered protective against suicide. Evidence supports that the experience of shame is pronounced in trauma survivors (Taylor, 2015) and in females with borderline personality disorder (Wiklander et al., 2012). These findings may explain some of the influencing factors for increased risk of suicide in these populations.

Sociological Theories

Sociological theories focus primarily on interpersonal factors that influence risk for suicide. Lack of connectedness with others is a unifying theme among these theories.

Durkheim's Theory

Durkheim classic work (1951) studied the interaction of individuals with the society in which they lived. He believed that the more cohesive the society and the more that individuals felt an integrated part of society, the less likely they were to carry out suicide. Durkheim described three social categories of suicide:

- ***Egoistic suicide*** is the response of the individual who feels separate and apart from the mainstream of society. Integration is lacking, and the individual does not feel a part of any cohesive group (such as a family or a church).
- ***Altruistic suicide*** is the opposite of egoistic suicide. The individual who is prone to altruistic suicide is excessively integrated into the group. The group is often governed by cultural, religious, or political ties, and allegiance is so strong that the individual will sacrifice their life for the group.
- ***Anomic suicide*** occurs in response to changes in an individual's life (e.g., divorce, loss of job) that disrupt feelings of relatedness to the group. An interruption in the customary norms of behavior instills feelings of "separateness" and fears of being without support from the formerly cohesive group.

Interpersonal Theory

Thomas Joiner's (2005) interpersonal theory of suicide supports some of the same principles advanced by Durkheim, which associated a lack of feeling of belonging with suicide risk. But Joiner's theory introduces the concept that suicide ideation and suicide attempts need to be understood as distinct processes. He proposed that low connectedness and a high sense of one's being a burden interact with each other to increase suicidal thoughts and desires, but those features in the presence of high capability for suicide are strongly associated with the move from ideation to lethal attempts. He advances the concept that people become less fearful (and therefore more capable) of self-destructive acts when they expose themselves repeatedly to painful or violent stimuli: a kind of "working up" to actually being capable of self-harm. The move from suicide ideation to attempts is not viewed as an impulsive act but rather a process of steps that, over time, create greater and greater risk.

The Three-Step Theory

Inspired by Joiner's theory, Klonsky and May (2015a) found that impulsivity is elevated both in people who have made suicide attempts and those who have thoughts and have never made an attempt. The researchers therefore sought to identify the factors that elevate suicide ideation to an active risk for attempts. Their research supported the following three-step trajectory:

1. Pain (usually psychological pain) when combined with hopelessness significantly increases suicide

ideation (for both men and women and across age-groups).
2. Connectedness prevents suicide ideation from escalating in those at risk, but when pain and hopelessness exceed one's sense of connectedness to others, suicide ideation becomes active.
3. When strong, active suicide ideation is present, it leads to an attempt only if one has the capacity to make an attempt.

Biological Theories

Biological theories attempt to understand the biochemical and genetic influences in the risk for suicidal behavior. Current theories recognize that the complexity of suicide risk and behavior is likely a complex interaction of biological, psychological, interpersonal, and environmental factors.

Genetics

Twin studies have shown a much higher concordance rate for monozygotic twins than for dizygotic twins. Some studies with people who have attempted suicide have focused on the genotypic variations in the gene for tryptophan hydroxylase, with results indicating significant association to suicidality (Zhang et al., 2010). Tryptophan hydroxylase is an enzyme associated with the synthesis of serotonin, and diminished serotonin has implications for both depression and suicidal behavior. Additional research has identified a genetic variation in prefrontal cortex tissue that may be a biomarker for suicide risk when vulnerable individuals are exposed to a significant stressor (Sudak, 2017). These findings suggest the potential for genetic predisposition toward suicidal behavior, but more research is needed.

Neurochemical Factors

Studies have revealed altered levels of serotonin, glutamate, gamma-aminobutyric acid (GABA), and dopamine, and increased levels of corticotropin-releasing hormone (CRH) (which triggers the release of cortisol) in individuals who died by suicide (Offord, 2020). These studies have supported the association of altered neurochemical levels with risk for suicide.

However, a recent meta-analysis examining biological factors found that they are, in general, weak predictors of a future suicide attempt or death by suicide (Chang et al., 2016). The only two biological factors that had statistical significance in this analysis were cytokines (anti-inflammatory response chemicals) and low levels of fish oil nutrients (including omega-3 fatty acids).

Application of the Nursing Process With the Suicidal Patient

Many research studies are being conducted that explore suicide from different vantage points to identify demographics, risk factors, predictors of risk for suicide attempts, and strategies for prevention. This research can help nurses become more aware of the phenomenon of suicide and understand the limitations of research in making a clinical judgment about a patient's actual risks versus statistical risks. Influential organizations across the nation are advancing the importance of improving the quality of care, documentation, and reporting of details around sentinel events related to acts of or deaths by suicide. In addition to government-endorsed national strategies for suicide prevention, The Joint Commission (2016) has advanced standards that include requiring organizations to conduct risk assessments "identifying specific patient characteristics and environmental features that may increase or decrease the risk of suicide." It is nurses practicing in general medical settings, including emergency departments and primary care practices, who are frontline practitioners in the fight to prevent suicide, so these assessment skills are critical wherever nurses are practicing. The American Psychiatric Nurses Association (APNA, 2020; Puntil et al., 2013) has taken a leadership role in identifying psychiatric mental health nurse essential competencies for assessment and management of individuals at risk for suicide. The CDC (2011) has advanced strategies for a uniform definition and reporting about acts of self-directed violence to improve data collection and ultimately improve our understanding and prevention of suicide. At the heart of this wealth of information is the necessity for accurate, comprehensive assessment that includes collaboration with the patient and other clinicians and is rooted in forming a therapeutic relationship of trust and open communication.

Assessment

When nurses assess a patient's suicide ideation, it is important to identify and distinguish ideas (thoughts), plans (intentions), and attempts (behavior). Each of these assessment factors can provide information about a patient's level of risk. When the patient has attempted self-injury, it is important to distinguish between *suicidal self-injury* and *nonsuicidal self-injury*. The latter injury is often used as a method to release emotions, but it may also be a way of communicating the severity of distress that the patient is experiencing (Nock et al., 2013). Dr. David Satcher, as Surgeon General of the United States (1998–2002), spoke of risk factors and protective factors in his *Call to Action to Prevent Suicide* (U.S. Public Health Service, 1999). This report initiated a national movement toward research designed to better understand predictors of suicide risk and develop more evidence-based interventions. Current models have clarified risk factors as different from warning signs associated with a greater potential for suicide and suicidal behavior. Protective factors have been identified that are associated with reduced potential for suicide. Examples of protective factors are outlined in Box 11–1. Figure 11–1 presents a model for differentiating low, high, and imminent suicide risks. The goal of such models is not to predict a suicide attempt but to assist in making a clinical judgment about the level of intervention needed to prevent an attempt. Further, while risk assessment is part of a *comprehensive psychosocial assessment and safety plan*, there is good evidence that risk assessment scales, when used alone, have not had strong predictive value, and may provide a false sense of reassurance (Chan et al., 2016; Large et al., 2016). The importance of a comprehensive and collaborative approach cannot be overstated.

BOX 11–1 Examples of Protective Factors

- Resilient temperament
- Social competency
- Skills in problem-solving, coping, and conflict resolution
- Perception of social support from adults and peers
- Positive expectations, optimism for the future; identification of future goals
- Connectedness to family, school, community
- Presence and involvement of caring adults (for adolescents)
- Integration in social networks
- Cultural and religious beliefs that discourage suicide and encourage preservation of life
- Access to quality social services and clinical health care for mental, physical, and substance use disorders
- Support through ongoing medical and mental health-care relationships
- Restricted access to highly lethal means of suicide

Source: Crosby et al. (2011).

Demographics

The following demographics should be noted when evaluating a patient for suicide risk. Although demographics alone do not directly increase a person's risk, they provide information as part of a comprehensive assessment of proximal or potentiating risk factors.

- ***Age:*** Adolescents and the elderly have been generally identified as high-risk groups, but recent statistics demonstrating the highest incidence in the 45-to-54-year-old age-group as well as increasing incidence among children suggests that nurses should assess for suicide risk in all age-groups.
- ***Sex:*** Males are at higher risk for death by suicide than females, but females attempt suicide more frequently.
- ***Ethnicity/race:*** The CDC reports that the "highest rates across the life span [are] occurring among non-Hispanic American Indian/Alaska Native and non-Hispanic White populations" (CDC, 2018).
- ***Marital status:*** Those with recent changes in marital or relationship status (such as a breakup, divorce, or recently widowed individuals) may be associated with increased risk for depression and suicide.
- ***Socioeconomic influences:*** Financial strain and unemployment are identified as risk factors for suicide.
- ***Occupation:*** Health-care professionals (especially physicians), law enforcement officers, dentists, artists, mechanics, lawyers, and insurance agents have all been identified as occupational groups believed to incur greater risks for suicide. Potential contributing factors include occupations that involve high stress, isolation, lack of access to health-care resources, and repeated exposure to painful or violent stimuli. The most recent data on suicide rates by occupation (Peterson et al., 2020) identified that highest rates were among construction workers, maintenance and repair workers, those in the arts and entertainment industry (including sports and the media), transportation workers, protective service workers, and health-care support staff (particularly personal care aides and registered nurses).
- ***Religion:*** People with close religious affiliation may be at less risk for attempting suicide if they believe, for example, that suicide is an unforgivable sin or that suicide is strictly forbidden within the religion. Conversely, people *without* close affiliations that impose restrictions about suicide may be at greater risk.

WARNING SIGNS:

- Threatening to harm or end one's life
- Seeking or access to means: seeking pills, weapons, or other means
- Evidence or expression of a suicide plan
- Expressing (writing or talking) ideation about suicide, wish to die or death
- Hopelessness
- Rage, anger, seeking revenge
- Acting recklessly, engaging impulsively in risky behavior
- Expressing feelings of being trapped with no way out
- Increasing or excessive substance use
- Withdrawing from family, friends, society
- Anxiety, agitation, abnormal sleep (too much or too little)
- Dramatic changes in mood
- Expresses no reason for living, no sense of purpose in life

POTENTIATING RISK FACTORS:

- Unemployed or recent financial difficulties
- Divorced, separated, widowed
- Social isolation
- Prior traumatic life events or abuse
- Previous suicide behavior
- Chronic mental illness
- Chronic, debilitating physical illness

Number of Warning Signs

Very High Risk: seek immediate help from emergency or mental health professional.

High Risk: seek help from mental health professional.

Low Risk: recommend counseling and monitor for development of warning signs.

FIGURE 11–1 Risk factors and warning signs for suicide. Reprinted with permission from the Ontario Hospital Association.

- ***Family history:*** A family history of suicide increases an individual's risk for suicide.
- ***Military history:*** Military personnel—active duty, veterans, and reserves—are at high risk for suicide. Firearms account for over 60% of all suicides among military members (Center for Deployment Psychology, n.d.).

Medical-Psychiatric Diagnosis

Assessment data to screen for suicide risk must be gathered for all clients regardless of the psychiatric or physical condition for which they are being treated. Mood disorders (major depression and bipolar disorders) are the most common disorders that precede suicide. Individuals with substance use disorders are also at high risk. Other psychiatric disorders in which suicide risks have been identified include anxiety disorders, schizophrenia, bipolar disorders, substance use disorders, anorexia nervosa, attention deficit-hyperactivity disorder, and borderline and antisocial personality disorders. Chronic and terminal physical illnesses have also been identified as potentiating risk factors.

Suicidal Ideas or Acts

An important part of the assessment of a patient's suicide risk is to determine the patient's intentions. How serious is the patient's intent to die by suicide? Does the person have a plan? If so, do they have the means? How lethal are the means? Do they intend to carry out this plan? Has the individual ever attempted suicide before? These questions must be asked by the person conducting the assessment of the patient who is expressing suicide ideation.

Individuals may provide both behavioral and verbal clues about their intentions to act. Examples of behavioral clues that may indicate a decision to carry out suicidal intent include giving away prized possessions, getting financial affairs in order, writing suicide notes, and a sudden shift in mood.

Verbal clues may be both direct and indirect. Examples of direct statements include "I want to die" and "I'm going to kill myself." Examples of indirect statements include "This is the last time you'll see me," "I won't be around much longer for the doctor to have to worry about," and "I don't have anything worth living for anymore."

Recent research (Rogers & Joiner, 2017) provides evidence that suicide-specific rumination, that is, fixation on one's thoughts, intentions, and plans, may be an important predictor of suicidal behavior. Asking how frequently the patient is thinking about suicide ideas, intentions, and plans helps to discern this level of risk.

The lethality of the method identified by an individual with suicide ideation or by one who has already made an attempt provides meaningful information about the patient's intent to die. Use of firearms, hanging, and suffocation, for example, are considered highly lethal methods. Other assessments include determining whether individuals have a plan, and if so, whether they have the means to carry out that plan. If the person states the suicide will be carried out with a gun, does the person have access to a gun? Bullets? If pills are planned, what kind of pills? Are they accessible? Asking the patient, "How likely are you to carry out this plan?" may provide verbal confirmation of their level of intent.

Interpersonal Support System

Does the individual have support persons on whom to rely during a crisis situation? Lack of a meaningful network of satisfactory relationships may indicate an individual has a higher risk for suicide during an emotional crisis.

Analysis of the Suicidal Crisis

Three aspects of assessment that enhance understanding of the patient's current suicidal crisis include an evaluation of the patient's precipitating stressors, relevant history, and life-stage issues.

- ***The precipitating stressor:*** Adverse life events in combination with other risk factors, such as depression, may lead to suicide. Life stresses accompanied by an increase in emotional disturbance include the loss of a loved person either by death or by divorce, problems in major relationships, changes in roles, or serious physical illness.
- ***Relevant history:*** Has the individual experienced multiple failures or rejections that might increase their vulnerability for a dysfunctional response to the current situation?
- ***Life-stage issues:*** The ability to tolerate losses and disappointments is often compromised if the individual is also struggling with the developmental tasks associated with different life stages (e.g., adolescence, midlife, old age).

Psychiatric, Medical, and Family History

The individual should be assessed for previous psychiatric treatment for depression or other mental disorders, substance use disorders, or previous suicide attempts. Medical history should be obtained to determine the presence of chronic, debilitating, or terminal illness. Is there a history of depressive disorder in the family, and has a close relative died by suicide in the past?

Coping Strategies

How has the individual handled previous crisis situations? How does this situation differ from previous ones?

Presenting Symptoms

Several acronyms have been developed as mnemonic devices to summarize important factors that may increase a person's risk for suicidal behavior. One of these is the acronym IS PATH WARM? (American Association of Suicidology, 2020; Juhnke et al., 2007). The assessment items and descriptors for each letter are as follows:

Ideation: Has suicide ideas that are current and active, especially with an identified plan

Substance abuse: Has current and/or excessive use of alcohol or other mood-altering drugs

---

Purposelessness: Expresses thoughts that there is no reason to continue living

Anger: Expresses uncontrolled anger or feelings of rage

Trapped: Expresses the belief that there is no way out of the current situation

Hopelessness: Expresses lack of hope and perceives little chance of positive change

---

Withdrawal: Expresses desire to withdraw from others or has begun withdrawing
Anxiety: Expresses anxiety, agitation, and/or changes in sleep patterns
Recklessness: Engages in reckless or risky activities with little thought of consequences
Mood: Expresses dramatic mood shifts

Mnemonic devices such as IS PATH WARM? can be helpful in remembering what types of presenting symptoms to assess for, but the overall assessment and management of suicidal behavior are far more complex and must consider available support systems, the patient's willingness to accept support, and the patient's ability to establish a trusting therapeutic alliance with health-care professionals intervening on their behalf. Ultimately, a clinical judgment must be made about the patient's degree of risk so that appropriate measures can be taken to prevent an attempt. The Columbia Suicide Severity Rating Scale (Posner et al., 2011) is an evidence-based tool that assists in this process (Figure 11–2).

The Collaborative Assessment and Management of Suicidality (CAMS) model is an evidence-based approach that focuses on the importance of patient-centered, problem-focused intervention to build an alliance with patients for collaboration in reducing risk for suicidal behavior (Jobes, 2012). This model focuses on assessment, which necessarily includes asking the patient to identify what is driving the desire to take their own life so that alternatives (identifying and capitalizing on motivations to live) can be explored. For all health-care professionals, this work begins with developing skill in asking basic and direct questions such as, "Are you having thoughts of hurting or killing yourself?"

Beyond the basic questions of whether or not a person has suicidal ideas, a plan, and access to

Columbia-Suicide Severity Rating Scale
Screen Version - Recent

	Past Month		Lifetime (Worst Point)	
Ask questions that are bolded and underlined.	**Yes**	**No**	**Yes**	**No**
Ask Questions 1 and 2				
1) ***Have you wished you were dead or wished you could go to sleep and not wake up?***				
2) ***Have you actually had any thought of killing yourself?***				
If YES to 2, ask questions 3, 4, 5, and 6. If NO to 2, go directly to question 6.				
3) ***Have you been thinking about how you might do this?*** E.g. *"I thought about taking an overdose but I never made a specific plan as to when where or how I would actually do it...and I would never go through with it."*				
4) ***Have you had these thoughts and had some intention of acting on them?*** *As opposed to "I have the thought but I definitely will not do anything about them."*				
5) ***Have you started to work out or worked out the details of how to kill yourself? Do you intend to carry out this plan?***				

How long ago did the Worst Point Ideation occur? _____

	Yes	No
6) ***Have you ever done anything, started to do anything, or prepared to do anything to end your life?*** Examples: Collected pills, obtained a gun, gave away valuables, wrote a will or suicide note, took out pills but didn't swallow any, held a gun but changed your mind or it was grabbed from your hand, went to the roof but didn't jump; or actually took pills, tried to shoot yourself, cut yourself, tried to hang yourself, etc...		
If YES, ask: ***Was this within the past three months?***		

Low risk Moderate risk High risk

FIGURE 11–2 Columbia Suicide Severity Rating Scale (C-SSRS). Reprinted with permission from The Columbia Lighthouse Project.

means, there must be recognition that patients are not always forthcoming or truthful in their answers to such questions. Several strategies for enhancing a collaborative, therapeutic relationship and communication about suicide assessment have been elaborated. Because nurses are often at the front line of this assessment in medical-surgical, emergency department, outpatient care, schools, and other health-care settings, they must be thoughtful, comprehensive, and conscientious in this pursuit regardless of the practice setting and whether or not the patient has been identified as having mental health issues. Shea (2009) states that nurses need to assess not only what the patient is directly stating about their suicidal intent (stated intent) but also the amount of thinking, planning, and behaviors associated with suicide ideation (reflected intent) and the suicide intent that is withheld from the nurse (withheld intent). A summary of guiding principles in suicide risk assessment is included in Table 11–2.

One model for enhancing communication in suicide assessment is the CASE (Chronological Assessment of Suicide Events) approach. It is described as a flexible guide for interviewing that includes communication techniques designed to elicit and enhance detailed, valid feedback from patients about sensitive topics such as suicide. Several examples, as elaborated by Shea (2009), follow:

- ***Normalizing*** communicates that the patient is not the only one who experiences suicidal ideation. *Example:* "Sometimes when people are in a lot of emotional pain, they have thoughts of killing themselves. Have you had any thoughts like that?"

TABLE 11–2 Guiding Principles for Suicide Risk Assessment

PRINCIPLES	EXPLANATIONS
Screening for suicide risk should be conducted as an essential component of health assessment, and risk factors, warning signs, and threats should be taken seriously.	This includes identifying through detailed assessment the individual's unique situation to discern additional resources, consults, and interventions needed to ensure patient safety.
Establishment of a therapeutic relationship is foundational to effective suicide risk assessment.	This includes establishing trust through empathy and respect, which provides a safe environment for the patient to tell their story.
Suicide risk assessment is complex and challenges the nurse to use many different communication strategies.	This includes exploring the patient's thoughts, feelings, and behaviors from a variety of perspectives.
Suicide risk assessment is an ongoing process, and level of risk can increase or decrease over time.	This includes assessing over time for fluctuations in risk factors, changes in stress level, changes in intensity of ideation, changes in intention to act on suicide ideation, and changes in support systems.
Collaboration with the patient and other sources of information facilitates confidence in clinical judgments.	This includes information provided by other people who are familiar with the patient from home, work, or school and other clinical team members. Collaboration also implies that all those involved in the patient's care are working together.
Suicide risk assessment uses direct rather than indirect language.	This includes using terminology such as "suicide" and "death" rather than "not happy with living" or other indirect statements. It also communicates to the patient that these are acceptable topics to discuss.
Suicide risk assessment attempts to discern the underlying message.	This includes attempting to discern when the patient is communicating unbearable distress, feeling trapped, feeling hopeless, and/or feeling driven to avoid additional emotional or physical pain.
Suicide risk assessment considers cultural context.	This includes recognizing that anyone regardless of race, religion, or culture may be at risk for suicide. Some cultural or religious prohibitions may influence someone's willingness to openly discuss personal feelings.
Suicide risk assessment is documented in detail.	This includes risk factors, warning signs, underlying themes, level of risk, clinical judgments, and recommended interventions.

Source: Adapted from Perlman et al. (2011).

- ***Asking about behavioral events*** rather than the patient's opinions may elicit more concrete information.
  Example: "What did you do when you had those thoughts?" "How many pills did you take?" "What happened next?"
- ***Gentle assumptions*** encourage further discussion by assuming there is more to tell.
  Example: "What other times have you attempted suicide?"
- ***Denial of the specific*** is helpful when a patient generally denies suicidal ideation. This strategy encourages more in-depth thought and response by asking questions that might trigger memories of specific events.
  Example: After the patient denies suicidal ideation in response to a general question, the nurse asks more specifically, "Have you ever had thoughts of overdosing?" "Have you ever had thoughts about shooting yourself?"
- ***Chronologically exploring*** the presenting suicide event, recent suicide events, past suicide events, and finally the immediate suicide events can broaden the nurse's understanding of the patient's immediate suicidal intent in the context of their behavior over time.
  Example: Ask the patient about the event that precipitated this episode of care: "Tell me about the event that led you to be hospitalized," and then ask about any other recent events: "When was the last time you attempted suicide prior to this event? Tell me more about that event" (as well as their history of suicidal behavioral over time). Finally, explore immediately current ideation and intent: "Tell me about your level of risk right now. Current ideas? Intensity? Intentions?"

Diagnosis and Outcome Identification

Nursing diagnoses for the suicidal patient may include the following:

- Risk for suicide related to feelings of hopelessness and desperation
- Hopelessness related to absence of support systems and perception of worthlessness
- Ineffective coping related to extreme stress, crisis, feeling trapped, poorly developed coping skills

Outcome Criteria

Outcome criteria include short- and long-term goals. Timelines are individually determined. The criteria that follow may be used for measurement of outcomes in the care of the suicidal patient.

The patient:

- Has experienced no physical harm to self.
- Sets realistic goals for self.
- Expresses some optimism and hope for the future.

Planning and Implementation

Table 11–3 provides a plan of care for the hospitalized suicidal patient. Nursing diagnoses are presented, along with outcome criteria, appropriate nursing interventions, and rationales for each.

Intervention With the Suicidal Client Following Discharge or in an Outpatient Setting

In some instances, it may be determined that suicidal intent is low and that hospitalization is not required. Instead, the client with suicidal ideation may be treated in an outpatient setting. Guidelines for treatment of the suicidal client on an outpatient basis include the following:

- The person should have immediate access to support systems and be tied to a system of care because the term following hospital discharge is a high-risk period. Arrangements must be made for the client to stay with family or friends. If this is not possible, hospitalization should be reconsidered.
- A detailed safety plan should be developed that is an outgrowth of a comprehensive assessment and a collaborative problem-solving discussion with the client. This intervention explores with clients what they will do to stay safe if there is a repeat or increase in suicidal thoughts or urges. See Box 11–2 for more on the essential components of a safety plan.
- A safety plan should not be confused with a no-suicide contract. See Boxes 11–3 and 11–4 to learn about issues associated with developing an appropriate safety plan.
- Enlist the help of family or friends to ensure that the home environment is safe from dangerous items, such as firearms or stockpiled drugs. Give support persons the telephone number of the counselor or an emergency contact person in the event that the counselor is not available.
- Appointments may need to be scheduled daily or every other day at first until the immediate suicidal crisis has subsided.
- Establish rapport and promote a trusting relationship. It is important for the suicide counselor to become a key person in the client's support system at this time.
- Accept the client's feelings in a nonjudgmental manner.

Table 11–3 | CARE PLAN FOR THE SUICIDAL PATIENT

NURSING DIAGNOSIS: RISK FOR SUICIDE

RELATED TO: Feelings of hopelessness and desperation

OUTCOME CRITERIA	NURSING INTERVENTIONS	RATIONALE
Patient will not harm self.	1. Ask directly: "Have you thought about harming yourself in any way? If so, what do you plan to do? Do you have the means to carry out this plan? How strong are your intentions to die? How often do you think about suicide?"	1. The risk of suicide is greatly increased if the patient has developed a plan and particularly if means are accessible for the patient to execute the plan. Suicide-specific rumination is associated with suicide attempts.
	2. Create a safe environment for patient. Remove all potentially harmful objects from patient's access (sharp objects, straps, belts, ties, glass items, alcohol). Supervise closely during meals and medication administration. Perform room searches as deemed necessary.	2. Patient safety is a nursing priority.
	3. Maintain close observation of patient. Depending on level of suicide precaution, provide one-to-one contact, constant visual observation, or every-15-minute checks. Place in room close to nurse's station; do not assign to private room. Accompany to off-unit activities if attendance is indicated. May need to accompany to bathroom.	3. Close observation is necessary to ensure that the patient does not harm self in any way. Being alert for suicidal and escape attempts facilitates being able to prevent or interrupt harmful behavior.
	4. Maintain special care in administration of medications.	4. Prevents saving up to overdose or discarding.
	5. Make rounds at frequent, *irregular* intervals (especially at night, toward early morning, at change of shift, or other predictably busy times for staff).	5. Prevents the patient from saving up to overdose or discarding medication. Prevents staff surveillance from becoming predictable. To be aware of the patient's location is important, especially when staff is busy and least available and observable.
	6. Encourage patient to express honest feelings, including anger. Provide activities for appropriate outlets for anger if needed.	6. Depression and suicidal behaviors may be viewed as anger turned inward on the self. If this anger can be verbalized in a nonthreatening environment, the patient may be able to eventually resolve these feelings.
Patient develops a safety plan for management of suicidal thoughts and urges.	1. Establish a trusting, therapeutic relationship to encourage open discussion of suicide.	1. Establishing trust and open communications encourages the patient to share thoughts and feelings.
	2. Collaborate with the patient to develop a safety plan that includes recognition of warning signs, coping strategies, supportive people and places, resources and contact information for crisis management, and plans to restrict access to lethal means.	2. Development of a comprehensive **collaborative safety plan** concretizes resources and management strategies. Actively engaging the patient in collaboration on the development of a safety plan promotes ownership and investment in the process.

Continued

Table 11–3 | CARE PLAN FOR THE SUICIDAL PATIENT—cont'd

OUTCOME CRITERIA	NURSING INTERVENTIONS	RATIONALE
	3. Assess verbal and nonverbal clues to identify the likelihood that patient intends to follow through with the established safety plan and evaluate the patient's follow-through with safety plan measures while still hospitalized.	3. Assessment of patient safety includes analyzing congruence of verbal communication, nonverbal communication, and behavior.

NURSING DIAGNOSIS: HOPELESSNESS

RELATED TO: Absence of support systems and perception of worthlessness

EVIDENCED BY: Verbal cues (despondent content, "I can't"); decreased affect; lack of initiative; suicidal ideas or attempts

OUTCOME CRITERIA	NURSING INTERVENTIONS	RATIONALE
Patient expresses hope and acceptance of life and situations over which the patient has no control.	1. Identify stressors in the patient's life that precipitated current crisis. Include assessing the degree of emotional pain and hopelessness in relationship to feelings of connectedness or lack of connectedness with others.	1. It is important to identify contributing factors to assist the patient with stress management.
	2. Determine coping behaviors previously used and the patient's perception of effectiveness then and now.	2. Identifying the patient's strengths encourages their use in current crisis situation.
	3. Encourage the patient to explore and verbalize feelings and perceptions related to reasons for wanting to die as well as reasons for wanting to live.	3. Identification of feelings underlying behaviors helps the patient to begin the process of taking control of own life and enables the nurse to help the patient focus on maximizing their reasons for wanting to live.
	4. Provide expressions of hope to patient in positive, low-key manner (e.g., "I know you feel you cannot go on, but I believe that things can get better for you. What you are feeling is temporary. It is okay if you don't see it just now." "You matter.").	4. Although patient feels hopeless, it is helpful to hear positive expressions from others. The patient's current state of mind may prevent identifying anything positive in life. It is important to accept the patient's feelings nonjudgmentally and to affirm personal worth and value.
	5. Help patient identify areas of life situation that are under own control.	5. Patient's emotional condition may interfere with ability to problem solve. Assistance may be required to perceive the benefits and consequences of available alternatives accurately.
	6. Identify sources that the patient may use after discharge when crises occur or feelings of hopelessness and possible suicidal ideation prevail. This includes local suicide hotlines and other available support services.	6. A collaboratively developed, concrete plan promotes hope in the face of a future crisis.
	7. Assist the patient to explore and identify future-oriented goals.	7. Identifying goals encourages the patient to focus on hopefulness for the future.

Table 11–3 | CARE PLAN FOR THE SUICIDAL PATIENT—cont'd

NURSING DIAGNOSIS: INEFFECTIVE COPING

RELATED TO: Extreme stress, crisis, altered mental status, poorly developed coping skills, feeling trapped or hopeless, impulsivity

EVIDENCED BY: Verbal cues (despondent content, "I can't"); decreased affect; lack of initiative; suicidal ideas or attempts

OUTCOME CRITERIA	NURSING INTERVENTIONS	RATIONALE
Patient identifies coping strategies and expresses commitment to incorporate these as part of a plan to maintain personal safety	1. Assist the patient to identify stressors and other warning signs that are associated with thoughts and plans for suicide.	1. Patient's awareness of triggers for increases in suicidal thinking, plans, and intentions promotes an understanding of situations requiring the implementation of the safety plan.
	2. Explore past coping skills that the patient identifies as effective	2. Exploring the patient's perception of effective coping skills promotes active engagement in the process of identifying and carrying out a safety plan.
	3. Maintain a nonjudgmental attitude when discussing the patient's suicide ideas, plans, and intentions.	3. A nonjudgmental attitude promotes open communication and collaboration.
	4. Assist the patient to identify internal coping strategies for immediate response to a trigger event.	4. This promotes the patient's ability to develop a sense of personal control in response to suicide ideas.
	5. Assist the patient in identifying support systems, resources, and social activities that the patient can use to support ongoing personal safety.	5. External coping strategies, such as eliciting support from a family member or friend, community resources, and social activities that may help the patient minimize rumination about suicide, are all positive coping skills essential to a comprehensive safety plan.

CLINICAL PEARL Be direct. Talk openly and matter-of-factly about suicide. Listen actively and encourage expression of feelings, including anger.

- Discuss the current crisis situation in the client's life. Use the problem-solving approach. Offer alternatives to suicide while at the same time empathizing with the client's pain that led to viewing suicide as an option (Jobes, 2012). An example of this kind of communication might be:

  "I understand how this emotional pain you've been experiencing led you to consider suicide, but I'd like to explore with you some alternative ways to decrease your pain and to identify some reasons for continuing to live."

- Help the client identify areas of the life situation that are within their control and those that the client does not have the ability to control. Discuss feelings associated with these control issues. It is important for the client to feel some control over their life situation in order to perceive a measure of self-worth.
- The physician or nurse practitioner may prescribe antidepressants for an individual who is experiencing suicidal depression. Initially a prescription is written for a small number of pills to minimize the risk of intentional overdose (potentially fatal consequences are a particular concern with tricyclic antidepressant overdose).
- Psychological interventions that have demonstrated effectiveness in reducing suicidal behavior include dialectical behavior therapy (DBT), cognitive behavior therapy, and CAMS (Jobes, 2015).

BOX 11–2 Essential Components of a Safety Plan

According to Stanley and Brown (2008, pp. 3–4), the essential components of a safety plan include nursing support and assistance for the following:

1. Recognizing warning signs that precede suicide crises
2. Identifying and employing internal coping strategies that the client can implement without needing to contact additional support people
3. Identifying supportive family members and friends with whom the client can discuss suicide and who may help resolve a potential crisis
4. Identifying people and healthy social settings that the client can use for general support and distraction from suicidal thoughts and urges
5. Identifying resources and contact information for mental health professionals and agencies when needed in an escalating crisis situation
6. Problem-solving with the client ways to reduce the potential for access to and use of lethal means

Once the safety plan is elaborated with the client, an evaluation of the appropriateness of the plan and a collaborative assessment of the likelihood that the client will implement this plan should be conducted.

Assessment for suicidal risk and responsive intervention must be ongoing, because suicidal ideas and intent may change over hours, days, or longer time periods. The need for revision of the safety plan may become evident. Critical times for reassessment of risk and reevaluation of the safety plan (Hoffman, 2013) include the following:

1. When there is a change in the client's clinical presentation or worsening of symptoms
2. When medications or treatments are changed
3. When significant others identify an increase in concern
4. When a client stops treatment

BOX 11–3 The Issue of No-Suicide Contracts

A critical issue that needs to be understood is that of no-suicide contracts, sometimes called *safety contracts*, a strategy used by some clinicians in the context of a long-term, therapeutic relationship in which the client "promises" to contact the clinician before acting on suicidal ideation. **No-suicide contracts are not the same as the development of a thorough safety plan. Contracting with a client is a controversial and often misused strategy** (Hoffman, 2013; Shea, 2009). **Evidence has not supported the efficacy of this method as a primary intervention** (Drew, 2001; Edwards, 2010; Freedenthal, 2013; Rudd et al., 2006). In fact, it may even be counterproductive in clients with borderline or passive-aggressive pathology (Shea, 2009). **Such contracts should *never* be used in short-term encounters with clients,** such as in emergency departments or during brief hospital stays, or with clients who are unknown, agitated, psychotic, impulsive, or under the influence of drugs and alcohol (Hoffman, 2013). **They should never be used with the presumption that they will deter a client from attempting suicide.** Shea adds that if clinicians use a safety contract with the belief that it will be a deterrent to suicide, they should understand that it **not only "guarantees nothing [but also] may yield a false sense of security" among clinicians** (2009, p. 21). The consequential danger is that clinicians may become less watchful or feel less need to reassess the client, thus missing critical signs of increasing suicide risk. Roberts (2020) cites American Psychiatric Association (APA) practice guidelines that advise against using no-suicide contracts independently or outside of a well-established patient-provider relationship. **Nurses should avoid no-suicide contracting altogether.** Even in the conduct of therapy by a skilled therapist, it should be used with great caution and for limited, specific assessment purposes.

In general, it is important to recognize that not all suicidal individuals are alike, so **interventions should be multifaceted and suicide prevention plans should be comprehensive.** Many models and tools for suicide assessment have been developed. One such model, SAFE-T (Suicide Assessment Five-Step Evaluation and Triage), summarizes the key elements in suicide assessment (see Box 11–4).

Single interventions, including hospitalization, medication, and no-suicide contracts, are not supported by evidence as being effective in reducing suicides (Jobes, 2015). Clients need to be actively engaged as partners in every step of the assessment and intervention process. Evidence does support that early follow-up phone calls with patients who have been treated for a suicide attempt is an effective strategy for reducing suicide risk (Exbrayat et al., 2017; Stanley et al., 2018).

Information for Family and Friends of the Suicidal Client

The following suggestions are made for family and friends of an individual who is suicidal:

- Take any hint of suicide seriously. Anyone expressing suicidal feelings needs immediate attention.

BOX 11–4 SAFE-T: Suicide Assessment Five-Step Evaluation and Triage

1. ***Identify risk factors.*** Note those that can be modified to reduce risk.
2. ***Identify protective factors.*** Note those that can be enhanced.
3. ***Conduct suicide inquiry.*** Evaluate suicidal thoughts, plans, behavior, and intent.
4. ***Determine risk level and intervention.*** Choose appropriate intervention to address and reduce level of risk.
5. ***Document.*** Record assessment of risk, rationale, intervention, and follow-up.

- Do not keep secrets. If a suicidal person says, "Promise you won't tell anyone," do not make that promise. Suicidal individuals are ambivalent about dying, and suicidal behavior is a cry for help. It is that ambivalence that leads the person to confide to you the suicidal thoughts. Get help for the person and for you. The national hotline 1-800-SUICIDE is available 24 hours a day.
- Be a good listener. If people express suicidal thoughts or feel depressed, hopeless, or worthless, be supportive. Let them know you are there for them and are willing to help them seek professional help.
- Many people find it awkward to put into words how another person's life is important for their own well-being, but it is important to stress that the person's life is important to you and to others. Emphasize in specific terms the ways in which the person's suicide would be devastating to you and to others.
- Express concern for individuals who express thoughts about suicide. Individuals may make veiled comments or comments that sound as if they are joking, or people may be withdrawn and reluctant to discuss what they are thinking. In each case ask questions, acknowledge the pain and feelings of hopelessness, and encourage individuals to talk to someone else if they do not feel comfortable talking with you.
- Familiarize yourself with suicide intervention resources, such as mental health centers and suicide hotlines.
- Ensure that access to firearms or other means of self-harm is restricted.
- Communicate caring and commitment to provide support. Fleener (n.d.) offers the following suggestions for interacting with people who are suicidal:
  - Acknowledge and accept their feelings and be an active listener.
  - Try to give them hope and remind them that what they are feeling is temporary.
  - Stay with them. Do not leave them alone. Go to where they are, if necessary.
  - Show love and encouragement. Hold them, hug them, touch them. Allow them to cry and express anger.
  - Help the person seek professional help.
  - Remove any items from the home with which the person may harm themselves.
  - If there are children present, try to remove them from the home. Perhaps friends or relatives can assist by taking the children to their home. This type of situation can be extremely traumatic for children.
  - DO NOT judge suicidal people, show anger toward them, provoke guilt in them, discount their feelings, or tell them to "snap out of it." This is a very real and serious situation to suicidal individuals. They are in real pain. They feel the situation is hopeless and that there is no other way to resolve it aside from taking their own life.

Intervention With Families and Friends of Suicide Victims

Suicide of a family member can induce a whole gamut of feelings in the survivors. It has long been recognized that the bereavement process for families in which a member has taken their own life is complicated and requires an understanding by health-care providers of some unique burdens of this type of loss. Macnab (1993) identified the following symptoms that may be evident in family and friends after the suicide of a loved one:

- A sense of guilt and responsibility
- Anger, resentment, and rage that can never find its "object"
- A heightened sense of emotionality, helplessness, failure, and despair
- A recurring self-searching: "If only I had done something," "If only I had not done something," "If only . . ."
- A sense of confusion and search for an explanation: "Why did this happen?" "What does it mean?" "What could have stopped it?" "What will people think?"

- A sense of inner injury; family feels wounded; does not know how they will ever get over it and get on with life
- A severe strain placed on relationships; a sense of impatience, irritability, and anger possible between family members
- A heightened feeling of vulnerability to illness and disease possible with this added burden of emotional stress

Read "Real People, Real Stories" for a better understanding of one person's lived experience of losing a child to suicide.

Real People, Real Stories

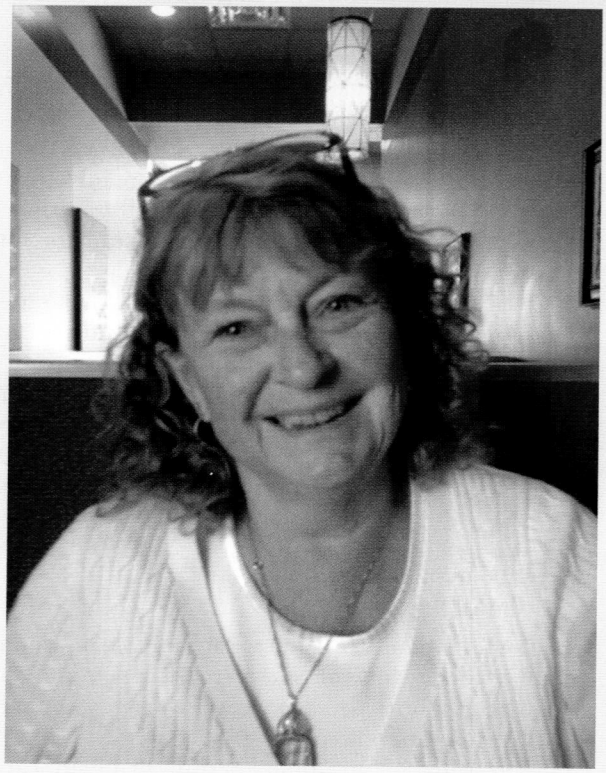

Losing a loved one to suicide results in a grief process often complicated by stigma, misinformation, lack of information, and sometimes a sense of alienation from others. Emmy's story describes her ongoing journey to grapple with the loss of her son to suicide.

Karyn: We've talked before but tell me more about your journey since Paul's death.

Emmy: My son Paul died in 1986 at age 17. The thing I remember most is that no one was talking about it. There were 10 students who died in his high school. Two others were known to be suicides.

Karyn: Do you mean no one was talking about it in the school system?

Emmy: Well, the students in Paul's class took up a collection that was for Paul, but the school couldn't decide how to use it, so it just sat there for the longest time. My other son heard they were going to use the money for supplies, so I went and talked to them to make sure that didn't happen. The school eventually built a memorial garden that became dedicated to all of the students who had died.

Paul died in June, and in August, when all the other students were returning to school, I got a call from a community suicide survivors counselor who told me she was holding a high school assembly to discuss suicide. I wanted her to talk to the ninth and tenth graders, but they wouldn't permit it. I thought the younger kids needed to talk about and learn about this too—they had been my younger son's classmates, and they were affected by it as well. When the suicide counselor intervened, the teachers were told to watch Paul's friends for any evidence of "copycat" behavior, but that was all. I felt the school administration thought there was a stigma in talking about the cause of his death. I found out later that the seniors were talking about and memorializing Paul in their study halls. They were remembering him as a friend who was missed.

Karyn: How has your family coped with Paul's death?

Emmy: We didn't talk about Paul for the longest time; it was as if he didn't exist. We were very separate; we all went in our own directions. My husband started taking long bicycle trips, and he worked on a suicide hotline. I got very involved with offering a program for high school students called Listening POST (People Offering Students Time), which allowed students to talk about anything they wanted to.

Karyn: I know you've told me that you're still close to several of Paul's peers.

Emmy: Oh yes, and their children too. But our family just became very separate. I don't even know how my other son got through his freshman year of high school. We went to a suicide survivors group as a family, and it was important to me as an outlet to talk, but we didn't talk as a family . . . and then we just stopped going, and the people who knew Paul didn't talk to us. I ***so*** wanted to talk to people who knew Paul.

After we stopped going to the survivors group, I started going to CoDA [Co-Dependents Anonymous] meetings,

Real People, Real Stories—cont'd

even though I don't think I'm codependent. It was more because I needed to talk . . . to understand how this happened. I felt like I wasn't there for him. . . . I was busy with my job and maybe I wasn't tuned in to his moods. I was always taught that boys don't like to talk about feelings.

Karyn: Yes, I guess I've been taught that, too.

Emmy: I just remember that night he told his dad and I that he loved us, he went to bed, and the next morning we found him. I just couldn't make sense of it. Years later, one of Paul's peers, who now has a teenage son, said he could finally tell me what he remembered. And there were signs. Apparently, he had said to some friends (while they were drinking alcohol), "Have you ever thought of killing yourself?" and they all laughed about it and nothing more was said. I also found out that he told an older peer, whom he had met at church camp, that he didn't want to live. The peer smacked him and told him if he ever had thoughts like that again that he [Paul] needed to come talk to him first. But they never told anyone else; they kept it among their peers. They thought they were all-knowing, and never told an adult. He was hysterical when he found out what happened.

On that last weekend, he had been partying with his friends . . . there was alcohol involved . . . and the friend that was with him told me that someday he would tell me what went down that day. But it's 30 years later, and I still don't know. I know he was at the party with a girl, but I've never been able to find her or talk with her. She went to a different school.

Karyn: And much of this information that you do know came 10 or more years after his death?

Emmy: Yes.

Karyn: What a long journey you've been on trying to put all the pieces together.

Emmy: (tearful) That's exactly it. Trying to put the pieces together, sort it out . . . but it never gets solved. . . . It's like being in a maze and you can't get out, and I had a lot of guilt. . . . Now I recognize that he just made some tragic bad choices.

Karyn: Appreciating that we don't "get over" such tremendous loss but rather amend our lives with some different understanding of love and loss, what has been most helpful in your healing?

Emmy: Yes, I think there was a point when I realized it was okay to feel some happiness. Being with people who don't know me makes it easier. My faith and fellowship group has been an important part of healing. CoDA was helpful because we talked about how different people process things, and I could understand better how people can get stuck. I used to say that my other son had lost his brother. I couldn't say that I had lost a son. When I had to fill out a health assessment at one point, and I had to respond to the question of how many pregnancies I'd had, that was the most difficult question . . . because I had to acknowledge . . . the reality. And I involved myself with all the boys who were on the track team with Paul and the Listening POST and just talked about everything.

Karyn: What is the most important thing that nurses need to know?

Emmy: By the time we would have had any contact with nurses, it was too late. There were no ER, medical, or mental health visits prior to that. If they were to have an impact, it would have been in prevention in the schools. For example, I didn't know at that time to ask questions like, "Are you having thoughts of hurting yourself?" and "Do you have a plan in mind?" And Paul put on a different face for me. He wasn't solitary; he had lots of friends; he was active on the track team. . . .

Karyn: I think you're not alone with not having been taught about things like suicide assessment. Because, as you've said, historically people haven't talked about it. There is an organization called Red Flags National that promotes mental health education for students, parents, and teachers as a standard part of health education in schools.

Emmy: Yes. It needs to be talked about. It's been helpful for me to talk about it even now. I've never had to try to explain the story before.

To learn more about Red Flags National, go to www.redflags.org.

Strategies for assisting survivors of suicide victims include the following:

- Encourage the survivors to talk to each other about the suicide and respond to each other's viewpoints and reconstructing of events. Share memories.
- Be aware of any blaming or scapegoating of specific family members. Discuss how each person fits into the family situation, both before and after the suicide.

- Listen to feelings of guilt and self-persecution. Gently move the individuals toward the reality of the situation.
- Encourage the family members to discuss individual relationships with the lost loved one. Focus on both positive and negative aspects of the relationships. Gradually, point out the irrationality of any idealized concepts of the deceased person. The family must be able to recognize both positive and negative aspects about the person before grief work can be resolved. No two people grieve in the same way. It may appear that some family members are "getting over" their grief faster than others. All family members must be educated that if this occurs, it is not because those family members "care less"—it is just that they "grieve differently." Variables that enter into this phenomenon include individual past experiences, personal relationship with the deceased person, and individual temperament and coping abilities.
- Recognize how the suicide has caused disorganization in family coping. Reassess interpersonal relationships in the context of the event. Discuss coping strategies that have been successful in times of stress in the past, and work to reestablish these strategies within the family. Identify new adaptive coping strategies that can be incorporated.
- Identify resources that provide support: religious beliefs and spiritual counselors, close friends and relatives, support groups for survivors of suicide. One online connection that puts individuals in contact with survivors groups specific to each state is the American Foundation for Suicide Prevention at www.afsp.org. A list of resources that provide information and help for issues regarding suicide is presented in Box 11–5.

BOX 11–5 Sources for Information Related to Issues of Suicide

National Suicide Hotline
1-800-SUICIDE (24/7)

National Suicide Prevention Lifeline
www.suicidepreventionlifeline.org
1-800-273-TALK (24/7)

American Association of Suicidology
www.suicidology.org

Depression and Bipolar Support Alliance (DBSA)
www.dbsalliance.org

American Foundation for Suicide Prevention
www.afsp.org

National Institute of Mental Health (NIMH)
www.nimh.nih.gov

American Psychiatric Association
www.psych.org

Mental Health America
www.nmha.org

American Psychological Association (APA)
www.apa.org

Screening for Mental Health

Stop a Suicide Today!
www.stopasuicide.org

Boys Town
Cares for troubled boys and girls and families in crisis.
www.boystown.org
1-800-448-3000 (24/7 national hotline)

Centre for Suicide Prevention (Canada)
www.suicideinfo.ca
1-833-456-4566 (24/7 helpline)

Samaritans (U.K. and Republic of Ireland)
www.samaritans.org
116-123 (24/7 helpline)

The Trevor Project
Confidential suicide hotline for LGBTQ youth
www.thetrevorproject.org
1-866-488-7386 (24/7 hotline)

Centers for Disease Control and Prevention (CDC)

National Center for Injury Prevention and Control Division of Violence Prevention
www.cdc.gov/injury/index.html

National Alliance on Mental Illness (NAMI)
www.nami.org

SAVE (Suicide Awareness Voices of Education)
www.save.org

Alliance of Hope: For Suicide Loss Survivors
www.allianceofhope.org

Evaluation

Evaluation of the client who is suicidal is an ongoing process accomplished through continuous reassessment and determination of goal achievement. Once the immediate crisis has been resolved, extended psychotherapy may be indicated. The long-term goals of individual or group psychotherapy for the suicidal client would be to:

- Develop and maintain a more positive self-concept and a sense of hopefulness.
- Learn more effective ways to express feelings to others.
- Achieve successful interpersonal relationships.
- Feel accepted by others and achieve a sense of belonging.

A person contemplating suicide feels worthless, hopeless, and oftentimes numb. These goals are directed toward promoting a sense of self-worth while offering a measure of hope and a purpose for living.

Summary and Key Points

- The majority of all persons who attempt or die by suicide have a diagnosed mental disorder.
- The highest current rates of suicide occur between the ages of 45 and 64 years (with the highest rates among those 52 to 59 years of age, and men 3.56 times more often than women). The second-highest rate was for those 85 or older. Suicide is the second-leading cause of death among young Americans ages 15 to 44 years and the eighth-leading cause of death for those ages 45 to 64.
- Evidence supports that recent change in relationship status (such as breakups, divorce, and widowhood) is a proximal risk factor.
- More women than men attempt suicide, but men succeed more often.
- Depressed men and women who consider themselves affiliated with a religion are less likely than their nonreligious counterparts to attempt suicide.
- Financial strain and unemployment are identified as risk factors for suicide.
- Among ethnic/racial groups the highest rates of suicide occur in white populations with the second-highest rate among American Indians and Alaska Natives. Much lower and roughly similar rates were found among black populations, Asians, and Pacific Islanders.
- Psychiatric disorders that are associated with higher risk for suicide include mood disorders, substance use disorders, schizophrenia, anorexia nervosa, borderline and antisocial personality disorders, anxiety disorders, and attention deficit-hyperactivity disorder.
- Predisposing factors include internalized anger, hopelessness and other symptoms of severe depression, history of aggression and violence, shame and humiliation, developmental stressors, sociological influences, genetics, and neurochemical factors.
- Suicide risk assessment should be a patient-centered, collaborative process in the context of a therapeutic relationship and should chronologically explore presenting suicide events, recent events, past events, and immediate intentions.
- Assessment of the level of intervention needed includes identifying the number of proximal or potentiating risks as well as the number of warning signs.
- It is important for the nurse to determine the seriousness of the patient's suicidal intentions, the existence of a plan, and the availability and lethality of the method.
- Many tools exist to screen for risk factors and warning signs for suicide. The Columbia Suicide Severity Rating Scale is an evidence-based tool for assessing the degree of risk and making clinical judgments about what level of treatment is needed to help the patient remain free from self-injury or death by suicide. Risk assessment scales should not be used alone but in combination with a comprehensive psychosocial assessment.
- The suicidal person should not be left alone.
- A safety plan is developed with the patient following a comprehensive suicide risk assessment and includes assisting the patient to recognize warning signs, identify and employ coping strategies, engage family members and friends as available support persons, identify people and social settings that can be used to distract from suicidal thoughts or urges, identify resources and contact information for crisis intervention, and problem-solve ways to restrict access to lethal means.
- Once the crisis intervention is complete, individuals may require long-term psychotherapy, during which they work to:
  - Develop and maintain a more positive self-concept.
  - Learn more effective ways to express feelings.
  - Improve interpersonal relationships.
  - Achieve a sense of belonging and a measure of hope for living.
- Evidence-based psychological interventions include dialectical behavior therapy, cognitive behavior therapy, and the Collaborative Assessment and Management of Suicidality (CAMS) approach.

Review Questions

Select the answer that is most appropriate for each of the following questions:

1. Which individual demonstrates the highest number of risk factors for suicide?
   a. A client who reports that they are in deep emotional pain, feels hopeless, and says "No one is there for me"
   b. A client who has been seeing a doctor for chronic, intractable pain and is taking pain medication
   c. An American Indian client who graduated from high school with honors
   d. A physician who reports feeling "burnt out" and is considering retirement
2. The nurse in the emergency department encounters a client who is expressing suicide ideation. The nurse recognizes which consideration as important to good suicide risk assessment? (Select all that apply.)
   a. Collaborating with the client
   b. Asking specific questions about leisure activities
   c. Establishing trust and open communication with the client
   d. Asking the client specific questions about the strength of their intention to die
   e. Identifying whether the client has thought about a plan for trying to kill themselves
3. A client is hospitalized following a suicide attempt after breaking up with her boyfriend. Freudian psychoanalytic theory would explain the client's suicide attempt in which of the following ways?
   a. She feels hopeless about her future without her boyfriend.
   b. Without her boyfriend, she feels like an outsider with her peers.
   c. She is feeling intense guilt because her boyfriend broke up with her.
   d. She is angry at her boyfriend for breaking up with her and has turned the anger inward on herself.
4. Which intervention is appropriate for a client on suicide precautions? (Select all that apply.)
   a. Remove all sharp objects, belts, and other potentially dangerous articles from the client's environment.
   b. Accompany the client to off-unit activities.
   c. Reassess intensity of suicidal thoughts and urges on a regular basis.
   d. Put all of the client's possessions in storage and explain that they will be returned when there is no longer a risk for suicide.
5. Success of long-term psychotherapy with a client (who attempted suicide following a breakup with his girlfriend) could be measured by which behavior?
   a. The client has a new girlfriend.
   b. The client has an increased sense of self-worth.
   c. The client does not take antidepressants anymore.
   d. The client told his old girlfriend how angry he was with her for breaking up with him.

Clinical Judgment Questions

6. A 27-year-old female client was admitted to the psychiatric unit from the medical intensive care unit where she was treated for taking a deliberate overdose of her antidepressant medication, trazodone (Desyrel). She says to the nurse, "My boyfriend broke up with me. We had been together for 6 years. I love him so much. I know I'll never get over him." Which is the best response by the nurse?
   a. "You'll get over him in time."
   b. "Forget him. There are other fish in the sea."
   c. "You must be feeling very sad about your loss."
   d. "Why do you think he broke up with you?"

7. The nurse identifies the primary nursing diagnosis for a client as "Risk for suicide related to feelings of hopelessness from loss of relationship." Which outcome criterion is most appropriate for this diagnosis?
   a. The client has experienced no self-harm.
   b. The client sets realistic goals.
   c. The client expresses some optimism and hope for the future.
   d. The client has reached a stage of acceptance in the loss of the relationship.
8. A client is hospitalized following a suicide attempt after breaking up with their boyfriend. The client says to the nurse, "When I get out of here, I'm going to try this again, and next time I'll choose a no-fail method." Which is the best response by the nurse?
   a. "You are safe here. We will make sure nothing happens to you."
   b. "You're just lucky your roommate came home when she did."
   c. "What exactly do you plan to do?"
   d. "I don't understand. You have so much to live for."
9. In determining degree of suicide risk with a suicidal client, the nurse assesses the following behavioral manifestations: severely depressed, withdrawn, statements of worthlessness, difficulty accomplishing activities of daily living, no close support systems. The nurse identifies the client's risk for suicide as which of the following?
   a. Low risk
   b. High risk
   c. Imminent risk
   d. Unable to be determined
10. A client who has been hospitalized following a suicide attempt is placed on suicide precautions on the psychiatric unit. The client admits that they are still feeling suicidal. Which of the following interventions is most appropriate in this instance? (Select all that apply.)
   a. Restrict access to any item that might be harmful by placing the client in a seclusion room.
   b. Check on the client every 15 minutes at irregular intervals or assign a staff person to stay with them on a one-to-one basis.
   c. Obtain an order from the physician to give the client a sedative to calm them and reduce suicide ideas.
   d. Do not allow the client to participate in any unit activities while they are on suicide precautions.
   e. Ask the client specific questions about their thoughts, plans, and intentions related to suicide.

Communication Exercises

1. Mr. J was brought to the emergency department by his brother who is concerned about Mr. J's worsening depression. During the assessment, Mr. J tells the nurse, "None of this matters. There's nothing that can make this any better." What would be an appropriate response by the nurse?
2. Mr. J admits to the nurse that he has had suicide ideas for the last couple of weeks. How would the nurse intervene with Mr. J at this point?
3. Mr. J tells the nurse that ever since his wife died 3 months ago, he doesn't want to go on living. What would be an example of empathic communication in response to this statement by Mr. J?

MOVIE CONNECTIONS

Dead Poet's Society ▪ *It's Kind of a Funny Story* ▪ *The Perks of Being a Wallflower* ▪ *Girl, Interrupted* ▪ *Cyberbully*

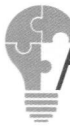

Go to **Davis Advantage** to complete your learning: strengthen understanding, apply your knowledge, and prepare for the Next Gen NCLEX®.

References

Ahmad, F. B., Cisewski, J. A., Miniño, A., & Anderson, R. N. (2021) Provisional mortality data—United States, 2020. *Morbidity and Mortality Weekly Report.* https://www.cdc.gov/mmwr/volumes/70/wr/mm7014e1.htm?s_cid=mm7014e1_w

Ahmedani, B. K., Peterson, E. L., Hu, Y., Rossom, R. C., Lynch, F., Lu, C. Y., Waitzfelder, B. E., Owen-Smith, A. A., Hubley, S., Prabhakar, D. L., Williams, L. K., Zeld, N., Mutter, E., Beck, A., Tolsma, D., & Simon, G. E. (2017). Major physical health conditions and risk of suicide. *American Journal of Preventive Medicine, 53*(3), 308–315. https://doi.org/10.1016/j.amepre.2017.04.001

Almendrala, A. (2015). *Native American youth suicide rates are at crisis levels.* http://www.huffingtonpost.com/entry/native-american-youth-suicide-rates-are-at-crisis-levels_us_560c3084e4b0768127005591

American Association of Suicidology. (2020). *Know the warning signs.* www.suicidology.org/resources/warning-signs

American Association of Suicidology. (2021). *Facts and statistics.* https://suicidology.org/facts-and-statistics/

American Foundation for Suicide Prevention. (2021). *Suicide statistics.* https://afsp.org/suicide-statistics

American Psychiatric Nurses Association. (2020). *Psychiatric-mental health nurse essential competencies for assessment and management of individuals at risk for suicide.* https://www.apna.org/i4a/pages/index.cfm?pageid=5684

Bauman, S., Toomey, R. B., & Walker, J. L. (2013). Associations among bullying, cyberbullying, and suicide in high school students. *Journal of Adolescence, 36*(2), 341–350. https://doi.org/10.1016/j.adolescence.2012.12.001

Bridge, J. A., Asti, L., Horowitz, L. M., Greenhouse, J. B., Fontanella, C. A., Sheftall, A. H., & Campo, J. V. (2015). Suicide trends among elementary school-aged children in the United States from 1993 to 2012. *JAMA Pediatrics, 169*(7), 673–677. https://doi.org/10.1001/jamapediatrics.2015.0465

Byron, W. J. (2016). Do people who commit suicide go to hell? *Catholic Digest.* http://www.catholicdigest.com/articles/faith/knowledge/2007/04-01/do-people-who-commit-suicide-go-to-hell

Cassels, C. (2011). "Striking" risk for suicidality, depression in gay teens. *Medscape Medical News.* http://www.medscape.com/viewarticle/740429

Center for Deployment Psychology. (n.d.). *Suicide in the military.* https://deploymentpsych.org/disorders/suicide-main

Centers for Disease Control and Prevention. (2011). *Self-directed violence surveillance; uniform definitions and recommended data elements.* https://stacks.cdc.gov/view/cdc/11997

Centers for Disease Control and Prevention (CDC). (2016). *Gay and bisexual men's health.* http://www.cdc.gov/msmhealth/suicide-violence-prevention.htm

Centers for Disease Control and Prevention. (2018). Preventing suicide. https://www.cdc.gov/violenceprevention/suicide/fastfact.html

Centers for Disease Control and Prevention. (2019a). *Deaths: Leading Causes for 2017. National Vital Statistics Reports, 68*(6). https://www.cdc.gov/nchs/data/nvsr/nvsr68/nvsr68_06-508.pdf

Centers for Disease Control and Prevention. (2019b). *Risk factors for Suicide.* https://www.cdc.gov/violenceprevention/suicide/riskprotectivefactors.html

Centers for Disease Control and Prevention. (2021a). *FastStats: Suicide and self-harm injury.* https://www.cdc.gov/nchs/fastats/suicide.htm

Centers for Disease Control and Prevention. (2021b). *FastStats: Adolescent health.* https://www.cdc.gov/nchs/fastats/adolescent-health.htm

Chan, M., Bhatti, H., Meader, N., Stockton, S., Evans, J., O'Connor, R., Kapur, N., & Kendall, T. (2016). Predicting suicide following self-harm: Systematic review of risk factors and risk scales. *British Journal of Psychiatry, 209*(4), 277–283. https://doi.org/10.1192/bjp.bp.115.170050

Chang, B. P., Franklin, J. C., Ribeiro, J. D., Fox, K. R., Bentley, K. H., Kleiman, E. M., & Nock, M. K. (2016). Biological risk factors for suicidal behaviors: A meta-analysis. *Translational Psychiatry, 6*(9), e887. https://doi.org/10.1038/tp.2016.165

Chung, D., Hadzi-Pavlovic, D., Wang, M., Swaraj, S., Olfson, M., & Large, M. (2019). Meta-analysis of suicide rates in the first week and the first month after psychiatric hospitalization. *BMJ Open, 9*(3), e023883. https://doi.org/10.1136/bmjopen-2018-023883

Crosby, A. E., Ortega, L., & Melanson, C. (2011). *Self-directed violence surveillance: Uniform definitions and recommended data elements, version 1.0.* Centers for Disease Control and Prevention, National Center for Injury Prevention and Control. http://www.cdc.gov/violenceprevention/pdf/Self-Directed-Violence-a.pdf

Drew, B. (2001). Self-harm and no-suicide contract in psychiatric inpatient settings. *Archives of Psychiatric Nursing, 15*(3), 99–106.

Duran, S., & McGuinness, T. M. (2016). Suicide in childhood. *Journal of Psychosocial Nursing, 54*(10), 27–30.

Edgerton, E., & Limber, S. (2013). *Research brief: Suicide and bullying.* https://www.stopbullying.gov/blog/2013/02/27/research-brief-suicide-and-bullying

Edwards, S. J. & Sachman, M. D. (2010). No-suicide contracts, no-suicide agreements, and no-suicide assurances: A study of their nature, utilization, perceived effectiveness, and potential to cause harm. *Crisis, 31*(6), 290–302.

Eisenberg, M. E., & Resnick, M. D. (2006). Suicidality among gay, lesbian and bisexual youth: The role of protective factors. *Journal of Adolescent Health, 39*(5), 662–668.

Exbrayat, S., Coudrot, C., Gourdon, X., Gay, A., Seos, J., Pellet, J., Trombert-Paviot, B., & Massoubre, C. (2017). Effect of telephone follow-up on repeated suicide attempt in patients discharged from an emergency psychiatry department: A controlled study. *BMC Psychiatry, 17*, 96. https://doi.org/10.1186/s12888-017-1258-6

Fleener, P. (n.d.). How to help a suicidal person. *Mental Health Today.* http://www.mental-health-today.com/suicide/sui2.htm

Forte, A., Buscajoni, A., Fiorillo, A., Pompili, M., & Baldessarini, R. J. (2019). Suicidal risk following hospital discharge: A review. *Harvard Review of Psychiatry, 27*(4), 209–216. https://doi.org/10.1097/HRP.0000000000000222

Freedenthal, S. (2013). *The use of no-suicide contracts.* https://www.speakingofsuicide.com/2013/05/15/no-suicide-contracts/

Fuller, K. (2020). *5 common myths about suicide debunked.* https://www.nami.org/Blogs/NAMI-Blog/September-2020/5-Common-Myths-About-Suicide-Debunked

Gordon, J. A. (2020). Addressing the crisis of black youth suicide. *Director's Messages.* https://www.nimh.nih.gov/about/director/messages/2020/addressing-the-crisis-of-black-youth-suicide.shtml

Hoffman, R. (2013). Contracting for safety: A misused tool. *Pennsylvania Patient Safety Advisory, 10*(2), 82–84.

Ivey-Stephenson, A. Z., Crosby, A. E., Jack, S. P., Haileyesus, T., & Kresnow-Sedacca, M. (2017). Suicide trends among and within urbanization levels by sex, race/ethnicity, age group, and mechanism of death—United States, 2001–2015. *MMWR Surveillance Summary, 66*(SS-18), 1–16.

Jobes, D. A. (2012). The Collaborative Assessment and Management of Suicidality (CAMS): An evolving evidence-based clinical approach to suicide risk. *Suicide and Life-Threatening Behavior, 42*(6), 640–653. https://doi.org/10.1111/j.1943-278X.2012.00119.x

Jobes, D. A. (2015, September). *Clinical suicidology: Innovations in assessment treatment of suicidal risk* [Paper presentation]. Psychiatric Grand Rounds, Summa Health Systems, Akron, OH.

John, A., Glendenning, A. C., Marchant, A., Montgomery, P., Stewart, A., Wood, S., Lloyd, K., & Hawton, K. (2018). Self-harm, suicidal behaviours, and cyberbullying in children and young people: Systematic review. *Journal of Medical Internet Research, 20*(4), e129. https://doi.org/10.2196/jmir.9044

Joiner, T. E. (2005). *Why people die by suicide.* Harvard University Press.

Juhnke, G. A., Granello, P. F., & Lebron-Striker, M. (2007). IS PATH WARM? A suicide assessment mnemonic for counselors. *ACA Professional Counseling Digest-03.* http://www.counseling.org/resources/library/ACA%20Digests/ACAPCD-03.pdf

Kim, J. L., Kim, J. M., Choi, Y., Lee, T., & Park, E. (2016). Effect of socioeconomic status on the linkage between suicidal ideation and suicide attempts. *Suicide and Life-Threatening Behavior, 46*(5), 588–597. https://doi.org/10.1111/sltb.12242

King, M., Semlyen, J., Tai, S. S., Killaspy, H., Osborn, D., Popelyuk, D., & Nazareth, I. (2008). A systematic review of mental disorder, suicide, and deliberate self-harm in lesbian, gay, and bisexual people. *BMC Psychiatry, 8*(70). http://www.biomedcentral.com/1471-244X/8/70

Klonsky, D. E., & May, A. M. (2015a). The three-step theory (3ST): A new theory of suicide rooted in the "ideation-to-action" framework. *International Journal of Cognitive Therapy, 8*(2), 114–129. https://doi.org/10.1521/ijct.2015.8.2.114

Klonsky, D. E., & May, A. M. (2015b). Impulsivity and suicide risk: Review and clinical implications. *Psychiatric Times, 32*(8). http://www.psychiatrictimes.com/specialreports/impulsivity-and-suicide-risk-review-and-clinical-implications/page/0/2

Kposowa, A. (2000). Marital status and suicide in the National Longitudinal Mortality Study. *Journal of Epidemiology and Community Health, 54*(4), 254–261. https://doi.org/10.1136/jech.54.4.254

Large, M., Kaneson, M., Myles, N., Myles, H., Gunaratne, P., & Ryan, C. (2016) Meta-analysis of longitudinal cohort studies of suicide risk assessment among psychiatric patients: Heterogeneity in results and lack of improvement over time. *PLoS ONE, 11*(6), e0156322. https://doi.org/10.1371/journal.pone.0156322

Lawrence, R. E., Oquendo, M. A., & Stanley, B. (2016). Religion and suicide risk: A systematic review. *Archives of Suicide Research, 20*(1), 1–21. https://doi.org/10.1080/13811118.2015.1004494

Lopez, C. T. (2019). *DOD Releases report on suicide among troops, military family members.* https://www.defense.gov/Explore/News/Article/Article/1972793/dod-releases-report-on-suicide-among-troops-military-family-members/

Mercado, M. C., Holland, K., Leemis, R. W., Stone, D. M., & Wang, J. (2017). Trends in emergency department visits for nonfatal self-inflicted injuries among youth aged 10 to 24 years in the United States, 2001–2015. *Journal of the American Medical Association, 318*(19), 1931–1933. https://doi.org/10.1001/jama.2017.13317

National Alliance on Mental Illness. (2021). *Risks of suicide.* www.nami.org/Learn-More/Mental-Health-Conditions/Related-Conditions/Risk-of-Suicide

National Indian Council on Aging. (2019). *American Indian suicide rate increases.* https://www.nicoa.org/national-american-indian-and-alaska-native-hope-for-life-day/

Nock, M. K., Deming, C. A., Fullerton, C. S., Gilman, S. E., Goldenberg, M., Kessler, R. C., McCarroll, J. E., & Ursan, R. J. (2013). Suicide among soldiers: A review of psychosocial risk and protective factors. *Psychiatry, 76*(2), 97–125. http://www.ncbi.nlm.nih.gov/pmc/articles/PMC4060831

Offord, C. (2020). What neurobiology can tell us about suicide. *The Scientist.* https://www.the-scientist.com/features/what-neurobiology-can-tell-us-about-suicide-66922

Olfson, M., Wall, M., Wang, S., Crystal, S., Shang-Min Liu, S.-M., Gerhard, T., & Blanco, C. (2016). Short-term suicide risk after psychiatric hospital discharge. *JAMA Psychiatry, 73*(11), 1119–1126. https://doi.org/10.1001/jamapsychiatry.2016.2035

Perlman, C. M., Neufeld, E., Martin, L., Goy, M., & Hirdes, J. P. (2011). *Risk assessment inventory: A resource guide for Canadian healthcare organizations.* Ontario Hospital Association and Canadian Patient Safety Institute.

Peterson, C., Sussell, A., Li, J., Schumacher, P. K., Yeoman, K., & Stone, D. M. (2020). Suicide rates by industry and occupation—national violent death reporting system, 32 states, 2016. *MMWR Morbidity & Mortality Weekly Report, 69,* 57–62. https://doi.org/10.15585/mmwr.mm6903a1external icon

Plöderl, M., Wagenmakers, E. J., Tremblay, P., Ramsay, R., Kralovek, K., Fartacek, C., & Fartacek, R. (2013). Suicide risk and sexual orientation: A critical review. *Archives of Sexual Behavior, 42*(5), 715–727.

Posner, K., Brown, G. K., Stanley, B., Brent, D. A., Yershova, K. V., Oquendo, M. A., Currier, G. W., Melvin, G. A., Greenhill, L., Shen, S., & Mann, J. J. (2011). The Columbia–Suicide Severity Rating Scale: Initial validity and internal consistency findings from three multisite studies with adolescents and adults. *American Journal of Psychiatry, 168*(12), 1266–1277. https://doi.org/10.1176/appi.ajp.2011.10111704

Puntil, C., York, J., Limandri, B., Greene, P., Arauz, E., & Hobbs, D. (2013). Competency-based training for PMH nurse generalists: Inpatient intervention and prevention of suicide. *Journal of the American Psychiatric Nurses Association, 19*(4), 205–210. https://doi.org/10.1177/1078390313496275

Rasic, D. T., Belik, S. L., Elias, B., Katz, L. Y., Enns, M., & Sareen, J. (2009). Spirituality, religion, and suicidal behavior in a nationally representative sample. *Journal of Affective Disorders, 114*(1), 32–40.

Reyes, M. S., Cayubit, F. O., Angala, M. H., Bries, S. C., Capalungan, J. T., & McCutcheon, L. E. (2015). Exploring the link between adolescent anger expression and tendencies for suicide: A brief report. *North American Journal of Psychology, 17*(1), 113–118.

Roberts, C. (2020). *No-suicide contracts: Can they work?* https://www.mdedge.com/psychiatry/article/226013/depression/no-suicide-contracts-can-they-work?sso=true

Rogers, M. L., & Joiner, T. E. (2017). Suicide-specific rumination relates to lifetime suicide attempts above and beyond a variety of other suicide risk factors. *Journal of Psychiatric Research, 98.* https://doi.org/10.1016/j.jpsychires.2017.12.017

Roškar, S., Podlesek, A., Kuzmanić, M., Demšar, L. O., Zaletel, M., & Marušič, A. (2011). Suicide risk and its relationship to change in marital status. *Crisis, 32*(1), 24–30. https://doi.org/10.1027/0227-5910/a000054

Rudd, D. M., Mandrusiak, M., & Joiner, T. E. (2006). The case against no-suicide contract: The commitment to treatment statement as a practice alternative. *Journal of Clinical Psychology, 62*(2), 243–251.

Shea, S. C. (2009). Suicide assessment: Part 1: Uncovering suicidal intent: A sophisticated art. Part 2: Uncovering suicidal intent using the chronological assessment of suicide events. *Psychiatric Times, 26*(12). https://www.psychiatrictimes.com/view/suicide-assessment-part-1-uncovering-suicidal-intent-sophisticated-art and https://www.psychiatrictimes.com/view/suicide-assessment-part-2-uncovering-suicidal-intent-using-case-approach

Stanley, B., Brown, G. K., Brenner, L. A., Galfalvy, H. C., Currier, G. W., Knox, K. L., Chaudhury S. R., Bush A. L., & Green, K. L. (2018). Follow-up vs usual care of suicidal patients treated in the emergency department. *JAMA Psychiatry, 75*(9), 894–900. https://doi.org/10.1001/jamapsychiatry.2018.1776

Stanley, B., & Brown, G. K. (2008). *The safety plan treatment manual to reduce suicide risk: Veteran version.* U.S. Department of Veterans Affairs.

Stroumsa, D. (2014). The state of transgender health care: Policy, law, and medical frameworks. *American Journal of Public Health, 104*(3), 31–37. https://doi.org/10.2105/AJPH.2013.301789

Substance Abuse and Mental Health Services Administration. (2020). *Suicide prevention.* https://www.samhsa.gov/suicide-prevention

Sudak, H. S. (2017). Suicide treatment. In B. J. Sadock, V. A. Sadock, & P. Ruiz (Eds.), *Comprehensive textbook of psychiatry* (pp. 2618–2622). Wolters Kluwer.

Swogger, M. T., Van Orden, K. A., & Conner, K. R. (2014). The relationship of outwardly-directed aggression to suicidal ideation and suicide attempts across two high-risk samples. *Psychology of Violence, 4*(2), 184–195. https://doi.org/10.1037/a0033212

Taylor, T. F. (2015). The influence of shame on posttrauma disorders: Have we failed to see the obvious? *European Journal of Psychotraumatology, 6.* https://doi.org/10.3402/ejpt.v6.28847

The Joint Commission. (2016). *Sentinel Event Alert 56: Detecting and treating suicide ideation in all settings.* https://www.jointcommission.org/sea_issue_56

The Samaritans. (2021). *Myths about suicide.* http://samaritansnyc.org/myths-about-suicide

The Trevor Project. (2021). *Facts about suicide.* https://www.thetrevorproject.org/resources/preventing-suicide/facts-about-suicide/

Whalen, D., Dixon-Gordon, K., Belden, A., Barch, D., & Luby, J. (2015). Correlates and consequences of suicidal cognitions and behaviors in children ages 3 to 7 years. *Journal of the American Academy of Child & Adolescent Psychiatry, 54*(11), 926–937. https://doi.org/10.1016/j.jaac.2015.08.009

Wiklander, M., Samuelsson, M., Jokinen, J., Nilsonne, A., Wilczek, A., Rylander, G., & Åsberg, M. (2012). Shame-proneness in attempted suicide patients. *BMC Psychiatry, 12.* https://doi.org/10.1186/1471-244X-12-50

Yamauchi, T., Fujita, T., Tachimori, H., Takeshima, T., Inagaki, M., & Sudo, A. (2013). Age-adjusted relative suicide risk by marital and employment status over the past 25 years in Japan. *Journal of Public Health, 35*(1), 49–56. https://doi.org/10.1093/pubmed/fds054

Zhang, Y., Zhang, C., Yuan, G., Yao, J., Cheng, Z., Liu, C., Liu, Q., Wan, G., Shi, G., Cheng, Y., Ling, Y., & Li, K. (2010). Effect of tryptophan hydroxylase-2 rs7305115 SNP on suicide attempts risk in major depression. *Behavioral and Brain Functions, 6*(49). https://doi.org/10.1186/1744-9081-6-49

Zweig, J., & Dank, M. (2013). *Technology, teen dating, violence and abuse, and bullying.* The Urban Institute. http://www.urban.org/sites/default/files/alfresco/publication-pdfs/412891

Classical References

Durkheim, E. (1951). *Suicide: A study of sociology.* Free Press.

Freud, S. (1957). *Mourning and melancholia.* In *Standard edition of the complete psychological works of Freud* (Vol. XIV). Hogarth Press.

MacDonald, M., & Murphy, T. R. (1991). *Sleepless souls: Suicide in early modern England.* Oxford University Press.

Macnab, F. (1993). *Brief psychotherapy: An integrative approach in clinical practice.* John Wiley & Sons.

Minois, G. (2001). *History of suicide: Voluntary death in Western culture.* Johns Hopkins University Press.

U.S. Public Health Service. (1999). *The Surgeon General's call to action to prevent suicide.*

UNIT 3

Care of Patients With Psychiatric Disorders

12 Caring for Patients With Mental Illness and Substance Use Disorders in General Practice Settings

CORE CONCEPTS

Health Promotion: Screening, Referral

Professional Behavior: Assessment, Stigmatization

Caring: Patient-centered care

CHAPTER OUTLINE

Objectives

Introduction

The Need for Education of Health-Care Providers

Screening

Priority Issues for Screening in Any Health-Care Setting

Referral

Stigma

The Role of the Nurse in Caring for Patients With Psychiatric and Substance Use Disorders in Nonpsychiatric Settings

Summary and Key Points

Review Questions

Clinical Judgment Questions

KEY TERMS

diagnostic overshadowing

nonsuicidal self-injuring behavior (NSSIB)

patient-centered care

referral

retraumatization

screening

screening, brief intervention, and referral to treatment (SBIRT)

social distancing

stigmatization

trauma-informed care

OBJECTIVES

After reading this chapter, the student will be able to:

1. Recognize the impact of inadequate assessment, treatment, and referral for the client with mental health and substance use disorders.
2. Discuss the evidence identifying the need for further mental health and substance use disorder education among health-care providers in primary care and other non-psychiatric settings.
3. Describe essential elements in appropriate screening and referral of mental health and substance abuse clients.
4. Analyze barriers that influence the screening, intervention, and referral process for clients with mental health and substance use concerns.
5. Describe essential aspects of the nurse's role in providing care for patients with psychiatric/mental health and substance use disorders in general practice.

Introduction

The client with mental illness has historically been misunderstood, misdiagnosed, and mistreated (see Chapter 1, "Mental Health and Mental Illness"). Current examples confirm that this problem is ongoing. In one case, a patient came into the emergency department setting with garbled speech that made their responses to questions difficult to comprehend. The patient was known to be a homeless person with chronic schizophrenia and was quickly transferred to a psychiatric hospital. Once there, their right-sided weakness, vital signs, and difficulty speaking were recognized as evidence of a cerebrovascular accident.

In another case, a hospitalized patient with schizophrenia reported to the nurse that there was a rock band playing music in their body and the drummer was playing in his chest; initially, these symptoms were identified as delusional thinking. However, after further assessment, it was determined that the patient was having a heart attack. Real examples of potentially fatal misdiagnoses like these are far too common.

Clients presenting with symptoms like pain, lack of energy, and feelings of helplessness could be experiencing a variety of medical conditions, but these can also be signs of depression. If effective screening is not conducted, the client may be at risk for worsening depression and suicide.

Nurses who choose to work in nonpsychiatric settings are *the* frontline responders in recognizing, intervening, and referring clients with neuropsychiatric illness for further treatment. Studies reveal, though, that attitudes, lack of education about the need for screening, and issues related to accessing services are all influential in lack of appropriate intervention to meet the needs of this population.

Clearly there are genetic, neurological, neurochemical, and environmental influences in the etiology of mental illness that differentiate clinical illness from the range of emotions and behavior that is a part of general human experience. However, without education and appreciation for these symptoms as distressing signs of neurological illness, clients will continue to remain at risk for lack of treatment or mistreatment of both psychiatric and other medical disorders. Nurses must take the lead in educating other health-care professionals and the public, combating stigmatization of clients with mental illness, recognizing neuropsychiatric symptoms, conducting appropriate screening, and collaborating effectively with other health-care providers to ensure appropriate referral when specialized mental health and addictions treatment are needed. This chapter explores the nurse's role and the evidence for education, screening, and referral needs in various nonpsychiatric settings.

The Need for Education of Health-Care Providers

Evidence supports that clients with significant mental illness die, on average, 25 years earlier than the general population and that 60% of those deaths are related to preventable or treatable causes (Gomes et al., 2015). The increased risk of mortality for individuals with mental illness may be related to **diagnostic overshadowing,** a phenomenon in which a person's physical symptoms are attributed to their mental illness. For example, Gomes and associates reviewed studies showing that patients with both mental illness and a cardiovascular condition received one-half as many follow-up interventions following a heart attack as those without a concurrent mental illness. This finding is significant because many patients with mental illnesses are at greater risk for cardiovascular disease due to genetic, lifestyle, or environmental issues or to adverse effects from psychotropic medications.

Other studies have demonstrated that clients with mental illness who present to general health-care settings are at risk for lack of treatment or appropriate referral, which may be related to lack of knowledge about symptom detection (by both patients and health-care providers), stigmatization, and lack of awareness about counseling and referral services (Bay et al., 2016; Betz et al., 2013; Ndetei et al., 2011). These realities have led many people with mental illness to avoid seeking health care altogether.

As we learn more about the progression and prognosis of illnesses like schizophrenia, it has become apparent that early intervention is critical because repeated psychotic episodes may have a cumulative damaging effect on the brain (see Chapter 15, "Schizophrenia Spectrum and Other Psychotic Disorders," for further discussion). The barriers to early intervention are compounded for individuals with schizophrenia because one of the neurological symptoms common in this disorder is *anosognosia* (a lack of awareness or recognition of symptoms). During acute psychotic episodes, these clients—who are often suspicious of people and the surrounding environment and unaware that they have a mental illness—may be brought to the emergency department against their will. It is not difficult to imagine how frightening this scenario might be for such an individual. Nurses in emergency settings play a key role in recognizing this patient as one who is experiencing significant neurological symptoms and requires immediate and ongoing care. Unfortunately, this patient may instead be stigmatized as one who is neither "really ill" nor requiring complex and compassionate intervention. The consequence of these attitudes for the patient is prolonged suffering and sometimes early death.

Nurses in any nonpsychiatric setting must also have a clear working knowledge of the impact of depressive disorders in treating other illnesses. Depression, a mental illness with multiple etiologies and symptoms, affects 1 in 5 women and 1 in 10 men during their lifetime, is increasingly being diagnosed in children and adolescents, and is demonstrating greater chronicity than previously thought (Akiskal, 2017) (see Chapter 16, "Depressive Disorders," for further discussion). In addition, Akiskal (2017) notes that there is evidence that bipolar disorder, which is characterized by bouts of depression and mania, accounts for up to 50% of all cases of depression (see Chapter 17, "Bipolar and Related Disorders," for further discussion of these disorders). Knowledge of the distinction between depressive disorder and bipolar disorder has important implications for medication management and ongoing treatment. With such a high prevalence, the potential disabling effects of untreated or mistreated illness, and the fact that suicide is a risk at all times in depressive illness, it seems apparent that all patients, in any encounter with health-care professionals, should be screened for evidence of depression and risk for suicide. But this has not been the case.

In addition, there are links between depression and many other diseases. Depression not only increases risk for other illnesses but also is associated with poorer outcomes when left untreated. Evidence has demonstrated that depression is a risk factor for cardiovascular disease, metabolic syndrome, diabetes, dementia, asthma, arthritis, and hyperlipidemia (Bica et al., 2017). The risk of poorer outcomes has implications for both the medical condition and the depression and, ultimately, for the risk of suicide. Across the nation, the incidence of suicide has reached such epidemic proportions that it should be an assessment skill that every nurse is confident in performing (see Chapter 11, "Suicide Prevention," for further discussion of this topic). The importance of this knowledge base and appropriate screening may seem to be an obvious need in primary care and community settings, but it is equally important in medical settings within hospitals. Suicide in hospital settings is a sentinel event that is frequently reported to The Joint Commission, an organization that accredits hospitals and health-care systems. Horowitz and associates (2013) found that 25% of all inpatient suicides occur in nonbehavioral health settings and that in 80% the root cause was lack of adequate assessment.

Individuals using opioids (a national epidemic) and those with other substance use disorders commonly seek care first in general medical and community practice settings before they are treated in psychiatric or substance abuse treatment settings. People often die of overdose before they ever reach an emergency department, which has prompted a nationwide effort to educate not only health-care professionals but also the general public about how to recognize symptoms of overdose and administer treatment, such as naloxone and rescue breathing, to treat associated respiratory depression. Nurses play key educational, screening, and referral roles in community, primary, medical, and long-term care settings (see Chapter 14, "Substance Use and Addictive Disorders," for further discussion of this topic).

Psychiatric nursing is an essential component of basic undergraduate nursing curricula. *Every* nurse needs education about recognition of mental illnesses to perform competently in *any* nursing role. Studies have shown that when health-care professionals in nonpsychiatric settings are trained to develop confidence in their ability to recognize the need for screening and how to utilize valid, reliable screening tools, rates of intervention and/or referral for mental health treatment improve. Although nurses typically enter general practice with a basic knowledge of mental illness recognition, communication strategies, and basic interventions, additional variables influence how these skills are put into practice. Three of these variables are availability of screening tools, knowledge and accessibility of referral sources, and attitudes about the client with mental illness or substance use disorders.

CORE CONCEPT

Screening

Screening is the evaluation of the patient for conditions before they are known to be clinically significant. The purpose of screening is early diagnosis and treatment of illness.

Screening

Many valid and reliable screening tools exist for identifying mental illnesses and substance use disorders. The purpose of screening is to identify clinically significant symptoms that require further assessment and intervention. Tools that are completed by patient self-report are time efficient, but their use depends on the clinician's recognition of symptoms that support the need for screening and a belief that screening is essential for adequate identification and management of mental health and substance use issues.

Evidence supports that use of screening tools is better than clinical judgment alone in diagnosis of mental illness (Jackman et al., 2016; Mitchell et al., 2011; Préville et al., 2004; Singer et al., 2011) and may help reduce the risk that an individual's illness is missed completely or incorrectly identified (i.e., a false-negative result).

In one study, Horowitz and associates (2013) developed a two-item nursing screen for suicide risk in any medical setting. The need was identified after The Joint Commission issued a "Sentinel Event" alert highlighting the importance of suicide risk assessment in all medical settings. The screen had nurses ask patients two questions: "In the past month, have you had thoughts about suicide?" and "Have you ever made a suicide attempt?" A yes response to either question prompted a third question, "Are you having thoughts of suicide right now?" The study demonstrated improvement in identification of medical-surgical patients who may be at risk for suicide (4% were referred for additional evaluation) and highlighted the time efficiency of such screening tools (this tool took about 2 minutes to complete). Again, critical to the success of any strategy is the nurse's belief that this kind of screening is essential. Endorsement for the necessity of this screening by accrediting bodies like The Joint Commission reinforces that this is an essential role for nurses.

Fortunately, more research is being done to identify the need for better screening for mental illness and substance abuse in nonpsychiatric settings. Screening tools for depression, anxiety, and suicide risk have been identified as priorities. Roberge and associates (2016) conducted a qualitative study based on the recognition that depression and anxiety in patients seeking primary care for chronic diseases is linked to morbidity and mortality. Both patients and clinicians in this study identified a need for holistic care that includes screening and management of mental illness. Another study (Mollard et al., 2016) identified an increase in the incidence of postpartum depression among women in rural areas (a trend also seen internationally), and they concluded that nurses should be the lead change agents in improving policy around screening for depression in this population. In a third study (Garcia de la Garza et al., 2021) noted that screening the general population for suicide risk is essential, because over a third of individuals making nonfatal suicide attempts do not seek mental health treatment. Research efforts have identified the need for improved neuropsychiatric screening in a variety of other settings as well, including home care, community care, long-term care, medical-surgical care, oncology, geriatrics, and child-adolescent care (Bica et al., 2017; Grundberg, 2016; Koposov et al., 2017; Langdon et al., 2013; McGovern & Selwyn, 2014; Thompson et al., 2008).

Nurse managers are integral in promoting the importance of mental health and substance use screening by educating and equipping their staff nurses with screening tools that are valid, reliable, time efficient, and user friendly. Staff nurses must adopt an attitude that screening for mental illness is critical to their success in interventions for the medical illness that brought the patient to their nonpsychiatric setting. Screening provides the foundation for referring patients to ongoing evaluation and treatment for the mental illness itself.

Many resources exist that identify valid and reliable screening tools for use in clinical practice settings. Moran and associates (2018), in a systematic review of the literature, identified 24 tools that are psychometrically tested and appropriate for use in primary care settings. The National Alliance on Mental Illness (NAMI, 2021) stresses the importance of screening youth and young adults:

> Approximately 50% of lifetime mental health conditions begin by age 14 and 75% begin by age 24. At the same time, the average delay between when symptoms first appear and intervention is approximately 11 years. Mental health screenings allow for early identification and intervention and help bridge the gap.

The American Academy of Pediatrics (2018) publishes a table of mental health screening and assessment tools for children, adolescents, and adults. These tools were chosen because of their evidence-based reliability and accessibility. Many screening tools are free to use and widely accessible, whereas others are copyrighted, proprietary, and associated with a fee for use.

Priority Issues for Screening in Any Health-Care Setting

The importance of screening for depression has already been discussed with regard to its prevalence, its link to the development of other diseases, and its association with poorer outcomes. Other issues that arise as part of a general health assessment may trigger the need for screening and further assessment, but some issues are considered so prevalent and so high risk that they are priorities to screen for in all patients. Three of these issues are trauma, suicide risk, and substance use disorders.

Trauma History

Screening for violence and trauma history is now well accepted as an essential psychosocial issue that should be conducted with patients when they first enter a health-care setting. Even in the early 1990s, violence and trauma were identified in nursing literature as growing areas of concern that were linked to a high risk for injury, unhealthy coping mechanisms, and other illnesses such as arthritis, irritable bowel syndrome, and chronic pain (Hoff & Rosenbaum, 1994), as well as having implications in surgical outcomes (Schofferman et al., 1992).

Hoff and Rosenbaum also noted that although violence and trauma cross gender boundaries (as well as racial, ethnic, class, and national boundaries), most individuals affected by violence are women and children. Hoff and Ross (1993) estimate that up to 75% of female psychiatric patients have a current or past history of abuse. The classic study on adverse childhood events (ACEs) linked trauma in childhood to significant cognitive, social, psychological, and neurobiological changes that contribute to a host of physical and mental problems and early death (Felitti et al., 1998). These studies identified the critical importance of screening for trauma history. However, because many individuals with this history may be in denial, frightened about the consequences of sharing information, or experiencing guilt or shame, they may be reluctant to disclose information about their circumstances and history unless direct screening takes place.

It is critical that nurses conduct screenings in private and communicate with a compassionate, nonjudgmental attitude. Pardee and associates (2017), in their review of ACE assessment tools, concluded that primary care nurse practitioners still need more education and more efficient assessment tools to ensure that this type of screening is accomplished in primary care settings.

As research and nursing practice have focused more attention on the importance of screening for trauma and interpersonal violence history, we have also learned a great deal more about the importance of **trauma-informed care**—care that incorporates sensitivity to the impact of trauma history on current behavior and relationships. Patients are at risk for **retraumatization** (a triggering of feelings associated with the previous trauma) if trauma screening is conducted without sensitivity to the impact of that trauma on an individual's current level of functioning (see Chapter 19, "Trauma- and Stressor-Related Disorders," and Chapter 25, "Survivors of Abuse or Neglect," for further discussion of these topics). Given the high prevalence of trauma, it is incumbent on nurses to practice trauma-informed care in every aspect of nursing intervention.

Risk for Suicide

National attention to the ever-alarming suicide rates across the life span, among military personnel, and within specific ethnic groups and communities has raised awareness of the critical needs for screening and intervention among laypeople and health-care providers alike. Military personnel with post-traumatic stress disorder may present in medical settings with physical complaints, reports of nightmares, and/or substance use, but unless health-care professionals specifically screen for suicide risk and warning signs, this potentially fatal risk may go undetected. The older adult with depression is another population that more often presents with physical complaints in primary care settings and may not even consider discussing depression, loneliness, or thoughts of suicide unless specifically asked.

Recent studies (Chen et al., 2020; Fuller-Thomson et al., 2020; Kõlves, 2021) have highlighted an increased risk for suicide among patients with Parkinson's disease, autism, and women with attention deficit-hyperactivity disorder, all of whom are more likely to be seen in primary care rather than in psychiatric settings. As with trauma victims, the fact that people at risk for suicide may not be forthcoming with this information; that suicide is a high-risk, potentially fatal problem; and that suicide is a highly prevalent concern reinforces the need for universal screening.

One very important caution about screening for suicide that we are learning from ongoing research in suicide prevention is that although brief screening may open a door for discussion with a client, it is not enough to prevent suicide in some individuals. In other words, just because a patient responds "no" to the question, "Are you having thoughts of taking your own life?" does not mean that they are risk free. Jobes (2015) suggests that in spite of the numerous brief screening tools that are available, they have perhaps been more often used as defensive medicine than actually contributing to suicide prevention. *Defensive medicine* refers to doing the minimum number of interventions needed to "meet the letter of the law." In this case, it would mean asking the patient the preceding question, documenting that the patient denies suicidal ideation, and then assuming that the health-care provider "covered the necessary bases." Current research, as Jobes points out, has demonstrated that brief screening may be inadequate because of the many variables that influence a person's decision to take their own life and the fact that ideation (as well as the intent to act on ideation) can change in intensity over time.

Patients in primary care settings with depression, substance abuse issues, and/or chronic pain should be recognized as having *identified risk factors* for suicide and should be screened carefully. In addition, given the current prevalence rates of suicide, nurses should develop the skill to carefully screen for suicide risk with every patient in every health-care setting. Establishing trust with the patient, developing a collaborative relationship, and displaying a willingness to discuss this issue from various vantage points (such as past history, recent history, immediate risk, and strength of the individual's intent to harm themselves) are all essential elements in identifying the need for referral and the level of care required for the patient's safety.

Nonsuicidal self-injuring behavior (NSSIB) is a related and complex phenomenon that is increasingly being seen in nonpsychiatric settings and challenges the nurse's skills to discern how to screen and when to refer for more intensive treatment. Colloquially, NSSIB is often associated with "cutting" (cutting oneself with a sharp object), but any other nonlethal method of self-injury, such as burning, self-hitting, or head banging, is also classified as NSSIB. Kameg and associates (2013) report that although NSSIB is typically a nonlethal, repetitive act used to reduce distress rather than end one's life, the individual who uses NSSIB is more likely to consider or attempt suicide than non-self-injurers. Therefore, individuals who exhibit NSSIB require screening for suicide risk. The authors also state that any patient who is identified as having comorbid psychiatric symptoms such as labile mood, dysphoria, anxiety, depersonalization, anhedonia, or borderline personality disorder should be referred to specialized mental health-care services. Those who exhibit NSSIB in response to command hallucinations should be considered in need of immediate medical attention. Several tools are available to screen for self-harm. Kameg and associates (2013) identify that the Self-Harm Inventory (Box 12–1) can be completed within 5 minutes and screens for borderline personality disorder symptoms as well as a variety of self-harm behaviors.

Substance Use Disorders

In the United States, rates of opioid abuse have reached epidemic levels, and rates of methamphetamine use have also increased significantly. Opioid addiction can lead to overdose, and methamphetamine withdrawal is associated with an increased risk for suicide. In addition, the numerous physical and psychological consequences of long-term alcohol use are well documented. All of these facts underscore the importance of screening for substance use disorders in nonpsychiatric settings. Although many tools exist to screen for substance abuse, the extent of their use in general practice settings varies. **Screening, brief intervention, and referral to treatment (SBIRT)** (Substance Abuse and Mental Health Service Administration [SAMHSA], 2020) is an evidence-based approach that can be used in emergency departments, trauma centers, primary care, and other community settings. SAMHSA (2020) describes the SBIRT approach as follows:

- **S**creening quickly assesses the severity of substance use and identifies the appropriate level of treatment.
- **B**rief **I**ntervention focuses on increasing insight and awareness regarding substance use and motivation toward behavioral change.
- **R**eferral to **T**reatment provides those identified as needing more extensive treatment with access to specialty care.

One study (Rahm et al., 2015) sought to identify why routine screening does not occur for an issue that has been so clearly identified as a public health concern. The authors, using SBIRT as the preferred model, asked primary care providers (including nurses, physicians, mental health specialists, and others) and patients to identify barriers to implementation of this approach. Although patients supported universal screening, they also noted that privacy concerns may be an issue. This is an important consideration for nurses who are screening patients for substances of abuse. Patients may deny using substances, particularly illegal substances, because they fear legal consequences. For example, many states consider substance use during pregnancy to be child abuse with legal consequences, and 25 states and the District of Columbia require health professionals

BOX 12–1 The Self-Harm Inventory

Instructions: Please answer the following questions by checking either, "Yes," or "No." Check "Yes" only to those items that you have intentionally, or on purpose, used to hurt yourself.

Yes	No	Have you ever intentionally, or on purpose, done any of the following:
___	___	1. Overdosed? (If yes, number of times _____)
___	___	2. Cut yourself on purpose? (If yes, number of times _____)
___	___	3. Burned yourself on purpose? (If yes, number of times _____)
___	___	4. Hit yourself? (If yes, number of times _____)
___	___	5. Banged your head on purpose? (If yes, number of times _____)
___	___	6. Abused alcohol?
___	___	7. Driven recklessly on purpose? (If yes, number of times _____)
___	___	8. Scratched yourself on purpose? (If yes, number of times _____)
___	___	9. Prevented wounds from healing?
___	___	10. Made medical situations worse on purpose (e.g., skipped medication)?
___	___	11. Been promiscuous (i.e., had many sexual partners)? (If yes, how many? _____)
___	___	12. Set yourself up in a relationship to be rejected?
___	___	13. Abused prescription medication?
___	___	14. Distanced yourself from God as punishment?
___	___	15. Engaged in emotionally abusive relationships? (If yes, number of relationships? _____)
___	___	16. Engaged in sexually abusive relationships? (If yes, number of relationships? _____)
___	___	17. Lost a job on purpose? (If yes, number of times _____)
___	___	18. Attempted suicide? (If yes, number of times _____)
___	___	19. Exercised an injury on purpose?
___	___	20. Tortured yourself with self-defeating thoughts?
___	___	21. Starved yourself to hurt yourself?
___	___	22. Abused laxatives to hurt yourself? (If yes, number of times _____)

Have you engaged in any other self-destructive behaviors not asked about in this inventory? If so, please describe below.

_____

_____

Source: Used with permission from Sansone, R., & Sansone, L. (2010). Measuring self-harm behavior with the Self-Harm Inventory. Psychiatry, *7(4), 16–20.*

to report suspected prenatal drug use (Guttmacher Institute, 2021), which may deter some women from ever seeking prenatal care. Establishment of trust, clear communication about why this information is being collected, and how it will be used are important first steps in the screening process.

The health-care providers in Rahm and associates' study (2015) noted that another barrier to implementation of screening processes for mental health issues and substance use disorders is competing workload demands. This finding suggests that the success of screening may be tied, at least in part, to workload issues or lack of clarity about how to prioritize tasks. Nurses face these concerns in most areas of practice. Recognizing the vital importance of screening and creating the structure to ensure that it occurs requires multidisciplinary collaboration, commitment, and support from health-care managers. Nurses are in a key position to educate others about the importance of screening for psychiatric and substance abuse issues in nonpsychiatric settings. Nurse leaders are in a key position to direct changes in screening requirements that address such critical public health-care needs.

CORE CONCEPT

Referral

Referral entails sending a patient to another health-care provider or specialty service for consultation or treatment when the need has been identified.

Referral

Although structured screening of mental health issues has been identified as a critical first step in improving care for both mental illness and other medical illnesses, controversy exists over how much care can be provided in nonpsychiatric settings and, therefore, when referral (sending a patient to another health-care provider or specialty service for consultation or treatment) is appropriate. Grundberg (2016) concluded that if nonpsychiatric nurses are to be involved in early detection and interventions for mental health–related issues, these activities must be explicitly stated work objectives and there must be effective collaboration between care providers. If nurses lack clarity about their roles and responsibilities and the vital importance of this type of screening, referring the patient to needed services is unlikely to happen.

Several studies have found that providing training and education about evidence-based screening tools and referral pathways improved the referral process for mental health services (Allen et al., 2011; Brooker et al., 2007; Bruce et al., 2007; Hasche et al., 2013; Thompson et al., 2008). The process for referral to specialized mental health services is one in which the nurse must collaborate effectively with physicians, social workers, and other health-care providers within their practice setting and with the setting to which they are referring a patient.

CORE CONCEPT

Patient-centered care

Patient-centered care is an approach to care provision that intends to "identify, respect, and care about patients' differences, values, preferences, and expressed needs; relieve pain and suffering; coordinate continuous care; listen to, clearly inform, communicate with, and educate patients; share decision making and management: and continuously advocate disease prevention, wellness, and promotion of healthy lifestyles, including a focus on population health" (Institute of Medicine, Committee on the Health Professions Education Summit, 2003).

The process of referral also involves collaboration with the patient. This is the essence of patient-centered care. The Institute of Medicine (2003) has stressed, in its landmark study of deaths associated with medical errors, that we must improve our understanding and application of this concept to improve the safety and quality of health care in the future. To apply the concepts of patient-centered care requires that nurses and other health-care professionals listen to the patient, empower them in decision making around their care, and establish a collaborative partnership.

There are some circumstances in which providing care for a psychiatric patient cannot be conducted collaboratively. Patients who are either strongly intent on hurting themselves or unaware that they have significant, life-threatening symptoms of mental illness need to be referred to a more restrictive environment even when it is against their will. Essential elements in this process include collaboration with other health-care professionals to increase confidence in the difficult clinical judgment to involuntarily hospitalize the patient and thoughtful communication with the patient about the reasons for this referral. Lauder and associates (2006), in their study of how nurses make clinical judgments about patients who are neglecting their self-care, caution that nurses need to be clear about the difference between severity of mental illness and capacity to make decisions. Just because a patient has a severe mental illness does not necessarily mean that the patient is incapable of making decisions. Nurses should be making referral (or any other) decisions *for* patients only when it is clear that the patients do not have the current capacity to make decisions in the interest of their personal safety and livelihood.

Two barriers to effective referral of patients with mental illness are lack of knowledge about available options for specialized treatment and difficulty accessing resources that are available. Some primary care settings and emergency departments have incorporated mental health specialists either to provide on-site intervention or to assist in the clinical judgment about needs for referral to more intensive treatment. Nurses in nonpsychiatric settings must be familiar with mental health services and facilities within the community in which they practice to effectively collaborate and refer patients appropriately for ongoing care. SAMHSA provides an online locator map to identify mental health and substance abuse treatment services in localities throughout the United States (https://findtreatment.samhsa.gov/locator). Box 12–2 lists some types of mental health and substance use disorder resources for referral.

CORE CONCEPT

Stigmatization

Stigmatization is the devaluing of a person because of a particular characteristic or illness. It is an attitude that is negative, discriminatory, and unethical. In the practice of health care, stigmatizing patients has the potential to inhibit the patient's ability to receive accurate diagnose and adequate treatment.

BOX 12–2 Types of Referral Resources for Mental Health and Substance Abuse Treatment

Self-Help Groups	12-step programs such as Alcoholics Anonymous (AA), Emotions Anonymous, and others provide ongoing peer support and education. Location and availability of AA meetings can be found online (www.aa.org). Some meetings are also conducted online.
Mental Health-Care Professionals	Psychiatrists (MDs) and psych-mental health nurse practitioners (PMH NPs) provide diagnostic, medication management, and counseling services and may conduct psychotherapy. Licensed independent social workers (LISWs) provide counseling, case management, and advocacy. Psychologists (PhDs) provide counseling, individual and group psychotherapy, and psychological testing services.
Community Mental Health Centers	Operated by community or county governments to provide public mental health services primarily to clients who cannot afford private services. Usually staffed with a broad range of mental health professionals and *peer support specialists* (individuals with mental illness who provide support in illness management and recovery), some of whom may have specialized training and certification. May provide a broad range of services for mental health and substance use disorders such as outpatient counseling, case management, intensive outpatient programs, and day programs. Often collaborate with and refer to area resources for support with employment, housing, and other care needs.
Substance Abuse and Addiction Treatment Centers	These treatment facilities usually have a broad range of mental health and addictions treatment health professionals including certified chemical dependency counselors and physicians certified in addictions medicine. Services usually include detoxification (for safe withdrawal from addictive substances), intensive outpatient services (intensive group therapy, 3 to 5 days per week, and support with establishing relapse prevention plans), and/or residential treatment (inpatient rehabilitation; lengths of stay may range from several weeks to several months).
Physician or Nurse Practitioner Primary Care	Some primary care practices have incorporated mental illness management within their practice settings, particularly in areas where specialists are not readily accessible.
Telemedicine	Some mental health organizations provide counseling and medication management via televideo interaction. Typically, these services are provided by psychiatrists and nurse practitioners.
General Hospital Inpatient Psychiatric Units	These units provide inpatient psychiatric care primarily for the purpose of assessment, monitoring and safety, medication management, and referral to outpatient mental health services for ongoing care. Typically staffed by a broad range of mental health professionals working as an interdisciplinary team that may include occupational or activities therapists, pastoral counselors, and mental health technicians in addition to psychiatrists, nurses, and social workers. Lengths of stay typically average 3 to 5 days.
State Psychiatric Hospitals	These are government-run inpatient treatment facilities with a broad range of mental health professionals, as listed previously. Provide public mental health services for those unable to afford private services. Lengths of stay vary from several days to months or even years, depending on patient needs.

Stigma

Even with accessible, evidence-based screening tools and clear pathways for referral to mental health specialists, interventions can be derailed when the mental health client is stigmatized. **Stigmatization** has been identified as a barrier to effective mental illness treatment in primary care, emergency departments, medical-surgical settings, and even at times in psychiatric settings.

One of the negative outcomes of stigma is that individuals with mental illnesses or addictions may not seek treatment at all, which can have devastating consequences on the progression of the illness and may leave many other physical illnesses undetected and untreated. This is an international problem, and in 2001, the World Health Organization (WHO, 2001) published a report recommending that mental health care be integrated in general health-care settings, including primary care settings, based on the premise that clients with mental illness may avoid mental health services because of the associated stigma. Since then, research has informed us that there are several concerns to be addressed when the mental health client seeks help in a nonpsychiatric setting as well, particularly knowledge gaps, clinical skills, and stigma (Beaulieu et al., 2017; Gwaikolo et al., 2017; J. Li et al., 2014; Ng et al., 2017). In one study, it was found that clients, on average, consulted more than three caregivers in a general hospital setting, and that 75% did not receive a diagnosis or treatment (X. Li et al., 2014). Knowledge gaps about mental illnesses and attitudes toward the client manifesting symptoms of mental illness or substance addiction are primary influences. Ng and associates (2017) specifically studied nurses' attitudes and found that previous psychiatric training, a desire to learn about neuropsychiatric illnesses, and positive contact with people who have mental illnesses were associated with less stigmatizing attitudes. It is difficult to understand the lack of desire to be knowledgeable about a group of illnesses that have such a significant impact on all aspects of nursing care, but sometimes it is related to myths, fear, and stigma. Efforts to increase social contact and understand the *person* are important strategies to reduce stigma, but it first requires the nurse's willingness to engage meaningfully with people who have mental illnesses and addictions.

Social distancing is an aspect of stigma that refers to the tendency of health-care workers and others to avoid people with mental illness or addiction. This is different from the usage of the term that has become popularized as a strategy to reduce the spread of coronavirus disease (COVID-19). In the context of mental health, social distancing refers to a stigmatizing avoidance of patients when confronted with symptoms that are poorly understood or difficult to manage. Symptoms like hallucinations, neglect of self-care, and agitation can be challenging symptoms for clinicians to manage when they feel frightened or ill equipped to intervene effectively. Reavely and Jorm (2015) found that mental health clients reported similar avoidance behaviors among family and friends. These findings clarify the extent of the marginalization and disenfranchisement experienced by many individuals with mental illness and substance use disorders.

In a study of nurses in primary care settings (Ihalainen-Tamlander et al., 2016), researchers found that nurses' attitudes toward mental health clients were generally positive, but that less-experienced nurses or those without additional mental health training were more fearful and more likely to think that mental health patients should be segregated. The authors highlight the importance of ongoing on-the-job training, especially for less-experienced nurses, to increase confidence, reduce fear, and prevent the development of stigmatizing and distancing attitudes. Several studies validate that education programs, consultation with mental health professionals to increase comfort and skill levels, and exposure to individuals with mental illness or substance use disorders are effective tools in reducing negative stereotyping, social distancing, and other stigmatizing attitudes and behaviors (Beaulieu et al., 2017; Flanagan et al., 2016; J. Li et al., 2014; Ng et al., 2017).

Student nurses who have been educated about mental illnesses, communication, and intervention strategies; have developed an awareness of the problems associated with stigma; and have had encounters with patients in treatment for mental illness and/or substance use disorders enter the workforce in a unique position to spearhead culture change. Many chapters within this text, particularly those with the "Real People, Real Stories" features, provide important information to improve the nurse's knowledge and confidence in caring for clients with mental illness in any practice setting. To effectively apply those skills and knowledge requires that the nurse have a clear understanding of their role in this regard.

The Role of the Nurse in Caring for Patients With Psychiatric and Substance Use Disorders in Nonpsychiatric Settings

The nurse's role in caring for patients with psychiatric and substance use disorders in nonpsychiatric settings includes the following:

- Examine one's personal beliefs and attitudes about individuals with mental illness and substance use disorders, focusing on contributing factors such as fear or lack of confidence in managing the patient's needs.
- Develop awareness of the negative impact of stigmatization on provision of appropriate care and actively seek knowledge and skills needed to increase confidence in patient care management.
- Identify patients with potentially high-prevalence, high-risk mental health issues who require universal screening in any health-care setting.
- Use evidence-based screening tools to identify patients needing further evaluation and/or referral to mental health or substance use disorder services.
- Provide for patient safety, up to and including continuous monitoring, while determinations are being made about referral needs.
- Establish a working knowledge of available mental health services for referral and collaborate with physicians and other members of the health-care team to identify the most appropriate resources.
- Engage the patient throughout the assessment and referral process using a patient-centered approach that empowers the patient in decision making about care recommendations to the best of their ability.

All nurses will encounter patients with mental illness and substance use disorders, regardless of the practice setting. It is imperative that each nurse recognize their role in reducing stigma personally and within the culture of the care team and provide the same attention to screening, intervention, and referral that is provided for patients with other chronic illnesses. This necessary foundation for nursing care addresses priority health-care needs, reduces poorer outcomes, improves individuals' quality of life, and minimizes the risks of premature death.

Summary and Key Points

- In the United States and globally, clients with psychiatric illness and substance use disorders are vulnerable to lack of or inadequate treatment, and this is associated with poorer outcomes with regard to the mental illness, undetected physical illnesses, and early death.
- *Diagnostic overshadowing* is a process of wrongly assuming that the patient's medical symptoms are attributable to their mental illness.
- Three variables that influence nurses' responses to the patient with mental health and substance use disorders are lack of education and recognition of symptoms, lack of appropriate screening, and nurses' attitudes about patients with these illnesses.
- Many evidence-based screening tools exist for detection of mental illness or substance use disorders. Some are easily accessible, free to use, and time efficient.
- Because of the high risk of morbidity and mortality, high prevalence, and risk that patients are not openly forthcoming about these issues, all patients should be screened for trauma history, substance use, and risk for suicide.
- One of the identified barriers to adequate screening of mental health issues in nonpsychiatric settings is competing workload demands. Nurses and nurse managers have a responsibility to prioritize mental illnesses and substance abuse as critical public health-care issues.
- Another identified barrier to appropriate screening and intervention is *social distancing*, which refers to the nurses' avoidance of patients with mental illnesses because of fear, lack of knowledge, lack of confidence in clinical skills, and stigma.
- Nurses in nonpsychiatric settings must have a working knowledge of available resources for referral when mental health and substance abuse are identified concerns. SAMHSA provides online information about available mental health and addictions services for every locality in the United States.
- *Referral* is a collaborative process with members of the health-care team, including the patient.
- *Patient-centered care* requires that nurses listen to the patient, empower the patient in decision making around their care, develop a collaborative partnership, and only make decisions for the patient (such as involuntary hospitalization) when they are clearly unable to and when it is necessary to protect their safety.
- *Stigmatization* is the devaluing, marginalizing, and disenfranchising of certain patients because of

symptoms or conditions. Stigmatizing patients with psychiatric and substance use disorders is an international concern contributing to patient neglect, inadequate treatment, avoidance of health-care professionals and treatment settings, and risk of early death.

- The first step for every nurse in accomplishing safe, effective care for the patient with mental health and substance use disorders is reflection on one's own beliefs, attitudes, and behaviors, and actively making efforts to reduce stigma personally and within the culture of their practice setting.

Review Questions

Select the answer that is most appropriate for each of the following questions:

1. A client enters the emergency department and reports, "My bed is on fire, and my stomach, and we're all dead." The nurse's initial response is to call the psychiatric unit to secure an inpatient bed for this patient. This is an example of:
   a. Prompt, appropriate referral
   b. Patient-centered care
   c. Stigmatization
   d. Collaboration
2. One of the outcomes of diagnostic overshadowing in clients with mental illness is:
   a. Better quality of life
   b. Increased access to resources
   c. More comprehensive care
   d. Increased risk for death
3. The nurse is reviewing discharge instructions with a client being discharged following a total knee replacement. Knowing that the client has a history of bipolar disorder, the nurse asks the client what needs they perceive they have related to this mental illness. This is an example of:
   a. Patient-centered care
   b. Diagnostic overshadowing
   c. Stigmatization
   d. Discrimination
4. Screening for substance use disorders and suicide risk should occur in which of the following practice settings?
   a. Emergency departments
   b. Primary care settings
   c. Medical units
   d. All of the above

Clinical Judgment Questions

5. A client presents in the emergency department loudly proclaiming with rapid speech, "If I don't get more pain medication right now, I'm going to call the attorney general and sue the entire health-care network." Which condition should be included in initial screening and assessment? (Select all that apply.)
   a. Substance use
   b. Pain
   c. Mental Illness
   d. Prior history of convictions
   e. Availability of an inpatient psychiatric bed

Continued

6. A client was admitted to the intensive care unit after a single car accident in which they struck a cement wall. The client is now responsive and wants to be discharged within the next couple of days. Which of the following are priorities for screening? (Select all that apply.)
   a. Traumatic brain injury
   b. Chronic pain
   c. Sexual dysfunction
   d. Depression and risk for suicide
7. The nurse manager recognizes a need to improve mental health and substance use screening and referral services for their clients in the public health clinic. Which of the following is a priority to begin an effective process for implementation?
   a. Provide a list of referral sources that is readily available to staff.
   b. Educate staff about the importance of prioritizing these public health concerns.
   c. Explore the literature for evidence-based screening tools.
   d. Inform the staff that they have been stigmatizing patients and this will not be tolerated.
8. A client on a medical unit is identified as having suicidal ideation. Which of the following is a priority in managing immediate care?
   a. Screen for depression
   b. Provide sedative medication
   c. Refer client to another setting
   d. Continuous monitoring and observation

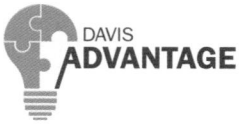

Go to **Davis Advantage** to complete your learning: strengthen understanding, apply your knowledge, and prepare for the Next Gen NCLEX®.

References

Akiskal, H. S. (2017). Mood disorders: Historical introduction and conceptual overview. In B. J. Sadock, V. A. Sadock, & P. Ruiz (Eds.), *Comprehensive textbook of psychiatry* (pp. 1599–1603). Wolters Kluwer.

Allen, J., Annells, M., Nunn, R., Petrie, E., Clark, E., Lang, L., & Robins, A. (2011). Evaluation of effectiveness and satisfaction outcomes of a mental health screening and referral clinical pathway for community nursing care. *Journal of Psychiatric and Mental Health Nursing, 18*(5), 375–385.

American Academy of Pediatrics. (2018). *Developmental, behavioral, psychosocial screening and assessment forms.* https://brightfutures.aap.org/materials-and-tools/tool-and-resource-kit/Pages/Developmental-Behavioral-Psychosocial-Screening-and-Assessment-Forms.aspx

Bay, N., Bjørnestad, J., Johannessen, J. O., Larsen, T. K., & Joa, I. (2016). Obstacles to care in first-episode psychosis patients with a long duration of untreated psychosis. *Early Intervention in Psychiatry, 10*(1), 71–76. https://doi.org/10.1111/eip.12152

Beaulieu, T., Patten, S., Knaak, S., Weinerman, R., Campbell, H., & Lauria-Horner, B. (2017). Impact of skill-based approaches in reducing stigma in primary care physicians: Results from a double-blind, parallel-cluster, randomized controlled trial. *The Canadian Journal of Psychiatry, 62*(5), 327–335.

Betz, M. E., Sullivan, A. F., Manton, A. P., Espinola, J. A., Miller, I., Camargo Jr, C. A., Boudreaux, E. D., & ED-SAFE Investigators. (2013). Knowledge, attitudes, and practices of emergency department providers in the care of suicidal patients. *Depression & Anxiety, 30*(10), 1005–1012.

Bica, T., Castelló, R., Toussaint, L. L., & Montesó-Curto, P. (2017). Depression as a risk factor of organic diseases: An international integrative review. *Journal of Nursing Scholarship, 49*(4), 389–399.

Brooker, C., Ricketts, T., Bennett, S., & Lemme, F. (2007). Admission decisions following contact with an emergency mental health assessment and intervention service. *Journal of Clinical Nursing, 16*(7), 1313–1322.

Bruce, M. L., Brown, E. L., Raue, P. J., Mlodzianowski, A. E., Meyers, B. S., Leon, A. C., & Nassisi, P. (2007). A randomized trial of depression assessment intervention in home health care. *Journal of the American Geriatrics Society, 55*(11), 1793–1800.

Chen, Y., Yu, S., Hu, Y., Li, R. C., Artaud, F., Carcaillon-Bentata, L., Elbaz, A., & Lee, P. (2020). Risk of suicide among patients with Parkinson disease. *JAMA Psychiatry.* Advance online publication. https://doi.org/10.1001/jamapsychiatry.2020.4001

Flanagan, E. H., Buck, T., Gamble, A., Hunter, C., Sewell, I., & Davidson, L. (2016). "Recovery speaks": A photovoice intervention to reduce stigma among primary care providers. *Psychiatric Services, 67*(5), 566–569. https://doi.org/10.1176/appi.ps.201500049

Fuller-Thomson, E., Rivière, R. N., Carrique, L., & Agbeyaka, S. (2020). The dark side of ADHD: Factors associated with suicide attempts among those with ADHD in a national representative Canadian sample. *Archives of Suicide Research,* 1–19. https://doi.org/10.1080/13811118.2020.1856258

Garcia de la Garza, A., Blanco, C., Olfson, M., & Wall, M. M. (2021). Identification of suicide attempt risk factors in a national US survey using machine learning. *JAMA Psychiatry, 78*(4), 398–406. https://doi.org/10.1001/jamapsychiatry.2020.4165

Gomes, J., Duraes, D., & Lima, G. (2015). Stigma kills. *European Psychiatry, 1*(30), 1863. https://doi.org/10.1016/S0924-9338(15)31427-9

Grundberg, Å. (2016). District nurses' perspectives on detecting mental health problems and promoting mental health among community-dwelling seniors with multimorbidity. *Journal of Clinical Nursing, 25*(17/18), 2590–2599.

Guttmacher Institute. (2021). *Substance use during pregnancy.* https://www.guttmacher.org/state-policy/explore/substance-use-during-pregnancy

Gwaikolo, W. S., Kohrt, B. A., & Cooper, J. L. (2017). Health system preparedness for integration of mental health services in rural Liberia. *BMC Health Services Research, 17*, 1–10.

Hasche, L. K., Lee, M. J., Proctor, E. K., & Morrow-Howell, N. (2013). Does identification of depression affect community long-term care services ordered for older adults? *Social Work Research, 37*(3), 255–262.

Horowitz, L. M., Snyder, D., Ludi, E., Rosenstein, D. L., Kohn-Godbout, J., Lee, L., Cartledge, T., Farrrar, A., & Pao, M. (2013). Ask suicide-screening questions to everyone in medical settings: The asQ'em Quality Improvement Project. *Psychosomatics 54*(3), 239–247.

Ihalainen-Tamlander, N., Vähäniemi, A., Löyttyniemi, E., Suominen, T., & Välimäki, M. (2016). Stigmatizing attitudes in nurses towards people with mental illness: A cross-sectional study in primary settings in Finland. *Journal of Psychiatric and Mental Health Nursing, 23*(6–7), 427–437. https://doi.org/10.1111/jpm.12319

Institute of Medicine, Committee on the Health Professions Education Summit. (2003). *Health professions education: A bridge to quality.* National Academy of Sciences.

Jackman, K., Honig, J., & Bockting, W. (2016). Nonsuicidal self-injury among lesbian, gay, bisexual and transgender populations: An integrative review. *Journal of Clinical Nursing, 25*(23/24), 3438–3453.

Jobes, D. A. (2015, September). *Clinical suicidology: Innovations in assessment treatment of suicidal risk* [Paper presentation]. Psychiatric Grand Rounds, Summa Health Systems, Akron, OH.

Kameg, K. M., Spencer Woods, A., Luther Szpak, J., & McCormick, M. (2013). Identifying and managing nonsuicidal self-injurious behavior in the primary care setting. *Journal of the American Association of Nurse Practitioners, 25*(4), 167–172.

Kölves, K., Fitzgerald, C., Nordentoft, M., Wood, S. J., & Erlangsen, A. (2021). Assessment of suicidal behaviors among individuals with autism spectrum disorder in Denmark. *JAMA Network Open. 4*(1), e2033565. https://doi.org/10.1001/jamanetworkopen.2020.33565

Koposov, R., Fossum, S., Frodl, T., NytrØ, O., Leventhal, B., Sourander, A., Quaglini, S., Molteni, M., Iglesia Vayá, M., Prokosch, H. U., Barbarini, N., Milham, M. P., Castellanos, F. X., & Skokauskas, N. (2017). Clinical decision support systems in child and adolescent psychiatry: A systematic review. *European Child & Adolescent Psychiatry, 26*(11), 1309–1317.

Langdon, R., Johnson, M., Carroll, V., & Antonio, G. (2013). Assessment of the elderly: It's worth covering the risks. *Journal of Nursing Management, 21*(1), 94–105.

Lauder, W., Ludwick, R., Zeller, R., & Winchell, J. (2006). Factors influencing nurses' judgements about self-neglect cases. *Journal of Psychiatric & Mental Health Nursing, 13*(3), 279–287.

Li, J., Li, J., Huang, Y., & Thornicroft, G. (2014). Mental health training program for community mental health staff in Guangzhou, China: Effects on knowledge of mental illness and stigma. *International Journal of Mental Health Systems, 8*(1), 49.

Li, X., Zhang, W., Lin, Y., Zhang, X., Qu, Z., Wang, X., Zhang, Y., Xu, H., Zhao, S., Li, Y., Tian, D. (2014). Pathways to psychiatric care of patients from rural regions: A general-hospital-based study. *International Journal of Social Psychiatry, 60*(3), 280–289. https://doi.org/10.1177/0020764013485364

McGovern, A., & Selwyn, J. (2014). A quality improvement project: Improving recognition of low mood and depression in elderly inpatients. *Age & Ageing, 43* (Suppl. 2), ii7–ii7.

Mitchell, A. J., Hussain, N., Grainger, L., & Symonds, P. (2011). Identification of patient-reported distress by clinical nurse specialists in routine oncology practice: A multicentre UK study. *Psycho-Oncology, 20*(10), 1076–1083.

Mollard, E., Brage Hudson, D., Ford, A., & Pullen, C. (2016). An integrative review of postpartum depression in rural U.S. communities. *Archives of Psychiatric Nursing, 30*(3), 418–424.

Moran, G. E., Daniels, A. S., & Ghose, S. S. (2018). Screening for behavioral health conditions in primary care settings: A systematic review of the literature. *Journal of General Internal Medicine, 33*(3), 335–346. https://doi.org/10.1007/s11606-017-4181-0

National Alliance on Mental Illness. (2021). *Mental health screening.* https://www.nami.org/Advocacy/Policy-Priorities/Intervene-Early/Mental-Health-Screening

Ndetei, D. M., Khasakhala, L. I., Mutiso, V., & Mbwayo, A. W. (2011). Knowledge, attitude and practice (KAP) of mental illness among staff in general medical facilities in Kenya: Policy implications. *African Journal of Psychiatry, 14*(3), 225–235.

Ng, Y. P., Rashid, A., & O'Brien, F. (2017). Determining the effectiveness of a video-based contact intervention in improving attitudes of Penang primary care nurses towards people with mental illness. *PloS ONE, 12*(11), 1–19.

Pardee, M. L., Kuzma, E., Dahlem, C. H., Boucher, N., & Darling-Fisher, C. (2017). Current state of screening high-ACE youth and emerging adults in primary care: Screening of high-ACE youth in primary care settings. *Journal of the American Association of Nurse Practitioners, 29.* https://doi.org/10.1002/2327-6924.12531

Préville, M., Côté, G., Boyer, R., & Hébert, R. (2004). Detection of depression and anxiety disorders by home care nurses. *Aging & Mental Health, 8*(5), 400–409.

Rahm, A. K., Boggs, J. M., Martin, C., Price, D. W., Beck, A., Backer, T. E., & Dearing, J. W. (2015). Facilitators and barriers to implementing screening, brief intervention, and referral to treatment (SBIRT) in primary care in integrated health care settings. *Substance Abuse, 36*(3), 281–288.

Reavely, N. J., & Jorm, A. F. (2015). Experiences of discrimination and positive treatment in people with mental health problems: Findings from an Australian national survey. *Australian and New Zealand Journal of Psychiatry, 49*(10), 906–913. https://doi.org/10.1177/0004867415602068

Roberge, P., Hudon, C., Pavilanis, A., Beaulieu, M., Benoit, A., Brouillet, H., Boulianne, I., De Pauw, A., Frigon, S., Gaboury, I., Gaudreault, M., Girard, A., Giroux, M, Grégoire, E., Langlois, L., Lemieux, M., Loignon, C., & Vanasse, A. (2016). A qualitative study of perceived needs and factors associated with the quality of care for common mental disorders in patients with chronic diseases: The perspective of primary care clinicians and patients. *BMC Family Practice, 17*, 1–14.

Sansone, R., & Sansone, L. (2010). Measuring self-harm behavior with the Self-Harm Inventory. *Psychiatry, 7*(4), 16–20.

Singer, S., Brown, A., Einenkel, J., Hauss, J., Hinz, A., Klein, A., Papsdorf, K., Stolzenburg, J. U., & Brähler, E. (2011). Identifying tumor patients' depression. *Supportive Care in Cancer, 19*(11), 1697–1703.

Substance Abuse and Mental Health Services Administration. (2020). *About screening, brief intervention, and referral to treatment (SBIRT).* https://www.samhsa.gov/sbirt/about

Thompson, P., Lang, L., & Annells, M. (2008). A systematic review of the effectiveness of in-home community nurse led interventions for the mental health of older persons. *Journal of Clinical Nursing, 17*(11), 1419–1427.

World Health Organization. (2001). *The World Health Report 2001. Mental health: New understanding, new hope.* http://www.who.int/whr/2001/en/whr01_en.pdf

Classical References

Felitti, V. J., Anda, R. F., Nordenberg, D., Williamson, D. F., Spitz, A. M., Edwards, V., Koss, M. P., & Marks, J. S. (1998). Relationship of childhood abuse and household dysfunction to many of the leading causes of death in adults—The adverse childhood experiences (ACE) study. *American Journal of Preventive Medicine, 14,* 245–258.

Hoff, L. A., & Rosenbaum, L. (1994). A victimization assessment tool: Instrument development and clinical implications. *Journal of Advanced Nursing, 20,* 627–634.

Hoff, L. A., & Ross, M. (1993). Curriculum guide for nursing: Violence against women and children. Ottawa, Canada: University of Ottawa, Faculty of Health Sciences, School of Nursing, Ottawa.

Schofferman, J., Anderson, D., Hines, R., Smith, G., & White, A. (1992). Childhood psychological trauma correlates with unsuccessful lumbar spine surgery. *Spine, 17*(Suppl.), 138–144.

Neurocognitive Disorders 13

CHAPTER OUTLINE

Objectives
Introduction
Delirium
Neurocognitive Disorder
Application of the Nursing Process
Treatment Modalities
Summary and Key Points
Review Questions
Clinical Judgment Questions
Test Your Clinical Reasoning and Clinical Judgment Skills
Communication Exercises
Movie Connections

CORE CONCEPTS

Intracranial Regulation: Delirium, Dementia (major neurocognitive disorder)
Professional Behavior: Nursing process in the care of patients with neurocognitive disorders
Safety
Clinical Judgment

KEY TERMS

aphasia
apraxia
ataxia
confabulation
delirium
dementia
neurocognitive disorders (NCDs)
pseudodementia
sundowning

OBJECTIVES

After reading this chapter, the student will be able to:

1. Define and differentiate among various neurocognitive disorders (NCDs).
2. Discuss predisposing factors implicated in the etiology of NCDs.
3. Describe clinical symptoms and use the information to assess patients with NCDs.
4. Identify nursing diagnoses common to patients with NCDs and select appropriate nursing interventions for each.
5. Identify topics for patient and family teaching relevant to NCDs.
6. Discuss criteria for evaluating nursing care of patients with NCDs.
7. Describe various treatment modalities relevant to care of patients with NCDs.

Introduction

Neurocognitive disorders (NCDs) include those in which a clinically significant deficit in cognition or memory exists, representing a significant change from a previous level of functioning. These disorders were previously identified in the *Diagnostic and Statistical Manual of Mental Disorders* (4th ed., text rev.; *DSM-IV-TR;* American Psychiatric Association [APA], 2000) as "Dementia, Delirium, Amnestic, and Other Cognitive Disorders." In the *DSM-5*, NCDs include delirium and the syndromes called major NCD or minor NCDs, which are further specified according to the underlying cause (such as Alzheimer's disease, Parkinson's disease, or others) (APA, 2013).

This chapter presents predisposing factors, clinical symptoms, and nursing interventions for care of patients with NCDs. The objective is to provide quality care, respect patients' dignity, and promote quality of life while offering guidance and support to their families or primary caregivers.

CORE CONCEPT

Delirium

Delirium is a mental state characterized by an acute disturbance of cognition, which is manifested by short-term confusion, excitement, disorientation, and a clouded consciousness. Hallucinations and illusions are common.

Delirium

Clinical Findings and Course

Delirium is characterized by a disturbance in attention and awareness and a change in cognition that develop rapidly over a short period (APA, 2013). Symptoms of delirium include difficulty sustaining and shifting attention. The person is very distractible and must be repeatedly reminded to focus attention. Disorganized thinking prevails and is reflected by speech that is rambling, irrelevant, pressured, and incoherent and that unpredictably switches from subject to subject. Reasoning ability and goal-directed behavior are impaired. Disorientation to time and place is common, and impairment of recent memory is invariably evident. Misperceptions of the environment (illusions) and false perceptions (hallucinations) are prominent. Disturbances in the sleep–wake cycle also occur.

The individual's state of awareness may range from that of hypervigilance (heightened awareness to environmental stimuli) to stupor or semicoma. Sleep may fluctuate between hypersomnolence (excessive sleepiness) and insomnia. Vivid dreams and nightmares are common.

Psychomotor activity may fluctuate between agitated, purposeless movements (e.g., restlessness, hyperactivity, striking out at nonexistent objects) and a vegetative state resembling catatonic stupor. Various forms of tremor are frequently present.

Emotional instability may be manifested by fear, anxiety, depression, irritability, anger, euphoria, or apathy. These various emotions may be evidenced by crying, calls for help, cursing, muttering, moaning, acts of self-destruction, fearful attempts to flee, or attacks on others who are falsely viewed as threatening. Autonomic manifestations, such as tachycardia, sweating, flushed face, dilated pupils, and elevated blood pressure, are common.

The symptoms of delirium usually begin quite abruptly (e.g., following a head injury or seizure). At other times, they may be preceded by several hours or days of prodromal symptoms (e.g., restlessness, difficulty thinking clearly, insomnia or hypersomnolence, and nightmares). The slower onset is more common if the underlying cause is systemic illness or metabolic imbalance.

The duration of delirium is usually brief (generally less than 1 week) and, upon elimination of the underlying causes, symptoms usually diminish over a 3- to 7-day period but in some instances may take as long as 2 weeks (Boland & Verduin, 2022). The age of the client and duration of the delirium influence rate of symptom resolution. Delirium is associated with a high mortality rate because of the seriousness of the precipitating medical conditions that precipitate delirium. At times, delirium may also shift into a more permanent cognitive disorder (e.g., major NCD).

Predisposing Factors

Delirium

Individuals most predisposed to developing delirium include those with serious medical, surgical, or neurological conditions, and sensory or cognitive impairments (such as dementia). People over 65 years of age are considered a high-risk group. Depression, falls, and elder abuse may also contribute to delirium. Other precipitating factors include the following (Boland & Verduin, 2022; Fabian & Solai, 2017):

- Systemic infections
- Febrile illness or hypothermia
- Metabolic disorders, such as electrolyte imbalances, hypercarbia, hypoglycemia, or hyponatremia
- Hypoxia and chronic obstructive pulmonary disease (COPD)
- Hepatic failure or renal failure
- Head trauma
- Seizures
- Migraine headaches
- Brain abscess or brain neoplasms
- Stroke
- Malnutrition or dehydration
- Uncontrolled pain
- Burns
- Heat stroke
- Orthopedic and cardiac surgeries
- Social isolation, emotional stress, physical restraints, admission to an intensive care unit

Other Causes of Delirium

Substance Intoxication Delirium

In this case, the symptoms of delirium are attributed to intoxication from certain substances, such as alcohol, amphetamines, cannabis, cocaine, hallucinogens, inhalants, opioids, phencyclidine, sedative, hypnotic, and anxiolytics, or other (or unknown) substance.

Substance Withdrawal Delirium

Withdrawal from certain substances can precipitate symptoms of delirium that are sufficiently severe to warrant clinical attention. These substances include alcohol, opioids, sedatives, hypnotics or anxiolytics, and others.

Medication-Induced Delirium

Medications that have been known to precipitate delirium include antibiotics, antivirals, antifungals, anticholinergics, antihypertensives, corticosteroids, anticonvulsants, cardiac glycosides, analgesics, anesthetics, antineoplastic agents, antiparkinson drugs, H_2-receptor antagonists (e.g., cimetidine), and others (Boland & Verduin, 2022; Fabian & Solai, 2017). In addition, polypharmacy is, at times, implicated in precipitating delirium.

Delirium Due to Another Medical Condition or to Multiple Etiologies

Evidence from the history, physical examination, or laboratory findings may indicate that the symptoms of delirium are associated with another medical condition or can be attributable to more than one cause. The current evidence supports that delirium is usually the result of many factors rather than one (Fabian & Solai, 2017).

CORE CONCEPT

Neurocognitive

A term that is used to describe cognitive functions closely linked to particular areas of the brain that have to do with thinking, reasoning, memory, learning, and speaking.

Neurocognitive Disorder

Neurocognitive disorder (NCD) is classified in the *DSM-5* (APA, 2013) as either *mild* or *major*, distinguished primarily by the severity of symptomatology. In some settings, mild NCD is called *mild cognitive impairment* and is a focus of early intervention, which is critical to preventing or slowing the progression of the disorder. Major NCD was previously described as *dementia* in the *DSM-IV-TR* (APA, 2000). In progressive neurodegenerative conditions, these two diagnoses (mild or major NCD) may serve to identify earlier and later stages of the same disorder. Either diagnosis may be appropriate (depending on severity of symptoms) for certain other NCDs that are the result of a reversible or temporary condition. *DSM-5* criteria for these disorders are presented in Box 13–1.

CORE CONCEPT

Dementia (major neurocognitive disorder)

Dementia is a general term for the impaired ability to remember, think, or make decisions that that is severe enough to interfere with social, behavioral, occupational, and emotional functioning. Several different disease processes can culminate in dementia. Unlike delirium, the progression of cognitive decline occurs slowly, over time. In some cases, dementia may be reversible.

Clinical Findings, Epidemiology, and Course

An estimated 5.8 million people in the United States currently have Alzheimer's disease (AD), the most common form of NCD, and the prevalence (the number of people with the disease at any one time) increases dramatically with age, affecting about 3% of individuals between 65 and 74, 17% of individuals between 75 and 84, and 32% of individuals 85 and older (Alzheimer's Association, 2020). Although a small percentage of those with AD are under age 65, the majority (80%) are over age 75. Despite these age-related increases, AD is not a normal part of aging. Almost two-thirds of Americans with AD are women, and there is a disproportionately higher prevalence in black/African American and Hispanics/Latinos than among non-Hispanic whites (Alzheimer's Association, 2020). It is projected that by 2050, the number of individuals age 65 and older with AD will nearly triple if current population trends continue and no preventive treatments become available (Alzheimer's Association, 2020).

The increase in AD incidence is not the result of an "epidemic." The greatest risk factor for AD is age, and the population of older adults in the United States continues to grow. Survival after diagnosis typically ranges from 4 to 8 years, with most of that time spent in the most severe stage. Despite the alarming

BOX 13–1 A Comparison of Diagnostic Criteria

Mild Neurocognitive Disorder	Major Neurocognitive Disorder
A. Evidence of modest cognitive decline from a previous level of performance in one or more cognitive domains (complex attention, executive function, learning and memory, language, perceptual-motor, or social cognition) based on: 1. Concern of the individual, a knowledgeable informant, or the clinician that there has been a mild decline in cognitive function; and 2. A modest impairment in cognitive performance, preferably documented by standardized neuropsychological testing, or, in its absence, another quantified clinical assessment. B. The cognitive deficits do not interfere with capacity for independence in everyday activities (i.e., complex instrumental activities of daily living such as paying bills or managing medications are preserved, but greater effort, compensatory strategies, or accommodation may be required). C. The cognitive deficits do not occur exclusively in the context of a delirium. D. The cognitive deficits are not better explained by another mental disorder (e.g., major depressive disorder, schizophrenia). Specify whether due to: ▪ Alzheimer's disease ▪ Frontotemporal lobar degeneration ▪ Lewy body disease ▪ Vascular disease ▪ Traumatic brain injury ▪ Substance/medication use ▪ HIV infection ▪ Prion disease ▪ Parkinson's disease ▪ Huntington's disease ▪ Another medical condition ▪ Multiple etiologies ▪ Unspecified Specify: ***Without behavioral disturbance:*** If the cognitive disturbance is not accompanied by any clinically significant behavioral disturbance. ***With behavioral disturbance*** *(specify disturbance):* If the cognitive disturbance is accompanied by a clinically significant behavioral disturbance (e.g., psychotic symptoms, mood disturbance, agitation, apathy, or other behavioral symptoms).	A. Evidence of significant cognitive decline from a previous level of performance in one or more cognitive domains (complex attention, executive function, learning and memory, language, perceptual-motor, or social cognition) based on: 1. Concern of the individual, a knowledgeable informant, or the clinician that there has been a significant decline in cognitive function; and 2. A substantial impairment in cognitive performance, preferably documented by standardized neuropsychological testing, or, in its absence, another quantified clinical assessment. B. The cognitive deficits interfere with independence in everyday activities (i.e., at a minimum, requiring assistance with complex instrumental activities of daily living such as paying bills or managing medications). C. The cognitive deficits do not occur exclusively in the context of a delirium. D. The cognitive deficits are not better explained by another mental disorder (e.g., major depressive disorder, schizophrenia). Specify whether due to: ▪ Alzheimer's disease ▪ Frontotemporal lobar degeneration ▪ Lewy body disease ▪ Vascular disease ▪ Traumatic brain injury ▪ Substance/medication use ▪ HIV infection ▪ Prion disease ▪ Parkinson's disease ▪ Huntington's disease ▪ Another medical condition ▪ Multiple etiologies ▪ Unspecified Specify: ***Without behavioral disturbance:*** If the cognitive disturbance is not accompanied by any clinically significant behavioral disturbance. ***With behavioral disturbance*** *(specify disturbance):* If the cognitive disturbance is accompanied by a clinically significant behavioral disturbance (e.g., psychotic symptoms, mood disturbance, agitation, apathy, or other behavioral symptoms). Specify current severity: ***Mild:*** Difficulties with instrumental activities of daily living (e.g., housework, managing money) ***Moderate:*** Difficulties with basic activities of daily living (e.g., feeding, dressing) ***Severe:*** Fully dependent

Source: Reprinted with permission from the Diagnostic and Statistical Manual of Mental Disorders, Fifth Edition *(Copyright 2013). American Psychiatric Association.*

statistics about AD, recent studies have indicated that dementia, in general, has declined in the United States over the past few years. This trend could be a temporary change or may be related to improved treatment and education about risk factors associated with heart disease and stroke, which are responsible for some forms of dementia (Langa et al., 2017).

NCDs can be classified as either primary or secondary. Primary NCDs are those, such as AD, in which the NCD itself is the major sign of some organic brain disease not directly related to any other organic illness. Secondary NCDs are caused by or related to another disease or condition, such as HIV disease or a cerebral trauma.

In NCD, impairment is evident in abstract thinking, judgment, and impulse control. The conventional rules of social conduct are often disregarded. Behavior may be uninhibited and inappropriate. Personal appearance and hygiene are often neglected. Language may or may not be affected. Some individuals may have difficulty naming objects, or the language may seem vague and imprecise. In severe forms of NCD, the individual may not speak at all **(aphasia)**. The client may know their needs but may not know how to communicate those needs to a caregiver.

Personality change is common in NCD and may be manifested by either an alteration or accentuation of premorbid characteristics. For example, an individual who was previously very socially active may become apathetic and socially isolated. A previously neat person may become markedly untidy in their appearance. Conversely, an individual who may have had difficulty trusting others prior to the illness may exhibit extreme fear and paranoia as manifestations of the disorder.

The reversibility of NCD is dependent on the basic etiology of the disorder. Truly reversible NCD occurs in only a small percentage of cases and might be more appropriately termed *temporary* NCD. Reversible causes of NCD (dementia or dementia-like symptoms) include some brain tumors, subdural hematomas, depression, medication reactions, normal pressure hydrocephalus, vitamin/nutritional deficiencies (especially B_1, B_6, and B_{12}), central nervous system (CNS) infections, thyroid disorders, too much or too little sodium or calcium, immune disorders (multiple sclerosis), and metabolic disorders (hypoglycemia) (Mayo Clinic, 2021a). In most clients, NCD runs a progressive, irreversible course.

As the disease progresses, **apraxia,** the inability to carry out purposeful motor activities despite intact motor function and the inability to use objects properly, may develop. The individual may be irritable or moody or may exhibit sudden outbursts over trivial issues. The ability to work or care for personal needs independently will no longer be possible. These individuals can no longer be left alone because they do not comprehend their limitations and are at serious risk for accidents. Wandering away from the home or care setting often becomes a problem. In advanced dementia, clinical features include profound memory deficits, minimal verbal communication, loss of ambulatory ability, inability to perform activities of daily living (ADLs), and incontinence. The most common clinical complications are eating problems and infections (Mitchell, 2015).

Several causes have been described for NCD (see section "Predisposing Factors"), but AD is the most common cause of dementia in older adults, accounting for 60% to 80% of all cases (Alzheimer's Association, 2020). The progressive nature of symptoms associated with AD has been described in seven stages (National Institute on Aging [NIA], 2017; WebMD, 2021):

Stage 1. No apparent symptoms: In the first stage of the illness, there is no apparent decline in memory despite changes that are beginning to occur in the brain; a positron emission tomography (PET) scan can be used to detect these changes.

Stage 2. Very mild change: The individual begins to lose things or forget names of people. Losses in short-term memory are common. The individual is aware of the intellectual decline and may feel ashamed, becoming anxious and depressed, which in turn may worsen the symptom. Maintaining organization with lists and a structured routine provides some compensation. These symptoms often are not noticed by others and do not interfere with the individual's ability to work or live independently.

Stage 3. Mild cognitive decline: In this stage there are changes in thinking and reasoning that interfere with work performance and become noticeable to coworkers. The individual may get lost when driving a car. Concentration may be interrupted. There is difficulty recalling names or words, which becomes noticeable to family and close associates. A decline occurs in the ability to plan or organize.

Stage 4. Moderate cognitive decline: At this stage, individuals may forget major events in personal history, such as their own child's birthday; experience declining ability to perform tasks, such as shopping, cooking, and managing personal finances; or be unable to understand current news events. They may deny that a problem exists by covering up memory loss with **confabulation** (creating imaginary events to fill in memory gaps). Depression and social withdrawal are common. At this stage the individual requires some assistance to maintain safety.

Stage 5. Moderately severe cognitive decline: At this stage, individuals lose the ability to perform some ADLs independently, such as hygiene, dressing, and grooming, and require some assistance to manage these tasks on an ongoing basis. They may forget addresses, phone numbers, and names of close relatives. They may become disoriented about place and time, but they maintain knowledge about themselves. Frustration, withdrawal, and self-absorption are common.

Stage 6. Severe cognitive decline: At this stage, individuals may be unable to recall the name of their spouse or may misidentify people (e.g., thinking a child is their spouse). Disorientation to surroundings is common, and the person may be unable to recall the day, season, or year. The person is unable to manage ADLs without assistance. Delusions often become apparent, such as maintaining the belief that one must go to work even though the person is no longer employed. Urinary and fecal incontinence is common. Sleeping becomes a problem. Psychomotor symptoms include wandering, obsessiveness, agitation, and aggression. Symptoms seem to worsen in the late afternoon and evening—a phenomenon termed **sundowning.** Communication becomes more difficult with increasing loss of language skills. Institutional care is usually required at this stage.

Stage 7. Very severe decline: In the end stages of AD, individuals are unable to recognize family members. They most commonly are bedfast and aphasic. Problems of immobility, such as pressure injuries and contractures, may occur.

The NIA (2017) describes some specific symptoms of the latest stage of AD and associated care needs:

- Muscle immobility may require assistance from health-care professionals to move, position, and exercise patients with the goal of preventing contractures and pressure injuries.
- Individuals lose interest in food, lack awareness of mealtimes, or can't remember if they have eaten and therefore will require assistance to maintain adequate nutrition. In addition, chewing and swallowing difficulties are common, so supervision and assistance to prevent choking or aspiration pneumonia are important interventions.
- Body jerking (myoclonus) increases risk for injury; the physician may prescribe medication to ease these symptoms.

Predisposing Factors

NCDs are differentiated by their etiology, although they share a common symptom presentation. Categories include NCDs due to:

- AD
- Frontotemporal lobar degeneration
- Lewy body disease
- Vascular disease
- Traumatic brain injury
- Substances/medications
- HIV infection
- Prion disease
- Parkinson's disease
- Huntington's disease
- Another medical condition
- Multiple etiologies
- Unspecified

Neurocognitive Disorder Due to Alzheimer's Disease

AD is characterized by the syndrome of symptoms identified as mild or major NCD and by those listed in the seven stages described previously. The disease begins many years before the onset of symptoms; when symptoms begin to appear, the course is slow and insidious, generally progressive, and deteriorating. Memory impairment is a prominent feature.

Refinement of diagnostic criteria now enables clinicians to use specific clinical features to identify the disease with considerable accuracy. Examination by computerized tomography (CT) scan or magnetic resonance imagery (MRI) reveals a degenerative pathology of the brain that includes atrophy, widened cortical sulci, and enlarged cerebral ventricles (Figs. 13–1 and 13–2). Diagnostic tests reveal specific biomarkers, tau neurofibrillary tangles, and amyloid beta plaques in the brains of clients with AD through specialized PET scans and in cerebrospinal fluid. These changes apparently occur as a part of the normal aging process. However, in clients with AD, they are found in dramatically increased numbers, and their profusion is concentrated in the hippocampus and certain parts of the cerebral cortex. Recent research points to a mutation in microtubule affinity regulating kinase (MARK 4) as contributing to an accumulation and toxicity of tau proteins leading to neurodegeneration and pathogenesis in AD (Oba et al., 2020).

In 2018, the NIA and Alzheimer's Association redefined AD as identified by three specific biomarkers

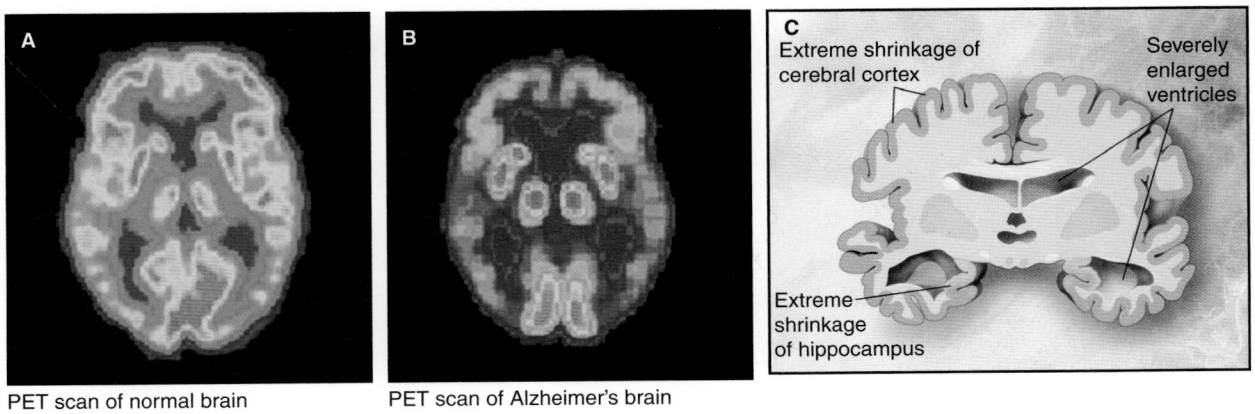

FIGURE 13–1 Changes in the Alzheimer's brain. A. Metabolic activity in a healthy brain. B. Diminished metabolic activity in the Alzheimer's diseased brain. C. Late-stage Alzheimer's disease with generalized atrophy and enlargement of the ventricles and sulci. (Source: Alzheimer's Disease Education & Referral Center, A Service of the National Institute on Aging.)

(amyloid beta plaques, tau neurofibrillary tangles, and neuronal damage) rather than by the progression of cognitive symptoms (Sullivan, 2018). It is believed that this redefinition will, in the short term, clarify research and clinical drug trials and in the long term may change the way AD is understood and treated. Other biomarkers, including lower levels of metabolites such as histamine, asparagine, aspartate, and citrulline (all involved in regulating inflammation), suggest that inflammation may be a key component in the pathology of this disease (Hampel et al., 2018). Because biomarkers are present before cognitive symptoms appear, the potential for preventive interventions will, no doubt, be the focus of ongoing research. Although researchers have identified evidence that mitochondrial dysfunction and inflammation are relevant in the development of AD, they are, as yet, unclear about the process (Perez Ortiz & Swerdlow, 2019).

Etiological Theories

The etiology of AD is unknown, but experts believe that with the exception of rare cases in which genetic mutations *cause* AD, multiple factors rather than a single cause influence the development of this illness (Alzheimer's Association, 2021a). It is known that genetic factors are influential in increasing *risk* for AD, and, particularly in late-onset AD, the risk is influenced by multiple genes and environmental factors and their interaction with amyloid beta proteins in the transition to AD (Graziane & Sweet, 2017). As previously mentioned, a recent research study highlighted the impact of a mutation in microtubule affinity regulating kinase (MARK 4) as contributing to an accumulation and toxicity of tau proteins leading to neurodegeneration and pathogenesis in AD (Oba et al., 2020). Several other findings in research studies have led to hypotheses about contributing or causative factors:

- ***Neurotransmitter alterations:*** Research indicates that in the brains of clients with AD, the enzyme required to produce acetylcholine is dramatically reduced (Boland & Verduin, 2022). The reduction seems to be greatest in the nucleus basalis, which lies in the basal forebrain area. This decrease in production of acetylcholine reduces the amount of the neurotransmitter that is released to cells in the cortex and hippocampus, resulting in cognitive process disturbances. Other neurotransmitters believed to be disrupted in AD include norepinephrine, serotonin, dopamine, and the amino acid glutamate. It has been proposed that in NCD, excess glutamate leads to overstimulation of the *N*-methyl-D-aspartate (NMDA) receptors, leading to increased intracellular calcium and subsequent neuronal degeneration and cell death. Decreased levels of somatostatin and corticotropin have also been found in individuals with AD.
- ***Plaques and tangles:*** As mentioned previously, an overabundance of structures called *plaques* and *tangles* appears in the brains of individuals with AD. The plaques are made of a peptide called amyloid beta (Aβ), which are fragments of a larger protein called amyloid precursor protein (APP). Plaques are formed when Aβ peptides clump together and mix with molecules and other cellular matter. Tangles are formed from a special kind of cellular protein called *tau protein*, whose function is to provide stability to the neuron. In AD, the tau protein is

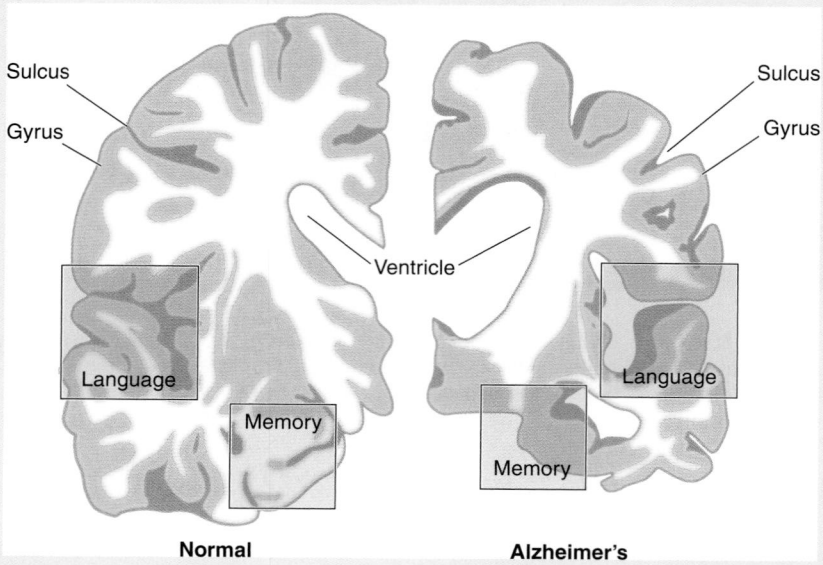

FIGURE 13–2 Neurobiology of Alzheimer's disease. Source: Copyright 2000 BrightFocus Foundation. https://www.brightfocus.org/alzheimers/infographic/brain-alzheimers-disease

NEUROTRANSMITTERS

A decrease in the neurotransmitter *acetylcholine* has been implicated in Alzheimer's disease. Cholinergic sources arise from the brainstem and the basal forebrain to supply areas of the basal ganglia, thalamus, limbic structures, hippocampus, and cerebral cortex.

Cell bodies of origin for the *serotonin* pathways lie within the raphe nuclei located in the brainstem. Those for *norepinephrine* originate in the locus ceruleus. Projections for both neurotransmitters extend throughout the forebrain, prefrontal cortex, cerebellum, and limbic system. *Dopamine* pathways arise from areas in the midbrain and project to the frontal cortex, limbic system, basal ganglia, and thalamus. Dopamine neurons in the hypothalamus innervate the posterior pituitary.

Glutamate, an excitatory neurotransmitter, has largely descending pathways, with highest concentrations in the cerebral cortex. It is also found in the hippocampus, thalamus, hypothalamus, cerebellum, and spinal cord.

AREAS OF THE BRAIN AFFECTED

Areas of the brain affected by Alzheimer's disease and associated symptoms include the following:

- ***Frontal lobe:*** Impaired reasoning ability; unable to solve problems and perform familiar tasks; poor judgment; inability to evaluate the appropriateness of behavior; aggressiveness.
- ***Parietal lobe:*** Impaired orientation ability; impaired visuospatial skills (unable to remain oriented within own environment).
- ***Occipital lobe:*** Impaired language interpretation; unable to recognize familiar objects.
- ***Temporal lobe:*** Inability to recall words; inability to use words correctly (language comprehension); in late stages, some clients experience delusions and hallucinations.
- ***Hippocampus:*** Impaired memory; short-term memory is affected initially; later, the individual is unable to form new memories.
- ***Amygdala:*** Impaired emotions: depression, anxiety, fear, personality changes, apathy, paranoia.
- ***Neurotransmitters:*** Alterations in acetylcholine, dopamine, norepinephrine, serotonin, and others may play a role in behaviors such as restlessness, sleep impairment, mood, and agitation.

MEDICATIONS AND THEIR EFFECTS ON THE BRAIN

1. Cholinesterase inhibitors (e.g., donepezil, rivastigmine, and galantamine) act by inhibiting acetylcholinesterase, which slows the degradation of acetylcholine, thereby increasing concentrations of the neurotransmitter in the brain. Most common side effects include dizziness, gastrointestinal upset, fatigue, and headache.
2. NMDA receptor antagonists (e.g., memantine) act by blocking NMDA receptors from excessive glutamate, preventing continuous influx of calcium into the cells, and ultimately slowing down neuronal degradation. Possible side effects include dizziness, headache, and constipation.

chemically altered. Strands of the protein become intertwined, interfering with the neuronal transport system. It should be noted that both plaques and neurofibrillary tangles are seen in other disorders and, to some extent, in the normal brain with increasing age (Boland & Verduin, 2022). Plaques and tangles are thought to contribute to the destruction and death of neurons, leading to memory failure, personality changes, inability to carry out ADLs, and other features of the disease. The plaques themselves can cause space-occupying lesions in the cortex, which contribute to inflammatory processes, synapse loss, and neuronal death (Graziane & Sweet, 2017). The number and density of these plaques (also called *amyloid plaques* or *senile plaques*) found in postmortem studies correlate with disease severity (Boland & Verduin, 2022).

- ***Head trauma:*** Individuals who have a history of head trauma are at risk for AD. Studies have shown that some individuals who had experienced head trauma subsequently (after years) developed AD. There is evidence that head trauma can increase inflammatory mediators, causing amyloid beta plaques to be deposited in the brain, and the effects of traumatic brain injury on amyloid beta plaque development may also be mediated by genetic factors (Graziane & Sweet, 2017).
- ***Genetic factors:*** A familial pattern is evident for some forms of AD, with as many as 40% of AD patients having a family history for the disease. Some families exhibit a pattern of inheritance that suggests possible autosomal-dominant gene transmission (Boland & Verduin, 2022). Some studies indicate that early-onset cases are more likely than late-onset cases to be familial, and that from one-third to one-half of all cases may be of the genetic form. Research indicates that there is a link between AD and gene mutations found on chromosomes 21, 14, and 1 (Graziane & Sweet, 2017). Mutations on chromosome 21 cause the formation of abnormal APP. Mutations on chromosome 14 cause abnormal presenilin 1 (PS-1) to be made, and mutations on chromosome 1 lead to the formation of abnormal presenilin 2 (PS-2). Each of these mutations results in an increased amount of the Aβ protein that is a major component of the plaques associated with AD. Individuals with Down's syndrome (who carry an extra copy of chromosome 21) have been found to be unusually susceptible to AD.

Late-onset AD is influenced by a gene known as apolipoprotein E (*APOE*) and particularly *APOE 4*, but in individuals with this genotype who do not have disease symptoms by the age of 65, only about 50% will develop AD (Graziane & Sweet, 2017). As research has continued, 20 additional influential genes have been identified, but their exact role in causing AD is still unclear. Although much of the research has focused on toxic amyloid and tau proteins in AD, current research is exploring other molecular and cellular pathways that may be involved in the development of this disease, including glial cell activation, inflammation, glucose transport systems, and abnormal neuronal circuit activity.

A study aimed at identifying biomarkers of AD before the onset of symptoms (Schindler et al., 2019) reports evidence that a blood test for amyloid levels, especially when considered along with age and presence of the *APOE4* gene variant, is 94% accurate in identifying people with early brain changes indicative of AD. Amyloid proteins begin to accumulate in the brain up to two decades before the onset of symptoms (Bhandari, 2019), and such a blood test, although not yet available for clinical use, could pave the way for identifying early prevention and treatment strategies. Other research found that individuals with the *APOE4* gene variant showed hippocampal atrophy and cortical thinning in early Alzheimer's disease, which suggests this may be a valuable biomarker and a target for research into medication that slows the processes of deterioration in these structures (Abushakra et al., 2020). Because previous research has demonstrated that ketone bodies have a protective effect on neurons, some research has focused on the impact of ketones in improving memory and learning. Several studies have reported the potential benefits of ketone-rich diets in slowing or improving cognitive decline in AD because blood sugar disorders have been associated with this disease (University Health News, 2019).

Vascular Neurocognitive Disorder

The cognitive symptoms in vascular NCD are caused by significant cerebrovascular disease. When blood flow in the brain is impaired, progressive intellectual deterioration occurs. Impairment may be located in large vessels or microvascular networks, and symptoms vary depending on the type, extent, and location of vascular lesion (APA, 2013). The disorder is more common in men than in women.

Vascular NCD differs from AD in that it has a more abrupt onset and a highly variable course. In vascular NCD, progression of the symptoms occurs in noticeable "steps" downward rather than as a gradual deterioration (Mayo Clinic, 2021b). At times the symptoms seem to subside and the individual exhibits fairly lucid thinking and better memory. The client may become optimistic that improvement is occurring, only to experience further decline of functioning in a fluctuating pattern of progression. This irregular pattern of decline can be an intense source of anxiety for clients with this disorder.

In vascular NCD, clients may suffer the equivalent of small strokes that destroy many areas of the brain. The pattern of deficits is variable, depending on which regions of the brain have been affected. Certain focal neurological signs are commonly seen with vascular NCD, including weaknesses of the limbs, small-stepped gait, and difficulty with speech. The disorder is more common in men than in women.

The cause of vascular NCD is directly related to an interruption of blood flow to the brain. Symptoms result from death of nerve cells in regions nourished by diseased vessels. Various diseases and conditions that interfere with blood circulation have been implicated.

High blood pressure is thought to be one of the most significant factors in the etiology of multiple small strokes or cerebral infarcts. Hypertension leads to damage to the lining of blood vessels. This damage can result in rupture of the blood vessel with subsequent hemorrhage or an accumulation of fibrin in the vessel with intravascular clotting and inhibited blood flow. NCD also can result from infarcts related to occlusion of blood vessels by particulate matter that travels through the bloodstream to the brain. These emboli may be solid (e.g., clots, cellular debris, platelet aggregates), gaseous (e.g., air, nitrogen), or liquid (e.g., fat, following soft tissue trauma or fracture of long bones).

Cognitive impairment can occur with multiple small infarcts (sometimes called "silent strokes") over time or with a single cerebrovascular event that occurs in a strategic area of the brain. An individual may have both vascular NCD and AD simultaneously, referred to as a *mixed* disorder, the prevalence of which is likely to increase as the population ages.

Frontotemporal Neurocognitive Disorder

Symptoms from frontotemporal NCD occur as a result of shrinking of the frontal and temporal anterior lobes of the brain. This type of NCD was identified as Pick's disease in the *DSM-IV-TR*. The cause of frontotemporal NCD is unknown, but a genetic factor appears to be involved because this disorder often runs in families. Symptoms tend to fall into two clinical patterns: (1) behavioral and personality changes and (2) speech and language problems. Common behavioral changes include "behavior that can be either impulsive (disinhibited) or bored and listless (apathetic) and includes inappropriate social behavior; lack of social tact; lack of empathy; distractibility; loss of insight into the behaviors of oneself and others; an increased interest in sex; changes in food preferences; agitation or, conversely, blunted emotions; neglect of personal hygiene; repetitive or compulsive behavior, and decreased energy and motivation" (National Institute of Neurological Disorders and Stroke [NINDS], 2019). Speech problems include impairment or loss of speech or increasing difficulty in using and understanding written and spoken language. Spatial skills and memory remain intact, but the disease progresses steadily and often rapidly, ranging from less than 2 years in some individuals to more than 10 years in others (NINDS, 2019).

Neurocognitive Disorder Due to Traumatic Brain Injury

According to *DSM-5* criteria, this disorder "is caused by an impact to the head or other mechanisms of rapid movement or displacement of the brain within the skull, with one or more of the following: loss of consciousness, posttraumatic amnesia, disorientation and confusion, or neurological signs (e.g., positive neuroimaging demonstrating injury, a new onset of seizures or a marked worsening of a preexisting seizure disorder, visual field cuts, anosmia, hemiparesis)" (APA, 2013). Amnesia is the most common neurobehavioral symptom following head trauma. Other symptoms may include confusion and changes in speech, vision, and personality. Depending on the severity of the injury, these symptoms may eventually subside or may become permanent. Severe head injuries increase one's risk for AD or other dementias, especially in those who carry the apolipoprotein E (*APOE*) gene, which increases anyone's risk for AD (Graff-Radford, 2021). Repeated head trauma, such as the type experienced by boxers, can result in *dementia pugilistica*, a syndrome characterized by emotional lability, dysarthria, ataxia, and impulsivity.

Neurocognitive Disorder Due to Lewy Body Dementia

Dementia with Lewy bodies is now identified as the second most common cause of dementia in the elderly after AD (Graziane & Sweet, 2017). Clinically, Lewy body NCD is fairly similar to AD; however, it tends to progress more rapidly, with earlier appearance of visual hallucinations and parkinsonian features.

Depression and delusions are also common symptoms in this population. Lewy body dementia recently gained public attention when an autopsy of famous comedian Robin Williams revealed that he had this disease. His widow reported that he had been seeking neurocognitive testing because he was aware of a decline in his mental capacities. He was also manifesting symptoms of depression and ultimately died by suicide.

This disorder is distinguished by the presence of Lewy bodies—eosinophilic inclusion bodies—seen in the cerebral cortex and brainstem. Three core features include significant variations in alertness and attention, detailed visual hallucinations, and spontaneous motor features of parkinsonism (Graziane & Sweet, 2017). Acetylcholinesterase (ACh) concentrations are reduced in the brains of people with Lewy body NCD, and, consequently, cholinesterase inhibitors are likely to be more effective for this population than for those with Alzheimer's dementia (Crystal, 2019). These patients are highly sensitive to extrapyramidal effects of antipsychotic medications. The disease is progressive and irreversible, with a survival time of up to 10 years, and may account for as many as 25% of all NCD cases.

Neurocognitive Disorder Due to Parkinson's Disease

NCD is observed in as many as 75% of clients with Parkinson's disease (APA, 2013). In this disease, there is a loss of nerve cells located in the substantia nigra, and dopamine activity is diminished, resulting in involuntary muscle movements, slowness, and rigidity. Tremor in the upper extremities is characteristic. In some instances, the cerebral changes that occur in NCD due to Parkinson's disease closely resemble those of AD.

Neurocognitive Disorder Due to HIV Infection

Infection with the human immunodeficiency virus type 1 (HIV-1) can result in an NCD called *HIV-1-associated cognitive/motor complex.* A less severe form, known as *HIV-1-associated minor cognitive/motor disorder,* also occurs. The severity of symptoms is correlated to the extent of brain pathology. The immune dysfunction associated with HIV disease can lead to brain infections by other organisms, and HIV-1 also appears to cause NCD directly. In the early stages, neuropsychiatric symptoms may be manifested by barely perceptible changes in a person's normal psychological presentation. Severe cognitive changes, particularly confusion, changes in behavior, and sometimes psychoses, are not uncommon in the later stages.

With the advent of the highly active antiretroviral therapies (HAART), incidence rates of NCD due to HIV infection have been on the decline. However, Moore and Marquine (2017) note that several studies have observed elevated rates of NCDs in older adults who are HIV positive, suggesting that there may be additive negative effects for older HIV-positive individuals.

Substance- or Medication-Induced Neurocognitive Disorder

NCD can occur as the result of substance reactions, overuse, or abuse. Symptoms are consistent with major or mild neurocognitive disorder and persist beyond the usual duration of intoxication and acute withdrawal (APA, 2013). Substances that have been associated with the development of NCDs include alcohol, sedatives, hypnotics, anxiolytics, and inhalants. Drugs that cause anticholinergic side effects and toxins such as lead and mercury have also been implicated.

Neurocognitive Disorder Due to Huntington's Disease

Huntington's disease is transmitted as a mendelian dominant gene. Damage occurs in the areas of the basal ganglia and the cerebral cortex. The onset of symptoms (i.e., involuntary twitching of the limbs or facial muscles, mild cognitive changes, depression or mood swings, and apathy) usually occurs between age 30 and 50 years. The client usually declines into a profound state of cognitive impairment and **ataxia** (muscular incoordination). The average duration of the disease is 10 to 25 years depending on the severity of symptoms. As the disease progresses, the weakened individual usually dies secondary to pneumonia, heart failure, choking, or other complications (Huntington's Disease Society of America [HDSA], 2021). About 10% of the cases occur in children and adolescents, and the progression is typically more rapid than it is in adult-onset Huntington's disease.

Neurocognitive Disorder Due to Prion Disease

Prion disease is a group of disorders caused by infectious agents called prions and characterized by insidious onset and rapid progression. Manifestations include problems with coordination and other movement disturbances along with rapidly progressing dementia. This type of NCD is diagnosed when there is evidence of characteristic biomarkers, including recognized lesions in the brain, specific types of proteins in the cerebrospinal fluid, and distinctive triphasic waves on electroencephalograms (APA, 2013). From 5% to 15% of cases of prion disease have a genetic component. Symptoms may develop at any age in adulthood but typically occur between ages 40 and 60 years. The clinical course is extremely rapid with progression from diagnosis to death in less than 2 years. The most common form of prion disease in humans is Creutzfeldt-Jakob's disease (Johns Hopkins Medicine, n.d.).

Neurocognitive Disorder Due to Another Medical Condition

A number of other general medical conditions can cause NCD. Some of these include structural lesions, hypothyroidism, hyperparathyroidism, pituitary insufficiency, uremia, hepatic or renal failure encephalitis, brain tumor, pernicious anemia, thiamine deficiency, pellagra, uncontrolled epilepsy, cardiopulmonary insufficiency, fluid and electrolyte imbalances, CNS and systemic infections, systemic lupus erythematosus, and multiple sclerosis.

The etiological factors associated with delirium and NCD are summarized in Box 13–2.

Application of the Nursing Process

Background Assessment Data

Nursing assessment of the patient with delirium or mild or major NCD is based on knowledge of the symptomatology associated with the various disorders previously described in this chapter. Subjective and objective data are gathered by various members of the health-care team. Clinicians report use of a variety of methods for obtaining assessment information.

Patient History

Nurses play a significant role in acquiring the patient history, including the specific mental and physical changes that have occurred and the age at which the changes began. If the patient is unable to relate information adequately, the data should be obtained from family members or others who would be aware of the patient's physical and psychosocial history.

From the patient history, nurses should assess the following areas of concern: (1) type, frequency, and severity of mood swings; personality and behavioral changes; and catastrophic emotional reactions; (2) cognitive changes such as problems with attention span, thinking process, problem-solving, and memory (recent and remote); (3) language difficulties; (4) orientation to person, place, time, and situation; and (5) appropriateness of social behavior.

BOX 13–2 Etiological Factors Implicated in the Development of Delirium and/or Mild or Major Neurocognitive Disorder

Biological Factors	Exogenous Factors
Hypoxia: Any condition leading to a deficiency of oxygen to the brain	***Birth trauma:*** Prolonged labor, damage from use of forceps, other obstetric complications
Nutritional deficiencies: Vitamins (particularly B and C); protein; fluid and electrolyte imbalances	***Cranial trauma:*** Concussion, contusions, hemorrhage, hematomas
Metabolic disturbances: Porphyria; encephalopathies related to hepatic, renal, pancreatic, or pulmonary insufficiencies; hypoglycemia	***Volatile inhalant compounds:*** Gasoline, glue, paint, paint thinners, spray paints, cleaning fluids, typewriter correction fluid, varnishes, and lacquers
Endocrine dysfunction: Thyroid, parathyroid, adrenal, pancreas, pituitary	***Heavy metals:*** Lead, mercury, manganese
Cardiovascular disease: Stroke, cardiac insufficiency, atherosclerosis	***Other metallic elements:*** Aluminum
Primary brain disorders: Epilepsy, Alzheimer's disease, frontotemporal NCD, Huntington's disease, multiple sclerosis, Parkinson's disease	***Organic phosphates:*** Various insecticides
Infections: Encephalitis, meningitis, pneumonia, septicemia, neurosyphilis (dementia paralytica), HIV, acute rheumatic fever, Creutzfeldt-Jakob disease	***Substance abuse/dependence:*** Alcohol, amphetamines, caffeine, cannabis, cocaine, hallucinogens, inhalants, nicotine, opioids, phencyclidine, sedatives, hypnotics, anxiolytics
Intracranial neoplasms: Glioblastomas, craniopharyngiomas, pituitary adenomas	***Other medications:*** Anticholinergics, antihistamines, antidepressants, antipsychotics, antiparkinsonians, antihypertensives, steroids, digitalis
Congenital defects: Prenatal infections such as first-trimester maternal rubella	

The nurse also should obtain information regarding current and past medication usage, history of other drug and alcohol use, and possible exposure to toxins. Knowledge regarding the history of related symptoms or specific illnesses (e.g., Huntington's disease, AD, frontotemporal NCD, or Parkinson's disease) in other family members may be useful.

Physical Assessment

Assessment of physical systems by both the nurse and the physician has two main emphases: signs of damage to the nervous system and evidence of diseases of other organs that could affect mental function. Diseases of various organ systems can induce confusion, loss of memory, and behavioral changes. These causes must be considered in diagnosing cognitive disorders. In the neurological examination, the patient is asked to perform maneuvers or answer questions that are designed to evaluate specific parts of the brain or peripheral nerves. Testing will assess mental status and alertness, muscle strength, reflexes, sensory perception, language skills, and coordination. Physical assessment should include looking for signs of abuse or neglect and screening for hearing or vision impairments and conducting a mental status examination. An example of a mental status examination for a patient with NCD is presented in Box 13–3.

BOX 13–3 Mental Status Examination for Neurocognitive Disorder

Patient Name _____ Date _____
Age _____ Sex _____ Diagnosis _____

	Maximum	Patient's Score
1. VERBAL FLUENCY		
Ask patient to name as many animals as they can. (Time: 60 seconds) (Score 1 point/2 animals)	10 points	_____
2. COMPREHENSION		
a. Point to the ceiling	1 point	_____
b. Point to your nose and the window	1 point	_____
c. Point to your foot, the door, and ceiling	1 point	_____
d. Point to the window, your leg, the door, and your thumb	1 point	_____
3. NAMING AND WORD FINDING		
Ask the patient to name the following as you point to them:		
a. Watch stem (winder)	1 point	_____
b. Teeth	1 point	_____
c. Sole of shoe	1 point	_____
d. Buckle of belt	1 point	_____
e. Knuckles	1 point	_____
4. ORIENTATION		
a. Date	2 points	_____
b. Day of week	2 points	_____
c. Month	1 point	_____
d. Year	1 point	_____
5. NEW LEARNING ABILITY		
Tell the patient: "I'm going to tell you four words, which I want you to remember." Have the patient repeat the four words after they are initially presented, and then say that you will ask them to remember the words later. Continue with the examination, and at intervals of 5 and 10 minutes, ask the patient to recall the words. Three different sets of words are provided here.		5 min. / 10 min.
a. Brown (Fun) (Grape)	2 points each:	_____ / _____
b. Honesty (Loyalty) (Happiness)	2 points each:	_____ / _____
c. Tulip (Carrot) (Stocking)	2 points each:	_____ / _____
d. Eyedropper (Ankle) (Toothbrush)	2 points each:	_____ / _____

Continued

BOX 13–3 Mental Status Examination for Neurocognitive Disorder—cont'd

6. VERBAL STORY FOR IMMEDIATE RECALL
Tell the patient: "I'm going to read you a short story, which I want you to remember. Listen closely to what I read because I will ask you to tell me the story when I finish." Read the story slowly and carefully, but without pausing at the slash marks. After completing the paragraph, tell the patient to retell the story as accurately as possible. Record the number of correct memories (information within the slashes) and describe confabulation if it is present. (1 point = 1 remembered item [13 maximum points])

It was July / and the Rogers family, mom, dad, and four children / were packing up their station wagon / to go on vacation.
They were taking their yearly trip / to the beach at Gulf Shores.
This year they were making a special 1-day stop / at The Aquarium in New Orleans.
After a long day's drive, they arrived at the motel / only to discover that in their excitement / they had left the twins / and their suitcases / in the front yard.

7. VISUAL MEMORY (HIDDEN OBJECTS)
Tell the patient that you are going to hide some objects around the office (desk, bed) and that you want them to remember where they are. Hide four or five common objects (e.g., keys, pen, reflex hammer) in various places in the patient's sight. After a delay of several minutes, ask the patient to find the objects. (1 point per item found)

a. Coin	1 point	_____
b. Pen	1 point	_____
c. Comb	1 point	_____
d. Keys	1 point	_____
e. Fork	1 point	_____

8. PAIRED ASSOCIATE LEARNING
Tell the patient that you are going to read a list of words two at a time. The patient will be expected to remember the words that go together (e.g., big—little). When they are clear on the directions, read the first list of words at the rate of one pair per second. After reading the first list, test for recall by presenting the first recall list. Give the first word of a pair and ask for the word that was paired with it. Correct incorrect responses and proceed to the next pair. After the first recall has been completed, allow a 10-second delay and continue with the second presentation and recall lists.

Presentation Lists

1	2
a. High—Low	a. Good—Bad
b. House—Income	b. Book—Page
c. Good—Bad	c. High—Low
d. Book—Page	d. House—Income

Recall Lists

1	2		
a. House _____	a. High _____	2 points	_____
b. Book _____	b. Good _____	2 points	_____
c. High _____	c. House _____	2 points	_____
d. Good _____	d. Book _____	2 points	_____

BOX 13–3 Mental Status Examination for Neurocognitive Disorder—cont'd

9. CONSTRUCTIONAL ABILITY
Ask patient to reconstruct this drawing and to draw the other two items: 3 points _____

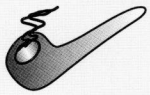

Draw a daisy in a flowerpot. 3 points _____

Draw a clock with all the numbers and set the clock at 2:30. 3 points _____

10. WRITTEN COMPLEX CALCULATIONS

a. Addition	108 +79	1 point	_____
b. Subtraction	605 −86	1 point	_____
c. Multiplication	108 ×36	1 point	_____
d. Division	559 ÷ 43	1 point	_____

11. PROVERB INTERPRETATION
Tell the patient to explain the following sayings. Record the answers.

a. Don't cry over spilled milk. 2 points _____
_____

b. Rome wasn't built in a day. 2 points _____
_____

c. A drowning man will clutch at a straw. 2 points _____
_____

d. A golden hammer can break down an iron door. 2 points _____
_____

e. The hot coal burns, the cold one blackens. 2 points _____
_____

12. SIMILARITIES
Ask the patient to name the similarity or relationship between each of the two items.

a. Turnip	Cauliflower	2 points	_____
b. Car	Airplane	2 points	_____
c. Desk	Bookcase	2 points	_____
d. Poem	Novel	2 points	_____
e. Horse	Apple	2 points	_____

Maximum: 100 points _____

Continued

BOX 13–3 Mental Status Examination for Neurocognitive Disorder—cont'd

Normal Individuals		Patients with Alzheimer's Disease	
Age Group	**Mean Score (standard deviation)**	**Stage**	**Mean Score (standard deviation)**
40–49	80.9 (9.7)	I	57.2 (9.1)
50–59	82.3 (8.6)	II	37.0 (7.8)
60–69	75.5 (10.5)	III	13.4 (8.1)
70–79	66.9 (9.1)		
80–89	67.9 (11.0)		

Source: Adapted from Strub, R. L., & Black, F. W. (2000). The mental status examination in neurology *(4th ed.), F. A. Davis. With permission.*

A battery of psychological tests may be ordered as part of the diagnostic examination. The results of these tests may be used to make a differential diagnosis between NCD and **pseudodementia** (depression). Depression is one of the most common mental illnesses in the elderly, but it is often misdiagnosed and treated inadequately. Cognitive symptoms of depression may mimic NCD, and because of the prevalence of NCD in the elderly, diagnosticians are often too eager to make this diagnosis. A comparison of symptoms of NCD and pseudodementia (depression) is presented in Table 13–1. Nurses can assist in this assessment by carefully observing and documenting these sometimes subtle differences.

Diagnostic Laboratory Evaluations

The nurse also may be required to help the patient fulfill the physician's orders for special diagnostic laboratory evaluations. Many of these tests are conducted to rule out other factors associated with dementia and include the following:

- Evaluation of blood and urine samples to test for various infections
- Liver function studies to rule out hepatic disease
- Glucose tests to rule out diabetes or hypoglycemia
- Electrolyte tests to rule out imbalances
- Thyroid tests to rule out hypothyroidism
- Vitamin B_{12} test to rule out nutritional deficiencies
- Drug and alcohol screening to rule out the presence of toxic substances.

A rapid plasma reagin (RPR) to test for syphilis and HIV testing should be included if the patient is at higher risk for these conditions. CT scanning produces an image of the size and shape of the brain and MRI is used to obtain a computerized image of soft tissue in the brain. Both CT and MRI scans are useful in identifying areas of atrophy such as those seen in AD and may identify other pathological processes needed for differential diagnosis. A lumbar puncture may be performed to examine the cerebrospinal fluid for evidence of CNS infection or hemorrhage if these conditions are suspected.

PET is used to reveal the metabolic activity of the brain, an evaluation some researchers believe is important for early diagnosis of AD. PET scan techniques can identify Aβ plaques and tau neurofibrillary tangles in the brain. Fluorodeoxyglucose (FDG) PET scans show areas of the brain in which nutrients are poorly metabolized, indicating areas of degeneration which can help distinguish between Alzheimer's disease and other types of dementia (Mayo Clinic, 2021c). Most recently, a blood test for Aβ plaques has become available and received certification in the United States by the Centers for Medicare & Medicaid Services to allow distribution on the market (Mayo Clinic, 2021c).

Nursing Diagnosis and Outcome Identification

Using information collected during the assessment, the nurse completes the patient database from which the selection of appropriate nursing diagnoses is determined. Table 13–2 presents a list of patient behaviors and the NANDA-I nursing diagnoses that correspond to those behaviors, which may be used in planning care for the patient with an NCD (Herdman et al., 2021).

Outcome Criteria

The following criteria may be used for measurement of outcomes in the care of the patient with an NCD. The patient:

- Has not experienced physical injury.
- Has not harmed self or others.
- Maintains reality orientation to the best of their capability.
- Is able to communicate with a consistent caregiver.
- Fulfills ADLs with assistance (or for the patient who is unable, has needs met, as anticipated by the caregiver).
- Discusses positive aspects about self and life.

TABLE 13–1 A Comparison of Neurocognitive Disorder (NCD) and Pseudodementia (Depression)

SYMPTOM ELEMENT	NCD	PSEUDODEMENTIA (DEPRESSION)
PROGRESSION OF SYMPTOMS	SLOW	RAPID
Memory	Progressive deficits; recent memory loss greater than remote; may confabulate for memory "gaps"; no complaints of loss	More like forgetfulness; no evidence of progressive deficit; recent and remote loss equal; complaints of deficits; no confabulation (will more likely answer "I don't know.")
Orientation	Disoriented to time and place; may wander in search of the familiar	Oriented to time and place; no wandering
Task performance	Consistently poor performance but struggles to perform	Performance is variable; little effort is put forth
Symptom severity	Worse as the day progresses	Better as the day progresses
Affective distress	Appears unconcerned	Communicates severe distress
Appetite	Unchanged initially, but as dementia progresses there may be loss of appetite, inability to recognize hunger, or loss of interest in food	Diminished
Attention and concentration	Impaired	Generally intact but sometimes depressed patient has significant impairment in concentration and speed of processing information

TABLE 13–2 Assigning Nursing Diagnoses to Behaviors Commonly Associated With Neurocognitive Disorders

BEHAVIORS	NURSING DIAGNOSES
Falls, wandering, poor coordination, confusion, misinterpretation of the environment (illusions, hallucinations), lack of understanding of environmental hazards, memory deficits	Risk for trauma Risk for falls
Disorientation, confusion, memory deficits, inaccurate interpretation of the environment, suspiciousness, paranoia	Disturbed thought processes* Impaired memory
Having hallucinations (hears voices, sees visions, feels crawling sensation on skin)	Disturbed sensory perception*
Aggressiveness (hitting, scratching, or kicking)	Risk for other-directed violence
Inability to name objects/people, loss of memory for words, difficulty finding the right word, confabulation, incoherent, screaming and demanding verbalizations	Impaired verbal communication
Inability to perform activities of daily living (ADLs): feeding, dressing, hygiene, toileting	Self-care deficit (specify)
Expressions of shame and self-degradation, progressive social isolation, apathy, decreased activity, withdrawal, depressed mood	Situational low self-esteem; Grieving

*These nursing diagnoses have been resigned from the NANDA-I list of approved diagnoses but are used for purposes of this text.

Planning and Implementation

Table 13–3 provides a plan of care for the patient with a cognitive disorder (irrespective of etiology). Selected nursing diagnoses are presented, along with outcome criteria, appropriate nursing interventions, and rationales for each.

Concept Care Mapping

The concept map care plan (see Chapter 6, "The Nursing Process in Psychiatric Mental Health Nursing") is a diagrammatic teaching and learning strategy that allows visualization of interrelationships between medical diagnoses, nursing diagnoses, assessment data, and treatments. An example of a concept map care plan for a patient with an NCD is presented in Figure 13–3.

Patient and Family Education

The role of patient teacher is important in the psychiatric area, as it is in all areas of nursing. A list of topics for patient and family education relevant to NCDs is presented in Box 13–5.

Evaluation

In the final step of the nursing process, reassessment occurs to determine whether the nursing interventions have been effective in achieving the intended goals of care. Evaluation of the patient with an NCD is based on a series of short-term goals rather than on long-term goals. Resolution of identified problems is unrealistic for this client. Instead, outcomes must be measured in terms of slowing down the process rather than stopping

Table 13–3 | CARE PLAN FOR THE PATIENT WITH A NEUROCOGNITIVE DISORDER (NCD)

NURSING DIAGNOSES: RISK FOR FALLS, RISK FOR TRAUMA

RELATED TO: Impairments in cognitive and psychomotor functioning

OUTCOME CRITERIA	NURSING INTERVENTIONS	RATIONALE
Short-Term Goals ■ Patient will call for assistance when ambulating or carrying out other activities (if it is within their cognitive ability). ■ Patient will maintain a calm demeanor, with minimal agitated behavior. ■ Patient will not experience physical injury. **Long-Term Goal** ■ Patient will not experience physical injury.	1. The following measures may be instituted: a. Arrange furniture and other items in the room to accommodate patient's disabilities. b. Store frequently used items within easy access. c. Do not keep bed in an elevated position. Pad siderails and headboard if client has history of seizures. Keep bedrails up when patient is in bed (if regulations permit). d. Assign room near nurses' station; observe frequently. e. Assist patient with ambulation. f. Keep a dim light on at night. g. Supervise the patient to assist with activity completion as needed and assess behavioral responses. h. Frequently orient to place, time, and situation. i. If patient is prone to wander, provide an area within which wandering can be carried out safely. j. Soft restraints may be required if patient is very disoriented and hyperactive.	1. To ensure patient safety.

Table 13–3 | CARE PLAN FOR THE PATIENT WITH A NEUROCOGNITIVE DISORDER (NCD)—cont'd

NURSING DIAGNOSIS: DISTURBED THOUGHT PROCESSES; IMPAIRED MEMORY

RELATED TO: Cerebral degeneration

EVIDENCED BY: Disorientation, confusion, memory deficits, and inaccurate interpretation of the environment

OUTCOME CRITERIA	NURSING INTERVENTIONS	RATIONALE
Short-Term Goals ■ Patient will utilize measures provided (e.g., clocks, calendars, room identification) to maintain reality orientation. ■ Patient will experience fewer episodes of acute confusion. **Long-Term Goal** ■ Patient will maintain reality orientation to the best of their cognitive ability.	1. Frequently orient patient to reality. Use clocks and calendars with large numbers that are easy to read. Notes and large, bold signs may be useful as reminders. Allow patient to have personal belongings. 2. Keep explanations simple. Use face-to-face interaction. Speak slowly and do not shout.	1. All of these items serve to help maintain orientation and aid in memory and recognition. **NOTE:** Some believe that repeated reality orientation for individuals with NCD contributes to problems with mood and self-esteem (see Box 13–4 for an alternative or adjunctive intervention; validation therapy). 2. These interventions facilitate comprehension. Shouting may create discomfort, and in some instances may provoke anger.
	3. Discourage rumination or delusional thinking. Talk about real events and real people. But remember that the patient's level of reality is different from the nurse's. Do not lie to the patient. May need to use validation therapy and redirection.	3. Rumination promotes disorientation. Reality orientation and validation therapy increase a sense of self-worth and personal dignity.
	4. Monitor for medication side effects.	4. Physiological changes in the elderly can alter the body's response to certain medications. Toxic effects may intensify altered thought processes.
	5. Encourage patient to view old photograph albums and utilize reminiscence therapy.	5. These are excellent ways to promote self-esteem and provide orientation to reality.

Continued

Table 13–3 | CARE PLAN FOR THE PATIENT WITH A NEUROCOGNITIVE DISORDER (NCD)—cont'd

NURSING DIAGNOSIS: DISTURBED SENSORY PERCEPTION

RELATED TO: Cerebral degeneration

EVIDENCED BY: Auditory and visual hallucinations

OUTCOME CRITERIA	NURSING INTERVENTIONS	RATIONALE
Short-Term Goal ■ Patient will exhibit fewer manifestations of disturbed sensory perception. **Long-Term Goal** ■ Patient will maintain reality orientation to the best of their cognitive ability.	1. Do not ignore reports of hallucinations when it is clear that the patient is experiencing them. It is important for the nurse to hear an explanation of the hallucination from the patient.	1. These perceptions are very real and often very frightening to the patient. Unless they are appropriately managed, hallucinations can escalate into disturbing and even hostile behaviors.
	2. Rule out the disturbed sensory perception as a possible side effect of certain physical conditions or medications.	2. Physical changes in the elderly result in less ability to metabolize medications, causing an increased risk of side effects. Some infections are also known to cause hallucinations in the elderly.
	3. Check to ensure that hearing aid is working properly and that faulty sounds are not being emitted.	3. Faulty sounds from a hearing aid defect could be misinterpreted for auditory hallucinations.
	4. Check eyeglasses to ensure that the individual is indeed wearing their own glasses.	4. Wearing the wrong prescription eyeglasses could cause the individual to misinterpret visual perceptions.
	5. Try to determine from where the visual hallucination is emanating and correct the situation by moving or covering the item.	5. Patients often see faces in patterns on fabrics or in pictures on the wall. A mirror can also be the culprit when there are false perceptions.
	6. Provide distractions for the patient. Focus on real situations and real people.	6. Hallucinations are less likely to occur when the person is occupied or involved in what is going on around them.
	7. Depending on the situation, it may be better at times to just listen to the patient rather than attempting to distract or reorient.	7. Not all hallucinations are upsetting, and there are times when trying to distract the person from the hallucination or reorient them may incur increased stress and agitation in the individual.

Table 13–3 | CARE PLAN FOR THE PATIENT WITH A NEUROCOGNITIVE DISORDER (NCD)—cont'd

NURSING DIAGNOSIS: SELF-CARE DEFICIT

RELATED TO: Disorientation, confusion, and memory deficits

EVIDENCED BY: Inability to fulfill ADLs

OUTCOME CRITERIA	NURSING INTERVENTIONS	RATIONALE
Short-Term Goal ■ Patient will participate in ADLs with assistance from caregiver. **Long-Term Goals** ■ Patient will accomplish ADLs to the best of their ability. ■ Unfulfilled needs will be met by caregivers.	1. Provide a simple, structured environment: a. Identify self-care deficits and provide assistance as required. Promote independent actions as able. b. Allow plenty of time for patient to perform tasks. c. Provide guidance and support for independent actions by talking the patient through the task one step at a time. d. Provide a structured schedule of activities that does not change from day to day. e. ADLs should follow usual routine as closely as possible. f. Provide for consistency in assignment of daily caregivers.	1. To minimize confusion.
	2. Perform ongoing assessment of patient's ability to fulfill nutritional needs, ensure personal safety, follow medication regimen, and communicate need for assistance with activities that cannot be accomplish independently.	2. Patient safety and security are nursing priorities.
	3. Assess prospective caregivers' ability to anticipate and fulfill patient's unmet needs. Provide information to assist caregivers with this responsibility. Ensure that caregivers are aware of available community support systems from which they may seek assistance when required. Examples include adult day care centers, housekeeping and homemaker services, respite care services, or the local chapter of a national support organization: a. For Parkinson's disease information: National Parkinson Foundation Inc. www.parkinson.org b. For Alzheimer's disease information: Alzheimer's Association www.alz.org	3. To ensure provision and continuity of patient care.

Continued

Table 13–3 | CARE PLAN FOR THE PATIENT WITH A NEUROCOGNITIVE DISORDER (NCD)—cont'd

NURSING DIAGNOSIS: IMPAIRED VERBAL COMMUNICATION

RELATED TO: Impairments in cognitive and psychomotor functioning

OUTCOME CRITERIA	NURSING INTERVENTIONS	RATIONALE
Short-Term Goals ■ Patient will be able to make needs known to primary caregiver. ■ Patient is able to understand basic communications in interactions with primary caregiver. **Long-Term Goal** ■ Unfulfilled needs will be met by caregivers.	1. The following communication techniques may be used: a. Keep interactions with the patient calm and reassuring. b. Use simple words, speak slowly and distinctly, and maintain face-to-face contact with the patient. c. Always identify yourself and call the patient by name at each meeting. d. Use nonverbal gestures to help the patient understand what you want to accomplish, if appropriate. e. Ask only one question/give only one direction at a time and give the patient plenty of time to process the information and respond. Rephrase question only if it is clear that the patient has not understood the meaning of the direction.	1. These interventions promote an effective communication process and facilitate the patient's comprehension.
	2. Approach the patient from the front whenever possible.	2. An unexpected approach/touch from behind may startle the patient and could promote aggressive behavior. When it is *clearly* appropriate, use touch and affection to communicate. Sometimes patients will respond to a hug or to a hand reaching for theirs when they will respond to nothing else.
	3. Provide for consistency in assignment of daily caregivers.	3. To minimize confusion and facilitate patient security.

or curing the problem. Evaluation questions may include the following:

- Has the patient experienced injury?
- Does the patient maintain orientation to time, person, place, and situation to the best of their cognitive ability?
- Is the patient able to fulfill basic needs? Have those needs unmet by the patient been fulfilled by caregivers?
- Is confusion minimized by familiar objects and structured, routine schedule of activities?
- Do the prospective caregivers have information regarding the progression of the patient's illness?
- Do caregivers have information regarding where to go for assistance and support in the care of the patient?
- Have the prospective caregivers received instruction in how to promote the patient's safety, minimize confusion and disorientation, and cope with difficult client behaviors (e.g., hostility, anger, depression, agitation)?

Quality and Safety Education for Nurses (QSEN)

The Institute of Medicine (IOM), in its 2003 report *Health Professions Education: A Bridge to Quality*, challenged faculties of medicine, nursing, and other

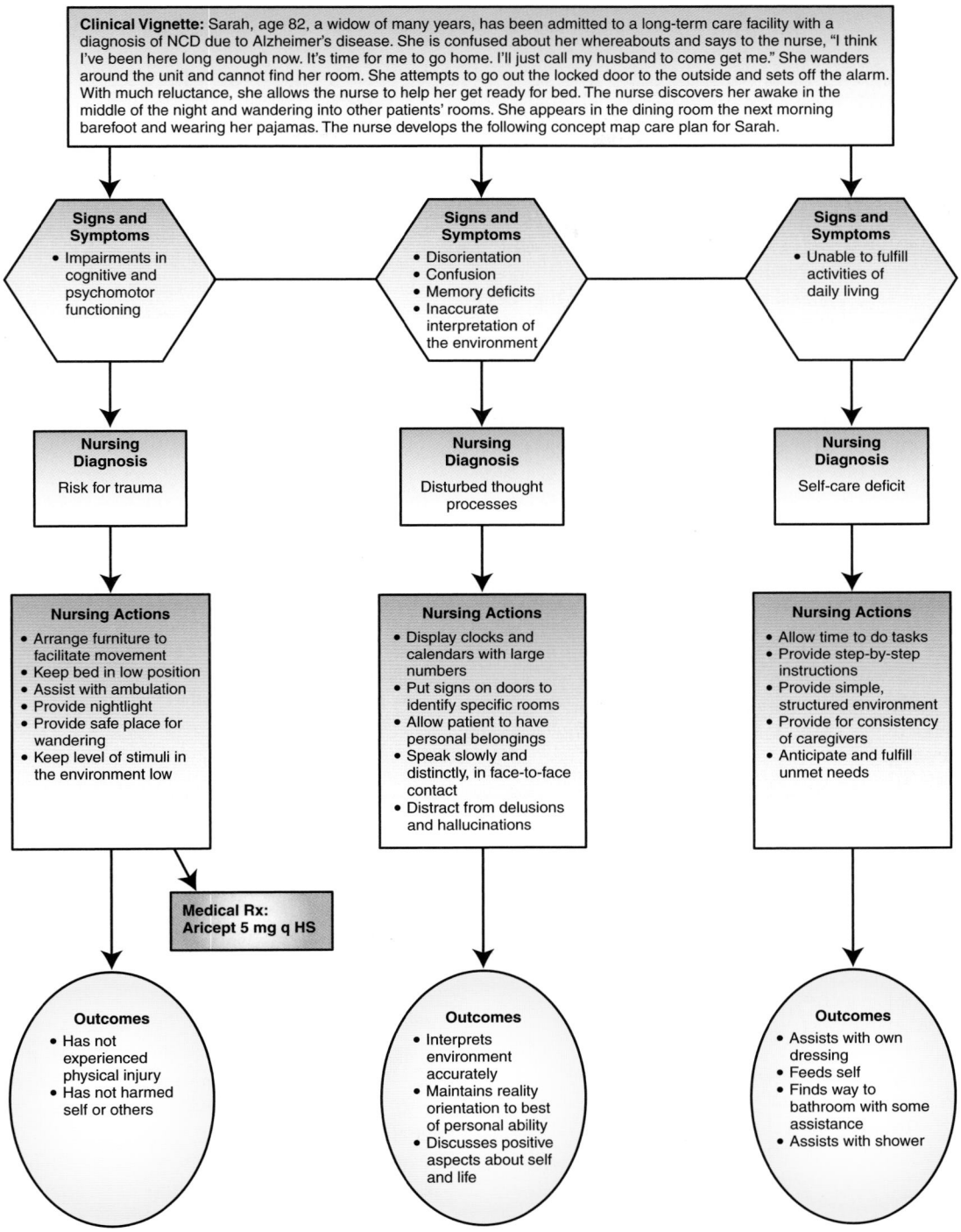

FIGURE 13–3 Concept map care plan for patient with major neurocognitive disorder.

BOX 13–4 Validation Therapy

Validation therapy (VT), originated by Naomi Feil, a gerontological social worker, is a "method of communicating and being with disoriented very old people. It is a practical way of working that helps reduce stress, enhance dignity, and increase happiness. Validation is built on an empathetic attitude and a holistic view of individuals" (Validation Training Institute, 2021). The caregiver's approach involves listening nonjudgmentally with an openness to hearing what the patient is communicating and without correction, reorientation, or dismissal. Validation therapy validates the feelings and emotions of a person with NCD and may also integrate redirection techniques. Other important communication strategies include not lying, arguing, or contradicting what the patient says. Instead, listen with curiosity and ask questions to better understand what the patient is trying to communicate. For example, if the patient begins talking about their deceased spouse as if they were still alive it is better not to communicate that the spouse is still alive (which would be a lie) but rather listen empathically and ask questions like "How did you meet your spouse?" or "What was your favorite thing to do together?"

EXAMPLES

Mrs. W (agitated): "That old lady stole my watch! I know she did. She goes into people's rooms and takes our things. We call her 'sticky fingers'!"

Nurse: "That watch is very important to you. Have you looked around the room for it?" ***(validating the patient's feelings)***

Mrs. W: "My husband gave it to me. He will be so upset that it is gone. I'm afraid to tell him."

Nurse: "I'm sure you miss your husband very much. Tell me what it was like when you were together. What kinds of things did you do for fun?" ***(listening with curiosity and asking questions)***

Mrs. W: "We did a lot of traveling. To Italy, and England, and France. We ate wonderful food."

Nurse: "Speaking of food, it is lunch time, and I will walk with you to the dining room." ***(redirection)***

Mrs. W: "Yes, I'm getting really hungry."

In this situation, the nurse validated Mrs. W's feelings about not being able to find her watch. She did not deny that it had been stolen, nor did she remind Mrs. W that her husband was deceased. *(Remember: A concept of VT is that on some level, Mrs. W knows that her husband is dead.)* The nurse validated the emotions Mrs. W was feeling about missing her husband. She brought up special times that Mrs. W and her husband had spent together, which served to elevate her mood and self-esteem. Finally, she redirected Mrs. W to the dining room to have her lunch. (The watch was eventually found in Mrs. W's medicine cabinet, where she had hidden it for safekeeping.) Through each of these communication strategies, the patient's perception of reality is validated and their self-esteem and dignity are preserved.

BOX 13–5 Topics for Patient and Family Education Related to Neurocognitive Disorders

1. Nature of the illness
   a. Possible causes
   b. What to expect
   c. Symptoms
2. Management of the illness
   a. Ways to ensure patient safety
   b. How to maintain reality orientation
   c. Providing assistance with ADLs
   d. Nutritional information
   e. Difficult behaviors
   f. Medication administration
   g. Matters related to hygiene and toileting
3. Support services
   a. Financial assistance
   b. Legal assistance
   c. Caregiver support groups
   d. Respite care
   e. Home health care

health professions to ensure that their graduates have achieved a core set of competencies in order to meet the needs of the 21st-century health-care system. These competencies include *providing patient-centered care, maintaining safety, working in interdisciplinary teams, employing evidence-based practice, incorporating quality improvement,* and *utilizing informatics.*

Several studies have demonstrated the positive outcomes associated with a *patient-centered care* approach for patients with dementia (Ballard et al., 2018; Ballard et al., 2020; Ballard et al., 2016; Whitaker et al., 2014). This program, called "Well-Being and Health for People With Dementia (WHELD)," is a nonpharmacological, psychosocial intervention that focuses on tailored person-centered activities, exercise, and social interaction for patients with dementia in long-term care settings. The evidence supported that training staff and incorporating these patient-centered interventions reduced patient agitation, reduced the need for antipsychotic medication, and improved quality of life in this population. Lack of medications to improve dementia and the

dangers associated with antipsychotic use in elderly patients with dementia make these evidence-based interventions an important tool for quality nursing care in this population.

Treatment Modalities

Delirium

The first step in the treatment of delirium should be the determination and correction of the underlying causes. Additional attention must be given to fluid and electrolyte status, hypoxia, anoxia, and diabetic problems. Staff members should remain with the patient at all times to monitor behavior and provide reorientation and assurance. A low level of stimuli should be maintained in the room.

Some physicians prefer not to prescribe medications for the patient with delirium, reasoning that additional agents may only compound the syndrome of brain dysfunction. However, psychosis with agitation and aggression demonstrated by the patient with delirium may require chemical and/or mechanical restraint for their personal safety. The choice of therapy is made with consideration for the patient's clinical condition and the underlying cause of the delirium. Low-dose antipsychotics are the pharmacological treatment of choice in most cases. However, two meta-analyses have found mixed results. One analysis of 15 studies concluded that second generation antipsychotics are beneficial (and preferable to haloperidol) in the treatment of delirium (Kishi et al., 2015), but a second meta-analysis of 19 studies concluded that the evidence does not support use of antipsychotics for prevention or treatment of delirium (Neufeld et al., 2016). Haloperidol (Haldol) is still used to treat psychotic features, but because it has been associated with prolongation of QT intervals, nurses should monitor the patient's cardiac status. A benzodiazepine (e.g., lorazepam) is commonly used when the etiology is substance withdrawal. Melatonin, an over-the-counter supplement, and ramelteon (Rozerem), a prescription medication for treatment of insomnia, have both been identified as potentially beneficial in prevention and treatment of delirium, because melatonin levels were found to be altered in patients with delirium (Alagiakrishnan, 2019).

Neurocognitive Disorder (NCD)

Once a definitive diagnosis of NCD has been made, a primary consideration in the treatment of the disorder is the etiology. Focus must be directed to the identification and resolution of potentially reversible processes. Boland and Verduin (2022) identify that once dementia is apparent, it is essential to complete a clinical workup to identify the syndrome and its causes because 10% to 15% of all patients with dementia have a potentially reversible condition if treatment is initiated before irreversible brain damage occurs.

The need for general supportive care (with provisions for security, stimulation, nutrition, and treating the individual with patience and respect) is recognized and accepted treatment. Several pharmaceutical agents have been tried, with varying degrees of success, in the treatment of clients with NCD. Some of these drugs are described in the following sections according to symptomatology for which they are indicated. A summary of selected medications for clients with NCD is provided in Table 13–4.

Cognitive Impairment

Cholinesterase inhibitors are often used for treatment of mild to moderate cognitive impairment in AD and have demonstrated efficacy in treating patients with Lewy body dementia (Crystal, 2019). Higher-dose donepezil has also been approved for severe AD. Some of the clinical manifestations of AD are thought to be the result of a deficiency of the neurotransmitter acetylcholine. In the brain, acetylcholine is inactivated by the enzyme acetylcholinesterase. Donepezil (Aricept), rivastigmine (Exelon), and galantamine (Razadyne) act by inhibiting acetylcholinesterase, which slows the degradation of acetylcholine, thereby increasing concentrations of the neurotransmitter in the cerebral cortex. Because their action relies on functionally intact cholinergic neurons, the effects of these medications may lessen as the disease process advances, and there is no evidence that these medications alter the course of the underlying degenerative process.

Another medication, an NMDA receptor antagonist, was approved by the Food and Drug Administration (FDA) in 2003. The medication, memantine (Namenda), was approved for the treatment of moderate to severe AD. A research meta-analysis (Meng et al., 2019) also identified memantine's benefits in the treatment of cognitive impairment in Parkinson's disease and dementia with Lewy bodies. High levels of glutamate in the brains of AD patients are thought to contribute to the symptomatology and decline in functionality. These high levels are caused by abnormal glutamate transmission. In normal neurotransmission, glutamate plays an essential role in learning and memory by triggering NMDA receptors to allow a controlled amount of calcium to flow into a nerve cell, creating the appropriate environment for information processing. In AD, there is a sustained release of glutamate, which results in a continuous influx of calcium

TABLE 13-4 Selected Medications Used in the Treatment of Clients With NCD

MEDICATION	CLASSIFICATION	FOR TREATMENT OF	DAILY DOSAGE RANGE (MG)	SIDE EFFECTS
Donepezil (Aricept)	Cholinesterase inhibitor	Cognitive impairment	5–10	Insomnia, dizziness, gastrointestinal (GI) upset, headache
Rivastigmine (Exelon) (Exelon transdermal)	Cholinesterase inhibitor	Cognitive impairment	6–12 4.6–13.3 / 24 hr	Dizziness, headache, GI upset, fatigue
Galantamine (Razadyne)	Cholinesterase inhibitor	Cognitive impairment	8–24	Dizziness, headache, GI upset
Memantine (Namenda)	NMDA receptor antagonist	Cognitive impairment	5–20	Dizziness, headache, constipation
Memantine, extended release + donepezil (Namzaric)	Anti-Alzheimer's agent	Moderate to severe Alzheimer's type dementia	Memantine ER 14–28 and donepezil 10 once daily	Headache, nausea, vomiting, dizziness, diarrhea, decreased appetite
Risperidone* (Risperdal)	Antipsychotic	Agitation, aggression, hallucinations, thought disturbances, wandering	1–4 (increase dosage cautiously)	Agitation, insomnia, headache, extrapyramidal symptoms
Olanzapine* (Zyprexa)	Antipsychotic	Agitation, aggression, hallucinations, thought disturbances, wandering	5 (increase dosage cautiously)	Hypotension, dizziness, sedation, constipation, weight gain, dry mouth
Quetiapine* (Seroquel)	Antipsychotic	Agitation, aggression, hallucinations, thought disturbances, wandering	Initial dose 25 (titrate slowly)	Hypotension, tachycardia, dizziness, drowsiness, headache, constipation, dry mouth
Haloperidol* (Haldol)	Antipsychotic	Agitation, aggression, hallucinations, thought disturbances, wandering	1–4 (increase dosage cautiously)	Dry mouth, blurred vision, orthostatic hypotension, extrapyramidal symptoms, sedation
Pimavanserin (Nuplazid)	Antipsychotic	Hallucinations and delusions specifically associated with Parkinson's disease psychosis **NOTE:** Pimavanserin is not approved for dementia-related psychosis unrelated to Parkinson's disease psychosis	34 daily (17 twice daily)	Peripheral edema, nausea, confusion, hallucinations, constipation, gait disturbance
Sertraline (Zoloft)	Antidepressant (selective serotonin reuptake inhibitors [SSRI])	Depression	50–100	Fatigue, insomnia, sedation, GI upset, headache, dizziness
Paroxetine (Paxil)	Antidepressant (SSRI)	Depression	10–40	Dizziness, headache, insomnia, somnolence, GI upset
Nortriptyline (Pamelor)	Antidepressant (Tricyclic)	Depression	30–50	Anticholinergic, orthostatic hypotension, sedation, arrhythmia

TABLE 13–4 Selected Medications Used in the Treatment of Clients With NCD—cont'd

MEDICATION	CLASSIFICATION	FOR TREATMENT OF	DAILY DOSAGE RANGE (MG)	SIDE EFFECTS
Lorazepam **(Ativan)	Antianxiety (Benzodiazepine)	Anxiety	1–2	Drowsiness, dizziness, GI upset, hypotension, tolerance, dependence
Oxazepam** (Serax)	Antianxiety (Benzodiazepine)	Anxiety	10–30	Drowsiness, dizziness, GI upset, hypotension, tolerance, dependence
Temazepam** (Restoril)	Sedative-hypnotic (Benzodiazepine)	Insomnia	15	Drowsiness, dizziness, GI upset, hypotension, tolerance, dependence
Zolpidem (Ambien)	Sedative-hypnotic (Nonbenzodiazepine)	Insomnia	5	Headache, drowsiness, dizziness, GI upset
Zaleplon (Sonata)	Sedative-hypnotic (Nonbenzodiazepine)	Insomnia	5	Headache, drowsiness, dizziness, GI upset
Eszopiclone (Lunesta)	Sedative-hypnotic (Nonbenzodiazepine)	Insomnia	1–2	Headache, drowsiness, dizziness, GI upset, unpleasant taste
Ramelteon (Rozerem)	Sedative-hypnotic (Nonbenzodiazepine)	Insomnia	8	Dizziness, fatigue, drowsiness, GI upset
Trazodone	Antidepressant (Heterocyclic)	Depression and Insomnia	50	Dizziness, drowsiness, dry mouth, blurred vision, GI upset
Mirtazapine (Remeron)	Antidepressant (Tetracyclic)	Depression and insomnia	7.5–15	Somnolence, dry mouth, constipation, increased appetite

*Although clinicians may still prescribe these medications in low-risk patients, no antipsychotics have been approved by the FDA for the treatment of patients with NCD-related psychosis. All antipsychotics include black box warnings about increased risk of death in elderly patients with NCD.
**Benzodiazepines should only be used for short-term treatment and NOT used in combination with opiate medication.

into the nerve cells. This increased intracellular calcium concentration ultimately leads to disruption and death of the neurons.

Memantine may protect cells against excess glutamate by partially blocking NMDA receptors. Although it does not stop or reverse the effects of the disease, it has been shown to slow down the progression of the decline in cognition and function. Because memantine's action differs from that of the cholinesterase inhibitors, consideration has been given to co-administration of these medications. In 2014 the FDA approved one such medication, Namzaric, which is a combination of memantine and donepezil.

A recent study (Coupland et al., 2019) found that anticholinergic drugs, including anticholinergic antidepressants, antipsychotics, antiepileptics, antiparkinsonian, and antimuscarinic drugs, *increased* the risk for dementia. The authors report that these findings highlight the importance of minimizing anticholinergic drug exposure in middle-aged and older adults. Anticholinergic side effects include confusion, blurred vision, constipation, dry mouth, dizziness, and difficulty urinating. Older people, and especially those with NCD, are particularly sensitive to these effects because of decreased cholinergic reserves. Many elderly individuals are also at increased risk for developing an anticholinergic toxicity syndrome because of the additive anticholinergic effects of multiple medications.

Current drug trials are under way to test for a vaccine against AD. Some researchers are focused on developing passive vaccines against amyloid and tau proteins that are then injected, whereas other researchers are focusing on active immunotherapies that trigger a body to produce its own antibodies (Newman, 2018). Vaccine trials have continued for the past several years without major breakthroughs. However, in 2016, a group of American and Australian researchers reported a "very promising" vaccine that affects amyloid and tau proteins, both of which are implicated in AD. It is clear that interest in such research is high, with government funding for AD research exceeding $1 billion in 2016 (LaVigne, 2016). Although some experts say they expect a vaccine will be available within the near future, other health experts suggest that it will be many years and possibly decades before a vaccine is available for humans (Ries, 2019). The rationales cited include that AD is a complex disease and the underlying pathology has not yet been clearly elucidated.

Antipsychotics have been associated with increased mortality in patients with dementia and no antipsychotics have been approved by the FDA for the treatment of patients with NCD-related psychosis. All antipsychotics have a black box warning about the increased risk of death in elderly patients with NCD. "The second-generation antipsychotics risperidone, aripiprazole, and olanzapine have the best evidence for NCD-associated agitation and psychosis, but concerns about adverse effects (cardio- and cerebrovascular, metabolic, extrapyramidal) and modest efficacy limit their use" (Elie & Rej, 2018, p. 69). Although clinicians may still prescribe these medications, American Psychiatric Association (APA) practice guidelines (2015) recommend prescribing antipsychotics only when the symptoms are severe and dangerous, the risks and benefits are discussed with patient and family, and the prescription is titrated up to the minimum effective dose.

Several herbs, vitamins, and other supplements have been studied for their potential benefits in the prevention and treatment of dementia. Of those studied, vitamin E has been advanced as potentially delaying the progression for those with mild to moderate disease, omega-3 fatty acids may lower the risk of developing dementia, while curcumin and gingko biloba have not demonstrated any benefits (Mayo Clinic, 2021c). More recent research has focused on the chemical resveratrol, found in grape skins, cacao, and other foods. It has been advanced as having anti-aging properties and neuroprotective functions as well as possibly reducing the buildup of amyloid plaques associated with AD. Turner and colleagues (2015) found promising evidence that high doses of resveratrol (up to 2,000 mg daily) have CNS effects on biomarkers for AD. Kou and Chen (2017, p. 927), in their review, report that "mounting evidence from in vitro and in vivo AD models has demonstrated that resveratrol, one of polyphenolic compounds, can exert neuroprotective role in neurodegenerative diseases especially AD." The researchers caution that more research is needed to fully understand the impact of these changes on the trajectory of AD.

Nonpharmacological treatments for cognitive impairment are also used for patients with NCD. Cognitive rehabilitation (which includes education about cognitive strengths and weaknesses, cognitive retraining, and compensatory strategies) has demonstrated some evidence of modest improvement in cognitive domains with the benefits of less dependence in activities and less caregiver burden even when global cognition declined (Germain et al., 2018).

Several studies support that mindfulness and meditation have significant benefits in a broad range of measures, "including a reduction of cognitive decline, reduction in perceived stress, increase in quality of life, as well as increases in functional connectivity, percent volume brain change and cerebral blood flow in areas of the cortex" (Russell-Williams et al., 2018, p. 791).

Rabin and colleagues (2019) found that reducing vascular risk factors and increased physical activity reduced Aβ-related cognitive decline and gray matter volume loss, suggesting that these interventions may be beneficial in slowing the progression of AD.

Agitation, Aggression, Hallucinations, Thought Disturbances, and Wandering

Historically, physicians have prescribed antipsychotic medications to control agitation, aggression, hallucinations, thought disturbances, and wandering in clients with NCD. The atypical antipsychotic medications, such as risperidone, olanzapine, quetiapine, and ziprasidone, are often favored because of their lessened propensity to cause anticholinergic and extrapyramidal side effects. In 2005, however, following review of a number of studies, the FDA ordered black box warnings on drug labels for all atypical antipsychotics, noting that the drugs are associated with an increased risk of death in elderly patients with psychotic behaviors associated with NCD. Most of the deaths appeared to be cardiovascular related. In July 2008, based on the results of several studies, the FDA extended this warning to include all first-generation antipsychotics as well, such as haloperidol and perphenazine. As previously mentioned, the APA has established detailed guidelines for their use in this population.

In 2016 a novel drug, pimavanserin (Nuplazid), was approved by the FDA specifically for treatment of hallucinations and delusions in Parkinson's disease psychosis. The mechanism of action is unknown, but it is thought to provide benefit through its serotonin agonist and antagonist activities. It also carries a black box warning for increased risk of death in elderly patients with dementia-related psychosis.

Many antipsychotic, antidepressant, and antihistaminic medications produce *anticholinergic side effects*, which include confusion, blurred vision, constipation, dry mouth, dizziness, and difficulty urinating. Older people, and especially those with NCD, are particularly sensitive to these effects because of decreased cholinergic reserves. Many elderly individuals are also at increased risk for developing an anticholinergic toxicity syndrome because of the additive anticholinergic effects of multiple medications.

As previously mentioned, the WHELD program of person-centered activities, social interaction, and exercise has demonstrated benefits for decreasing agitation, decreasing use of antipsychotic medication, and improving quality of life for patients with dementia in long-term care settings (Ballard et al., 2020).

Depression

It is estimated that up to 40% of people with AD also suffer from major depression (Alzheimer's Association, 2021b). Recognizing the symptoms of depression in these individuals is often a challenge. Depression—which affects thinking, memory, sleep, and appetite and interferes with daily life—is sometimes difficult to distinguish from NCD. Clearly, the presence of depression in the client with NCD complicates and worsens the individual's functioning.

Antidepressant medication is sometimes used in treatment of depression in NCD. The selective serotonin reuptake inhibitors (SSRIs) are considered by many to be the first-line drug treatment for depression in the elderly because of their favorable side effect profile, although patients should be assessed for hyponatremia. Trazodone may be a good choice, used at bedtime, for depression and insomnia. Dopaminergic agents (e.g., methylphenidate, amantadine, bromocriptine, and bupropion) may be helpful in the treatment of severe apathy. Tricyclic antidepressants are often avoided because of cardiac and anticholinergic side effects.

Not only is depression common in AD, but evidence supports that individuals with depression—especially recurrent and chronic depression—are about two times more likely to develop AD than those who do not have depression (Herbert, 2016). Possible explanations for this increased risk have included common genetic links (which so far looks unlikely); disturbance in glucocorticoids that occurs in both AD and some forms of depression that inhibit hippocampal neurogenesis and plasticity; and cytokines, which are elevated in some forms of depression and are a known risk factor for AD (Herbert & Lucassen, 2016). The authors note that more research is needed to better understand subtypes of depression and their distinct connections to risk for AD.

Anxiety

The progressive loss of mental functioning is a significant source of anxiety in the early stages of NCD. It is important that clients be encouraged to verbalize their feelings and fears associated with this loss. These interventions may be useful in reducing the anxiety of clients with NCD. Some research suggests that anxiety may also be an early indicator of developing brain disease, and one study cited by Norton (2021) suggests that older adults with mild cognitive impairment may progress more rapidly to Alzheimer's disease when anxiety symptoms are also significant.

Nonpharmacological treatments for anxiety include mindfulness meditation and other relaxation exercises. Antianxiety medications may be helpful but should not be used routinely or for prolonged periods. Benzodiazepines with shorter half-lives (e.g., lorazepam and oxazepam) are preferred to those longer-acting medications (e.g., diazepam), which promote a higher risk of oversedation and falls. Barbiturates are not appropriate as antianxiety agents because they frequently induce confusion and paradoxical excitement in elderly individuals.

Sleep Disturbances

Sleep problems are common in clients with NCD and often intensify as the disease progresses. Wakefulness and nighttime wandering create much distress and anguish in family members who are charged with protection of their loved one. Sleep disturbances are among the problems that most frequently initiate the need for placement of the client in a long-term care facility.

Some physicians treat sleep problems with sedative-hypnotic medications. The benzodiazepines may be useful for some clients but are indicated for relatively brief periods only. Examples include flurazepam (Dalmane), temazepam (Restoril), and triazolam (Halcion). Daytime sedation and cognitive impairment, in addition to paradoxical agitation in elderly clients, are of particular concern with these medications. The nonbenzodiazepine sedative-hypnotics zolpidem (Ambien), zaleplon (Sonata), eszopiclone (Lunesta), and ramelteon (Rozerem) and the antidepressants trazodone (Desyrel) and mirtazapine (Remeron) may also be prescribed. Daytime sedation is a potential problem with these medications as well. As previously stated, barbiturates should not be used in elderly clients. Sleep problems are usually ongoing, and most clinicians prefer to use medications only to help an individual through a short-term stressful situation. Rising at the same time each morning; minimizing daytime sleep; participating in regular physical exercise (but no later

CASE STUDY AND SAMPLE CARE PLAN

NURSING HISTORY AND ASSESSMENT

Carmen is an 81-year-old widow who has lived in the same small town in the same house that she shared with her husband until his death 16 years ago. She and her husband reared two daughters, Joan and Nancy, who have been living with their husbands in a large city about 2 hours away from Carmen. They have always visited Carmen every 1 or 2 months. She has four grown grandchildren who live in distant states and who see their grandmother on holidays.

About a year ago, Carmen's daughters began to receive reports from friends and other family members about incidents in which Carmen was becoming forgetful (e.g., forgetting to go to a cousin's birthday party, taking a wrong turn and getting lost on the way to a niece's house [where she had driven many times], returning to church to search for something she thought she had forgotten [although she could not explain what it was], sending birthday gifts to people when it was not their birthday). During routine visits, the elder daughter, Joan, found bills left unpaid, sometimes months overdue. Housekeepers and yard workers reported to Joan that Carmen would forget she had paid them and try to pay them again and sometimes a third time. She became very confused when she would attempt to fill her weekly pillboxes, a task she had completed in the past without difficulty. Hundreds of dollars would disappear from her wallet, and she could not tell Joan what happened to them.

Joan and her husband subsequently moved to the small town where Carmen lived. They bought a home, and Joan visited her mother every day, took care of finances, and ensured that Carmen took her daily medications, although Joan worked at a job that required occasional out-of-town travel. As the months progressed, Carmen's cognitive abilities deteriorated. She burned food on the stove, left the house with the broiler-oven on, forgot to take her medication, got lost in her car, missed appointments, and forgot the names of her neighbors whom she had known for many years. She began to lose weight because she was forgetting to eat her meals.

Carmen was evaluated by a neurologist, who diagnosed her with Neurocognitive Disorder due to Alzheimer's Disease. Because they believed that Carmen needed 24-hour care, Joan and Nancy made the painful decision to place Carmen in long-term care. In the nursing home, her condition has continued to deteriorate. Carmen wanders up and down the halls (day and night), and she has fallen twice, once while attempting to get out of bed. She requires assistance to shower and dress and has become incontinent of urine. The nurses found her attempting to leave the building, saying, "I'm going across the street to visit my daughter." One morning at breakfast she appeared in her pajamas in the communal dining room, not realizing that she had not dressed. She is unable to form new memories and sometimes uses confabulation to fill in the blanks. She asks the same questions repeatedly, sometimes struggling for the right word. She can no longer provide the correct names of items in her environment. She has no concept of time.

Joan visits Carmen daily, and Nancy visits weekly, each offering support to the other in person and by phone. Carmen always seems pleased to see them but can no longer call either of them by name. They are unsure if she knows who they are.

NURSING DIAGNOSES AND OUTCOME IDENTIFICATION

From the assessment data, the nurse develops the following nursing diagnoses for Carmen:

1. Risk for trauma related to impairments in cognitive and psychomotor functioning; wandering; falls.
   a. Outcome criteria: Carmen will remain injury free during her nursing home stay.
   b. Short-term goals:
      - Carmen will not fall while wandering the halls.
      - Carmen will not fall out of bed.

CASE STUDY AND SAMPLE CARE PLAN—cont'd

2. Disturbed thought processes related to cerebral degeneration evidenced by disorientation, confusion, and memory deficits.
   a. Outcome criteria: Carmen will maintain reality orientation to the best of her cognitive ability.
   b. Short-term goals:
      - Carmen will be able to find her room.
      - Carmen will be able to communicate her needs to staff.
3. Self-care deficit related to cognitive impairments, disorientation, confusion, and memory deficits.
   a. Outcome criteria: Carmen will accomplish ADLs to the best of her ability.
   b. Short-term goals:
      - Carmen will assist with dressing herself.
      - Carmen will cooperate with trips to the bathroom.
      - Carmen will wash herself in the shower with help from the nurse.

PLANNING AND IMPLEMENTATION

RISK FOR TRAUMA

The following nursing interventions may be implemented *to ensure patient safety*:

1. Arrange the furniture in Carmen's room so that it will accommodate her moving around freely.
2. Store frequently used items within her easy reach.
3. Provide a "low bed," or possibly move her mattress from the bed to the floor, to prevent falls from the bed.
4. Attach a bed alarm to alert the nurse's station when Carmen has alighted from her bed.
5. Keep a dim light on in her room at night.
6. During the day and evening, provide a well-lighted area where Carmen can safely wander.
7. Ensure that all outside doors are electronically controlled.
8. Play soft music and maintain a low level of stimuli in the environment.

DISTURBED THOUGHT PROCESSES

The following nursing interventions may be implemented *to help maintain orientation and aid in memory and recognition*:

1. Use clocks and calendars with large numbers that are easy to read.
2. Put a sign on Carmen's door with her name on it and hang a personal item of hers on the door.
3. Ask Joan to bring some of Carmen's personal items for her room, even a favorite comfy chair, if possible. Ask also for some old photograph albums if they are available.
4. Keep staff and caregivers to a minimum to promote familiarity.
5. Speak slowly and clearly while looking into Carmen's face.
6. Use reminiscence therapy with Carmen. Ask her to share happy times from her life with you. This technique helps decrease depression and boost self-esteem.
7. Mention the date and time in casual conversation. Refer to "spring rain," "summer flowers," "fall leaves." Emphasize holidays.
8. Correct misperceptions gently and matter-of-factly and focus on real events and real people if false ideas should occur. Validate her feelings associated with current and past life situations.
9. Monitor for medication side effects because toxic effects from certain medications can intensify altered thought processes.

SELF-CARE DEFICIT

The following nursing interventions may be implemented *to ensure that Carmen's personal care needs are fulfilled*.

1. Assess what Carmen can do independently and with what she needs assistance.
2. Allow plenty of time for her to accomplish tasks that are within her ability. Clothing that allows easy removal or replacement, such as Velcro fasteners, facilitates independence.
3. Provide guidance and support for independent actions by talking her through tasks one step at a time.
4. Provide a structured schedule of activities that does not change from day to day.
5. Ensure that Carmen has snacks between meals.
6. Take Carmen to the bathroom regularly (according to her usual pattern, e.g., after meals, before bedtime, on arising).
7. To minimize nighttime wetness, offer fluid every 2 hours during the day and restrict fluid after 6:00 p.m.
8. To promote more restful nighttime sleep (and less wandering at night), reduce naps during late afternoon and encourage sitting exercises, walking, and ball toss. Carbohydrate snacks at bedtime may also be helpful.

EVALUATION

The outcome criteria identified for Carmen have been met. She has experienced no injury. She has not fallen out of bed. She continues to wander in a safe area. She can find her room by herself but occasionally requires some assistance when she is anxious and more confused. She has some difficulty communicating her needs to the staff, but those who work with her on a consistent basis are able to anticipate her needs. All ADLs are being fulfilled, and Carmen assists with dressing and grooming, accomplishing about half on her own. Nighttime wandering has been minimized. Soft bedtime music helps to relax her.

than 4 hours before bedtime); getting proper nutrition; avoiding alcohol, caffeine, and nicotine; and retiring at the same time each night are behavioral approaches to sleep problems that may eliminate the need for sleep aids, particularly in the early stages of NCD. Because of the increased risk of adverse drug reactions in the elderly, many of whom are already taking multiple medications, pharmacological treatment of insomnia should be considered only after attempts at nonpharmacological strategies have failed.

Summary and Key Points

- Neurocognitive disorders (NCDs) constitute a large and growing public health concern.
- Delirium is a disturbance of awareness and a change in cognition that develop rapidly over a short period. Level of consciousness is often affected, and psychomotor activity may fluctuate between agitated purposeless movements and a vegetative state resembling catatonic stupor.
- The symptoms of delirium usually begin quite abruptly and often are reversible and brief.
- Delirium may be caused by a general medical condition, substance intoxication or withdrawal, or ingestion of a medication or exposure to a toxin.
- NCD is a syndrome of acquired, persistent intellectual impairment with compromised function in multiple spheres of mental activity, such as memory, language, visuospatial skills, emotion or personality, and cognition.
- Dementia (also described as major NCD in the *DSM-5*) is a progressive decline of cognitive abilities in the presence of clear consciousness.
- Symptoms of major NCD are insidious and develop slowly over time. In most patients, the disorder runs a progressive, irreversible course.
- NCD may be caused by genetics, cardiovascular disease, infections, neurophysiological disorders, and other general medical conditions.
- Nursing care of the patient with an NCD is presented around the six steps of the nursing process.
- Objectives of care for the patient experiencing an acute syndrome are aimed at eliminating the etiology, promoting patient safety, and a return to the highest possible level of functioning.
- Objectives of care for the patient experiencing a chronic, progressive disorder are aimed at preserving the dignity of the individual, promoting deceleration of the symptoms, and maximizing functional capabilities.
- "Well-Being and Health for People With Dementia (WHELD)" is an evidence-based intervention for patients with dementia in long-term care settings that has demonstrated effectiveness in decreasing agitation, decreasing the need for antipsychotic medication, and improving the quality of life in this population.
- Nursing interventions are also directed toward helping the patient's family or primary caregivers learn about a chronic, progressive neurocognitive disorder.
- Education is provided about the disease process, expectations of patient behavioral changes, methods for facilitating care, and sources of assistance and support as they struggle, both physically and emotionally, with the demands brought on by a disease process that is slowly taking their loved one away from them.

Review Questions

Select the answer that is most appropriate for each of the following questions:

1. An example of a treatable (reversible) form of NCD is one that is caused by which of the following? (Select all that apply.)
   a. Multiple sclerosis
   b. Multiple small brain infarcts
   c. Electrolyte imbalances
   d. HIV disease
   e. Folate deficiency
2. NCD due to Alzheimer's disease is associated with the presence of which anomaly?
   a. Multiple small brain infarcts
   b. Lewy bodies
   c. Cerebral abscess
   d. Amyloid beta plaques and neurofibrillary tangles

3. Which medications have been indicated for improvement in cognitive functioning in mild to moderate Alzheimer's disease? (Select all that apply.)
   a. Donepezil (Aricept)
   b. Rivastigmine (Exelon)
   c. Risperidone (Risperdal)
   d. Sertraline (Zoloft)
   e. Galantamine (Razadyne)
4. Which factor is not associated with an increased incidence of neurocognitive disorder due to Alzheimer's disease?
   a. Multiple small strokes
   b. Family history of Alzheimer's disease
   c. Head trauma
   d. Advanced age
5. In addition to disturbances in cognition and orientation, individuals with Alzheimer's disease may also show changes in which of the following? (Select all that apply.)
   a. Personality
   b. Vision
   c. Speech
   d. Hearing
   e. Mobility

Clinical Judgment Questions

6. A client, who has NCD due to Alzheimer's disease, says to the nurse, "I have a date tonight. I always have a date on Christmas." Which of the following is the most appropriate response?
   a. "Don't be silly. It's not Christmas."
   b. "Today is Tuesday, October 21st. We will have supper soon, and then your daughter will come to visit."
   c. "Who is your date with?"
   d. "I think you need some more medication. I'll bring it to you now."
7. A client, who has NCD due to Alzheimer's disease, has trouble sleeping and wanders around at night. Which of the following nursing actions would be *best* to promote sleep in this client?
   a. Ask the doctor to prescribe flurazepam (Dalmane).
   b. Ensure that the client gets an afternoon nap so they will not be overtired at bedtime.
   c. Make the client a cup of tea with honey before bedtime.
   d. Ensure that the client gets regular physical exercise during the day.
8. The night nurse finds a client with Alzheimer's disease wandering the hallway at 4 a.m. and trying to open the door to the side yard. Which statement is the best initial response by the nurse?
   a. "That door leads out to the patio. It's nighttime. You don't want to go outside now."
   b. "You look confused. What is bothering you?"
   c. "This is the patio door. Are you looking for the bathroom?"
   d. "Are you lonely? Perhaps you'd like to go back to your room and talk for a while."
9. A client with neurocognitive disease due to Alzheimer's disease is admitted to the hospital. Which action by the nurse is a priority?
   a. Ensuring that the client receives food they like to prevent anxiety
   b. Ensuring that the environment is safe to prevent injury
   c. Ensuring that the client meets the other patients to prevent social isolation
   d. Ensuring that the client takes care of their own ADLs to prevent dependence

Continued

10. Which intervention is most appropriate for helping a client with Alzheimer's disease with ADLs?
    a. Perform ADLs for the hospitalized client.
    b. Provide a written list of activities the client is expected to perform.
    c. Provide step-by-step instructions and plenty of time to perform independently as many ADLs as possible.
    d. Tell the client that if morning care is not completed by 9:00 a.m., it will be performed by the nurse's aide in order to be on time for group therapy.

TEST YOUR CLINICAL REASONING AND CLINICAL JUDGMENT SKILLS

Joe, a 62-year-old accountant, began having difficulty remembering details necessary to perform his job. He was also having trouble at home, failing to keep his finances straight and forgetting to pay bills. It became increasingly difficult for him to function properly at work, and eventually he was forced to retire. Cognitive deterioration continued, and behavioral problems soon began. He became stubborn, verbally and physically abusive, and suspicious of almost everyone in his environment. His wife and son convinced him to see a physician, who recommended hospitalization for testing.

At Joe's initial evaluation, he was fully alert and cooperative but obviously anxious and fidgety. He thought he was at his accounting office, and he could not state what year it was. He could not say the names of his parents or siblings, nor did he know who the current President of the United States was. He could not perform simple arithmetic calculations, write a proper sentence, or copy a drawing. He interpreted proverbs concretely and had difficulty stating similarities between related objects.

Laboratory serum studies revealed no abnormalities, but a CT scan showed marked cortical atrophy. The physician's diagnosis was Neurocognitive Disorder due to Alzheimer's Disease.

Answer the following questions related to Joe:

1. What are the pertinent assessment data from which nursing care will be devised?
2. What is the primary nursing diagnosis for Joe?
3. How would outcomes be identified?

Communication Exercises

1. **Mrs. B is a patient on the Alzheimer's unit. The nurse hears her yelling, "Waitress! Waitress! Why can't I get some service around here?!" How would the nurse respond appropriately to this statement by Mrs. B?**
2. **Mrs. B, who had breakfast an hour ago, says to the nurse, "I've been waiting and waiting for my breakfast. On the farm, we always had breakfast by six o'clock. Those were the good old days." How would the nurse respond appropriately to this statement by Mrs. B?**

MOVIE CONNECTIONS

The Notebook (Alzheimer's disease) ▪ *Away From Her* (Alzheimer's disease) ▪ *Iris* (Alzheimer's disease) ▪ *Still Alice* (Early-onset Alzheimer's disease)

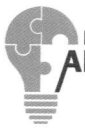

Go to **Davis Advantage** to complete your learning: strengthen understanding, apply your knowledge, and prepare for the Next Gen NCLEX®.

References

Abushakra, S., Porsteinsson, A. P., Sabbagh, M., Bracoud, L., Schaerer, J., Power, A., Hey, J. A., Scott, D., Suhy, J., & Tola, M. (2020). APOE ε4/ε4 homozygotes with early Alzheimer's disease show accelerated hippocampal atrophy and cortical thinning that correlates with cognitive decline. *Alzheimer's & Dementia: Translational Research & Clinical Interventions, 6*(1), e12117.

Alagiakrishnan, K. (2019). *Delirium medications.* http://emedicine.medscape.com/article/288890-medication

Alzheimer's Association. (2020). *2020 Alzheimer's disease facts and figures.* https://www.alz.org/media/Documents/alzheimers-facts-and-figures.pdf

Alzheimer's Association. (2021a). *Causes and risk factors for Alzheimer's disease.* https://www.alz.org/alzheimers-dementia/what-is-alzheimers/causes-and-risk-factors

Alzheimer's Association. (2021b). *Depression.* http://www.alz.org/care/alzheimers-dementia-depression.asp

American Psychiatric Association. (2000). *Diagnostic and statistical manual of mental disorders* (4th ed., text rev.).

American Psychiatric Association. (2013). *Diagnostic and statistical manual of mental disorders* (5th ed.).

American Psychiatric Association. (2015). *The American Psychiatric Association practice guideline on the use of antipsychotics to treat agitation or psychosis in patients with dementia.* http://psychiatryonline.org/doi/book/10.1176/appi.books.9780890426807

Ballard, C., Corbett, A., Orrell, M., Williams, G., Moniz-Cook, E., Romeo, R., Woods, B., Garrod, L., Testad, I., Woodward-Carlton, B., Wenborn, J., Knapp, M., & Fossey J. (2018). Impact of person-centred care training and person-centred activities on quality of life, agitation, and antipsychotic use in people with dementia living in nursing homes: A cluster-randomised controlled trial. *PLoS Med, 15*(2), e1002500. https://doi.org/10.1371/journal.pmed.1002500

Ballard, C., Orrell, M., Moniz-Cook, E., Woods, R., Whitaker, R., Corbett, A., Aarsland, D., Murray, J., Lawrence, V., Testad, I., Knapp, M., Romeo, R., Zala, D., Stafford, J., Hoare, Z., Garrod, L., Sun, Y., McLaughlin, E., Woodward-Carlton, B., Williams, G., & Fossey, J. (2020). Improving mental health and reducing antipsychotic use in people with dementia in care homes: The WHELD research programme including two RCTs. *Programme Grants for Applied Research, 8*(6). https://doi.org/10.3310/pgfar08060

Ballard, C., Orrell, M., Yong Zhong, S., Moniz-Cook, E., Stafford, J., Whittaker, R., Woods, B., Corbett, A., Garrod, L., Khan, Z., Woodward-Carlton, B., Wenborn, J., & Fossey, J. (2016). Impact of antipsychotic review and nonpharmacological intervention on antipsychotic use, neuropsychiatric symptoms, and mortality in people with dementia living in nursing homes: A factorial cluster-randomized controlled trial by the well-being and health for people with dementia (WHELD) program. *American Journal of Psychiatry, 173*(3), 252–262. https://doi.org/10.1176/appi.ajp.2015.15010130

Bhandari, T. (2019, August 1). *Blood test is highly accurate at identifying Alzheimer's before symptoms arise* [Press release]. Washington University School of Medicine, St. Louis.

Boland, R., & Verduin, M. L. (2022). *Kaplan & Sadock's synopsis of psychiatry* (P. Ruiz, Ed.). (12th ed.). Wolters Kluwer.

Coupland, C. A., Hill, T., Dening, T., Morriss, R., Moore, M., & Hippisley-Cox, J. (2019). Anticholinergic drug exposure and the risk of dementia: A nested case-control study. *JAMA Internal Medicine, 179*(8), 1084–1093. https://doi.org/10.1001/jamainternmed.2019.0677

Crystal, H. A. (2019). Dementia with Lewy bodies: Treatment and management. *Medscape.* emedicine.medscape.com/article/1135041-medication#2

Elie, D., & Rej, S. (2018). Pharmacological management of neuropsychiatric symptoms in patients with major neurocognitive disorders. *Journal of Psychiatry & Neuroscience, 43*(1), 69–70. https://doi.org/10.1503/jpn.170117

Fabian, T. J., & Solai, L. K. (2017). Neurocognitive disorders. In B. J. Sadock, V. A. Sadock, & P. Ruiz (Eds.), *Comprehensive textbook of psychiatry* (pp. 1178–1191). Wolters Kluwer.

Germain, S., Wojtasik,V., Lekeu, F., Quittre, A., Olivier, C., Godichard, V., & Salmon, E. (2018). Efficacy of cognitive rehabilitation in Alzheimer disease: A 1-year follow-up study. *Journal of Geriatric Psychiatry and Neurology, 32*(1), 16–23. https://doi.org/10.1177/0891988718813724

Graff-Radford, J. (2021). *Can a head injury cause or hasten Alzheimer's disease or other types of dementia?* https://www.mayoclinic.org/diseases-conditions/alzheimers-disease/expert-answers/alzheimers-disease/faq-20057837

Graziane, J. A., & Sweet, R. A. (2017). Dementia. In B. J. Sadock, V. A. Sadock, & P. Ruiz (Eds.), *Comprehensive textbook of psychiatry* (pp. 1191–1221). Wolters Kluwer.

Hampel, H., O'Bryant, S. E., Molinuevo, J. L., Zetterberg, H., Masters, C. L., Lista, S., Kiddle, S. J., Batrla, R., & Blennow, K. (2018). Blood-based biomarkers for Alzheimer disease: Mapping the road to the clinic. *Nature Reviews Neurology, 14*(11), 639–652. https://doi.org/10.1038/s41582-018-0079-7

Herbert, J. (2016). Depression is a risk for Alzheimer's: We need to know why. *Psychology Today.* https://www.psychologytoday.com/us/blog/hormones-and-the-brain/201604/depression-is-risk-alzheimer-s-we-need-know-why

Herbert, J., & Lucassen, P. J. (2016). Depression as a risk factor for Alzheimer's disease: Genes, steroids, cytokines and neurogenesis—What do we need to know? *Frontiers in Neuroendocrinology, 41,* 153–171. https://doi.org/10.1016/j.yfrne.2015.12.001

Herdman, T. H., Kamitsuru, S., & Lopes, C. T. (Eds.). (2021). *NANDA-I nursing diagnoses: Definitions and classification, 2021–2023* (12th ed.). Thieme.

Huntington's Disease Society of America. (2021). *What is Huntington's disease?* http://hdsa.org/what-is-hd/overview-of-huntingtons-disease/

Institute of Medicine. (2003). *Health professions education: A bridge to quality.*

Johns Hopkins Medicine. (n.d.). Prion diseases. *Health Library.* https://www.hopkinsmedicine.org/healthlibrary/conditions/nervous_system_disorders/prion_diseases_134,56

Kishi, T., Hirota, T., Matsunaga, S., & Iwata, N. (2015). Antipsychotic medications for the treatment of delirium: A systematic review and meta-analysis of randomised controlled trials. *Journal of Neurology, Neurosurgery, and Psychiatry, 87*(7), 767–774. https://doi.org/10.1136/jnnp-2015-311049

Kou, X., & Chen, N. (2017). Resveratrol as a natural autophagy regulator for prevention and treatment of Alzheimer's disease. *Nutrients, 9*(9), 927. https://doi.org/10.3390/nu9090927

Langa, K. M., Larson, E. B., Crimmins, E. M., Faul, J. D., Levine, D. A., Kabeto, M. U., & Weir, D. R. (2017). A comparison of the prevalence of dementia in the United States in 2000 and 2012. *JAMA Internal Medicine, 177*(1), 51–58. https://doi.org/10.1001/jamainternmed.2016.6807

LaVigne, P. (2016). *Alzheimer's vaccine: Researchers target brain proteins in mouse study.* http://www.thevaccinereaction.org/2016/08/alzheimers-vaccineresearchers-target-brain-proteins-in-mouse-study

Mayo Clinic. (2021a). *Dementia: Symptoms and causes.* https://www.mayoclinic.org/diseases-conditions/dementia/symptoms-causes/syc-20352013

Mayo Clinic. (2021b). *Vascular dementia.* https://www.mayoclinic.org/diseases-conditions/vascular-dementia/symptoms-causes/syc-20378793

Mayo Clinic. (2021c). *Alzheimer's disease: Diagnosis and treatment.* https://www.mayoclinic.org/diseases-conditions/alzheimers-disease/diagnosis-treatment/drc-20350453%99s-disease-vaccine-be-reality

Meng, Y. H., Wang, P. P., Song, Y. X., & Wang, J. H. (2019). Cholinesterase inhibitors and memantine for Parkinson's disease dementia and Lewy body dementia: A meta-analysis. *Experimental and Therapeutic Medicine, 17*(3), 1611–1624. https://doi.org/10.3892/etm.2018.7129

Mitchell, S. (2015). Advanced dementia. *New England Journal of Medicine, 372*(26), 2533–2540.

Moore, R. C., & Marquine, M. J. (2017). HIV and aging. In B. J. Sadock, V. A. Sadock, & P. Ruiz (Eds.), *Comprehensive textbook of psychiatry* (pp. 4268–4274). Wolters Kluwer.

National Institute of Neurological Disorders and Stroke. (2019). *NINDS frontotemporal dementia information page.* https://www.ninds.nih.gov/Disorders/All-Disorders/Frontotemporal-Dementia-Information-Page

National Institute on Aging. (2017). *Coping with late-stage Alzheimer's disease.* https://www.nia.nih.gov/health/coping-late-stage-alzheimers-disease

Neufeld, K. J., Yue, J., Robinson, T. N., Inouye, S. K., & Needham, D. M. (2016). Antipsychotic medication for prevention and treatment of delirium in hospitalized adults: A systematic review and meta-analysis. *Journal of the American Geriatrics Society, 64*(4), 705–714. https://doi.org/10.1111/jgs.14076

Newman, T. (2018). *Alzheimer's vaccine draws closer.* https://www.medicalnewstoday.com/articles/323734.php

Norton, A. (2021). *Anxiety might speed Alzheimer's: Study.* https://www.webmd.com/alzheimers/news/20201124/anxiety-might-speed-alzheimers-study

Oba, T., Saito, T., Asada, A., Shimizu, S., Iijima, K. M., & Ando, K. (2020). Microtubule affinity–regulating kinase 4 with an Alzheimer's disease-related mutation promotes tau accumulation and exacerbates neurodegeneration. *Molecular Bases of Disease Neurobiology, 295*(50), P17138–17147. https://doi.org/10.1074/jbc.RA120.014420

Perez Ortiz, J. M., & Swerdlow, R. H. (2019). Mitochondrial dysfunction in Alzheimer's disease: Role in pathogenesis and novel therapeutic opportunities. *British Journal of Pharmacology,* 1–19. https://doi.org/10.1111/bph.14585

Rabin, J. S., Klein, H., Kirn, D. R., Schultz, A. P., Yang, H. S., Hampton, O., Jiang, S., Buckley, R. F., Viswanathan, A., Hedden, T., Pruzin, J., Yau, W. W., Guzmán-Vélez, E., Quiroz, Y. T., Properzi, M., Marshall, G. A., Rentz, D. M., Johnson, K. A., Sperling, R. A., & Chhatwal, J. P. (2019). Associations of physical activity and β-amyloid with longitudinal cognition and neurodegeneration in clinically normal older adults. *JAMA Neurology, 76*(10), 1203–1210. https://doi.org/10.1001/jamaneurol.2019.1879

Ries, J. (2019). *An Alzheimer's vaccine won't be approved anytime soon, here's why.* https://www.healthline.com/health-news/dont-bet-on-an-alzheimers-vaccine-anytime-soon#Alzheimer%E2%80%99s-is-a-complex-disease-and-difficult-to-treat

Russell-Williams, J., Jaroudi, W., Perich, T., Hoscheidt, S., El Haj, M., & Moustafa, A. A. (2018). Mindfulness and meditation: Treating cognitive impairment and reducing stress in dementia. *Reviews in the Neurosciences, 29*(7), 791–804. https://doi.org/10.1515/revneuro-2017-0066

Schindler, S. E., Bollinger, J. G., Ovod, V., Mawuenyega, K. G., Li, Y., Gordon, B. A., Holtzman, D. M., Morris, J. C., Benzinger, T. L. S., Xiong, C., Fagan, A. M., & Bateman, R. J. (2019). High-precision plasma β-amyloid 42/40 predicts current and future brain amyloidosis. *Neurology, 93*(17), e1647–e1659. https://doi.org/10.1212/WNL.0000000000008081

Strub, R. L., & Black, F. W. (2000). *The mental status examination in neurology* (4th ed.). F.A. Davis.

Sullivan, M. (2018). Alzheimer's: Biomarkers, not cognition, will now define disorder. *Clinical Psychiatry News.* https://www.mdedge.com/clinicalpsychiatrynews/article/163073/alzheimers-cognition/alzheimers-biomarkers-not-cognition-will/page/0/6

Turner, R. S., Thomas, R. G., Craft, S., van Dyck, C. H., Mintzer, J., Reynolds, B. A., Brewer, J. B., Rissman, R. A., Raman, R., Aisen, P. S., Alzheimer's Disease Cooperative Study. (2015). A randomized, double-blind, placebo-controlled trial of resveratrol for Alzheimer disease. *Neurology, 85*(16), 1383–1391. https://doi.org/10.1212/WNL.0000000000002035

University Health News. (2019). Ketogenic diet shows promising results for all dementia stages. https://universityhealthnews.com/daily/memory/ketogenic-diet-shows-promising-results-for-all-dementia-stages/

WebMD. (2021). *7 stages of Alzheimer's disease.* https://www.webmd.com/alzheimers/guide/alzheimers-disease-stages#2

Whitaker, R., Fossey, J., Ballard, C., Orrell, M., Moniz-Cook, E., Woods, R. T., Murray, J., Stafford, J., Knapp, M., Romeo, R., Carlton, B.W., Testad, I., & Khan, Z. (2014). Improving well-being and health for people with dementia (WHELD): Study protocol for a randomised controlled trial. *BioMed Central, 15*(284). https://doi.org/10.1186/1745-6215-15-284

Validation Training Institute. (2021). *What is validation?* https://vfvalidation.org/get-started/what-is-validation/

Substance Use and Addiction Disorders 14

CHAPTER OUTLINE

Objectives
Introduction
Substance Use Disorder, Defined
Substance-Induced Disorder, Defined
Classes of Psychoactive Substances
Predisposing Factors to Substance-Related Disorders
The Dynamics of Substance-Related Disorders
Application of the Nursing Process
The Chemically Impaired Nurse
Codependency
Treatment Modalities
Nonsubstance Addictions
Summary and Key Points
Review Questions
Clinical Judgment Questions
Implications for Evidence-Based Practice
Test Your Clinical Reasoning and Clinical Judgment Skills
Communication Exercises
Movie Connections

CORE CONCEPTS

Addiction
Behaviors: Maladaptive behavior
Safety: Intoxication, Withdrawal
Professional Behavior: Nursing process in the care of patients with substance use disorders
Clinical Judgment

KEY TERMS

addiction
Alcoholics Anonymous
amphetamines
ascites
cannabis
codependency
detoxification
disulfiram
dual diagnosis
esophageal varices
Gamblers Anonymous
hepatic encephalopathy
intoxication
Korsakoff's psychosis
medication-assisted treatment
misuse
opioid
peer assistance programs
Wernicke's encephalopathy
withdrawal

OBJECTIVES

After reading this chapter, the student will be able to:

1. Define *addiction, intoxication*, and *withdrawal*.
2. Discuss predisposing factors implicated in the etiology of substance-related and addictive disorders.
3. Identify symptomatology and use the information in assessment of clients with various substance-related and addictive disorders.
4. Identify nursing diagnoses common to patients with substance-related and addictive disorders and select appropriate nursing interventions for each.
5. Identify topics for patient and family teaching relevant to substance-related and addictive disorders.
6. Describe relevant outcome criteria for evaluating nursing care of patients with substance-related and addictive disorders.

Continued

OBJECTIVES—cont'd
After reading this chapter, the student will be able to:

7. Discuss the issue of substance-related and addictive disorders within the profession of nursing.
8. Define *codependency* and identify behavioral characteristics associated with the disorder.
9. Discuss treatment of codependency.
10. Describe various modalities relevant to treatment of individuals with substance-related and addictive disorders.

Introduction

Substance-related disorders comprise two groups: the substance use disorders (addiction) and the substance-induced disorders (intoxication, withdrawal, delirium, neurocognitive disorder, psychosis, bipolar disorder, depressive disorder, obsessive-compulsive disorder, anxiety disorder, sexual dysfunction, and sleep disorders). This chapter discusses addiction, intoxication, and withdrawal. The remainder of the substance-induced disorders are included in the chapters with which they share symptomatology (e.g., substance-induced depressive disorder is discussed in Chapter 16, "Depressive Disorders"; substance-induced anxiety disorder is discussed in Chapter 18, "Anxiety, Obsessive-Compulsive, and Related Disorders"). Also included in this chapter is a discussion of gambling disorder, a nonsubstance addiction disorder.

Drugs are a pervasive part of our society. Certain mood-altering substances are quite socially acceptable and are used moderately by many adult Americans. They include alcohol, caffeine, and nicotine. Society has even developed a relative indifference to an occasional misuse of these substances despite documentation of their negative impact on health.

A wide variety of substances are produced for medicinal purposes. These include central nervous system (CNS) stimulants (e.g., amphetamines), CNS depressants (e.g., sedatives, tranquilizers), as well as numerous over-the-counter preparations designed to relieve nearly every kind of human ailment, real or imagined.

Some historically illegal substances have achieved a degree of social acceptance by certain societal subcultures. These drugs, such as marijuana and hashish, are by no means harmless even though they are becoming legalized in some states. The long-term effects are still being studied, whereas the dangerous effects of other illegal substances (e.g., lysergic acid diethylamide [LSD], phencyclidine, cocaine, and heroin) have been well documented. Opiate use has increased dramatically in both prescriptions for medicinal purposes and those purchased illegally. Currently this substance use disorder has been identified as a national epidemic and is associated with an alarming number of deaths.

This chapter discusses the physical and behavioral manifestations and personal and social consequences related to the **misuse** (overuse with potentially harmful consequences) of or **addiction** (physical, mental, and behavioral reliance) to alcohol, other CNS depressants, CNS stimulants, opioids, hallucinogens, cannabinols, and the nonsubstance addiction to gambling. The term *misuse* is equivalent to *abuse* but is replacing the latter term in many contexts to reduce the shaming and stigmatization associated with individuals being described as *abusers*. Variations in attitudes regarding substance consumption and patterns of use are explored. For example, drinking alcohol is considered by many to be part of the culture of college life while, at the same time, substance *misuse* is especially prevalent among individuals between the ages of 18 and 24. Substance-related disorders are diagnosed more commonly in men than in women, but the gender ratios vary with the class of the substance.

Codependency is described in this chapter, as are aspects of treatment for the disorder. The issue of substance impairment within the profession of nursing is also explored. Nursing care for individuals with substance use and addictive disorders is presented in the context of the six steps of the nursing process. Various medical and other treatment modalities are also discussed.

Substance Use Disorder, Defined

CORE CONCEPT
Addiction
A compulsive or chronic requirement. The need is so strong as to generate distress (physical or psychological) if left unfulfilled.

Substance Addiction

The *Diagnostic and Statistical Manual of Mental Disorders, Fifth Edition, Text Revision (DSM-5-TR)* (American Psychiatric Association [APA], 2022) lists diagnostic criteria for addiction to specific substances, including alcohol, cannabis, hallucinogens, inhalants, opioids, sedative-hypnotics, stimulants, and tobacco. These are identified as substance use disorders. Individuals are considered to have a substance use disorder when use of the substance interferes with their ability to fulfill role obligations, such as at work, school, or home. Often the individual would like to cut down or control use of the substance, but attempts fail, and use of the substance continues to increase. There is an intense craving for the substance, and an excessive amount of time is spent trying to procure more of the substance or recover from the effects of its use. Use of the substance causes problems with interpersonal relationships, and the individual may become socially isolated. Individuals with substance use disorders often participate in hazardous activities when they are impaired by the substance and continue to use the substance despite knowing that its use is contributing to a physical or psychosocial problem. Addiction is evident when tolerance develops, the amount required to achieve the desired effect continues to increase, and the priority focus of behavior is obtaining the substance. A syndrome of symptoms, characteristic of the specific substance, occurs when the individual with the addiction attempts to discontinue use of the substance.

Substance-Induced Disorder, Defined

CORE CONCEPT

Intoxication

A state of disturbance in cognition, perception, behavior, level of consciousness, judgment, and other functions that is directly attributable to the effects of a psychoactive drug. It may be marked by a physical and mental state of exhilaration and emotional frenzy or lethargy and stupor.

Substance Intoxication

Substance **intoxication** is defined as the development of a reversible syndrome of symptoms following excessive use of a substance. The symptoms are drug specific and occur during or shortly after the ingestion of the substance. The CNS is directly affected, and disruption in physical and psychological functioning occurs. Judgment is disturbed, resulting in inappropriate and maladaptive behavior, and social and occupational functioning are impaired.

CORE CONCEPT

Withdrawal

Withdrawal is the physiological and mental readjustment that accompanies the discontinuation of an addictive substance.

Substance Withdrawal

Substance **withdrawal** occurs upon abrupt reduction or discontinuation of a substance that has been used regularly over a prolonged period. The substance-specific syndrome includes clinically significant physical signs and symptoms as well as psychological changes such as disturbances in thinking, feeling, and behavior.

Classes of Psychoactive Substances

The following classes of psychoactive substances are associated with substance use and substance-induced disorders:

1. Alcohol
2. Caffeine
3. Cannabis
4. Hallucinogens
5. Inhalants
6. Opioids
7. Sedative-hypnotics
8. Stimulants
9. Tobacco (nicotine)

Predisposing Factors to Substance-Related Disorders

A number of factors have been implicated in the predisposition to misuse and become addicted to substances. At present, there is no single theory that can adequately explain the etiology of this problem. No doubt the interaction between various elements forms a complex collection of determinants that influence a person's susceptibility.

Biological Factors

Genetics

Hereditary factors appear to be involved in the development of substance use disorders, especially alcoholism. Children of alcoholics are four times more likely than other children to become alcoholics (American Academy of Child and Adolescent Psychiatry, 2019). Studies of monozygotic and dizygotic twins have demonstrated that monozygotic (one egg, genetically identical) twins have a higher rate for concordance of alcoholism than dizygotic (two eggs, genetically nonidentical) twins (Schuckit, 2017). Furthermore, biological offspring of alcoholic parents have a significantly greater incidence of alcoholism than offspring of nonalcoholic parents whether the child was reared by the biological parents or by nonalcoholic adoptive parents (Schuckit, 2017). Although there is no single factor that determines whether someone will develop a substance use disorder, scientists estimate that genetics accounts for 40% to 60% of a person's vulnerability (National Institute on Drug Abuse [NIDA], 2020a). Some of this vulnerability may be related to heritable personality traits, such as high novelty seeking and low harm avoidance, both of which have been linked to substance use disorders (Iannucci & Weiss, 2017). Other variables include lifestyle influences such as diet, exercise, and types of social activities (e.g., frequency of engaging in social activities that include regular substance use).

Biochemical

There is good evidence that changes in brain structure and brain neurochemistry occur in the process of addiction, but whether these changes wholly explain etiology remains controversial. Alcohol has demonstrated effects on almost all neurotransmitters, but those most strongly linked to substance overuse include opioid, catecholamine (especially dopamine), glutamate (especially those binding to *N*-methyl-D-aspartate [NMDA]), and gamma-aminobutyric acid (GABA) systems (Volkow & Boyle, 2018; Wang et al., 2019). Once activated, the neuronal pathways that are responsible for sensing pleasure and reward are believed to be responsible for pleasurable sensations associated with addictive substances as well as creating a "memory" that triggers desire for repeated use of the substance. These pathways are referred to as the *brain-reward circuitry*. Over time, the brain tries to compensate for this excessive activation by lowering levels of these neurotransmitters, and the result is that an individual begins to feel sick. At this point, the substance user may be drawn to continue use of the substance simply to feel less sick.

Skeptics of the biochemical theories of addiction argue that because substance-dependent individuals have the capacity to change their behavior, addiction is more likely a complex interaction of several factors than strictly a single biochemical process. While ongoing research will continue to shed light on specific mechanisms in addiction, both the American Society of Addiction Medicine (ASAM, 2015) and the Surgeon General (U.S. Department of Health and Human Services [HHS], Office of the Surgeon General, 2016) agree that addiction is a disease of the brain.

Psychological Factors

Developmental Influences

The psychodynamic approach to the etiology of substance misuse focuses on a punitive superego and fixation at the oral stage of psychosexual development. Thus, individuals with punitive superegos turn to drugs to diminish unconscious anxiety and increase feelings of power and self-worth. Boland and Verduin (2022) state, "As a form of self-medication, alcohol may be used to control panic, opioids to diminish anger, and amphetamines to alleviate depression. Some addicts have great difficulty recognizing their inner emotional states, a condition called *alexithymia*" (p. 275).

Personality Factors

Certain personality traits have been associated with an increased tendency toward addictive behavior. Some clinicians believe that low self-esteem, frequent depression, passivity, antisocial personality traits, high risk-taking traits, the inability to relax or to defer gratification, and the inability to communicate effectively are common in individuals who misuse substances. These personality characteristics cannot be called *predictive* of addictive behavior, yet for reasons not completely understood, they have been found to accompany addiction in many instances. In some cases, the substance user may be self-medicating to treat symptoms of depression or anxiety.

Cognitive Factors

Irrational thinking patterns have long been identified as a problem that is central in addictions. Whether these thought patterns contribute to the development or simply perpetuate an existing addiction is an unanswered question, but their influence is widely accepted. Twerski (1997) describes these thought patterns as "addictive thinking" and suggests that when these thought patterns are unchallenged, they may culminate in additional addictions (drugs, sex, gambling, etc.) even when individuals stop using the substance to which they first became addicted. Some examples of irrational thinking patterns often associated with addiction include denial ("I'm not really addicted"), projection ("It's my wife's fault that I take drugs"), and rationalization ("I have to take drugs because I am in pain"). Exploring these thought patterns and their influence on problematic behavior, which is the basis of cognitive behavior therapy (CBT), has been identified as beneficial in addictions treatment (NIDA, 2020b).

Sociocultural Factors

Social Learning

The effects of modeling, imitation, and identification on behavior can be observed from early childhood onward. The family appears to be an important influence in individuals with substance use disorders. Various studies have shown that children and adolescents are more likely to use substances if they have parents who provide a model for substance use. Peers often exert substantial influence in the life of the child or adolescent who is being encouraged to use substances for the first time. Modeling may continue to be a factor in the use of substances once the individual enters the workforce, particularly if the work setting provides plenty of leisure time with coworkers and drinking is valued as a way to express group cohesiveness.

Conditioning

Conditioning is a learned response that occurs after repeated exposure to a stimulus. Substance misuse can become a learned response from the substance itself as well as from the environment where use occurs. Many substances create a pleasurable experience that encourages the user to repeat it; thus, it is the intrinsically reinforcing properties of addictive drugs that "condition" the individual to repeatedly seek out their use.

The environment in which the substance is taken also contributes to the reinforcement. If the environment is pleasurable, substance use is usually increased. In addition, as the substance induces a state of pleasure, the user may begin to associate that environment with these feelings and thus with drug use. Aversive stimuli within an environment are thought to be associated with a decrease in substance use within that environment.

Cultural and Ethnic Influences

Factors within an individual's culture may contribute to establishing patterns of substance use by molding attitudes, influencing patterns of consumption based on cultural acceptance, and determining the availability of the substance. However, it is important to remember that a person's risk for addiction is multifaceted and cannot be tied solely to ethnic or cultural factors. For centuries, the French and Italians have considered wine an essential part of the family meal, even for the children. The incidence of alcohol addiction is low, and acute intoxication from alcohol is not common. Conversely, alcohol problems in Ireland, where alcohol is a part of the social culture and pubs are considered a hub for social activity, are among the highest internationally; the National Alcohol Diary Survey (Alcohol Action Ireland, 2021) found that 54% of the population were classified as harmful drinkers.

Some races and ethnic groups (notably Asian or American Indian individuals) have a higher risk for genetic variations that affect the activity of isoenzymes involved in alcohol metabolism. These changes cause alcohol to be converted quickly to acetaldehyde as well as a decrease in the rate at which acetaldehyde is oxidized. As a result of these changes, acetaldehyde rapidly accumulates in the body, producing unpleasant symptoms such as flushing, headaches, nausea, and palpitations when alcohol is consumed (Hanley, 2017). However, whether these genetic variations influence higher or lower prevalence of substance use disorders is unclear.

The Dynamics of Substance-Related Disorders

Alcohol Use Disorder

Profile of the Substance

Alcohol is a natural substance formed by the reaction of fermenting sugar with yeast spores. Although there are many alcohols, the type in alcoholic beverages is known scientifically as ethyl alcohol and chemically as C_2H_5OH. Its abbreviation, ETOH, is sometimes seen in medical records and in various other documents and publications.

By strict definition, alcohol is classified as a food because it contains calories; however, it has no nutritional value. Different alcoholic beverages are produced by using different sources of sugar for the fermentation process. For example, beer is made from malted barley, wine from grapes or berries, whiskey from malted grains, and rum from molasses. Distilled beverages (e.g., whiskey, scotch, gin, vodka, and other "hard" liquors) derive their name from further concentration of the alcohol through a process called *distillation.*

The alcohol content varies by type of beverage. For example, most American beers contain 3% to 6% alcohol, wines average 10% to 20% alcohol, and distilled beverages range from 40% to 50% alcohol. For consistency, the average-sized drink, regardless of beverage, is considered to have 0.5 ounces (14 grams) of alcohol. This amount is present in 12 ounces of beer, 5 ounces of wine, and 1.5 ounces of whiskey. If consumed at the same rate, all would have an equivalent effect on one's body.

Alcohol exerts a depressant effect on the CNS, resulting in behavioral and mood changes. The effects of alcohol on the CNS are proportional to the alcoholic concentration in the blood. Most states consider that an individual is legally intoxicated with a blood alcohol level of 0.08%.

The body burns alcohol at the rate of about 0.5 ounce per hour, so behavioral changes would not be expected to occur in an individual who slowly consumed only one average-sized drink per hour. Other factors do influence these effects, however, such as individual size and whether or not the stomach contains food at the time the alcohol is consumed. Alcohol is also thought to have a more profound effect when an individual is emotionally stressed or fatigued.

Most alcohol is metabolized in the liver, and the outcome of this process is the production of acetaldehyde. Acetaldehyde is then broken down by aldehyde dehydrogenase. Increased exposure to acetaldehyde leads to CNS depression, and prolonged exposure is associated with many detrimental health effects. At high levels, acetaldehyde causes the release of histamines and catecholamines, which can affect blood pressure and produce flushing, nausea, and vomiting. Although acetaldehyde oxidation generally occurs rapidly, in individuals who have genetic variations that affect alcohol dehydrogenase and aldehyde dehydrogenase, the process occurs more slowly, which may result in negative physical reactions to alcohol. These genetic variations are more common in Asian (Japanese, Chinese, and Korean) individuals (Schuckit, 2017).

Historical Perspectives

The use of alcohol can be traced back to the Neolithic age. Beer and wine are known to have been used around 6400 BC. With the introduction of distillation by the Arabs in the Middle Ages, alchemists believed that alcohol was the answer to all of their ailments. The word *whiskey*, meaning "water of life," became widely known.

In America, American Indian and Alaska Native (AI/AN) peoples had been drinking beer and wine prior to the arrival of the first European immigrants. Refinement of the distillation process made beverages with high alcohol content readily available. By the early 1800s, one renowned physician of the time, Benjamin Rush, identified excessive, chronic alcohol consumption as a disease and an addiction. The strong religious mores on which the United States was founded soon led to the Temperance movement, which sought to prohibit the sale of alcoholic beverages. By the middle of the 19th century, 13 states had passed prohibition laws. The most widespread prohibition of alcohol in the United States was from 1920 to 1933. The mandatory restrictions on national social habits resulted in the creation of profitable underground markets, which in turn led to flourishing criminal enterprises. Conversely, millions of dollars in federal, state, and local revenues from taxes and import duties on alcohol were lost. Although today alcohol is legal in the United States and the majority of people do not become physically addicted, there is a high prevalence of physical illness, injury, and loss of life secondary to alcohol misuse.

Patterns of Use

According to the 2019 National Survey of Drug Use and Health (Substance Abuse and Mental Health Services Administration [SAMHSA], 2020) the prevalence of alcohol use is 9.4% among those ages 12 to 17 years, and 54% to 55% for adults 18 years and older. There has been a significant decline in alcohol use among young adults (18–26 years) since 2016. Overall, about 14.1 million Americans meet criteria for an alcohol use disorder.

Why do people drink? In the United States people use alcoholic beverages to enhance the flavor of food with meals; at social gatherings to encourage relaxation and conviviality among the guests; and to promote a feeling of celebration at special occasions such as weddings, birthdays, and anniversaries. An alcoholic beverage (wine) is also used as part of the sacred ritual in some religious ceremonies. Therapeutically, alcohol is the major ingredient in many over-the-counter and prescription medicines that are prepared in concentrated form. Therefore, alcohol can be harmless and enjoyable—sometimes even beneficial—if it is used responsibly and in moderation.

Like any other mind-altering drug, however, alcohol has the potential for abuse. Indeed, it currently accounts for the largest percentage (73.1%) of substance use disorders in the United States (SAMHSA, 2020). It is estimated that, annually, 95,000 deaths are related to excessive alcohol use, and it is the third-leading lifestyle-related cause of death in the United States (the first is tobacco and the second is poor diet and physical inactivity) (National Institute on Alcohol Abuse and Alcoholism [NIAAA], 2021). In addition, it is a factor in more than one-half of all homicides, suicides, and motor vehicle crashes. Incidents of domestic violence are commonly alcohol related. Heavy drinking contributes to illness in each of the top three causes of death: heart disease, cancer, and stroke. An emerging trend is a phenomenon called high-intensity drinking, which is defined as consuming alcohol at levels that are two or more times the gender-specific binge drinking thresholds. Compared with people who did not binge drink, people who drank alcohol at twice the gender-specific binge drinking thresholds were 70 times more likely to have an alcohol-related emergency department (ED) visit, and those who consumed alcohol at three times the gender-specific binge thresholds were 93 times more likely to have an alcohol-related ED visit (NIAAA, 2021). It is estimated that up to 40% of hospital beds in the United States are being used to treat health conditions related to alcohol consumption. Fetal alcohol syndrome, caused by prenatal exposure to alcohol, is the leading known cause of intellectual disability in the United States (Vaux, 2016).

Development of an Alcohol Use Disorder

Jellinek's classic work (1952) outlined four phases through which the pattern of drinking progresses to becoming an alcohol use disorder (commonly referred to as alcoholism). Some variability among individuals is to be expected within this model of progression.

Phase I. Prealcoholic Phase

This phase is characterized by the use of alcohol for its effects in relieving the everyday stress and tensions of life. As a child, the individual may have observed parents or other adults drinking alcohol and enjoying the effects; societally the individual learns that use of alcohol is an acceptable method of coping with stress. Tolerance develops, and the amount required to achieve the desired effect increases steadily.

Phase II. Early Alcoholic Phase

This phase begins with blackouts—brief periods of amnesia that occur during or immediately following a period of drinking. Now the alcohol is no longer a source of pleasure or relief for the individual but rather a drug that is *required* by the individual. Common behaviors include sneaking drinks or secret drinking, preoccupation with drinking and maintaining the supply of alcohol, rapid gulping of drinks, and further blackouts. The individual feels enormous guilt and becomes very defensive about their drinking. Excessive use of denial and rationalization is evident.

Phase III. Crucial Phase

In this phase, the individual has lost control, and physiological addiction is clearly evident. This loss of control has been described as the inability to choose whether or not to drink. Binge drinking, lasting from a few hours to several weeks, is common. The NIAAA defines binge drinking as a pattern of drinking that brings blood alcohol concentration (BAC) levels to 0.08 g/dL in about 2 hours, which typically occurs after 4 drinks for women and 5 drinks for men (NIAAA, 2021). These episodes are characterized by sickness, loss of consciousness, squalor, and degradation. In this phase, the individual is extremely ill. Anger and aggression are common manifestations. Drinking is the total focus, and individuals are willing to risk losing everything that was once important in an effort to maintain the addiction. By this phase of the illness, it is not uncommon for the individual to have experienced the loss of a job, marriage, family, friends, and most especially, self-respect.

Phase IV. Chronic Phase

This phase is characterized by emotional and physical disintegration. Individuals are usually intoxicated more than they are sober. Emotional disintegration is evidenced by profound helplessness and self-pity. Impairment in reality testing may result in psychosis. Life-threatening physical manifestations may be evident in virtually every system of the body. Unmanaged withdrawal from alcohol results in a terrifying syndrome of symptoms that include hallucinations, tremors, convulsions, severe agitation, and panic. Depression and ideas of suicide are not uncommon. For long-term, heavy drinkers, abrupt withdrawal of alcohol can be fatal.

Effects on the Body

Alcohol can induce a general, nonselective, reversible depression of the CNS. About 20% of a single dose of alcohol is absorbed directly and immediately into the bloodstream through the stomach wall. Unlike other "foods," alcohol does not have to be digested. The blood carries alcohol directly to the brain, where it acts on the brain's central control areas, slowing or depressing brain activity. The other 80% of the alcohol in one drink is processed only slightly more slowly through the upper intestinal tract and into the bloodstream. Only moments after alcohol is consumed, it can be found in all tissues, organs, and secretions of the body. Rapidity of absorption is influenced by various factors. For example, absorption is delayed when the drink is sipped rather than gulped, when the stomach contains food rather than being empty, and when the drink is wine or beer rather than distilled beverages.

At low doses, alcohol produces relaxation, loss of inhibitions, lack of concentration, drowsiness, slurred speech, and sleep. Chronic misuse results in multisystem physiological impairments. These complications include (but are not limited to) those outlined in the following sections.

Peripheral Neuropathy

Peripheral neuropathy, characterized by peripheral nerve damage, results in pain, burning, tingling, or prickly sensations of the extremities. Researchers believe that it is the direct result of deficiencies in the B vitamins, particularly thiamine. Nutritional deficiencies are common in chronic alcoholics because of insufficient intake of nutrients as well as the toxic effect of alcohol that results in malabsorption of nutrients. The process is often reversible with abstinence from alcohol and restoration of nutritional deficiencies, but for some individuals, pain and numbness may be permanent (Schuckit, 2017). With chronic alcohol use permanent muscle wasting and paralysis can occur.

Alcoholic Myopathy

Alcoholic myopathy may occur as an acute or chronic condition. In the acute condition, also called *alcoholic necrotizing myopathy* or *alcoholic rhabdomyolysis*, the individual experiences a sudden onset of muscle pain, swelling, and weakness along with myoglobinuria evidenced by a red tinge in the urine. Creatine kinase may be elevated before the appearance of symptoms. Experimental studies have suggested that alcohol use and malnourishment are necessary to produce this syndrome (Lanska, 2020). Muscle symptoms are usually generalized, but pain and swelling may selectively involve the calves or other muscle groups. Laboratory studies show elevations of the enzymes creatine phosphokinase (CPK), lactate dehydrogenase (LDH), aldolase, and aspartate aminotransferase (AST). The symptoms of chronic alcoholic myopathy include a gradual wasting and weakness in skeletal muscles. Neither the pain and tenderness nor the elevated muscle enzymes seen in acute myopathy are evident in the chronic condition.

Alcoholic myopathy is thought to be a result of the same B vitamin deficiency that contributes to peripheral neuropathy and to the general injurious effects of acetaldehyde. Improvement is observed with abstinence from alcohol and the return to a nutritious diet with vitamin supplements.

Wernicke's Encephalopathy

Wernicke's encephalopathy represents the most serious form of thiamine deficiency in alcoholics. Symptoms include paralysis of the ocular muscles, diplopia, ataxia, somnolence, and stupor. If thiamine replacement therapy is not undertaken quickly, death will ensue.

Korsakoff's Psychosis

Korsakoff's psychosis is identified by a syndrome of confusion, loss of recent memory, and confabulation in alcoholics. It is frequently encountered in clients recovering from Wernicke's encephalopathy. In the United States, the two disorders are usually considered together and are called *Wernicke-Korsakoff syndrome.* Treatment is with parenteral or oral thiamine replacement.

Alcoholic Cardiomyopathy

The effect of alcohol on the heart is an accumulation of lipids in the myocardial cells, resulting in enlargement and a weakened condition. The clinical findings of alcoholic cardiomyopathy generally relate to congestive heart failure or arrhythmia. Symptoms include decreased exercise tolerance, tachycardia, dyspnea, edema, palpitations, and nonproductive cough. Laboratory studies may show elevation of the enzymes CPK, AST, alanine aminotransferase (ALT), and LDH. Changes may be observed by electrocardiogram, and congestive heart failure may be evident on chest x-ray films.

Treatment involves total, permanent abstinence from alcohol. Specific treatment of the congestive heart failure may include rest, oxygen, digitalization, sodium restriction, and diuretics. Prognosis is encouraging if treated in the early stages. The death rate is high for individuals with advanced symptomatology.

Esophagitis

Esophagitis—inflammation and pain in the esophagus—occurs because of the toxic effects of alcohol on the esophageal mucosa. It also occurs because of frequent vomiting associated with alcohol misuse.

Gastritis

The effects of alcohol on the stomach include inflammation of the stomach lining characterized by epigastric distress, nausea, vomiting, and distention. Alcohol breaks down the stomach's protective mucosal barrier, allowing hydrochloric acid to erode the stomach wall. Damage to blood vessels may result in hemorrhage.

Pancreatitis

Pancreatitis may be categorized as *acute* or *chronic*. Acute pancreatitis usually occurs 1 or 2 days after a binge of excessive alcohol consumption. Symptoms include constant, severe epigastric pain; nausea and vomiting; and abdominal distention. Chronic pancreatitis leads to pancreatic insufficiency, resulting in steatorrhea, malnutrition, weight loss, and diabetes mellitus.

Alcoholic Hepatitis

Alcoholic hepatitis is inflammation of the liver caused by long-term heavy alcohol use. Clinical manifestations include an enlarged and tender liver, nausea and vomiting, lethargy, anorexia, elevated white blood cell count, fever, and jaundice. Ascites and weight loss may be evident in more severe cases. With treatment—which includes strict abstinence from alcohol, proper nutrition, and rest—the individual can experience complete recovery. Severe cases can lead to cirrhosis or hepatic encephalopathy.

Cirrhosis of the Liver

Cirrhosis of the liver may be caused by anything that results in chronic injury to the liver. It is the end-stage of alcoholic liver disease and results from long-term chronic alcohol abuse. There is widespread destruction of liver cells, which are replaced by fibrous (scar) tissue. Clinical manifestations include nausea and vomiting, anorexia, weight loss, abdominal pain, jaundice, edema, anemia, and blood coagulation abnormalities. Treatment includes abstention from alcohol, correction of malnutrition, and supportive care to prevent complications of the disease. Complications of cirrhosis include the following:

- ***Portal hypertension:*** Elevation of blood pressure through the portal circulation results from defective blood flow through the cirrhotic liver.
- ***Ascites:*** **Ascites**, a condition in which an excessive amount of serous fluid accumulates in the abdominal cavity, occurs in response to portal hypertension. The increased pressure results in the seepage of fluid from the surface of the liver into the abdominal cavity.
- ***Esophageal varices:*** **Esophageal varices** are veins in the esophagus that become distended because of excessive pressure from defective blood flow through the cirrhotic liver. As this pressure increases, these varicosities can rupture, resulting in hemorrhage and sometimes death.
- ***Hepatic encephalopathy:*** **Hepatic encephalopathy** is a serious complication that occurs in response to the inability of the diseased liver to convert ammonia to urea for excretion. The continued rise in serum ammonia results in progressively impaired mental functioning, apathy, euphoria or depression, sleep disturbance, increasing confusion, and progression to coma and eventual death. Treatment includes complete abstention from alcohol; reduction of protein in the diet; avoidance of medications broken down by the liver or medications with ammonium (including certain antacids); and reduction of intestinal ammonia using neomycin, rifaximin, or lactulose (National Library of Medicine, 2019).

Leukopenia

The production, function, and movement of the white blood cells are impaired in chronic alcoholics. This condition, called *leukopenia*, places the individual at high risk for contracting infectious diseases and for complicated recovery.

Thrombocytopenia

Platelet production and survival are impaired as a result of the toxic effects of alcohol, which increases the risk of hemorrhage. Abstinence from alcohol rapidly reverses this deficiency.

Sexual Dysfunction

Alcohol interferes with the normal production and maintenance of female and male hormones, and long-term alcohol use can interfere with the liver's ability to metabolize estrogenic compounds (Boland & Verduin, 2022). For women, this can mean changes in the menstrual cycle and a decreased or loss of ability to become pregnant. For men, decreased testosterone levels result in a diminished libido, decreased sexual performance, and impaired fertility, and gynecomastia may develop secondary to testicular atrophy.

Use During Pregnancy

Fetal Alcohol Spectrum Disorders

Prenatal exposure to alcohol can result in a broad range of disorders to the fetus, known as *fetal alcohol spectrum disorders* (FASDs), the most involved of which is fetal alcohol syndrome (FAS). People with FAS have central nervous system problems, minor facial features, and growth problems. They often have a hard time in school and trouble getting along with others (CDC, 2021a). There may be problems with learning, memory, attention span, communication, vision, hearing, or a combination of these. Other FASDs include alcohol-related neurodevelopmental disorder (ARND) and alcohol-related birth defects (ARBD) which might include problems with the heart, kidneys, bones, or hearing (CDC, 2021a).

No amount of alcohol during pregnancy is considered safe, and alcohol can damage a fetus at any stage of pregnancy (CDC, 2021a; Vaux, 2016). Therefore, drinking alcohol should be avoided by women who are pregnant and by women who could become pregnant. Few estimates of the prevalence for FASDs are available, but experts estimate that the numbers may be as high as 1% to 5% of the population (CDC, 2021a). Vaux (2016) adds that FASDs cross all races and ethnic groups. The common feature in the development of FASDs is women who drink heavily during pregnancy. Maier and West (2013) state:

> The number of women who engage in heavy alcohol consumption during pregnancy surpasses the total number of children diagnosed with either FAS or ARND, meaning that not every child whose mother drank alcohol during pregnancy develops FAS or ARND. Moreover, the degree to which people with FAS or ARND are impaired differs from person to person. Several factors may contribute to this variation in the consequences of maternal drinking.
>
> These factors include, but are not limited to, the following:
>
> - Maternal drinking pattern
> - Differences in maternal metabolism
> - Differences in genetic susceptibility
> - Timing of the alcohol consumption during pregnancy
> - Variation in the vulnerability of different brain regions

Boland and Verduin (2022) report that women with alcohol-related disorders have a 35% risk of having a child with defects. Children with FASDs may have the following characteristics or exhibit the following behaviors (CDC, 2021a):

- Abnormal facial features (Fig. 14–1)
- Small head size
- Shorter-than-average height
- Low body weight
- Poor coordination
- Hyperactive behavior
- Difficulty paying attention
- Poor memory
- Difficulty in school
- Learning disabilities
- Speech and language delays
- Intellectual disability or low IQ
- Poor reasoning and judgment skills
- Sleep and sucking problems as a baby
- Vision or hearing problems
- Problems with the heart, kidneys, or bones

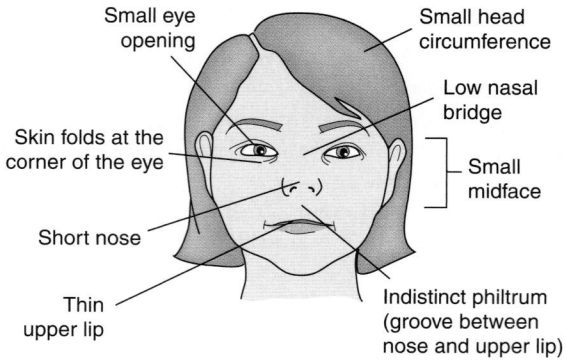

FIGURE 14–1 Facial features of fetal alcohol syndrome. (From the National Institute of Alcohol Abuse and Alcoholism of the National Institutes of Health, Washington, DC.)

Neuroimaging of children with FASDs shows abnormalities in multiple regions of the brain, particularly structural anomalies in white matter tracts within different parts of the corpus callosum (Zhang et al., 2019). Studies show that children with FASDs are often at risk for psychiatric disorders, most commonly attention deficit-hyperactivity disorder, mood disorders, and oppositional defiant disorder (Denny et al., 2017).

Children with FASDs require lifelong care and treatment. There is no cure for FASDs, but it can be prevented. The Collaborative for Alcohol-Free Pregnancy, a joint effort of the CDC along with FASDs Practice and Implementation Centers and National Partners (CDC, 2021a), stresses the importance of using evidence-based tools such as alcohol screening and brief intervention (SBI) to prevent alcohol-exposed pregnancy and risky alcohol use. Nurses who work with women of childbearing age or who are pregnant can play a vital role in ensuring that this type of screening is conducted. Online training and resources for nurses and other healthcare professionals are available at https://nccd.cdc.gov/FASD/

Alcohol Intoxication

Symptoms of alcohol intoxication include disinhibition of sexual or aggressive impulses, mood lability, impaired judgment, impaired social or occupational functioning, slurred speech, incoordination, unsteady gait, nystagmus, and flushed face. Intoxication usually is evident at blood alcohol levels between 100 and 200 mg/dL. Several physical symptoms associated with alcohol intoxication include CNS depression, hypoglycemia, hypothermia, hyper- or hypotension, and vomiting, among others. Death has been reported at levels ranging from 400 to 700 mg/dL.

Alcohol Withdrawal

Within 4 to 12 hours of cessation of or reduction in heavy and prolonged (several days or longer) alcohol use, the following withdrawal symptoms may appear: coarse tremor of hands, tongue, or eyelids; nausea or vomiting; malaise or weakness; tachycardia; sweating; elevated blood pressure; anxiety; depressed mood or irritability; transient hallucinations or illusions; headache; and insomnia. About 5% of hospital patients with alcohol-related disorders develop *alcohol withdrawal delirium,* also known as DTs (delirium tremens), a medical emergency that, if left untreated, confers a 20% mortality rate (Boland & Verduin, 2022). Concomitant medical problems may increase the risk. Onset of delirium is usually on the second or third day following cessation of or reduction in prolonged, heavy alcohol use. Symptoms include those described under the syndrome of delirium in Chapter 13, "Neurocognitive Disorders."

Sedative, Hypnotic, or Anxiolytic Use Disorder

Profile of the Substance

The sedative, hypnotic, and anxiolytic compounds are drugs of diverse chemical structures that are all capable of inducing varying degrees of CNS depression, from tranquilizing relief of anxiety to anesthesia, coma, and even death. They are generally categorized as (1) barbiturates, (2) nonbarbiturate hypnotics, and (3) antianxiety agents. Effects produced by these substances depend on size of dose and potency of drug administered.

Table 14–1 presents a selected list of drugs included in these categories. Generic names are followed in parentheses by the trade names. Common street names for each category are also included.

TABLE 14–1 Sedative, Hypnotic, and Anxiolytic Drugs

CATEGORIES	GENERIC (TRADE) NAMES	COMMON STREET NAMES
Barbiturates	Amobarbital (Amytal) Pentobarbital (Nembutal) Secobarbital (Seconal) Butabarbital (Butisol) Phenobarbital Mephobarbital (Mebaral)	Bluebirds; blue angels (amobarbital); yellow jackets; yellow birds (pentobarbital); GBs; red birds; red devils (secobarbital)
Nonbarbiturate hypnotics	Chloral hydrate Diphenhydramine Estazolam Flurazepam Temazepam (Restoril) Triazolam (Halcion) Quazepam (Doral) Eszopiclone (Lunesta) Ramelteon (Rozerem) Zaleplon (Sonata) Zolpidem (Ambien) Suvorexant (Belsomra) Tasimelteon (Hetlioz)	Peter, Mickey (chloral hydrate); sleepers
Antianxiety agent	Alprazolam (Xanax) Chlordiazepoxide (Librium) Clonazepam (Klonopin) Clorazepate (Tranxene) Diazepam (Valium) Lorazepam (Ativan) Oxazepam (Serax) Meprobamate (Miltown)	Green and whites, roaches (Librium); candy, downers (benzodiazepines); Vs (Valium; color designates strength); dolls, dollies (meprobamate)
Club drugs	Flunitrazepam (Rohypnol) Gamma-hydroxybutyric acid (gamma hydroxybutyrate; GHB)	Date-rape drug; roofies, R-2, rope (Rohypnol); G, liquid X, grievous bodily harm, easy lay (GHB)

Several principles have been identified that apply fairly uniformly to all CNS depressants:

1. ***The effects of CNS depressants are additive with one another and with the behavioral state of the user.*** For example, when these drugs are used in combination with each other or in combination with alcohol, the depressive effects are compounded. These intense depressive effects are often unpredictable and can even be fatal. Similarly, a person who is mentally depressed or physically fatigued may have an exaggerated response to a dose of the drug that would only slightly affect a person in a normal or excited state. The U.S. Food and Drug Administration (FDA, 2016) began requiring black box warnings, its strongest warning label, for opioid analgesics, opioid cough products, and benzodiazepines based on evidence that the combination of opioids and benzodiazepines carries a particularly high risk for excessive sleepiness, respiratory depression, coma, and death.
2. ***CNS depressants are capable of producing physiological addiction.*** If large doses of CNS depressants are repeatedly administered over a prolonged duration, a period of CNS hyperexcitability occurs upon withdrawal of the drug. The response can be quite severe, even leading to convulsions and death.
3. ***CNS depressants are capable of producing psychological addiction.*** CNS depressants have the potential to generate within the individual a psychic drive for periodic or continuous administration of the drug to achieve a maximum level of functioning or feeling of well-being.
4. ***Cross-tolerance and cross-dependence may exist between various CNS depressants.*** Cross-tolerance refers to a condition in which individuals become resistant to the effects of one drug because they have developed tolerance to another drug with similar pharmacological activity. Cross-dependence is a condition in which an individual can become dependent on more than one substance because of their similar activity and effects.

Historical Perspectives

Anxiety and insomnia, two of the most common human afflictions, were treated during the 19th century with opiates, bromide salts, chloral hydrate, paraldehyde, and alcohol (Julien, 2014). Because the opiates were known to produce physical addiction, bromides carried the risk of chronic bromide poisoning, and chloral hydrate and paraldehyde had an objectionable taste and smell, alcohol became the prescribed depressant drug of choice. However, some people refused to use alcohol either because they did not like the taste or for moral reasons, and others tended to take more than was prescribed. Therefore, a search for a better sedative drug continued.

Although barbituric acid was first synthesized in 1864, it was not until 1912 that phenobarbital was introduced into medicine as a sedative drug, the first of the structurally classified group of drugs called barbiturates (Julien, 2014). Since that time, more than 2,500 barbiturate derivatives have been synthesized, but, currently, fewer than a dozen remain in medical use. Illicit use of the drugs for recreational purposes grew throughout the 1930s and 1940s.

Efforts to create depressant medications that were not barbiturate derivatives accelerated. By the mid-1950s, the market for depressants had been expanded by the appearance of the nonbarbiturates glutethimide, ethchlorvynol, methyprylon, and meprobamate. Benzodiazepines were introduced around 1960 with the marketing of chlordiazepoxide (Librium), followed shortly by its derivative diazepam (Valium). The use of these drugs and others within their group grew very rapidly, and they are prescribed widely in medical practice. Their margin of safety is greater than that of barbiturates and the other nonbarbiturates. However, prolonged use of even moderate doses is likely to result in physical and psychological addiction with a characteristic syndrome of withdrawal that can be severe.

Patterns of Use

Boland and Verduin (2022) reported that about 15% of all persons in the United States have had a benzodiazepine prescribed by a physician. Of all the drugs used in clinical practice, the sedative, hypnotic, and anxiolytic drugs are among the most widely prescribed.

Two patterns of addiction are described. The first pattern is one of an individual whose physician originally prescribed the CNS depressant as treatment for anxiety or insomnia. Independently, the individual has increased the dosage or frequency from that which was prescribed. Use of the medication is justified on the basis of treating symptoms, but as tolerance grows, more and more of the medication is required to produce the desired effect. Substance-seeking behavior is evident as the individual seeks prescriptions from several physicians in order to maintain sufficient supplies.

The second pattern involves young people in their teens or early 20s who, in the company of their peers, use substances that are obtained illegally. The initial objective is to achieve a feeling of euphoria. The drug is usually used intermittently during recreational gatherings. This pattern of intermittent use leads to regular use and extreme levels of tolerance. Combining use with other substances is not uncommon. Physical and psychological addiction leads to intense substance-seeking behaviors, most often through illegal channels.

Effects on the Body

The sedative, hypnotic, and anxiolytic compounds induce a general depressant effect; that is, they depress the activity of the brain, nerves, muscles, and heart tissue. The primary action of sedatives, hypnotics, and anxiolytics is on nervous tissue. However, large doses may affect other organ systems. They reduce the rate of metabolism in a variety of tissues throughout the body, and in general, they depress any system that uses energy. Large doses are required to produce these effects. In lower doses, these drugs appear to be more selective in their depressant actions by exerting their action on the centers within the brain that are concerned with arousal (e.g., the ascending reticular activating system, in the reticular formation, and the diffuse thalamic projection system).

These drugs are capable of producing all levels of CNS depression—from mild sedation to death. The level is determined by dosage and potency of the drug used. In Figure 14–2, a continuum demonstrates how increasing doses of the drugs affect the level of CNS depression.

Following is a discussion of the physiological effects of these medications.

Effects on Sleep and Dreaming

Barbiturate use decreases the amount of sleep time spent in dreaming. During drug withdrawal, dreaming becomes vivid and excessive. Rebound insomnia and increased dreaming (termed *REM rebound*) are not uncommon with abrupt withdrawal from long-term use of these drugs as sleeping aids.

Respiratory Depression

Barbiturates are capable of inhibiting the reticular activating system, resulting in respiratory depression, and can be lethal in overdose. In addition, additive effects can occur with the concurrent use of other CNS depressants, also effecting a life-threatening situation.

Cardiovascular Effects

Hypotension may be a problem with large doses. Only a slight decrease in blood pressure is noted with normal oral dosage. High dosages of barbiturates also compromise cardiac contractility and vascular tone, which may result in cardiovascular collapse. Individuals with congestive heart failure are more susceptible to these effects (Lafferty, 2017).

Renal Function

In doses high enough to produce anesthesia and in overdose, barbiturates may reduce urine output (oliguria). At the usual sedative-hypnotic dosage, there is no evidence of direct action on the kidneys.

Hepatic Effects

Barbiturates stimulate the production of liver enzymes. Increases in cytochrome P450 isoenzymes inhibit the metabolism of many medications including antipsychotics, antidepressants, anticonvulsants, and steroid hormones, and accelerate metabolism of the barbiturates themselves (Dubovsky, 2017). Pre-existing liver disease may predispose an individual to additional liver damage with excessive barbiturate use.

Body Temperature

High doses of barbiturates can greatly decrease body temperature. Body temperature is not significantly altered with normal dosage levels.

Sexual Function

CNS depressants have a tendency to produce a biphasic response. There is an initial increase in libido, presumably from the primary disinhibitory effects of the

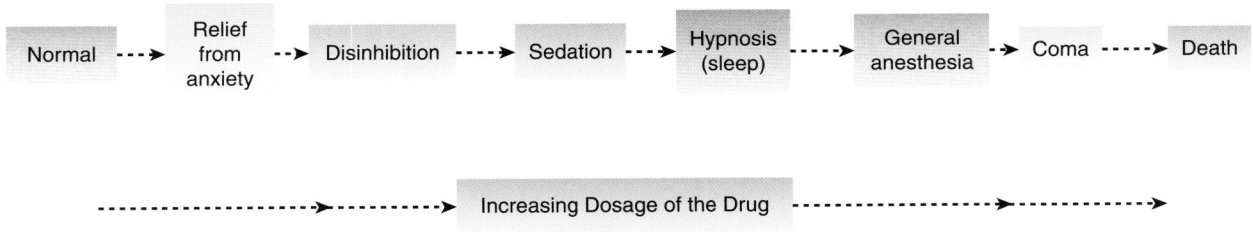

FIGURE 14–2 Continuum of CNS depression with increasing doses of sedative-hypnotic drugs.

drug. In men, this initial response is then followed by a decrease in the ability to maintain an erection.

Sedative, Hypnotic, or Anxiolytic Intoxication

The *DSM-5-TR* (APA, 2022) describes sedative, hypnotic, or anxiolytic intoxication as the presence of clinically significant maladaptive behavioral or psychological changes that develop during or shortly after use of one of these substances. These maladaptive changes may include inappropriate sexual or aggressive behavior, mood lability, impaired judgment, or impaired social or occupational functioning. Other symptoms that may develop with excessive use of CNS depressants include slurred speech, incoordination, unsteady gait, nystagmus, impairment in attention or memory, and stupor or coma.

"Club drugs" in this category include gamma-hydroxybutyric acid (GHB) and flunitrazepam (Rohypnol). Like all of the depressants, they can produce a state of disinhibition, excitement, drunkenness, and amnesia. They have been widely implicated as "date rape" drugs, their presence being easily disguised in drinks. They produce anterograde amnesia, the inability to remember events experienced while under their influence.

Sedative, Hypnotic, or Anxiolytic Withdrawal

Withdrawal from sedatives, hypnotics, or anxiolytics produces a characteristic syndrome of symptoms that develops after a marked decrease in or cessation of intake after several weeks or more of regular use (APA, 2022). Onset and duration of withdrawal symptoms depend on the half-life of the drug from which the individual is withdrawing. With short-acting sedative-hypnotics (e.g., alprazolam, lorazepam), symptoms may begin between 12 and 24 hours after the last dose, reach peak intensity between 24 and 72 hours, and subside in 5 to 10 days. Withdrawal symptoms from substances with longer half-lives (e.g., diazepam, phenobarbital, chlordiazepoxide) may begin within 2 to 7 days, peak on the 5th to 8th day, and subside in 10 to 16 days.

Severe withdrawal is most likely to occur when a substance has been used at high dosages for prolonged periods. However, withdrawal symptoms also have been reported with moderate dosages taken over a relatively short duration. Withdrawal symptoms associated with sedative-hypnotics include autonomic hyperactivity (e.g., sweating or pulse rate greater than 100), increased hand tremor, insomnia, nausea or vomiting, hallucinations, illusions, depersonalization, psychomotor agitation, anxiety, grand mal seizures, and delirium.

Stimulant Use Disorder

Profile of the Substance

CNS stimulants are identified by the behavioral stimulation and psychomotor agitation that they induce. They differ widely in their molecular structures and in their mechanisms of action. The amount of CNS stimulation caused by a certain drug depends on both the area in the brain or spinal cord that is affected by the drug and the cellular mechanism fundamental to the increased excitability. The *DSM-5-TR* (APA, 2022) categorizes caffeine-related disorders and tobacco-related disorders as separate and distinct diagnoses. For purposes of this text, these substances are discussed with the stimulant-related disorders.

Groups within this category are classified according to similarities in mechanism of action. The *psychomotor stimulants* induce stimulation by augmentation or potentiation of the neurotransmitters norepinephrine, epinephrine, or dopamine. The *general cellular stimulants* (caffeine and nicotine) exert their action directly on cellular activity. Caffeine inhibits the enzyme phosphodiesterase, allowing increased levels of 3′,5′-cyclic adenosine monophosphate (cAMP), a chemical substance that promotes increased rates of cellular metabolism. Nicotine stimulates ganglionic synapses. This results in increased acetylcholine, which stimulates nerve impulse transmission to the entire autonomic nervous system. A selected list of drugs included in these categories is presented in Table 14–2.

The two most prevalent and widely used stimulants are caffeine and nicotine. Caffeine is readily available in every supermarket and grocery store as a common ingredient in coffee, tea, colas, and chocolate. Nicotine is the primary psychoactive substance found in tobacco products. When used in moderation, these stimulants tend to relieve fatigue and increase alertness. They are a generally accepted part of our culture; however, with increased social awareness regarding the health risks associated with tobacco products, their use has become stigmatized in some circles.

The more potent stimulants, because of their potential for physiological addiction, are under regulation by the Controlled Substances Act. These controlled stimulants are available for therapeutic purposes by prescription only; however, they are also clandestinely manufactured and widely distributed on the illicit market. More recently, the synthetic stimulants mephedrone, 3,4-methylenedioxypyrovalerone (MDPV), methylone, and others have become available, and because their chemical structures had been altered, they were not initially identifiable as a

TABLE 14–2 Central Nervous System (CNS) Stimulants

CATEGORIES	GENERIC (TRADE) NAMES	COMMON STREET NAMES
Amphetamines	Dextroamphetamine (Dexedrine) Methamphetamine (Desoxyn) 3,4-Methylenedioxyamphetamine (MDMA)* Amphetamine + dextroamphetamine (Adderall)	Dexies, uppers, truck drivers Meth, speed, crystal, ice, crank, chalk, fire, glass Adam, ecstasy, EVE, XTC, Molly Beans, pep pills, speed, uppers, study buddies, smart pills
Synthetic stimulants	3,4-Methylenedioxypyrovalerone* (MDPV) 4-Methylmethcathinone (mephedrone, 4-MMC)* Methylone* Ethylone Dibutylone Alpha-PVP	Bath salts (also called blue silk, cloud 9, ivory wave, vanilla sky, white lightning, white knight, and others) flakka, gravel
Nonamphetamine stimulants	Phendimetrazine (Bontril) Benzphetamine (Didrex) Diethylpropion (Tenuate) Phentermine (Adipex-P; Ionamin) Sibutramine (Meridia)† Methylphenidate (Ritalin, Concerta) Dexmethylphenidate (Focalin) Modafinil (Provigil)	Diet pills Speed, uppers
Cocaine	Cocaine hydrochloride	Coke, blow, toot, snow, lady, flake, crack
Caffeine	Coffee, tea, colas, chocolate	Java, mud, brew, cocoa
Nicotine	Cigarettes, cigars, pipe tobacco, snuff	Weeds, fags, butts, chaw, cancer sticks

*Cross-listed with the hallucinogens.
†No longer marketed in the United States.

controlled substance or regulated by the federal government. Known as "bath salts," their street names include, among others, blue silk, cloud 9, ivory wave, vanilla sky, white knight, white lightning stardust, and purple wave. In October 2011, the U.S. Drug Enforcement Administration (DEA) issued emergency scheduling of these substances to make their possession and sales illegal (except as authorized by law). They are currently designated as Schedule I substances, the most restrictive category under the Controlled Substances Act. This action was taken in response to reports of episodes of violent behavior associated with use of the substance.

Another synthetic cathinone, alpha-PVP (commonly known as flakka, gravel, $5 insanity, or the zombie drug), whose chemical structure is similar but not identical to bath salts, was seen in the United States in 2014 and 2015. This drug can be snorted, injected, eaten, and vaporized for inhalation in e-cigarettes, for example. Vaporization is a particularly dangerous route because of its immediate absorption, and deaths have been reported secondary to overdose, suicide, and heart attack. Flakka has been considered a particularly dangerous drug because of reports of violent aggression, homicide, and suicide related to its use.

Flakka was considered a significant threat in the United States in 2014 and 2015, but no deaths were reported in 2016 after China (the singular provider of the drug) banned the production and exportation of alpha-PVP (Storrs, 2016). Although flakka use has diminished, flakka-related erratic behavior and sometimes criminal activity continue to surface in some areas of the United States. Storrs (2016) additionally reports that when one synthetic substance is banned, it is often replaced by another. For example, when China banned methylone (a drug similar to flakka), in 2014, it was replaced by ethylone; after ethylone was banned, a similar drug called dibutylone surfaced. This pattern creates an ongoing challenge for the FDA and DEA to identify and take action on each new synthetic substance as it comes to public attention (usually through significant health consequences or deaths). New synthetic drugs may also be difficult to identify because standard drug screens do not recognize these chemicals.

Historical Perspectives

Cocaine is the most potent stimulant derived from nature. It is extracted from the leaves of the coca plant, which has been cultivated in the Andean highlands of South America since prehistoric times. Natives of the region chew the leaves of the plant for refreshment and relief from fatigue.

The coca leaves must be mixed with lime to release the cocaine alkaloid. The chemical formula for the pure form of the drug was developed in 1960. Physicians began using the drug as an anesthetic in eye, nose, and throat surgeries. It has also been used therapeutically in the United States in a morphine-cocaine elixir designed to relieve the suffering associated with terminal illness. These therapeutic uses are now obsolete.

Cocaine has achieved a degree of acceptability within some social circles. It is illicitly distributed as a white crystalline powder, often mixed with other ingredients to increase its volume and thereby create more profits. The drug is most commonly "snorted," and chronic users may manifest symptoms that resemble the congested nose of a common cold. The intensely pleasurable effects of the drug create the potential for extraordinary psychological addiction.

Another form of cocaine commonly used in the United States is made by processing powdered cocaine with ammonia or sodium bicarbonate and water and heating it to remove the hydrochloride. The term *crack*, which is the street name for this form of the drug, refers to the crackling sound heard when the mixture is smoked. Because this type of cocaine can be easily vaporized and inhaled, its effects have an extremely rapid onset. See "Real People, Real Stories" to learn more about Alan's experience with crack cocaine and alcohol addiction.

Amphetamine was first produced in 1887. Various derivatives of the drug soon followed, and clinical use of the drug began in 1927. **Amphetamines** were used extensively for medical purposes through the 1960s, but recognition of their abuse potential has sharply decreased clinical use. Today, they are prescribed only to treat narcolepsy (a rare disorder resulting in an uncontrollable desire for sleep), hyperactivity disorders in children, and in certain cases of obesity. Clandestine production of amphetamines for distribution on the illicit market has become a thriving business. Methamphetamine can be smoked, snorted, injected, or taken orally. The effects include an intense rush from smoking or IV injection to a slower onset of euphoria as a result of snorting or oral ingestion. Another form of the drug, crystal methamphetamine, is produced by slowly recrystallizing powder methamphetamine from a solvent such as methanol, ethanol, isopropanol, or acetone. It is a colorless, odorless, large-crystal form of *d*-methamphetamine and is commonly called *glass* or *ice* because of its appearance. Crystal meth is usually smoked in a glass pipe like crack cocaine.

Although methamphetamine use is widespread, particularly on college campuses, its use has perhaps been overshadowed by the nationwide opiate epidemic with its associated deaths. An alarming recent trend has been the increasing use of methamphetamines in combination with opiates. Ellis and associates, as cited by Dotinga (2018), report that the use of crystal meth increased by 82% in the past decade and combined use of opioids and methamphetamine almost doubled during the same time period. Ellis notes that individuals with opiate-use disorder sometimes use amphetamines to create a state of arousal to counteract the sedative effects of opiates. The use of combinations of drugs increases the risk for adverse effects and overdose. It also underscores the importance of assessing for multisubstance use in any individual presenting with substance use issues.

The earliest history of caffeine is unknown and is shrouded by legend and myth. Caffeine was first isolated in coffee in 1820 and in tea 7 years later. Both beverages have been widely accepted and enjoyed as a "pick-me-up" by many cultures.

Tobacco was used by the aborigines from remote times. Introduced in Europe in the mid-16th century, its use grew rapidly and soon became prevalent in Asia. Tobacco came to America with the settlement of the earliest colonies. Today, it is grown in many countries of the world, and although smoking is decreasing in most industrialized nations, it continues to be a serious problem in developing areas.

Patterns of Use

Because of their pleasurable effects, CNS stimulants have a high abuse potential. In 2019 the National Survey on Drug Use and Health (NSDUH) estimated 5.5 million people age 12 or older were past users of cocaine, including about 778,000 users of crack and 2 million users of methamphetamine in the past year (SAMHSA, 2021). Additionally, recent research (Roehler et al., 2021) reports that nonfatal stimulant overdoses have increased in all agegroups under 25 years of age including those under 10 years of age. Approximately 1 million people had a methamphetamine use disorder. Overdose deaths have increased for both cocaine and methamphetamines; methamphetamine overdose deaths quadrupled from 2011 to 2017, and in 2020 during the COVID-19 pandemic, overdose deaths from psychostimulants (like methamphetamine) increased by almost 35% (CDC, 2020b).

Many individuals who misuse or are addicted to CNS stimulants began using the substance for the appetite-suppressant effect in an attempt at weight control. Increasingly higher doses are consumed in an effort to maintain the pleasurable effects. With continued use, these pleasurable effects diminish as dysphoric effects increase. A persistent craving for the substance remains even in the face of unpleasant adverse effects from continued use.

CNS stimulant use is usually characterized by either episodic or chronic daily, or almost daily, use. Individuals who use the substances on an episodic basis often "binge" on the drug with very high dosages followed by a day or two of recuperation. This recuperation period is characterized by extremely intense and unpleasant symptoms, often called a "crash."

The daily user may take large or small doses and may use the drug several times a day or only at a specific time during the day. The amount consumed usually increases over time as tolerance develops. Chronic users tend to rely on CNS stimulants to feel more powerful, more confident, and more decisive. They often fall into a pattern of taking "uppers" in the morning and "downers," such as alcohol or sleeping pills, at night.

Real People, Real Stories: Alan Brunner on Substance Use Disorder

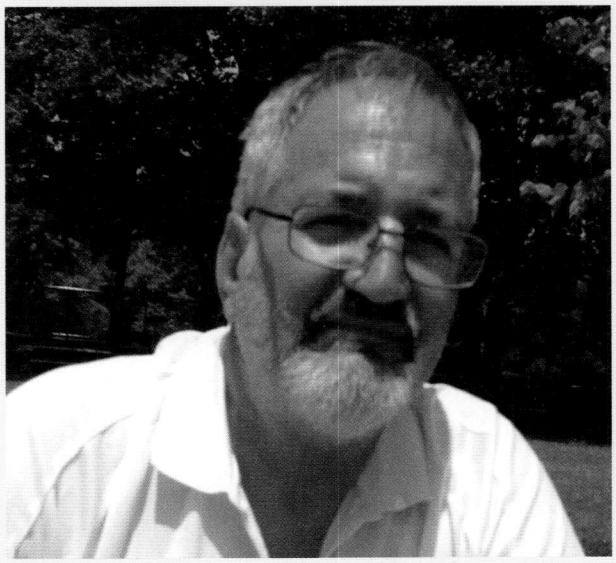

Substance use disorders often follow a progressive pattern that develops over a long period. Alan's story is an example of that process. See also Chapter 5, "Relationship Development and Therapeutic Communication," for an interaction with Alan that incorporates motivational interviewing. Reflect on important issues for primary prevention education. Consider examples of interventions that are ineffective or unhealthy for the user and the care provider. Incorporate an understanding of codependency in this reflection.

Karyn: Tell me about when you first used drugs or alcohol.

Alan: I was 15 years old when I first started smoking pot and 16 when I had my first drink. The pot use went from occasional use to several times a week by the time I was a senior in high school. I knew that was a problem, but the drinking progressed much more gradually. For years, I only drank on weekends. For a while, my buddy and I would share a quart on the weekend. Eventually, we each had our own quart, then two quarts each. I only drank beer. Once when I was a teenager, I drank a fifth of vodka and I got extremely sick. My mom didn't try to rescue me or help me feel better or cover for me. I just had to live through the consequences, and that was probably a good thing; I never drank vodka again. But the beer drinking became more often and at higher amounts. Even so, it took another 35 years to recognize that it was a problem!

Karyn: Was there any history of alcoholism in your family?

Alan: Oh yeah . . . several relatives. My dad had a drinking problem, and that led to my parents divorcing when I was 14 years old. When I was 19, I moved in with my dad, and then I started drinking during the week, too—because he did. My dad always worked and had a strong work ethic, even though he was a heavy drinker, so I thought, "As long as I'm able to drink and it's not interfering with work, then it's not a problem." I also remember thinking, "It's just beer, and I would never use the 'strong' or 'bad' drugs, like cocaine—I would NEVER do that."

Karyn: So your beer drinking increased while you were living with your father?

Alan: Initially, yes, but then I was surrounding myself with people and friends who liked to drink. I moved in with a friend, and we usually drank a case of beer each night. Then I started an auto repair business with a friend who

Continued

Real People, Real Stories: Alan Brunner on Substance Use Disorder—cont'd

was a heavy drinker, and we had beer at the shop. Pretty soon we weren't leaving the shop until all the beer was gone. Then I got involved with auto racing, and that was an environment with lots of alcohol and cocaine.

Karyn: I remember you said you were using cocaine. Is that when the use started?

Alan: No, actually I had become friends with a deacon at my church, probably because we both liked to drink. He was the one that introduced me to cocaine.

Karyn: So you started using cocaine along with drinking?

Alan: Yeah, even though I had said I would never do that. But I discovered that if I did cocaine, I had a lot more energy and I could stay awake longer, so I could be a much "better" drinker. (chuckles)

Karyn: Tell me about when you recognized that your use was a problem.

Alan: Well, eventually, I was drinking at home because it was a waste of "good drinking time" to get together with other people. So largely, I was sitting at home in the dark drinking by myself, and the beer never even made it into the fridge. The cocaine was putting me in the company of some very bad people. I knew I had to somehow get away from that . . . and when I started using cocaine, I said, "One thing I'll never do is crack," but then I started doing that, and that's when things completely fell apart.

Karyn: Fell apart?

Alan: I was racking up a lot of legal problems. I had some DUIs and reckless operation charges before that, but now I'm getting drug possession charges, paraphernalia charges, driving with a suspended license, driving with expired license plates, more DUIs, disorderly conduct charges. And the crack—that drug rips out your soul! You're always chasing the high that you got the first time you used it, and you never find that, so you keep using more. That's why one of my friends called crack "gotta" because you gotta have it. . . . And you don't care about ANYTHING else—you don't care if you die.

Karyn: You told me you've been clean and sober for seven years. How did you turn the corner?

Alan: I had such a huge legal mess that my lawyer was recommending I just accept the jail time (3 to 10 days) and be done with it, but the judge offered treatment in lieu of jail, and I told him that's what I wanted because I knew I needed it. I was told, though, that if I violated the treatment program, I would spend a year in jail, so I knew I was taking a big risk by going into treatment. But I knew it was the only way out—and I knew I needed it.

Karyn: So what is your relapse prevention plan?

Alan: I have an AA sponsor, and I go to meetings sometimes, but not as often as I used to. I never allow myself to become too proud about my sobriety because I know all it would take is one drink. As long as I remember that, I'm vulnerable. . . . I don't get too cocky. I've also had a lot of support from family, especially my mom. She supported me every step of the way in treatment. Having supportive people around you is essential. The relationship I had been in for many years broke up largely because she was telling my counselors that she wanted me to cut down but she wasn't in favor of abstinence—she was quite a partier, too. Staying in that relationship, I believed (and my counselors believed), was putting my sobriety at risk.

Karyn: What do you think is important for health-care providers to know or to do to help someone who has a substance use problem?

Alan: First of all, a person has to want help. You can't fix another person, and you can't help someone who doesn't want help.

Karyn: I agree, that is so important. I think health-care providers (and family caregivers) are vulnerable sometimes to thinking they can fix any health problem, which can culminate in interventions that are ineffective and unhealthy for the user and for the care provider.

Alan: Yes, and I would also say that health-care providers need to know how to recognize symptoms of problematic substance use.

Karyn: Like?

Alan: Like someone having "the shakes," someone not looking at you when they are answering questions, blaming other people for their circumstances and consequences, talking in circles. Don't ever ask someone, "Are you an alcoholic or a drug addict?" because we'll always say no unless we're in recovery—the denial is so strong. I also think not being too judgmental is important so you can find ways to open the door to discuss the issues. If someone is too "hard-nosed" and judgmental, I think it reinforces the denial. Asking a question like "Have you ever been drinking and couldn't remember events around that time?" is good because having blackouts is a good indication of an alcohol problem. You may not be able to "fix" someone but you can "plant seeds" and hope that the information and education will have an impact at some point. I think that's why people who are recovering themselves can be so effective as health-care providers because they can share their own story of addiction and, since most people think they are completely unique, hearing someone else's story about having been in the same place you are now may turn on a light switch and help people recognize their own need for treatment.

The average American consumes two cups of coffee (about 200 mg of caffeine) per day. Caffeine is consumed in various amounts by about 90% of the population. At a level of 500 to 600 mg of daily caffeine consumption, symptoms of anxiety, insomnia, and depression are not uncommon. It is also at this level that caffeine dependence and withdrawal can occur. Caffeine consumption is prevalent among children as well as adults. Energy drinks have some of the highest caffeine contents of all beverages, and a Consumer Reports study (2012) found that several energy drinks had over 20% more caffeine than reported on the label. In addition, many beverages have multiple servings in one bottle and some beverages do not list the caffeine content on the label. Individuals may be at risk for consuming far more caffeine than they expected. Table 14–3 lists some common sources of caffeine.

Next to caffeine, nicotine (the active ingredient in tobacco) is the most widely used psychoactive substance in U.S. society. According to the 2019 NSDUH, 58.1 million Americans currently use tobacco, and it is the leading cause of preventable death (SAMHSA, 2021). Since 1964, when the results of the first public health report on smoking were issued, the percentage of total smokers has declined. However, the percentage of women and teenage smokers has declined more slowly than that of adult men. Even though tobacco use is on the decline, people with severe mental illness and those in addiction treatment continue to have higher rates than the general population (SAMHSA, 2021).

The dangers of secondhand smoke continue to be identified as a significant health hazard. The CDC (2021b) reports that, annually, secondhand smoke claims the lives of over 49,000 nonsmokers from heart disease and lung cancer, and exposure to smoke after birth increases the risk of infant mortality from sudden infant death syndrome.

Vaping, the use of a device to heat and release chemicals that can then be inhaled, is a current trend. One such device is the e-cigarette, which typically contains nicotine. In addition to its addiction potential, nicotine is known to be harmful to developing brains and, therefore, particularly dangerous to teens and pregnant women. Its use has become common among young people, now surpassing conventional cigarette smoking (CDC, 2020a).

The National Institute on Drug Abuse (NIDA, 2020c) reported significant increases in vaping among teenagers, with as high as 40.6% admitting use within the past year. Vaping of marijuana among teenagers has doubled in the past 2 years. Reports of serious respiratory illness secondary to vaping have raised additional safety concerns. The CDC (2020a) reports:

> E-cigarette aerosol generally contains fewer toxic chemicals than the deadly mix of 7,000 chemicals in smoke from regular cigarettes. However, e-cigarette aerosol is not harmless. It can contain harmful and potentially harmful substances, including nicotine, heavy metals like lead, volatile organic compounds, and cancer-causing agents.

TABLE 14–3 Common Sources of Caffeine

SOURCE	CAFFEINE CONTENT (mg)
FOOD AND BEVERAGES	
8 oz. brewed coffee	90–165
8 oz. instant coffee	63–110
8 oz. decaffeinated coffee	2–5
1 oz. espresso	47–64
8 oz. brewed tea	25–48
6 oz. instant tea	30
8 oz. green tea	25–29
8–12 oz. cola drinks	22–54
8–24 oz. energy drinks	142–375
2 oz. high-energy drinks	215–240
1.93 oz. 10-hr energy shot	215–422
5–6 oz. cocoa	20
8 oz. chocolate milk	2–7
1 oz. chocolate bar	22
PRESCRIPTION MEDICATIONS	
APCs (aspirin, phenacetin, caffeine)	32
Cafergot	100
Fiorinal	40
Migralam	100
OVER-THE-COUNTER ANALGESICS	
Anacin, Empirin, Midol, Vanquish	32
Excedrin Migraine (aspirin, acetaminophen, caffeine)	65
OVER-THE-COUNTER STIMULANTS	
NoDoz	100
Vivarin	200
Caffedrine	250

Sources: Compiled from Juliano & Griffiths (2017); Mayo Clinic (2020).

Effects on the Body

The CNS stimulants are a group of pharmacological agents that are capable of exciting the entire nervous system. This is accomplished by increasing the activity or augmenting the capability of the neurotransmitter agents known to be directly involved in physical and behavioral stimulation. Physiological responses vary markedly according to the potency and dosage of the drug.

Central Nervous System Effects

Stimulation of the CNS results in tremor, restlessness, anorexia, insomnia, agitation, and increased motor activity. Amphetamines, nonamphetamine stimulants, and cocaine produce increased alertness, decrease in fatigue, elation and euphoria, and subjective feelings of greater mental agility and muscular power. Chronic use of these drugs may result in compulsive behavior, paranoia, hallucinations, and aggressive behavior.

Cardiovascular and Pulmonary Effects

Amphetamines can induce increased systolic and diastolic blood pressure, increased heart rate, and cardiac arrhythmias. These drugs also relax bronchial smooth muscle.

Cocaine intoxication typically produces an increase in myocardial demand for oxygen and an increased heart rate. Severe vasoconstriction may occur and can result in myocardial infarction, ventricular fibrillation, and sudden death. Inhaled cocaine can cause pulmonary hemorrhage, chronic bronchiolitis, and pneumonia. Nasal rhinitis is a result of chronic cocaine snorting.

Caffeine ingestion can result in increased heart rate, palpitations, extrasystoles, and cardiac arrhythmias. Caffeine induces dilation of pulmonary and general systemic blood vessels and constriction of cerebral blood vessels.

Nicotine stimulates the sympathetic nervous system, resulting in an increase in heart rate, blood pressure, and cardiac contractility, thereby increasing myocardial oxygen consumption and demand for blood flow. Contractions of gastric smooth muscle associated with hunger are inhibited, thereby producing a mild anorectic effect.

Gastrointestinal and Renal Effects

Gastrointestinal (GI) effects of amphetamines are somewhat unpredictable; however, a decrease in GI tract motility commonly results in constipation. Contraction of the bladder sphincter makes urination difficult. Caffeine exerts a diuretic effect on the kidneys. Nicotine stimulates the hypothalamus to release antidiuretic hormone, reducing the excretion of urine. Because nicotine increases the tone and activity of the bowel, it may occasionally cause diarrhea.

Most CNS stimulants induce a small increase in metabolic rate and various degrees of anorexia. Amphetamines and cocaine can cause a rise in body temperature.

Sexual Function

CNS stimulants appear to increase sexual urges in both men and women. Women, more than men, report that stimulants make them feel sexier and have more orgasms. Some men may experience sexual dysfunction with the use of stimulants. For the majority of individuals, however, these drugs exert a powerful aphrodisiac effect.

Stimulant Intoxication

Stimulant intoxication produces maladaptive behavioral and psychological changes that develop during or shortly after use of these drugs. Amphetamine and cocaine intoxication typically produces euphoria or affective blunting; changes in sociability; hypervigilance; interpersonal sensitivity; anxiety, tension, or anger; stereotyped behaviors; or impaired judgment. In severe amphetamine intoxication, symptoms may include memory loss, psychosis, and violent aggression. Physical effects include tachycardia or bradycardia, pupillary dilation, elevated or lowered blood pressure, perspiration or chills, nausea or vomiting, weight loss, psychomotor agitation or retardation, muscular weakness, respiratory depression, chest pain, cardiac arrhythmias, confusion, seizures, dyskinesias, dystonias, or coma (APA, 2022).

Intoxication from caffeine usually occurs following consumption well in excess of 250 mg, but may occur with low doses in children, elderly, or those not previously exposed to caffeine. Symptoms include restlessness, nervousness, excitement, insomnia, flushed face, diuresis, GI disturbance, muscle twitching, rambling flow of thought and speech, tachycardia or cardiac arrhythmia, periods of inexhaustibility, and psychomotor agitation (APA, 2022).

Stimulant Withdrawal

Stimulant withdrawal is the presence of a characteristic withdrawal syndrome that develops within a few hours to several days after cessation of or marked reduction in prolonged (generally high dose) stimulant use (APA, 2022). This syndrome is often referred to as *crashing*, an apt description because the symptoms include fatigue, cramps, depression, headaches, and nightmares. The dysphoria can be intense enough to result in increased risk for suicide. Peak withdrawal symptoms usually occur within 2 to 4 days of abstinence.

Caffeine withdrawal syndrome can occur with abrupt cessation (or substantial reduction in) of caffeine intake after a prolonged daily use of the substance (APA, 2022). The symptoms begin within 24 hours after last consumption and may include the following symptoms: headache, fatigue, drowsiness, dysphoric mood, irritability, difficulty concentrating, flu-like symptoms, nausea, vomiting, and/or muscle pain and stiffness.

Withdrawal from nicotine results in dysphoric or depressed mood; insomnia; irritability, frustration, or anger; anxiety; difficulty concentrating; restlessness; decreased heart rate; and increased appetite or weight gain (APA, 2022). A mild syndrome of nicotine withdrawal can appear when a smoker switches from regular cigarettes to low-nicotine cigarettes (Boland & Verduin, 2022).

Inhalant Use Disorder

Profile of the Substance

Inhalant disorders are induced by inhaling the aliphatic and aromatic hydrocarbons found in substances such as fuels, solvents, adhesives, aerosol propellants, and paint thinners. Specific examples of these substances include gasoline, varnish remover, lighter fluid, airplane glue, rubber cement, cleaning fluid, spray paint, shoe conditioner, and typewriter correction fluid. Toluene (methylbenzene, toluol, phenylmethane) is a common ingredient in many of the substances that are inhaled, including paints, glues, and gasoline, and it is responsible for the mind-altering effects that occur after inhalation.

Patterns of Use

Inhalant substances are readily available, legal, and inexpensive—three factors that make them attractive to children, teens, and young adults. Younger teens more commonly inhale glue, gasoline, and spray paints. In older teens, nitrous oxide (also known as "whippets") use is more common, and in adults, nitrites, such as amyl nitrites (also called "poppers") are common inhalants used for mind-altering effects.

Inhalant use among teenagers has been increasing over the last several years (NIDA, 2020d) with significant increases among eighth graders. Johnston and associates (2018) note that because inhalant use had been declining for over a decade, this trend reversal bears watching. Another finding in the national survey was a decline in the number of adolescents who believe that use of inhalants is harmful. Past education and advertising campaigns about the risks associated with inhalant use have contributed to the decline in use over the past decade (Johnston et al., 2018), and this education may need to be reintroduced and reinforced with today's adolescents. Nurses who work with children and adolescents can play a significant role in providing that education.

Methods of use include "huffing"—a procedure in which a rag soaked with the substance is applied to the mouth and nose and the vapors breathed in. Another common method is called "bagging," in which the substance is placed in a paper or plastic bag and inhaled from the bag by the user. The substance may also be inhaled directly from the container ("sniffing") or sprayed in the mouth or nose ("snorting").

Boland and Verduin (2022) reported that

> inhalant use among adolescents may be most common in those whose parents or older siblings use illegal substances. Inhalant use among adolescents is also associated with an increased likelihood of conduct disorder or antisocial personality disorder. (p. 327)

Tolerance to inhalants has been reported with heavy use. A mild withdrawal syndrome has been documented but does not appear to be clinically significant. Among children with inhalant disorder, the products may be used several times a week, often on weekends and after school. Adults with inhalant addiction may use the substance at varying times during each day, or they may binge on the substance during a period of several days.

Effects on the Body

Inhalants are absorbed through the lungs and reach the CNS very rapidly. Inhalants initially create rapid excitation followed by drowsiness, incoordination, and disinhibition. The effects are relatively brief, lasting from several minutes to a few hours, depending on the specific substance and amount consumed.

Central Nervous System Effects

Inhalants can cause both central and peripheral nervous system damage. Neurological damage, such as ataxia, peripheral and sensorimotor neuropathy, speech problems, and tremor, can occur. Other CNS effects that have been reported with heavy inhalant use include ototoxicity, encephalopathy, parkinsonism, and damage to the protective sheath around certain nerve fibers in the brain and peripheral nervous system. These effects are particularly damaging to youths because their nervous systems are still developing.

Chronic use has been associated with the development of several mental illnesses, including anxiety and psychotic disorders. Inhalant use in pregnant women has been linked to fetal development disorders, malformations, and death. Infants are at risk for *fetal solvent syndrome*, (similar to FAS) a syndrome of behavioral, language, and developmental impairments that may include hyperactivity and aggression (Howard et al., 2017).

Respiratory Effects

Respiratory effects of inhalant use range from coughing and wheezing to dyspnea, emphysema, and pneumonia. There is increased airway resistance due to inflammation of the passages. Death can occur from asphyxiation, suffocation when plastic bags are put over one's head to inhale substances, and from *sudden sniffing death*, a sudden fatal heart failure secondary to rapid and irregular heart rhythms.

Gastrointestinal Effects

Abdominal pain, nausea, and vomiting may occur. A rash may be present around the individual's nose and mouth. Unusual breath odors are common. Chronic inhalant use has been associated with liver failure (and renal failure) as well as liver tumors.

Renal System Effects

Acute and chronic renal failure and hepatorenal syndrome have occurred. Renal toxicity from toluene exposure has been reported, manifesting in renal tubular acidosis, hypokalemia, hypophosphatemia, hyperchloremia, azotemia, sterile pyuria, hematuria, and proteinuria (McKeown, 2019).

Inhalant Intoxication

The *DSM-5-TR* defines *inhalant intoxication* as "clinically significant problematic behavioral or psychological changes that developed during or immediately after intended or unintended inhalation of a volatile hydrocarbon substance" (APA, 2022; p. 606). Symptoms are similar to alcohol intoxication and may include the following (APA, 2022; Howard et al., 2017):

- Dizziness, ataxia
- Euphoria, excitation, disinhibition
- Nystagmus, blurred vision, double vision
- Slurred speech
- Hypoactive reflexes
- Psychomotor retardation, lethargy
- Generalized muscle weakness
- Stupor or coma (at higher doses)

Inhalant Withdrawal

Mild withdrawal symptoms may occur after chronic, long-term use. Reported symptoms include restlessness, nausea and vomiting, runny nose and watery eyes, poor attention and concentration, and mood changes. The *DSM-5-TR*, however, does not include inhalant withdrawal as a diagnosis because they believe the symptoms are considered either too mild or too inconsistent to be included (Patterson, 2020).

Opioid Use Disorder

Profile of the Substance

The term **opioid** refers to a group of compounds that includes opium, opium derivatives, and synthetic substitutes. Opioids exert both sedative and analgesic effects, and their major medical uses are for the relief of pain, treatment of diarrhea, and relief of coughing. Under close supervision, opioids are indispensable in the practice of medicine. They are the most effective agents known for the relief of intense pain. They also induce a pleasurable effect that promotes misuse. And because opioids are capable of inducing tolerance, their use may lead to physiological and psychological addiction. The physiological and psychological addiction that occurs with opioids, as well as the development of profound tolerance, contributes to the addicted individual's ongoing quest for more of the substance, regardless of the means. The United States is currently facing an unprecedented opiate epidemic and death toll.

Opioids are popular drugs of abuse because they desensitize an individual to both psychological and physiological pain and induce a sense of euphoria. Lethargy and indifference to the environment are common manifestations.

Individuals who are addicted to opiates usually spend much of their time acquiring the drug to sustain their addiction. They are seldom able to hold a steady job that will support their need and must therefore secure funds from friends, relatives, or whomever they have not yet alienated with their addiction-related behavior. It is not uncommon for individuals who are addicted to opioids to resort to illegal means of obtaining funds, such as burglary, robbery, prostitution, or selling drugs.

Methods of administration of opioid drugs include orally, snorting, or smoking, and by subcutaneous, intramuscular, and intravenous injection. A selected list of opioid substances is presented in Table 14–4.

Historical Perspectives

In its crude form, opium is a brownish-black, gummy substance obtained from the ripened pods of the opium poppy. References have been found to the use of opiates in the Egyptian, Greek, and Arabian cultures as early as 3000 BC. The drug became widely used both medicinally and recreationally throughout

TABLE 14–4 Opioids and Related Substances

CATEGORIES	GENERIC (TRADE) NAMES	COMMON STREET NAMES
Opioids of natural origin	Opium (ingredient in various antidiarrheal agents) Morphinan (Astramorph) Codeine (ingredient in various analgesics and cough suppressants) Kratom (opioid-like)	Black stuff, poppy, tar, big O M, white stuff, Miss Emma Terp, schoolboy, syrup, cody
Opioid derivatives	Heroin Hydromorphone (Dilaudid) Oxycodone (Percodan; OxyContin) Hydrocodone (Vicodin)	H, horse, junk, brown sugar, smack, skag, TNT, Harry DLs, 4s, lords, little D Perks, perkies, Oxy, O.C. Vike
Synthetic opiate-like drugs	Meperidine (Demerol) Methadone (Dolophine) Pentazocine (Talwin) Fentanyl (Fentora) Carfentanil Desomorphine U-47700 Sufentanil Tramadol	Doctors Dollies, done T's Apache, China girl, China town, dance fever, goodfella, jackpot Krokodil Pink, pinky, U4

Europe during the 16th and 17th centuries. Most of the opium supply came from China, where the drug was introduced by Arabic traders in the late 17th century. Morphine, the primary active ingredient of opium, was isolated in 1803 by the European chemist Friedrich Sertürner. Since that time, morphine, rather than crude opium, has been used throughout the world for the medical treatment of pain and diarrhea. This process was facilitated in 1853 by the development of the hypodermic syringe, which made it possible to deliver the undiluted morphine quickly into the body for rapid relief from pain.

This development also created a new variety of opioid user in the United States: one who was able to self-administer the drug by injection. During this time, there was also a large influx into the United States of Chinese immigrants, who introduced opium smoking to this country. By the early part of the 20th century, opium addiction was widespread.

In response to the concerns over widespread addiction, in 1914 the U.S. government passed the Harrison Narcotic Act, which created strict controls on the accessibility of opiates. Until that time, these substances had been freely available to the public without a prescription. The Harrison Act banned the use of opiates for other than medicinal purposes and drove the use of heroin underground. To this day, the beneficial uses of these substances are widely acclaimed within the medical profession, but the illicit trafficking of the drugs for recreational purposes continues to resist most efforts aimed at control. Historically, the term *opiate* referred to naturally occurring (or slightly modified) components of opium and the term *opioid* described synthetic opiates. However, more recently, the term *opioid* has been used to describe the entire class of drugs. For the purposes of this discussion, these terms are used interchangeably.

Patterns of Use

The development of opioid addiction may follow one of two typical behavior patterns. The first occurs in individuals who have obtained the drug by prescription from a physician for the relief of a medical problem. Misuse and addiction occur when individuals increase the amount and frequency of use, justifying the behavior as symptom treatment. They become obsessed with obtaining more and more of the substance and may see several physicians in order to replenish and maintain supplies.

The second pattern of behavior associated with addiction to opioids occurs among individuals who use the drugs for recreational purposes and obtain them from illegal sources. Opioids may be used alone to induce the euphoric effects or in combination with stimulants or other drugs to enhance the euphoria or to counteract the depressant effects of the opioid. Tolerance develops and addiction occurs, leading the individual to procure the substance by whatever means is required to support the habit.

The CDC reports that, on average, 128 Americans die per day from an opioid overdose (CDC, 2020c). Efforts have been made in some states to exert stricter controls on opiate prescription practices, and 2012 marked the first year of a trend toward a decline in prescription rates nationally. However, beginning in 2010, an increase in heroin use and in 2013 an increase in the use of synthetic opioids (like illicitly manufactured fentanyl and carfentanil) are evidence that the opiate epidemic and associated deaths are ongoing problems. The chemical structure of illegally manufactured fentanyl continues to change and is sometimes found mixed with heroin, counterfeit pills, and cocaine (CDC, 2020c).

The mixture of fentanyl with heroin is particularly lethal. When heroin is mixed with fentanyl, it may cause accidental overdose because fentanyl is 30 to 50 times more potent than pure heroin. Carfentanil (carfentanyl), a potent drug used mainly in the capture of wild animals, is 100 times more potent than fentanyl and 10,000 times more potent than morphine. It has been responsible for rapid overdose and often death when ingested along with heroin (National Institutes of Health [NIH], 2021).

Late in 2018, the FDA approved a sublingual tablet form of sufentanil (5 to 10 times more potent than fentanyl) and, although it is intended for the treatment of severe acute pain in certified, medically supervised health-care settings, critics argue that it adds one more very potent opioid to the arsenal of those that may be diverted, easily administered, and potentially fatal (Brooks, 2018).

Similar to the trend in development of synthetic amphetamines discussed earlier in this chapter, a new synthetic opioid, U-47700 (discovered in the 1970s), surfaced in 2015 and was responsible for 46 fatalities in 2016 before the substance underwent emergency classification as a Schedule I drug (Duffy, 2016). U-47700 is 10 times more potent than morphine. It is found in counterfeit oxycodone tablets and is the key ingredient in a street drug called "gray death" (Kyei-Baffour & Lindsley, 2020).

Kratom, a plant from Southeast Asia that triggers opiate-like effects, also surfaced in the United States and was subsequently banned; however, this decision was reversed when researchers argued that it may help them develop tools to overcome opioid and alcohol addiction as well as chronic pain (MPR, 2016). Two of the over 40 alkaloids that have been isolated from kratom leaves (mitragynine and 7-hydroxymitragynine) have opioid-like properties, and potency at the mu opioid receptors for these has been found to exceed that of morphine (Stanciu et al., 2020). The FDA has not yet approved or regulated kratom, and as of 2018, the FDA received reports of 44 deaths associated with its use (FDA, 2018). Currently, the DEA lists kratom as a chemical of concern. It is being evaluated for placement into controlled substance scheduling, although some states have already banned its use and identified it as a Schedule I substance (Drugs.com, 2021).

At present, the opioid epidemic remains a national epidemic, with overdose deaths increasing 38.4% in the 12-month period through May 2020 (CDC, 2020c). But several national initiatives to address this public health crisis have been identified. A National Practice Guideline for use of medications to treat opioid use disorder has been established (ASAM, 2015). For the first time in U.S. history, in 2016, the Surgeon General declared illicit drug use and misuse of prescription drugs a national health-care priority and committed to the need for additional research and treatment options. In 2018, the Surgeon General advanced a public health advisory urging more Americans to carry naloxone kits to assist (along with rescue breathing) in preventing opiate overdose and death. Some state programs, like Project Dawn in Ohio, are providing naloxone education and distribution free of charge to individuals who are willing to carry naloxone kits for responding to opioid overdose victims. In 2018, the NIH launched the HEAL (Helping to End Addiction Long-term) Initiative, identifying 15 areas of critical focus for research and development to address the opiate epidemic. These areas include research on longer-acting naloxone-type drugs, better responses to chronic pain management, better management of neonatal opiate withdrawal (NIDA [2019a] reports that every 15 minutes a baby is born in opiate withdrawal), and better access to and efficacy of treatment options (Twachtman, 2018). All of these efforts underscore the gravity of this ongoing national public health issue.

Effects on the Body

Opiates are sometimes classified as *narcotic analgesics.* They exert their major effects primarily on the CNS, eyes, and GI tract. Chronic morphine use or acute morphine toxicity is manifested by a syndrome of sedation, chronic constipation, decreased respiratory rate, and pinpoint pupils. Intensity of symptoms is largely dose dependent. The following physiological effects are common with opioid use.

Central Nervous System Effects

All opioids, opioid derivatives, and synthetic opioid-like drugs affect the CNS. Common manifestations include euphoria, mood changes, and mental clouding. Other common CNS effects include drowsiness and pain reduction. Pupillary constriction occurs in response to stimulation of the oculomotor nerve. CNS depression of the respiratory centers within the medulla results in respiratory depression. The antitussive response is due to suppression of the cough center within the medulla. The nausea and vomiting commonly associated with opiate ingestion are related to the stimulation of the centers within the medulla.

Gastrointestinal Effects

These drugs exert a profound effect on the GI tract. Both stomach and intestinal tone are increased, whereas peristaltic activity of the intestines is diminished. These effects lead to a marked decrease in the movement of food through the GI tract. This is a notable therapeutic effect in the treatment of severe diarrhea. In fact, no drugs have yet been developed that are more effective than the opioids for this purpose. However, constipation and even fecal impaction may be a serious problem for the chronic opioid user. Loperamide (Imodium), an antidiarrheal drug with small amounts of opioids, has surfaced as a drug of abuse, with users taking anywhere from 50 to over 100 pills to achieve a high. Not only does this increase the risk for significant constipation and other GI effects, but it has also been associated with deaths secondary to overdose.

Cardiovascular Effects

In therapeutic doses, opioids have minimal effect on the action of the heart. Morphine is used extensively to relieve pulmonary edema and the pain of myocardial infarction in clients experiencing a heart attack. At high doses, opioids induce hypotension, which may be caused by direct action on the heart or by opioid-induced histamine release. Although most opioids do not affect cardiac conductivity, "methadone and buprenorphine can prolong QTc, especially when used in patients at risk for QTc prolongation" (Chen & Ashburn, 2015, p. S27). Abuse of loperamide is a growing problem that has been linked to cardiac dysrhythmias and death, because at very high doses (needed to achieve other than antidiarrheal effects) this medication is highly cardiotoxic (Davenport, 2016).

Sexual Function

Opioid use causes decreased sexual function and diminished libido, and long-term use has been associated with erectile dysfunction (Deyo et al., 2013). Delayed ejaculation, impotence, and orgasm failure (in both men and women) may occur.

Opioid Intoxication

Opioid intoxication constitutes clinically significant problematic behavioral or psychological changes that develop during or shortly after opioid use (APA, 2022). Symptoms include initial euphoria followed by apathy, dysphoria, psychomotor agitation or retardation, and impaired judgment. Physical symptoms include pupillary constriction (or dilation due to anoxia from severe overdose), drowsiness, slurred speech, and impairment in attention or memory (APA, 2022). Symptoms are consistent with the half-life of most opioid drugs and usually last for several hours. Severe opioid intoxication can lead to respiratory depression, coma, and death.

Opioid Withdrawal

Opioid withdrawal produces a syndrome of symptoms that develops after cessation of or reduction in heavy and prolonged use of an opiate or related substance. Symptoms include dysphoric mood, nausea or vomiting, muscle aches, lacrimation or rhinorrhea, pupillary dilation, piloerection, sweating, diarrhea, yawning, fever, and insomnia (APA, 2022). With short-acting drugs such as heroin, withdrawal symptoms occur within 6 to 8 hours after the last dose, peak within 1 to 3 days, and gradually subside over a period of 5 to 10 days. With longer-acting drugs such as methadone, withdrawal symptoms begin within 1 to 3 days after the last dose, peak between days 4 and 6, and are complete in 14 to 21 days. Withdrawal from the ultra-short-acting meperidine begins quickly, reaches a peak in 8 to 12 hours, and is complete in 4 to 5 days.

Hallucinogen Use Disorder

Profile of the Substance

Hallucinogenic substances are capable of distorting an individual's perception of reality. They have the ability to alter sensory perception and induce hallucinations. For this reason, they have sometimes been referred to as "mind-expanding drugs." Some of the manifestations have been likened to a psychotic break. The hallucinations experienced by an individual with schizophrenia, however, are most often auditory, whereas substance-induced hallucinations are usually visual. Perceptual distortions have been reported by some users as spiritual, as giving a sense of depersonalization (observing oneself having the experience), or as being at peace with self and the universe. Others, who describe their experiences as "bad trips," report feelings of panic and a fear of dying or going insane. A common danger reported with hallucinogenic drugs is that of "flashbacks," or a spontaneous recurrence of the hallucinogenic state without ingestion of the drug. These can occur months after the drug was last taken.

Recurrent use can produce tolerance, encouraging users to resort to higher and higher dosages. No evidence of physical dependence (withdrawal syndrome) is detectable when the drug is withdrawn; however, psychological dependence, although rare, may occur (Boland & Verduin, 2022). This psychological addiction varies according to the drug, the dose, and the individual user. Hallucinogens are highly unpredictable in the effects they may induce each time they are used.

Many of the hallucinogenic substances have structural similarities. Some are produced synthetically; others are natural products of plants and fungi. A selected list of hallucinogens is presented in Table 14–5.

Historical Perspectives

Hallucinogens have been used throughout history in many cultures for religious and mystical experiences, including in Aztec, Mexican Indian, and Hindu ceremonies. Use of the peyote cactus as part of religious ceremonies in the southwestern part of the United States still occurs today, although this ritual use has greatly diminished.

Lysergic acid diethylamide (LSD) was first synthesized in 1943 by Dr. Albert Hoffman. It was used as a clinical research tool to investigate the biochemical etiology of schizophrenia. It soon reached the illicit market, however, and its abuse began to overshadow the research effort.

The use of hallucinogens reached a peak in the late 1960s, waned during the 1970s, and returned to favor in the 1980s with the so-called designer drugs (e.g., 3,4-methylene-dioxymethamphetamine [MDMA], also known as "Molly" or "ecstasy," and 3,4-methylenedioxyamphetamine [MDA]). Another hallucinogen, PCP (phencyclidine), originally was developed in the 1950s as an anesthetic, but this use was discontinued because of serious adverse effects. It continues to be used illegally and is often combined with cannabis. A number of deaths have been directly attributed to the use of PCP, and numerous accidental deaths have occurred as a result of overdose and behavioral changes the drug precipitates. A derivative of PCP, ketamine, which is also used as a preoperative anesthetic, is misused for its psychedelic properties. It produces effects similar to, but somewhat less intense than, those of PCP. In 2019, the FDA approved a nasal

TABLE 14–5 Hallucinogens

CATEGORIES	GENERIC (TRADE) NAMES	COMMON STREET NAMES
Naturally occurring hallucinogens	Mescaline (primary active ingredient of the peyote cactus)	Cactus, mesc, mescal, half moon, big chief, bad seed, peyote
	Psilocybin and psilocin (active ingredients of *Psilocybe* mushrooms)	Magic mushroom, God's flesh, shrooms
	Ololiuqui (morning glory seeds)	Heavenly blue, pearly gates, flying saucers
	Salvia divinorum	Salvia
Synthetic compounds	Lysergic acid diethylamide (LSD)—synthetically produced from a fungal substance found on rye or a chemical substance found in morning glory seeds	Acid, cube, big D, California sunshine, microdots, blue dots, sugar, orange wedges, peace tablets, purple haze, cupcakes
	Dextromethorphan (DXM)	Robo
	Dimethyltryptamine (DMT) and diethyltryptamine (DET)—chemical analogs of tryptamine	Businessman's trip
	2,5-Dimethoxy-4-methylamphetamine (DOM)	STP (serenity, tranquility, peace)
	Phencyclidine (PCP)	Angel dust, hog, peace pill, rocket fuel
	Ketamine (Ketalar)	Special K, vitamin K, kit kat
	3,4-Methylene-dioxyamphetamine (MDMA)*	XTC, ecstasy, Adam, Eve
	Methoxy-amphetamine (MDA)	Love drug, molly
	3,4-Methylenedioxypyrovalerone (MDPV)*	Bath salts (also called blue silk, cloud 9, ivory wave, vanilla sky, white knight, and others)
	4-Methylmethcathinone (mephedrone, 4-MMC)*	
	Methylone*	

*Cross-listed with the CNS stimulants.

spray formulation of esketamine (Spravato), for use in treatment-resistant depression. Its use is restricted to certified medical clinics and requires a risk evaluation and mitigation strategy (REMS). Several therapeutic uses of LSD have been proposed, including the treatment of depression, anxiety, chronic alcoholism, and the reduction of intractable pain such as occurs in malignant disease. In one systematic review of research on the therapeutic benefits of LSD for depression and anxiety, the authors concluded that evidence supports immediate antidepressant and antianxiety effects that endured for several months when taken in a controlled setting (Muttoni et al., 2019). They caution, though, that the number and size of the studies thus far have been small. In another systematic review, the authors conclude that the evidence is strongest for the use of LSD in alcohol treatment (Fuentes et al., 2020). Clearly there is current interest in the potential benefits of LSD in psychiatry, but more research is needed.

Patterns of Use

Use of hallucinogens is usually episodic. Because cognitive and perceptual abilities are so markedly affected by these substances, the user must set aside time from normal daily activities for their use. According to the most recent NSDUH survey in 2018, 2% of Americans 12 years and older reported using hallucinogens in the past year (NIDA, 2020e).

LSD, like other hallucinogens, does not lead to the development of physical addiction or withdrawal symptoms. However, tolerance for LSD and other hallucinogens develops quickly and to a high degree. In fact, tolerance is complete after 3 to 4 consecutive days of use. Recovery from the tolerance also occurs very rapidly (in 4 to 7 days), so that the individual is able to achieve the desired effect from the drug repeatedly and often.

PCP is usually taken episodically, in binges that can last for several days. However, some chronic users take the substance daily. Physical addiction does not occur with PCP; however, psychological addiction characterized by craving for the drug has been reported in chronic users, as has the development of tolerance. Tolerance apparently develops quickly with frequent use.

Psilocybin is an ingredient of the *Psilocybe* mushroom indigenous to the United States and Mexico. Ingestion of these mushrooms produces an effect similar to that of LSD but of a shorter duration. This hallucinogenic chemical can now be produced synthetically.

Mescaline is the only hallucinogenic compound used legally for religious purposes today by members of the Native American Church of the United States. It is the primary active ingredient of the peyote cactus. Neither physical nor psychological addiction occurs with the use of mescaline, although, as with other hallucinogens, tolerance can develop quickly with frequent use.

Salvia is an herb from the mint family that has hallucinogenic effects when dried leaves are chewed, extracted juices are consumed, or smoke from the leaves is inhaled. This particular hallucinogen is advertised and sold over the Internet because it is not regulated by the Controlled Substances Act, but some states have limited or banned its use. Currently, in most states, salvia is legal but some states, including Delaware, Louisiana, Maine, Missouri, Oklahoma, and Tennessee, have banned its use or possession. The DEA labels it a "drug of concern" (WebMD, 2021a).

Among the very potent hallucinogens of the current drug culture are those that are categorized as amphetamine derivatives. These include 2,5-dimethoxy-4-methylamphetamine (DOM [street name "STP"]), MDMA, and MDA. At lower doses, these drugs produce the "high" associated with CNS stimulants. At higher doses, hallucinogenic effects occur. These drugs have existed for many years but were "rediscovered" in the mid-1980s. Because of the rapid increase in recreational use, the DEA imposed an emergency classification of MDMA as a Schedule I drug in 1985. MDMA, or ecstasy, is a synthetic drug with both stimulant and hallucinogenic qualities. It has a chemical structure similar to methamphetamine and mescaline and has become widely available throughout the world. Because of its growing popularity, the demand for this drug has led to tablets and capsules being sold as "ecstasy" that are not pure MDMA. Many contain drugs such as methamphetamine, PCP, amphetamine, ketamine, and *p*-methoxyamphetamine (PMA, a stimulant with hallucinogenic properties; more toxic than MDMA). This practice has increased the dangers associated with MDMA use.

Effects on the Body

The effects produced by the various hallucinogens are highly unpredictable. The variety of effects may be related to dosage, the mental state of the individual, and the environment in which the substance is used. Some common effects have been reported (APA, 2022; Boland & Verduin, 2022; Julien, 2014) as discussed next.

Physiological Effects

- Nausea and vomiting
- Chills
- Pupil dilation
- Increased pulse, blood pressure, and temperature
- Mild dizziness
- Trembling
- Loss of appetite
- Insomnia
- Sweating
- Slowing of respirations
- Elevation in blood sugar

Psychological Effects

- Heightened response to color, texture, and sounds
- Heightened body awareness
- Distortion of vision
- Sense of slowing of time
- All feelings magnified: love, lust, hate, joy, anger, pain, terror, despair
- Fear of losing control
- Paranoia, panic
- Euphoria, bliss
- Projection of self into dreamlike images
- Serenity, peace
- Depersonalization
- Derealization
- Increased libido

The effects of hallucinogens are not always pleasurable for the user. Two types of toxic reactions are known to occur. The first is the *panic reaction*, or "bad trip." Symptoms include an intense anxiety, fear, and stimulation. The individual hallucinates and fears going insane. Paranoia and acute psychosis may be evident.

The second type of toxic reaction to hallucinogens is the *flashback*. This phenomenon refers to the transient, spontaneous repetition of a previous LSD-induced experience that occurs without taking the substance. The *DSM-5-TR* (APA, 2022) refers to this as *hallucinogen persisting perception disorder*. Various studies have reported that from 15% to 80% of hallucinogen users report having experienced flashbacks (Boland & Verduin, 2022). These episodes typically last for a few minutes or less.

Hallucinogen Intoxication

Symptoms of hallucinogen intoxication develop during or shortly after hallucinogen use. Maladaptive behavioral or psychological changes include marked anxiety or depression, ideas of reference (a type of delusional thinking that all activity within one's environment is "referred to" [about] oneself), fear of losing one's mind, paranoid ideation, and impaired judgment. Perceptual changes occur while the individual is fully awake and alert and include intensification of perceptions, depersonalization, derealization, illusions, hallucinations, and synesthesias (APA, 2022). Because hallucinogens are sympathomimetics, they can cause tachycardia, hypertension, sweating, blurred vision, papillary (pupil) dilation, and tremors.

Symptoms of PCP intoxication are unpredictable. Specific symptoms are dose related and may be manifested by impulsiveness, impaired judgment, assaultiveness, and belligerence, or the individual may appear calm, stuporous, or comatose. Physical symptoms include vertical or horizontal nystagmus, hypertension, tachycardia, ataxia, diminished pain sensation, muscle rigidity, and seizures. Symptoms of ketamine intoxication appear similar to those of PCP.

General effects of MDMA (ecstasy) include increased heart rate, blood pressure, and body temperature; dehydration; confusion; insomnia; and paranoia. Overdose can result in panic attacks, hallucinations, severe hyperthermia, dehydration, and seizures. Death can occur from kidney or cardiovascular failure.

Cannabis Use Disorder

Profile of the Substance

Marijuana is the most commonly used psychotropic drug in the United States after alcohol (NIDA, 2020f). The major psychoactive ingredient of this class of substances is delta-9-tetrahydrocannabinol (THC). It occurs naturally in the plant *Cannabis sativa*, which grows readily in warm climates. Technically, the term **cannabis** refers to all products from the cannabis sativa plant that contains roughly 540 chemical substances, but it is often used interchangeably with marijuana (NIH, 2019). *Cannabinoids* is a term that refers to active constituents of the cannabis plant, and the primary cannabinoids are THC and cannabidiol (CBD). Marijuana, the most prevalent type of cannabis preparation, is composed of the dried leaves, stems, and flowers of the plant. Hashish is a more potent concentrate of the resin derived from the flowering tops of the plant. Hash oil is a very concentrated form of THC made by boiling hashish in a solvent and filtering out the solid matter. NIDA (2019b) reports that smoking THC-rich resins is on the rise. The practice, called "dabbing," can deliver very large amounts of THC to the body and has been associated with contributing to various medical emergencies. Cannabis products are usually smoked in the form of loosely rolled cigarettes. Cannabis can also be taken orally when it is prepared in food, but about two to three times the amount of cannabis must be ingested orally to equal the potency of that obtained by the inhalation of its smoke (Boland & Verduin, 2022). Vaping THC has become more prevalent among teenagers with the rising popularity of vaping devices (NIH, 2019), and one study found that the majority of lung injuries associated with vaping, some of which were fatal, were among those vaping marijuana or cannabis oils (Butt et al., 2019).

At moderate dosages, cannabis produces effects resembling alcohol and other CNS depressants. By depressing higher brain centers, it releases lower centers from inhibitory influences. There has been some controversy in the past over the classification of these substances. They are not narcotics, although they are legally classified as controlled substances. They are not hallucinogens, although in very high dosages they can induce hallucinations. They are not sedative-hypnotics, although they most closely resemble these substances. Like sedative-hypnotics, their action occurs in the ascending reticular activating system.

Psychological addiction has been shown to occur with cannabis, and tolerance can occur. Controversy has existed about whether physiological addiction occurs with cannabis. In the past, symptoms of cannabis withdrawal were considered less than clinically significant to include the diagnosis in the *DSM*. However, the *DSM-5* Substance-Related Disorders Work Group determined that subsequent research has provided significant data to support cannabis withdrawal as a valid and reliable syndrome that can negatively impact abstinence attempts of heavy cannabis users. The diagnosis of cannabis withdrawal is included in the *DSM-5-TR*.

Synthetic cannabinoids, on the other hand, have been clearly identified as potentially addictive (NIDA, 2020g). Although some of these chemicals are illegal to buy, sell, or possess, manufacturers often sidestep the laws by altering their chemical formulas. Standard drug tests cannot easily detect many of these chemicals.

Common cannabis and synthetic cannabinoid preparations are presented in Table 14–6.

TABLE 14–6 Cannabinoids

CATEGORY	COMMON PREPARATIONS	STREET NAMES
Cannabis	Marijuana	Joint, weed, pot, grass, Mary Jane, Texas tea, loco-weed, MJ, hay, stick
	Hashish	Hash, bhang, ganja, charas
Synthetic cannabinoids	NPS (new psychoactive substances) powders or liquids to be inhaled	K2, Spice, Black Mamba, Joker, Kush, Kronic

Historical Perspectives

Products of *Cannabis sativa* have been used therapeutically for nearly 5,000 years (Julien, 2014). Cannabis was first employed in China and India as an antiseptic and an analgesic. Its use later spread to the Middle East, Africa, and Eastern Europe.

In the United States, medical interest in the use of cannabis arose during the early part of the 19th century. Many articles were published espousing its use for varied reasons. The drug was almost as commonly used for medicinal purposes as aspirin is today, and it could be purchased without a prescription in any drug store. It was purported to have antibacterial and anticonvulsant capabilities, to decrease intraocular pressure and decrease pain, to help in the treatment of asthma, to increase appetite, and generally was thought to raise one's morale.

The drug went out of favor primarily because of the large variation in potency across batches of medication caused by the variations in the THC content of different plants. Other medications were favored for their greater degree of solubility and faster onset of action than cannabis products. A federal law put an end to its legal use in 1937, after an association between marijuana and criminal activity became evident. In the 1960s, marijuana became the symbol of the "antiestablishment" generation, at which time it reached its peak as a drug of abuse.

Research continues in regard to the possible therapeutic uses of cannabis. It has been shown to be an effective agent for relieving the nausea and vomiting associated with cancer chemotherapy when other antinausea medications fail. It has also been used in the treatment of chronic pain, glaucoma, multiple sclerosis, AIDS, and epilepsy. Cannabidiol (CBD), a chemical in cannabis that has very small amounts of THC and that may block the psychoactive properties of THC, is being studied for its potential use in many medical disorders, including schizophrenia, dystonia, and Parkinson's disease.

Advocates who praise the therapeutic usefulness and support the legalization of the cannabinoids persist in the United States today. Groups such as the Alliance for Cannabis Therapeutics (ACT) and the National Organization for the Reform of Marijuana Laws (NORML) have lobbied extensively to allow disease sufferers easier access to the drug. The medical use of marijuana has been legalized in several states, as has recreational use. However, the DEA still considers marijuana a Schedule I controlled substance. Even the Farm Bill of 2018, which legalized the sale of hemp and hemp products in the United States, does not legalize all hemp-derived cannabidiol products (WebMD, 2021b).

Two medications that have components of the marijuana plant or related synthetic compounds are currently approved by the FDA. Dronabinol, a synthetic compound in the medication Marinol, is approved for nausea and vomiting associated with cancer treatment and for severe weight loss associated with AIDS. Nabilone, a chemical similar to THC and found in the medication Cesamet, is a similar FDA-approved drug. A third medication, nabiximols (Sativex), which is an oromucosal spray containing THC and cannabidiol, has been approved for use in several countries to treat pain and spasticity associated with multiple sclerosis but is not yet approved in the United States. In 2018, the first cannabis-based drug (Epidiolex) became FDA approved for the treatment of epilepsy.

Patterns of Use

NSDUH data from 2019 indicate that 48.2 million Americans age 12 or older, 17.5% of the population, used marijuana in the past year (SAMHSA, 2021). Many people incorrectly regard cannabis as a substance of low abuse potential. This lack of knowledge has promoted use of the substance by some individuals who believe it to be harmless. Tolerance, although it tends to decline rapidly, does occur with chronic use. As tolerance develops, physical addiction also occurs, resulting in a withdrawal syndrome upon cessation of drug use.

One controversy that exists regarding marijuana (particularly because of several statewide efforts toward legalization) is whether its use leads to the use of other illicit drugs. NIDA (2020f) reports that although some research shows that marijuana use is likely to precede use of other drugs and the development of addiction to other substances (including nicotine), "the majority of people who use marijuana do not go on to use other, 'harder' substances." More research is needed to clarify these associations as well as the impact of social environments on increasing one's tendency to try other drugs.

Effects on the Body

Following is a summary of some of the effects that have been attributed to marijuana in recent years. Undoubtedly, as research continues, evidence of additional physiological and psychological effects will be made available.

Cardiovascular Effects

Cannabis ingestion induces tachycardia and orthostatic hypotension; in some cases, it may elevate blood pressure (NIDA, 2020f). With the decrease in blood pressure, myocardial oxygen supply is decreased. Tachycardia in turn increases oxygen demand. Marijuana raises the heart rate for up to 3 hours after a person has smoked.

Respiratory Effects

Marijuana produces a greater amount of "tar" than its equivalent weight in tobacco. Because of the method by which marijuana is smoked—that is, the smoke is held in the lungs for as long as possible to achieve the desired effect—larger amounts of tar are deposited in the lungs, promoting deleterious effects to the respiratory system.

Although the initial reaction to the marijuana is bronchodilation, thereby facilitating respiratory function, chronic use results in obstructive airway disorders. Frequent marijuana users often have laryngitis, bronchitis, cough, and hoarseness.

Reproductive Effects

Some studies have shown that, with heavy marijuana use, men may have a decrease in sperm count, motility, and structure. In women, heavy marijuana use may result in a suppression of ovulation, disruption in menstrual cycles, and alteration of hormone levels. Marijuana use in pregnant women has been associated increased risk of brain and behavioral problems in infants. Children exposed to marijuana during fetal development have a higher incidence of attention, problem-solving, and memory problems than do unexposed children (NIDA, 2020f).

Central Nervous System Effects

Acute CNS effects of marijuana are dose related. Many people report a feeling of being high—the equivalent of being "drunk" on alcohol. Symptoms include feelings of euphoria, relaxed inhibitions, disorientation, depersonalization, and relaxation. At higher doses, sensory alterations may occur, including impairment in judgment of time and distance, recent memory, and learning ability. Physiological symptoms may include tremors, muscle rigidity, and conjunctival redness. Toxic effects are generally characterized by panic reactions. Very heavy usage has been shown to precipitate an acute psychosis that is self-limited and short-lived once the drug is removed from the body (Julien, 2014).

Heavy, long-term cannabis use is also associated with a condition called *amotivational syndrome*, which is defined as lack of motivation to persist in or complete a task that requires ongoing attention. Persons with the syndrome are described as "apathetic, anergic, usually gaining weight, and appearing slothful" (Boland & Verduin, 2022, p. 289). Evidence supports that long-term use also impairs cognitive functions of memory, attention, and organization, and these impairments may also contribute to some of the symptoms apparent in amotivational syndrome.

Sexual Function

Marijuana is reported to enhance the sexual experience in both men and women. The intensified sensory awareness and the subjective slowness of time perception are thought to increase sexual satisfaction. Marijuana also enhances sexual function by releasing inhibitions for certain activities that would normally be restrained.

Cannabis Intoxication

Cannabis intoxication is evidenced by the presence of clinically significant behavioral or psychological changes that develop during or shortly after cannabis use. Symptoms include impaired motor coordination, euphoria, anxiety, a sensation of slowed time, impaired judgment and memory, and social withdrawal. Physical symptoms include conjunctival injection (red eyes), increased appetite, dry mouth, and tachycardia (APA, 2022). The impairment of motor skills lasts for 8 to 12 hours and interferes with the operation of motor vehicles. These effects are additive to those of alcohol, which is often used in combination with cannabis. Cannabis intoxication delirium is marked by significant cognitive impairment and difficulty performing tasks. Higher doses also impair level of consciousness.

Marijuana when taken alone is not associated with death from overdose, but large amounts of THC (and THC content has been increasing over the past decade) can result in symptoms such as anxiety, paranoia, and (in rare cases) extreme psychotic reactions (NIDA, 2019b). Synthetic cannabinoids, on the other hand, are associated with toxic reactions, toxic reactions, elevated blood pressure, reduced blood supply to the heart, kidney damage, and seizures, all of which may be life threatening; the risk of fatality is increased when combined with synthetic opioids (NIDA, 2020g). Because the strengths are variable (up to 100 times more potent than THC), the risks of using these substances are unpredictable.

Cannabis Withdrawal

The *DSM-5-TR* describes a syndrome of symptoms that occurs upon cessation of cannabis use that has been heavy and prolonged (APA, 2022). Symptoms occur within a week following cessation of use and may include any of the following:

- Irritability, anger, or aggression
- Nervousness, restlessness, or anxiety
- Sleep difficulty (e.g., insomnia, disturbing dreams)
- Decreased appetite or weight loss
- Depressed mood
- Physical symptoms, such as abdominal pain, tremors, sweating, fever, chills, or headache

Tables 14–7 and 14–8 include summaries of the psychoactive substances, including symptoms of intoxication, withdrawal, use, overdose, possible therapeutic uses, and trade and common names by which they may be referred.

Application of the Nursing Process

Background Assessment Data

In the pre-introductory phase of relationship development, the nurse must examine their feelings about working with a patient who misuses substances. If these behaviors are viewed as morally wrong and the nurse has internalized these attitudes from very early in life, it may be very difficult to suppress judgmental feelings. The role that alcohol or other substances has played (or plays) in the life of the nurse most certainly will affect the way in which the nurse interacts with a patient who has a substance use disorder.

How are attitudes examined? Some individuals may have sufficient ability for introspection to be able to recognize on their own whether they have unresolved issues related to substance abuse. For others, it may be more helpful to discuss these issues in a group situation, where insight may be gained from feedback regarding the perceptions of others.

Whether alone or in a group, the nurse may gain a greater understanding about attitudes and feelings related to substance abuse by responding to the following types of questions. As written here, the

Text continued on page 334

TABLE 14–7 **Psychoactive Substances: A Profile Summary**

CLASS OF DRUGS	SYMPTOMS OF USE	THERAPEUTIC USES	SYMPTOMS OF OVERDOSE	TRADE NAMES OR CHEMICAL NAMES	COMMON STREET NAMES
CNS DEPRESSANTS					
Alcohol	Relaxation, loss of inhibitions, lack of concentration, drowsiness, slurred speech, sleep	Antidote for methanol consumption; ingredient in many pharmacological concentrates	Nausea, vomiting; shallow respirations; cold, clammy skin; weak, rapid pulse; coma; possible death	Ethyl alcohol, beer, gin, rum, vodka, bourbon, whiskey, liqueurs, wine, brandy, sherry, champagne	Booze, alcohol, liquor, drinks, cocktails, highballs, nightcaps, moonshine, white lightning, firewater
Other (barbiturates and nonbarbiturates)	Same as alcohol	Relief from anxiety and insomnia; as anticonvulsants and anesthetics	Anxiety, fever, agitation, hallucinations, disorientation, tremors, delirium, convulsions, possible death	Seconal, amytal, Nembutal, Valium, Librium, Noctec, Miltown	Red birds, yellow birds, blue birds, blues, yellows, green & whites mickeys, downers
CNS STIMULANTS					
Amphetamines and related drugs	Hyperactivity, agitation, euphoria, insomnia, loss of appetite	Management of narcolepsy, hyperkinesia, and weight control	Cardiac arrhythmias, headache, convulsions, hypertension, rapid heart rate, coma, possible death	Dexedrine, Didrex, Tenuate, Bontril, Ritalin, Focalin, Meridia, Provigil	Uppers, pep pills, wakeups, bennies, eye-openers, speed, black beauties, sweet A's
Cocaine	Euphoria, hyperactivity, restlessness, talkativeness, increased pulse, dilated pupils, rhinitis		Hallucinations, convulsions, pulmonary edema, respiratory failure, coma, cardiac arrest, possible death	Cocaine hydrochloride	Coke, flake, snow, dust, happy dust, gold dust, girl, Cecil, C, toot, blow, crack
Synthetic stimulants	Agitation, insomnia, irritability, dizziness, decreased ability to think clearly, increased heart rate, chest pains	Treatment-resistant depression Treatment-resistant post-traumatic stress disorder (PTSD) (MDMA)	Increased heart rate, increased blood pressure, nosebleeds, hallucinations, aggressive behavior	MDMA (3,4 methylenedioxy-methamphetamine, mephedrone, MDPV (3,4-methylene-di oxypyrovalerone), 4-methylmethcathinone (mephedrone, 4-MMC),* Methylone,* Ethylone, Dibutylone, Alpha-PVP	Bath salts, bliss, vanilla sky, ivory wave, purple wave, molly, flakka, gravel

OPIOIDS					
	Euphoria, lethargy, drowsiness, lack of motivation, constricted pupils	As analgesics; antidiarrheals, and antitussives; methadone in medication-assisted treatment; heroin has no therapeutic use	Shallow breathing, slowed pulse, clammy skin, pulmonary edema, respiratory arrest, convulsions, coma, possible death	Heroin Morphine Codeine Dilaudid Demerol Dolophine Percodan Talwin Opium Fentanyl Carfentanyl Sufentanil	Snow, stuff, H, harry, horse M, morph, Miss Emma Schoolboy Lords Doctors Dollies Perkies Ts Big O, black stuff
HALLUCINOGENS					
	Visual hallucinations, disorientation, confusion, paranoid delusions, euphoria, anxiety, panic, increased pulse	LSD has been proposed in the treatment of chronic alcoholism, depression, anxiety, and in the reduction of intractable pain	Agitation, extreme hyperactivity, violence, hallucinations, psychosis, convulsions, possible death	LSD PCP Mescaline DMT STP, DOM MDMA Ketamine MDPV	Acid, cube, big D Angel dust, hog, peace pill Mesc Businessman's trip Serenity and peace Ecstasy, XTC Special K, vitamin K, kit kat Bath salts
CANNABINOIDS					
	Relaxation, talkativeness, lowered inhibitions, euphoria, mood swings	Marijuana has been used for relief of nausea and vomiting associated with antineoplastic chemotherapy and to reduce eye pressure in glaucoma	Fatigue, paranoia, delusions, hallucinations, possible psychosis	Cannabis Hashish	Marijuana, pot, grass, joint, Mary Jane, MJ Hash, rope, sweet Lucy
Synthetic cannabinoids	Highly variable from elevated mood and relaxation to extreme anxiety, confusion, paranoia, hallucinations	Pain management in multiple sclerosis, diabetic neuropathy, nausea and vomiting	Rapid heart rate, vomiting, violent behavior, suicidal thoughts	Many chemical names	Fake weed, K2, Spice (over 500 street names for various chemical formulas)

TABLE 14–8 **Summary of Symptoms Associated With the Syndromes of Intoxication and Withdrawal**

CLASS OF DRUGS	INTOXICATION	WITHDRAWAL	COMMENTS
Alcohol	Aggressiveness, impaired judgment, impaired attention, irritability, euphoria, depression, emotional lability, slurred speech, incoordination, unsteady gait, nystagmus, flushed face	Tremors, nausea/vomiting, malaise, weakness, tachycardia, sweating, elevated blood pressure, anxiety, depressed mood, irritability, hallucinations, headache, insomnia, seizures	Alcohol withdrawal begins within 4–6 hours after last drink. May progress to delirium tremens on 2nd or 3rd day. Use of Librium or Serax is common for medication-assisted treatment.
Amphetamines and related substances	Fighting, grandiosity, hypervigilance, psychomotor agitation, impaired judgment, tachycardia, pupillary dilation, elevated blood pressure, perspiration or chills, nausea and vomiting	Anxiety, depressed mood, irritability, craving for the substance, fatigue, insomnia or hypersomnia, psychomotor agitation, paranoid, and suicidal ideation	Withdrawal symptoms usually peak within 2–4 days, although depression and irritability may persist for months. Antidepressants may be used.
Caffeine	Restlessness, nervousness, excitement, insomnia, flushed face, diuresis, GI complaints, muscle twitching, rambling flow of thought and speech, cardiac arrhythmia, periods of inexhaustibility, psychomotor agitation	Headache	Caffeine is contained in coffee, tea, colas, cocoa, chocolate, some over-the-counter analgesics, "cold" preparations, and stimulants.
Cannabis	Euphoria, anxiety, suspiciousness, sensation of slowed time, impaired judgment, social withdrawal, tachycardia, conjunctival redness, increased appetite, hallucinations	Restlessness, irritability, insomnia, loss of appetite, depressed mood, tremors, fever, chills, headache, stomach pain	Intoxication occurs immediately and lasts about 3 hours. Oral ingestion is more slowly absorbed and has long-lasting effects.
Cocaine	Euphoria, fighting, grandiosity, hypervigilance, psychomotor agitation, impaired judgment, tachycardia, elevated blood pressure, pupillary dilation, perspiration or chills, nausea/vomiting, hallucinations, delirium	Depression, anxiety, irritability, fatigue, insomnia or hypersomnia, psychomotor agitation, paranoid or suicidal ideation, apathy, social withdrawal	Large doses of the drug can result in convulsions or death from cardiac arrhythmias or respiratory paralysis.

Inhalants	Belligerence, assaultiveness, apathy, impaired judgment, dizziness, nystagmus, slurred speech, unsteady gait, lethargy, depressed reflexes, tremor, blurred vision, stupor or coma, euphoria, irritation around eyes, throat, and nose	Restlessness, body aches, nausea, vomiting, runny nose, watery eyes, poor attention and concentration, mood changes, tremors, panic attacks, seizures	Intoxication occurs within 5 minutes of inhalation. Symptoms last 60–90 minutes. Large doses can result in death from CNS depression or cardiac arrhythmia.
Nicotine		Craving for the drug, irritability, anger, frustration, anxiety, difficulty concentrating, restlessness, decreased heart rate, increased appetite, weight gain, tremor, headaches, insomnia	Symptoms of withdrawal begin within 24 hours of last drug use and decrease in intensity over days, weeks, or sometimes longer.
Opioids	Euphoria, lethargy, somnolence, apathy, dysphoria, impaired judgment, pupillary constriction, drowsiness, slurred speech, constipation, nausea, decreased respiratory rate and blood pressure	Craving for the drug, nausea/vomiting, muscle aches, lacrimation or rhinorrhea, pupillary dilation, piloerection or sweating, diarrhea, yawning, fever, insomnia	Withdrawal symptoms appear within 6–8 hours after last dose, reach a peak in the 2nd or 3rd day, and subside in 5–10 days. Times are shorter with meperidine and longer with methadone.
Phencyclidine and related substances	Belligerence, assaultiveness, impulsiveness, psychomotor agitation, impaired judgment, nystagmus, increased heart rate and blood pressure, diminished pain response, ataxia, dysarthria, muscle rigidity, seizures, hyperacusis, delirium	Irritability, anxiety, depression	Delirium can occur within 24 hours after use of phencyclidine or may occur up to a week following recovery from an overdose of the drug.
Sedatives, hypnotics, and anxiolytics	Disinhibition of sexual or aggressive impulses, mood lability, impaired judgment, slurred speech, incoordination, unsteady gait, impairment in attention or memory disorientation, confusion	Nausea/vomiting, malaise, weakness, tachycardia, sweating, anxiety, irritability, orthostatic hypotension, tremor, insomnia, seizures	Withdrawal may progress to delirium, usually within 1 week of last use. Long-acting barbiturates or benzodiazepines may be used in withdrawal medication-assisted treatment.

questions are specific to alcohol, but they could be adapted for any substance:

- What are my drinking patterns?
- If I drink, why do I drink? When, where, and how much?
- If I don't drink, why do I abstain?
- Am I comfortable with my drinking patterns?
- If I decided not to drink any more, would that be a problem for me?
- What did I learn from my parents about drinking?
- Have my attitudes changed as an adult?
- What are my feelings about people who become intoxicated?
- Does it seem more acceptable for some individuals than for others?
- Do I ever use terms like *sot, drunk,* or *boozer* to describe some individuals who overindulge yet overlook it in others?
- Do I ever overindulge?
- Has the use of alcohol (by me or others) affected my life in any way?
- Do I see alcohol/drug misuse (abuse) as a sign of weakness? A moral problem? An illness?

Unless nurses fully understand and accept their own attitudes and feelings, they cannot be empathetic toward patients' problems. Clients in recovery need to know they are accepted for themselves, regardless of past behaviors. Nurses must be able to separate the patient from the behavior and to accept that individual with unconditional positive regard.

Motivational Interviewing

Motivational interviewing is an approach that can be used in the assessment and intervention process for clients with any disorder, although it first gained popularity in treatment of substance use disorders. Its focus is on using skills such as empathy and reflection to explore the client's motivation, strengths, and readiness for change. Some of the previously mentioned questions could easily be reframed to explore the client's attitudes and feelings. Through this process, clients are empowered to become active partners in treatment goals while exploring reasons for any resistance to behavior change. For example, rather than telling clients that they must abstain from alcohol and must attend 12-step meetings, the health-care professional helps clients articulate what they want to achieve and then facilitates the process of exploring advantages and disadvantages of desired behavior change. See Chapter 5, "Relationship Development and Therapeutic Communication," for more discussion of this approach and a sample interview using motivational interviewing.

This is a patient-centered approach that encourages empowerment and active engagement, and as such, it articulates well with two current trends in psychiatric mental health nursing care: recognizing the importance of patient-centered care as an essential nursing competency (Institute of Medicine, 2003) and the recovery model (see Chapter 10, "The Recovery Model," for more discussion of this model).

Assessment Tools

Nurses often perform the admission interview. A variety of assessment tools are appropriate for use in chemical dependency units. A nursing history and assessment tool is presented in Chapter 6, "The Nursing Process in Psychiatric Mental Health Nursing." With some adaptation, it is an appropriate instrument for creating a database on clients who misuse substances. Box 14–1 presents a drug history and assessment that could be used in conjunction with the general biopsychosocial assessment.

The Clinical Institute Withdrawal Assessment of Alcohol Scale, Revised (CIWA-Ar) is an excellent tool that is used by many hospitals to assess risk and severity of withdrawal from alcohol. It may be used for initial assessment as well as ongoing monitoring of alcohol withdrawal symptoms. A copy of the CIWA-Ar is presented in Box 14–2.

Many screening tools exist for determining whether an individual has a problem with substances. SAMHSA recommends an integrated public health approach known as SBIRT to accomplish early intervention and identifying people at risk for substance use disorders. SBIRT is an acronym for Screening, Brief Intervention, Referral, and Treatment. Many screening tools and other resources to accomplish this approach are available on SAMHSA's Web site at https://www.samhsa.gov/sbirt/resources. Some psychiatric units administer these surveys to all admitted clients to help determine whether there is a secondary alcoholism problem in addition to the psychiatric problem for which the client is being admitted (sometimes called **dual diagnosis**). These tools can be adapted for use in diagnosing problems with other drugs as well.

Dual Diagnosis

The NIH (2018) reports that 7.7 million adults with a substance use disorder also have a co-occurring mental illness, which represents 37.9% of all adults with a substance use disorder. If it is determined that a

BOX 14–1 Drug History and Assessment*

1. When you were growing up, did anyone in your family drink alcohol or take other kinds of drugs?
2. If so, how did the substance use affect the family situation?
3. When did you have your first drink/drugs?
4. How long have you been drinking/taking drugs on a regular basis?
5. What is your pattern of substance use?
   a. When do you use substances?
   b. What do you use?
   c. How much do you use?
   d. Where are you and with whom when you use substances?
6. When did you have your last drink/drug? What was it, and how much did you consume?
7. Does using the substance(s) cause problems for you? Describe. Include family, friends, job, school, other.
8. Have you ever experienced injury as a result of substance use?
9. Have you ever been arrested or incarcerated for drinking/using drugs?
10. Have you ever tried to stop drinking/using drugs? If so, what was the result? Did you experience any physical symptoms, such as tremors, headache, insomnia, sweating, or seizures?
11. Have you ever experienced loss of memory for times when you have been drinking/using drugs?
12. Describe a typical day in your life.
13. Are there any changes you would like to make in your life? If so, what are they?
14. What plans or ideas do you have for seeing that these changes occur?

*To be used in conjunction with general biopsychosocial nursing history and assessment tool.

BOX 14–2 Clinical Institute Withdrawal Assessment of Alcohol Scale, Revised (CIWA-Ar)

Patient: _____ **Date:** _____

Time: _____ (24-hour clock, midnight = 00:00)

Pulse or heart rate, taken for one minute: _____ **Blood pressure:** _____

NAUSEA AND VOMITING—Ask "Do you feel sick to your stomach? Have you vomited?" Observation. 0 no nausea and no vomiting 1 mild nausea with no vomiting 2 3 4 intermittent nausea with dry heaves 5 6 7 constant nausea, frequent dry heaves and vomiting	TACTILE DISTURBANCES—Ask "Have you any itching, pins and needles sensations, any burning, any numbness, or do you feel bugs crawling on or under your skin?" Observation. 0 none 1 very mild itching, pins and needles, burning or numbness 2 mild itching, pins and needles, burning or numbness 3 moderate itching, pins and needles, burning or numbness 4 moderately severe hallucinations 5 severe hallucinations 6 extremely severe hallucinations 7 continuous hallucinations
TREMOR—Arms extended and fingers spread apart. Observation. 0 no tremor 1 not visible, but can be felt fingertip to fingertip 2 3 4 moderate, with patient's arms extended 5 6 7 severe, even with arms not extended	AUDITORY DISTURBANCES—Ask "Are you more aware of sounds around you? Are they harsh? Do they frighten you? Are you hearing anything that is disturbing to you? Are you hearing things you know are not there?" Observation. 0 not present 1 very mild harshness or ability to frighten 2 mild harshness or ability to frighten 3 moderate harshness or ability to frighten 4 moderately severe hallucinations 5 severe hallucinations 6 extremely severe hallucinations 7 continuous hallucinations

Continued

BOX 14–2 Clinical Institute Withdrawal Assessment of Alcohol Scale, Revised (CIWA-Ar)—cont'd

PAROXYSMAL SWEATS—Observation. 0 no sweat visible 1 barely perceptible sweating, palms moist 2 3 4 beads of sweat obvious on forehead 5 6 7 drenching sweats	VISUAL DISTURBANCES—Ask "Does the light appear to be too bright? Is its color different? Does it hurt your eyes? Are you seeing anything that is disturbing to you? Are you seeing things you know are not there?" Observation. 0 not present 1 very mild sensitivity 2 mild sensitivity 3 moderate sensitivity 4 moderately severe hallucinations 5 severe hallucinations 6 extremely severe hallucinations 7 continuous hallucinations
ANXIETY—Ask "Do you feel nervous?" Observation. 0 no anxiety, at ease 1 mildly anxious 2 3 4 moderately anxious, or guarded, so anxiety is inferred 5 6 7 equivalent to acute panic states as seen in severe delirium or acute schizophrenic reactions	HEADACHE, FULLNESS IN HEAD—Ask "Does your head feel different? Does it feel like there is a band around your head?" Do not rate for dizziness or lightheadedness. Otherwise, rate severity. 0 not present 1 very mild 2 mild 3 moderate 4 moderately severe 5 severe 6 very severe 7 extremely severe
AGITATION—Observation. 0 normal activity 1 somewhat more than normal activity 2 3 4 moderately fidgety and restless 5 6 7 paces back and forth during most of the interview, or constantly thrashes about	ORIENTATION AND CLOUDING OF SENSORIUM—Ask "What day is this? Where are you? Who am I?" 0 oriented and can do serial additions 1 cannot do serial additions or is uncertain about date 2 disoriented for date by no more than 2 calendar days 3 disoriented for date by more than 2 calendar days 4 disoriented for place/or person
	Total CIWA-Ar Score _____ Rater's Initials _____ Maximum Possible Score 67
The CIWA-Ar is not copyrighted and may be reproduced freely. This assessment for monitoring withdrawal symptoms requires approximately 5 minutes to administer. The maximum score is 67 (see instrument). Patients scoring less than 10 do not usually need additional medication for withdrawal.	

Source: Sullivan et al. (1989).

client has a coexisting substance disorder and mental illness, the client may be assigned to a specialized program that targets both disorders. Most dual diagnosis programs take a more supportive and less confrontational approach.

Peer support groups, psychodynamic therapy to explore how psychiatric disorders and substance abuse have reinforced one another and how the cycle can be broken, and cognitive and behavioral therapies may be included in treatment. Teaching patients about coping skills and stress management offers skills that promote abstinence and dealing with substance cravings. (See Chapter 21, "Eating Disorders," for Vic's discussion of his dual diagnosis, alcohol use disorder and anorexia nervosa, in "Real People, Real Stories.")

A dually diagnosed individual in a psychiatric facility or day treatment program may attend a chemical dependency group periodically in lieu of another scheduled activity therapy. Topics are directed toward areas that are unique to clients with a mental illness, such as mixing medications with other substances, as well as topics that are common to primary substance use disorders.

Continued attendance at 12-step group meetings is encouraged on discharge from treatment. Family involvement is enlisted, and preventive strategies are outlined. Individual case management is common, and success is often promoted by this close supervision.

Diagnosis and Outcome Identification

The next step in the nursing process is to identify appropriate nursing diagnoses by analyzing the data collected during the assessment phase. The individual who misuses or is dependent on substances undoubtedly has many unmet physical and emotional needs. Table 14–9 presents a list of patient behaviors and the NANDA-I nursing diagnoses (Herdman et al., 2021) that correspond to those behaviors, which may be used in planning care for the patient with a substance use disorder.

TABLE 14–9 Assigning Nursing Diagnoses to Behaviors Commonly Associated With Substance Use Disorders

BEHAVIORS	NURSING DIAGNOSES
Makes statements such as, "I don't have a problem with [substance]. I can quit any time I want to." Delays seeking assistance; does not perceive problems related to use of substances; minimizes use of substances; unable to admit impact of disease on life pattern	Denial
Misuse of chemical agents; destructive behavior toward others and self; inability to meet basic needs; inability to meet role expectations; risk taking	Ineffective coping
Loss of weight, pale conjunctiva and mucous membranes, decreased skin turgor, electrolyte imbalance, anemia, drinks alcohol or takes drugs instead of eating	Imbalanced nutrition: Less than body requirements Deficient fluid volume
Risk factors: malnutrition, altered immune system, failing to avoid exposure to pathogens	Risk for infection
Criticizes self and others, self-destructive behavior (use of substances as a coping mechanism), family conflicts	Chronic low self-esteem
Denies that substance is harmful; continues to use substance in light of obvious consequences	Deficient knowledge
FOR PATIENT WITHDRAWING FROM CNS DEPRESSANTS	
Risk factors: CNS agitation (tremors, elevated blood pressure, nausea and vomiting, hallucinations, illusions, tachycardia, anxiety, seizures)	Risk for injury/Risk for or Acute substance withdrawal syndrome
FOR PATIENT WITHDRAWING FROM CNS STIMULANTS	
Risk factors: intense feelings of lassitude and depression; "crashing," suicidal ideation	Risk for suicide/Risk for or Acute substance withdrawal syndrome

Outcome Criteria

The following criteria may be used for measurement of outcomes in the care of the patient with substance-related disorders. The patient:

- Has not experienced physical injury.
- Has not caused harm to self or others.
- Accepts responsibility for own behavior.
- Acknowledges association between personal problems and use of substance(s).
- Demonstrates adaptive coping mechanisms that can be used in stressful situations (instead of taking substances).
- Shows no signs or symptoms of infection or malnutrition.
- Exhibits evidence of increased self-worth by attempting new projects without fear of failure and by demonstrating less defensive behavior toward others.
- Verbalizes importance of abstaining from use of substances in order to maintain optimal wellness.

Planning and Implementation

Implementation of care with patients who misuse substances is a long-term process, often beginning with **detoxification** and progressing to total abstinence. The following are common priority interventions for each phase of this process.

Detoxification

- Provide a safe and supportive environment for detoxification.
- Administer medication-assisted treatment (see section on "Treatment Modalities for Substance-Related Disorders" for definition and discussion) as ordered.

Intermediate Care

- Provide explanations of physical symptoms.
- Promote understanding and identify the causes of substance dependency.
- Provide education and assistance in course of treatment to patient and family.

Rehabilitation

- Encourage continued participation in long-term treatment.
- Promote participation in outpatient support system (e.g., Alcoholics Anonymous [AA]).
- Assist patient to identify alternative sources of satisfaction.
- Provide support for health promotion and maintenance.

Table 14–10 provides a plan of care for the patient with substance-related disorders. Selected nursing diagnoses are presented, along with outcome criteria, appropriate nursing interventions, and rationales for each.

Text continued on page 342

Table 14–10 | CARE PLAN FOR THE PATIENT WITH A SUBSTANCE-RELATED DISORDER

NURSING DIAGNOSIS: RISK FOR INJURY

RELATED TO: Central nervous system (CNS) agitation secondary to intoxication or withdrawal from alcohol or other CNS depressant

OUTCOME CRITERIA	NURSING INTERVENTIONS	RATIONALE
Short-Term Goal ■ Patient's condition will stabilize within 72 hours. **Long-Term Goal** ■ Patient will not experience physical injury.	1. Assess patient's level of disorientation.	1. Determination of specific requirements for safety must be made.
	2. Obtain a drug history, if possible. It is important to determine the type of substance(s) used, the time and amount of last use, the length and frequency of use, and the amount used on a daily basis.	2. This information is essential to know what to expect during the withdrawal process and to establish an appropriate plan of care.
	3. Obtain a urine sample for laboratory analysis of substance content.	3. A subjective history is often not accurate.
	4. Keep the patient in as quiet an environment as possible. A private room is ideal.	4. Excessive stimuli may increase patient agitation.

Table 14–10 | CARE PLAN FOR THE PATIENT WITH A SUBSTANCE-RELATED DISORDER—cont'd

	5. Observe the patient's behaviors frequently. If seriousness of the condition warrants, it may be necessary to assign a staff person on a one-to-one basis.	5. Patient safety is a nursing priority.
	6. Accompany and assist the patient when ambulating and use a wheelchair for transporting the patient long distances.	6. In weakened condition, patient will require assistance to prevent falls.
	7. Pad the headboard and side rails of the bed with thick towels.	7. Individuals in withdrawal from CNS depressants are at risk for seizures. Padding will offer protection from injury should a seizure occur.
	8. Ensure that smoking materials and other potentially harmful objects are stored away from the patient's access. Institute suicide precautions, if necessary, for patients withdrawing from CNS stimulants.	8. A patient in withdrawal has impaired judgment. The environment must be made safe for the patient.
	9. Monitor the patient's vital signs every 15 minutes, and less frequently as acute symptoms subside.	9. Accurate assessment is vital for the provision of safe and effective nursing care.
	10. Follow the medication regimen as ordered by the physician.	10. Medication-assisted treatment will be prescribed to ease the symptoms of withdrawal from substances. (See section on "Medication-Assisted Treatment.")

NURSING DIAGNOSIS: DENIAL

RELATED TO: Lack of coping skills to manage anxiety

EVIDENCED BY: Statements denying a problem with substance use in the presence of objective evidence to the contrary.

OUTCOME CRITERIA	NURSING INTERVENTIONS	RATIONALE
Short-Term Goal ■ Patient will focus on behavioral outcomes associated with substance use rather than using deflection to focus on external issues.	1. Begin by working to develop a trusting nurse-patient relationship. Be honest. Keep all promises.	1. Trust is the basis of a therapeutic relationship.
	2. Convey an attitude of acceptance. Ensure that the patient understands "It is not *you* but your *behavior* that is unacceptable."	2. An attitude of acceptance promotes feelings of dignity and self-worth.

Continued

Table 14–10 | CARE PLAN FOR THE PATIENT WITH A SUBSTANCE-RELATED DISORDER—cont'd

OUTCOME CRITERIA	NURSING INTERVENTIONS	RATIONALE
Long-Term Goal ■ Patient will verbalize acceptance of responsibility for own behavior and acknowledge association between substance use and personal problems.	3. Provide information to correct misconceptions about substance misuse.	3. Many myths abound regarding use of specific substances. In addition, the patient may rationalize their behavior with statements such as, "I'm not an alcoholic. I can stop drinking any time I want. Besides, I only drink beer." Or "I only smoke pot to relax before class. So what? I know lots of people who do. Besides, you can't get hooked on pot." Factual information presented in a matter-of-fact, nonjudgmental way explaining what behaviors constitute substance-related disorders may help the patient focus on their own behaviors as an illness that requires help.
	4. Identify recent maladaptive behaviors or situations that have occurred in the patient's life and discuss how use of substances may have been a contributing factor.	4. The first step in decreasing use of denial is for the patient to see the relationship between substance use and personal problems.
	5. Use confrontation with caring. Do not allow patient to fantasize about their lifestyle (e.g., "It is my understanding that the last time you drank alcohol, you . . ." or "The laboratory report shows that you were under the influence of alcohol when you had the accident that injured three people").	5. Confrontation interferes with patient's ability to use denial; a caring attitude preserves self-esteem and avoids putting the patient on the defensive.
	6. Do not accept rationalization or projection as patient attempts to make excuses for or blame their behavior on other people or situations.	6. Rationalization and projection prolong denial that problems exist in the patient's life because of substance use.
	7. Encourage participation in group activities.	7. Peer feedback is often more accepted than feedback from authority figures. Peer pressure can be a strong factor, as well as association with individuals who are experiencing or who have experienced similar problems.
	8. Offer immediate positive recognition of the patient's expressions of insight gained regarding illness and acceptance of responsibility for their own behavior.	8. Positive reinforcement enhances self-esteem and encourages repetition of desirable behaviors.
	9. Employ motivational interviewing techniques to begin an exploration of the patient's motivations and readiness for change.	9. Using a patient-centered approach that includes techniques such as reflection, open-ended questions, clarification, and validation encourages the patient to actively engage in problem-solving.

Table 14–10 | CARE PLAN FOR THE PATIENT WITH A SUBSTANCE-RELATED DISORDER—cont'd

NURSING DIAGNOSIS: INEFFECTIVE COPING

RELATED TO: Inadequate coping skills

EVIDENCED BY: Use of substances as coping mechanism; manipulative behavior

OUTCOME CRITERIA	NURSING INTERVENTIONS	RATIONALE
Short-Term Goal ■ Patient will express true feelings about using substances as a method of coping with stress. **Long-Term Goal** ■ Patient will be able to verbalize adaptive coping mechanisms to use, instead of substance misuse, in response to stress (and demonstrate, as applicable).	1. Spend time with the patient to establish a trusting relationship.	1. Establishing trust is the foundation for therapeutic intervention and relationship development.
	2. Set limits on manipulative behavior. Be sure that the patient knows what is acceptable, what is not, and the consequences for violating the limits set. Ensure that all staff maintains consistency with this intervention.	2. The patient is unable to establish their own limits, so limits must be set for them. Unless administration of consequences for violation of limits is consistent, manipulative behavior will not be eliminated.
	3. Encourage the patient to verbalize feelings, fears, and anxieties. Answer any questions the patient may have regarding the disorder.	3. Verbalization of feelings in a nonthreatening environment may help the patient come to terms with long-unresolved issues.
	4. Explain the effects of substance misuse on the body. Emphasize that the prognosis is closely related to abstinence.	4. Many patients lack knowledge regarding the deleterious effects of substance misuse on the body.
	5. Explore options available to assist with stressful situations rather than resorting to substance misuse (e.g., contacting various members of Alcoholics Anonymous or Narcotics Anonymous; physical exercise; relaxation techniques; meditation).	5. The patient may have persistently resorted to chemical misuse and thus may possess little or no knowledge of adaptive responses to stress.
	6. Provide positive reinforcement for evidence of gratification delayed appropriately. Encourage the patient to be as independent as possible in performing their self-care. Provide positive feedback for independent decision making and effective use of problem-solving skills.	6. Positive reinforcement increases self-esteem and encourages repetition of adaptive behaviors.

Continued

Table 14–10 | CARE PLAN FOR THE PATIENT WITH A SUBSTANCE-RELATED DISORDER—cont'd

NURSING DIAGNOSIS: IMBALANCED NUTRITION: LESS THAN BODY REQUIREMENTS/DEFICIENT FLUID VOLUME

RELATED TO: Use of substances instead of eating

EVIDENCED BY: Loss of weight, pale conjunctiva and mucous membranes, poor skin turgor, electrolyte imbalance, anemias (and/or other signs and symptoms of malnutrition/dehydration)

OUTCOME CRITERIA	NURSING INTERVENTIONS	RATIONALE
Short-Term Goal ■ Abnormal laboratory values will be restored to normal. ■ Patient will gain weight on a regular, nutritious diet. **Long-Term Goal** ■ Patient will be free of signs/symptoms of malnutrition/dehydration.	1. Parenteral support may be required initially.	1. To correct fluid and electrolyte imbalance, hypoglycemia, and some vitamin deficiencies.
	2. Encourage cessation of smoking.	2. To facilitate repair of damage to GI tract.
	3. Consult dietitian. Determine the number of calories required based on body size and level of activity. Document intake and output and calorie count, and weigh patient daily.	3. These interventions are necessary to maintain an ongoing nutritional assessment.
	4. Ensure that the amount of protein in the diet is correct for the individual patient's condition. Protein intake should be adequate to maintain nitrogen equilibrium but should be drastically decreased or eliminated if there is potential for hepatic coma.	4. Diseased liver may be incapable of properly metabolizing proteins, resulting in an accumulation of ammonia in the blood that circulates to the brain and can result in altered consciousness.
	5. Sodium may need to be restricted.	5. To minimize fluid retention (e.g., ascites and edema).
	6. Provide foods that are nonirritating to patients with esophageal varices.	6. To avoid irritation and bleeding of these swollen blood vessels.
	7. Provide small frequent feeding of patient's favorite foods. Supplement nutritious meals with multiple vitamin and mineral tablet.	7. To encourage intake and facilitate patient's achievement of adequate nutrition and correct vitamin deficiencies

Concept Care Mapping

The concept map care plan (see Chapter 6) is a diagrammatic teaching and learning strategy that allows visualization of interrelationships between medical diagnoses, nursing diagnoses, assessment data, and treatments. An example of a concept map care plan for a patient with a substance use disorder is presented in Figure 14–3.

Patient and Family Education

The role of patient-teacher is important in all areas of nursing. In caring for the patient with a substance use disorder, educating family members about common dysfunctional family processes, such as enabling and codependency are core components of treatment. Referral to support groups designed for family members, such as Al-Anon or Co-Dependents Anonymous, may provide longer term support. A list of topics for patient and family education relevant to substance-related disorders is presented in Box 14–3.

Evaluation

The final step of the nursing process involves reassessment to determine whether the nursing interventions have been effective in achieving the intended

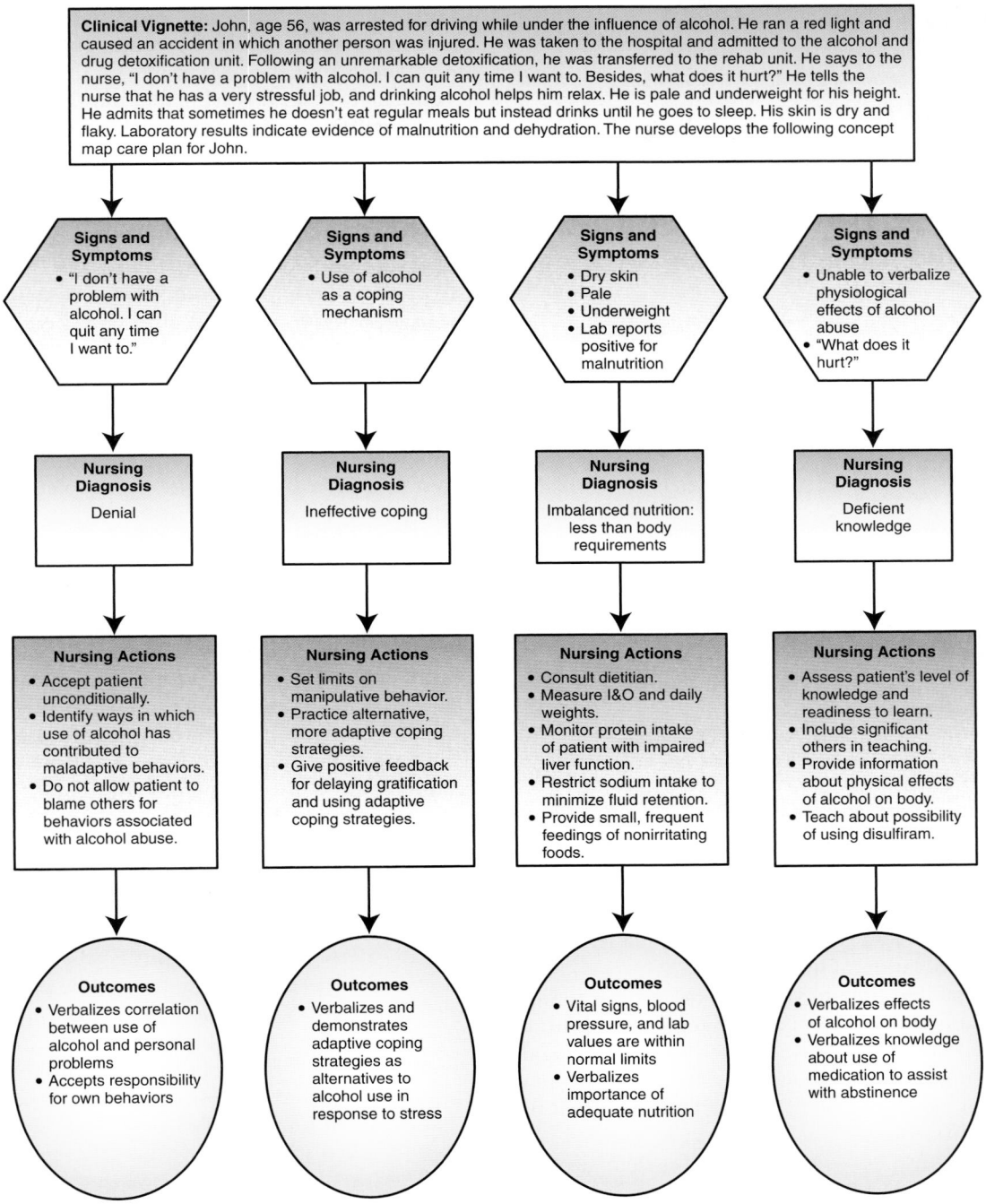

FIGURE 14–3 Concept map care plan for patient with alcoholism.

goals of care. Evaluation of the patient with a substance-related disorder may be accomplished by using information gathered from the following reassessment questions:

- Has detoxification occurred without complications?
- Is the patient no longer in denial?
- Does the patient accept responsibility for their own behavior? Has the patient acknowledged a personal problem with substances?
- Has a correlation been made between personal problems and the use of substances?
- Has the patient remained substance free during treatment?

BOX 14–3 Topics for Patient and Family Education Related to Substance Use Disorders

NATURE OF THE ILLNESS

1. Effects of (substance) on the body
   a. Alcohol
   b. Other CNS depressants
   c. CNS stimulants
   d. Hallucinogens
   e. Inhalants
   f. Opioids
   g. Cannabinols
2. Ways in which use of (substance) affects life.

MANAGEMENT OF THE ILLNESS

1. Activities to substitute for (substance) in times of stress
2. Relaxation techniques
   a. Progressive relaxation
   b. Tense and relax
   c. Deep breathing
   d. Autogenics
3. Problem-solving skills
4. The essentials of good nutrition
5. Medication-assisted treatment
6. Dysfunctional family dynamics

SUPPORT SERVICES

1. Financial assistance
2. Legal assistance
3. Alcoholics Anonymous, Al-Anon, Co-Dependents Anonymous (or other support group specific to another substance)
4. One-to-one support person

- Does the patient cooperate with treatment?
- Does the patient refrain from manipulative behavior and violation of limits?
- Is the patient able to verbalize motivation toward alternative adaptive coping strategies to substitute for substance use? Has the use of these strategies been demonstrated? Does positive reinforcement encourage repetition of these adaptive behaviors?
- Has nutritional status been restored? Does the patient consume a diet adequate for their size and level of activity? Is the patient able to discuss the importance of adequate nutrition?
- Has the patient remained free of infection during hospitalization?
- Is the patient able to verbalize the effects of substance misuse on the body?

The Chemically Impaired Nurse

Substance abuse and addiction are problems that have the potential for impairment in an individual's social, occupational, psychological, and physical functioning. They become especially serious problems when the impaired person is responsible for the lives of others on a daily basis. It is estimated that 10% of nurses have substance use disorders, which is the same as the prevalence in the general public (Worley, 2017). Alcohol is the most widely misused drug, followed closely by narcotics. Nurses who misuse substances have an added vulnerability because they often handle controlled substances when providing patient care.

For years, the impaired nurse was protected, promoted, transferred, ignored, or fired. These types of responses promoted the growth of the problem. Programs are needed that involve early reporting and treatment of chemical addiction as a disease with a focus on public safety and rehabilitation of the nurse.

How does one identify the impaired nurse? It is still easiest to overlook what *might* be a problem. Denial, on the part of the impaired nurse as well as nurse colleagues, is still the strongest reason for not dealing with a substance use disorder. Some states have mandatory reporting laws that require observers to report nurses to the state board of nursing when there is suspicion of substance misuse or impairment. They are difficult laws to enforce, and hospitals are not always compliant with mandatory reporting. Some hospitals may choose not to report to the state board of nursing if the impaired nurse is actively seeking treatment and is not placing patients in danger.

A number of clues for recognizing substance impairment in nurses have been identified (Ellis & Hartley, 2012). Signs of substance impairment are not easy to detect, and they vary according to the substance being used. There may be high absenteeism if the person's source is outside the work area, or the individual may rarely miss work if the substance source is at work. There may be an increase in "wasting" of drugs, increased incidences of incorrect narcotic counts, and a higher record of signing out drugs than for other nurses.

Poor concentration, difficulty meeting deadlines, inappropriate responses, and poor memory or recall usually occur late in the disease process. The person may also have problems with relationships. Some other possible signs are irritability, mood swings, tendency to isolate, elaborate excuses for behavior, unkempt appearance, impaired motor coordination, slurred speech, flushed face, inconsistent job performance, and frequent use of the restroom. Impaired nurses may frequently medicate other nurses' patients, and there may be patient complaints of inadequate pain control. Discrepancies in documentation may occur. Ideally, suspicious behavior has been recognized by peers and intervention sought before the impaired nurse reaches late stages of the disease process. As uncomfortable as it may seem to tell a supervisor about suspected impairment in a peer, it is in the interest of the nurse's health and most critically important to ensuring patient safety.

If suspicious behavior occurs, it is important to keep careful, objective records. Confrontation with the impaired nurse will undoubtedly result in hostility and denial. Confrontation should not occur solely between peers but rather should involve a supervisor or other nurse manager and should include the offer of assistance in seeking treatment. If a report is made to the state board of nursing, it should be a factual documentation of specific events and actions, not a diagnostic statement of impairment.

State boards generally decide each case on an individual basis. A state board may deny, suspend, or revoke a license when there is evidence of substance misuse or addiction by a nurse. Several state boards of nursing have passed diversionary laws that allow impaired nurses to avoid disciplinary action by agreeing to seek treatment. Some of these state boards administer the treatment programs themselves, and others refer the nurse to community resources or state nurses' association assistance programs. Treatment may entail successful completion of inpatient, outpatient, group, or individual counseling treatment program(s); evidence of regular attendance at nurse support groups or a 12-step program; random negative drug screens; and employment or volunteer activities during the suspension period. When a nurse is deemed safe to return to practice, the nurse may be closely monitored for several years and required to undergo random drug screenings. The nurse also may be required to practice under specifically circumscribed conditions for a designated period.

In 1982, the American Nurses Association (ANA) House of Delegates adopted a national resolution to provide assistance to impaired nurses. Since that time, the majority of state nurses' associations have developed (or are developing) programs for nurses who are impaired by substances or psychiatric illness. The individuals who administer these efforts are nurse members of the state associations as well as nurses who are in recovery themselves. For this reason, they are called **peer assistance programs.**

Peer assistance programs strive to intervene early, reduce hazards to patients, and increase prospects for the nurse's recovery. Most states provide either a hot-line number that the impaired nurse or intervening colleague may call or phone numbers of peer assistance committee members, which are made available for the same purpose. Typically, a contract is drawn up detailing the method of treatment, which may be obtained from various sources, such as employee assistance programs, Alcoholics Anonymous, Narcotics Anonymous, private counseling, or outpatient clinics. Guidelines for monitoring the course of treatment are established. Peer support is provided through regular contact with the impaired nurse, usually for a period of 2 years. Peer assistance programs serve to assist impaired nurses to recognize their impairment, to obtain necessary treatment, and to regain accountability within their profession.

Codependency

The concept of **codependency** arose out of a need to define the dysfunctional behaviors that are evident among members of the family of a chemically addicted person. The term has been expanded to include all individuals from families who harbor secrets of physical or emotional abuse, other cruelties, or pathological conditions. Living under these conditions results in unmet needs for autonomy and self-esteem and a profound sense of powerlessness. The codependent person is able to achieve a sense of control only through fulfilling the needs of others. Personal identity is relinquished, and boundaries with the other person become blurred. The codependent person disowns their own needs and wants in order to respond to external demands and the demands of others. Codependence has been called "a dysfunctional relationship with oneself."

The traits associated with a codependent personality are varied. In a relationship, the codependent person derives self-worth from that of the partner, whose feelings and behaviors determine how the codependent should feel and behave. In order for codependents to feel good, their partner must be happy and behave in appropriate ways. If partners are not happy, codependents feels responsible for *making* their partners happy. The codependent's home life is fraught with stress. Ego boundaries are weak, and behaviors are often enmeshed with those of the pathological partner. Denial that problems exist is common. Feelings are kept in control, and anxiety may be released in the form of stress-related illnesses or compulsive behaviors such as eating, spending, working, or use of substances.

Selected characteristics of the codependent individual (Beatty, 2011) include:

- Taking care of others at the expense of one's own needs
- Feeling responsible for fixing other people's problems

- Having low self-esteem; expecting to perform perfectly but never feeling "good enough"
- Desperately seeking approval from others; often identified as "people pleasers"
- Generally unhappy and seeking things outside oneself to attempt to fulfil unmet needs
- Tending to have come from dysfunctional families where there was abuse or neglect
- Having weak boundaries that lead to feelings of resentment, lack of trust, and anger toward others

The Codependent Nurse

Certain characteristics of codependence have been associated with the profession of nursing. A shortage of nurses combined with the increasing ranks of seriously ill patients may result in nurses providing care and fulfilling everyone's needs but their own. Many health-care workers who are reared in homes with a chemically addicted person or otherwise dysfunctional family are at risk for having unresolved codependent tendencies activated. Nurses who as children assumed the "fixer" role in their dysfunctional families of origin may attempt to resume that role in their caregiving professions. They are attracted to a profession in which they are needed, but they nurture feelings of resentment for receiving so little in return. Their emotional needs go unmet; however, they continue to deny that these needs exist. Instead, these unmet emotional needs may be manifested through use of compulsive behaviors, such as working or spending excessively, or addictions, such as to food or substances.

Codependent nurses have a need to be in control. They often strive for an unrealistic level of achievement. Their self-worth comes from the feeling of being needed by others and of maintaining control over their environment. They nurture the dependence of others and accept the responsibility for the happiness and contentment of others. They rarely express their true feelings, and they do what is necessary to preserve harmony and maintain control. They are at high risk for physical and emotional burnout.

Treating Codependency

Cermak (1986) identified four stages in the recovery process for individuals with codependent personality:

- ***Stage I: The survival stage:*** In this first stage, codependent persons must begin to let go of the denial that problems exist or that their personal capabilities are unlimited. This initiation of abstinence from blanket denial may be a very emotional and painful period.
- ***Stage II: The reidentification stage:*** Reidentification occurs when the individuals are able to glimpse their true selves through a break in the denial system. They accept the label of codependent and take responsibility for their own dysfunctional behavior. Codependents tend to enter reidentification only after being convinced that it is more painful not to. They accept their limitations and are ready to face the issues of codependence.
- ***Stage III: The core issues stage:*** In this stage, the recovering codependent must face the fact that relationships cannot be managed by force of will. Each partner must be independent and autonomous. The goal of this stage is to detach from the struggles of life that exist because of prideful and willful efforts to control those things that are beyond the individual's power to control.
- ***Stage IV: The reintegration stage:*** This is a stage of self-acceptance and willingness to change when codependents relinquish the power *over others* that was not rightfully theirs but reclaim the *personal* power that they do possess. Integrity is achieved out of awareness, honesty, and being in touch with one's spiritual consciousness. Control is achieved through self-discipline and self-confidence.

Self-help groups have been found to be helpful in the treatment of codependency. Groups developed for families of chemically addicted people, such as Al-Anon, may be of assistance. Groups specific to the problem of codependency also exist. One of these groups, which bases its philosophy on the Twelve Steps of Alcoholics Anonymous (see the section that follows) is:

Co-Dependents Anonymous (CoDA)
P.O. Box 33577
Phoenix, AZ 85067-3577P: (602) 277-7991
(888) 444-2359 (Toll free)
(888) 444-2379 (Spanish toll free)
www.coda.org

Treatment Modalities

Self-Help Groups: Alcoholics Anonymous

Alcoholics Anonymous (AA) is a major self-help organization for the treatment of alcoholism. It was founded in 1935 by two alcoholics—a stockbroker, Bill Wilson, and a physician, Dr. Bob Smith—who discovered that they could remain sober through mutual support. They accomplished sobriety not as professionals but as peers who were able to share their common experiences. Soon they were working with other alcoholics, who in turn worked with others. The movement grew, and, remarkably, individuals who had been treated unsuccessfully by professionals were able to maintain sobriety through helping one another.

Today AA chapters exist in virtually every community in the United States. The self-help groups are based on the concept of peer support—acceptance and understanding from others who have experienced the same problems in their lives. The only requirement for membership is a desire on the part of the alcoholic person to stop drinking. Each new member is assigned a support person from whom they may seek assistance when the temptation to drink occurs.

A survey by the General Service Office of Alcoholics Anonymous in 2014 (Alcoholics Anonymous, 2021) revealed the following statistics: Members ages 30 and younger composed 12% of the membership, and the average age of AA members was 50; women composed 38%; 89% were white, 4% were black, 3% were Hispanic, 1% were American Indian/Alaska Native, and 3% were Asian American and other minorities. Almost one-half (49%) of people involved in AA were referred by a health-care professional or treatment facility. The sole purpose of AA is to help members stay sober. When sobriety has been achieved, members in turn are expected to help other alcoholic persons. The Twelve Steps that embody the philosophy of AA provide specific guidelines on how to attain and maintain sobriety (Box 14–4).

AA accepts alcoholism as an illness and promotes total abstinence as the only cure, emphasizing that the alcoholic person can never safely return to social drinking. They encourage the members to seek sobriety, taking one day at a time. The Twelve Traditions are the statements of principles that govern the organization.

AA has been the model for various other self-help groups associated with addiction problems. Some of these groups and the memberships for which they are organized are listed in Table 14–11. Nurses need to be fully and accurately informed about available self-help groups and their importance as a treatment resource on the health-care continuum so they can be used as a referral source for patients with substance use disorders.

Pharmacotherapy

Disulfiram (Antabuse): Deterrent Therapy

Disulfiram (Antabuse) is a drug that can be administered as a deterrent to drinking to individuals who misuse alcohol. Ingestion of alcohol while disulfiram is in the body results in a syndrome of symptoms that can produce a great deal of discomfort for the individual. It can even result in death if the blood alcohol level is high. The reaction varies according to the sensitivity of the individual and how much alcohol was ingested.

Disulfiram works by inhibiting the enzyme aldehyde dehydrogenase, thereby blocking the oxidation of alcohol at the stage when acetaldehyde is converted to acetate. This results in an accumulation of acetaldehyde in the blood, which is thought to produce the symptoms associated with the disulfiram-alcohol reaction. These symptoms persist as long as alcohol is being metabolized. The rate of alcohol elimination does not appear to be affected.

Symptoms of disulfiram-alcohol reaction can occur within 5 to 10 minutes of ingestion of alcohol. Mild reactions can occur at blood alcohol levels as low as 5 to 10 mg/dL. Symptoms are fully developed at approximately 50 mg/dL and may include flushed skin, throbbing in the head and neck, respiratory difficulty, dizziness, nausea and vomiting, sweating, hyperventilation, tachycardia, hypotension, weakness, blurred vision, and confusion. With a blood alcohol level of approximately 125 to 150 mg/dL, severe reactions can occur, including respiratory depression, cardiovascular collapse, arrhythmias, myocardial infarction, acute congestive heart failure, unconsciousness, convulsions, and death.

Disulfiram should not be administered until it has been ascertained that the client has abstained from alcohol for at least 12 hours. If disulfiram is discontinued, it is important for the client to understand that the sensitivity to alcohol may last for as long as 2 weeks. Consuming alcohol or alcohol-containing substances during this 2-week period could result in the disulfiram- alcohol reaction.

Clients receiving disulfiram therapy should be aware of the large number of alcohol-containing substances. These products, such as liquid cough and cold preparations, vanilla extract, aftershave lotions, colognes, mouthwash, nail polish removers, and isopropyl alcohol, if ingested or even rubbed on the skin, are capable of producing the symptoms described. Individuals must read labels carefully and must inform any doctor, dentist, or other health-care professional from whom assistance is sought that they are taking disulfiram. In addition, it is important that clients carry a card explaining participation in disulfiram therapy, possible consequences of the therapy, and symptoms that may indicate an emergency situation.

The client must be assessed carefully before beginning disulfiram therapy. A thorough medical

BOX 14–4 Alcoholics Anonymous

The Twelve Steps

1. We admitted we were powerless over alcohol—that our lives have become unmanageable.
2. Came to believe that a Power greater than ourselves could restore us to sanity.
3. Made a decision to turn our will and our lives over to the care of God as we understood Him.
4. Made a searching and fearless moral inventory of ourselves.
5. Admitted to God, to ourselves, and to another human being the exact nature of our wrongs.
6. Were entirely ready to have God remove all these defects of character.
7. Humbly asked Him to remove our shortcomings.
8. Made a list of all persons we had harmed and became willing to make amends to them all.
9. Made direct amends to such people wherever possible except when to do so would injure them or others.
10. Continued to take personal inventory and when we were wrong promptly admitted it.
11. Sought through prayer and meditation to improve our conscious contact with God as we understood Him, praying only for knowledge of His will for us and the power to carry that out.
12. Having had a spiritual awakening as the result of these steps, we tried to carry this message to alcoholics and to practice these principles in all our affairs.

The Twelve Traditions

1. Our common welfare should come first; personal recovery depends upon AA unity.
2. For our group purpose there is but one ultimate authority—a loving God as He may express Himself in our group conscience. Our leaders are but trusted servants; they do not govern.
3. The one requirement for AA membership is a desire to stop drinking.
4. Each group should be autonomous except in matters affecting other groups or AA as a whole.
5. Each group has but one primary purpose—to carry its message to the alcoholic who still suffers.
6. An AA group ought never endorse, finance, or lend the AA name to any related facility or outside enterprise, lest problems of money, property, and prestige divert us from our primary purpose.
7. Every AA group ought to be fully self-supporting, declining outside contributions.
8. Alcoholics Anonymous should remain forever nonprofessional, but our service centers may employ special workers.
9. Alcoholics Anonymous, as such, ought never be organized; but we may create service boards of committees directly responsible to those they serve.
10. Alcoholics Anonymous has no opinion on outside issues; hence, the Alcoholics Anonymous name ought never be drawn into public controversy.
11. Our public relations policy is based on attraction rather than promotion; we need always maintain personal anonymity at the level of press, radio, and films.
12. Anonymity is the spiritual foundation of all our traditions, ever reminding us to place principles before personalities.

Source: The Twelve Steps and Twelve Traditions are reprinted with permission of Alcoholics Anonymous World Services, Inc. (AAWS). Permission to reprint the Twelve Steps and Twelve Traditions does not mean that AAWS has reviewed or approved the contents of this publication, or that AA necessarily agrees with the views expressed herein. AA is a program of recovery from alcoholism only. Use of the Twelve Steps and Twelve Traditions in connection with programs and activities which are patterned after AA, but which address other problems, or in any other non-AA context, does not imply otherwise.

screening is performed before starting therapy, and written informed consent is usually required. The drug is contraindicated for clients who are at high risk for alcohol ingestion. It is also contraindicated for psychotic clients and clients with severe cardiac, renal, or hepatic disease.

Disulfiram therapy is not a cure for alcoholism. It provides a measure of control for the individual who desires to avoid impulse drinking. Clients receiving disulfiram therapy are encouraged to seek other assistance with their problem, such as AA or other support group, to aid in the recovery process.

Vitamin Replacement in Alcohol Use Disorder

Multivitamin therapy in combination with daily injections or oral administration of thiamine is common protocol. Thiamine is commonly deficient in chronic alcoholics. Replacement therapy is required to prevent neuropathy, confusion, and encephalopathy.

Medication-Assisted Treatment

Various medications have been used to decrease the intensity of symptoms in an individual who is withdrawing from, or who is experiencing the effects of excessive use of, alcohol and other drugs and

TABLE 14–11 Addiction Self-Help Groups

GROUP	MEMBERSHIP
Adult Children of Alcoholics (ACOA)	Adults who grew up with an alcoholic in the home
Al-Anon	Families of alcoholics
Alateen	Adolescent children of alcoholics
Children Are People	School-age children with an alcoholic family member
Cocaine Anonymous	Individuals with cocaine addiction
Co-Dependents Anonymous (CoDA)	Families of alcohol or other substance misusers
Families Anonymous	Parents of children who misuse substances
Fresh Start	Individuals with nicotine addiction
Gamblers Anonymous	Individuals with gambling addiction
Narcotics Anonymous	Individuals with narcotics addiction
Nar-Anon	Families of individuals with narcotics addiction
Overeaters Anonymous	Individuals with food addiction
Pills Anonymous	Individuals with polysubstance addictions
Pot Smokers Anonymous	Individuals with marijuana addiction
SMART (Self-Management And Recovery Training) and CRAFT (Community Reinforcement and Family Training) group meetings	Individuals, family, and friends with many types of addictions, e.g., alcohol, eating disorders, marijuana, gambling, prescription drugs, heroin, sex addiction, smoking
Smokers Anonymous	Individuals with nicotine addiction
Women for Sobriety	Women with alcohol addictions

to decrease cravings by administering a controlled dose of another medication. This is referred to as **medication-assisted treatment.** A discussion of the types of medication-assisted treatment for specific withdrawal symptoms follows.

Alcohol Withdrawal

Benzodiazepines are the most widely used group of drugs for medication-assisted treatment in alcohol withdrawal. Benzodiazepines act similarly to alcohol in their effects but can be administered in controlled doses to prevent adverse effects of alcohol withdrawal. Chlordiazepoxide (Librium), oxazepam (Serax), lorazepam (Ativan), and diazepam (Valium) are the most commonly used agents. The approach to treatment with benzodiazepines for alcohol withdrawal is to start with relatively high doses and reduce the dosage by 20% to 25% each day until withdrawal is complete. Additional doses may be given for breakthrough signs or symptoms. In clients with liver disease, accumulation of the longer-acting agents (chlordiazepoxide and diazepam) may be problematic, and use of the shorter-acting benzodiazepines (lorazepam or oxazepam) is more appropriate.

Some physicians may order anticonvulsant medication (e.g., carbamazepine, valproic acid, phenobarbital, or gabapentin) for prevention of withdrawal seizures. These drugs are particularly useful in individuals who have had repeated episodes of alcohol withdrawal. Repeated episodes of withdrawal appear to "kindle" even more serious withdrawal episodes, including the production of withdrawal seizures that can result in brain damage (Julien, 2014). These anticonvulsants have been used successfully in acute withdrawal and to reduce longer-term craving. Rosenson and associates (2013) found that a single IV dose of phenobarbital along with symptom-guided lorazepam for management of acute withdrawal reduced intensive care unit (ICU) admissions and did not have any adverse effects.

Alcohol Abstinence

The narcotic antagonist naltrexone (Revia [oral], Vivitrol [injection]) was approved by the FDA in 1994 for the treatment of alcohol addiction. Naltrexone, which was approved in 1984 for the treatment of heroin abuse, works on the same receptors in the brain that produce the feelings of pleasure when heroin or other opiates bind to them, but it does not produce the "narcotic high" and is not habit forming. Although alcohol does not bind to these same brain receptors, a meta-analysis of research studies (Del Re et al., 2013) concluded that naltrexone affords a small but significant effect in percent days of abstinence and relapse to drinking. They also concluded that naltrexone had a larger effect on reducing heavy drinking than did abstinence.

In August 2004, the FDA approved acamprosate (Campral), which is indicated for the maintenance of abstinence from alcohol in patients with alcohol addiction who are abstinent at treatment initiation. The mechanism of action of acamprosate in maintenance of alcohol abstinence is not completely understood. It is thought to restore the normal balance between neuronal excitation and inhibition by interacting with glutamate and GABA neurotransmitter systems. Acamprosate is ineffective in clients who have not undergone detoxification and not achieved alcohol abstinence prior to beginning treatment. It is recommended for concomitant use with psychosocial therapy.

An over-the-counter antioxidant, *N*-acetylcysteine (which has been used to treat select respiratory illnesses and acetaminophen overdose) has demonstrated in animal studies to be beneficial in reducing alcohol-seeking and withdrawal symptoms and preventing alcohol toxicity. However, only one study in humans has shown that it may decrease use in adolescents who are using alcohol and marijuana concurrently (Tomko et al., 2018). More research is needed, and *N*-acetylcysteine is currently not approved by the FDA for treatment of substance use disorders.

Opiate Intoxication

Examples of drugs in the opioid classification include opium, morphine, codeine, heroin, hydromorphone, oxycodone, and hydrocodone. Synthetic opiate-like narcotic analgesics include meperidine, methadone, pentazocine, tramadol, fentanyl, carfentanil, sufentanil, and U-47700.

Narcotic antagonists include naloxone (Narcan) to treat opiate intoxication and naltrexone (Revia [oral], Vivitrol [injection]) to prevent relapse. In 2015, the FDA approved an intranasal form of naloxone hydrochloride under a fast-track approval process in response to the continued increase in deaths associated with drug overdose, particularly from respiratory depression and arrest. It is reported to work within 2 minutes but must be given quickly to prevent death (Brown, 2015). Naloxone nasal spray can cause severe withdrawal in patients who are opioid dependent. A current concern identified by the recent NIH initiative, HEAL, is a need for stronger, more effective naloxone options, because overdoses secondary to fentanyl and carfentanil do not always respond to existing medications.

Naltrexone is used after opioid intoxication to prevent relapse, but because it is a potent blocker of opioids, the client must be free of opioids for at least 7 to 14 days to avoid sudden withdrawal symptoms. The physician may order a naloxone challenge test before use of naltrexone to ensure a negative challenge test.

Opiate Withdrawal

Opiate withdrawal symptoms, as discussed previously, last for varying amounts of time depending on the type of opiate. Withdrawal therapy includes rest, adequate nutritional support, and medication-assisted treatment with drugs such as methadone or buprenorphine. Although not all patient treatment plans will include medication-assisted treatment (the administration of a controlled opiate agonist in substitution for the substance that was being used), there is evidence that they are beneficial in reducing withdrawal symptoms, and recent studies have supported that addition of this treatment reduces overall mortality risks (Jancin, 2018). Methadone, if ordered, is given on the first day in a dose sufficient to suppress withdrawal symptoms. The dose is then gradually tapered over a specified time. As the dose of methadone diminishes, renewed abstinence symptoms may be ameliorated by the addition of clonidine. Some patients are maintained on medication-assisted treatment indefinitely, although this was not the original intent for these drugs. Grossman, as cited by Jancin (2018), reports that studies repeatedly demonstrate that when treatment stops, the risk of relapse increases. Methadone can only be administered in methadone clinics that are overseen at state and federal levels.

In October 2002, the FDA approved two forms of the drug buprenorphine for treating opiate addiction. Buprenorphine is an opioid partial agonist (where methadone is an opioid agonist, similar to morphine) and is considered to be somewhat safer and cause fewer side effects, making it especially attractive for clients who are mildly or moderately addicted. Individuals are able to access treatment with buprenorphine in office-based settings, providing an alternative to methadone clinics. Physicians are deemed qualified to prescribe buprenorphine if they hold an addiction certification from the American Society of Addiction Medicine, the American Academy of Addiction Psychiatry, the American Psychiatric Association, or other associations deemed appropriate. The number of patients to whom individual physicians may provide outpatient buprenorphine treatment was previously limited to 100 but in response to the growing opioid epidemic, a new federal rule became effective in August 2016, increasing the allowable number to 275 patients with stipulations about necessary credentialing in addictions medicine or addictions psychiatry and allowable practice settings. Some exceptions are permissible in emergency situations. Currently, buprenorphine/naloxone combinations (in sublingual tablets or film, buccal film, extended release, and long-acting injectable forms) and injectable naltrexone are all options for medication-assisted treatment of opioid addiction.

Clonidine (Catapres) also has been used to suppress opiate withdrawal symptoms. As monotherapy, it is not as effective as substitution with methadone, but it is nonaddicting and serves effectively as a bridge to enable the client to stay opiate free long enough to facilitate termination of methadone maintenance.

Barbiturate Withdrawal

Medication-assisted treatment for CNS depressant withdrawal (particularly barbiturates) is most commonly used with the long-acting barbiturate phenobarbital (Luminal). The dosage required to suppress withdrawal symptoms is administered. When stabilization has been achieved, the dose is gradually decreased by 30 mg/day until withdrawal is complete. Long-acting benzodiazepines are commonly used for medication-assisted treatment when the substance of abuse is a nonbarbiturate CNS depressant.

Stimulant Intoxication

Treatment of stimulant intoxication usually begins with minor tranquilizers such as chlordiazepoxide and progresses to major tranquilizers such as haloperidol (Haldol). Antipsychotics should be administered with caution because of their propensity to lower seizure threshold. Repeated seizures are treated with IV diazepam.

Stimulant Withdrawal

Withdrawal from CNS stimulants does not constitute a medical emergency such as that observed with CNS depressants like alcohol or benzodiazepines. Treatment is usually aimed at reducing drug craving and managing severe depression. The client is placed in a quiet atmosphere and allowed to sleep and eat as much as is needed or desired. Suicide precautions may need to be instituted. Antidepressant therapy may be helpful in treating symptoms of depression.

Hallucinogens and Cannabinols

Medication-assisted treatment is not required with these drugs and there are no FDA-approved medications for treatment of these substance use disorders. When adverse reactions such as anxiety or panic occur, benzodiazepines (e.g., diazepam or chlordiazepoxide) may be prescribed to prevent harm to the client or others. Psychotic reactions may be treated with antipsychotic medications.

Counseling

Counseling on a one-to-one basis is often used to help the client who misuses substances. The relationship is goal directed, and the length of the counseling may vary from weeks to years. The focus is on current reality, development of a working treatment relationship, and strengthening ego assets. The counselor must be warm, kind, and nonjudgmental yet able to set limits firmly. Research consistently demonstrates that personal characteristics of counselors are highly predictive of client outcome. In addition to technical counseling skills, many important therapeutic qualities affect the outcome of counseling, including insight, respect, genuineness, concreteness, and empathy (SAMHSA, 2014). Often counselors in substance use disorders treatment are themselves engaged in an ongoing recovery program from alcohol or drug addiction, or both. Having the shared experience of addiction is considered an opportunity to develop connection and compassion with the client, and there is typically more self-disclosure about the counselor's own journey than is typical in psychiatric settings.

Counseling of the client who misuses substances passes through various phases, each of which is of indeterminate length. In the first phase, an assessment is conducted. Factual data are collected to determine whether the client does have a problem with substances—that is, that substances are regularly impairing effective functioning in a significant life area.

Following the assessment, in the working phase of the relationship the counselor assists the individual to work on acceptance of the fact that the use of substances causes problems in significant life areas and that the client has not been able to make adaptive changes. The client states a desire to make changes. The strength of the denial system is determined by the duration and extent of substance-related adverse effects in the person's life. Thus, those individuals with rather minor substance-related problems of recent origin have less difficulty with this stage than those with long-term extensive impairment. The individual also works to gain self-control and abstain from substances.

Once the problem has been identified and sobriety is achieved, the client must have a concrete and workable plan for getting through the early weeks of abstinence. Anticipatory guidance through role-play helps the individual practice how to respond when substances are readily obtainable and the impulse to partake is strong.

Counseling often includes the family or specific family members. In family counseling the therapist tries to help family members see how they have affected, and been affected by, the client's substance use. Family strengths are mobilized, and family members are encouraged to move in a positive direction. Referrals are often made to self-help groups such as Al-Anon, Nar-Anon, Alateen, Families Anonymous, and Adult Children of Alcoholics.

Group Therapy

Group therapy with substance users has long been regarded as a powerful agent of change. In groups, individuals are able to share their experiences with others who are going through similar problems. They are able to "see themselves in others" and thus confront their defenses about giving up the substance. They may confront similar attitudes and defenses in others. Groups also give individuals the capacity for communicating needs and feelings directly.

Some groups may be task-oriented education groups in which the leader is charged with presenting material associated with substance abuse and its various effects on the person's life. Psychoeducational groups employ strategies such as CBT, assertiveness education, and relaxation training that have demonstrated efficacy with individuals who misuse substances. Psychoeducational groups typically involve education *and* opportunities to process feelings and practice new coping skills.

Therapy groups and self-help groups such as AA are complementary to each other. Whereas the self-help group focus is on achieving and maintaining sobriety, in the therapy group, the individual may learn more adaptive ways of coping, how to deal with problems that may have arisen or were exacerbated by the former substance use, and ways to improve quality of life and to function more effectively without substances.

Nonsubstance Addictions

Gambling Disorder

This disorder is defined by the *DSM-5-TR* as persistent and recurrent problematic gambling behavior leading to clinically significant impairment or distress (APA, 2022). The preoccupation with gambling and the impulse to gamble often intensify when the individual is under stress. Many impulsive gamblers describe a physical sensation of restlessness and anticipation that can only be relieved by placing a bet. Winning stimulates reward centers in the brain, increasing feelings of power and decreasing anxiety. The problem gambler increasingly uses gambling to try to cope with stress and regain a sense of control.

As the need to gamble increases, the individual is forced to obtain money by any means available, which may include borrowing money from illegal sources or pawning personal items (or items that belong to others). As gambling debts accrue, or out of a need to continue gambling, the individual may desperately resort to forgery, theft, or even embezzlement. Family relationships are disrupted, and impairment in occupational functioning may occur because of absences from work in order to gamble.

Gambling behavior usually begins in adolescence; however, compulsive behaviors rarely occur before young adulthood. The disorder generally runs a chronic course, with periods of waxing and waning, largely dependent on periods of psychosocial stress. Although comprehensive statistics are lacking, available information estimates that 1% to 2% of the general population are problem gamblers (Boland & Verduin, 2022). It is more common among men than women.

Various personality disorder traits have been associated with pathological gambling. In a systematic review and meta-analysis (Dowling et al., 2015), the most prevalent included narcissistic, antisocial, avoidant, obsessive-compulsive, and borderline traits. The researchers concluded that in any treatment setting for gambling disorders, screening and treatment for these common comorbid conditions must be addressed. Other common comorbidities include depression, suicide ideation, substance use disorders, and post-traumatic stress disorder. Gambling problems may be episodic and increase during periods of stress or depression, or the behavior may be persistent (APA, 2022).

Predisposing Factors to Gambling Disorder

Biological Influences

- ***Genetic:*** Familial and twin studies show an increased prevalence of pathological gambling in family members of individuals diagnosed with the disorder. Black and associates (2014) found that first-degree relatives of pathological gamblers were eight times more likely to develop the same condition, suggesting an underlying genetic predisposition.
- ***Physiological:*** Studies of dopamine receptor systems have implicated this neurotransmitter in the development of addictive personality traits, including pathological gambling (Weiss & Pontone, 2014). Support for this association comes from studies that demonstrated a correlation between the development of pathological gambling behaviors after individuals were treated with dopamine receptor agonist drugs (Lanteri et al., 2018; Moore et al., 2014; Scavone et al., 2019). Biochemical theories suggest that, ironically, both winning and losing (perhaps related to the excitement of taking a risk) stimulate the reward and pleasure centers in the brain. This could contribute to persistent and repeated desire to gamble even when one is not winning.

Psychosocial Influences

Boland and Verduin (2022) report that the following may be predisposing factors to the development of pathological gambling: "loss of a parent by death, separation, divorce, or desertion before the child is 15 years of age; inappropriate parental discipline (absence, inconsistency, or harshness); exposure to and availability of gambling activities for the adolescent; a family emphasis on material and financial symbols; and a lack of family emphasis on saving, planning, and budgeting" (p. 332).

Treatment Modalities for Gambling Disorder

Because most pathological gamblers deny that they have a problem, treatment is difficult. In fact, most gamblers only seek treatment due to legal difficulties, family pressures, or other psychiatric complaints. Behavior therapy, cognitive therapy, motivational interviewing, 12-step programs (Gamblers Anonymous), and self-help strategies such as bibliotherapy have all been used with varying degrees of success. About one-third of individuals with gambling disorders recover without need for treatment (Rash et al., 2016). Some medications have been used with effective results in the treatment of pathological gambling. Selective serotonin reuptake inhibitors and clomipramine have been used to treat obsessive-compulsive disorders and may have benefits for those with gambling disorders who have comorbid obsessive-compulsive traits. Lithium, carbamazepine, and naltrexone have also demonstrated some effectiveness.

Possibly the most effective treatment of pathological gambling is participation by the individual in **Gamblers Anonymous** (GA). This self-help group is modeled after Alcoholics Anonymous.

CASE STUDY AND SAMPLE CARE PLAN

NURSING HISTORY AND ASSESSMENT

The police bring Dan to the emergency department of the local hospital around 9:00 p.m. His wife, Cassandra, called 911 when Dan became violent and she began to fear for her safety. Dan was fired from his job as a foreman in a manufacturing plant for refusing to follow his supervisor's directions on a project. When cleaning up after his move, several half-empty bottles of liquor were found in his work area.

Cassandra reports that Dan has been drinking since he came home shortly after noon today. He bloodied her nose and punched her in the stomach when she poured the contents of a bottle from which he was drinking down the kitchen sink. The police responded to her call and brought Dan to the hospital in handcuffs. By the time they arrive at the hospital, Dan has calmed down and appears drugged and drowsy. His blood alcohol level measures 247 mg/dL. He is admitted to the detoxification unit of the hospital with a diagnosis of Alcohol Intoxication.

Cassandra tells the admitting nurse that she and Dan have been married for 12 years. He was a social drinker before they were married, but his drinking has increased over the years. He has been under a lot of stress at work; hates his job, his boss, and his coworkers; and is depressed much of the time. He never had a loving relationship with his parents, who are now deceased. For the past few years, his pattern has been to come home, start drinking immediately, and drink until he passes out for the night. She states that she has tried to get him to go for help with his drinking, but he refuses and says that he doesn't have a problem. Cassandra begins to cry and says to the nurse, "We can't go on like this. I don't know what to do!"

Continued

CASE STUDY AND SAMPLE CARE PLAN—cont'd

NURSING DIAGNOSES AND OUTCOME IDENTIFICATION

From the assessment data, the nurse develops the following nursing diagnoses for Dan:

1. **Risk for injury** related to CNS agitation from alcohol withdrawal
   a. **Short-term goal:** Dan's condition will stabilize within 72 hours.
   b. **Long-term goal:** Dan will not experience physical injury.
2. **Denial** related to low self-esteem, weak ego development, and underlying fears and anxieties
   a. **Short-term goal:** Dan will focus immediate attention on behavioral changes required to achieve sobriety.
   b. **Long-term goal:** Dan will accept responsibility for his drinking behaviors and acknowledge the association between his drinking and personal problems.

PLANNING AND IMPLEMENTATION

RISK FOR INJURY

The following nursing interventions may be implemented *in an effort to ensure patient safety:*

1. Assess his level of disorientation; frequently orient him to reality and his surroundings.
2. Obtain a drug history.
3. Obtain a urine sample for analysis.
4. Place Dan in a quiet room (private, if possible).
5. Ensure that smoking materials and other potentially harmful objects are stored away.
6. Observe Dan frequently. Take vital signs every 15 to 30 minutes.
7. Monitor for signs of withdrawal within a few hours after admission. Watch for signs of
   a. Increased heart rate
   b. Tremors
   c. Headache
   d. Diaphoresis
   e. Agitation; restlessness
   f. Nausea
   g. Fever
   h. Convulsions
8. Follow medication regimen, as ordered by physician (commonly a benzodiazepine, thiamine, multivitamin).

DENIAL

The following nursing interventions may be implemented *in an effort to help Dan accept responsibility for the behavioral consequences associated with his drinking:*

1. Develop Dan's trust by spending time with him, being honest, and keeping all promises.
2. Ensure that Dan understands that it is not *him* but his *behavior* that is unacceptable.
3. Provide Dan with accurate information about the effects of alcohol. Do this in a matter-of-fact, nonjudgmental way.
4. Point out recent negative events that have occurred in Dan's life, and associate the use of alcohol with these events. Help him to see the association.
5. Use confrontation with caring: "Yes, your wife called the police. You were physically abusive. She was afraid. And your blood alcohol level was 247 when you were brought in. You were obviously not in control of your behavior at the time."
6. Don't accept excuses for his drinking. Point out rationalization and projection behaviors. These behaviors prolong denial that he has a problem. He must directly accept responsibility for his drinking (not make excuses and blame it on the behavior of others). He must come to understand that only *he* has control of his behavior.
7. Encourage Dan to attend group therapy during treatment and Alcoholics Anonymous following treatment. Peer feedback is a strong factor in helping individuals recognize their problems and to ultimately remain sober.
8. Encourage Cassandra to attend Al-Anon meetings. She can benefit from the experiences of others who have experienced and are experiencing the same types of problems as she.
9. Help Dan to identify ways that he can cope besides using alcohol, such as exercise, sports, and relaxation. He should choose what is most appropriate for him and should be given positive feedback for efforts made toward change.

EVALUATION

The outcome criteria identified for Dan have been met. He experienced an uncomplicated withdrawal from alcohol and exhibits no evidence of physical injury. He verbalizes understanding of the relationship between his personal problems and his drinking, and he accepts responsibility for his own behavior. He verbalizes understanding that alcohol addiction is an illness that requires ongoing support and treatment, and he regularly attends AA meetings. Cassandra regularly attends Al-Anon meetings.

Summary and Key Points

- Individuals are considered to be addicted to a substance when they are unable to control its use, even knowing that it interferes with normal functioning; when more and more of the substance is required to produce the desired effects; and when characteristic withdrawal symptoms develop upon cessation or drastic decrease in use of the substance.
- *Substance intoxication* is defined as the development of a reversible syndrome of maladaptive cognitive, behavioral, or psychological changes that are due to the direct physiological effects of a substance on the central nervous system (CNS) and develop during or shortly after ingestion of (or exposure to) a substance.
- *Substance withdrawal* is the development of substance-specific maladaptive symptoms, with physiological, cognitive, and behavioral concomitants, that is due to the cessation of, or reduction in, heavy and prolonged substance use.
- The etiology of substance use disorders is unknown. Various contributing factors have been implicated, such as genetics, biochemical changes, developmental influences, personality factors, social learning, conditioning, and cultural and ethnic influences.
- Although multiple factors influence the development of a substance use disorder, it is clearly a disease of the brain.
- Seven classes of substances are presented in this chapter in terms of a profile of the substance, historical perspectives, patterns of use and abuse, and effects on the body. They include alcohol, other CNS depressants, CNS stimulants, opioids, hallucinogens, inhalants, and cannabinoids.
- The nurse uses the nursing process as the vehicle for delivery of care of the patient with a substance-related disorder.
- The nurse must first examine their own feelings regarding personal substance use and substance use by others. Only the nurse who can be accepting and nonjudgmental of substance use behaviors will be effective in working with these clients.
- Patients with dual diagnoses of mental illness and substance use disorders are often referred to specialized dual diagnosis treatment programs which focus on treating both disorders.
- Addiction to substances is a problem for many members of the nursing profession. Most state boards of nursing and state nurses' associations have established avenues for peer assistance to provide help to impaired members of the profession.
- Individuals who are reared in families with chemically addicted persons learn patterns of dysfunctional behavior that carry over into adult life. One of these dysfunctional behavior patterns is *codependence.* Codependent persons sacrifice their own needs for the fulfillment of others in order to achieve a sense of control. Many nurses also have codependent traits.
- Treatment modalities for substance-related disorders include self-help groups, deterrent therapy, individual counseling, and group therapy. Medication-assisted treatment is frequently implemented with clients experiencing substance intoxication and substance withdrawal and to prevent relapse. Treatment modalities are implemented on an inpatient basis or in outpatient settings, depending on the severity of the impairment.
- Gambling disorder is defined by the *DSM-5-TR* as persistent and recurrent problematic gambling behavior leading to clinically significant impairment or distress. The etiology of gambling disorders has been theorized to include genetic vulnerability and abnormalities in the serotonergic, noradrenergic, and dopaminergic neurotransmitter systems and to be influenced by number of psychosocial factors including dysfunctional family patterns.

Review Questions

Select the answer that is most appropriate for each of the following questions:

1. A client is admitted to the hospital after an extended period of binge alcohol drinking. His wife reports that he has been a heavy drinker for a number of years. Laboratory reports reveal that he has a blood alcohol level of 250 mg/dL. He is placed on the chemical addiction unit for detoxification. When would the first signs of alcohol withdrawal symptoms be expected to occur?
   a. Several hours after the last drink
   b. 2 to 3 days after the last drink
   c. 4 to 5 days after the last drink
   d. 6 to 7 days after the last drink
2. Symptoms of alcohol withdrawal include which of the following?
   a. Euphoria, hyperactivity, and insomnia
   b. Depression, suicidal ideation, and hypersomnia
   c. Diaphoresis, nausea and vomiting, and tremors
   d. Unsteady gait, nystagmus, and profound disorientation
3. Which of the following medications is the physician most likely to order for a client experiencing alcohol withdrawal syndrome?
   a. Haloperidol (Haldol)
   b. Chlordiazepoxide (Librium)
   c. Methadone (Dolophine)
   d. Cannabidiol (Epidiolex)
4. A client who has been admitted to the alcohol rehabilitation unit after being fired for drinking on the job states to the nurse, "I don't have a problem with alcohol. I can handle my booze better than anyone I know." Which defense mechanism is the client using?
   a. Denial
   b. Projection
   c. Rationalization
   d. Displacement

Clinical Judgment Questions

5. A client who has been admitted to the alcohol rehabilitation unit after being fired for drinking on the job, states to the nurse, "I don't have a problem with alcohol. My boss is a jerk! I haven't missed any more days than my coworkers." What is the nurse's most therapeutic response?
   a. "Maybe your boss is mistaken."
   b. "You are here because your drinking was interfering with your work."
   c. "Get real! You're an alcoholic and you know it."
   d. "Why do you think your boss is a jerk?"
6. A client who has been admitted to intensive outpatient treatment for substance use disorder arrives for group therapy and appears groggy with constricted pupils. The client denies using substances. Which of the following would be the best intervention at this time?
   a. Ask the client to empty their pockets.
   b. Smell the client's breath for evidence of alcohol.
   c. Conduct a drug screen to assess for the presence of opioids.
   d. Discharge the client for failure to comply with treatment expectations.

7. A client admitted to the inpatient detoxification program for alcohol withdrawal approaches the nurse and complains of nausea and feeling shaky. The nurse notices that the client has hand tremors and appears diaphoretic. Which of these nursing interventions is a priority?
   a. Check the client's temperature.
   b. Send a urine specimen to the laboratory for a random drug screen.
   c. Ask the client if there is anything they are particularly stressed about.
   d. Administer the prn benzodiazepine that was ordered for management of withdrawal symptoms.
8. A client comes into the emergency department stating they are "crashing" and feels like they'd "be better off dead." Which of these nursing interventions is a priority?
   a. Instruct the client not to worry. These are temporary signs of withdrawal that should go away in a few days.
   b. Request an order for amphetamines to ease the client's withdrawal symptoms.
   c. Assess the client's risk for suicide.
   d. Instruct the physician that the client may need naloxone.
9. An unconscious client is brought to the emergency department by a friend who says the client was injecting heroin. The client is assessed to have a weak pulse. Which of these interventions are priorities?
   a. Administer naloxone and rescue breathing.
   b. Administer IV benzodiazepines and perform continuous monitoring of vital signs.
   c. Ask the friend how much heroin the client took and confirm with a laboratory drug screen.
   d. Initiate cardiopulmonary resuscitation and prepare to use an external defibrillator.
10. A client admitted to the emergency department smells strongly of alcohol, and their husband reports that the client has been a heavy drinker for the last 25 years. After the nurse completes the assessment, the physician asks if there are any physical signs of long-term chronic alcohol misuse. Which of these findings should the nurse include in reporting to the physician? (Select all that apply.)
    a. The client reports weak leg muscles, and their gait is unsteady.
    b. The client's abdomen is distended.
    c. The client reports that they were coughing up some blood.
    d. The client reports that they have double vision.
    e. Blood tests reveal a low white blood cell count.

IMPLICATIONS FOR EVIDENCE-BASED PRACTICE

Sherk, A., Thomas, G., Churchill, S., & Stockwell, T. (2020). Does drinking within low-risk guidelines prevent harm? Implications for high-income countries using the international model of alcohol harms and policies. *Journal of Studies on Alcohol and Drugs, 81*(3), 352–361. https://doi.org/10.15288/jsad.2020.81.352

DESCRIPTION OF THE STUDY: Record-level death and hospital stay data for Canada were accessed. The researchers note that many countries have proposed low-risk drinking guidelines (LRDGs) to mitigate alcohol-related harms and that North America has higher LRDGs by international standards. The study sought to estimate the number of hospital stays and alcohol-attributable deaths experienced by people who drink within the LRDGs. They applied the International Model of Alcohol Harms and Policies (Inter-MAHP) to quantify the experiences of alcohol-caused harms among those drinking within versus exceeding the established guidelines.

- The primary finding was that "low-risk" drinking was not without harms. Among those drinking within the LRDGs, there were 140 more deaths and 3,663 more hospital stays than among abstainers from alcohol, and the lowest risk was associated with a consumption level of 10 grams per day. For all consumption levels, men had a higher relative risk than women.
- Greater than 50% of alcohol-caused cancer deaths were experienced by those drinking within weekly limits.
- The authors conclude that low-risk drinking guidelines should reflect a consumption level of no more than 10 grams of alcohol per day (or roughly one drink).

IMPLICATIONS FOR NURSING PRACTICE: Nurses play an active role in educating patients about health-related behaviors. Studies such as this guide the nurse in making evidence-based recommendations.

TEST YOUR CLINICAL REASONING AND CLINICAL JUDGMENT SKILLS

Kelly, age 23, is a first-year law student. She is engaged to a surgical resident at the local university hospital. She has been struggling to do well in law school because she wants to make her parents, two prominent local attorneys, proud of her. She had never aspired to do anything but go into law, and that is also what her parents expected her to do.

Kelly's mid-term grades were not as high as she had hoped, so she increased the number of hours of study time, staying awake all night several nights a week to study. She started drinking large amounts of coffee to stay awake but still found herself falling asleep as she tried to study at the library and in her apartment. As final exams approached, she began to panic that she would not be able to continue the pace of studying she felt she needed in order to make the grades she hoped for.

One of Kelly's classmates told her that she needed some "speed" to give her that extra energy to study. Her classmate said, "All the kids do it. Hardly anyone I know gets through law school without it." She gave Kelly the name of a source.

Kelly contacted the source, who supplied her with enough amphetamines to see her through final exams. Kelly was excited because she had so much energy, did not require sleep, and was able to study the additional hours she thought she needed for the exams. However, when the results were posted, Kelly had failed two courses and would have to repeat them in summer school if she was to continue with her class in the fall. She continued to replenish her supply of amphetamines from her "contact" until he told her that he could no longer supply her with them. She became frantic and stole a prescription blank from her fiancé and forged his name for more pills.

She started taking more and more of the medication in order to achieve the "high" she wanted to feel. Her behavior became erratic. Yesterday, her fiancé received a call from a pharmacy to clarify an order for amphetamines that Kelly had written. He insisted that she admit herself to the chemical addiction unit for detoxification.

On the unit, she appears tired and depressed, moves very slowly, and wants to sleep all the time. She keeps saying to the nurse, "I'm a real failure. I'll never be an attorney like my parents. I'm too dumb. I just wish I could die."

Answer the following questions related to Kelly:

1. What is the primary nursing diagnosis for Kelly?
2. Describe important nursing interventions to be implemented with Kelly.
3. In addition to physical safety, what are the primary short-term goals the nurses would strive to achieve with Kelly?

Communication Exercises

1. **Tom is a patient on the alcohol treatment unit. He says to the nurse, "My boss and my wife ganged up on me. They think I have a drinking problem. I don't have a drinking problem! I can quit any time I want to!"**
   How would the nurse respond appropriately to this statement by Tom?

2. Tom says to the nurse, "My head hurts. I didn't sleep very well last night. I'm getting shaky, and it's hot in here! I could sure use a cup of coffee and a cigarette."
   How would the nurse respond appropriately to this statement by Tom?
3. Tom says, "Sure, I missed a couple days of work. Everyone gets sick now and then. I don't think my wife cares about what happens to me. She and my boss got together and decided I needed to be here, or I lose my job!"
   How would the nurse respond appropriately to this statement by Tom?

MOVIE CONNECTIONS

Affliction (Alcoholism) ▪ *Days of Wine and Roses* (Alcoholism) ▪ *I'll Cry Tomorrow* (Alcoholism) ▪ *When a Man Loves a Woman* (Alcoholism) ▪ *Clean and Sober* (Cocaine addiction) ▪ *28 Days* (Alcoholism) ▪ *Lady Sings the Blues* (Heroin addiction) ▪ *I'm Dancing as Fast as I Can* (Sedatives addiction) ▪ *The Rose* (Polysubstance addiction) ▪ *Ben Is Back* (Polysubstance addiction) ▪ *Beautiful Boy* (Amphetamine addiction) ▪ *Six Balloons* (Heroin addiction) ▪ *A Star Is Born* (Alcoholism)

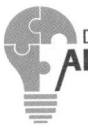

Go to **Davis Advantage** to complete your learning: strengthen understanding, apply your knowledge, and prepare for the Next Gen NCLEX®.

References

Alcohol Action Ireland. (2021). *Alcohol facts: How much do we drink?* http://alcoholireland.ie/facts/how-much-do-we-drink/

Alcoholics Anonymous. (2021). *Alcoholics Anonymous 2014 membership survey.* https://www.aa.org/assets/en_US/aa-literature/p-48-aa-membership-survey

American Academy of Child and Adolescent Psychiatry. (2019). *Children of alcoholics.* https://www.aacap.org/AACAP/Families_and_Youth/Facts_for_Families/FFF-Guide/Children-Of-Alcoholics-017.aspx

American Psychiatric Association. (2022). *Diagnostic and statistical manual of mental disorders* (5th ed., text rev.).

American Society of Addiction Medicine. (2015). *The ASAM national practice guideline for the use of medications in the treatment of addiction involving opioid use.* http://www.asam.org/docs/default-source/practice-support/guidelines-and-consensus-docs/asam-national-practiceguideline-supplement.pdf

Beatty, M. (2011). *Codependent no more.* Hazelden.

Black, D., Coryell, W., Crowe, R., McCormick, B., Shaw, M., & Allen, J. A. (2014). Direct, controlled, blind family study of DSM-IV pathological gambling. *Journal of Clinical Psychiatry, 75*(3), 215–221. https://doi.org/10.4088/JCP.13m08566

Boland, R., & Verduin, M. L. (2022). *Kaplan & Sadock's synopsis of psychiatry* (P. Ruiz, Ed.). (12th ed.). Wolters Kluwer.

Brooks, M. (2018). *FDA goes ahead with approval of sufentanil despite controversy.* http:www.medscape.com/viewarticle/904330

Brown, T. (2015). *FDA approves Narcan nasal spray to treat opioid overdose.* http://www.medscape.com/view article/854716

Butt, Y. M., Smith, M. L., Tazelaar, H. D., Vaszer, L. T., Swanson, K. L., & Mayo Clinic. (2019). Pathology of vaping-associated lung injury. *New England Journal of Medicine, 381,* 1780–1781. https://doi.org/10.1056/NEJMc1913069

Centers for Disease Control and Prevention. (2020a). *Youth and tobacco use.* https://www.cdc.gov/tobacco/data_statistics/fact_sheets/youth_data/tobacco_use/index.htm

Centers for Disease Control and Prevention. (2020b). *Overdose deaths accelerating during covid-19.* https://www.cdc.gov/media/releases/2020/p1218-overdose-deaths-covid-19.html

Centers for Disease Control and Prevention. (2020c). *Opiate overdose: Understanding the epidemic.* https://www.cdc.gov/drugoverdose/epidemic/index.html

Centers for Disease Control and Prevention. (2021a). *Facts about FASDs.* http://www.cdc.gov/ncbddd/fasd/facts.html

Centers for Disease Control and Prevention. (2021b). *Secondhand smoke (SHS) facts.* https://www.cdc.gov/tobacco/data_statistics/fact_sheets/secondhand_smoke/general_facts/index.htm

Chen, A., & Ashburn, M. A. (2015). Cardiac effects of opioid therapy. *Pain Medicine, 16,* S27–31. https://doi.org/10.1111/pme.12915

Consumer Reports. (2012). *The buzz on energy-drink caffeine.* https://www.consumerreports.org/cro/magazine/2012/12/the-buzz-on-energy-drink-caffeine/index.htm

Davenport, L. (2016). Abuse of OTC antidiarrheal meds linked to cardiac deaths. *Medscape.* https://www.medscape.com/viewarticle/863232

Del Re, A. C., Maisel, N., Blodgett, J., & Finney, J. (2013). The declining efficacy of naltrexone pharmacotherapy for alcohol use disorders over time: A multivariate meta-analysis. *Alcoholism: Clinical and Experimental Research, 37*(6), 1064–1068.

Denny, L., Coles, S., & Blitz, R. (2017). Fetal alcohol syndrome and fetal alcohol spectrum disorders. *American Family Physician, 96*(8):515–522A.

Deyo, R. A., Smith, D. H., Johnson, E. S., Tillotson, C. J., Donovan, M., Yang, X., & Dobscha, S. K. (2013). Prescription opioids for back pain and use of medications for erectile dysfunction. *Spine, 38*(11), 909–915. https://doi.org/10.1097/BRS.0b013e3182830482

Dotinga, R. (2018). Methamphetamine use climbing among opioid users. *Clinical Psychiatry News.* https://www.mdedge.com/psychiatry/article/169254/addiction-medicine/methamphetamine-use-climbing-among-opioid-users?utm_source=News_CPN_eNL_070418_F&utm_medium=email&utm_content=Opioid%20users%20turn%20to%20meth

Dowling, N. A., Cowlishaw, S., Jackson, A. C., Merkouris, S. S., Francis, K. L., & Christensen, D. R. (2015). The prevalence of comorbid personality disorders in treatment-seeking problem gamblers: A systematic review and meta-analysis. *Journal of Personality Disorders, 29*(6), 735–754. https://doi.org/10.1521/pedi_2014_28_168

Drugs.com. (2021). *Kratom.* https://www.drugs.com/illicit/kratom.html

Dubovsky, S. L. (2017). Barbiturates and similar acting substances. In B. A. Sadock, V. A. Sadock, & P. Ruiz (Eds.), *Comprehensive textbook of psychiatry* (10th ed., pp. 2984–2991). Wolters Kluwer.

Duffy, S. (2016). *DEA classifies deadly synthetic opioid as Schedule I.* http://www.empr.com/news/dea-classifies-deadly-syntheticopioid-as-schedule-i/article/572194

Ellis, J. R., & Hartley, C. L. (2012). *Nursing in today's world: Trends, issues, and management* (10th ed.). Lippincott Williams & Wilkins.

Fuentes, J. J., Fonseca, F., Elices, M., Farré, M., & Torrens, M. (2020). Therapeutic use of LSD in psychiatry: A systematic review of randomized-controlled clinical trials. *Frontiers in Psychiatry, 10*(943). https://doi.org/10.3389/fpsyt.2019.00943

Hanley, C. E. (2017). Navajos. In J. N. Giger (Ed.), *Transcultural nursing: Assessment and intervention* (7th ed.). Mosby.

Herdman, T. H., Kamitsuru, S., & Lopes, C. T. (Eds.). (2021). *NANDA International nursing diagnoses: Definitions and classification: 2021–2023* (12th ed.). Thieme.

Howard, M. O., Bowen, S. E., & Garland, E. L. (2017). Inhalant-related disorders. In B. J. Sadock, V. A. Sadock, & P. Ruiz (Eds.), *Comprehensive textbook of psychiatry* (10th ed., pp. 1328–1342). Wolters Kluwer.

Iannucci, R. A., & Weiss, R. D. (2017). Stimulant-related disorders. In B. A. Sadock, V. A. Sadock, & P. Ruiz (Eds.), *Comprehensive textbook of psychiatry* (10th ed., pp. 1280–1290). Wolters Kluwer.

Institute of Medicine. (2003). *Health professions education: A bridge to quality.*

Jancin, B. (2018). How to prescribe effectively for opioid use disorder. *Family Practice News.* https://www.mdedge.com/familypracticenews/article/171003/addiction-medicine/how-prescribe-effectively-opioid-use-disorder

Johnston, L. D., Miech, R. A., O'Malley, P. M., Bachman, J. G., Schulenberg, J. E., & Patrick, M. E. (2018). *Monitoring the future national survey results on drug use: 1975–2017: Overview, key findings on adolescent drug use.* Institute for Social Research, University of Michigan.

Juliano, L. M., & Griffiths, R. R. (2017). Caffeine-related disorders. In B. A. Sadock, V. A. Sadock, & P. Ruiz (Eds.), *Comprehensive textbook of psychiatry* (10th ed., pp. 1291–1303). Wolters Kluwer.

Julien, R. M. (2014). *A primer of drug action: A comprehensive guide to actions, uses and side effects of psychoactive drugs* (13th ed.). Worth.

Kyei-Baffour, K. & Lindsley, C. W. (2020). DARK classics in chemical neuroscience: U-47700. *ACS Chemical Neuroscience, 11*(23), 3928–3936. https://doi.org/10.1021/acschemneuro.0c00330

Lafferty, K. A. (2017). Barbiturate toxicity. *Medscape.* https://emedicine.medscape.com/article/813155-overview#a5

Lanska, D. (2020). Alcoholic myopathy. *Medlink Neurology.* http://www.medlink.com/article/alcoholic_myopathy

Lanteri, P. F., Leguia, A., Doladé, N. G., García, G. C., & Figueras, A. (2018). Drug-induced gambling disorder: A not so rare but underreported condition. *Psychiatry Research, 269,* 593–595. https://doi.org/10.1016/j.psychres.2018.09.008

Maier, S. E., & West, J. R. (2013). *Drinking patterns and alcohol-related birth defects.* http://pubs.niaaa.nih.gov/publications/arh25-3/168-174.htm

Mayo Clinic. (2020). *Caffeine content for coffee, tea, soda, and more.* https://www.mayoclinic.org/healthy-lifestyle/nutrition-and-healthy-eating/in-depth/caffeine/art-20049372

McKeown, N. J. (2019). Toluene toxicity. *Medscape.* http://emedicine.medscape.com/article/818939-overview

Moore, T. J., Glenmullen, J., & Mattison, D. R. (2014). Reports of pathological gambling, hypersexuality, and compulsive shopping associated with dopamine receptor agonist drugs. *JAMA Internal Medicine, 174*(12), 1930–1933. https://doi.org/10.1001/jamainternmed.2014.5262

MPR. (2016). *DEA reverses decision to ban kratom.* http://www.empr.com/news/dea-reverses-decision-to-ban-kratom/article/559547

Muttoni, S., Ardissino, M., & John, C. (2019). Classical psychedelics for the treatment of depression and anxiety: A systematic review. *Journal of Affective Disorders, 258,* 11–24. https://doi.org/10.1016/j.jad.2019.07.076.

National Institute on Alcohol Abuse and Alcoholism. (2021). *Alcohol facts and statistics.* https://www.niaaa.nih.gov/publications/brochures-and-fact-sheets/alcohol-facts-and-statistics

National Institute on Drug Abuse. (2019a). *Dramatic increases in maternal opioid use and neonatal abstinence syndrome.* https://www.drugabuse.gov/drug-topics/trends-statistics/infographics/dramatic-increases-in-maternal-opioid-use-neonatal-abstinence-syndrome

National Institute on Drug Abuse. (2019b). *Marijuana: Drug facts.* https://www.drugabuse.gov/publications/drugfacts/marijuana

National Institute on Drug Abuse. (2020a). *Drug misuse and addiction.* https://www.drugabuse.gov/publications/drugs-brains-behavior-science-addiction/drug-misuse-addiction

National Institute on Drug Abuse. (2020b). *Cognitive-Behavioral therapy (alcohol, marijuana, cocaine, methamphetamine, nicotine).* https://www.drugabuse.gov/publications/principles-drug-addiction-treatment-research-based-guide-third-edition/evidence-based-approaches-to-drug-addiction-treatment/behavioral-therapies/cognitive-behavioral-therapy

National Institute on Drug Abuse. (2020c). *Vaping.* https://www.drugabuse.gov/related-topics/vaping

National Institute on Drug Abuse. (2020d). *Monitoring the future study: Trends in prevalence of various drugs.* https://www.drugabuse.gov/drug-topics/trends-statistics/monitoring-future/monitoring-future-study-trends-in-prevalence-various-drugs

National Institute on Drug Abuse. (2020e). *Hallucinogens trends and statistics.* https://www.drugabuse.gov/drug-topics/hallucinogens/hallucinogens-trends-statstics

National Institute on Drug Abuse (2020f). *Marijuana research report.* https://www.drugabuse.gov/publications/research-reports/marijuana/what-marijuana

National Institute on Drug Abuse. (2020g). *Synthetic cannabinoids.* https://www.drugabuse.gov/publications/drugfacts/synthetic-cannabinoids-k2spice

National Institutes of Health. (2018). *Comorbidities: Substance use and other mental disorders.* https://www.drugabuse.gov/drug-topics/trends-statistics/infographics/comorbidity-substance-use-other-mental-disorders

National Institutes of Health. (2019). *Cannabis (marijuana) and cannabinoids: What you need to know.* https://www.nccih.nih.gov/health/cannabis-marijuana-and-cannabinoids-what-you-need-to-know

National Institutes of Health. (2021). *Carfentanil.* https://pubchem.ncbi.nlm.nih.gov/compound/carfentanil

National Library of Medicine. (2019). *Loss of brain function—Liver disease.* http://www.nlm.nih.gov/medlineplus/ency/article/000302.htm

Patterson. E. (2020). *What is inhalant withdrawal and detoxification like?* https://www.withdrawal.net/inhalant/

Rash, C. J., Weinstock, J., & Van Patten, R. (2016). A review of gambling disorder and substance use disorders. *Dovepress, 7,* 3–13. https://doi.org/10.2147/SAR.S83460

Roehler, D. R., Olsen, E. O., Mustaquim, D., & Vivolo-Kantor, A. M. (2021). Suspected nonfatal drug-related overdoses among youth in the US: 2016-2019. *Pediatrics 147*(1), e2020003491. https://doi.org/10.1542/peds.2020-003491

Rosenson, J., Clements, C., Simon, B., Vieaux, J., Graffman, S., Vahidnia, F., Cisse, B., Lam, J., & Alter, H. (2013). Phenobarbital for acute alcohol withdrawal: A prospective randomized double-blind placebo-controlled study. *The Journal of Emergency Medicine, 44*(3), 592–598.

Scavone, C., Stelitano, B., Rafaniello, C., Rossi, F., Sportiello, L., & Capuano, A. (2019). Drugs-induced pathological gambling: An analysis of Italian spontaneous reporting system. *Journal of Gambling Studies.* https://doi.org/10.1007/s10899-019-09828-1

Schuckit, M. A. (2017). Alcohol-related disorders. In B. A. Sadock, V. A. Sadock, & P. Ruiz (Eds.), *Comprehensive textbook of psychiatry* (10th ed., pp. 1264–1279). Wolters Kluwer.

Stanciu, C. N., Hybki, B. G., & Penders, T. M. (2020). Kratom: What we know and what to tell your patients. *Current Psychiatry, 19*(3), 37–42.

Storrs, C. (2016). *Is street drug flakka gone for good?* http://www.cnn.com/2016/04/18/health/flakka-drugdisappearance/index.html

Substance Abuse and Mental Health Services Administration. (2014). *Clinical supervision and professional development of the substance abuse counselor* (Treatment Improvement Protocol [TIP] Series 52, DHHS Publication No. SMA 09-4435).

Substance Abuse and Mental Health Services Administration. (2020). *2019 national survey of drug use and health.* https://www.samhsa.gov/data/sites/default/files/reports/rpt29392/Assistant-Secretary-nsduh2019_presentation/Assistant-Secretary-nsduh2019_presentation.pdf

Substance Abuse and Mental Health Services Administration. (2021). *Find help: Alcohol, tobacco, and other drugs.* https://www.samhsa.gov/find-help/atod

Tomko, R. L., Jones, J. L., Gilmore, A. K., Brady, K. T., Back, S. E., & Gray, K. M. (2018). N-acetylcysteine: A potential treatment for substance use disorders. *Current Psychiatry, 17*(6), 31–41.

Twachtman, G. (2018). *NIH launches HEAL initiative to combat opioid crisis.* https://www.mdedge.com/psychiatry/article/167889

U.S. Department of Health and Human Services, Office of the Surgeon General. (2016). *Facing addiction in America: The Surgeon General's report on alcohol, drugs, and health.*

U.S. Food and Drug Administration. (2016). *FDA requires strong warnings for opioid analgesics, prescription opioid cough products, and benzodiazepine labeling related to serious risks and death from combined use.* https://www.fda.gov/NewsEvents/Newsroom/PressAnnouncements/ucm518697.htm

U.S. Food and Drug Administration. (2018). *Statement from FDA Commissioner Scott Gottlieb, M.D., on the agency's scientific evidence on the presence of opioid compounds in kratom, underscoring its potential for abuse.* https://www.fda.gov/news-events/press-announcements/statement-fda-commissioner-scott-gottlieb-md-agencys-scientific-evidence-presence-opioid-compounds

Vaux, K. K. (2016). *Fetal alcohol syndrome.* http://emedicine.medscape.com/article/974016-overview

Volkow, N. D., & Boyle, M. (2018). Neuroscience of addiction: Relevance to prevention and treatment. *American Journal of Psychiatry, 175*(8), 729–740. https://doi.org/10.1176/appi.ajp.2018.17101174

Wang, W., Zeng, F., Hu, Y., & Li, X. (2019). A mini-review of the role of glutamate transporter in drug addiction. *Frontiers in Neurology.* https://doi.org/10.3389/fneur.2019.01123

WebMD. (2021a). *Salvia divinorum.* https://www.webmd.com/vitamins/ai/ingredientmono-1043/salvia-divinorum

WebMD. (2021b). *Cannabidiol.* https://www.webmd.com/vitamins/ai/ingredientmono-1439/cannabidiol-cbd

Weiss, H. D., & Pontone, G. M. (2014). Dopamine receptor agonist drugs and impulse control disorders. *JAMA Internal Medicine, 174*(12), 1935–1937. https://doi.org/10.1001/jamainternmed. 2014.4097

Worley, J. (2017). Nurses with substance use disorders: Where we are and what needs to be done. *Journal of Psychosocial Nursing and Mental Health Services, 55*(12), 11–14. https://doi.org/10.3928/02793695-20171113-02

Zhang, C., Paolozza, A., Tseng, P. H., Reynolds, J. N., Munoz, D. P. & Itti, L. (2019). Detection of children/youth with fetal alcohol spectrum disorder through eye movement, psychometric, and neuroimaging data. *Frontiers in Neurology, 10*(80). https://doi.org/10.3389/fneur.2019.00080

Classical References

Cermak, T. L. (1986). *Diagnosing and treating co-dependence.* Hazelton.

Jellinek, E. M. (1952). Phases of alcohol addiction. *Quarterly Journal of Studies on Alcohol, 13,* 673–684.

Sullivan, J. T., Sykora, K., Schneiderman, J., Naranjo, C. A., & Sellers, E. M. (1989). Assessment of alcohol withdrawal: The revised Clinical Institute Withdrawal Assessment for Alcohol scale (CIWA-Ar). *British Journal of Addiction, 84,* 1353–1357.

Twerski, A. (1997). *Addictive thinking: Understanding self-deception* (2nd ed.). Hazeldon.

15 Schizophrenia Spectrum and Other Psychotic Disorders

CORE CONCEPTS

Cognition: Psychosis

Professional Behavior: Nursing process in the care of patients with schizophrenia

Safety

Clinical Judgment

CHAPTER OUTLINE

Objectives
Introduction
Nature of the Disorder
Predisposing Factors
Other Schizophrenia Spectrum and Psychotic Disorders
Application of the Nursing Process
Treatment Modalities
Summary and Key Points
Review Questions
Clinical Judgment Questions
Implications for Evidence-Based Practice
Test Your Clinical Reasoning and Clinical Judgment Skills
Communication Exercises
Movie Connections

KEY TERMS

anhedonia
anosognosia
catatonia
circumstantiality
clang association
delusions
echolalia
echopraxia
hallucinations
illusion
loose associations
negative symptoms
neologism
neuroleptic malignant syndrome
paranoid delusions
perseveration
positive symptoms
psychosis
schizophrenia
serious mental illness (SMI)
social skills training
tangentiality
waxy flexibility
word salad

OBJECTIVES

After reading this chapter, the student will be able to:

1. Discuss the conceptualization of schizophrenia and other psychotic disorders.
2. Identify predisposing factors in the development of these disorders.
3. Describe various types of schizophrenia and other psychotic disorders.
4. Identify symptomatology associated with these disorders and use this information in patient assessment.
5. Formulate nursing diagnoses and outcomes of care for patients with schizophrenia and other psychotic disorders.
6. Identify topics for patient and family teaching relevant to schizophrenia and other psychotic disorders.
7. Describe appropriate nursing interventions for behaviors associated with these disorders.
8. Describe relevant criteria for evaluating nursing care of patients with schizophrenia and other psychotic disorders.
9. Discuss various modalities relevant to treatment of schizophrenia and other psychotic disorders.

Introduction

The term *schizophrenia* was coined in 1908 by the Swiss psychiatrist Eugen Bleuler. The word was derived from the Greek "skhizo" (split) and "phren" (mind).

Over the years, much debate has surrounded the concept of schizophrenia. Various definitions of the disorder have evolved, and numerous treatment strategies have been proposed, but none has proven to be uniformly effective or sufficient.

Evidence suggests that schizophrenia is probably not a homogeneous disease entity. The *Diagnostic and Statistical Manual of Mental Disorders, Fifth Edition, Text Revision; (DSM-5-TR;* American Psychiatric Association [APA], 2022) supports this concept by describing schizophrenia as one of the schizophrenia spectrum disorders. Although current consensus points to schizophrenia as a neurodevelopmental disorder (Álvarez et al., 2015), schizophrenia spectrum disorders may have several etiological influences including genetic predisposition, biochemical dysfunction, physiological factors, and psychosocial stress. Tripathi and colleagues (2018) believe that the neurodevelopmental hypothesis falls short in explaining the magnitude of brain changes that occur in schizophrenia. They suggest that these changes can better be explained as "the cumulative effect of neurodevelopmental abnormality, change in neuroplasticity, and alteration in neuronal maturation" (p. 8).

Although research is ongoing, there may never be a single treatment that cures the disorder. Effective treatment requires a comprehensive, multidisciplinary effort, including pharmacotherapy and various forms of psychosocial care, such as housing, living skills, **social skills training** (training in verbal and nonverbal skills needed for effective interpersonal relationships), rehabilitation and recovery, and family therapy. Emerging evidence indicates that early intervention and a comprehensive, patient-centered approach offer hope for a recovery process and improved quality of life for this population.

Of all the mental illnesses that cause suffering in society, schizophrenia is likely responsible for longer hospitalizations, greater chaos in family life, more exorbitant costs to individuals and governments, and more fear than any other. Studies have shown that people with a **serious mental illness (SMI)** like schizophrenia have, on average, a 25-year shorter life span than the general population (Chesney et al., 2014; Druss et al., 2011; Roberts et al., 2017). SMI is defined as a mental, behavioral, or emotional disorder resulting in serious functional impairment, which substantially interferes with or limits one or more major life activities. Because schizophrenia is such an enormous threat to life and happiness and because its causes are an unsolved puzzle, it has probably been studied more than any other mental disorder.

Risk for suicide is a significant concern among patients with schizophrenia. About 20% to 40% of people with schizophrenia attempt suicide, and current evidence suggests that about 5% die by suicide (Lewis et al., 2017). This chapter explores various theories of predisposing factors that have been implicated in the development of schizophrenia. Symptomatology associated with different diagnostic categories of the disorder is discussed. Nursing care is presented in the context of the six steps of the nursing process. Various dimensions of medical treatment are explored.

Nature of the Disorder

CORE CONCEPT

Psychosis

Psychosis is a severe mental condition in which there is disorganization of the personality, deterioration in social functioning, and loss of contact with or distortion of reality. There may be evidence of hallucinations (false sensory perceptions not associated with real external stimuli) and delusions (fixed, false beliefs). Psychosis can occur with or without the presence of organic impairment.

Schizophrenia is a disabling mental disorder. In untreated clients or those not responsive to treatment, the disturbances in thought processes, perception, affect, and behavior invariably result in a severe deterioration of social and occupational functioning.

The lifetime prevalence of schizophrenia is about 0.7% in the general population. Symptoms generally appear in late adolescence or early adulthood, although they may occur in middle or late adult life. Early-onset schizophrenia refers to symptoms that begin in childhood and adolescence before age 18 years. This condition, although rare, is recognized as a progressive neurodevelopmental disorder with a chronic and severely symptomatic course. Some studies have indicated that schizophrenia occurs more often and earlier in men than in women (B. Miller, 2020).

Phases of Schizophrenia

The pattern of development of schizophrenia may be viewed in four phases: premorbid, prodromal, active psychotic (acute schizophrenic episode), and residual phases.

Phase I: The Premorbid Phase

Premorbid signs are those that occur before there is clear evidence of illness and may include distinctive personality traits or behaviors. Premorbid personality and behavioral measurements that have been noted include being very shy and withdrawn, having poor peer relationships, doing poorly in school, and demonstrating asocial behavior. Boland and Verduin (2022) stated:

> In the typical, but not invariable, premorbid history of schizophrenia, patients had schizoid or schizotypal personalities characterized as quiet, passive, and introverted; as children, they had few friends. Preschizophrenic adolescents may have no close friends and no dates and may avoid team sports. They may enjoy [solitary activities] to the exclusion of social activities. (p. 349)

Current research is focused on the premorbid stage in hopes that identifying biomarkers and at-risk individuals may prevent transition to illness and provide greater opportunity for early intervention (Clark et al., 2016).

Phase II: The Prodromal Phase

Prodromal signs are differentiated from premorbid signs in that prodromal symptoms more clearly manifest as signs of developing schizophrenia than do premorbid signs. The prodromal phase of schizophrenia begins with a change from premorbid functioning and extends until the onset of frank psychotic symptoms. This phase can be as brief as a few weeks or months but for some it may last several years. During this phase, the individual begins to show signs of significant deterioration in function. Fifty percent complain of depressive symptoms (APA, 2022). Social withdrawal is not uncommon, and signs of cognitive impairment may begin to emerge. Some adolescent patients develop sudden onset of obsessive-compulsive behavior during the prodromal phase (Boland & Verduin, 2022).

Recognition of the behaviors associated with the prodromal phase provides an opportunity for early intervention with a possibility for improvement in long-term outcomes. Current treatment guidelines suggest therapeutic interventions that offer support with identified problems, cognitive therapies to minimize functional impairment, family interventions to improve coping, and involvement with the schools to reduce the possibility of failure. Some controversy exists about the benefits of pharmaceutical therapy during the prodromal phase; however, evidence supports that comprehensive treatment begun at the time of the first psychotic episode is associated with better outcomes (Kane et al., 2015).

Phase III: Active Psychotic Phase (Acute Schizophrenic Episode)

Schizophrenia is a chronic illness that is characterized by acute episodes in which symptoms are more pronounced. During acute episodes, psychotic symptoms are typically prominent. Box 15–1 describes the *DSM-5-TR* (APA, 2022) diagnostic criteria for schizophrenia.

Phase IV: Residual Phase

Schizophrenia is characterized by periods of remission and exacerbation. A residual phase usually follows an active phase of the illness (symptoms described in Phase III). During the residual phase, symptoms of the acute stage are either absent or no longer prominent. Positive symptoms (like delusions and hallucinations) are often ameliorated, but negative symptoms (see Box 15–2) may remain. Flat affect and impairment in role functioning are common in this phase. It has long been thought that these negative symptoms are pervasive and stable, but current research has challenged that belief with evidence that negative symptoms can improve over time (Savill et al., 2015), although admittedly they are difficult to treat. Residual impairment often increases with additional episodes of active psychosis.

Prognosis

Outcomes in schizophrenia are difficult to predict and are highly variable, but long-term follow-up studies indicate that significant clinical improvement occurs in about 44% of patients with schizophrenia (Os & Reininghaus, 2017). Several factors have been associated with a more positive outcome. These factors include good premorbid functioning, later age at onset, female sex, abrupt onset of symptoms with an obvious precipitating factor (as opposed to gradual, insidious onset of symptoms), lower depression scores, low baseline levels of aggression, rapid resolution of active-phase symptoms, minimal residual symptoms, absence of structural brain abnormalities, ability to live independently at baseline, no family history of schizophrenia and good family support (Boland & Verduin, 2022; Frankenburg, 2020; Shrivastava et al., 2010).

BOX 15–1 *DSM-5-TR* Criteria for Schizophrenia

A. Two (or more) of the following, each present for a significant portion of time during a 1-month period (or less if successfully treated). At least one of these must be (1), (2), or (3):
   1. **Delusions**
   2. **Hallucinations**
   3. **Disorganized speech (e.g., frequent derailment or incoherence)**
   4. Grossly disorganized or catatonic behavior
   5. Negative symptoms (i.e., diminished emotional expression or avolition)

B. For a significant portion of the time since the onset of the disturbance, level of functioning in one or more major areas, such as work, interpersonal relations, or self-care, is markedly below the level achieved prior to the onset (or when the onset is in childhood or adolescence, there is failure to achieve expected level of interpersonal, academic, or occupational functioning).

C. Continuous signs of the disturbance persist for at least 6 months. This 6-month period must include at least 1 month of symptoms (or less if successfully treated) that meet Criterion A (i.e., active-phase symptoms) and may include periods of prodromal or residual symptoms. During these prodromal or residual periods, the signs of the disturbance may be manifested by only negative symptoms or by two or more symptoms listed in Criterion A present in an attenuated form (e.g., odd beliefs, unusual perceptual experiences).

D. Schizoaffective disorder and depressive or bipolar disorder with psychotic features have been ruled out because either (1) no major depressive or manic episodes have occurred concurrently with the active-phase symptoms; or (2) if mood episodes have occurred during active-phase symptoms, they have been present for a minority of the total duration of the active and residual periods of the illness.

E. The disturbance is not attributable to the physiological effects of a substance (e.g., a drug of abuse, a medication) or another medical condition.

F. If there is a history of autism spectrum disorder or a communication disorder of childhood onset, the additional diagnosis of schizophrenia is made only if prominent delusions or hallucinations, in addition to the other required symptoms of schizophrenia, are also present for at least 1 month (or less if successfully treated).

Specify if: First episode, currently in acute, partial, or full remission; Multiple episodes, currently in acute, partial or full remission; Continuous; Unspecified; With catatonia

Specify current severity.

Source: Reprinted with permission from the Diagnostic and Statistical Manual of Mental Disorders, Fifth Edition, Text Revision (Copyright 2022). American Psychiatric Association.

Predisposing Factors

The cause of schizophrenia is still uncertain. Most likely, no single factor can be implicated in the etiology; rather, the disease probably results from a combination of influences, including biological, psychological, and environmental factors.

Biological Factors

Refer to Chapter 2, "Biological Implications," for a more thorough review of the biological implications of psychiatric illness.

Genetics

The body of evidence for genetic vulnerability to schizophrenia is growing. Studies show that relatives of individuals with schizophrenia have a much higher probability of developing the disease than does the general population. Whereas the lifetime risk for developing schizophrenia is about 0.7%, studies have shown that first degree relatives of an identified patient have up to a 9% greater risk of developing schizophrenia than relatives of controls (Os & Reininghaus, 2017).

The most compelling evidence for a genetic component in schizophrenia comes from twin studies. In monozygotic (identical) twins there is a 50% concordance rate for schizophrenia, which is four to five times the concordance rate in dizygotic twins or other first degree relatives (Boland & Verduin, 2022). Identical twins reared apart have the same rate of development of the illness as do those reared together. Because in about one-half of the cases only one of a pair of identical twins develops schizophrenia, genetic makeup cannot be solely responsible for causing this disease. Os and Reininghaus (2017) suggest that additive and interacting combinations of genes, environmental factors, and the moderation of gene expression through interaction with environmental factors are probably all influential.

How schizophrenia is inherited is uncertain. Current research is focused on determining which gene or genes are important in the predisposition to schizophrenia and what other biomarkers may predict risk

BOX 15–2 Positive and Negative Symptoms of Schizophrenia*

POSITIVE SYMPTOMS

Delusions (Fixed, False Beliefs)
(examples)

Persecutory—belief that one is going to be harmed by other(s)

Referential—belief that cues in the environment are specifically referring to them

Grandiose—belief that they have exceptional greatness

Somatic—beliefs that center on one's body functioning

Hallucinations (Sensory Perceptions Without External Stimuli)
Auditory (most common in schizophrenia)

Visual

Tactile

Olfactory

Gustatory

(NOTE: Hallucinations may be a normal part of religious experience in some cultural contexts.)

Disorganized Thinking (Manifested in Speech)
Loose association

Tangentiality

Circumstantiality

Incoherence (includes word salad)

Neologisms

Clang associations

Echolalia

Grossly Disorganized or Abnormal Motor Behavior (Including Catatonia)
Hyperactivity

Hypervigilance

Hostility

Agitation

Childlike silliness

Catatonia (ranging from rigid or bizarre posture and decreased responsivity to complete lack of verbal or behavioral response to the environment)

Catatonic excitement (excessive and purposeless motor activity)

Stereotyped, repetitive movements

Unusual mannerisms or postures

NEGATIVE SYMPTOMS

Lack of Emotional Expression
Blunted affect

Lack of movement in head and hands that adds expression in communication

Lack of intonation in speech

Decreased or Lack of Motivation to Complete Purposeful Activities (Avolition)
Neglect of activities of daily living

Decreased Verbal Communication (Alogia)
Decreased Interest in Social Interaction and Relationship (Asociality)

Withdrawal

Poor rapport

Diminished Ability for Abstract Thinking
Concrete interpretation of events and communication from others

*Positive symptoms refer to symptoms that are present ("added") in people with schizophrenia and not typically present in people without the disease. Negative symptoms are referred to as *deficits* or *impairments* (things "taken away" by the illness) in individuals with schizophrenia.

Sources: Compiled from APA (2022); Kay et al. (1987).

for this illness. Okazaki and associates (2016) studied gene expression in peripheral blood samples of patients admitted with acute psychosis and found that a specific combination of genes (*CDK4, MCM7,* and *POLD 4*) differentiated these patients from controls. This finding suggests that the combination could be a genetic biomarker for schizophrenia and may also influence certain pathophysiological aspects of schizophrenia. The authors conclude that messenger ribonucleic acid (mRNA) expression changes occurring in *CDK4* are potentially biomarkers for both trait (stable features) and state (temporary changes) symptoms in schizophrenia. The strongest genetic associations to date have been variations in the major histocompatibility complex (MHC), particularly C4 alleles that are involved in synaptic pruning that occurs during adolescence and young adulthood (Boland & Verduin, 2022). Research is ongoing to identify genetic influences in schizophrenia that will hone our understanding of the multivariate influences in the development of this disease and perhaps identify treatment implications.

Biochemical Factors

The oldest and most thoroughly explored biological theory in the explanation of schizophrenia attributes a pathogenic role to abnormal brain biochemistry. Notions of a "chemical disturbance" as an explanation for insanity were suggested by some theorists as early as the mid-19th century.

The Dopamine Hypothesis

This theory suggests that schizophrenia (or schizophrenia-like symptoms) may be caused by an excess of dopamine-dependent neuronal activity in the brain (Fig. 15–1). This excess activity may be related to increased production or release of the substance at nerve terminals, increased receptor sensitivity, too many dopamine receptors, or a combination of these mechanisms.

Pharmacological support for this hypothesis came from the observation that amphetamines, which increase levels of dopamine, induced symptoms that mimic those of psychosis. First generation antipsychotics (e.g., chlorpromazine or haloperidol) lower brain levels of dopamine by blocking dopamine receptors (particularly at D_2 receptors), thus reducing psychotic symptoms, including those induced by amphetamines.

Postmortem brain studies of individuals with schizophrenia reveal alterations in the presynaptic and postsynaptic dopaminergic system, and more recent in vivo studies using positron emission tomography (PET) and single photon emission computed tomography (SPECT) imaging have revealed increased dopamine synthesis capacity in patients with schizophrenia (Howes et al., 2015). Clients with **positive symptoms** such as delusions and hallucinations (referred to as *positive symptoms* because they are "added" to the clinical picture) respond with greater efficacy to dopamine-reducing drugs than do clients with **negative symptoms** (deficits such as apathy, poverty of ideas, and loss of drive). Positive and negative symptoms are listed in Box 15–2.

Over time we have learned that there are several different types of dopamine receptors (D_1, D_2, D_3, D_4, and D_5), and research continues to identify the specific role of each in the course of schizophrenia as well the implications for treatment. Clozapine, for example, an atypical antipsychotic with a unique clinical profile, has more affinity for D_4 receptors. D_3 receptors, found in several areas of the brain, have been identified as relevant in the expression of negative symptoms. While dopamine receptors have been a large focus of research, at least in part because of their relevance in drug pharmacological treatment, there are several other neurotransmitter dysregulations apparent in individuals with schizophrenia. These are discussed below.

Other Biochemical Hypotheses

Abnormalities in the neurotransmitters norepinephrine, serotonin, acetylcholine, and gamma-aminobutyric acid and in the neuroregulators, such as prostaglandins and endorphins, have all been implicated in the predisposition to schizophrenia. Excess of serotonin has been hypothesized to be responsible for both positive and negative symptoms of schizophrenia, and the effectiveness of medications such as clozapine (a strong serotonin antagonist) lends support to this hypothesis.

Recent research has implicated the neurotransmitter glutamate in the etiology of schizophrenia. The *N*-methyl-D-aspartate (NMDA) receptor is activated by the neurotransmitters glutamate and glycine. Psychopharmacological studies have shown that the drug class of glutamate antagonists (e.g., phencyclidine [PCP]; ketamine) can produce schizophrenia-like symptoms in individuals without the disorder (Hashimoto, 2006; Stahl, 2013). In one study, participants experiencing ketamine-induced schizophrenia-like psychotic symptoms were treated with a drug trial of a glycine transporter-1 inhibitor (D'Souza et al., 2012). This medication was shown to reduce the psychotic symptoms induced by the NMDA receptor antagonism of ketamine, so it is hoped it may also have benefits in schizophrenia treatment. Despite evidence of a glutamate link in schizophrenia (Hu et al., 2014), more research is needed on the implications for treatment. Previous studies have focused on reducing glutamate levels in patients who have advanced illness, but current research has identified that glutamate levels may be more important in the *transition* to psychosis, which is supported by the fact that first episodes of psychosis are often precipitated by stress, and glutamate increases under stress (Nauert, 2015). When glutamate levels are very high, the hippocampus becomes hypermetabolic and then begins to atrophy. Hippocampal atrophy has been identified as a significant finding in many individuals with schizophrenia. Future research may find that interventions targeting glutamate are beneficial in high-risk individuals or those in early stages of illness to prevent onset or slow the progression of the disease (Nauert, 2015).

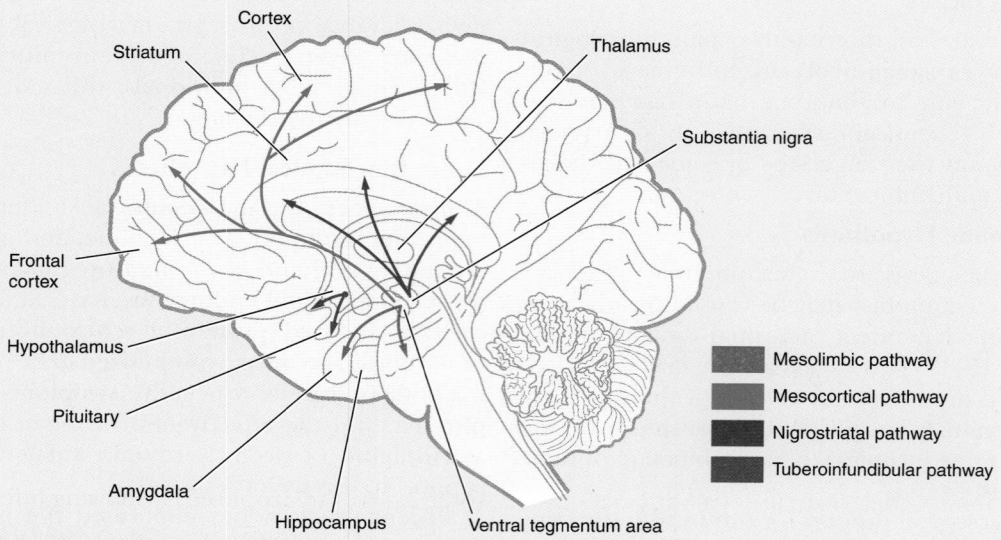

FIGURE 15–1 Neurobiology of schizophrenia.

NEUROTRANSMITTERS

A number of neurotransmitters have been implicated in the etiology of schizophrenia: dopamine, norepinephrine, serotonin, glutamate, and gamma-aminobutyric acid (GABA). The dopaminergic system has been most widely studied and closely linked to the symptoms associated with the disease.

AREAS OF THE BRAIN AFFECTED

Four major dopaminergic pathways (the pathways that transmit dopamine to different areas of the brain) have been identified:

- ***Mesolimbic pathway:*** Originates in the ventral tegmentum area (VTA) and projects to areas of the limbic system, including the nucleus accumbens, amygdala, and hippocampus. The mesolimbic pathway is associated with functions of memory, emotion, arousal, and pleasure. Excess activity in the mesolimbic tract has been implicated in the positive symptoms of schizophrenia (e.g., hallucinations, delusions). Dopamine blockade in this pathway is the target of antipsychotic medication to reduce hallucinations and delusions.
- ***Mesocortical pathway:*** Originates in the VTA and projects into the cortex. The mesocortical pathway is concerned with cognition, social behavior, planning, problem-solving, motivation, and reinforcement in learning. Negative symptoms of schizophrenia (e.g., flat affect, apathy, lack of motivation, and anhedonia) have been associated with diminished activity in the mesocortical tract, particularly at D_3 receptors.
- ***Nigrostriatal pathway:*** Originates in the substantia nigra and terminates in the striatum of the basal ganglia. This pathway is associated with the function of motor control. Degeneration in this pathway is associated with Parkinson's disease, and because typical antipsychotics may also block dopamine here, drug-induced Parkinson-like extrapyramidal side effects and tardive dyskinesia can occur.
- ***Tuberoinfundibular pathway:*** Originates in the hypothalamus and projects to the pituitary gland. It is associated with endocrine function, digestion, metabolism, hunger, thirst, temperature control, and sexual arousal. Dopamine blockade in this pathway is associated with an increase in prolactin levels (hyperprolactinemia), which can result in galactorrhea (milk discharge from the nipples) in both men and women, erectile disorder, and anorgasmia.

ANTIPSYCHOTIC MEDICATIONS

Type	Receptor Affinity	Associated Side Effects
First Generation (Typical) Antipsychotics		
Phenothiazines Haloperidol (ease positive symptoms such as hallucinations and delusions but worsen negative symptoms)	Strong D_2 (dopamine) Varying degrees of affinity for: ACh (acetylcholine) α_1 (norepinephrine) H_1 (histamine) Weak 5-HT (serotonin)	Extrapyramidal symptoms (EPS), hyperprolactinemia, **neuroleptic malignant syndrome** Anticholinergic effects Tachycardia, tremors, insomnia, postural hypotension

ANTIPSYCHOTIC MEDICATIONS—cont'd

Second Generation (Atypical) Antipsychotics Clozapine, olanzapine, quetiapine, aripiprazole, risperidone, iloperidone, ziprasidone, paliperidone, asenapine, lurasidone, and cariprazine (ameliorate positive symptoms with some improvement in negative symptoms—particularly cariprazine)	Strong 5-HT Low to moderate D_2 Varying degrees of affinity for: ACh α-adrenergic H_1 Partial agonist at D_2, D_3, and HT_{1A} (associated with more improvement in negative symptoms than other atypical antipsychotics)	Weight gain, sedation Low potential for ejaculatory difficulty Sexual dysfunction, GI disturbance, headache Low potential for EPS Anticholinergic effects Tachycardia, tremors, insomnia, postural hypotension

Typical (first generation) antipsychotic medications largely target the dopamine receptors in the brain. Newer, atypical (second generation) antipsychotics have a weaker affinity for dopamine receptors and a stronger affinity for serotonergic receptors. The glutamate model of schizophrenia suggests possibilities for new biomarkers signaling early illness and for new approaches to prevention and early treatment.

Physiological Factors

A number of potential physiological factors have been identified in the medical literature. However, their specific mechanisms and implications in the etiology of schizophrenia are unclear. Current theories suggest that it "is likely that these genetic risks, environmental risks and vulnerability factors are cumulative and interactive with each other and with critical periods of neurodevelopmental vulnerability" (Davis et al., 2016, p. 185).

Viral Infection

Boland and Verduin (2022) report that epidemiological data indicate a high incidence of schizophrenia after prenatal exposure to influenza. They stated:

> Other data supporting a viral hypothesis are an increased number of physical anomalies at birth, an increased rate of pregnancy and birth complications, seasonality of birth consistent with viral infection, geographical clusters of adult cases, and seasonality of hospitalizations. (p. 360)

The effect of autoimmune antibodies in the brain is being studied within the field of psychoneuroimmunology, and evidence suggests that such antibodies may be influential in the development of at least some cases of schizophrenia following infection from a neurotoxic virus (particularly prenatal exposure to *Toxoplasma gondii*) (Matheson et al., 2014). Symptoms of NMDA glutamate receptor autoimmune encephalopathy mimic the psychotic symptoms in schizophrenia, which supports the impact of immune system involvement in mental symptoms. The role of cytokines in inflammation and the specific effects of these chemicals in the brain are still being explored through ongoing research.

Anatomical Abnormalities

With the use of neuroimaging technologies, structural brain abnormalities have been observed in individuals with schizophrenia. Ventricular enlargement is the most consistent finding; however, some reductions in gray matter are also reported. As previously discussed, reduction in the volume of the hippocampus has also been identified in neuroimaging studies and may signal transition to a first psychotic episode (Harrisberger et al., 2016). Studies that focus on risks for a first psychotic episode are important, as early treatment is associated with better outcomes. Ultimately it is hoped that these studies will also point to preventive strategies.

Magnetic resonance imaging (MRI) has revealed reduced symmetry in several lobes of the brain and reductions in size of structures within the limbic system of individuals with schizophrenia. Considerable evidence from postmortem studies has shown abnormalities in the prefrontal cortex, and people who have had prefrontal lobotomies are reported to manifest many symptoms common to schizophrenia (Boland & Verduin, 2022), including flat affect and cognitive deterioration.

Diffusion tensor imaging studies have identified widespread white matter abnormalities in schizophrenia (Viher et al., 2016). These abnormalities in white matter microstructure appear to be primarily associated with negative symptoms and psychomotor behavior abnormalities.

Long-term studies of patients with schizophrenia have noted brain volume reduction, particularly in the temporal and preventricular areas (Veijola et al., 2014). It has been postulated that long-term antipsychotic medication use may contribute to this reduction, but the implications are unclear. Veijola and associates found that symptom severity, level of functional ability, and decline in cognitive abilities were not correlated with this reduction in brain volume.

Electrophysiology

Several studies have evaluated 40 Hz auditory steady-state response, a measure of electrical activity in the brain, and identified neural circuit dysfunctions in people with schizophrenia. A recent meta-analysis (Thunè et al., 2016) of these studies demonstrates robust evidence of such dysfunction in schizophrenia. The meaning of these circuit dysfunctions is not well understood but may indicate another biomarker for identifying risk or illness.

Physical Conditions

Several medical conditions are known to cause acute psychotic episodes, including Huntington's disease, hyperthyroidism or hypothyroidism, hypoglycemia, calcium imbalances, temporal lobe epilepsy, Wilson's disease, central nervous system (CNS) neoplasms, encephalitis, meningitis, neurosyphilis, and stroke (Mathews et al., 2013). See Box 15–3 for a list of many medical conditions associated with psychosis.

BOX 15–3 General Medical Conditions That May Cause Psychotic Symptoms

- Acute intermittent porphyria
- Brain abscesses
- Cerebrovascular disease
- CNS infections
- CNS trauma
- Cushing's syndrome
- Deafness
- Encephalitis
- Fluid or electrolyte imbalances
- Hepatic disease
- Herpes encephalitis
- Huntington's disease
- Hypoadrenocorticism
- Hypo- or hyperparathyroidism
- Hypo- or hyperthyroidism
- Meningitis
- Metabolic conditions (e.g., hypoxia; hypercarbia; hypoglycemia)
- Migraine headache
- Neoplasms
- Neurosyphilis
- NMDA glutamate receptor autoimmune encephalopathy
- Normal pressure hydrocephalus
- Renal disease
- Systemic lupus erythematosus
- Temporal lobe epilepsy
- Vitamin deficiency (e.g., B_{12})
- Wilson's disease

Sources: Compiled from APA (2022); Freudenreich (2010); Boland & Verduin (2022).

Psychological Factors

Early conceptualizations of schizophrenia focused on family relationship factors as major influences in the development of the illness, probably in light of the conspicuous absence of information related to a biological connection. These early theories implicated poor parent-child relationships, particularly condemning the mother as "schizophrenogenic" (inducing schizophrenia in her child) related to a troublesome communication style known as *double bind communication*. This theory is no longer considered credible. Researchers now focus on schizophrenia as a brain disorder. Although family relationships are not the cause of the illness, the symptoms in schizophrenia can contribute to significant disruption in communication and relationships among family members, so psychosocial factors should always be part of a comprehensive assessment. Furthermore, evidence suggests that childhood traumas, particularly multiple traumatizations, are associated (among many other influences) with the development of schizophrenia in vulnerable individuals (Álvarez et al., 2015; Davis et al., 2016; Matheson et al., 2014). Trauma-informed care is an important part of comprehensive assessment and intervention for this client.

Environmental Influences

Sociocultural Factors

Many studies have attempted to link schizophrenia to social class. Epidemiological statistics have shown that greater numbers of individuals from the lower socioeconomic classes (in urban neighborhoods) experience symptoms associated with schizophrenia than do those from higher socioeconomic groups (Os & Reininghaus, 2017). These studies consistently find that lack of material resources (including housing and access to health care) and fragmented social relationships increase the risk for schizophrenia, whereas social cohesion and ethnic density (the concentration of a given ethnic group in a particular area) are protective.

An alternative view is the *downward drift hypothesis*, which suggests that because of the characteristic symptoms of the disorder, individuals with schizophrenia have difficulty maintaining gainful employment and "drift down" to a lower socioeconomic level (or fail to rise out of a lower socioeconomic group). Proponents of this view consider poor social conditions to be a consequence rather than a cause of schizophrenia.

Stressful Life Events

No scientific evidence indicates that stress causes schizophrenia. It is probable, however, that stress may contribute to the severity and course of the illness. It is known that extreme stress can precipitate psychotic episodes, so it may also precipitate symptoms in an individual who possesses a genetic vulnerability to schizophrenia. Stressful life events also may be associated with exacerbation of schizophrenic symptoms and increased rates of relapse.

Cannabis and Genetic Vulnerability

Studies of genetic vulnerability for schizophrenia have linked certain genes (*COMT* and *ATK1*) to increased risk for psychosis and particularly for adolescents with this genetic vulnerability who use cannabinoids (Radhakrishnan et al., 2014). Longitudinal studies suggest an up to 40% greater risk of psychosis in individuals who have ever used cannabis. Both cannabis and synthetic cannabinoids can induce many schizophrenia-like symptoms. In individuals with a pre-existing psychosis, cannabinoids can exacerbate symptoms. Individuals with schizophrenia who continue to use cannabis experience shorter periods of remission and more frequent relapses (J. Miller, 2020). More importantly, the increased risk for psychotic disorders such as schizophrenia with cannabis use suggests the influence of lifestyle factors in the expression of genes and supports the theory that multiple factors play a role in the causality of this illness.

Theoretical Integration

Accumulating evidence supports the concept of multiple causation in the development of schizophrenia. Evidence gathered from a systematic review of the literature on schizophrenia (Matheson et al., 2014) suggests that schizophrenia is a widespread neural dysfunction accompanied by various psychological effects that respond moderately well to psychosocial and biomedical therapy:

> Patients have relatively poor cognitive functioning, and subtle, but diverse, structural brain alterations, altered electrophysiological functioning and sleep patterns, minor physical anomalies, neurological soft signs, and sensory alterations. There are markers of infection, inflammation or altered immunological parameters; and there is increased mortality from a range of causes. Risk for schizophrenia is increased with cannabis use, pregnancy and birth complications, prenatal exposure to *T. gondii*, childhood central nervous system viral infections, childhood adversities, urbanicity, and immigration (first and second generation), particularly in certain ethnic groups. Developmental motor delays and lower intelligence quotient in childhood and adolescence are apparent. (p. 3387)

Despite the wealth of research and knowledge that we have about schizophrenia, much more investigation is needed before we will fully understand this illness.

Other Schizophrenia Spectrum and Psychotic Disorders

The *DSM-5-TR* (APA, 2022) identifies a spectrum of psychotic disorders that are organized to reflect a gradient of psychopathology from least to most severe. Degree of severity is determined by the level, number, and duration of psychotic signs and symptoms.

Several disorders may carry the additional specifier of *With Catatonic Features*. **Catatonia** refers to a significant motor disturbance that may range from stupor (no motor activity) to excessive motor activity and agitation. The disorders in which catatonia may appear include brief psychotic disorder, schizophreniform disorder, schizophrenia, schizoaffective disorder, substance-induced psychotic disorder, neurodevelopmental disorder, major depressive disorder, and bipolar disorders I and II (APA, 2022).

The *DSM-5-TR* initiates the spectrum of disorders with Schizotypal Personality Disorder. For purposes of this textbook, this disorder is presented in Chapter 22, "Personality Disorders."

Delusional Disorder

Delusional disorder is characterized by the presence of delusions that have been experienced by the individual for at least 1 month. Although the individual with schizophrenia may experience similar delusions, this disorder does not meet the diagnostic criteria for schizophrenia (APA, 2022). If present at all, hallucinations are not prominent, and behavior is not bizarre. The subtype of delusional disorder is based on the predominant delusional theme. The *DSM-5* states that a specifier may be added to denote whether the delusions include *bizarre* content (i.e., whether the thought is "clearly implausible, not understandable, and not derived from ordinary life experiences") (p. 105). Subtypes of delusional disorders include erotomanic, grandiose, jealous, persecutory, somatic, and mixed. These are discussed further in the section "Application of the Nursing Process."

Brief Psychotic Disorder

This disorder is identified by the sudden onset of psychotic symptoms that may or may not be preceded by a severe psychosocial stressor. These symptoms last at least 1 day but less than 1 month, and there is an eventual full return to the premorbid level of functioning (APA, 2022). The individual experiences emotional turmoil or overwhelming perplexity or confusion. Evidence of impaired reality testing may include incoherent speech, delusions, hallucinations, bizarre behavior, and disorientation. Catatonic features also may be associated with this disorder.

Substance- and Medication-Induced Psychotic Disorder

The prominent hallucinations and delusions associated with substance-induced or medication-induced disorder are found to be directly attributable to substance intoxication or withdrawal or after exposure to a medication or toxin. This diagnosis is made when delusions and/or hallucinations predominate during or soon after intoxication, withdrawal, or exposure to a substance or medication and they are severe enough to warrant clinical attention (APA, 2022). The medical history, physical examination, and laboratory findings provide evidence that the appearance of the symptoms occurred in association with a substance intoxication or withdrawal or exposure to a medication or toxin. Substances that are believed to induce psychotic disorders are presented in Box 15–4. Catatonic features may also be associated with this disorder.

BOX 15–4 Substances That May Cause Psychotic Disorders

DRUGS OF ABUSE
- Alcohol
- Amphetamines and related substances
- Cannabis
- Cocaine
- Hallucinogens
- Inhalants
- Opioids
- Phencyclidine and related substances
- Sedatives, hypnotics, and anxiolytics

MEDICATIONS
- Anesthetics and analgesics
- Anticholinergic agents
- Anticonvulsants
- Antidepressant medication
- Antihistamines
- Antihypertensive agents
- Antimicrobial medications
- Antineoplastic medications
- Antiparkinsonian agents
- Cardiovascular medications
- Corticosteroids
- Disulfiram
- Gastrointestinal medications
- Muscle relaxants
- NSAIDs

TOXINS
- Anticholinesterase
- Carbon dioxide
- Carbon monoxide
- Nerve gases
- Organophosphate insecticides
- Volatile substances (e.g., fuel, paint, gasoline, toluene)

Sources: Compiled from APA (2022); Freudenreich (2010).

Psychotic Disorder Due to Another Medical Condition

The essential features of this disorder are prominent hallucinations and delusions that can be directly attributed to another medical condition (APA, 2022). The diagnosis is not made if the symptoms occur during the course of a delirium. Refer to Box 15–3 for a number of medical conditions that can cause psychotic symptoms.

Catatonic Disorder Due to Another Medical Condition

This diagnosis is made when catatonic features are evidenced from medical history, physical examination, or laboratory findings to be directly attributable to the physiological consequences of another medical condition (APA, 2022). Types of medical conditions that have been associated with catatonic disorder include metabolic disorders (e.g., hepatic encephalopathy, diabetic ketoacidosis, hypo- and hyperthyroidism, hypo- and hyperadrenalism, and vitamin B_{12} deficiency) and neurological conditions (e.g., epilepsy, tumors, cerebrovascular disease, head trauma, and encephalitis) (APA, 2022; Mathews et al., 2013).

Schizophreniform Disorder

The essential symptoms of schizophreniform disorder are identical to those of schizophrenia (Criterion A), but the duration, including prodromal, active, and residual phases, is at least 1 month but less than 6 months (APA, 2022). If the diagnosis is made while the individual is still symptomatic but has been so for less than 6 months, it is qualified as "provisional." The diagnosis is changed to schizophrenia if the clinical picture persists beyond 6 months. Schizophreniform disorder is thought to have a good prognosis if two of the following features are present: the individual's affect is not blunted or flat, there is a rapid onset of psychotic symptoms from the time the unusual behavior is noticed, there is confusion or perplexity, or the premorbid social and occupational functioning was satisfactory (APA, 2022). Catatonic features also may be associated with this disorder.

Schizoaffective Disorder

This disorder is manifested by signs and symptoms of schizophrenia, along with a strong element of symptomatology associated with the mood disorders (depression or mania). The client may appear depressed with psychomotor retardation and suicidal ideation, or symptoms may include euphoria, grandiosity, and hyperactivity (see the "Real People, Real Stories" interview with Josh, who describes his diagnosis and experience with schizoaffective disorder in Chapter 16, "Depressive Disorders"). A defining factor in the diagnosis of schizoaffective disorder is the presence of hallucinations and/or delusions that occur for at least 2 weeks in the absence of a major mood episode (APA, 2022). However, prominent mood disorder symptoms must be evident for the majority of the time. The prognosis for schizoaffective disorder is generally better than that for other schizophrenic disorders but worse than that for mood disorders alone. Catatonic features also may be associated with this disorder.

Application of the Nursing Process

Background Assessment Data

The diagnostic criteria for schizophrenia were presented Box 15–1. As previously stated, symptoms may present in phases with schizophrenia representing the active phase of the disorder. Symptoms associated with the active phase are discussed in this section.

In the first step of the nursing process, the nurse gathers a database from which nursing diagnoses are derived and a plan of care is formulated. This first step of the nursing process is extremely important because problem identification, objectives of care, and outcome criteria cannot be accurately determined without an accurate assessment.

Assessment of the patient with schizophrenia may be a complex process based on information gathered from a number of sources. Patients in an acute episode of their illness may not be able to make significant contributions to their history. Data may be obtained from family members if possible, from old medical records if available, or from other individuals who are able to report on the progression of the patient's symptoms.

The nurse must be familiar with symptoms common to the disorder to be able to obtain an adequate assessment of the patient with schizophrenia. This includes positive and negative symptoms. Most but not all clients exhibit a mixture of both types of symptoms.

The seven domains of cognitive dysfunction that are common in schizophrenia are working memory, attention, speed of processing thoughts, and verbal learning, with substantial deficit in reasoning, abstract thinking, and problem-solving. Tripathi and associates (2018) estimate the 98% of patients with schizophrenia have these cognitive deficits, which can aggravate other symptoms and dramatically interfere with quality of life. To date, pharmacological treatments have generally been ineffective in treating these symptoms.

It is important to note that not all patients with schizophrenia experience all of these symptoms. Bora (2015) notes that in individuals who develop cognitive deficits, the age of onset is variable, and

MacCabe and associates (2013) identify that a subgroup of individuals with schizophrenia have no cognitive impairment, even in adulthood. Many factors contribute to functional impairment and decline beyond the symptoms themselves, including comorbid metabolic conditions, chronic substance use, stress, frequency and intensity of episodes, residual symptoms, and social defeat (Bora, 2015). A summary of positive and negative symptoms was presented in Box 15–2 and is described in more detail in the following section.

Positive Symptoms

Positive symptoms are abnormal symptoms that are common manifestations of schizophrenia and referred to as positive because they are "added to" rather than deficits in the clinical picture.

Disturbances in Thought Content

Delusions are fixed false beliefs that are irrational and that the individual maintains as true despite evidence to the contrary. These beliefs are not explainable as part of the person's usual religious or cultural precepts. Delusions are subdivided according to their content. Some of the more common ones are listed here:

- ***Persecutory delusions:*** These are the most common type of delusion in which individuals believe they are being persecuted or malevolently treated in some way. Frequent themes include being plotted against, cheated or defrauded, followed and spied on, poisoned, or drugged. The individual may obsess about and exaggerate a slight rebuff (either real or imagined) until it becomes the focus of a delusional system. Repeated complaints may be directed at legal authorities. The individual feels threatened and believes that others intend harm or persecute them in some way (e.g., "The FBI has 'bugged' my room and intends to kill me"; "The government put a chip in my brain to erase my memories"). These may also be referred to as **paranoid delusions,** which describes the extreme suspiciousness of others and of their actions or perceived intentions (e.g., "I won't eat this food; I know it has been poisoned"). Aggression or violence may occur because the individuals believe that they must defend themselves against someone or something perceived to be a threat.
- ***Grandiose delusions:*** The individual with grandiose delusions has an exaggerated feeling of importance, power, knowledge, or identity. These individuals may believe that they have a special relationship with a famous person or even assume the identity of a famous person (believing that the actual person is an imposter). Grandiose delusions of a religious nature may lead to assumption of the identity of a deity or religious leader (e.g., "I am Jesus Christ").
- ***Delusions of reference:*** Events in the environment are assumed by individuals with delusions of reference to be referring to themselves (e.g., "Someone is trying to get a message to me through the articles in this magazine [or newspaper or TV program]; I must break the code so that I can receive the message") and these beliefs become fixed (as with other delusions) despite evidence to the contrary. *Ideas of reference* are less rigid than delusions of reference. For example, an individual with ideas of reference may think that other people in the room who are giggling must be laughing about them but with additional information can acknowledge that there could be other explanations for their laughter.
- ***Delusions of control or influence:*** Individuals believe that certain objects or persons have control over their behavior (e.g., "The dentist put a filling in my tooth; I now receive transmissions through the filling that control what I think and do") or they believe that their thoughts or behaviors have control over specific situations or people (e.g., the mother who believed that if she scolded her son in any way, he would die). This is similar to magical thinking, which is common in children (e.g., "The sky is raining because I'm sad").
- ***Somatic delusions:*** Individuals have a false idea about the functioning of their body. This may be a false belief that they have some type of general medical condition or that there has been an alteration in a body organ or its function (e.g., "The doctor says I'm not pregnant, but I know I am"; "There is an alien force that is eating my brain").
- ***Nihilistic delusions:*** The individual has a false idea that the self, a part of the self, others, or the world is nonexistent (e.g., "The world no longer exists"; "I have no heart").
- ***Erotomanic delusions:*** Individuals with erotomanic delusions falsely believe that someone, usually of a higher status, is in love with them. Famous persons are often the subjects of erotomanic delusions. Sometimes the delusion is kept secret, but some individuals may follow, contact, or otherwise try to pursue the object of their delusion.
- ***Jealous delusions:*** The content of jealous delusions centers on the idea that the person's sexual partner is unfaithful. The idea is irrational and

without cause, but the individual with the delusion searches for evidence to justify the belief. The sexual partner is confronted (and sometimes physically attacked) regarding the imagined infidelity. The imagined "lover" of the sexual partner also may be the object of the attack. Attempts to restrict the autonomy of the sexual partner in an effort to stop the imagined infidelity are common.

Disturbances in Thought Processes Manifested in Speech

- **Loose associations** are characterized by speech in which ideas shift from one unrelated subject to another. Typically, the individual with loose associations is unaware that the topics are unconnected. When the condition is severe, speech may be incoherent (e.g., "We wanted to take the bus, but the airport took all the traffic. The FBI is watching me. We have it all in our pockets").
- **Neologisms** are newly invented words that are meaningless to others but have symbolic meaning to the individual (e.g., "She wanted to give me a ride in her new *uniphorum*").
- **Clang associations** are words governed by sounds, often taking the form of rhyming (e.g., "It is very cold. I am cold and bold. The gold has been sold").
- **Word salad** is a group of words that are put together randomly, without any logical connection (e.g., "Most forward action grows life double plays circle uniform").
- **Circumstantiality** occurs when the individual delays in reaching the point of a communication because of unnecessary and tedious details. The point or goal is usually met but only with numerous interruptions by the interviewer to keep the person on track of the topic being discussed.
- **Tangentiality** refers to a veering away from the topic of discussion and difficulty maintaining focus and attention.
- **Perseveration** occurs when the individual persistently repeats the same word or idea in response to different questions. It is a manifestation of a thought-processing disturbance in which the person gets stuck on a particular thought.
- **Echolalia** refers to repeating words or phrases spoken by another. In toddlers this is a normal phase in development, but in children with autism, echolalia may persist beyond the toddler years. In adulthood, echolalia is a significant neurological symptom of thought disturbance that occurs in schizophrenia, strokes, and other neurological disorders.

Disturbances in Perception

- **Hallucinations,** or false sensory perceptions not associated with real external stimuli, may involve any of the five senses. Types of hallucinations include the following:
  - ***Auditory:*** Auditory hallucinations are false perceptions of sound. Most commonly they are of voices, but the individual may report clicks, rushing noises, music, and other noises. *Command hallucinations* are "voices" that issue commands to the individual. They are potentially dangerous when the commands are directing violence toward self or others. Auditory hallucinations are the most common type in schizophrenia.
  - ***Visual:*** These hallucinations are false visual perceptions that may consist of formed images, such as of people, or of unformed images, such as flashes of light. Visual hallucinations occur about 27% of the time in individuals with schizophrenia (and 15% of the time in affective psychoses). They typically co-occur with auditory hallucinations and are associated with poorer outcomes (Waters et al., 2014).
  - ***Tactile:*** Tactile hallucinations are false perceptions of the sense of touch, often of something on or under the skin. One specific tactile hallucination is *formication*, the sensation that something is crawling on or under the skin.
  - ***Gustatory:*** This type of hallucination is a false perception of taste. Most commonly, gustatory hallucinations are described as unpleasant tastes.
  - ***Olfactory:*** Olfactory hallucinations are false perceptions of the sense of smell.
- **Illusions** are misperceptions or misinterpretations of real external stimuli. These may occur in the prodromal, active, and residual phases of schizophrenia and may co-occur with delusions.
- **Echopraxia** occurs when a client imitates movements made by others. The mechanisms underlying echopraxia in schizophrenia are not well understood, but current evidence suggests that it may involve a disturbance in mirror neuron activity in the presence of social cognition impairments and self-monitoring deficits culminating in imitative behavior (Urvakhsh et al., 2014).

Negative Symptoms

Negative symptoms refer to a group of symptoms that are deficits commonly noted in the clinical picture of schizophrenia.

- ***Disturbances in affect:*** *Affect* describes the behavior associated with an individual's feeling state or emotional tone. In *inappropriate affect,* the individual's emotional tone is incongruent with the circumstances (e.g., a young woman who laughs when told of the death of her mother). In *bland (blunted) or flat affect,* the emotional tone is very weak. The individual with flat affect appears to be devoid of emotional tone (or overt expression of feelings).
- ***Apathy:*** The client with schizophrenia often demonstrates an indifference to or uninterest in the environment. The bland or flat affect is a manifestation of the emotional apathy.
- ***Avolition:*** Impaired volition has to do with the inability to initiate goal-directed activity. In the individual with schizophrenia, this may take the form of inadequate interest, lack of motivation, neglect of activities of daily living including personal hygiene and appearance, or inability to choose a logical course of action in a given situation.
- ***Lack of interest or skills in interpersonal interaction:*** Impairment in social functioning may be reflected in social isolation, emotional detachment, and lack of regard for social convention. Some clients with acute schizophrenia cling to others and intrude on the personal space of others, exhibiting behaviors that are not socially and culturally acceptable. Others may exhibit ambivalence in social relationships. Still others may withdraw from relationships altogether (asociality).
- ***Lack of insight:*** Some individuals lack awareness of there being any illness or disorder even when symptoms appear obvious to others. The term for this is **anosognosia.** The *DSM-5-TR* identifies this symptom as the "most common predictor of nonadherence to treatment, and it predicts higher relapse rates, increased number of involuntary treatments, poorer psychosocial functioning, aggression, and poorer course of illness" (APA, 2022, p. 116).
- ***Anergia*** is a deficiency of energy. The individual with schizophrenia may lack sufficient energy to carry out activities of daily living or to interact with others.
- ***Inability to experience pleasure:*** This distressing symptom, called **anhedonia,** may increase one's risk for suicide.
- ***Lack of abstract thinking ability:*** Concrete thinking, or literal interpretations of the environment, represents a regression to an earlier level of cognitive development. Abstract thinking becomes impaired in some individuals with schizophrenia. For example, the client with this deficit would have great difficulty describing the abstract meaning of sayings such as "I'm climbing the walls" or "It's raining cats and dogs."

Associated Features

- ***Waxy flexibility*** describes a condition in which the client with schizophrenia allows body parts to be placed in bizarre or uncomfortable positions. This symptom is associated with catatonia. Once placed in position, the arm, leg, or head remains in that position for long periods, regardless of how uncomfortable it is for the client. For example, the nurse may position the client's arm in an outward position to take a blood pressure measurement. When the cuff is removed, the client may maintain the arm in the position in which it was placed to take the reading.
- ***Posturing*** is manifested by the voluntary assumption of inappropriate or bizarre postures.
- ***Pacing back and forth and body rocking*** (a slow, rhythmic, backward-and-forward swaying of the trunk from the hips, usually while sitting) are common psychomotor behaviors of the client with schizophrenia.
- ***Regression*** is the retreat to an earlier level of development. Regression, a primary defense mechanism of schizophrenia, is a dysfunctional attempt to reduce anxiety. It provides the basis for many of the behaviors associated with schizophrenia.
- ***Eye movement abnormalities*** may manifest in several ways including difficulty maintaining focus on a stationary object and difficulty with smooth pursuit of a moving object. Research (Benson et al., 2012) has found that simple eye movement tests can distinguish the abnormalities common in schizophrenia with exceptional accuracy.

Diagnosis and Outcome Identification

Using information collected during the assessment, the nurse completes the client database from which the selection of appropriate nursing diagnoses is determined. Table 15–1 presents a list of patient behaviors and the NANDA International, Inc. (NANDA-I) nursing diagnoses (Herdman et al., 2021) that correspond to those behaviors, which may be used in planning care for patients with schizophrenia.

Outcome Criteria

The following criteria may be used for measurement of outcomes in the care of the patient with schizophrenia. The patient:

- Demonstrates an ability to relate satisfactorily with others.
- Recognizes distortions of reality.

TABLE 15–1 Assigning Nursing Diagnoses to Behaviors Commonly Associated With Psychotic Disorders

BEHAVIORS	NURSING DIAGNOSES
Impaired communication (inappropriate responses), disordered thought sequencing, rapid mood swings, poor concentration, disorientation, stops talking in midsentence, tilts head to side as if to be listening	Disturbed sensory perception*
Delusional thinking; inability to concentrate; impaired volition; inability to problem-solve, abstract, or conceptualize; extreme suspiciousness of others; inaccurate interpretation of the environment	Disturbed thought processes
Withdrawal, sad dull affect, need-fear dilemma, preoccupation with own thoughts, expression of feelings of rejection or of aloneness imposed by others, uncommunicative, seeks to be alone	Social isolation
Risk factors: Aggressive body language (e.g., clenching fists and jaw, pacing, threatening stance); verbal aggression; catatonic excitement; command hallucinations; rage reactions; history of violence; overt aggressive acts; goal-directed destruction of objects in the environment; self-destructive behavior; active, aggressive suicidal acts	Risk for violence: Self-directed or other-directed
Loose association of ideas, neologisms, word salad, clang associations, echolalia, verbalizations that reflect concrete thinking, poor eye contact, difficulty expressing thoughts verbally, inappropriate verbalization	Impaired verbal communication
Difficulty carrying out tasks associated with hygiene, dressing, grooming, eating, and toileting	Self-care deficit
Neglectful care of client in regard to basic human needs or illness treatment, extreme denial or prolonged overconcern regarding client's illness, depression, hostility and aggression	Interrupted Family Processes
Inability to take responsibility for meeting basic health practices, history of lack of health-seeking behavior, lack of expressed interest in improving health behaviors, demonstrated lack of knowledge regarding basic health practices, anosognosia (lack of insight about illness)	Ineffective health maintenance
Unsafe, unclean, disorderly home environment; household members express difficulty in maintaining their home in a safe and comfortable condition	Ineffective home maintenance

*This diagnosis has been resigned from the NANDA-I list of approved diagnoses. It is retained here because it is most compatible with the identified behaviors.
Source: Adapted from Herdman et al. (2021).

- Has not harmed self or others.
- Perceives self realistically.
- Demonstrates the ability to perceive the environment correctly.
- Maintains anxiety at a manageable level.
- Relinquishes the need for delusions and hallucinations.
- Demonstrates the ability to trust others.
- Uses appropriate verbal communication in interactions with others.
- Performs self-care activities independently.

Planning and Implementation

Table 15–2 provides a plan of care for the patient with schizophrenia. Selected nursing diagnoses are presented, along with outcome criteria, appropriate nursing interventions, and rationales for each. In general, nursing interventions should be geared toward establishing trust because suspiciousness is a common symptom in this disorder.

Use of a passive rather than a directive communication approach, which offers the client with paranoia the opportunity to make decisions about activities, treatment goals, and other aspects of care, helps establish trust while incorporating a patient-centered approach.

Nurses must be aware of their own attitudes in order to avoid perpetuating stigmatization of this patient because this concern has often been responsible for individuals avoiding treatment from healthcare professionals.

Text continued on page 383

Table 15–2 | CARE PLAN FOR THE PATIENT WITH SCHIZOPHRENIA

NURSING DIAGNOSIS: DISTURBED SENSORY PERCEPTION: AUDITORY/VISUAL

RELATED TO: Panic anxiety, extreme loneliness and withdrawal into the self

EVIDENCED BY: Inappropriate responses, disordered thought sequencing, rapid mood swings, poor concentration, disorientation, patient reports hearing voices that no one else can hear

OUTCOME CRITERIA	NURSING INTERVENTIONS	RATIONALE
Short-Term Goal ■ Patient will discuss content of hallucinations with nurse or therapist within 1 week. **Long-Term Goals** ■ Patient is able to define and test reality, reducing or eliminating the occurrence of hallucinations. (This goal may not be realistic for the individual with severe and persistent illness who has experienced auditory hallucinations for many years.) A more realistic goal may be: ■ Patient will verbalize understanding that the voices are a result of the illness and demonstrate ways to interrupt the hallucination.	1. Assess for signs of hallucinations (listening pose, laughing or talking to self, stopping in midsentence). Ask, "Are you hearing something else?" or "Are you hearing other voices?" If the patient is experiencing command hallucinations, assess the content for evidence of risk of violence toward self or others.	1. Early intervention may prevent aggressive response to command hallucinations. Since the patient may not recognize these voices as hallucinations, it is better to ask the patient what they are hearing rather than use the word *hallucinations*.
	2. Avoid touching the patient without warning them that you are about to do so.	2. Patient may perceive touch as threatening and may respond in an aggressive manner.
	3. An attitude of acceptance will encourage the patient to share the content of the hallucination with you. Ask, "What do you hear the voices saying to you?"	3. Touch is often perceived as threatening to a patient who is already anxious and suspicious.
	4. Do not reinforce the hallucination. Use "the voices" instead of words like *they* that imply validation. Let patient know that you do not share the perception. Say, "Even though I realize the voices are real to you, I do not hear any voices speaking."	4. It is important for the nurse to be honest, and the patient must accept the perception as unreal before hallucinations can be eliminated.
	5. Help the patient understand the connection between increased anxiety and the presence of hallucinations.	5. If the patient can learn to interrupt escalating anxiety, hallucinations may be prevented.
	6. Try to distract the patient from the hallucination. Encourage the patient to listen to music or audiobooks with headphones.	6. Involvement in interpersonal activities and explanation of the actual situation facilitates reality orientation.
	7. For some patients, auditory hallucinations persist after the acute psychotic episode has subsided. Listening to the radio or watching television helps distract some patients from attention to the voices. Others have benefited from an intervention called *voice dismissal*. With this technique, the patient is taught to say loudly, "Go away!" or "Leave me alone!" in a conscious effort to dismiss the auditory perception.	7. These activities assist the patient to exert some conscious control over the hallucination. Listening to music or other content distracts the patient's focus away from auditory hallucinations and may help to decrease associated anxiety.

Table 15–2 | CARE PLAN FOR THE PATIENT WITH SCHIZOPHRENIA—cont'd

NURSING DIAGNOSIS: DISTURBED THOUGHT PROCESSES

RELATED TO: Inability to trust, panic anxiety, possible hereditary and biochemical factors

EVIDENCED BY: Delusional thinking; inability to concentrate; impaired volition; inability to problem-solve, abstract, or conceptualize; extreme suspiciousness of others

OUTCOME CRITERIA	NURSING INTERVENTIONS	RATIONALE
Short-Term Goal ■ By the end of 2 weeks, patient will recognize and verbalize that false ideas occur at times of increased anxiety. **Long-Term Goals** ■ By time of discharge from treatment, patient's verbalizations will reflect reality-based thinking with no evidence of delusional ideation. ■ By time of discharge from treatment, the patient will be able to differentiate between delusional thinking and reality.	1. Convey acceptance of patient's need for the false belief but indicate that you do not share the belief.	1. Patient must understand that you do not view the idea as real.
	2. Do not argue or deny the belief. Use *reasonable doubt* as a therapeutic technique: "I understand that you believe this is true, but I personally find it hard to accept."	2. Arguing with the patient or denying the belief serves no useful purpose; these beliefs are very real to the patient delusional ideas are not eliminated by this approach, and the development of a trusting relationship may be impeded.
	3. Reinforce and focus on reality. Although initially encouraging the patient to describe their thoughts may help to understand the patient's experience, discourage long ruminations about the irrational thinking. Talk about real events and real people.	3. Repeated discussions that focus on the false ideas are purposeless and useless and may even aggravate the psychosis.
	4. If patient is highly suspicious, the following interventions may be helpful: a. Use same staff as much as possible; be honest and keep all promises. b. Avoid physical contact; ask the patient before touching to perform a procedure, such as taking a blood pressure. c. Avoid laughing, whispering, or talking quietly where patient can see but cannot hear what is being said. d. Provide canned food with can opener or serve food family style. e. Mouth checks may be necessary following medication administration to verify whether the patient is actually swallowing the pills. f. Provide activities that encourage a one-to-one relationship with the nurse or therapist. g. Maintain an assertive, matter-of-fact, yet genuine approach.	4. To decrease patient's suspiciousness: a. Familiar staff and honesty promote trust. b. Patients with suspicious ideation often perceive touch as threatening and may respond in an aggressive or defensive manner. c. Patients may have ideas of reference and believe they are being talked about. d. Suspicious patients may believe they are being poisoned and refuse to eat food from an individually prepared tray. e. Suspicious patients may believe they are being poisoned with their medication and attempt to discard the tablets or capsules. f. Competitive activities may exacerbate suspicious ideation. g. Patients with suspicious ideation are prone to distrust and are hypervigilant of people's behavior and communication. Approaches that are overly directive or cheerful may increase the patient's suspiciousness.

Continued

Table 15–2 | CARE PLAN FOR THE PATIENT WITH SCHIZOPHRENIA—cont'd

NURSING DIAGNOSIS: SOCIAL ISOLATION

RELATED TO: Inability to trust, panic anxiety, delusional thinking, regression, lack of interest or skills in interpersonal interaction

EVIDENCED BY: Withdrawal, sad, dull affect, preoccupation with own thoughts, expression of feelings of rejection or of aloneness imposed by others

OUTCOME CRITERIA	NURSING INTERVENTIONS	RATIONALE
Short-Term Goal ■ Patient will willingly attend therapy activities accompanied by trusted staff member within 1 week. **Long-Term Goal** ■ Patient will voluntarily spend time with other patients and staff members in group therapeutic activities.	1. Convey an accepting attitude by making brief, frequent contacts. 2. Show unconditional positive regard. 3. Offer to be with patient during group activities that the patient finds frightening or difficult. 4. Give recognition and positive reinforcement for patient's voluntary interactions with others.	1. An accepting attitude increases feelings of self-worth and facilitates trust. 2. This conveys a belief in the patient as a worthwhile human being. 3. The presence of a trusted individual provides emotional security for the patient. 4. Positive reinforcement enhances self-esteem and encourages repetition of acceptable behaviors.

NURSING DIAGNOSIS: RISK FOR VIOLENCE: SELF-DIRECTED OR OTHER-DIRECTED

RISK FACTORS: Extreme suspiciousness, panic anxiety, catatonic excitement, rage reactions, command hallucinations, overt and aggressive acts, goal-directed destruction of objects in the environment, self-destructive behavior or active aggressive suicidal acts

OUTCOME CRITERIA	NURSING INTERVENTIONS	RATIONALE
Short-Term Goals ■ Within [a specified time], patient will recognize signs of increasing anxiety and agitation and report to staff (or other care provider) for assistance with intervention. ■ Patient will not harm self or others. **Long-Term Goal** ■ Patient will not harm self or others.	1. Maintain low level of stimuli in patient's environment (low lighting, few people, simple decor, low noise level). 2. Observe behavior frequently. Do this while carrying out routine activities. 3. Remove all dangerous objects from patient's environment. Assess for risk of violence toward others or suicidal ideation. 4. Intervene at the first sign of increased anxiety, agitation, or verbal or behavioral aggression. Offer empathetic response to the patient's feelings: "You seem anxious [or frustrated or angry] about this situation. How can I help?"	1. Anxiety level rises in a stimulating environment. A suspicious, agitated patient may perceive individuals as threatening. 2. Observation during routine activities avoids creating suspiciousness on the part of the patient. Close observation is necessary so that intervention can occur if required to ensure patient (and others') safety. 3. Removal of dangerous objects prevents patient, in an agitated, confused state, from using them to harm self or others. 4. Validation of the patient's feelings conveys a caring attitude and offering assistance reinforces trust.

Table 15–2 | CARE PLAN FOR THE PATIENT WITH SCHIZOPHRENIA—cont'd

OUTCOME CRITERIA	NURSING INTERVENTIONS	RATIONALE
	5. It is important to maintain a calm attitude toward the patient. As the patient's anxiety increases, offer some alternatives: participating in a physical activity (e.g., physical exercise), talking about the situation, taking some antianxiety medication.	5. Offering alternatives to the patient gives them a feeling of some control over the situation.
	6. Have sufficient staff available to indicate a show of strength to the patient if it becomes necessary.	6. This shows the patient evidence of control over the situation and provides some physical security for staff.
	7. If patient is not calmed by "talking down" or by medication, use of mechanical restraints may be necessary.	7. The avenue of the "least restrictive alternative" must be selected when planning interventions for a violent patient. Restraints should be used only as a last resort after all other interventions have been unsuccessful and the patient is clearly at risk of harm to self or others.
	8. If restraint is deemed necessary, ensure that sufficient staff is available to assist. Follow the protocol established by the institution.	8. These interventions are necessary for the protection of patient and staff.
	9. Ensure that the patient in restraints is assessed at least every 15 minutes to ensure that circulation to extremities is not compromised (check temperature, color, pulses); to assist the patient with needs related to nutrition, hydration, and elimination; and to position the patient so that comfort is facilitated, and aspiration is prevented. Maintain continuous one-to-one monitoring of restrained patients, to assess level of agitation and to prevent injury.	9. Patient safety is a nursing priority.
	10. As agitation decreases, assess the patient's readiness for restraint removal or reduction. Remove one restraint at a time while assessing the patient's response.	10. This minimizes the risk of injury to patient and staff.

Continued

Table 15–2 | CARE PLAN FOR THE PATIENT WITH SCHIZOPHRENIA—cont'd

NURSING DIAGNOSIS: IMPAIRED VERBAL COMMUNICATION

RELATED TO: Panic anxiety, regression, withdrawal, disordered and delusional thinking

EVIDENCED BY: Loose association of ideas, neologisms, word salad, clang association, echolalia, verbalizations that reflect concrete thinking, poor eye contact

OUTCOME CRITERIA	INTERVENTION	RATIONALE
Short-Term Goal ■ Patient will demonstrate the ability to remain on one topic using appropriate, intermittent eye contact for 5 minutes with the nurse or therapist.	1. Attempt to decode incomprehensible communication patterns. Seek validation and clarification by asking, "Is it that you mean . . .?" or "I don't understand what you mean by that. Would you please explain it to me?"	1. These techniques reveal how the patient is being perceived by others and convey the nurse's desire to establish meaningful communication.
	2. Maintain staff assignments as consistently as possible.	2. This facilitates trust and understanding between patient and nurse.
Long-Term Goal ■ By time of discharge from treatment, the patient will demonstrate ability to carry on a verbal communication in a socially acceptable manner with health-care providers and peers.	3. The technique of *verbalizing the implied* is used with the patient who is struggling to communicate thoughts and feelings. Example: "That must be frightening to worry that others are wiretapping your house."	3. This approach conveys empathy and may encourage the patient to disclose thoughts and feelings.
	4. Anticipate and fulfill patient's needs until functional communication pattern returns.	4. Patient safety and comfort are nursing priorities.
	5. Orient patient to reality as needed. Call the patient by name. Validate those aspects of communication that help differentiate between what is real and not real.	5. These techniques may facilitate restoration of functional communication patterns in the patient.
	6. Explanations must be provided at the patient's level of comprehension. Example: "Pick up the spoon, scoop some mashed potatoes into it, and put it in your mouth."	6. Because concrete thinking may be a symptom, abstract phrases and clichés must be avoided because they are likely to be misinterpreted.

NURSING DIAGNOSIS: SELF-CARE DEFICIT

RELATED TO: Withdrawal, regression, panic anxiety, perceptual or cognitive impairment, inability to trust

EVIDENCED BY: Difficulty carrying out tasks associated with hygiene, dressing, grooming, eating, toileting

OUTCOME CRITERIA	NURSING INTERVENTIONS	RATIONALE
Short-Term Goal ■ Patient will verbalize a desire to perform activities of daily living (ADLs) by end of 1 week.	1. Provide assistance with self-care needs as required. Some patients who are severely withdrawn may require total care.	1. Patient safety and comfort are nursing priorities.
	2. Encourage the patient to perform as many activities as possible independently. Provide positive reinforcement for independent accomplishments.	2. Independent accomplishment and positive reinforcement enhance self-esteem and promote repetition of desirable behaviors.

Table 15–2 | CARE PLAN FOR THE PATIENT WITH SCHIZOPHRENIA—cont'd

OUTCOME CRITERIA	NURSING INTERVENTIONS	RATIONALE
Long-Term Goal ■ Patient will perform ADLs in an independent manner and demonstrate a willingness to do so by time of discharge from treatment.	3. Use concrete communication to show the patient what is expected and to minimize misinterpretation by the patient. Provide step-by-step instructions for assistance in performing ADLs. Example: "Take your pajamas off and put them in the drawer. Take your shirt and pants from the closet and put them on. Comb your hair and brush your teeth."	3. Because concrete thinking may be a symptom, explanations must be provided at the patient's concrete level of comprehension.
	4. Creative approaches may need to be taken with the patient who is not eating, such as allowing patient to open own canned or packaged foods; family-style serving may also be an option.	4. These techniques may be helpful with the patient who is paranoid and may be suspicious about being poisoned with food or medication.
	5. If toileting needs are not being met, establish a structured schedule for the patient.	5. A structured schedule will help the patient establish a pattern to develop a habit of toileting independently.

Real Nurses, Real Advice

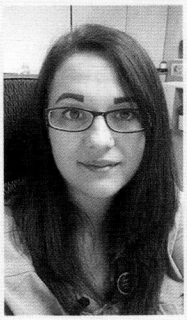

"The delusions, paranoia, and voices are very real to the patient with schizophrenia, so making sure not to devalue their experience is very important. It can also be a frightening experience so approaching slowly, staying at least an arm's length away, and speaking in a calming voice lets them know that you are there to help. Many times they just want someone to listen and treat them like a person first instead of always seeing their illness first."

–**Sarah Taylor,** Psychiatric Nursing Supervisor

One way to reduce stigma is to become familiar with real people who suffer from this disorder rather than relying on fictitious representations (and sometimes misrepresentations) of this population in popular media. (See the "Real People, Real Stories" introduction to Dr. Fred Frese.)

A case management model (see Chapter 6, "The Nursing Process in Psychiatric Mental Health Nursing") may be used to coordinate care. In general, team approaches to the care of the patient with schizophrenia have been identified as essential to positive outcomes and recovery.

Concept Care Mapping

The concept map care plan is a diagrammatic teaching and learning strategy that allows visualization of interrelationships between medical diagnoses, nursing diagnoses, assessment data, and treatments (see Chapter 6, "The Nursing Process in Psychiatric Mental Health Nursing"). An example of a concept map care plan for a patient with schizophrenia is presented in Figure 15–2.

Patient and Family Education

The role of patient and family educator is important in the psychiatric area, as it is in all areas of nursing. A list of topics for patient and family education relevant to schizophrenia is presented in Box 15–5.

Evaluation

In the final step of the nursing process, a reassessment is conducted in order to determine whether the nursing actions have been successful in achieving the objectives of care. Evaluation of the nursing actions for the patient with exacerbation of schizophrenic

Real People, Real Stories: Dr. Fred Frese

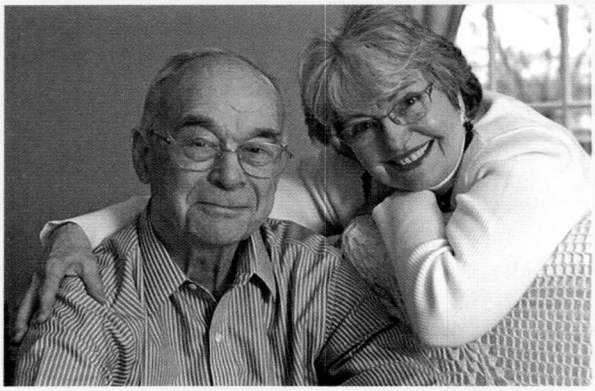

People with schizophrenia continue to be disenfranchised, misunderstood, and stigmatized. Even within health care, evidence has shown that some settings have been very hostile to people with serious mental illnesses. One way to begin combating stigmatization of people with mental illness is to get to know them personally. Dr. Fred Frese is a licensed psychologist and an internationally renowned speaker, writer, and advocate in the field of mental illness.

Karyn: Could you share a little bit about your history with the illness of schizophrenia?

Dr. Frese: I was 25 when I had my first episode. I was in the Marines and—I know I had seen the movie *The Manchurian Candidate* previously—and I began to think that the Vietnamese were using the same strategies from the movie to control us. When I let my commanding officer know my theories, I was hospitalized involuntarily, and for the next 10 years I was in and out of hospitals—mostly involuntarily—taking various medications, living many different places, and not employed.

Karyn: Were you getting any treatments or intervention that you thought were helpful to your recovery?

Dr. Frese: Well, at that time it was thought that schizophrenia was not an illness from which one could recover. Even recently, I've heard some folks who have a family member with schizophrenia say, "There's no way that anyone with this illness can get better." But that's starting to change, and now that the government, through SAMHSA (Substance Abuse and Mental Health Services Administration) is backing the recovery model approach, I think health care will improve. I remember being told that my brain was going to progressively deteriorate and that I would never be able to function on my own. All in all, I probably spent about a year of my life in hospitalizations. Once the laws changed and I knew you had to be of imminent harm to yourself or others in order to be hospitalized involuntarily, I talked some of the health professionals out of admitting me. During the last attempt to hospitalize me, I actually escaped and ran away, even though I was in pretty bad shape.

Karyn: So since you were knowledgeable about the laws, you could essentially be your own self-advocate and argue your case, so to speak?

Dr. Frese: Yes, and by that time, I was in grad school and had secured a job at what is now the Department of Mental Health and Addiction Services. I remember I was living in the hallway of some university housing, and one of the students, who saw me day after day just hanging around and not really doing anything, suggested that I might be eligible for a government job because of my military background. When I applied, the receptionist saw my history of mental health commitments and said I would never get the job, but I did. The last time I went to the hospital, I went voluntarily because I knew I needed more medication, but they thought I needed to be hospitalized and I didn't; so I ran away.

Karyn: Sounds like you were managing a lot of stuff—grad school, working—and, at the same time, episodically struggling with symptoms of illness. You were working in the field of mental health, too. Was the work environment supportive?

Dr. Frese: Not always. It seemed like even among my coworkers, when something strange happened, they thought it was something wrong with me.

Karyn: What do you mean by "something strange"?

Dr. Frese: Like one time when they perceived I was spending too much time interacting with patients, they assumed I was "going off again," and next thing I knew, they called a "blue alert" and wanted to hospitalize me. But that time, the medical director just told me to take some time off. I never did find out why they called that blue alert.

Karyn: So you haven't been hospitalized for a very long time, and you are internationally renowned for all of your work and advocacy in the field of mental health. What do you think has contributed most to your recovery?

Dr. Frese: No, I haven't been hospitalized since I got married. I think that has been central in my recovery: having a person who you trust to give you feedback and let me know when I need more medication.

Karyn: What role do medications play in recovery?

Dr. Frese: It's very individual. We need more research to identify who, among people with schizophrenia, will benefit most by continuous medication versus episodic, reduced doses, or no medication. Genetic research is hopeful, but we're not there yet. It's hard to advise any individual what to do without knowing their individual circumstances, and even knowing, it can be very hard.

Karyn: What do you think is most important for future nurses to know about what they should do or say when they encounter someone with schizophrenia in a healthcare setting, such as ER, for example?

Real People, Real Stories: Dr. Fred Frese—cont'd

Dr. Frese: Even though Freud's theories about psychoanalysis and insight-oriented therapy have been shown in research to be not only *not* helpful in the treatment of people with schizophrenia but potentially harmful, these ideas continue to influence the thinking of health-care professionals. I would tell nurses to wean themselves away from psychoanalytic concepts in treating people with schizophrenia. There continue to be assumptions that something bad must have happened in this patient's childhood, and the family is probably to blame. It's not a good way to forge relationships and may prejudge or isolate the people that can provide invaluable support.

So I would say to future nurses, don't make assumptions about me because you see a diagnosis or the kind of medication I'm on, and don't try to blame anyone for my symptoms. Treat me with civility and respect, don't respond to me with shock and disbelief, bullying, or laughing at me. Listening to the patient is the best way to establish and maintain a relationship. Even if the patient is saying something that doesn't make any sense to you, the best response is, "That's very interesting; tell me more."

To learn more about Dr. Frese, go to www.fredfrese.com.

psychosis may be facilitated by gathering information utilizing the following types of questions:

- Has the patient established trust with at least one staff member?
- Is anxiety maintained at a manageable level?
- Is delusional thinking still prevalent?
- Is hallucinogenic activity evident? Does the patient share content of hallucinations, particularly if commands are heard?
- Is the patient able to manage escalating anxiety with adaptive coping mechanisms?
- Is the patient easily agitated?
- Is the patient able to interact with others appropriately?
- Does the patient voluntarily attend therapy activities?
- Is verbal communication comprehensible?
- Is the patient compliant with medication? Does the patient verbalize the importance of taking medication regularly and on a long-term basis? Does the patient verbalize understanding of possible side effects and when to seek assistance from the physician?
- Does the patient spend time with others rather than isolating self?
- Is the patient able to carry out all activities of daily living independently?
- Is the patient able to verbalize resources for seeking assistance outside the hospital?
- Does the family have information regarding support groups in which they may participate and from which they may seek assistance in dealing with their family member who is ill?
- If the patient lives alone, do they have a source for assistance with home maintenance and health management?

Quality and Safety Education for Nurses (QSEN)

The Institute of Medicine (IOM), in its 2003 report *Health Professions Education: A Bridge to Quality*, challenged faculties of medicine, nursing, and other health professions to ensure that their graduates have achieved a core set of competencies in order to meet the needs of the 21st-century health-care system. These competencies include *providing patient-centered care, maintaining safety, working in interdisciplinary teams, employing evidence-based practice, incorporating quality improvement,* and *utilizing informatics.*

Patient-centered care is foundational to the recovery model (see Chapter 10, "The Recovery Model"), which has been advanced as an important framework for empowering clients with serious mental illnesses like schizophrenia. This model promotes active patient engagement in treatment with a focus on achieving their full recovery potential. However, in order to maintain *patient safety* and because some patients lack insight about their need for treatment, decisions may need to be made for these patients in their best interest. Supporting the patient's recovery necessitates the use of several resources and disciplines, which may include housing and financial assistance, medication management, peer support, spiritual counsel, and case management services. It is essential that nurses working with this population have a good understanding of the available support services for patients with schizophrenia and that they effectively work within *interdisciplinary teams* to meet this patient's complex needs.

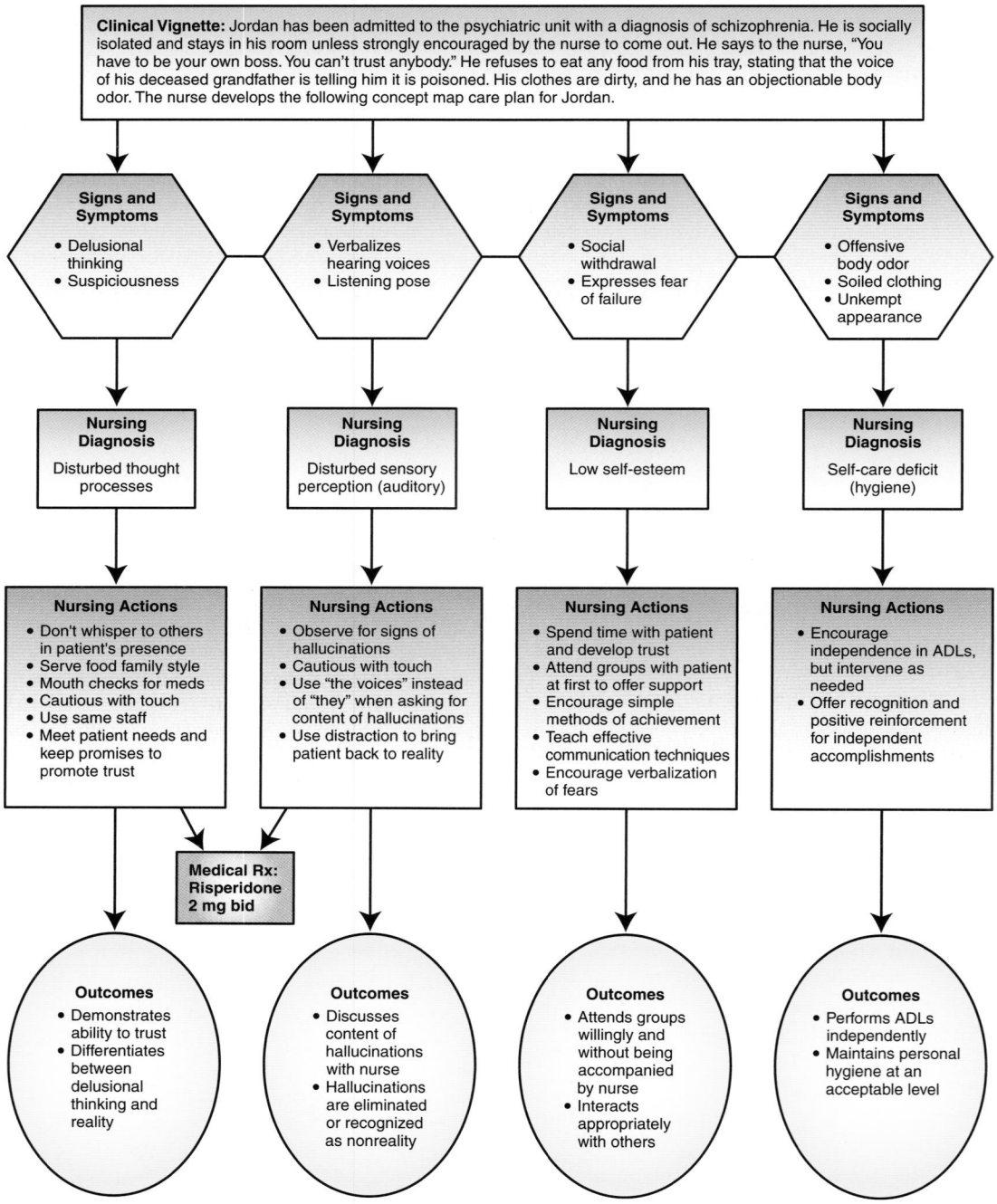

FIGURE 15–2 Concept map care plan for a patient with schizophrenia.

Treatment Modalities

The prognosis for schizophrenia has often been reported in a paradigm of thirds. About one-third of the people achieve significant and lasting improvement. They may never experience another episode of psychosis following the initial occurrence. One-third may achieve some improvement with intermittent relapses and residual disability. Their occupational level may have decreased because of their illness, or they may be socially isolated. Finally, one-third experience severe and permanent incapacity. They often

BOX 15–5 Topics for Patient and Family Education Related to Schizophrenia

NATURE OF THE ILLNESS
1. What to expect as the illness progresses
2. Symptoms associated with the illness
3. Ways for family to respond to behaviors associated with the illness

MANAGEMENT OF THE ILLNESS
1. Connection of exacerbation of symptoms to times of stress
2. Appropriate medication management
3. Side effects of medications
4. Importance of not stopping medications
5. When to contact health-care provider
6. Relaxation techniques
7. Social skills training
8. Daily living skills training

SUPPORT SERVICES
1. Financial assistance
2. Housing
3. Legal assistance
4. Caregiver support groups
5. Respite care
6. Home health care
7. Residential treatment options

do not respond to medication and remain severely ill for much of their lives. Men typically have poorer outcomes than women do; women respond better to treatment with antipsychotic medications. Although the paradigm of thirds provides a general guideline for understanding the variable course and prognosis in schizophrenia, Jablensky (2017) notes that with each successive decade there has been a trend toward a less deteriorating course in schizophrenia, which may be attributed to both treatment advances and changes in attitudes about this illness.

Psychological Treatments

Individual Psychotherapy

Individual recovery-oriented psychotherapy and cognitive therapies are evidence-based interventions in the treatment of the client with schizophrenia, but they should be adjuncts to a multifaceted team approach. The primary focus in all cases must reflect efforts to decrease anxiety and increase trust.

Establishing a relationship is often particularly difficult because the individual with schizophrenia is desperately lonely yet defends against closeness and trust. The individual is likely to respond to attempts at closeness with suspiciousness, anxiety, aggression, or regression. Successful intervention may be achieved with honesty, simple directness, and a manner that respects the client's privacy and human dignity. Exaggerated warmth and professions of friendship are likely to be met with confusion and suspicion.

Once a therapeutic interpersonal relationship has been established, reality orientation is maintained through exploration of the client's behavior in relationships. Education is provided to help the client identify sources of real or perceived danger and ways of reacting appropriately. Methods for improving interpersonal communication, emotional expression, and frustration tolerance are attempted.

Group Therapy

Group therapy for individuals with schizophrenia has been shown to be effective, particularly with outpatients and when combined with drug treatment.

Boland and Verduin (2022) stated:

> Group therapy for persons with schizophrenia generally focuses on real-life plans, problems, and relationships. Some investigators doubt that dynamic interpretation and insight therapy are valuable for typical patients with schizophrenia. But group therapy is effective in reducing social isolation, increasing the sense of cohesiveness, and improving reality testing for patients with schizophrenia. (p. 355)

Group therapy in inpatient settings is less productive. Inpatient treatment usually occurs when symptomatology and social disorganization are at their most intense. At this time, having the least stimuli possible is most beneficial for the patient. Because group therapy can be intensive and highly stimulating, it may be counterproductive early in treatment.

Group therapy for schizophrenia has been most useful over the long-term course of the illness. The social interaction, sense of cohesiveness, identification, and reality testing achieved within the group setting have proven to be highly therapeutic processes for individuals with this illness. Groups that offer a supportive environment appear to be more helpful than those that follow a more confrontational approach.

Behavior Therapy

Behavior modification has a history of qualified success in reducing the frequency of bizarre, disturbing, and deviant behaviors and increasing appropriate behaviors. Features that have led to the most positive results include the following:

- Clearly defining goals and how they will be measured
- Attaching positive, negative, and aversive reinforcements to adaptive and maladaptive behavior
- Using simple, concrete instructions and prompts to elicit the desired behavior

In the treatment setting, the health-care provider can use praise and other positive reinforcements to help the patient with schizophrenia reduce the frequency of maladaptive or deviant behaviors. A limitation of this type of therapy is the inability of some individuals with schizophrenia to generalize what they have learned from the treatment setting to the community setting.

Social Treatments

Social Skills Training

Social skills training is used to help clients manage struggles with interpersonal relationships and communication, which are often complicated by clients' inability to accurately perceive responses in others. Mueser and colleagues (2001) describe this training as follows:

> The basic premise of social skills training is that complex interpersonal skills involve the smooth integration of a combination of simpler behaviors, including *nonverbal behaviors* (e.g., facial expression, eye contact); *paralinguistic features* (e.g., voice loudness and affect); *verbal content* (i.e., the appropriateness of what is said); and *interactive balance* (e.g., response latency, amount of time talking). These specific skills can be systematically taught, and, through the process of *shaping* (i.e., rewarding successive approximations toward the target behavior), complex behavioral repertoires can be acquired.

Social dysfunction is a hallmark of schizophrenia. Impairment in interpersonal relations is included as part of the defining diagnostic criteria for the condition in the *DSM-5-TR* (APA, 2022). Considerable attention is now being given to enhancement of social skills for this population.

The educational procedure in social skills training focuses on role-play. A series of brief scenarios are selected. These should be typical of situations that clients experience in their daily lives and be graduated in terms of level of difficulty. The health-care provider may serve as a role model for some behaviors,—for example, "See how I sort of nod my head up and down and look at your face while you talk." This demonstration is followed by the client's role-playing. Immediate feedback is provided regarding the client's presentation. Only by countless repetitions does the response gradually become smooth and effortless.

Progress is geared toward the individual's needs and limitations. The focus is on small units of behavior, and the training proceeds very gradually. Highly threatening issues are avoided, and emphasis is placed on functional skills that are relevant to activities of daily living. *Milieu therapy*, which focuses on the client's interaction within a social environment, may provide opportunities for social skills training.

Cognitive Remediation Therapy

As mentioned previously, many of the cognitive deficits common in schizophrenia have not been particularly responsive to existing pharmacological treatments. However, some evidence suggests that cognitive therapies, which include social cognition training, can be an effective treatment. Cognitive remediation is based on behavioral training aimed at helping the client to mend areas of cognitive dysfunction, including attention, memory, social cognition, and executive functions. The intervention entails repetitive drills and practice. The evidence supports that this training results in significant improvements in memory, attention, problem-solving, cognition, social cognition, independent living skills, and social adjustment (Tripathi et al., 2018).

Family Therapy

Schizophrenia is an illness that can puzzle, disrupt, and sometimes tear apart families. Even when families appear to cope well, there is a notable impact on the mental and physical health of relatives when a family member has the illness.

The importance of the expanded role of family in the aftercare of relatives with schizophrenia has been recognized, thereby stimulating interest in family intervention programs designed to support the family system, prevent or delay relapse, and help maintain the client in the community. These psychoeducational programs treat the family as a resource rather than a stressor, with the focus on concrete problem-solving and specific helping behaviors for coping with stress. These programs recognize the biological basis for schizophrenia and the impact that stress has on the client's ability to function. By providing the family with information about the illness and suggestions for effective coping, psychoeducational programs reduce the likelihood of the client's relapse and the possible emergence of mental illness in previously nonaffected relatives.

Mueser and associates (2001) stated that although models of family intervention with schizophrenia differ in their characteristics and methods, effective treatment programs share a number of common features:

- All programs are long term (usually 9 months to 2 years or longer).
- They all provide the client and family with information about the illness and its management.
- They focus on improving adherence to prescribed medications.
- They strive to decrease stress in the family and improve family functioning.

Asen (2002) suggested the following interventions with families of individuals with schizophrenia:

- Forming a close alliance with the caregivers
- Lowering the emotional intrafamily climate by reducing stress and burden on relatives
- Increasing the ability of relatives to anticipate and solve problems
- Reducing the expressions of anger and guilt by family members
- Maintaining reasonable expectations for how the ill family member should perform
- Encouraging relatives to set appropriate limits while maintaining some degree of separateness
- Promoting desirable changes in the relatives' behaviors and belief systems

Family therapy typically consists of a brief program of family education about schizophrenia and a more extended program of family contact designed to reduce overt manifestations of conflict and to improve patterns of family communication and problem-solving. The response to this type of therapy has been very dramatic. Studies have clearly revealed that a more positive outcome in the treatment of the client with schizophrenia can be achieved by including the family system in the program of care (Caqueo-Urízar et al., 2015).

Assertive Community Treatment

Assertive community treatment (ACT) is an evidence-based program of case management that takes a team approach in providing comprehensive, community-based psychiatric treatment, rehabilitation, and support to persons with serious and persistent mental illness such as schizophrenia. Other terms for this type of treatment include *mobile treatment teams* and *community support programs.* Assertive programs of treatment are individually tailored for each client, intended to be proactive, and include the teaching of basic living skills, helping clients work with community agencies, and assisting clients in developing a social support network. Vocational expectations are emphasized, and supportive work settings (i.e., sheltered workshops) are an important part of the treatment program. Other services include substance abuse treatment, psychoeducational programs, family support and education, mobile crisis intervention, and attention to health-care needs.

Responsibilities are shared by multiple team members, including psychiatrists, nurses, social workers, vocational rehabilitation therapists, and substance abuse counselors. Services are provided in the person's home; within the neighborhood; in local restaurants, parks, stores; or wherever assistance by the client is required. These services are available to the client 24 hours a day, 365 days a year, and ACT is considered a long-term intervention strategy. One recent study looked at the impact of a *Housing First* intervention (an intervention that prioritizes rapid re-housing for homeless individuals with schizophrenia) and found that when this type of intervention was combined with ACT, medication adherence improved from below 50% to 78%. Additionally, these combined interventions improved clients' integration into the community, increased residential stability, and decreased criminal convictions (Rezansoff et al., 2016).

ACT has been shown to reduce the number of hospitalizations and decrease costs of care. Although it has been called "paternalistic" and "coercive" by its critics, ACT has provided much-needed services and improved quality of life for many clients who are unable to manage in a less-structured environment. One limitation is that treatment programs of this kind are time and labor intensive.

The Recovery Model

Research provides support for recovery as an obtainable objective for individuals with schizophrenia (Lysaker et al., 2010). Lysaker and associates state:

> Recovery from schizophrenia, in the sense of a state in which persons experience no difficulties associated with the illness, can occur but the modal outcome seems to be one in which difficulties linked to symptoms, social function, and work appear periodically but can be successfully confronted. (p. 40)

Conceptual models of recovery from mental illness are presented in Chapter 10, "The Recovery Model."

The recovery model has been used primarily in caring for individuals with serious mental illness, such as schizophrenia and bipolar disorder. However, concepts of the model are amenable to use with all individuals experiencing emotional conditions with which they require assistance and who have a desire to take control and manage their lives more independently.

Weiden (2010) identifies two types of recovery with schizophrenia: functional and process. *Functional recovery* focuses on the individual's level of functioning in such areas as relationships, work, independent living, and other kinds of life functioning. The individual may or may not be experiencing active symptoms of schizophrenia.

Weiden (2010) suggests that recovery can also be considered as a process. With *process recovery*, there is no defined end point, but recovery is viewed as a process that continues throughout the individual's life and involves collaboration between client and clinician. The individual identifies goals based on personal values or what they define as giving meaning and purpose to life. The clinician and client work together to develop a treatment plan that is in alignment with the goals set forth by the client. In the process recovery model, the individual may still be experiencing symptoms. Weiden states:

> Patients do not have to be in remission, nor does remission automatically have to be a desired (or likely) goal when embarking on a recovery-oriented treatment plan. As long as the patient (and family) understands that a process recovery treatment plan is not to be confused with a promise of "cure" or even "remission," then one does not overpromise.

The concept of recovery in schizophrenia remains controversial among clinicians, and many challenges lie ahead for continued study. Recovery models have similarities with ACT in that they both necessarily engage the support of multiple resources, but recovery models also highlight the dimension of active engagement and empowerment of the client in decision making. Some argue that this approach is difficult to implement when clients lack insight about their illness or the need for treatment. Furthermore, there is a lack of consistency in what constitutes "recovery," and many concepts exist.

One of the identified QSEN competencies is *patient-centered care* and despite the controversies about the recovery model approach, the hope is that as these models become better studied and more clearly defined, they will provide a treatment approach that is comprehensive, protective, and supportive of patient-centered care.

RAISE (Recovery After an Initial Schizophrenia Episode)

The RAISE approach to treatment for schizophrenia is based on a large National Institute of Mental Health (NIMH) initiative that began in 2008. Research findings published in 2015 have demonstrated several benefits of this approach. Kane and associates (2015, p. 2) describe the RAISE approach as follows:

> The premise of the NIMH RAISE-ETP (Early Treatment Program) is to combine state-of-the-art pharmacologic and psychosocial treatments delivered by a well-trained, multidisciplinary team, in order to significantly improve the functional outcome and quality of life for first episode psychosis patients.

The RAISE approach incorporates many elements from other treatment approaches, including community treatment, recovery model approaches, family approaches, and comprehensive care models. It adds the dimension of early intervention at the first episode of psychosis. The research findings after 5 years of studying this approach look very promising for improving care to this population when intervention begins at the earliest onset of psychotic symptoms. Positive outcomes have included greater adherence to treatment programs; greater improvement in symptoms, interpersonal relationships, and quality of life; more involvement in employment or educational pursuits; and less frequent hospitalizations than are seen for clients involved in more traditional treatment approaches (Kane et al., 2015).

The hope for this approach to treatment is that, through early and comprehensive intervention, the long-term, debilitating consequences of schizophrenia can be averted or minimized.

Psychopharmacological Treatment

Chlorpromazine (Thorazine) was first introduced in the United States in 1952. At that time, it was used in conjunction with barbiturates in surgical anesthesia. With increased use, the drug's psychic properties were recognized, and by 1954 it was marketed as an antipsychotic medication in the United States. The manufacture and sale of other antipsychotic drugs followed in rapid succession.

Antipsychotic medications are also called *neuroleptics* and historically were referred to as *major tranquilizers*. They are effective in the treatment of acute and chronic manifestations of schizophrenia and in maintenance therapy to prevent exacerbation of schizophrenic symptoms. A meta-analysis of studies (Takeuchi et al., 2017) evaluating the benefits of maintenance antipsychotic medication found that there was a significant worsening of symptoms over the course of a year in patients who did not continue on medication.

As mentioned earlier, the efficacy of antipsychotic medications is enhanced by adjunct psychosocial therapy. Because the psychotic manifestations of the illness subside with use of the drugs, clients are generally more cooperative with the psychosocial therapies. However, although the sedative effects are relatively immediate, it takes several weeks for the antipsychotics to effectively treat positive symptoms, a fact that often leads to discontinuation of the medication. Clients and families need to be educated about the importance of waiting, often for several weeks, to determine whether the drug will be effective.

These medications are classified as either typical antipsychotics (first generation with more dopaminergic activity) or atypical antipsychotics (second generation with more serotonergic activity). In 2019 a newer novel drug (that does not bind to D_2 or 5-HT_{2A}) was given U.S. Food and Drug Administration (FDA) "breakthrough therapy" approval for investigation, and early results indicate that it may be effective in treating both positive and negative symptoms (Ernst, 2019). Examples of commonly used antipsychotic agents are presented in Table 15–3. A description of these medications follows. More detailed information is available in Chapter 4, "Psychopharmacology."

Indications

Antipsychotic medications are used in the treatment of schizophrenia and other psychotic disorders. Selected agents are used in the treatment of bipolar mania (olanzapine, aripiprazole, chlorpromazine, quetiapine, risperidone, asenapine, ziprasidone).

Action

Typical antipsychotics work by blocking postsynaptic dopamine (D_2) receptors in the basal ganglia, hypothalamus, limbic system, brainstem, and medulla. They also demonstrate varying affinity for cholinergic, $alpha_1$-adrenergic, and histaminic receptors. Antipsychotic effects may also be related to inhibition of dopamine-mediated transmission of neural impulses at the synapses.

Atypical antipsychotics are weaker dopamine receptor antagonists than the conventional antipsychotics but are more potent antagonists of the serotonin (5-hydroxytryptamine) type 2A (5-HT_{2A}) receptors. They also exhibit antagonism for cholinergic, histaminic, and adrenergic receptors.

Positive symptoms respond relatively well to treatment with both typical (first generation) and atypical (second generation) antipsychotic medication. Boland and Verduin (2022) identify that positive symptoms tend to become less severe over time, whereas the negative or "deficit" symptoms are socially debilitating and may increase in severity. Atypical antipsychotics have been advanced as being somewhat more effective than first generation antipsychotics in treating negative symptoms (particularly cariprazine), but researchers continue to search for medications that will specifically treat the several cognitive deficits that are most problematic for patients with schizophrenia. These deficits include memory, attention, language, and executive functions, and they can dramatically impact an individual's overall functional ability.

A detailed discussion of contraindications, precautions, side effects, and drug interactions associated with antipsychotic medications is available in Chapter 4, "Psychopharmacology."

Side Effects

The effects of these medications are related to blockage of a number of receptors for which they exhibit various degrees of affinity. Blockade of the dopamine receptors is thought to be responsible for controlling positive symptoms of schizophrenia. Dopamine blockade also results in extrapyramidal symptoms (EPS) and prolactin elevation (galactorrhea; gynecomastia). (A list of medications commonly used to treat EPS is included in Table 15–4.) Cholinergic blockade causes anticholinergic side effects (dry mouth, blurred vision, constipation, urinary retention, and tachycardia). Blockage of the $alpha_1$-adrenergic receptors produces dizziness, orthostatic hypotension, tremors, and reflex tachycardia. Histamine blockade is associated with weight gain and sedation.

The plan of care should include monitoring for the side effects from antipsychotic medications and educating the patient and family about safety precautions when taking antipsychotic medication. (A list of side effects and relevant nursing interventions is included in Chapter 4, "Psychopharmacology.")

There have been two recent and novel developments in psychopharmacological treatments for patients with schizophrenia. The first is a formulation of aripiprazole (AbilifyMyCite) with a tracking sensor that allows the client (and others) to monitor whether the medication was taken. Approved in late 2017, this formulation has spurred controversy and debate about the benefits versus the potential intrusiveness of such a monitoring device. The second

TABLE 15-3 Antipsychotic Agents

CATEGORY	GENERIC (TRADE NAME)	DAILY DOSAGE RANGE (MG)
Typical antipsychotic agents (first generation; conventional)	Chlorpromazine	40–400
	Fluphenazine	2.5–10
	Haloperidol (Haldol)	1–100
	Loxapine	20–250
	Perphenazine	12–64
	Pimozide (Orap)	1–10
	Prochlorperazine	15–150
	Thioridazine	150–800
	Thiothixene (Navane)	6–30
	Trifluoperazine	4–40
Atypical antipsychotic agents (second generation; novel)	Aripiprazole (Abilify)	10–30
	(Abilify MyCite; with tracking sensor)	2–30
	Aripiprazole lauroxil (Aristada)	441–662 monthly, 882 every 6 weeks, 1064 every 2 months (IM injection)
	Asenapine (Saphris) (SL)	10–20
	(Secuado) (transdermal)	3.8–7.6 every 24 hr
	Brexpiprazole (Rexulti)	2–4
	Lumateperone (Caplyta)	42 daily
	Cariprazine (Vraylor)	1.5–6
	Clozapine (Clozaril)	300–900
	Iloperidone (Fanapt)	12–24
	Lurasidone (Latuda)	40–80
	Olanzapine (Zyprexa)	5–20
	Paliperidone (Invega)	6–12
	(Invega Sustenna—once a month)	39–234 (IM injection)
	(Invega Trinza—once every 3 months)	273–819 (IM injection)
	Quetiapine (Seroquel)	300–400
	Risperidone (Risperdal)	4–8
	Long-acting risperidone (Perseris)	90 or 120 subcutaneously (once a month)
	Ziprasidone (Geodon)	40–160

novel treatment is valbenazine (Ingrezza), a drug for the treatment of tardive dyskinesia. Tardive dyskinesia, a movement disturbance that is more prevalent with typical antipsychotics, is particularly troubling because it has been a permanent, incurable side effect. Valbenazine works by reducing dopamine release at the synaptic cleft and has demonstrated effectiveness in reducing abnormal involuntary movements such as tardive dyskinesia. Future research will determine its long-term effectiveness. Currently, the cost for this treatment is over $125,000 annually, which may limit its accessibility for many with chronic, serious mental illness.

Patient and Family Education Related to Antipsychotics

The patent receiving antipsychotic medication should:

- Use caution when driving or operating dangerous machinery. Drowsiness and dizziness can occur.
- Not stop taking the drug abruptly after long-term use. To do so might produce withdrawal symptoms, such as nausea, vomiting, dizziness, gastritis, headache, tachycardia, insomnia, tremulousness.
- Use sunblock lotion and wear protective clothing when spending time outdoors. Skin is more susceptible to sunburn, which can occur after only 30 minutes.
- Report weekly (if receiving clozapine therapy) to have blood levels drawn and to obtain a weekly supply of the drug.
- Immediately report to the physician the occurrence of any of the following symptoms: sore throat, fever, malaise, unusual bleeding, easy bruising, persistent nausea and vomiting, severe headache, rapid heart rate, difficulty urinating, muscle twitching, tremors, darkly colored urine, excessive urination, excessive thirst, excessive hunger, weakness, pale stools, yellow skin or eyes, muscular incoordination, or skin rash.

TABLE 15–4 Agents Used to Treat Extrapyramidal Side Effects of Antipsychotic Drugs

Indication	Antiparkinsonian agents: Used to treat parkinsonism of various causes and drug-induced extrapyramidal reactions. VMAT2 inhibitors: Used to treat tardive dyskinesia
Action	Antiparkinsonian agents: Restores the natural balance of acetylcholine and dopamine in the CNS. The imbalance is a deficiency in dopamine that results in excessive cholinergic activity. VMAT2 inhibitors: mechanism of action unknown
Contraindications/ Precautions	Antiparkinsonian agents are contraindicated in individuals with hypersensitivity. Anticholinergics should be avoided by individuals with angle-closure glaucoma; pyloric, duodenal, or bladder neck obstructions; prostatic hypertrophy; or myasthenia gravis. Caution should be used in administering these drugs to clients with hepatic, renal, or cardiac insufficiency; elderly and debilitated clients; those with a tendency toward urinary retention; and those exposed to high environmental temperatures. VMAT2 inhibitors are contraindicated in individuals with hypersensitivity. Warnings include risk for somnolence and prolongation of QT interval; may cause parkinsonism in patients with tardive dyskinesia.
Common Side Effects	Anticholinergic effects (dry mouth, blurred vision, constipation, paralytic ileus, urinary retention, tachycardia, elevated temperature, decreased sweating), nausea/GI upset, sedation, dizziness, orthostatic hypotension, exacerbation of psychoses. Side effects with VMAT2 inhibitors include hypersensitivity, somnolence, QT interval prolongation, parkinsonian symptoms, weight gain, increased blood glucose, anxiety.

CHEMICAL CLASS	GENERIC (TRADE) NAME	DAILY DOSAGE RANGE (MG)
Anticholinergics	Benztropine (Cogentin) Biperiden (Akineton) Trihexyphenidyl	1–8 2–6 1–15
Antihistamines	Diphenhydramine (Benadryl)	25–200
Dopaminergic Agonists	Amantadine	200–300
VMAT2 inhibitor	Valbenazine Deutetrabenazine	40–80 6–48

CNS: central nervous system; GI: gastrointestinal; VMAT2: vesicular monoamine transporter type 2.

- Rise slowly from a sitting or lying position to prevent a sudden drop in blood pressure.
- Take frequent sips of water, chew sugarless gum, or suck on hard candy, if dry mouth is a problem. Good oral care (frequent brushing, flossing) is very important.
- Consult the physician regarding smoking while on antipsychotic therapy. Smoking increases the metabolism of antipsychotics, requiring an adjustment in dosage to achieve a therapeutic effect.
- Dress warmly in cold weather and avoid extended exposure to very high or low temperatures. Body temperature is harder to maintain with this medication.
- Avoid drinking alcohol while on antipsychotic therapy. These drugs potentiate each other's effects.
- Avoid taking other medications (including over-the-counter products) without the physician's approval. Many medications contain substances that interact with antipsychotics in a way that may be harmful.
- Be aware of possible risks of taking antipsychotics during pregnancy. Antipsychotics are thought to cross the placental barrier; if so, a fetus could experience adverse effects of the drug. Neonates are at increased risk for EPS and withdrawal after delivery when exposed to antipsychotics in the third trimester. Inform the physician immediately if pregnancy occurs, is suspected, or is planned.
- Be aware of side effects of antipsychotic drugs. Refer to written materials furnished by health-care providers for safe self-administration.
- Continue to take the medication even if feeling well and as though it is not needed. Symptoms may return if medication is discontinued.
- Carry a card or other identification at all times describing medications being taken.

Smoking Cessation

Smoking cigarettes has long been identified as a particular health risk for clients with schizophrenia because the prevalence is three times that of the general population; it is estimated that as many as 88% of those with schizophrenia and 70% of those with bipolar disorder are smokers (Kranjac, 2016). Some clients report increased ability to concentrate when smoking tobacco, which has led to clinical trials of drugs that increase nicotine levels. However, to date, these drugs have not been proven to be effective. In addition to the obvious health risks of chronic lung diseases and cancers, smoking decreases the effectiveness of some psychotropic medications. Varenicline (Chantix), a nicotine agonist used as a smoking deterrent, was once thought to increase symptoms and even suicide risk in those with serious mental illness. However, a recent meta-analysis (Wu et al., 2016) concluded that varenicline is effective for assisting with smoking cessation in this population and that "there was no clear evidence of neuropsychiatric or other adverse events compared with placebo" (p. 1554). In any scenario, assessing the client's motivation to stop smoking and exploring viable treatment options, including psychological interventions, are important components of treatment.

CASE STUDY AND SAMPLE CARE PLAN

NURSING HISTORY AND ASSESSMENT

Frank is 22 years old. He joined the Marines just out of high school at age 18 for a 3-year enlistment. His final year was spent in Afghanistan. When his 3-year enlistment was up, he returned to his hometown and married a young woman who had been a high school classmate. Frank has always been quiet and somewhat withdrawn, and he had very few friends. He was the only child of a single mom who never married, and he does not know his father. His mother was killed in an automobile accident the spring before he enlisted in the Marines.

During the past year, he has become increasingly isolated and withdrawn. He is without regular employment but finds work as a day laborer when he can. His wife, Suzanne, works as a secretary and is the primary wage earner. Lately, Frank has become very suspicious of her and sometimes follows her to work. He also drops in on her at work and accuses her of having affairs with some of the men in the office.

Last evening, when Suzanne got home from work, Frank was hiding in the closet. She didn't know he was home. When she started to undress, he jumped out of the closet holding a large kitchen knife and threatened to kill her "for being unfaithful." Suzanne managed to flee their home and ran to the neighbor's house and called the police.

Frank told the police that he received a message over the radio from his Marine commanding officer telling him that he couldn't allow his wife to continue to commit adultery, and the only way he could stop it was to kill her. The police took Frank to the emergency department of the VA hospital, where he was admitted to the psychiatric unit. Suzanne is helping with the admission history.

Suzanne tells the nurse that she has never been unfaithful to Frank, and she doesn't know why he believes that she has. Frank tells the nurse that he has been "taking orders from my commanding officer through my car radio ever since I got back from Afghanistan." He survived a helicopter crash in Afghanistan in which all were killed except Frank and one other man. Frank says, "I have to follow my CO's orders. God saved me to annihilate the impure."

Following an evaluation, the psychiatrist diagnoses Frank with Schizophrenia and orders olanzapine 10 mg PO to be given daily and olanzapine 10 mg IM q6h prn for agitation.

NURSING DIAGNOSES AND OUTCOME IDENTIFICATION

From the assessment data, the nurse develops the following nursing diagnoses for Frank:

1. **Risk for self-directed or other-directed violence** related to unresolved grief over loss of mother; survivor's guilt associated with helicopter crash; command hallucinations; and history of violence
   a. **Short-Term Goals:**
      - Frank will seek out staff when anxiety and agitation start to increase.
      - Frank will not harm self or others.
   b. **Long-Term Goal:** Frank will not harm self or others.
2. **Disturbed sensory perception: Auditory** related to increased anxiety and agitation, withdrawal into self, and stress of sufficient intensity to threaten an already weak ego
   a. **Short-Term Goals:**
      - Frank will discuss the content of the hallucinations with the nurse.
      - Frank will maintain anxiety at a manageable level.
   b. **Long-Term Goal:** Frank will be able to define and test reality, reducing or eliminating the occurrence of hallucinations.

CASE STUDY AND SAMPLE CARE PLAN—cont'd

PLANNING AND IMPLEMENTATION

RISK FOR SELF-DIRECTED OR OTHER-DIRECTED VIOLENCE

1. Keep the stimuli as low as possible in Frank's environment.
2. Monitor Frank's behavior frequently but in a manner of carrying out routine activities so as not to create suspiciousness on his part.
3. Watch for the following signs (considered the prodrome to aggressive behavior): increased motor activity, pounding, slamming, tense posture, defiant affect, clenched teeth and fists, arguing, demanding, and challenging or threatening staff.
4. If Frank should become aggressive, maintain a calm attitude. Try talking. Offer medication. Provide physical activities.
5. If these interventions fail, indicate a show of strength with a team of staff members.
6. Utilize restraints only as a last resort and if Frank is clearly at risk of harm to himself or others.
7. Help Frank recognize unresolved grief and fixation in denial or anger stage of grief process.
8. Encourage him to talk about the loss of his mother and of fellow Marines in Afghanistan.
9. Encourage him to talk about guilt feelings associated with survival when others died.
10. Assess for presence of suicide risk and collaborate with the patient to develop a personal safety plan.

DISTURBED SENSORY PERCEPTION: AUDITORY

1. Monitor Frank's behavior for signs that he is hearing voices: listening pose, talking and laughing to self, stopping in midsentence.
2. If these behaviors are observed, ask Frank, "Are you hearing the voices again?"
3. Encourage Frank to share the content of the hallucinations. This information is important for early intervention in case the content contains commands to harm himself or others.
4. Say to Frank, "I understand that the voice is real to you, but I do not hear any voices speaking." It is important for him to learn the difference between what is real and what is not real.
5. Try to help Frank recognize that the voices often appear at times when he becomes anxious about something and his agitation increases.
6. Help him to recognize this increasing anxiety, and teach him methods to keep it from escalating.
7. Use distracting activities to bring him back to reality. Involvement with real people and real situations will help to distract him from the hallucination.
8. Teach him to use *voice dismissal*. When he hears the CO's (or others') voice, he should shout, "Go away!" or "Leave me alone!" These commands may help to diminish the sounds and give him a feeling of control over the situation.

EVALUATION

The outcome criteria identified for Frank have been met. When feeling especially anxious or becoming agitated, he seeks out staff for comfort and for assistance in maintaining his anxiety at a manageable level. He currently denies suicide ideation and has collaborated to develop a personal safety plan. He is experiencing fewer auditory hallucinations and has learned to use voice dismissal to interrupt the behavior. He is beginning to recognize his position in the grief process and is working toward resolution at his own pace.

Summary and Key Points

- Of all of the mental illnesses, schizophrenia undoubtedly results in the greatest amount of personal, emotional, and social costs. It presents an enormous threat to life and happiness.
- For many years, there was little agreement as to a definition of the concept of schizophrenia. The *DSM-5-TR* (APA, 2022) identifies specific criteria for diagnosis of the disorder.
- The initial symptoms of schizophrenia most often occur in early adulthood. Development of the disorder can be viewed in four phases: (I) the premorbid phase, (II) the prodromal phase, (III) the active psychotic phase (schizophrenia), and (IV) the residual phase.
- The cause of schizophrenia remains unclear. Most likely, no single factor can be implicated; rather, the disease probably results from a complex interaction of genetic, biochemical, psychological, and environmental factors.
- A spectrum of schizophrenic and other psychotic disorders has been identified. These include (on a gradient of psychopathology from least to most severe): schizotypal personality disorder, delusional disorder, brief psychotic disorder, substance-induced psychotic disorder, psychotic disorder associated with another medical condition,

catatonic disorder associated with another medical condition, schizophreniform disorder, schizoaffective disorder, and schizophrenia.

- Nursing care of the patient with schizophrenia is accomplished using the six steps of the nursing process.
- Nursing assessment is based on knowledge of symptomatology related to thought content and processes, perception, affect, volition, interpersonal functioning and relationship to the external world, and psychomotor behavior.
- Symptoms of schizophrenia are categorized as *positive* (an excess or distortion of normal functions) or *negative* (a diminution or loss of normal functions).
- Antipsychotic medications remain the mainstay of pharmacological treatment for psychotic disorders. Atypical antipsychotics have become the first line of therapy. They have a more favorable side effect profile than the conventional (typical) antipsychotics.
- Individuals with schizophrenia require long-term integrated treatment with pharmacological and other interventions. Some of these include individual psychotherapy, group therapy, behavior therapy, social skills training, milieu therapy, family therapy, and assertive community treatment. For the majority of clients, the most effective treatment appears to be a combination of psychotropic medication and psychosocial therapy.
- Some clinicians are choosing a course of therapy based on a model of recovery, somewhat like that which has been used for many years with problems of addiction. The basic premise of a recovery model is empowerment of the patient. The recovery model is designed to allow consumers primary control over decisions about their own care and to enable persons with mental health problems to live a meaningful life in a community of their choice while striving to achieve their full potential.
- Families generally require support and education about psychotic illnesses. The focus is on coping with the diagnosis, understanding the illness and its course, teaching about medication, and learning ways to manage symptoms.
- The most current, evidence-based approach to treatment, RAISE (Recovery After an Initial Schizophrenia Episode), demonstrates that early intervention at the first episode of psychosis can significantly improve outcomes.

Review Questions

Select the answer that is most appropriate for each of the following questions:

1. Recent research on the RAISE approach to treatment of schizophrenia incorporates which of the following elements as important to improving outcomes? (Select all that apply.)
   a. Early intervention at the first episode of psychosis
   b. Support for employment and/or educational pursuits
   c. Rapid, high-dose loading with antipsychotic medication
   d. Court-ordered sanctions for treatment
   e. Recovery-focused psychotherapy
2. Which of the following is the primary goal in working with an actively psychotic, suspicious client?
   a. Promote interaction with others.
   b. Decrease the client's anxiety and increase trust.
   c. Improve the client's relationship with their parents.
   d. Encourage participation in therapy activities.
3. A client with schizophrenia has physician's orders for haloperidol (Haldol) 5 mg. IM STAT and then 3 mg PO tid; 2 mg benztropine PO bid prn. Why is benztropine ordered?
   a. To treat extrapyramidal symptoms
   b. To prevent neuroleptic malignant syndrome
   c. To decrease psychotic symptoms
   d. To induce sleep

4. A client on the psychiatric unit tells the nurse that the CIA is looking for him and will kill him if they find him. The client's false belief is an example of a delusion of:
   a. Persecution
   b. Reference
   c. Control or influence
   d. Grandeur
5. The primary focus of family therapy for clients with schizophrenia and their families is:
   a. To discuss problem-solving and adaptive behaviors for coping with stress
   b. To introduce the family to others with the same problem
   c. To keep the client and family in touch with the health-care system
   d. To promote family interaction and increase understanding of the illness
6. A client recently admitted to the hospital reports to the nurse, "I don't understand why I was brought here. I was simply hanging out in my apartment and the police said I had to come with them." This is an example of what symptom of schizophrenia?
   a. Delusions of reference
   b. Loose association
   c. Anosognosia
   d. Auditory hallucinations

Clinical Judgment Questions

7. Which of the following assessments by the nurse would convey a need for prn benztropine?
   a. Increased level of agitation
   b. Complaints of a sore throat
   c. A yellowish cast to the skin
   d. Muscle spasms
8. A client on the psychiatric unit has been diagnosed with schizophrenia. The client tells the nurse that the CIA is looking for them and will kill them if they find them. The most appropriate response by the nurse is:
   a. "That's ridiculous. No one is going to hurt you."
   b. "The CIA isn't interested in people like you."
   c. "Why do you think the CIA wants to kill you?"
   d. "I know you believe that, but it's really hard for me to believe."
9. The nurse is interviewing a client on the psychiatric unit. The client tilts their head to the side, stops talking in midsentence, and listens intently. Which is the most appropriate follow-up assessment based on this information?
   a. Ask the client if they are experiencing loose associations.
   b. Ask the client if they need more medication.
   c. Ask the client if they are hearing something or someone other than the nurse's voice.
   d. Ask the client if their neck is stiff.
10. A client reports to the nurse that their foot is on fire, and they think the demons are trying to burn off their flesh. The priority nursing intervention for this symptom is to:
    a. Administer prn haloperidol as ordered
    b. Evaluate the client's foot to rule out physical causes for their complaint
    c. Administer prn benztropine as ordered
    d. Ask the client if they would like to speak with a chaplain

Continued

11. When a client suddenly becomes aggressive and violent on the unit, which of the following approaches would be best for the nurse to use first?
    a. Provide large motor activities to relieve the client's pent-up tension.
    b. Administer a dose of prn olanzapine to keep the client calm.
    c. Call for sufficient help to control the situation safely.
    d. Convey to the client that their behavior is unacceptable and will not be permitted.
12. A client has been diagnosed with schizophrenia. The client has been socially isolated and hearing voices telling them to kill their parents. The client has been admitted to the psychiatric unit from the emergency department. Which is the most important initial intervention for this client?
    a. Give the client an injection of haloperidol.
    b. Assess the client to evaluate their safety toward themself and others.
    c. Place the client in restraints.
    d. Order the client a nutritious diet.

IMPLICATIONS FOR EVIDENCE-BASED PRACTICE

Stroup, T. S., Olfson, M., Huang, C., Wall, M. M., Goldberg, T., Devanand, D. P., & Gerhard, T. P. (2021). Age-specific prevalence and incidence of dementia diagnoses among older US adults with schizophrenia. *JAMA Psychiatry, 78*(6), 632–641. https://doi.org/10.1001/jamapsychiatry.2021.0042

DESCRIPTION OF THE STUDY: This study sought to estimate the age-specific prevalence and incidence of dementia in older adults with schizophrenia by comparing them to older adults without schizophrenia. This was a retrospective cohort study of 8,011,773 Medicare recipients 66 years and older. It is known that the risk of dementia among those with schizophrenia is high, and this study sought to clarify the magnitude and timing of this increased risk.

RESULTS OF THE STUDY: At 66 years of age, the prevalence of diagnosed dementia was 27.9% among individuals with schizophrenia compared with 1.3% in the group without serious mental illness (SMI). By 80 years of age, the prevalence of dementia diagnoses rose to 70.2% in the group with schizophrenia and 11.3% in the group without SMI. The annual incidence of dementia diagnoses per 1,000 person-years at 66 years of age was 52.5 among individuals with schizophrenia and 4.5 among individuals without SMI and increased to 216.2 and 32.3, respectively, by 80 years of age.

IMPLICATIONS FOR NURSING PRACTICE: Several symptoms of schizophrenia overlap with those of dementia, so differential diagnosis can be a challenge. One of the most prominent symptoms in dementia, however, is recent memory loss, and when nurses assess this to be prominent in the older adult with schizophrenia the nurse can play an active role in collaborating with team members to recommend further testing. Nurses also play an active role in educating patients and families regarding lifestyle factors that may decrease risks for dementia such as weight management, diabetes management, and strategies to reduce risk for cardiovascular disease. Careful assessment and collaboration with team members has treatment implications as well, because antipsychotic medication use in the patient with dementia has been associated with many risks, including sudden death.

TEST YOUR CLINICAL REASONING AND CLINICAL JUDGMENT SKILLS

Sara, a 23-year-old single woman, has just been admitted to the psychiatric unit by her parents. They explain that over the past few months, she has become increasingly withdrawn. She stays in her room alone but lately has been heard talking and laughing to herself.

Sara left home for the first time at age 18 to attend college. She performed well during her first semester, but when she returned after Christmas, she began to accuse her roommate of stealing her possessions. She started writing to her parents that her roommate wanted to kill her and that her roommate was turning everyone against her. She said she feared for her life. She started missing classes and stayed in her bed most of the time. Sometimes she locked herself in her closet. Her parents took her home, and she was hospitalized and diagnosed with schizophrenia. Sara has since been maintained on antipsychotic medication while taking a few classes at the local community college.

Sara tells the admitting nurse that she quit taking her medication 4 weeks ago because the pharmacist who fills the prescriptions is plotting to have her killed. She believes he is trying to poison her. She says she got this information from a television message. As Sara speaks, the nurse notices that she sometimes stops in midsentence and listens; sometimes she cocks her head to the side and moves her lips as though she is talking.

Answer the following questions related to Sara:

1. From the assessment data, what would be the most immediate nursing concern in working with Sara?
2. What is the nursing diagnosis related to this concern?
3. What interventions must be accomplished before the nurse can be successful in working with Sara?

Communication Exercises

1. Hal, a patient on the psychiatric unit, has a diagnosis of schizophrenia. He lives in a halfway house, where last evening he began yelling that "aliens were on the way to take over our bodies! The message is coming through loud and clear!" The residence supervisor became frightened and called 911. As Hal was being admitted to the psychiatric unit, he told the nurse, "I'm special! I get messages from a higher being! We are in for big trouble!"
   How would the nurse respond appropriately to this statement by Hal?
2. The nurse notices that Hal is sitting off by himself in a corner of the dayroom. He appears to be talking to himself and tilts his head to the side as if listening to something.
   How would the nurse intervene with Hal in this situation?
3. Hal says to the nurse, "We must choose to take a ride. All alone we slip and slide. Now it's time to take a bride."
   How would the nurse respond appropriately to these statements by Hal?

MOVIE CONNECTIONS

I Never Promised You a Rose Garden (Schizophrenia) ▪ *A Beautiful Mind* (Schizophrenia) ▪ *The Fisher King* (Schizophrenia) ▪ *Bennie & Joon* (Schizophrenia) ▪ *Out of Darkness* (Schizophrenia) ▪ *Conspiracy Theory* (Paranoia) ▪ *The Fan* (Delusional disorder) ▪ *The Soloist* (Schizophrenia) ▪ *Of Two Minds* (Schizophrenia)

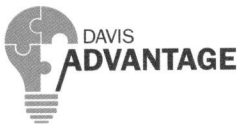

Go to **Davis Advantage** to complete your learning: strengthen understanding, apply your knowledge, and prepare for the Next Gen NCLEX®.

References

Álvarez, M. J., Masramon, H., Peña, C., Pont, M., Gourdier, C., Roura-Poch, P., & Arrufat, F. (2015). Cumulative effects of childhood traumas: Polytraumatization, dissociation, and schizophrenia. *Community Mental Health Journal, 51*(1), 54–62. https://doi.org/10.1007/s10597-014-9755-2

American Psychiatric Association. (2022). *Diagnostic and statistical manual of mental disorders* (5th ed., text rev.).

Asen, E. (2002). Outcome research in family therapy: Family intervention for psychosis. *Advances in Psychiatric Treatment, 8*, 230–238.

Benson, P. J., Beedie, S. A., Shephard, E., Giegling, I., Rujescu, G., & St. Clair, D. (2012). Simple viewing tests can detect eye movement abnormalities that distinguish schizophrenia cases from controls with exceptional accuracy. *Biological Psychiatry, 72*(9), 716–724.

Boland, R., & Verduin, M. L. (2022). *Kaplan & Sadock's synopsis of psychiatry* (P. Ruiz, Ed.). (12th ed.). Wolters Kluwer.

Bora, E. (2015). Neurodevelopmental origin of cognitive impairment in schizophrenia. *Psychological Medicine, 45*(1), 1–9. https://doi.org/10.1017/S0033291714001263

Caqueo-Urízar, A., Rus-Calafell, M., Urzúa, A., Escudero, J., & Gutiérrez-Maldonado, J. (2015). The role of family therapy in the management of schizophrenia: Challenges and solutions. *Neuropsychiatric Disease and Treatment, 11*, 145–151. https://doi.org/10.2147/NDT.S51331

Chesney, E., Goodwin, G. M., & Fazel, S. (2014). Risks of all-cause and suicide mortality in mental disorders: A meta-review. *World Psychiatry*. https://doi.org/10.1002/wps.20128

Clark, S. R., Baune, B. T., Schubert, K. O., Lavoie, S., Smesny, S., Rice, S. M., & Amminger, G. P. (2016). Prediction of transition from ultra-high risk to first-episode psychosis using a probabilistic model combining history, clinical assessment and fatty-acid biomarkers. *Translational Psychiatry, 6*(9), e897. https://doi.org/10.1038/tp.2016.170

Davis, J., Eyre, H., Jacka, F. N., Dodd, S., Dean, O., McEwen, S., Debnath, M., McGrath, J., Maes, M., Amminger, P., McGorry, P. D., Pantelis, C., & Berk, M. (2016). A review of vulnerability and risks for schizophrenia: Beyond the two hit hypothesis. *Neuroscience and Biobehavioral Reviews, 65*, 185–194. https://doi.org/10.1016/j.neubiorev.2016.03.017

D'Souza, D. C., Singh, N., Elander, J., Carbuto, M., Pittman, B., Udo de Haes, J., Sjogren, M., Peeters, P., Ranganathan, M., & Schipper, J. (2012). Glycine transporter inhibitor attenuates the psychotomimetic effects of ketamine in healthy males: Preliminary evidence. *Neuropsychopharmacology, 37*(4), 1036–1046. https://doi.org/10.1038/npp.2011.295

Druss, B. G., Zhao, L., Von Esenwein, S., Morrato, E. H., & Marcus, S. C. (2011). Understanding excess mortality in persons with mental illness: 17-year follow up of a nationally representative US survey. *Medical Care, 49*(6), 599–604.

Ernst, D. (2019). Novel treatment for schizophrenia gets FDA's breakthrough therapy designation. https://www.psychiatryadvisor.com/home/topics/schizophrenia-and-psychoses/novel-treatment-for-schizophrenia-gets-fdas-breakthrough-therapy-designation/

Frankenburg, F. R. (2020). What factors affect the prognosis of schizophrenia? *Medscape*. https://www.medscape.com/answers/288259-13995/what-factors-affect-the-prognosis-of-schizophrenia

Freudenreich, O. (2010). Differential diagnosis of psychotic symptoms: Medical "mimics." *Psychiatric Times, 27*(12), 52–61.

Harrisberger, F., Smieskova1, R., Vogler, C., Egli, T., Schmidt, A., Lenz, C., Simon, A. E., Riecher-Rössler, A., Papassotiropoulos, A., & Borgwardt, S. (2016). Impact of polygenic schizophrenia-related risk and hippocampal volumes on the onset of psychosis. *Translational Psychiatry, 6*, e868. https://doi.org/10.1038/tp.2016.143

Hashimoto, K. (2006). Glycine transporter inhibitors as therapeutic agents for schizophrenia. *Recent Patents on CNS Drug Discovery, 1*, 43–53.

Herdman, T. H., Kamitsuru, S., & Lopes, C. T. (Eds.). (2021). *NANDA International, Inc. nursing diagnoses: Definitions and classification, 2021–2023* (12th ed.). Thieme.

Howes, O., McCutcheon, R., & Stone, J. (2015). Glutamate and dopamine in schizophrenia: An update for the 21st century. *Journal of Psychopharmacology (Oxford, England), 29*(2), 97–115. https://doi.org/10.1177/0269881114563634

Hu, W., MacDonald, M. L., Elswick, D. E., & Sweet, R. A. (2014). The glutamate hypothesis of schizophrenia: Evidence from human brain tissue studies [Abstract]. *Annals of the New York Academy of Sciences, 1338*, 38–57. https://doi.org/10.1111/nyas

Institute of Medicine. (2003). *Health professions education: A bridge to quality.*

Jablensky, A. (2017). Worldwide burden of schizophrenia. In B. J. Sadock, V. A. Sadock, & P. Ruiz (Eds.), *Comprehensive textbook of psychiatry* (11th ed., pp. 1425–1437). Wolters Kluwer.

Kane, J. M., Schooler, N. R., Marcy, P., Correll, C. U., Brunette, M. F., Mueser, K. T., Rosenheck, R. A., Addington, J., Estroff, S. E., Robinson, J., Penn, D. L., & Robinson, D. G. (2015). The RAISE early treatment program for first-episode psychosis: Background, rationale, and study design. *The Journal of Clinical Psychiatry, 76*(3), 240–246. https://doi.org/10.4088/JCP.14m09289

Kranjac, D. (2016). *Pharmacotherapy for smoking cessation in adults with neuropsychiatric illness.* http://www.psychiatryadvisor.com/addiction/smoking-cessation-in-adults-with-neuropsychiatric-illness/article/518385

Lewis, S. F., Escalona, R., & Keith, S. J. (2017). The phenomenology of schizophrenia. In B. J. Sadock, V. A. Sadock, & P. Ruiz (Eds.), *Comprehensive textbook of psychiatry* (11th ed., pp. 1406–1425). Wolters Kluwer.

Lysaker, P. H., Roe, D., & Buck, K. D. (2010). Recovery and wellness amidst schizophrenia: Definitions, evidence, and the implications for clinical practice. *Journal of the American Psychiatric Nurses Association, 16*(1), 36–42.

MacCabe, J. H., Wicks, S., Löfving, S., David, A. S., Berndtsson, Å., Gustafsson, J-E, Allebeck, P., & Dalman, C. (2013). Decline in cognitive performance between ages 13 and 18 years and the risk for psychosis in adulthood: A Swedish longitudinal cohort study in males. *JAMA Psychiatry 70*(3), 261–270. https://doi.org/10.1001/2013.jamapsychiatry.43

Matheson, S. L., Shepherd, A. M., & Carr, V. J. (2014). How much do we know about schizophrenia and how well do we know it? Evidence from the Schizophrenia Library. *Psychological Medicine—London, 44*(6), 3387–3405. https://doi.org/10.1017/S0033291714000166

Mathews, M., Tesar, G. E., Fattal, O., & Muzina, D. J. (2013). *Schizophrenia and acute psychosis.* http://www.clevelandclinicmeded.com/medicalpubs/diseasemanagement/psychiatry-psychology/schizophrenia-acute-psychosis

Miller, B. (2020). Schizophrenia: Clinical considerations in men versus women. *Psychiatric Times.* https://www.psychiatrictimes.com/view/schizophrenia-clinical-considerations-men-versus-women

Miller, J. (2020). Schizophrenia: A Broad Rx. *Psychiatric Times.* https://www.psychiatrictimes.com/view/schizophrenia-a-broad-rx

Mueser, K. T., Bond, G. R., & Drake, R. E. (2001). Community-based treatment of schizophrenia and other severe mental disorders: Treatment outcomes. *Medscape General Medicine 3*(1) [formerly published in Medscape Psychiatry & Mental Health eJournal *6*(1), 2001]. http://www.medscape.com/viewarticle/430529

Nauert, R. (2015). Excess neurotransmitter in brain may trigger schizophrenia. *Psych Central.* http://psychcentral.com/news/2013/04/19/excess-neurotransmitter-in-brain-may-trigger-schizophrenia/53880.html

Okazaki, S., Boku, S., Otsuka, I., Mouri, K., Aoyama, S., Shiroiwa, K., Sora, I., Fujita, A., Shirai, Y., Shirakawa, O., Kokai, M., & Hishimoto, A. (2016). The cell cycle-related genes as biomarkers for schizophrenia. *Progress Neuropsychopharmacology and Biological Psychiatry, 70*(Suppl. 9), 85–91. https://doi.org/10.1016/j.pnpbp.2016.05.005

Os, J. V., & Reininghaus, U. (2017). The clinical epidemiology of schizophrenia. In B. J. Sadock, V. A. Sadock., & P. Ruiz (Eds.), *Comprehensive textbook of psychiatry* (10 ed., pp. 1445–1457). Wolters Kluwer.

Radhakrishnan, R., Wilkinson, S. T., & D'Souza, D. C. (2014). Gone to pot—A review of the association between cannabis and psychosis. *Frontiers in Psychiatry, 5*(54). https://doi.org/10.3389/fpsyt.2014.00054

Rezansoff, S., Moniruzzaman, A., Fazel, S., McCandless, L., Procyshyn, R., & Somers, J. M. (2016). Housing First improves adherence to antipsychotic medication among formerly homeless adults with schizophrenia: Results of a randomized controlled trial. *Schizophrenia Bulletin.* https://doi.org/10.1093/schbul/sbw136

Roberts, L. W., Louie, A. K., Guerrero, A., Balon, R., Beresin, E. V., Brenner, A., & Coverdale, J. (2017). Premature mortality among people with mental illness: Advocacy in academic psychiatry. *Academic Psychiatry, 41*, (4), 441–446.

Savill, M., Banks, C., Khanom, H., & Priebe, S. (2015). Do negative symptoms of schizophrenia change overtime?

A meta-analysis of longitudinal data. *Psychological Medicine, 45*, 1613-1627. https://doi.org/10.1017/S0033291714002712

Shrivastava, A., Shah, N., Johnston, M., Stitt, L., & Thakar, M. (2010). Predictors of long-term outcome of first-episode schizophrenia: A ten-year follow-up study. *Indian Journal of Psychiatry, 52*(4), 320–326. https://doi.org/10.4103/0019-5545.74306

Stahl, S. M. (2013). *Stahl's essential psychopharmacology: Neuroscientific basis and practical applications* (4th ed.). Cambridge University Press.

Stroup, T. S., Olfson, M., Huang, C., Wall, M. M., Goldberg, T., Devanand, D. P., & Gerhard, T. P. (2021). Age-specific prevalence and incidence of dementia diagnoses among older us adults with schizophrenia. *JAMA Psychiatry, 78*(6), 632–641. https://doi.org/10.1001/jamapsychiatry.2021.0042

Takeuchi, H., Kantor, N., Sanches, M., Fervaha, G., Agid, O., & Remington, G. (2017). One-year symptom trajectories in patients with stable schizophrenia maintained on antipsychotics versus placebo: Meta-analysis. *British Journal of Psychiatry, 211*(3). https://doi.org/10.1192/bjp.bp.116.186007

Thunè, H., Recasens, M., & Uhlhaas, P. J. (2016). The 40-Hz auditory steady-state response in patients with schizophrenia: A meta-analysis. *JAMA Psychiatry, 78(11), 1145–1153.* http://jamanetwork.com/journals/jamapsychiatry/article-abstract/2566207

Tripathi, A., Kar, S. K., & Shukla, R. (2018). Cognitive deficits in schizophrenia: Understanding the biological correlates and remediation strategies. *Clinical Psychopharmacology and Neuroscience, 16*(1), 7–17. https://doi.org/10.9758/cpn.2018.16.1.7

Urvakhsh, M. M., Thirthalli, J., Aneelraj, D., Jadhav, P., Gangadhar, B. N., & Keshavan, M. S. (2014). Mirror neuron dysfunction in schizophrenia and its functional implications: A systematic review. *Schizophrenia Research, 160*(1–3), 9–19. https://doi.org/http://dx.doi.org/10.1016/j.schres.2014.10.040

Veijola, J., Guo, J. Y., Moilanen, J. S., Jaaskelainen, E., Miettunen, J., Kyllonen, M., Haapea, M., Huhtaniska, S., Alaräisänen, A., Mäki, P., Kiviniemi, V., Nikkinen, J., Starck, T., Remes, J. J., Tanskanen, P., Tervonen, O., Wink, A. M., Kehagia, A., Suckling, J., . . . Murray, G. (2014). Longitudinal changes in total brain volume in schizophrenia: Relation to symptom severity, cognition and antipsychotic medication. *PLoS ONE, 9*(7), e101689. https://doi.org/10.1371/journal.pone.0101689

Viher, P. V., Stegmayer, K., Giezendanner, S., Federspiel, A., Bohlhalter, S., Vanbellingen, T., Weist, R., Strik, W., & Walthera, S. (2016). Cerebral white matter structure is associated with DSM-5 schizophrenia symptom dimensions. *Neuroimage: Clinical, 12*(Suppl. 7), 93–99. https://doi.org/10.1016/j.nicl.2016.06.013

Waters, F., Collerton, D., Ffytche, D. H., Jardri, R., Pins, D., Dudley, R., Blom, J. D., Mosimann, U. P., Eperjesi, F., Ford, S., & Laroi, F. (2014). Visual hallucinations in the psychosis spectrum and comparative information from neurodegenerative disorders and eye disease. *Schizophrenia Bulletin, 40*(Suppl. 4), 233–245. https://doi.org/10.1093/schbul/sbu036

Weiden, P. J. (2010). Is recovery attainable in schizophrenia? *Medscape Psychiatry & Mental Health.* http://www.medscape.com/viewarticle/729750

Wu, Q., Gilbody, S., Peckham, E., Brabyn, S., & Parrott, S. (2016). Varenicline for smoking cessation and reduction in people with severe mental illnesses: Systematic review and meta-analysis. *Addiction, 111*(9), 1554–1567. Advance online publication. https://doi.org/10.1111/add.13415

Classical Reference

Kay, S. R., Fiszbein, A., & Opler, L. A. (1987). The positive and negative syndrome scale (PANSS) for schizophrenia. *Schizophrenia Bulletin, 13*(2), 261–276.

16 Depressive Disorders

CORE CONCEPTS

Mood and Affect: Depression

Professional Behavior: Nursing process in the care of patients with depressive disorders

Safety

Clinical Judgment

CHAPTER OUTLINE

Objectives
Introduction
Historical Perspective
Epidemiology
Types of Depressive Disorders
Predisposing Factors
Developmental Implications
Application of the Nursing Process
Treatment Modalities
Summary and Key Points
Review Questions
Clinical Judgment Questions
Implications for Evidence-Based Practice
Test Your Clinical Reasoning and Clinical Judgment Skills
Communication Exercises
Movie Connections

KEY TERMS

affect
cognitive behavior therapy
depression
dysthymia
melancholia
mood
postpartum depression
premenstrual dysphoric disorder
psychomotor retardation

OBJECTIVES

After reading this chapter, the student will be able to:

1. Recount historical perspectives of depression.
2. Discuss the epidemiology of depression.
3. Describe various types of depressive disorders.
4. Identify predisposing factors in the development of depression.
5. Discuss implications of depression related to developmental stage.
6. Identify symptomatology associated with depression and use this information in patient assessment.
7. Formulate nursing diagnoses and goals of care for patients with depression.
8. Identify topics for patient and family teaching relevant to depression.
9. Describe appropriate nursing interventions for behaviors associated with depression.
10. Describe relevant criteria for evaluating nursing care of patients with depression.
11. Discuss various modalities relevant to treatment of depression.

Introduction

Depression is likely the oldest and still one of the most frequently diagnosed psychiatric illnesses. Symptoms of depression have been described almost as far back as there is evidence of written documentation.

An occasional bout with the "blues," a feeling of sadness or downheartedness, is common among healthy people and is considered to be a normal response to everyday disappointments in life. These episodes are short lived as the individual adapts to the loss, change, or failure (real or perceived) that has been experienced. Pathological depression occurs when adaptation is ineffective and the symptoms are significant enough to impair functioning.

CORE CONCEPT

Mood and Affect

Mood is a pervasive and sustained emotion that may have a major influence on a person's perception of the world. Examples of mood include depression, joy, elation, anger, and anxiety. **Affect** is described as the external, observable emotional reaction associated with an experience. A *flat affect* describes someone who lacks emotional expression and it is often seen in severely depressed clients.

This chapter focuses on the different manifestations of depressive illness and implications for nursing intervention. A historical perspective and epidemiology of depression are presented. Predisposing factors that have been implicated in the etiology of depression provide a framework for studying the dynamics of the disorder. Similarities and differences between depressive disorders and grief are discussed.

Depressive illnesses specific to individuals at various developmental stages are reviewed. An explanation of the symptomatology is presented as background knowledge for assessing the client with depression. Nursing care is described in the context of the six steps of the nursing process. Various medical treatment modalities are explored.

CORE CONCEPT

Depression

Depression is an alteration in mood that is expressed by feelings of sadness, despair, and pessimism. In clinically significant depression, there is a loss of interest in usual activities, and somatic symptoms may be evident. Changes in appetite, sleep patterns, and cognition are common. Severe depression may be accompanied by suicide ideation and/or attempts.

Historical Perspective

Many ancient cultures (e.g., Babylonian, Egyptian, Hebrew) believed in the supernatural or divine origin of mood disorders. The Old Testament states in the Book of Samuel that King Saul's depression was inflicted by an "evil spirit" sent from God to "torment" him.

A clearly nondivine point of view regarding depression was held by the Greek medical community from the 5th century BC through the 3rd century AD and represented the thinking of Hippocrates, Celsus, and Galen, among others. They strongly rejected the idea of divine origin and considered the brain as the seat of all emotional states. Hippocrates believed that **melancholia** was caused by an excess of black bile, a heavily toxic substance produced in the spleen or intestine, which affected the brain. Melancholia is currently used to describe a severe form of major depressive disorder in which symptoms are exaggerated and interest or pleasure in virtually all activities is lost.

During the Renaissance, several new theories evolved. Depression was viewed by some as being the result of obstructed air circulation, excessive brooding, or helpless situations beyond the individual's control. Depression was reflected in major literary works of the time, including Shakespeare's *King Lear, Macbeth,* and *Hamlet.*

Contemporary thinking has been substantially shaped by the works of Sigmund Freud, Emil Kraepelin, and Adolf Meyer. Having evolved from these early 20th-century models, current thinking about mood disorders generally encompasses the intrapsychic, behavioral, and biological perspectives. These various perspectives support the notion of multiple causation in the development of mood disorders.

Epidemiology

Major depressive disorder (MDD) is one of the leading causes of disability in the United States. In addition to the disability posed by the disorder itself, recent research links depression to an increased risk for several other medical conditions, including coronary artery disease (another leading cause of death), especially in women younger than age 65 (Jiang et al., 2016). In 2019, 4.7% of adults age 18 and older reported regular feelings of depression, 18.5% reported feelings of depression in the past 2 weeks, and women were more likely than men to have experienced depressive symptoms (Centers for Disease Control and Prevention, [CDC], 2021b). In a national survey (Hasin et al., 2018) the lifetime prevalence of major depressive disorder was found to be 20.6% and commonly associated with comorbid disorders, making it not only highly prevalent but often disabling. Akiskal (2017) reports that as diagnostic evaluation of bipolar disorders (alternating episodes of depression and manic or hypomanic symptoms) has improved, there are convincing data that up to 50% of all depressions may actually be bipolar illness.

There is evidence that the incidence of depression is increasing among American teens and young adults, particularly adolescent girls. In 2019, 3.8 million (15.7%) American teens ages 12 to 17 reported having had at least one major depressive episode within the last year, and 11.1% of those had severe impairment (over double the percentages reported for 2006) (Substance Abuse and Mental Health Services Administration [SAMHSA], 2020). Teens with depression were also more likely than those without depression to use substances. The reasons for these increases are unclear, but there is a correlation between these statistics and the increasing suicide rates among teens, and it is recognized as a major public health issue.

Age and Sex

Although the lifetime prevalence of depressive disorders is higher in those age 45 years or younger (Merikangas & Rihmer, 2017), it is difficult to pinpoint a single age correlate because many factors influence age-related depressive symptoms. Depression is more common in women than men. Boland and Verduin (2022) report that this is "an almost universal observation, independent of country or culture" (p. 394). The gender difference is less pronounced between ages 45 and 65, but after 65, women again are more likely than men to experience depression. Many biological explanations have been suggested, including that women have higher concentrations of monoamine oxidase (a neurotransmitter associated with depression); greater vulnerability to thyroid dysfunctions; and hormone changes that occur during the menstrual cycle, postpartum, and at menopause (Akiskal, 2017). Psychosocial factors contributing to depression in women may include increased sensitivity to stress (and higher prevalence of anxiety disorders), multiple social roles, and poorer coping mechanisms (Merikangas & Rihmer, 2017). In general, this gender-related increased risk for depression is influenced by many factors in complex interactions that are not yet clearly understood.

Socioeconomic Factors

Historically, depression was viewed as a "disease of affluence," but Ridley and associates (2020) found that the evidence supports a bicausal relationship between poverty and mental illness (particularly depression and anxiety). That is, mental illness may present economic burdens culminating in poverty, and conversely economic hardship can contribute to mental illness. Merikangas and Rihmer (2017) cite that depression is three times more prevalent among those without employment than those with one. Whether these findings are related to lack of access to resources and early treatment, difficulty managing multiple stressors associated with socioeconomic well-being, or a combination of many factors requires more research.

Race and Culture

Studies have not yet identified a consistent relationship between race and affective disorders. One problem encountered in reviewing racial comparisons involves the multiple variables that contribute to depression in minority groups such as access to health services and accurate diagnosis, U.S. region at birth, immigrant versus nonimmigrant nativity, and discrimination (Akincigil et al., 2012; Budhwani et al., 2015; Chang et al., 2016). In other words, some factors contributing to depression may be matters of public policy rather than biological factors associated with one's race. Boland and Verduin (2022) add that racial and ethnic differences are also challenging to measure because they are highly dependent on the methods and approaches used.

Marital Status

A number of studies have suggested that marriage has a positive effect on the psychological well-being of an individual as compared to those who are single or do not have a close relationship with another person (Liu et al., 2010; Marcussen, 2005; Uecker, 2012). Other studies have suggested that marital status alone is not a valid indicator of risk for depression (Lapate et al., 2014; LaPierre, 2004). Some of those studies have identified age as an important variable in risk for depression among married and single individuals. Lapate and associates (2014) report that marital *stress* was associated with increased risk for depression suggesting that social stress may also be an important variable to consider.

In a broader context, it may be that lack of social connectedness rather than marital status is associated with higher incidence of depression. Holt-Lundstat and colleagues (2017) cite studies that associate lack of social connections (including high divorce rates, among others) with morbidity for many diseases (including cardiovascular disease, which has been associated with depression) and mortality. These authors suggest that there are so many factors that influence lack of social connectedness and illness that it is difficult to pinpoint one of those (such as marital status) as a singular cause.

Seasonality

Studies exploring whether seasonality is a cause of depression have yielded varying results. The *Diagnostic and Statistical Manual of Mental Disorders, Fifth Edition, Text Revision (DSM-5-TR)* (American Psychiatric Association [APA], 2022) uses the term *seasonal pattern* to describe and specify any depressive disorder that occurs at "characteristic times of the year" (p. 187). The authors note that episodes are most common in fall or winter, but some clients have recurrent summer episodes. Authors of one large study report that prevalence rates of depression with seasonal patterns have varied from 1% to 12%, but in their study of 5,549 patients from primary care settings, there was no evidence of seasonal patterns for MDD (Winthorst et al., 2011). Another study (Cobb et al., 2014) found that a small but significant peak in depression symptoms occurred in winter months, but in over 20 years of following those clients, the winter seasonal pattern was not stable. Seasonal affective disorder (SAD) continues to be popularly referred to as a separate condition, although the *DSM-5-TR* does not list it as a distinct diagnosis. The reported benefits of bright light therapy seem to support a seasonal cause for depression during winter months when there may be less exposure to natural sunlight, but in a meta-analysis of the research on benefits of bright white light in treating depression, the authors found that the evidence was not consistent or conclusive (Mårtensson et al., 2015).

Types of Depressive Disorders

Major Depressive Disorder

Major depressive disorder (MDD) is characterized by depressed mood or loss of interest or pleasure in usual activities. Evidence will show impaired social and occupational functioning that has existed for at least 2 weeks, no history of manic behavior, and symptoms that cannot be attributed to use of substances or a general medical condition. Additionally, the diagnosis of MDD is specified according to whether it is a *single episode* (the individual's first encounter with a major depressive episode) or *recurrent* (the individual has a history of previous major depressive episodes). The diagnosis will also identify the degree of severity of symptoms (mild, moderate, or severe) and whether there is evidence of psychotic, catatonic, or melancholic features. The presence of anxiety and severity of suicide risk may also be noted. MDD is differentiated from schizoaffective disorder, a condition in which the individual expresses symptoms of a mood disorder as well as symptoms of schizophrenia. Read Josh's story on his experience with depression and an eventual diagnosis of schizoaffective disorder in the "Real People, Real Stories" feature that follows. The *DSM-5-TR* (APA, 2022) diagnostic criteria for major depressive episode are presented in Box 16–1.

Persistent Depressive Disorder (Dysthymia)

Characteristics of **dysthymia** are similar to, if somewhat milder than, those ascribed to MDD. Individuals with this mood disturbance describe their mood as sad or "down in the dumps." There is no evidence of psychotic symptoms. The essential feature is a chronically depressed mood (or possibly an irritable mood in children or adolescents) for most of the day, more days than not, for at least 2 years (1 year for children and adolescents). The diagnosis is identified as *early onset* (occurring before age 21 years) or *late onset* (occurring at age 21 years or older). The *DSM-5-TR* diagnostic criteria for dysthymia are presented in Box 16–2.

Premenstrual Dysphoric Disorder

The essential features of **premenstrual dysphoric disorder** (PMDD) include markedly depressed mood, excessive anxiety, mood swings, and decreased interest in activities during the week prior to menses, improving shortly after the onset of menstruation, and becoming minimal or absent in the week postmenses (APA, 2022). The major difference between the diagnosis of premenstrual dysphoric disorder and the premenstrual mood changes that many women experience is a matter of intensity and frequency of symptoms. The symptoms of premenstrual dysphoric disorder are severe enough to interfere with one's ability to function

Real People, Real Stories: Josh's Experience With Depression and the Eventual Diagnosis of Schizoaffective Disorder

(This individual preferred to remain anonymous, so his name has been changed.)

Consider reflecting on factors that may contribute to Josh's perceptions about his illness and his perceptions about the contributions of health-care providers in his recovery process.

Karyn: Tell me about the time when you first became aware that you had a mood disorder. [Josh had told me he had depression. I was unaware when we began the interview that his actual diagnosis was schizoaffective disorder.]

Josh: I was in senior high school and was doing well. I was in advanced placement [AP] courses, and suddenly I got an F in AP English. Nothing like that had ever happened before. I started becoming more withdrawn. I was smoking pot with my friends, and I wonder now if that had an impact. I graduated high school, then attended college for two years until the symptoms really surfaced. I was cut from the soccer team, so there were some disappointments, but I became very withdrawn and depressed. I had suicide ideas and a plan. I had to take a break from school, and I just wasn't doing anything; I was just very withdrawn. Four years later I was diagnosed with schizoaffective disorder.

Karyn: What did you think about that diagnosis?

Josh: I thought it was wrong. I did have some difficulty tracking objects with my eyes, and I still do when I don't get enough sleep [difficulty tracking objects with one's eyes is a common neurological symptom in schizophrenia]. I guess now that I think of it, there was a time in college when I thought my roommates were talking about me, and then I started thinking people in the next room were talking about me. I would read into things a lot. Sometimes I thought I saw something out of the corner of my eye, and sometimes I heard voices.

Karyn: It seems like that would be difficult, maybe even frightening, to have these symptoms and get this diagnosis. What was that like for you?

Josh: Yeah, it was, but I was glad to get a diagnosis because then I knew what I had to deal with. At the same time, though, I thought it was too quickly made and they were too quick to prescribe pills. If I had it to do over, I would have just trusted the doctors, but I rebelled against the drugs several times; sometimes because I was having side effects like tardive dyskinesia; one time because I was convinced the meds were holding me back and even hurting me; and one time because I just gave up, since I didn't have any of the things I wanted, like marriage, a college degree, or a career. Sometimes I thought, "I can just be smarter than this, and I'll get over it." But I was very disorganized and incoherent. Each time I didn't take the pills, I became withdrawn, depressed, and hearing voices, and eventually I just couldn't find anything else to blame it on. I tried to hide the fact that I had stopped taking the pills, but it always became evident eventually. I stay on the medications now because I know I have to.

Karyn: You've come so far since then!

Josh: (smiles) Yeah, it took me eight years to finish my college degree, but now I have a good job in information technology at a large hospital system, and I live on my own. I was engaged, and although it didn't work out, I'm dating again and hopeful about pursuing a committed relationship.

Karyn: What do you think has been most important in supporting your recovery?

Josh: My parents supported me through all of it. They were my only support, and I didn't want other people to know my "stuff." I was able to stay with my parents until I got back on my feet, and that was really important. The last time I stopped taking my meds, I'd have to consult court records to remember everything that happened, but I know there were trespassing charges. I had run-ins with the police. I also had run-ins with my parents, who eventually called in a crisis team, and I was hospitalized against my will. I was in the hospital for around 30 days, and I saw people who were homeless and had no one supporting them, and they were really doing poorly. Knowing I had some place to live really helped me.

Also, I had a job and some successes at work, so that gave me focus. My job is largely mathematical and doesn't require a lot of social skills challenges. That was helpful for me because, while some people may be self-taught with social skills, I've always struggled with that. My job allows me to develop great insights, be quirky, and not have to try to figure people out.

Karyn: What are your thoughts about the impact of the health-care providers with whom you've interacted?

Josh: I work in a hospital, so I have a great appreciation for their hard work. I saw an NP [nurse practitioner] who gave me good advice and was very supportive. She asked some probing questions and confronted me at times, and that was challenging, but she was just doing her job and I was trying to hide from my illness. She told me the medications might end up being less effective if I didn't take them or stay on them early in my illness, so that may have encouraged me to keep taking them.

I had good community health services—a case worker, a psychiatrist, and a behavioral health specialist that I found to be particularly supportive because we talked about spiritual things, and that made it okay to explore other issues. In the hospital, the nurses mostly worked at the station, and that was probably better for their safety,

Real People, Real Stories: Josh's Experience With Depression and the Eventual Diagnosis of Schizoaffective Disorder—cont'd

but still, I could talk to them and they made it seem like it was okay that I was there. That was important because I wasn't sure what was happening to me, and they just talked about normal, everyday stuff. They seemed more like warm people than cold or clinical.

I go to NAMI [National Alliance on Mental Illness] meetings now because I want to share the message with people who have a mental illness (and with their family members) that the professionals could see things I was unable to see at the time I was symptomatic, so it's important to trust the process. I also want families to know that having ongoing support from family members was a lifeline for me even when we were having run-ins and they were facilitating hospitalization against my will.

BOX 16–1 Diagnostic Criteria for Major Depressive Disorder

A. Five (or more) of the following symptoms have been present during the same 2-week period and represent a change from previous functioning; at least one of the symptoms is either (1) depressed mood or (2) loss of interest or pleasure. **NOTE:** Do not include symptoms that are clearly due to another medical condition.

1. Depressed mood most of the day, nearly every day, as indicated by either subjective report (e.g., feels sad, empty, or hopeless) or observation made by others (e.g., appears tearful) (**NOTE:** In children and adolescents, can be irritable mood.)
2. Markedly diminished interest or pleasure in all, or almost all, activities most of the day, nearly every day (as indicated by either subjective account or observation)
3. Significant weight loss when not dieting or weight gain (e.g., a change of more than 5% of body weight in a month), or decrease or increase in appetite nearly every day (**NOTE:** In children, consider failure to make expected weight gain.)
4. Insomnia or hypersomnia nearly every day
5. Psychomotor agitation or retardation nearly every day (observable by others, not merely subjective feelings of restlessness or being slowed down)
6. Fatigue or loss of energy nearly every day
7. Feelings of worthlessness or excessive or inappropriate guilt (which may be delusional) nearly every day (not merely self-reproach or guilt about being sick)
8. Diminished ability to think or concentrate, or indecisiveness, nearly every day (either by subjective account or as observed by others)
9. Recurrent thoughts of death (not just fear of dying), recurrent suicidal ideation without a specific plan, or a suicide attempt or a specific plan for committing suicide

B. The symptoms cause clinically significant distress or impairment in social, occupational, or other important areas of functioning.

C. The episode is not attributable to the physiological effects of a substance or another medical condition.

NOTE: Criteria A, B, and C represent a major depressive episode.

NOTE: Responses to a significant loss (e.g., bereavement, financial ruin, losses from a natural disaster, a serious medical illness or disability) may include feelings of intense sadness, rumination about the loss, insomnia, poor appetite, and weight loss noted in Criterion A, which may resemble a depressive episode. Although such symptoms may be understandable or considered appropriate to the loss, the presence of a major depressive episode in addition to the normal response to a significant loss should also be carefully considered. This decision inevitably requires the exercise of clinical judgment based on the individual's history and the cultural norms for the expression of distress in the context of loss.

D. At least one major depressive episode is not better explained by schizoaffective disorder, and is not superimposed on schizophrenia, schizophreniform disorder, delusional disorder, or other specified and unspecified schizophrenia spectrum and other psychotic disorders.

E. There has never been a manic episode or a hypomanic episode. **NOTE:** This exclusion does not apply if all of the manic-like or hypomanic-like episodes are substance-induced or are attributable to the physiological effects of another medical condition.

Specify:

With anxious distress
With mixed features
With melancholic features
With atypical features
With mood-congruent psychotic features
With mood-incongruent psychotic features
With catatonia
With peripartum onset
With seasonal pattern

Reprinted with permission from American Psychiatric Association. (2022). *Diagnostic and statistical manual of mental disorders, fifth edition, text revision.* American Psychiatric Association.

BOX 16–2 Diagnostic Criteria for Persistent Depressive Disorder (Dysthymia)

A. Depressed mood for most of the day, for more days than not, as indicated by either subjective account or observation by others, for at least 2 years. **NOTE:** In children and adolescents, mood can be irritable and duration must be at least 1 year.
B. Presence, while depressed, of two (or more) of the following:
   1. Poor appetite or overeating
   2. Insomnia or hypersomnia
   3. Low energy or fatigue
   4. Low self-esteem
   5. Poor concentration or difficulty making decisions
   6. Feelings of hopelessness
C. During the 2-year period (1 year for children or adolescents) of the disturbance, the individual has never been without the symptoms in Criteria A and B for more than 2 months at a time.
D. Criteria for a major depressive disorder may be continuously present for 2 years.
E. There has never been a manic episode or a hypomanic episode.
F. The disturbance is not better explained by a persistent schizoaffective disorder, schizophrenia, delusional disorder, or other specified or unspecified schizophrenia spectrum and other psychotic disorder.
G. The symptoms are not attributable to the physiological effects of a substance (e.g., a drug of abuse, a medication) or another medical condition (e.g., hypothyroidism).
H. The symptoms cause clinically significant distress or impairment in social, occupational, or other important areas of functioning.

Specify if:
With anxious distress
With atypical features

Specify if:
With pure dysthymic syndrome
With persistent major depressive episode
With intermittent major depressive episodes, with current episode
With intermittent major depressive episodes, without current episode

Specify if:
In partial remission
In full remission

Specify if:
Early onset if onset is before age 21 years
Late onset if onset is at age 21 years or older

Specify if:
Mild
Moderate
Severe

Reprinted with permission from American Psychiatric Association. (2022). *Diagnostic and statistical manual of mental disorders, fifth edition, text revision.* American Psychiatric Association.

socially, at work, or at school and they are recurrent for the majority of menstrual cycles over the course of a year.

Substance/Medication-Induced Depressive Disorder

The symptoms associated with a substance/medication-induced depressive disorder are considered to be the direct result of physiological effects of a substance (e.g., a drug of abuse, a medication, or toxin exposure). This disorder causes clinically significant distress or impairment in social, occupational, or other important areas of functioning. The depressed mood is associated with *intoxication* or *withdrawal* from substances such as alcohol, amphetamines, cocaine, hallucinogens, opioids, phencyclidine-like substances, sedatives, hypnotics, or anxiolytics and the symptoms meet the full criteria for a relevant depressive disorder (APA, 2022).

Many medications have been known to evoke mood symptoms. Classifications include anesthetics, analgesics, anticholinergics, anticonvulsants, antihypertensives, antiparkinsonian agents, antiulcer agents, cardiac medications, oral contraceptives, psychotropic medications, muscle relaxants, steroids, and sulfonamides. Some specific examples are included in the discussion of predisposing factors to depressive disorders.

Depressive Disorder Due to Another Medical Condition

This disorder is characterized by symptoms associated with a major depressive episode that are the direct physiological consequence of another medical condition (APA, 2022). The depression causes clinically significant distress or impairment in social, occupational, or other important areas of functioning. Examples of medical conditions that influence depression include stroke, myocardial infarction, traumatic brain injuries, thyroid disorders, Cushing's disease, Huntington's disease, Parkinson's disease, and multiple sclerosis.

Predisposing Factors

The etiology of depression is unclear. No single theory or hypothesis has been postulated that substantiates a clear-cut explanation for the disease. Evidence continues to mount in support of multiple causations, recognizing the combined effects of genetic, biochemical, and psychosocial influences on an individual's susceptibility to depression. A number of theoretical postulates are presented here.

Biological Theories

Genetics

Affective illness has been the subject of considerable research on the relevance of hereditary factors. A genetic link has been suggested in numerous studies; however, a definitive mode of genetic transmission has yet to be demonstrated. In addition, recent studies have focused on genetic variants that are associated with depression (Lipp et al., 2020). For example, one genetic variant (an *MTHFR C677T* gene mutation) has been associated with impaired folate metabolism that may lead to decreased synthesis of neurotransmitters.

Twin Studies

Twin studies suggest a strong genetic factor in the etiology of affective illness, including depressive disorders and bipolar disorders. When compared to dizygotic twins, monozygotic twins have a two to four times greater incidence of depression but between monozygotic twins there is only a 70% to 80% chance of both twins having the illness (Kelsoe & Greenwood, 2017). These findings suggest that although twin studies do identify genetic risk, genetics does not explain all depressions. Environmental risks are not only an important variable but are also uniquely individual.

Family Studies

Family studies have shown that major depression is seven times more common among first-degree biological relatives of people with the disorder than among the general population (Kelsoe & Greenwood, 2017). The evidence to support an increased risk of depressive disorder in individuals with positive family history is quite compelling. It is unlikely that random environmental factors could cause the concentration of illness that is seen within families.

Adoption Studies

Further support for heritability as an etiological influence in depression comes from studies of the adopted offspring of affectively ill biological parents. These studies have indicated that biological children of parents with mood disorders are at increased risk of developing a mood disorder, even when they are reared by adoptive parents who do not have the disorder (Kelsoe & Greenwood, 2017). Conversely, adoption studies have also been used to look at the effects of being reared by an adoptive parent (particularly the maternal parent) with depression and the risks for depression in nongenetically similar children. Interestingly, these studies have demonstrated an increased risk of depression (as well as oppositional defiant disorder and conduct disorder) in adopted children that cannot be explained by genetics (Natsuaki et al., 2014). Again, this finding suggests that environmental factors also play a role in the etiology of depressive illnesses.

Biochemical Influences

Biogenic Amines

It has been hypothesized that depressive illness may be related to a deficiency of the neurotransmitters norepinephrine, serotonin, and dopamine at functionally important receptor sites in the brain. Historically, the biogenic amine hypothesis of mood disorders grew out of the observation that reserpine, an antihypertensive, which depletes the brain of amines such as norepinephrine, was associated with the development of a depressive syndrome. The catecholamine norepinephrine has been identified as a key component in the mobilization of the body to deal with stressful situations. Cortisol levels are increased in patients with depression. Neurons that contain serotonin are critically involved in the regulation of many psychobiological functions, such as mood, anxiety, arousal, vigilance, irritability, thinking, cognition, appetite, aggression, sleep–wake cycles, eating, and intestinal motility. Low levels of serotonin have been noted in depression and in some patients with suicidal impulses (Boland & Verduin, 2022). Tryptophan, the amino acid precursor of serotonin, has been shown to enhance the efficacy of antidepressant medications and, on occasion, to be effective as an antidepressant itself. The level of dopamine in the mesolimbic system of the brain is thought to exert a strong influence over human mood and behavior. A diminished supply of these biogenic amines inhibits the transmission of impulses from one neuronal fiber to another, causing a failure of the cells to fire or become charged (Fig. 16–1).

Abnormal levels of acetylcholine, glutamate, glycine, and gamma-aminobutyric acid (GABA) have

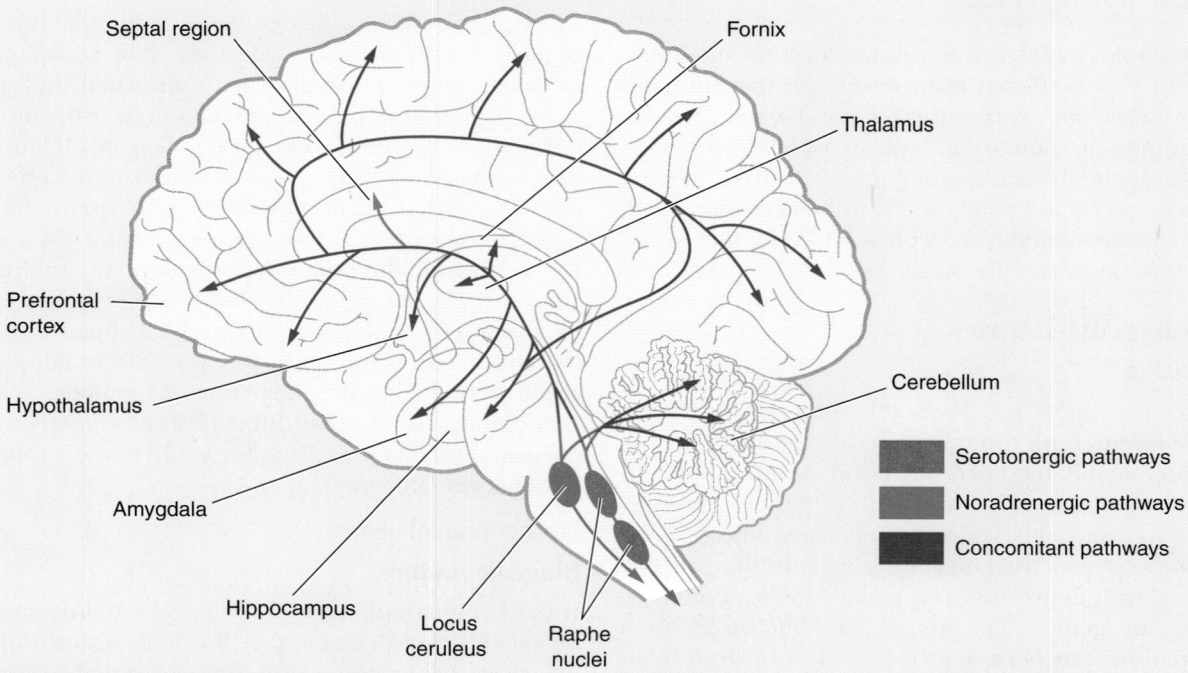

FIGURE 16–1 Neurobiology of depression.

NEUROTRANSMITTERS

Although other neurotransmitters have also been implicated in the pathophysiology of depression, disturbances in serotonin and norepinephrine have been the most extensively scrutinized.

Cell bodies of origin for the serotonin pathways lie within the raphe nuclei located in the brainstem. Those for norepinephrine originate in the locus ceruleus. Projections for both neurotransmitters extend throughout the forebrain, prefrontal cortex, cerebellum, and limbic system.

AREAS OF THE BRAIN AFFECTED

Areas of the brain affected by depression and the symptoms that they mediate include the following:

- ***Hippocampus:*** Memory impairments, feelings of worthlessness, hopelessness, and guilt
- ***Amygdala:*** Anhedonia, anxiety, reduced motivation
- ***Hypothalamus:*** Increased or decreased sleep and appetite; decreased energy and libido
- ***Other limbic structures:*** Emotional alterations
- ***Frontal cortex:*** Depressed mood; problems concentrating
- ***Cerebellum:*** Psychomotor retardation/agitation

MEDICATIONS AND THEIR EFFECTS ON THE BRAIN

All medications that increase serotonin or norepinephrine, or both, can improve the emotional and vegetative symptoms of depression. Medications that produce these effects include those that block the presynaptic reuptake of the neurotransmitters or block receptors at nerve endings (tricyclics, SSRIs, SNRIs) and those that inhibit monoamine oxidase, an enzyme that is involved in the metabolism of the monoamines serotonin, norepinephrine, and dopamine (MAOIs).

Side effects of these medications relate to their specific neurotransmitter receptor-blocking action. Tricyclic and tetracyclic drugs (e.g., imipramine, amitriptyline, mirtazapine) block reuptake and/or receptors for serotonin, norepinephrine, acetylcholine, and histamine. SSRIs are selective serotonin reuptake inhibitors. Others, such as bupropion, venlafaxine, and duloxetine, block serotonin and norepinephrine reuptake and also are weak inhibitors of dopamine.

Blockade of norepinephrine reuptake results in side effects of tremors, cardiac arrhythmias, sexual dysfunction, and hypertension. Blockade of serotonin reuptake results in side effects of gastrointestinal disturbances, increased agitation, and sexual dysfunction. Blockade of dopamine reuptake results in side effects of psychomotor activation. Blockade of acetylcholine reuptake results in dry mouth, blurred vision, constipation, and urinary retention. Blockade of histamine reuptake results in sedation, weight gain, and hypotension.

also been associated with depression. Because cholinergic agents have profound effects on mood, electroencephalograms, sleep, and neuroendocrine function, it has been suggested that the problem in depression and mania may be an imbalance between the biogenic amines and acetylcholine. Glutamate and glycine bind at *N*-methyl-D-aspartate (NMDA) receptors, and recent evidence suggests that drugs that antagonize NMDA receptors have antidepressant effects (Boland & Verduin, 2022). Reductions in GABA appear in depression, and antidepressants upregulate GABA receptors.

The precise role that any neurotransmitters play in the etiology of depression is unknown because these chemicals cannot be directly measured in the human brain outside of postmortem studies. It has been theorized that because selective serotonin reuptake inhibitors (SSRIs) are drugs that elevate serotonin levels, low serotonin levels in the brain must be responsible for depression. However, SSRIs also seem to be beneficial in the treatment of anxiety, leading to the hypothesis that low serotonin levels are responsible for anxiety. Further, too much serotonin has also been implicated in anxiety states and in schizophrenia. Boland and Verduin (2022) state:

> It is unclear to what extent serotonin acts as a true synaptic or "private" neurotransmitter versus action as a local endocrine hormone or "social transmitter" or whether its roles differ depending on the fiber type from which it is released. (p. 955)

Newer antidepressants that act on both serotonergic and noradrenergic receptors suggest that the dysregulation of biogenic amines in depression is far more complex than can be explained by single neurotransmitter hypotheses (Akiskal, 2017). Ongoing research will hopefully clarify what are, at present, only hypotheses about the etiology of depression.

Neuroendocrine Disturbances

Neuroendocrine disturbances may play a role in the pathogenesis or persistence of depressive illness. This notion has arisen in view of the marked disturbances in mood observed with the administration of certain hormones or in the presence of spontaneously occurring endocrine disease.

Hypothalamic-Pituitary-Adrenocortical Axis

In individuals who are depressed, the normal system of hormonal inhibition fails, resulting in a hypersecretion of cortisol. This elevated serum cortisol is the basis for the dexamethasone suppression test that is sometimes used to determine whether an individual has somatically treatable depression.

Hypothalamic-Pituitary-Thyroid Axis

Thyrotropin-releasing factor (TRF) from the hypothalamus stimulates the release of thyroid-stimulating hormone (TSH) from the anterior pituitary gland. In turn, TSH stimulates the thyroid gland. Diminished TSH response to administered TRF is observed in approximately 20% to 30% of patients with depression and appears to be associated with increased risk for relapse despite treatment with antidepressants (Boland & Verduin, 2022). Individuals with hypothyroidism often manifest with signs of depression (in addition to a host of other symptoms), and nearly 20 million people in the United States (women are five to eight times more likely than men) suffer from thyroid conditions (American Thyroid Association, 2021). Laboratory testing to evaluate TSH is relevant to distinguish between depressive disorders and thyroid disorders because in thyroid disorders the symptoms of depression are treated with hormone replacement rather than antidepressants.

Although there is not a single diagnostic test for depression, several findings from tests that may indicate depression but are nonspecific, such as increased corticotropin-releasing factor in cerebrospinal fluid, steroid overproduction (evidenced by the dexamethasone suppression test), and thyroid dysregulation (evidenced by thyrotropin challenge tests), have led Akiskal (2017) to conclude that there is clear evidence of midbrain disturbance (and thus, evidence of a legitimate disease process) in clinical depression.

Physiological Influences

Depressive symptoms that occur as a consequence of a non–mood disorder or as an adverse effect of certain medications are called *secondary depression.* Secondary depression may be related to medication side effects, neurological disorders, electrolyte or hormonal disturbances, nutritional deficiencies, and other physiological or psychological conditions.

Medication Side Effects

A number of drugs, either alone or in combination with other medications, can produce a depressive syndrome. Most common among these drugs are those that have a direct effect on the central nervous system. Examples of these include the anxiolytics, antipsychotics, sedative-hypnotics (including barbiturates and opioids), and anticonvulsant mood stabilizers. Many drugs that are used to treat general medical conditions have also been associated with inducing depression and several are listed here:

- Antibacterial, antifungal, and antiviral agents
- Anticonvulsants

- Antihypertensives (including beta blockers and calcium blockers)
- Antimalarials (including mefloquine)
- Antineoplastics (including vincristine and zidovudine)
- Dermatologics (including Accutane and finasteride)
- Hormones (including contraceptives)
- Nonnucleoside reverse transcriptase inhibitors (HIV medications)
- Respiratory agents (leukotriene inhibitors)
- Smoking cessation agents (varenicline)
- Statins
- Steroids

Neurological Disorders

An individual who has had a cerebrovascular accident (CVA) may experience despondency unrelated to the severity of the CVA. These are true mood disorders, and antidepressant drug therapy may be indicated. Brain tumors, particularly in the area of the temporal lobe, often cause symptoms of depression. Agitated depression may be part of the clinical picture associated with Alzheimer's disease, Parkinson's disease, and Huntington's disease. Agitation and restlessness may also represent an underlying depression in the individual with multiple sclerosis.

Electrolyte Disturbances

Excessive levels of sodium bicarbonate or calcium can produce symptoms of depression, as can deficits in magnesium and sodium. Potassium is also implicated in the syndrome of depression. Symptoms have been observed with excesses of potassium in the body as well as in instances of potassium depletion. Interestingly, *hypo*natremia is a side effect of serotonergic antidepressants, especially in the elderly.

Hormonal Disturbances

Depression is associated with dysfunction of the adrenal cortex and is commonly observed in individuals with Addison's disease or Cushing's syndrome. Other endocrine conditions that may result in symptoms of depression include hypoparathyroidism, hyperparathyroidism, hypothyroidism, and hyperthyroidism.

An imbalance of the hormones estrogen and progesterone has been implicated in the predisposition to PMDD, although the exact etiology is unknown. The interaction of these hormonal changes also has an impact on serotonin levels, which may contribute to the depression associated with this disorder. It is also noted that individuals with PMDD often have underlying depression and anxiety, so it is possible that the hormone changes are exacerbating an already existing condition (Burnett, 2021).

Nutritional Deficiencies

Deficiencies in proteins, carbohydrates, vitamin B_1 (thiamine), vitamin B_2 (riboflavin), vitamin B_6 (pyridoxine), vitamin B_9 (folate), vitamin B_{12}, iron, zinc, calcium, chromium, iodine, lithium, selenium, and potassium have all been associated with producing symptoms of depression (Kubala, 2021; Sathyanarayana et al., 2008). A recent large study also found that vitamin D deficiency was linked to depressive symptoms (Shin et al., 2016), although another study concluded that vitamin D_3 supplementation did not change the incidence or recurrence of depressive symptoms (Okereke et al., 2020). Individuals with anorexia nervosa who have significant nutritional deficiencies commonly have comorbid depression.

Other Physiological Conditions

Other conditions that have been associated with secondary depression include collagen disorders, such as systemic lupus erythematosus (SLE) and polyarteritis nodosa; cardiovascular disease, such as cardiomyopathy, congestive heart failure, and myocardial infarction; infections, such as encephalitis, hepatitis, mononucleosis, pneumonia, and syphilis; and metabolic disorders, such as diabetes mellitus and porphyria.

The Role of Inflammation

The role of inflammation in the development of depression is an area of current research. The function of the immune system in the development of disease is being explored with regard to a host of illnesses including cancer, autoimmune disorders, and several psychiatric disorders. Not all patients with depression have signs of inflammation, but individuals with treatment-resistant depression manifest with high C-reactive protein levels (CRP) and tumor necrosis factor (TNF), which are biomarkers of inflammation (Miller, 2018). Cytokines, part of the inflammatory response, have specific activities in the brain, including impacting neurotransmitters associated with depression (monoamines) and dopamine. Stress, another inflammatory process, has been shown to increase the permeability of the blood-brain barrier and consequently may have an impact on the development of depression when inflammatory responses in the brain trigger chemical changes. Recent research (Slezak, 2021) demonstrates, through state-of-the-art imaging, that chronic stress creates permanent changes in the brain, particularly dysregulated astrocyte metabolism, and that this is a major hallmark of depression.

Does depression trigger inflammation or is inflammation one potential cause of depression? Much more research is needed, but there is current evidence that elevated inflammation biomarkers can predict a patient's response to conventional antidepressants, psychotherapy, ketamine, and anti-cytokine immunotherapy (Miller, 2018). This research reinforces the complex interactions and dynamics associated with the disease of depression.

Psychosocial Theories

Psychoanalytical Theory

Freud (1957) presented his classic paper "Mourning and Melancholia" in 1917. He defined the distinguishing features of melancholia as

> a profoundly painful dejection, cessation of interest in the outside world, loss of the capacity to love, inhibition of all activity, and a lowering of the self-regarding feelings to a degree that finds utterances in self-reproaches and self-revilings, and culminates in a delusional expectation of punishment. (p. 242)

He observed that melancholia occurs after the loss of a loved object, either actually by death or emotionally by rejection, or the loss of some other abstraction of value to the individual. Freud indicated that in melancholia, the depressed patient's rage is internally directed because of identification with the lost object.

Freud believed that the individual predisposed to melancholia experienced ambivalence in love relationships. He postulated, therefore, that once the loss had been incorporated into the self (ego), the hostile part of the ambivalence that had been felt for the lost object is then turned inward against the ego.

Learning Theory

The model of "learned helplessness" arises out of Seligman's (1973) experiments with dogs. The animals were exposed to electrical stimulation from which they could not escape. Later, when they were given the opportunity to avoid the traumatic experience, they reacted with helplessness and made no attempt to escape. A similar state of helplessness exists in humans who have experienced numerous failures (either real or perceived). The individual abandons any further attempt to succeed. Seligman theorized that learned helplessness predisposes individuals to depression by imposing a feeling of lack of control over their life situation. They become depressed because they feel helpless; they have learned that whatever they do is futile. This can be especially damaging very early in life because the sense of mastery over one's environment is an important foundation for future emotional development.

Object Loss Theory

The theory of object loss suggests that depressive illness occurs as a result of having been abandoned by or otherwise separated from a significant other during the first 6 months of life. Because during this period the mother represents the child's main source of security, she is considered to be the "object." This absence of attachment, which may be either physical or emotional, leads to feelings of helplessness and despair that contribute to lifelong patterns of depression in response to loss.

The concept of "anaclitic depression" was introduced in 1946 by psychiatrist René Spitz to refer to children who became depressed after being separated from their mothers for an extended period during the first year of life. The condition included behaviors such as excessive crying, anorexia, withdrawal, **psychomotor retardation** (sluggish physical movements), stupor, and a generalized impairment in the normal process of growth and development. Object loss theory suggests that loss in adult life afflicts people much more severely in the form of depression if the individuals have suffered early childhood loss.

Cognitive Theory

Beck and colleagues (1979) proposed a theory suggesting that the primary disturbance in depression is cognitive rather than affective. The underlying cause of the depression is cognitive distortions that result in negative, defeated attitudes. Beck and colleagues identified three cognitive distortions that they believe serve as the basis for depression:

1. Negative expectations of the environment
2. Negative expectations of the self
3. Negative expectations of the future

These cognitive distortions arise out of a defect in cognitive development, and the individual feels inadequate, worthless, and rejected by others. Outlook for the future is one of pessimism and hopelessness.

Cognitive theorists believe that depression is the product of negative thinking. This is in contrast to the suggestions by other theorists that negative thinking occurs when an individual is depressed. **Cognitive behavior therapy** (CBT) focuses on helping individuals to alter mood and behavior by changing the way they think. The individual is taught to control negative thought distortions that lead to pessimism, lethargy, procrastination, indecisiveness, and low self-esteem.

The Transactional Model of Stress and Adaptation

No single theory or hypothesis exists to substantiate a clear-cut explanation for depressive disorder.

Evidence continues to mount in support of multiple causation. The transactional model of stress and adaptation recognizes the combined effects of genetic, biochemical, and psychosocial influences on an individual's susceptibility to depression (for more information on the transactional model of stress and adaptation, see Chapter 19, "Trauma- and Stressor-Related Disorders").

Developmental Implications

Childhood

Only in recent years has a consensus developed among investigators identifying MDD as an entity in children and adolescents that can be identified using criteria similar to those used for adults. It is not uncommon, however, for the symptoms of depression to be manifested differently in childhood. In addition to some of the classic symptoms of depression (mood, appetite, sleep and energy changes, and withdrawal), children may present with irritable mood, excessive self-reproach, and excessive clinging to parents (Anxiety and Depression Association of America, 2021; Boland & Verduin, 2022). In school-age children, changes in grades, getting into trouble at school, refusal to go to school, and school phobias may be symptomatic of depression.

Other symptoms of childhood and adolescent depression may include hyperactivity, delinquency, psychosomatic complaints, sleeping and eating disturbances, social isolation, delusional thinking, and suicidal thoughts or actions. Wagner and Brent (2017) note that youths with depression are more often irritable rather than dysphoric and consequently less likely to identify themselves as depressed. Additionally, they cite that anywhere from 40% to 90% of youths with depression have other comorbid psychiatric conditions, so comprehensive assessment is essential.

The APA (2022) has included a diagnostic category in the "Depressive Disorders" chapter of the *DSM-5-TR*. This childhood disorder is called *disruptive mood dysregulation disorder*. The diagnostic criteria for disruptive mood dysregulation disorder are presented in Box 16–3.

BOX 16–3 Diagnostic Criteria for Disruptive Mood Dysregulation Disorder

A. Severe recurrent temper outbursts manifested verbally (e.g., verbal rages) and/or behaviorally (e.g., physical aggression toward people or property) that are grossly out of proportion in intensity or duration to the situation or provocation.
B. The temper outbursts are inconsistent with developmental level.
C. The temper outbursts occur, on average, three or more times per week.
D. The mood between temper outbursts is persistently irritable or angry most of the day, nearly every day, and is observable by others (e.g., parents, teachers, peers).
E. Criteria A–D have been present for 12 or more months. Throughout that time, the individual has not had a period lasting 3 or more consecutive months without all of the symptoms of Criteria A–D.
F. Criteria A and D are present in at least two of three settings (i.e., at home, at school, with peers) and are severe in at least one of these.
G. The diagnosis should not be made for the first time before age 6 or after age 18 years.
H. By history or observation, the age at onset of Criteria A–E is before 10 years.
I. There has never been a distinct period lasting more than 1 day during which the full symptom criteria, except duration, for a manic or hypomanic episode have been met. *Note:* Developmentally appropriate mood elevation, such as occurs in the context of a highly positive event or its anticipation, should not be considered as a symptom of mania or hypomania.
J. The behaviors do not occur exclusively during an episode of major depressive disorder and are not better explained by another mental disorder (e.g., autism spectrum disorder, post-traumatic stress disorder, separation anxiety disorder, persistent depressive disorder [dysthymia]).

NOTE: This diagnosis cannot coexist with oppositional defiant disorder, intermittent explosive disorder, or bipolar disorder, though it can coexist with others, including major depressive disorder, attention-deficit/hyperactivity disorder, conduct disorder, and substance use disorders. Individuals whose symptoms meet criteria for both disruptive mood dysregulation disorder and oppositional defiant disorder should only be given the diagnosis of disruptive mood dysregulation disorder. If an individual has ever experienced a manic or hypomanic episode, the diagnosis of disruptive mood dysregulation disorder should not be assigned.

K. The symptoms are not attributable to the physiological effects of a substance or to another medical or neurological condition.

Reprinted with permission from American Psychiatric Association. (2022). *Diagnostic and statistical manual of mental disorders, fifth edition, text revision.* American Psychiatric Publishing.

Children may become depressed for various reasons. In many depressed children, there is a genetic predisposition toward the condition, which is then precipitated by a stressful situation. Common precipitating factors include physical or emotional detachment by the primary caregiver, parental separation or divorce, death of a loved one (person or pet), a move, academic failure, or physical illness. In any event, the common denominator is loss.

The focus of therapy for depressed children is to alleviate the child's symptoms and strengthen the child's coping and adaptive skills with the hope of possibly preventing future psychological problems. Some studies have shown that untreated childhood depression may lead to subsequent problems in adolescence and adult life. Most children are treated on an outpatient basis. Hospitalization of depressed children usually occurs only if they are actively suicidal, when the home environment precludes adherence to a treatment regimen, or if a child needs to be separated from the home because of psychosocial deprivation.

Parental therapy and family therapy are commonly used to help the younger depressed child. Recovery is facilitated by emotional support and guidance to family members. Children older than age 8 years usually participate in family therapy. In some situations, individual treatment may be appropriate for older children. Medications, such as antidepressants, can be important in the treatment of children, especially for the more serious and recurrent forms of depression. The SSRIs have been used with success, particularly in combination with psychosocial therapies. However, because there has been some concern that the use of antidepressant medications may cause suicidal behavior in young people, the U.S. Food and Drug Administration (FDA) has applied a black box warning (described in the next section) to all antidepressant medications. The National Institute of Mental Health (NIMH, 2018) stated:

> In some cases, children, teenagers, and young adults under 25 may experience an increase in suicidal thoughts or behavior when taking antidepressants, especially in the first few weeks after starting or when the dose is changed. This warning from the U.S. Food and Drug Administration (FDA) also says that patients of all ages taking antidepressants should be watched closely, especially during the first few weeks of treatment.

Adolescence

Depression may be even harder to recognize in an adolescent than in a younger child. Feelings of sadness, loneliness, anxiety, and hopelessness associated with depression may be perceived as the normal emotional stresses of growing up. Therefore, many young people whose symptoms are attributed to the "normal adjustments" of adolescence do not get the help they need. Depression is a major cause of suicide among teens, and suicide is the second-leading cause of death in the 15-to-19-year-old age-group (National Center for Health Statistics, 2021).

Common symptoms of depression in the adolescent are inappropriately expressed anger, aggressiveness, running away, delinquency, social withdrawal, sexual acting out, substance abuse, restlessness, and apathy. Loss of self-esteem, sleeping and eating disturbances, and psychosomatic complaints are also common.

What, then, differentiates mood disorder from the typical turbulent behavior of adolescence? A visible manifestation of *behavioral change that lasts for several weeks* is the best clue for a mood disorder. Examples include the normally outgoing and extroverted adolescent who becomes withdrawn and isolates herself, the good student who previously received consistently high marks but is now failing and skipping classes, and the usually self-confident teenager who is now inappropriately irritable and defensive with others.

Adolescents become depressed for the same reasons that were discussed under childhood depression. In adolescence, however, depression is a common manifestation of the stress and independence conflicts associated with the normal maturation process. Depression may also be the response to death of a parent, other relative, or friend or to a breakup with a boyfriend or girlfriend. This perception of abandonment by parents or closest peer relationship is thought to be the most frequent immediate precipitant to adolescent suicide.

Treatment of the depressed adolescent is often conducted on an outpatient basis. Hospitalization may be required in cases of severe depression or threat of imminent suicide, when a family situation is such that treatment cannot be carried out in the home, when the physical condition precludes self-care of biological needs, or when the adolescent has indicated possible harm to self or others in the family.

In addition to supportive psychosocial intervention, antidepressant therapy may be part of the treatment of adolescent mood disorders. However, as mentioned previously, the FDA has issued a public health advisory warning the public about the increased risk of suicidal thoughts and behavior in children and adolescents being treated with antidepressant medications. The black box warning on all antidepressant medications describes this risk and emphasizes the need for close monitoring of adolescents and young adults started on these medications. The advisory language does not prohibit the use of antidepressants in children, adolescents, and young adults. Rather, it warns of the risk of suicidality and encourages prescribers to balance this risk with clinical need.

Fluoxetine (Prozac) has been approved by the FDA to treat depression in children and adolescents, and escitalopram (Lexapro) was approved in 2009 for treatment of MDD in adolescents ages 12 to 17 years. The other SSRI medications, such as sertraline, citalopram, and paroxetine, and the serotonin-norepinephrine reuptake inhibitor (SNRI) antidepressants duloxetine, venlafaxine, and desvenlafaxine have not been approved for treatment of depression in children or adolescents, although they have been prescribed to children by physicians in "off-label use" (use other than the FDA-approved use). In June 2003, the FDA recommended that paroxetine not be used in children and adolescents for the treatment of MDD. The FDA analysis of antidepressant medications, as reported by the Mayo Clinic (2019), identified that a small number of those taking antidepressants had a worsening in suicidal thoughts or behavior and that none of the children in the study actually took their own life. Nonetheless, the potential risk is considered significant enough to carefully evaluate risks versus benefits before prescribing antidepressants to children and adolescents.

Senescence

Depression (along with dementia) is one of the most common psychiatric disorders among the elderly. Estimates are that about 1% to 5% of older adults living in the community have depression but that incidence increases to 13.5% for those requiring home health care and 11.5% for older adults who are hospitalized (CDC, 2021a). Depression is also more common in older adults with other medical conditions, such as heart disease and those with functional limitations.

Depression among the elderly may be influenced by the value our society places on youth, vigor, and uninterrupted productivity. These societal attitudes reinforce feelings of low self-esteem, helplessness, and hopelessness that become more pervasive and intensive with advanced age. Further, the aging individual's adaptive coping strategies may be seriously challenged by major stressors, such as financial problems, physical illness, changes in bodily functioning, and an increasing awareness of approaching death. The problem is often intensified by the numerous losses that individuals experience during this period in life, such as spouse, friends, children, home, and independence. A phenomenon called *bereavement overload* occurs when individuals experience so many losses in their lives that they are not able to resolve one grief response before another one begins. Bereavement overload predisposes older individuals to depressive illness. Evidence-based treatments for depression will continue to be a focal point of care for this population.

Although they make up only about 14.5% of the population, the elderly account for a proportionately larger percentage of the suicides in the United States. Suicide rates increase during the life course and are as high as 48.7/100,000 among older white men in the United States (Conejero et al., 2018). For all ages and races, including the elderly, the suicide rate among white men is almost four times the national rate.

Some symptoms of depression in the elderly are similar to those in younger adults. However, depressive syndromes are often confused with those of other illnesses associated with the aging process. Symptoms of depression are often misdiagnosed as neurocognitive disorder (NCD) when, in fact, the memory loss, confused thinking, or apathy symptomatic of NCD may be the result of depression. This is referred to as *pseudodementia.* The early awakening and reduced appetite typical of depression are common among many older people who are not depressed. Compounding this situation is that many medical conditions, including endocrinological, neurological, nutritional, and metabolic disorders, often present with classic symptoms of depression. Many medications commonly used by the elderly, such as antihypertensives, corticosteroids, and analgesics, can also produce a depressant effect.

Depression accompanies many of the illnesses that affect older people, such as Parkinson's disease, cancer, arthritis, and the early stages of Alzheimer's disease. Treating depression in these situations can reduce unnecessary suffering and help individuals cope with their medical problems.

The most effective treatment for depression in the elderly individual is thought to be a combination of psychosocial and biological approaches.

Antidepressant medications are administered with consideration for age-related physiological changes in absorption, distribution, elimination, and brain receptor sensitivity. Because of these changes, plasma concentrations of these medications can reach very high levels despite moderate oral doses. Anticholinergic side effects associated with tricyclic antidepressants can be problematic for the elderly, and SSRIs have been associated with inducing significant hyponatremia in this population. Careful evaluation and monitoring are essential.

Electroconvulsive therapy (ECT) is an important alternative for treatment of major depression in the elderly, especially considering the problematic side effects of antidepressants in this population. The response to ECT may be slower with advancing age, and the therapeutic effects are of limited duration, but in a systematic review, researchers concluded that use of ECT in the elderly is "highly effective, safe, and well tolerated" in the geriatric population (Geduldig & Kellner, 2016, p. 40). It may be considered the treatment of choice for the elderly individual who is an acute suicidal risk or is unable to tolerate antidepressant medications. Confusion, a side effect of ECT that typically lasts a few minutes to several hours, is generally more pronounced in the elderly (Mayo Clinic, 2021).

Other therapeutic approaches include interpersonal, behavioral, cognitive, group, and family psychotherapies. Appropriate treatment of the depressed elderly individual can bring relief from suffering and offer a new lease on life with a feeling of renewed productivity.

Postpartum Depression

The severity of depression in the postpartum period varies from a feeling of the blues to moderate depression to severe depression with psychotic features. About 50% of these episodes actually begin prior to delivery, so the *DSM-5-TR* collectively classifies episodes that occur during pregnancy and in the postpartum period as *peripartum* episodes (APA, 2022). The onset of symptoms during pregnancy increases risk for major depression in the postpartum period. Major depression with psychotic features occurs in about 1 or 2 out of 1,000 postpartum women.

Symptoms of the "baby blues" include worry, sadness, and fatigue after having a baby. These symptoms affect about 80% of mothers and usually subside within a week or two (National Institute of Mental Health, n.d.).

Symptoms of moderate **postpartum depression** have been described as depressed mood varying from day to day, with more bad days than good, tending to be worse toward evening and associated with fatigue, irritability, loss of appetite, sleep disturbances, and loss of libido. In addition, the new mother expresses a great deal of concern about her inability to care for her baby. These symptoms begin somewhat later than those described in the maternity blues and take from a few weeks to several months to abate.

Postpartum depression with psychotic features is characterized by depressed mood, agitation, indecision, lack of concentration, guilt, and an abnormal attitude toward bodily functions. The symptoms can be severe and incapacitating. There may be lack of interest in or rejection of the baby or a morbid fear that the baby may be harmed, accompanied by delusions and hallucinations. Risks of suicide and infanticide should not be overlooked. There is a 30% to 50% likelihood of postpartum psychosis recurring with subsequent pregnancies (APA, 2022).

The etiology of postpartum depression remains unclear. Maternity blues may be associated with hormonal changes, tryptophan metabolism, or alterations in membrane transport during the early postpartum period. Besides being exposed to these same somatic changes, the woman who experiences moderate to severe symptoms probably possesses a vulnerability to depression related to heredity, upbringing, early life experiences, personality, or social circumstances. A history of depression appears to be a risk factor for postpartum depression (NIMH, 2018) and family history of psychiatric disorders, including schizophrenia, bipolar, depression, and other psychiatric disorders, also increases risk (Bauer et al., 2018). The etiology of postpartum depression may very likely be a combination of hormonal, metabolic, and psychosocial influences.

Treatment of postpartum depression varies with the severity of the illness. Psychotic depression may be treated with antidepressant medication, along with supportive psychotherapy, group therapy, and possibly family therapy. In 2019, the FDA approved the first novel drug for the treatment of postpartum depression. Brexanolone (Zulresso) is administered in an IV transfusion over 2.5 days and is only available through a restricted distribution program in a certified health agency. In addition, because there is a risk of severe side effects, including sedation and sudden loss of consciousness, this drug requires a Risk Evaluation and Mitigation Strategy (REMS). Pulse oximetry must be continuously monitored, and patients must be accompanied during interactions with children while receiving the infusion (FDA, 2019a).

Moderate depression may be relieved with supportive psychotherapy and continuing assistance with home management until the symptoms subside. The individual with baby blues, the sadness and mood swings occurring in the immediate postpartum period, usually needs no treatment beyond reassurance from the physician or nurse that these feelings are common (up to 80% of new moms experience these symptoms) and will soon pass. Support and comfort from significant others is also important.

Application of the Nursing Process

Background Assessment Data

Symptomatology of depression can be viewed on a continuum from transient symptoms to severe depression according to severity of the illness. All individuals become depressed from time to time in response to life's disappointments, and these symptoms tend to be transient. Severe depression, however, is marked by significant distress that interferes with social, occupational, cognitive, and emotional functioning.

The individual who is severely depressed may also demonstrate a loss of contact with reality. This level is associated with a complete lack of pleasure in all activities, and ruminations about suicide are common. MDD is an example of severe depression. A continuum of depression is presented in Figure 16–2.

A number of assessment rating scales are available for measuring severity of depressive symptoms. Some are meant to be clinician administered, whereas others may be self-administered. Examples of self-rating scales include the Zung Self-Rating Depression Scale and the Beck Depression Inventory. One of the most widely used clinician-administered scales is the Hamilton Depression Rating Scale (HDRS) (Box 16–4). It has been reviewed and revised over the years and exists today in several versions. The original version contains seventeen items and is designed to measure mood, guilty feelings, suicidal ideation, sleep disturbances, anxiety levels, and weight loss.

Symptoms of depression can be described as alterations in four spheres of human functioning: (1) affective, (2) behavioral, (3) cognitive, and (4) physiological. Alterations within these spheres differ according to degree of severity of symptomatology.

Transient Depression

Symptoms at this level of the continuum are not necessarily dysfunctional; in fact, they may be considered part of the broad range of typical human emotional responses that accompany everyday disappointments in life. Transient depression subsides quickly, and the individual is able to refocus on other goals and achievements. Alterations include the following:

- ***Affective:*** Sadness, dejection, feeling downhearted, having the blues
- ***Behavioral:*** Some crying
- ***Cognitive:*** Some difficulty getting mind off one's disappointment
- ***Physiological:*** Feeling tired and listless

Mild Depression

Symptoms at the mild level of depression are like those associated with grieving. Alterations at the mild level include the following:

- ***Affective:*** Denial of feelings, anger, anxiety, guilt, helplessness, hopelessness, sadness, despondency
- ***Behavioral:*** Tearfulness, regression, restlessness, agitation, withdrawal
- ***Cognitive:*** Preoccupation with the loss, self-blame, ambivalence, blaming others
- ***Physiological:*** Anorexia or overeating, insomnia or hypersomnia, headache, backache, chest pain, or other symptoms associated with the loss of a significant other

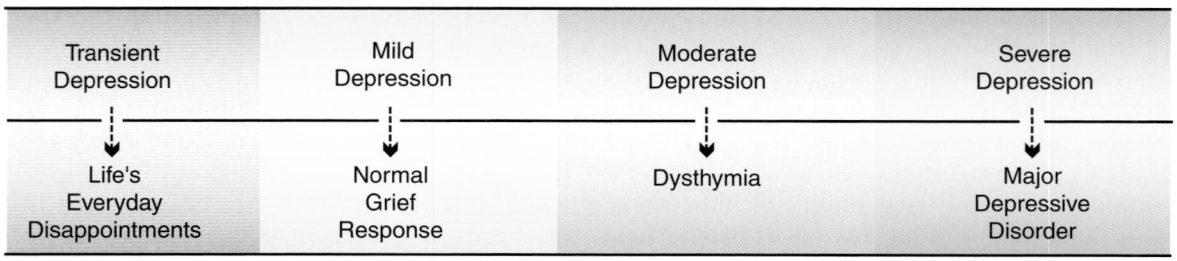

FIGURE 16–2 A continuum of depression.

BOX 16–4 Hamilton Depression Rating Scale (HDRS)

Instructions: For each item, circle the number to select the one "cue" that best characterizes the patient.

1. Depressed Mood (sadness, hopeless, helpless, worthless)
- 0 = Absent
- 1 = These feeling states indicated only on questioning
- 2 = These feeling states spontaneously reported verbally
- 3 = Communicates feeling states nonverbally (e.g., through facial expression, posture, voice, tendency to weep)
- 4 = Patient reports virtually only these feeling states in spontaneous verbal and nonverbal communication

2. Feelings of Guilt
- 0 = Absent
- 1 = Self-reproach; feels he/she has let people down
- 2 = Ideas of guilt or rumination over past errors or sinful deeds
- 3 = Present illness is a punishment; delusions of guilt
- 4 = Hears accusatory or denunciatory voices and/or experiences threatening visual hallucinations

3. Suicide
- 0 = Absent
- 1 = Feels life is not worth living
- 2 = Wishes he/she were dead or any thoughts of possible death to self
- 3 = Suicidal ideas or gesture
- 4 = Attempts at suicide (any serious attempt rates 4)

4. Insomnia: Early in the Night
- 0 = No difficulty falling asleep
- 1 = Complains of occasional difficulty falling asleep (i.e., more than ½ hour)
- 2 = Complains of nightly difficulty falling asleep

5. Insomnia: Middle of the Night
- 0 = No difficulty
- 1 = Complains of being restless and disturbed during the night
- 2 = Waking during the night—any getting out of bed rates 2 (except for purposes of voiding)

6. Insomnia: Early Hours of the Morning
- 0 = No difficulty
- 1 = Wakes in early hours of the morning but goes back to sleep
- 2 = Unable to fall asleep again if he/she get out of bed

7. Work and Activities
- 0 = No difficulty
- 1 = Thoughts and feelings of incapacity, fatigue, or weakness related to activities, work, or hobbies
- 2 = Loss of interest in activity, hobbies, or work—either directly reported by patient or indirectly in listlessness, indecision, and vacillation (feels he/she has to push self to work or do activities)
- 3 = Decrease in actual time spent in activities or decrease in productivity. Rate 3 if patient does not spend at least 3 hours a day in activities (job or hobbies), excluding routine chores
- 4 = Stopped working because of present illness. Rate 4 if patient engages in no activities except routine chores or does not perform routine chores unassisted

8. Psychomotor Retardation (slowness of thought and speech, impaired ability to concentrate, decreased motor activity)
- 0 = Normal speech and thought
- 1 = Slight retardation during the interview
- 2 = Obvious retardation during the interview
- 3 = Interview difficult
- 4 = Complete stupor

9. Agitation
- 0 = None
- 1 = Fidgetiness
- 2 = Playing with hands, hair, etc.
- 3 = Moving about, can't sit still
- 4 = Hand wringing, nail biting, hair pulling, biting of lips

10. Anxiety (Psychic)
- 0 = No difficulty
- 1 = Subjective tension and irritability
- 2 = Worrying about minor matters
- 3 = Apprehensive attitude apparent in face or speech
- 4 = Fears expressed without questioning

11. Anxiety (Somatic): Physiological concomitants of anxiety (e.g., dry mouth, indigestion, diarrhea, cramps, belching, palpitations, headache, tremor, hyperventilation, sighing, urinary frequency, sweating, flushing)
- 0 = Absent
- 1 = Mild
- 2 = Moderate
- 3 = Severe
- 4 = Incapacitating

12. Somatic Symptoms (Gastrointestinal)
- 0 = None
- 1 = Loss of appetite, but eating without encouragement; heavy feelings in abdomen
- 2 = Difficulty eating without urging from others; requests or requires medication for constipation or gastrointestinal symptoms

13. Somatic Symptoms (General)
- 0 = None
- 1 = Heaviness in limbs, back or head; backaches, headache, muscle aches; loss of energy and fatigability
- 2 = Any clear-cut symptom rates 2

14. Genital Symptoms (e.g., loss of libido, impaired sexual performance, menstrual disturbances)
- 0 = Absent
- 1 = Mild
- 2 = Severe

15. Hypochondriasis
- 0 = Not present
- 1 = Self-absorption (bodily)
- 2 = Preoccupation with health
- 3 = Frequent complaints, requests for help, etc.
- 4 = Hypochondriacal delusions

Continued

BOX 16–4 Hamilton Depression Rating Scale (HDRS)—cont'd

16. Loss of Weight (rate *either* A *or* B)

A. According to subjective patient history:

0 = No weight loss
1 = Probably weight loss associated with present illness
2 = Definite weight loss associated with present illness

B. According to objective weekly measurements:

0 = Less than 1 lb. weight loss in week
1 = Greater than 1 lb. weight loss in week
2 = Greater than 2 lb. weight loss in week

17. Insight

0 = Acknowledges being depressed and ill
1 = Acknowledges illness but attributes cause to bad food, climate, overwork, virus, need for rest, etc.
2 = Denies being ill at all

SCORING:

0–6 = No evidence of depressive illness
7–17 = Mild depression
18–24 = Moderate depression
>24 = Severe depression

TOTAL SCORE _____

Source: Hamilton (1960). The HDRS is in the public domain.

Moderate Depression

Dysthymia (also called *persistent depressive disorder*) is an example of moderate depression and represents a more chronic disturbance that, according to the *DSM-5-TR*, is characterized by symptoms that are enduring for at least 2 years (APA, 2022). Symptoms associated with this disorder include the following:

- ***Affective:*** Feelings of sadness, dejection, helplessness, powerlessness, hopelessness; gloomy and pessimistic outlook; low self-esteem; difficulty experiencing pleasure in activities
- ***Behavioral:*** Psychomotor retardation; slumped posture; slowed speech; limited verbalizations, possibly consisting of ruminations about life's failures or regrets; social isolation with a focus on the self; increased use of substances possible; self-destructive behavior possible; decreased interest in personal hygiene and grooming
- ***Cognitive:*** Slowed thinking processes; difficulty concentrating and directing attention; obsessive and repetitive thoughts, generally portraying pessimism and negativism; verbalizations and behavior reflecting suicidal ideation
- ***Physiological:*** Anorexia or overeating; insomnia or hypersomnia; sleep disturbances; amenorrhea; decreased libido; headaches; backaches; chest pain; abdominal pain; low energy level; fatigue and listlessness; feeling best early in the morning and continually worse as the day progresses (this may be related to the diurnal variation in the level of neurotransmitters that affect mood and level of activity)

Severe Depression

Severe depression (also called *major depressive disorder*) is characterized by an intensification of the symptoms described for moderate depression (see Box 16–1). Symptoms at the severe level of depression include the following:

- ***Affective:*** Feelings of total despair, hopelessness, and worthlessness; flat (unchanging) affect, appearing devoid of emotional tone; prevalent feelings of nothingness and emptiness; apathy; loneliness; sadness; inability to feel pleasure
- ***Behavioral:*** Psychomotor retardation so severe that physical movement may literally come to a standstill, or psychomotor behavior manifested by rapid, agitated, purposeless movements; slumped posture; sitting in a curled-up position; walking slowly and rigidly; virtually nonexistent communication (when verbalizations do occur, they may reflect delusional thinking); no personal hygiene and grooming; social isolation is common, with virtually no inclination toward interaction with others
- ***Cognitive:*** Prevalent delusional thinking with delusions of persecution and somatic delusions being most common; confusion, indecisiveness, and an inability to concentrate; hallucinations reflecting misinterpretations of the environment; excessive self-deprecation, self-blame, and thoughts of suicide

NOTE: Because of the low energy level and slow thought processes, the individual may be unable to follow through on suicidal ideas. However, the desire is strong at this level.

- ***Physiological:*** A general slowdown of the entire body, reflected in sluggish digestion, constipation, and urinary retention; amenorrhea; impotence; diminished libido; anorexia; weight loss; difficulty falling asleep and awakening very early in the morning; feeling worse early in the morning and somewhat better as the day progresses (as with moderate depression, this may reflect the diurnal variation in the level of neurotransmitters that affect mood and activity); pain syndromes.

Diagnosis and Outcome Identification

Using information collected during the assessment, the nurse completes the patient database from which the selection of appropriate nursing diagnoses is determined. Table 16–1 presents a list of behaviors and the NANDA International nursing diagnoses (Herdman et al., 2021) that correspond to those behaviors, which may be used in planning care for the depressed patient.

Outcome Criteria

The following criteria may be used for measurement of outcomes in the care of the depressed patient. The patient:

- Has experienced no physical harm to self.
- Discusses feelings with staff and family members.
- Expresses hopefulness.
- Sets realistic goals for self.
- Is no longer afraid to attempt new activities.
- Is able to identify aspects of self-control over life situation.
- Expresses personal satisfaction and support from spiritual practices.
- Interacts willingly and appropriately with others.
- Is able to maintain reality orientation.
- Is able to concentrate, reason, solve problems, and make decisions.
- Eats a well-balanced diet with snacks to prevent weight loss and maintain nutritional status.

TABLE 16–1 Assigning Nursing Diagnoses to Behaviors Commonly Associated With Depression

BEHAVIORS	NURSING DIAGNOSES
Depressed mood; feelings of hopelessness and worthlessness; anger turned inward in the self; misinterpretations of reality; suicidal ideation, plan, and available means	Risk for suicidal behavior
Depression, preoccupation with thoughts of loss, self-blame, grief avoidance, inappropriate expression of anger, decreased functioning in life roles	Maladaptive grieving
Expressions of helplessness, uselessness, guilt, and shame; hypersensitivity to slight or criticism; negative, pessimistic outlook; lack of eye contact; self-negating verbalizations	Low self-esteem
Apathy, verbal expressions of having no control, dependence on others to fulfill needs	Powerlessness
Expresses anger toward God, expresses lack of meaning in life, sudden changes in spiritual practices, refuses interactions with significant others or with spiritual leaders	Spiritual distress
Withdrawn, uncommunicative, seeks to be alone, dysfunctional interaction with others, discomfort in social situations	Social isolation/Impaired social interaction
Inappropriate thinking, confusion, difficulty concentrating, impaired problem-solving ability, inaccurate interpretation of environment, memory deficit	Disturbed thought processes
Weight loss, poor muscle tone, pale conjunctiva and mucous membranes, poor skin turgor, weakness	Imbalanced nutrition: Less than body requirements
Difficulty falling asleep, difficulty staying asleep, lack of energy, difficulty concentrating, verbal reports of not feeling well rested	Insomnia
Uncombed hair, disheveled clothing, offensive body odor	Self-care deficit (hygiene, grooming)

- Sleeps 6 to 8 hours per night and reports feeling well rested.
- Bathes, washes and combs hair, and dresses in clean clothing without assistance.

Planning and Implementation

Table 16–2 presents a plan of care for the depressed patient. Selected nursing diagnoses are presented, along with outcome criteria, appropriate nursing interventions, and rationales for each.

Some institutions use a case management model to coordinate care (see Chapter 6 for more detailed explanation). In case management models, the plan of care may take the form of a critical pathway.

Concept Care Mapping

The concept map care plan is an approach to planning and organizing nursing care (see Chapter 6). It is a diagrammatic teaching and learning strategy that allows visualization of interrelationships between medical diagnoses, nursing diagnoses, assessment data, and treatments. An example of a concept map care plan for a patient with depression is presented in Figure 16–3.

Patient and Family Education

The role of patient teacher is important in the psychiatric area, as it is in all areas of nursing. A list of topics for patient and family education relevant to depression is presented in Box 16–5.

Evaluation of Care for the Depressed Patient

In the final step of the nursing process, a reassessment is conducted to determine whether the nursing actions have been successful in achieving the objectives of care. Evaluation of the nursing actions for the depressed patient may be facilitated by gathering information using the following types of questions:

- Has self-harm to the individual been avoided?
- Have suicidal ideations subsided?
- Does the individual know where to seek assistance outside the hospital when suicidal thoughts occur?
- Has the patient discussed the recent loss with staff and family members?
- Is the patient able to verbalize feelings and behaviors associated with each stage of the grieving process and recognize own position in the process?
- Have obsession with and idealization of the lost object subsided?
- Is anger toward the lost object expressed appropriately?
- Does the patient set realistic goals for self?
- Is the patient able to verbalize positive aspects about self, past accomplishments, and future prospects, including a desire to live?
- Can the patient identify areas of life situation that are controllable?
- Is the patient able to participate in usual religious practices and feel satisfaction and support from them?
- Is the patient seeking interaction with others in an appropriate manner?
- Does the patient maintain reality orientation with no evidence of delusional thinking?
- Is the patient able to concentrate and make decisions concerning own self-care?
- Is the patient selecting and consuming foods sufficiently high in nutrients and calories to maintain weight and nutritional status?
- Does the patient sleep without difficulty and wake feeling rested?
- Does the patient attend to personal hygiene and grooming?
- Have somatic complaints subsided?

Real Nurses, Real Advice

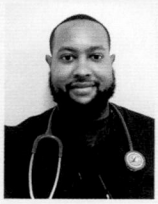

"The anhedonia, psychomotor retardation, and anergia in acute depression can make assessment a challenge. It's important to offer hope to a client who may be uncertain about how to navigate their present state of deep depression and to remain diligent while not making the patient feel pressured to speak. Paraphrasing what the patient has said to you conveys understanding and provides validation. Open-ended questions encourage the patient to elaborate rather than just answer 'yes' or 'no.'"

—Larry Johnson, RN

Treatment Modalities

Interpersonal Psychotherapy

Research has documented the importance of close, satisfactory attachments in the prevention of depression with over double the risk among those with the lowest quality of social relationships (Teo et al., 2013). With this concept in mind, interpersonal psychotherapy focuses on the client's current interpersonal relations. Interpersonal psychotherapy with the depressed person proceeds through three phases.

Text continued on page 428

Table 16–2 | CARE PLAN FOR THE DEPRESSED PATIENT

NURSING DIAGNOSIS: RISK FOR SUICIDE

RELATED TO: Depressed mood, feelings of hopelessness and worthlessness, anger turned inward on the self, misinterpretations of reality

OUTCOME CRITERIA	NURSING INTERVENTIONS	RATIONALE
Short-Term Goals ■ Patient will seek out staff when feeling urge to harm self. ■ Patient will not harm self.	1. Ask the patient directly: "Have you thought about killing yourself?" or "Have you thought about harming yourself in any way? If so, what do you plan to do? Do you have the means to carry out this plan? How strong are your intentions to die?"	1. The risk of suicide is greatly increased if the patient has developed a plan, has strong intentions to die, and particularly if means exist for the patient to execute the plan.
Long-Term Goal ■ Patient will not harm self.	2. Create a safe environment for the patient. Remove all potentially harmful objects from patient's access (sharp objects, straps, belts, ties, glass items, alcohol). Supervise closely during meals and medication administration. Perform room searches as deemed necessary.	2. Patient safety is a nursing priority.
	3. Convey an attitude of unconditional acceptance of the patient as a worthwhile individual. Encourage the patient to actively participate in establishing a safety plan.	3. A relationship founded on trust and acceptance is essential for collaboration with the patient in developing a plan for their ongoing safety. Suicidal patients are often ambivalent about their feelings related to suicide and discussion (and "buy in") about strategies for maintaining safety. Empower the patient to collaborate in preventing a crisis situation.
	4. Maintain close observation of the patient. Depending on level of suicide precaution, provide one-to-one contact, constant visual observation, or every-15-minute checks. Place in room close to nurse's station; do not assign to private room. Accompany to off-unit activities if attendance is indicated and, if necessary, to the bathroom.	4. Close observation is necessary to ensure that patient does not harm self in any way. Being alert for suicidal and escape attempts facilitates being able to prevent or interrupt harmful behavior.
	5. Maintain special care in administration of medications.	5. Prevents saving up to overdose or discarding and not taking.
	6. Make rounds at frequent, *irregular* intervals (especially at night, toward early morning, at change of shift, or other predictably busy times for staff).	6. Prevents staff surveillance from becoming predictable. To be aware of the patient's location is important, especially when staff is busy, unavailable, or less observable.

Continued

Table 16–2 | CARE PLAN FOR THE DEPRESSED PATIENT—cont'd

OUTCOME CRITERIA	NURSING INTERVENTIONS	RATIONALE
	7. Encourage the patient to express honest feelings, including anger. Provide hostility release if needed. Help the patient to identify the true source of anger and to work on adaptive coping skills for use outside the treatment setting.	7. Depression and suicidal behaviors may be viewed as anger turned inward on the self. If this anger can be verbalized in a nonthreatening environment, the patient may eventually be able to resolve these feelings.
	8. Identify community resources that the patient can access for support and assistance as needed post-discharge.	8. Having a concrete plan for seeking assistance should suicidal ideation recur or intensify post-discharge assists the patient to manage symptoms and prevent self-destructive behaviors.

NURSING DIAGNOSIS: MALADAPTIVE GRIEVING

RELATED TO: Real or perceived loss, bereavement overload

EVIDENCED BY: Denial of loss, inappropriate expression of anger, idealization of or obsession with lost object, inability to carry out activities of daily living

OUTCOME CRITERIA	NURSING INTERVENTIONS	RATIONALE
Short-Term Goals ■ Patient will express anger about the loss. ■ Patient will verbalize behaviors associated with normal grieving. **Long-Term Goal** ■ Patient will be able to recognize their position in the grief process, while progressing at own pace toward resolution.	1. Determine the stage of grief in which the patient is fixed. Identify behaviors associated with this stage.	1. Accurate baseline assessment data are necessary to effectively plan care for the grieving patient.
	2. Develop a trusting relationship with the patient. Show empathy, concern, and unconditional positive regard. Be honest and keep all promises.	2. Trust is the basis for a therapeutic relationship.
	3. Convey an accepting attitude and enable the patient to express feelings openly.	3. An accepting attitude conveys to the patient that you believe them to be a worthwhile person. Trust is enhanced.
	4. Encourage the patient to express anger. Do not become defensive if the initial expression of anger is displaced on the nurse or therapist. Help the patient explore angry feelings so that they may be directed toward the actual intended person or situation.	4. Verbalization of feelings in a nonthreatening environment may help the patient come to terms with unresolved issues.
	5. Help the patient to discharge pent-up anger through participation in large-motor activities (e.g., brisk walks, jogging, physical exercise, volleyball, exercise bike).	5. Physical exercise provides a safe and effective method for discharging pent-up tension.
	6. Teach the normal stages of grief and behaviors associated with each stage. Help the patient to understand that feelings such as guilt and anger toward the lost concept are appropriate and acceptable during the grief process and should be expressed rather than held inside.	6. Knowledge of acceptability of the feelings associated with normal grieving may help to relieve some of the guilt that these responses generate.

Table 16–2 | CARE PLAN FOR THE DEPRESSED PATIENT—cont'd

OUTCOME CRITERIA	NURSING INTERVENTIONS	RATIONALE
	7. Encourage the patient to review the relationship with the lost entity. With support and sensitivity, point out the reality of the situation in areas where misrepresentations are expressed.	7. The patient must give up an idealized perception and be able to accept both positive and negative aspects about the lost entity before the grief process is complete.
	8. Communicate to the patient that crying is acceptable. Use of touch may also be therapeutic.	8. Some individuals believe it is important to remain stoic and refrain from crying openly, and some are uncomfortable with touch. It is important to be aware of individual preferences before employing these interventions.
	9. Encourage the patient to reach out for spiritual support during this time in whatever form is desirable. Assess spiritual needs of the patient (see online Chapter 31) and assist as necessary in the fulfillment of those needs.	9. Patient may find comfort in religious rituals with which they are familiar.

NURSING DIAGNOSIS: LOW SELF-ESTEEM

RELATED TO: Learned helplessness, feelings of abandonment by significant other, impaired cognition fostering negative view of self

EVIDENCED BY: Expressions of worthlessness, hypersensitivity to slights or criticism, negative and pessimistic outlook

OUTCOME CRITERIA	NURSING INTERVENTIONS	RATIONALE
Short-Term Goals ■ Patient will verbalize areas they like about self. ■ Patient will attempt new activities without fear of failure. **Long-Term Goal** ■ By time of discharge from treatment, patient will exhibit increased feelings of self-worth as evidenced by verbal expression of positive aspects of self, past accomplishments, and future prospects.	1. Be accepting of and spend time with the patient even though pessimism and negativism may seem objectionable. Focus on strengths and accomplishments and minimize limitations and failures.	1. Interventions that focus on the positive contribute toward feelings of self-worth.
	2. Promote attendance in therapy groups that offer the patient simple methods of accomplishment. Encourage the patient to be as independent as possible.	2. Success and independence promote feelings of self-worth.
	3. Encourage the patient to recognize areas of change and provide assistance toward this effort.	3. Patients may need assistance with problem-solving. Indecisiveness is a common symptom in depression.
	4. Teach assertiveness techniques: the ability to recognize the differences among passive, assertive, and aggressive behaviors; and the importance of respecting the human rights of others while protecting one's own basic human rights.	4. Self-esteem is enhanced by the ability to interact with others in an assertive manner.
	5. Teach effective communication techniques, such as the use of "I" messages (e.g., "I feel hurt when you say those things").	5. "I" statements help to avoid making judgmental statements.

Continued

Table 16–2 | CARE PLAN FOR THE DEPRESSED PATIENT—cont'd

NURSING DIAGNOSIS: POWERLESSNESS

RELATED TO: Dysfunctional grieving process, lifestyle of helplessness

EVIDENCED BY: Feelings of lack of control over life situation, overdependence on others to fulfill needs

OUTCOME CRITERIA	NURSING INTERVENTIONS	RATIONALE
Short-Term Goal ■ Patient will participate in decision making regarding own care within 5 days. **Long-Term Goal** ■ Patient will be able to effectively problem-solve ways to take control of life situations by time of discharge from treatment, thereby decreasing feelings of powerlessness.	1. Encourage patient to take as much responsibility as possible for their own self-care practices. In the most acute stage of severe depression, patients may have extreme difficulty making decisions. It may be more helpful to use active communication to help the patient accomplish even basic ADLs. For example, "It's time to eat lunch," rather than, "Would you like to eat lunch now?" Ongoing assessment is important so that the patient can be encouraged to make choices as soon as possible. Examples: a. Include the patient in setting the goals of care they want to achieve. b. Allow the patient to establish own schedule for self-care activities. c. Provide privacy as need is determined. d. Provide positive feedback for decisions made. Respect the patient's right to make those decisions independently, and refrain from attempting to influence the patient toward decisions that may seem more logical.	1. Providing the patient with simple choices, when they are able to tolerate decision making, will increase their feelings of control.
	2. Help the patient set realistic goals.	2. Realistic goals will avoid setting the patient up for failure and reinforcing feelings of powerlessness.
	3. Help the patient identify those areas of life situations that can be controlled.	3. The patient's emotional condition interferes with their ability to solve problems. Assistance is required to perceive the benefits and consequences of available alternatives accurately.
	4. Help the patient identify areas of life situations that are not within their ability to control. Encourage verbalization of feelings related to this inability.	4. Verbalization of unresolved issues may help the patient accept what cannot be changed.

Table 16–2 | CARE PLAN FOR THE DEPRESSED PATIENT—cont'd

NURSING DIAGNOSIS: SPIRITUAL DISTRESS

RELATED TO: Maladaptive grieving over loss of valued object

EVIDENCED BY: Anger toward God, questioning meaning of own existence, inability to participate in usual religious practices

OUTCOME CRITERIA	NURSING INTERVENTIONS	RATIONALE
Short-Term Goal ■ Patient will identify meaning and purpose in life, moving forward with hope for the future. **Long-Term Goal** ■ Patient will express achievement of support and personal satisfaction from spiritual practices.	1. Be accepting and nonjudgmental when the patient expresses anger and bitterness toward God. Stay with the patient.	1. The nurse's presence and nonjudgmental attitude increase the patient's feelings of self-worth and promote trust in the relationship.
	2. Encourage the patient to express feelings related to meaning of their own existence in the face of current loss.	2. The patient may believe they cannot go on living without the lost entity. Catharsis can provide relief and put life back into realistic perspective.
	3. Encourage the patient as part of grief work to reach out to previous religious practices for support. Encourage the patient to discuss these practices and how they provided support in the past.	3. The patient may find comfort in familiar religious rituals.
	4. Reassure the patient that many feel inadequate in the search for life's answers.	4. Validation of the patient's feelings and the assurance that others share them offer reassurance and an affirmation of acceptability.
	5. Contact the spiritual leader of the patient's choice, if requested.	5. These individuals serve to provide relief from spiritual distress and often can do so when other support persons cannot.

NURSING DIAGNOSIS: HOPELESSNESS

RELATED TO: Absence of support systems and perception of worthlessness

EVIDENCED BY: Verbal cues (despondent content, "I can't"); decreased affect; lack of initiative; suicidal ideas or attempts

OUTCOME CRITERIA	NURSING INTERVENTIONS	RATIONALE
Short-Term Goals ■ Patient will express acceptance of life and situations over which there is no control. **Long-Term Goal** ■ Patient will verbalize a measure of hope for the future by identifying reachable goals and ways to achieve them.	1. Identify stressors in the patient's life that precipitated the current crisis.	1. It is important to identify causative or contributing factors in order to plan appropriate assistance.
	2. Determine coping behaviors previously used and the patient's perception of effectiveness then and now.	2. Reviewing coping behaviors assists the patient to recognize personal strengths that have been helpful in the past.
	3. Encourage the patient to explore and verbalize feelings and perceptions.	3. Identification of feelings underlying behaviors helps the patient to begin the process of taking control of their own life.

Continued

Table 16–2 | CARE PLAN FOR THE DEPRESSED PATIENT—cont'd

OUTCOME CRITERIA	NURSING INTERVENTIONS	RATIONALE
	4. Provide expressions of hope to the patient in a positive, low-key manner (e.g., "I know you feel you cannot go on, but I believe that things can get better for you. What you are feeling is temporary. It is okay if you don't see it just now. You are very important to the people who care about you").	4. Even though the patient feels hopeless, it is helpful to hear positive expressions from others. The patient's current state of mind may prevent identifying anything positive in life. It is important to accept the patient's feelings nonjudgmentally and to affirm the individual's personal worth and value.
	5. Help the patient identify areas of life situation that are under their own control.	5. The patient's emotional condition may interfere with their ability to problem-solve. Assistance may be required to perceive the benefits and consequences of available alternatives accurately.
	6. Identify sources that the patient may use after discharge when crises occur or feelings of hopelessness and possible suicidal ideation prevail.	6. Providing information about local suicide hotlines or other local support services from which to seek assistance following discharge from the hospital promotes follow-through with an ongoing safety plan.

Phase I

During the first phase, the client is assessed to determine the extent of the illness. Complete information is then given to the individual regarding the nature of depression, symptom pattern, frequency, clinical course, and alternative treatments. If the level of depression is severe, interpersonal psychotherapy has been shown to be more effective if conducted in combination with antidepressant medication. The client is encouraged to continue working and participating in regular activities during therapy. A mutually agreeable therapeutic contract is negotiated.

Phase II

Treatment at this phase focuses on helping the client resolve maladaptive grief reactions, which may include resolving the ambivalence with a lost relationship and assistance with establishing new relationships. Other areas of treatment focus may include interpersonal disputes between the client and a significant other, difficult role transitions at various developmental life cycles, and correction of interpersonal deficits that may interfere with the client's ability to initiate or sustain interpersonal relationships.

Phase III

During the final phase of interpersonal psychotherapy, the therapeutic alliance is terminated. With emphasis on reassurance, clarification of emotional states, improvement of interpersonal communication, testing of perceptions, and performance in interpersonal settings, interpersonal psychotherapy has been successful in helping depressed persons recover enhanced social functioning.

Group Therapy

Group therapy forms an important dimension of multimodal treatment for the depressed client. Once an acute phase of the illness is passed, groups can provide an atmosphere in which individuals may discuss issues in their lives that cause, maintain, or arise out of having a serious affective disorder. The element of peer support provides a feeling of security, because troublesome or embarrassing issues are discussed and resolved. Some groups have other specific purposes, such as helping to monitor medication-related issues or serving as an avenue for promoting education related to the affective disorder and its treatment. Therapy groups

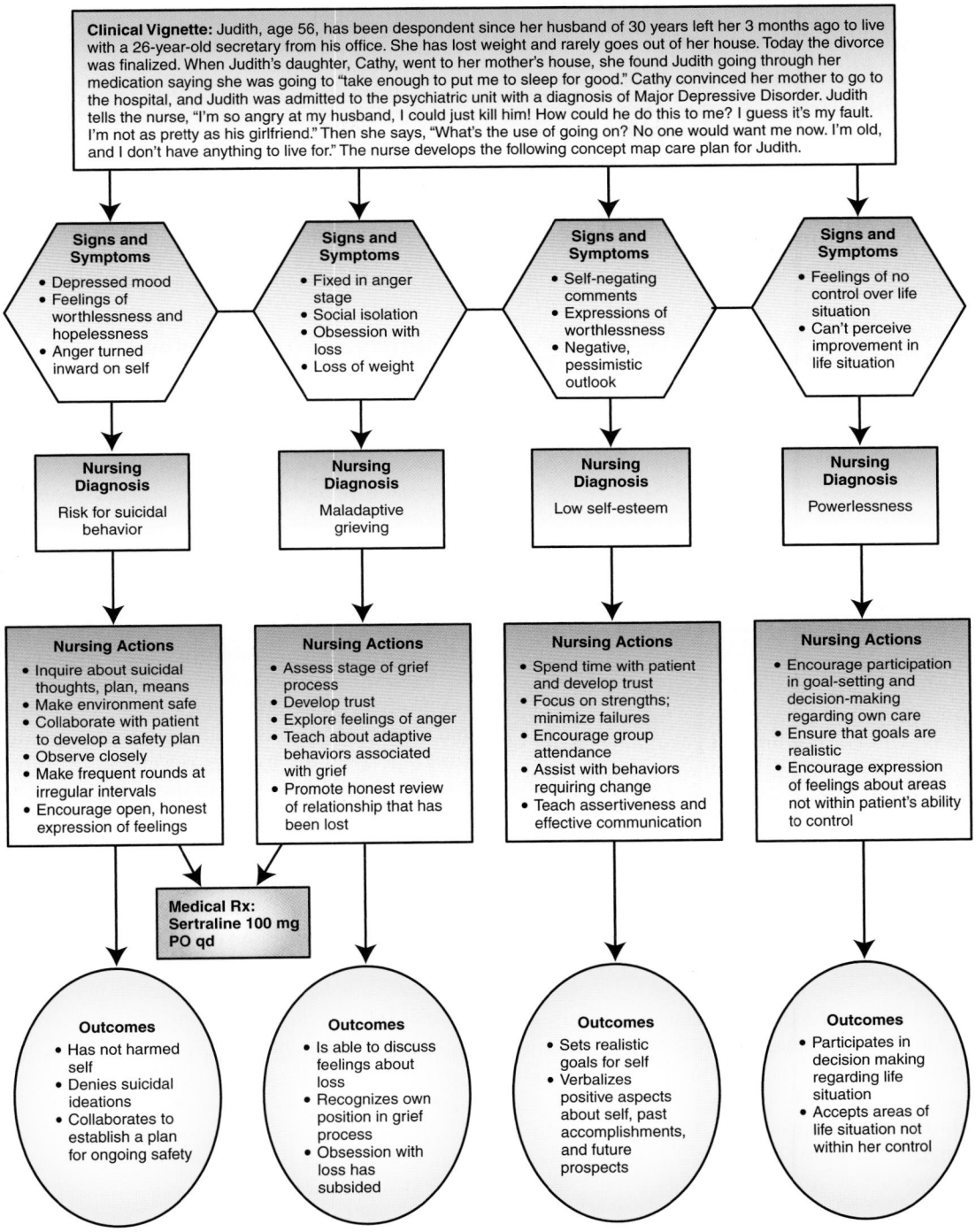

FIGURE 16–3 Concept map care plan for a patient with depression.

BOX 16–5 Topics for Patient and Family Education Related to Depression

NATURE OF THE ILLNESS

1. Stages of grief and symptoms associated with each stage
2. What is depression?
3. Why do people get depressed?
4. What are the symptoms of depression?

MANAGEMENT OF THE ILLNESS

1. Medication management
   a. Nuisance side effects
   b. Side effects to report to physician
   c. Importance of taking regularly
   d. Length of time to take effect
   e. Diet (related to MAOIs)
2. Assertiveness techniques
3. Stress-management techniques
4. Ways to increase self-esteem
5. Electroconvulsive therapy

Support Services

1. Suicide hotline
2. Support groups
3. Legal/financial assistance

help members gain a sense of perspective on their condition and tangibly encourage them to link up with others who have common problems. A sense of hope is conveyed when members are able to see that they are not alone or unique in experiencing affective illness.

Self-help groups offer another avenue of support for the depressed client. These groups are usually peer led and are not meant to substitute for or compete with professional therapy. They offer supplementary support that frequently enhances compliance with the medical regimen. Examples of self-help groups are the Depression and Bipolar Support Alliance (DBSA), Depressed Anonymous, Recovery International, Mental Health America, and NAMI Connection. Although self-help groups are not psychotherapy groups, they do provide important adjunctive support experiences, which often have therapeutic benefit for participants.

Family Therapy

The ultimate objectives in working with families of clients with mood disorders are to resolve the symptoms and initiate or restore adaptive family functioning. Similar to group therapy, the most effective approach appears to be a combination of psychotherapeutic and pharmacotherapeutic treatments. Boland and Verduin (2022) state that family therapy is indicated

> if the disorder jeopardizes the patient's marriage or family functioning or if the mood disorder is promoted or maintained by the family situation. Family therapy examines the role of the mood-disordered member in the overall psychological well-being of the whole family; it also examines the role of the entire family in the maintenance of the patient's symptoms. (p. 393)

Cognitive Behavior Therapy

In cognitive behavior therapy (CBT), the individual is taught to control thought distortions that are considered to be a factor in the development and maintenance of mood disorders. In the cognitive model, depression is characterized by a triad of negative distortions related to expectations of the environment, self, and future. The environment and activities within it are viewed as unsatisfying, the self is unrealistically devalued, and the future is perceived as hopeless.

The general goals in CBT are to obtain symptom relief as quickly as possible, to assist the client in identifying dysfunctional patterns of thinking and behaving, and to guide the client to evidence and logic that effectively test the validity of the dysfunctional thinking. Therapy focuses on changing "automatic thoughts" that occur spontaneously and contribute to the distorted affect. Following are examples of automatic thoughts that may be common cognitive distortions in depression:

- ***Personalizing:*** "I'm the only one who failed."
- ***All or nothing:*** "I'm a complete failure."
- ***Mind reading:*** "He thinks I'm foolish."
- ***Discounting positives:*** "The other questions were so easy. Any dummy could have gotten them right."

The client is asked to describe evidence that both supports and disputes the automatic thought. The logic underlying the inferences is then reviewed with the client. Another technique involves evaluating what would most likely happen if the client's automatic thoughts were true. Implications of the consequences are then discussed.

Clients should not become discouraged if one technique seems not to be working. No single technique works with all clients. They should be reassured that any of a number of techniques may be used, and both the therapist and client may explore these possibilities.

CBT has offered encouraging results in the treatment of depression. In fact, the results of several studies with depressed clients show that in some cases CBT even more effective than antidepressant medication alone (Amick et al., 2015; Gautam et al., 2020; Grosse Holtforth et al., 2019).

Electroconvulsive Therapy

Electroconvulsive therapy (ECT) is the induction of a grand mal (generalized) seizure through the application of electrical current to the brain. ECT is effective with clients who are acutely suicidal and in the treatment of severe depression, particularly in those clients who are also experiencing psychotic symptoms and those with psychomotor retardation and neurovegetative changes, such as disturbances in sleep, appetite, and energy. It is often considered for treatment only after a trial of therapy with antidepressant medication has proved ineffective.

Mechanism of Action

The exact mechanism by which ECT effects a therapeutic response is unknown. Many parts of the central nervous system are affected by ECT, including hormones, neuropeptides, neurotrophic factors, and nearly every neurotransmitter (Mankad, 2019). Affected neurotransmitters include serotonin, norepinephrine, and dopamine, the same biogenic amines that are affected by antidepressant drugs. Research on serotonin has yielded mixed results and the effect of ECT on serotonin levels remains controversial (Boland & Verduin, 2022). Other possible mechanisms of action, based on changes that occur during ECT, include an increase in GABA transmission and an increase of endogenous opioids, both of which may raise the seizure threshold (Mankad, 2019; Sharma et al., 2018).

A longitudinal study of imaging research shows that the therapeutic ECT response is associated with several effects on the brain, including decreased frontal perfusion and decreases in cerebral metabolism, functional connectivity, volume, and neuronal chemical metabolites, all of which support anticonvulsant and neurotrophic effects of ECT (Abbott et al., 2014). Other studies have demonstrated increased GABA levels, increased sensitization of 5-HT_{1A} serotonin receptors, increased dopamine binding, and normalized dexamethasone suppression tests in patients who received ECT (Sharma et al., 2018). In another study, the researchers conclude that therapeutic response from ECT may be related to neuroplasticity in white matter microstructures, which are altered in major depression (Lyden et al., 2014).

Several studies have identified an increase in gray matter, particularly in the hippocampal and amygdala areas, following ECT (Depping et al., 2016; Pirnia et al., 2016; Sartorius et al., 2015). Because these areas of the brain show a decrease in volume in major depression, the study findings are being looked at with interest as an indication of neuroplasticity and the neurorestorative effects of ECT.

The results of studies relating to the mechanism underlying the effectiveness of ECT continue to be mixed and controversial. Its effectiveness may be a complex dynamic of several effects interacting with one another.

Side Effects

The most common side effects of ECT are temporary memory loss (retrograde and anterograde amnesia) and confusion. Critics of the therapy argue that these changes represent irreversible brain damage. Proponents insist that they are temporary and reversible. Other cognitive deficits in the immediate post-ECT period include processing speed, attention, verbal and visual memory, spatial problem-solving, and executive functioning deficits, but Semkovska and McLoughlin's meta-analysis (2010) demonstrated that most of those resolve within 3 days after treatment and some improve beyond baseline after 15 days. It has been argued that bilateral electrode placement may be more effective than right unilateral (RUL) placement but is associated with more cognitive side effects. However, evidence supports that a more aggressive stimulus in RUL placement improves its efficacy (Pulia et al., 2013).

Risks Associated With ECT

Mortality

In 2011, the American Psychiatric Nurses Association (APNA) advanced a position statement in support of ECT for "severe depression that has been shown to be refractory to medication administration" (APNA, 2011). The APNA cites a mortality rate less than that of childbirth. Studies indicate that the mortality rate from ECT is about 0.002% per treatment and 0.01% for each patient (Boland & Verduin, 2022). Although the occurrence is rare, the major cause of death with ECT is from cardiovascular complications (e.g., acute myocardial infarction or CVA), usually in individuals with previously compromised cardiac status. Assessment and management of cardiovascular disease prior to treatment is vital in the reduction of morbidity and mortality rates associated with ECT.

Memory Loss

Memory impairment almost always occurs to some degree during the course of ECT treatments, but follow-up studies indicate that most patients return to their cognitive baselines after 6 months (Boland & Verduin, 2022). Some clients do report persistent memory impairment, and, in most cases, this impairment occurs among patients who showed little improvement with ECT (Boland & Verduin, 2022). Stimulation produced by sine wave (continuous) current resulted in greater short- and long-term deficits than that produced by short-pulse wave (intermittent) current. Sine waveforms are no longer recommended and have primarily been replaced by brief and, more recently, ultrabrief pulse stimulations (Prudic & Duan, 2017). The risk of post-ECT cognitive deficits is also increased when there are baseline impairments in global cognitive functioning and concurrent use of lithium or medications with anticholinergic effects (Prudic & Duan, 2017). Although the overall risks of enduring memory loss are minimal, the physician should discuss this risk factor with all patients when obtaining informed consent.

Brain Damage

The question of brain damage secondary to ECT treatments has been advanced as a concern by critics of the procedure. The subject has been studied using a variety of brain imaging modalities, and virtually all conclude that there is no evidence of brain damage caused by ECT treatments (Boland & Verduin, 2022; McClintock & Husain, 2011). Previously cited studies on the *neurorestorative* effects of ECT have argued that this, too, is evidence in contradiction to ideas about brain-damaging effects of ECT.

Medications Used With ECT

Several medications are associated with ECT. A pretreatment medication, such as atropine sulfate or glycopyrrolate (Robinul), is administered intramuscularly (IM) approximately 30 minutes before the treatment. Either of these medications may be ordered to decrease secretions (to prevent aspiration) and counteract the effects of vagal stimulation (bradycardia) induced by the ECT.

In the treatment room, the anesthesiologist administers IV a short-acting anesthetic, such as propofol (Diprivan) or etomidate (Amidate). A muscle relaxant, usually succinylcholine chloride (Anectine), is given IV to prevent severe muscle contractions during the seizure, thereby reducing the possibility of fractured or dislocated bones. Because succinylcholine paralyzes respiratory muscles as well, the client is oxygenated with pure oxygen during and after the treatment, except for the brief interval of electrical stimulation, until spontaneous respirations return.

Clients and families must also understand that ECT is voluntary and that consent may be withdrawn at any time (APA, 2001; Fetterman & Ying, 2011). This kind of education supports patient-centered care.

Repetitive Transcranial Magnetic Stimulation (rTMS)

Repetitive transcranial magnetic stimulation (rTMS) is a noninvasive procedure that is used to treat depression by stimulating nerve cells in the brain. rTMS involves the use of very short pulses of magnetic energy to stimulate nerve cells at localized areas in the cerebral cortex, similar to the electrical activity observed with ECT. However, unlike with ECT, the electrical waves generated by rTMS do not result in generalized seizure activity (George et al., 2013). The waves are passed through a coil placed on the scalp to areas of the brain involved in mood regulation. It is noninvasive and generally considered safe. High-frequency waves are used to stimulate the left prefrontal cortex, and low-frequency waves are used to stimulate the right prefrontal cortex. This combination has been shown most effective in treating depression (Sharma et al., 2018). A typical course of treatment consists of 40-minute sessions, three to five times a week for 4 to 6 weeks (Raposelli, 2015). In rare instances, seizures have been triggered with the use of TMS therapy, particularly with high-frequency rTMS, but more common adverse effects include tinnitus, headache, or facial twitching (Sharma et al., 2018).

Gaynes and associates (2014) conducted a meta-analysis demonstrating that rTMS had a remission rate of 30%. Effectiveness ratings for ECT have varied from 17% to 70%. Although the effectiveness ratings may seem small or highly variable, both treatments provide an option for patients who are otherwise treatment resistant. Magnezi and associates (2016) compared ECT to rTMS and found that although ECT was more effective than rTMS and additionally relieved anxiety symptoms, ECT had a much higher incidence (60%) of adverse effects, mostly related to memory loss. From the client's perspective, rTMS was still deemed preferable to ECT (if it was covered by insurance), which may be related to the stigma associated with ECT.

George and associates (2013) stated:

> Since FDA approval, TMS has been generally safe and well tolerated with a low incidence of treatment discontinuation, and the therapeutic effects once obtained appear at least as durable as other antidepressant treatments. TMS also shows promise in several other psychiatric disorders, particularly treating acute and chronic pain. (p. 17)

More recently, researchers compared rTMS to pharmacotherapy and found them both effective but identified rTMS as more cost effective (Raposelli, 2015). Currently, not all insurance companies cover this treatment, so from the client's standpoint, this may be a more expensive alternative. Raposelli reports that up to 40% of patients with MDD do not respond to pharmacotherapy, so alternatives such as ECT and rTMS may offer some hope of recovery for treatment-resistant conditions.

Vagus Nerve Stimulation and Deep Brain Stimulation

During studies for the treatment of epilepsy, researchers found that vagus nerve stimulation (VNS) improved mood. This treatment involves implanting an electronic device in the skin to stimulate the vagus nerve. Chronic stimulation of these nerve fibers changes activity in the brainstem nuclei that alters serotonin activity and has anticonvulsant effects (Boland & Verduin, 2022). Positive emission tomography studies performed during treatment demonstrate metabolic changes in areas of the brain associated with mood disorders (Sharma et al., 2018), including the amygdala, hippocampus, and cingulate gyrus. Response rates vary from 13% to 40% and remission rates are around 13%. Success rates are lower than those for ECT (Boland & Verduin, 2022) but it provides an alternative for those individuals who have not responded to less invasive treatments.

A novel approach is deep brain stimulation (DBS), which is a form of psychosurgery. In this procedure, as in VNS, an electrode is implanted with the intent of stimulating brain function. The implant is deeper than that used in VNS and requires craniotomy. DBS has been well studied to determine its safety and effectiveness for other conditions, and controlled trials are ongoing. The procedure is reversible and stimulation levels can easily be adjusted (Sharma et al., 2018). There is no consensus on the best area of the brain for implantation, but studies have reported improvement regardless of the site of electrode placement (Sharma et al., 2018). Berlim and associates (2014) conducted a systematic review of several studies using DBS and determined a response rate of approximately 40% and a remission rate of approximately 26%. Currently, DBS is reserved for patients with intractable, debilitating depression or obsessive-compulsive disorder who have not responded to any other more conservative treatments.

Bright Light Therapy

The prevalence of depression with a seasonal pattern is reported to be up to 10% but varies on the basis of geographic location (Kurlansik & Ibay, 2013). The *DSM-5-TR* identifies this disorder as Major Depressive Disorder, Recurrent, With Seasonal Pattern (APA, 2022). It is commonly known as seasonal affect disorder (SAD). One theory suggests that SAD is related to the presence of the hormone melatonin (Cotterell, 2010), which is produced by the pineal gland. Melatonin plays a role in the regulation of biological rhythms for sleep and activation. It is produced during the cycle of darkness and shuts off in the light of day. During the months of longer hours of darkness, production of melatonin increases, which seems to trigger the symptoms of SAD in susceptible people. Other research has pointed to seasonal serotonin transporter fluctuations associated with variation in exposure to daylight (McMahon et al., 2016).

Bright light therapy, or exposure to light, has been shown, in several studies, to be an effective short-term treatment for SAD. The light therapy is administered by a 10,000-lux light box, which contains white fluorescent light tubes covered with a plastic screen that blocks ultraviolet rays. The individual sits in front of the box with the eyes open (although the client should not look directly into the light). Therapy usually begins with 10- to 15-minute sessions and gradually progresses to 30 to 45 minutes. The mechanism of action is believed to be related to retinal stimulation, which triggers a reduction of melatonin and an increase in serotonin in the brain (Rodriguez, 2015). Studies have demonstrated benefits of bright light therapy in the treatment of nonseasonal, unipolar depression as well (Cunningham et al., 2019; Lam et al., 2015; Sikkens et al., 2019). Some people notice improvement rapidly, within a few days, whereas others may take several weeks to feel better. Side effects appear to be dosage related and include headache, eyestrain, nausea, irritability, photophobia (eye sensitivity to light), insomnia (when light therapy is used late in the day), and (rarely) hypomania (Kurlansik & Ibay, 2013).

Light therapy and antidepressants have shown comparable efficacy in studies of SAD treatment. One study compared the efficacy of light therapy for SAD to daily treatment with 20 mg of fluoxetine (Lam et al., 2015). The authors concluded that "light treatment showed earlier response onset and lower rate of some adverse events relative to fluoxetine, but there were no other significant differences in outcome between light therapy and antidepressant medication" (p. 805). Sikkens and associates (2019), noting that depression is often accompanied by sleep disorders, used bright light therapy to reset patients' circadian rhythm. The study subjects were maintained on antidepressant medication as well, and overall response was around 35%. Although improvement is often noted within 2 weeks, most clients relapse in the short term. Treatment should therefore be continued until an expected time of spontaneous remission, such as the change in season to spring or summer (Kurlansik & Ibay, 2013). Another study demonstrated that CBT is as effective as bright light therapy with the added benefit of preventing recurrences over time (Rohan et al., 2016).

Psychopharmacology

Antidepressant medication is generally considered first-line treatment for severe clinical depression, but antidepressants are also used in the treatment of other depressive disorders. These include tricyclic, tetracyclic, monoamine oxidase inhibitors (MAOIs); SSRIs; SNRIs; and SSRI/SNRI combination drugs. Examples of commonly used antidepressant medications are presented in Table 16–3. A detailed description of these medications can be found in Chapter 4, Psychopharmacology. In addition to the side effects and safety issues addressed in Chapter 4, it is important to highlight that antidepressant medication can be lethal in overdose. Depressed, suicidal patients must be observed closely and suicide risk assessed frequently in the use of this treatment modality.

Atypical antipsychotics have been advanced as an add-on treatment for patients who are not responding to antidepressant medication. Antipsychotics carry a black box warning for risk of sudden death in elderly patients with neurocognitive disorders and a recent population-based cohort study identified that there is a similar increased risk of mortality in middle-aged adults (Gerhard et al., 2020). The risk was determined to be higher in the 55-to-64-year-old age-group and among women. The researchers report that while the causes of increased mortality are not clear, cardiac and infectious causes are likely. Their findings suggest that atypical antipsychotics should only be added in treatment-resistant cases and after careful evaluation of risks versus benefits.

In 2019 the FDA approved a nasal spray formulation of esketamine (Spravato) for limited distribution (certified doctor's offices and clinics) to treat patients with refractory (treatment-resistant) depression. Early clinical trials of intranasal esketamine reported improved depression and suicide symptoms within 4 hours, a revolutionary claim (Canuso et al., 2018). More recent studies have indicated that some benefits are seen within 2 days of treatment (FDA, 2019b). This option is particularly attractive considering the substantial lag period in the therapeutic effect of other antidepressants. It is intended for use along with an oral antidepressant. Concerns that will need continued evaluation include side effects of sedation, dissociation, and addiction potential associated with the use of ketamine preparations. But there is hope that its use will provide an option for individuals with treatment-resistant depression and recurrent suicide risk. Other ketamine-like medications are being investigated in clinical trials.

Latest research has focused on the potential benefits of classic psychedelic drugs, such as psilocybin and LSD, in treating major depressive disorder (Holoyda, 2021). These drugs activate the serotonin 5-HT_{2A} receptors. Previous research has demonstrated benefits of psilocybin for cancer treatment among patients with depression and for treatment-resistant depression (Davis et al., 2020). Davis and associates' research support that two sessions with psilocybin administration demonstrated efficacy in treating MDD. Research is ongoing.

CLINICAL PEARL All antidepressants carry an FDA black box warning for increased risk of suicidality in children and adolescents.

CLINICAL PEARL As antidepressant drugs take effect and mood begins to lift, the individual may have increased energy with which to implement a suicide plan. Suicide potential often increases as level of depression decreases. The nurse should be particularly alert to sudden lifts in mood.

TABLE 16–3 **Selected Medications Used in the Treatment of Depression**

CHEMICAL CLASS	GENERIC (TRADE) NAME*	DAILY ADULT DOSAGE RANGE (mg)†	THERAPEUTIC PLASMA RANGE (mg)
TRICYCLICS	Amitriptyline	50–300	110–250 (including metabolite)
	Amoxapine	50–300	200–500
	Clomipramine (Anafranil)	25–250	80–100
	Desipramine (Norpramin)	25–300	125–300
	Doxepin	25–300	100–200 (including metabolite)
	Imipramine (Tofranil)	30–300	200–350 (including metabolite)
	Nortriptyline (Aventyl; Pamelor)	30–100	50–150
	Protriptyline (Vivactil)	15–60	100–200
	Trimipramine (Surmontil)	50–300	180 (including metabolite)
SELECTIVE SEROTONIN REUPTAKE INHIBITORS (SSRIS)	Citalopram (Celexa)	20–40	Not well established
	Escitalopram (Lexapro)	10–20	Not well established
	Fluoxetine (Prozac; Serafem)	20–80	Not well established
	Fluvoxamine (Luvox)	50–300	Not well established
	Paroxetine (Paxil)	10–50 (CR: 12.5–75)	Not well established
	Sertraline (Zoloft)	25–200	Not well established
	Vilazodone (Viibryd) (also acts as a partial serotonergic agonist)	40	Not well established
	Vortioxetine (Brintellix)	10–20	
MONOAMINE OXIDASE INHIBITORS	Isocarboxazid (Marplan)	20–60	Not well established
	Phenelzine (Nardil)	45–90	Not well established
	Tranylcypromine (Parnate)	30–60	Not well established
	Selegiline Transdermal System (Emsam)	6/24 hr–12/24 hr patch	Not well established
ATYPICAL ANTIDEPRESSANTS	Bupropion (Wellbutrin)	200–450	Not well established
	Maprotiline	25–225	200–300 (including metabolite)
	Mirtazapine (Remeron)	15–45	Not well established
	Nefazodone	200–600	Not well established
	Trazodone	150–600	800–1600
SEROTONIN-NOREPINEPHRINE REUPTAKE INHIBITORS (SNRIS)	Desvenlafaxine (Pristiq)	50–400	Not well established
	Duloxetine (Cymbalta)	40–60	Not well established
	Venlafaxine (Effexor)	75–375	Not well established
PSYCHOTHERAPEUTIC COMBINATIONS	Olanzapine and fluoxetine (Symbyax)	6/25–12/50	Not well established
	Chlordiazepoxide and fluoxetine (Limbitrol)	20/50–40/100	Not well established
	Perphenazine and amitriptyline (Etrafon)	6/30–16/200	Not well established

Patient and Family Education Related to Antidepressants

The patient should:

- Continue to take the medication even though the symptoms have not subsided. The therapeutic effect may not be seen for as long as 4 weeks. If after this length of time no improvement is noted, the physician may prescribe a different medication.
- Use caution when driving or operating dangerous machinery. Drowsiness and dizziness can occur. If these side effects become persistent or interfere with activities of daily living (ADLs), the patient should report them to the physician. Dosage adjustment may be necessary.
- Do not discontinue use of the drug abruptly. To do so might produce withdrawal symptoms, such as nausea, vertigo, insomnia, headache, malaise, nightmares, and return of symptoms for which the medication was prescribed.
- Use sunblock lotion and wear protective clothing when spending time outdoors. The skin may be sensitive to sunburn.
- Report occurrence of any of the following symptoms to the physician immediately: sore throat, fever, malaise, yellowish skin, unusual bleeding, easy bruising, persistent nausea/vomiting, severe headache, rapid heart rate, difficulty urinating, anorexia/weight loss, seizure activity, stiff or sore neck, and chest pain.
- Rise slowly from a sitting or lying position to prevent a sudden drop in blood pressure.
- Take frequent sips of water, chew sugarless gum, or suck on hard candy if dry mouth is a problem. Good oral care (frequent brushing, flossing) is very important.
- Do not consume the following foods or medications while taking MAOIs: aged cheese, wine (especially Chianti), beer, chocolate, colas, coffee, tea, sour cream, smoked and processed meats, beef or chicken liver, canned figs, soy sauce, overripe and fermented foods, pickled herring, raisins, caviar, yogurt, yeast products, broad beans, cold remedies, diet pills. To do so could cause a life-threatening hypertensive crisis.
- Avoid smoking while receiving tricyclic therapy. Smoking increases the metabolism of tricyclics, requiring an adjustment in dosage to achieve the therapeutic effect.
- Avoid drinking alcohol while taking antidepressant therapy. These drugs potentiate the effects of each other.
- Avoid use of other medications (including over-the-counter medications) without the physician's approval while receiving antidepressant therapy. Many medications contain substances that, in combination with antidepressant medication, could precipitate a life-threatening hypertensive crisis.
- Notify the physician immediately if inappropriate or prolonged penile erections occur while taking trazodone. If the erection persists longer than 1 hour, seek emergency department treatment. This condition is rare but has occurred in some men who have taken trazodone. If measures are not instituted immediately, impotence can result.
- Not "double up" on medication if a dose of bupropion (Wellbutrin) is missed, unless advised to do so by the physician. Taking bupropion in divided doses will decrease the risk of seizures and other adverse effects.
- Follow the correct procedure for applying the selegiline transdermal patch:
  a. Apply to dry, intact skin on upper torso, upper thigh, or outer surface of upper arm.
  b. Apply approximately same time each day to new spot on skin after removing and discarding old patch.
  c. Wash hands thoroughly after applying the patch.
  d. Avoid exposing application site to direct heat (e.g., heating pads, electric blankets, heat lamps, hot tub, or prolonged direct sunlight).
  e. If patch falls off, apply new patch to a new site and resume previous schedule.
- Be aware of possible risks of taking antidepressants during pregnancy. Safe use during pregnancy and lactation has not been fully established. These drugs are believed to readily cross the placental barrier; if so, the fetus could experience adverse effects of the drug. Inform the physician immediately if pregnancy occurs, is suspected, or is planned.
- Be aware of the side effects of antidepressants. Refer to written materials furnished by health-care providers for safe self-administration.
- Carry a card or other identification at all times describing the medications being taken.

Pharmacogenomics

Recent genetic studies have demonstrated that variations in genes can predict whether someone will respond to SSRIs (Lee, 2015), which may offer clinicians important guidance in prescribing antidepressants according to a client's genetic makeup. As Lee reports, between 30% and 50% of people don't respond to the first antidepressant they are prescribed. Patients and family members often express frustration as prescriptions are changed in an effort to find the right antidepressant and dose that are most effective for each individual. Genotyping has also demonstrated benefits in identifying which individuals may be more prone to certain side effects.

One study cited by Lee demonstrated that Asian populations with a specific genotype were at increased risk for sexual dysfunction side effects associated with SSRIs. This information could be useful because sexual dysfunction is a primary reason that many people choose to stop taking these medications. Currently, this area of study is in its infancy, and further study is needed to identify benefits of routine genotyping, its cost-effectiveness, and the ability to provide timely results so that therapy can be initiated promptly.

CASE STUDY AND SAMPLE CARE PLAN

NURSING HISTORY AND ASSESSMENT

Seth is a 45-year-old white male admitted to the psychiatric unit of a general medical center by his family physician, Dr. Jones, who reported that Seth had become increasingly despondent over the past month. His wife reported that he had made statements such as "Life is not worth living" and "I think I could just take all those pills Dr. Jones prescribed at one time; then it would all be over." Seth says he loves his wife and children and does not want to hurt them, but he feels they no longer need him. He states, "They would probably be better off without me." His wife appears to be very concerned about his condition, although in his despondency, he seems oblivious to her feelings. His mother (a widow) lives in a neighboring state, and he sees her infrequently. His father was an alcoholic and physically abused Seth and his siblings. He admits that he is somewhat bitter toward his mother for allowing him and his siblings to "suffer from the physical and emotional brutality of their father." His siblings and their families live in distant states, and he sees them rarely, during holiday gatherings.

Seth earned a college degree working full time at night to pay his way. He is employed in the administration department of a large corporation. Over the past 12 years, Seth has watched while a number of his peers were promoted to management positions. Seth has been considered for several of these positions but has never been selected. Last month, a management position became available for which Seth felt he was qualified. He applied for this position, believing he had a good chance of being promoted. However, when the announcement was made, the position had been given to a younger man who had been with the company for only 5 years. Seth seemed to accept the decision, but over the past few weeks, he has become increasingly withdrawn. He speaks to very few people at the office and is falling behind in his work. At home, he eats very little, talks to family members only when they ask a direct question, withdraws to his bedroom early in the evenings, and does not come out until it is time to leave for work the next morning. Today, he refused to get out of bed or to go to work. His wife convinced him to talk to their family doctor, who admitted him to the hospital. The referring psychiatrist diagnosed Seth with Major Depressive Disorder.

NURSING DIAGNOSES AND OUTCOME IDENTIFICATION

From the assessment data, the nurse develops the following nursing diagnoses for Seth:

1. **Risk for suicide** related to depressed mood and expressions of having nothing to live for
   a. **Short-Term Goals:**
      - Seth will discuss suicide ideation and intentions with staff.
      - Seth will collaborate with the nurse to identify a plan for maintaining safety.
   b. **Long-Term Goal:** Seth will not harm himself during his hospitalization.
2. **Maladaptive grieving** related to unresolved losses (job promotion and unsatisfactory parent/child relationships) evidenced by anger turned inward on self and desire to end his life
   a. **Short-Term Goal:** Seth will discuss anger toward boss and parents within 1 week.
   b. **Long-Term Goal:** Seth will verbalize his position in the grief process and begin movement in the progression toward resolution by time of discharge from treatment.

PLANNING AND IMPLEMENTATION

RISK FOR SUICIDE

The following nursing interventions have been identified for Seth:

1. Develop a trusting relationship with Seth that facilitates open, nonjudgmental discussion of suicide ideation and related thoughts and feelings.
2. Ask Seth directly, "Have you thought about killing yourself? If so, what do you plan to do? Do you have the means to carry out this plan?"

Continued

CASE STUDY AND SAMPLE CARE PLAN—cont'd

3. Create a safe environment. Remove all potentially harmful objects from immediate access (sharp objects, straps, belts, ties, glass items).
4. Assess suicide risk each shift and identify any changes in level of hopelessness. Encourage honest verbalization of feelings. Through discussion and exploration, assist Seth to identify symbols of hope in his life (reasons for wanting to live).
5. Allow Seth to express angry feelings within appropriate limits. Encourage use of the exercise room and other activities for releasing energy appropriately. Help him to identify the true source of his anger, and work on adaptive coping skills for use outside the hospital (e.g., jogging, using the exercise club available to employees of his company).
6. Identify community resources that he may use as a support system and from whom he may request help if feeling suicidal (e.g., suicidal or crisis hotline, psychiatrist or social worker at community mental health center, hospital "HELP" line).
7. Introduce Seth to support and education groups for adult children of alcoholics (ACoA).
8. Spend time with Seth. Doing so will help him to feel safe and secure while conveying the message that he is a worthwhile person.

MALADAPTIVE GRIEVING

The following nursing interventions have been identified for Seth:

1. Discuss with Seth the stages in the grief process and encourage him to explore his feelings so that he may come to realize the connection between grief and his anger.
2. Develop a trusting relationship with Seth. Show empathy and caring. Be honest and keep all promises.
3. Convey an accepting attitude—one in which Seth is not afraid to express feelings openly.
4. Facilitate Seth's verbalization of feelings of anger. The initial expression of anger may be displaced onto the health-care provider. Do not become defensive if this should occur. Assist him to explore these angry feelings so that they may be directed toward the intended persons (boss, parents). Help Seth write letters *(not to be mailed)* expressing his feelings toward his boss and his parents. Discuss the "letters" and then destroy them.
5. Assist Seth to discharge pent-up anger through participation in large motor activities (brisk walks, jogging, physical exercises, volleyball, exercise bike, or other equipment).
6. Help Seth to understand that feelings such as guilt and anger toward his boss and parents are appropriate and acceptable during this stage of the grieving process. Help him also to understand that he must work through these feelings and move past this stage in order to eventually feel better. Knowledge of acceptability of the feelings associated with normal grieving may help to relieve some of the guilt that these responses generate. Knowing why he is experiencing these feelings may also help to resolve them.
7. Encourage Seth to review the relationship with his parents. Educate Seth about the common roles and behaviors of members in families with alcoholic parents. Encourage Seth to explore his roles and behavior within his family of origin.
8. Assist Seth in problem-solving as he attempts to determine methods for more adaptive coping. Suggest alternatives to automatic negative thinking patterns (e.g., thought-stopping techniques). Provide positive feedback for strategies identified and decisions made.
9. Encourage Seth to reach out for spiritual support during this time in whatever form is desirable to him. Assess spiritual needs (see online Chapter 31, "Cultural Concepts Relevant to Psychiatric Mental Health Nursing," for an assessment tool), and assist as necessary in the fulfillment of those needs. Seth may find comfort in religious rituals with which he is familiar.

EVALUATION

The outcome criteria identified for Seth have been met. He sought out staff when feelings of suicide surfaced and identified a safety plan for which he reports willingness to engage. He has not harmed himself in any way. He verbalizes no further thought of suicide and expresses hope for the future. He is able to verbalize names of resources outside the hospital from whom he may request help if thoughts of suicide return. He is able to verbalize normal stages of the grief process and behaviors associated with each stage. He is able to identify his own position in the grief process and express honest feelings related to the loss of the job promotion and satisfactory parent/child relationships. He expresses willingness to continue exploring behaviors and coping mechanisms through a local ACoA meeting.

Summary and Key Points

- Depression is one of the oldest recognized psychiatric illnesses that is still prevalent today. It is associated with increased risk for suicide and is recognized a significant public health issue.
- The cause of depressive disorders is not entirely known. A number of factors, including genetics, biochemical influences, and psychosocial experiences, likely enter into the development of the disorder.
- Secondary depression occurs in response to other physiological disorders and may be induced by a variety of substances or medications.
- Symptoms of depression occur along a continuum according to the degree of severity from transient to severe.
- Depression occurs at all developmental levels, including childhood, adolescence, senescence, and during the puerperium.
- Treatment of depression may include individual therapy, group and family therapy, cognitive therapy, electroconvulsive therapy, bright light therapy, repetitive transcranial magnetic stimulation, vagal nerve or deep brain stimulation, and psychopharmacology.
- Nursing care of the depressed patient is provided using the six steps of the nursing process.

Review Questions

Select the answer that is most appropriate for each of the following questions:

1. A client, age 68, is a widow of 6 months. Over the past month they have become socially withdrawn, has lost weight, and told their sister today that they "don't have anything more to live for." The client has been hospitalized with a diagnosis of major depressive disorder. The *priority* nursing diagnosis for this client is:
   a. Imbalanced nutrition: Less than body requirements
   b. Maladaptive grieving
   c. Risk for suicide
   d. Social isolation
2. The goal of cognitive behavior therapy with depressed clients is to:
   a. Identify and change dysfunctional patterns of thinking.
   b. Resolve the symptoms and initiate or restore adaptive family functioning.
   c. Alter the neurotransmitters that are creating the depressed mood.
   d. Provide feedback from peers who are having similar experiences.
3. A client expresses interest in alternative treatments for depression with seasonal variations and asks the nurse about bright light therapy. Which evidence-based teaching points should the nurse share with the client? (Select all that apply.)
   a. Bright light therapy has demonstrated effectiveness that is comparable to antidepressants.
   b. Bright light therapy should be used regularly until the season changes.
   c. Bright light therapy should only be used when ECT has proven to be ineffective.
   d. Side effects such as headache, nausea, or agitation, when they occur, are usually mild and transient.
   e. Bright light therapy can cause sedation so the best time to use it is before bedtime.
4. A client has just been admitted to the psychiatric unit with a diagnosis of major depressive disorder. Which manifestation might the nurse expect to assess? (Select all that apply.)
   a. Slumped posture
   b. Hallucinations
   c. Feelings of despair
   d. Appears to have boundless energy
   e. Anorexia
5. A client with depression asks the nurse, "Why would they be checking my thyroid function when I clearly have depression and I'm not overweight?" Which is an accurate response?
   a. An underactive thyroid gland can manifest as depression.
   b. Depression has been proven to be a hormonal illness.
   c. Thyroid hormone replacement is a first-line treatment for most people with depression.
   d. Abnormal thyroid function predicts positive response to antidepressant medication.

Continued

6. An acutely depressed client isolates themselves in their room and just sits and stares into space. Which is the best example of an active communication approach with this client?
   a. "Do you like exercise?"
   b. "Come with me. I will go with you to group therapy."
   c. "Would you like to go to group therapy, stay in bed, or come out to the day lounge for some activities?"
   d. "Why do you stay in your room all the time?"

Clinical Judgment Questions

7. A client who has been taking sertraline (Zoloft) 50 mg PO bid for depression tells the nurse, "I've been on this medication for almost a week and I don't feel a bit better." What is the most appropriate response by the nurse?
   a. "Cheer up. You have so much to be happy about."
   b. "Sometimes it takes a few weeks for the medicine to bring about an improvement in symptoms."
   c. "I'll report that to the physician. Maybe he will order something different."
   d. "Try not to dwell on your symptoms. Why don't you join the others down in the dayroom?"
8. A client reports to the mental health clinic with complaints of feeling more depressed over the last few weeks. The client's score on the Hamilton Depression Rating Scale is 40. What is the priority nursing action at this finding?
   a. Assess the client's history of treatment for depression.
   b. Encourage the client to keep weekly follow-up appointments at the clinic.
   c. Educate the client about treatment options for mild, moderate, and severe depression.
   d. Assess the client's current risk for suicide.
9. A client whose husband died 6 months ago is diagnosed with major depressive disorder. She says to the nurse, "I start feeling angry that Harold died and left me all alone; he should have stopped smoking years ago! But then I start feeling guilty for feeling that way." What is an appropriate response by the nurse?
   a. "Yes, he should have stopped smoking. Then he probably wouldn't have gotten lung cancer."
   b. "I can understand how you must feel."
   c. "Those feelings are a normal part of the grief response."
   d. "Just think about the good times that you had while he was alive."
10. A client is admitted to the hospital with major depressive disorder and repeatedly makes negative statements about themself. Which intervention will promote positive self-esteem in the client? (Select all that apply.)
   a. Teach assertive communication skills.
   b. Make observations to the client when they complete a goal or task.
   c. Instruct the client that you will not talk with them unless they stop talking negatively about themself.
   d. Offer to spend time with the client using a nonjudgmental, accepting approach.
11. What is the priority nursing intervention before starting ECT therapy?
   a. Take vital signs and record.
   b. Have the client void.
   c. Administer succinylcholine.
   d. Ensure that the consent form has been signed.

IMPLICATIONS FOR EVIDENCE-BASED PRACTICE

Kauffman, K., Davey, C. H., Dolata, J., Figueroa, M., Gunzler, D., Huml, A. Pencak, J., Sajatovic, M., & Sehgal, A. R. (2021). Changes in self-reported depressive symptoms among adults in the United States from 2005 to 2016. *Journal of the American Psychiatric Nurses Association*, *27*(2), 148–155.

DESCRIPTION OF THE STUDY: The aim of this study was to evaluate national trends in self-reported depressive symptoms over an 11-year period. Interview data from the National Health and Nutrition Examination Survey, Patient Health Questionnaire (PHQ-9) were examined to identify trends in depressive symptomatology (n = 31,191).

RESULTS OF THE STUDY: The authors found that the proportion of individuals with clinically significant PHQ-9 scores increased from 6.2% to 8.1% over the period being studied. The odds of having a PHQ-9 score that indicated greater severity of depression increased by 27%. The associated symptoms demonstrating the greatest increases include anhedonia, guilt/worthlessness, changes in appetite, and changes in activity levels.

IMPLICATIONS FOR NURSING PRACTICE: The reasons for the increases in self-reported depressive symptoms were not clarified in this study, but the finding that self-reported depressive symptoms are increasing and demonstrating greater severity highlights the importance of screening for depression in all health-care settings and making appropriate referrals to mental health services as needed.

TEST YOUR CLINICAL REASONING AND CLINICAL JUDGMENT SKILLS

Emma is a 17-year-old high school senior. She will graduate in 1 month and has plans to attend the state university a few hours from her home. Emma has always made good grades in school, has participated in many activities, and has been a pep squad cheerleader. She had been dating the star quarterback, Alan, since last summer, and they had spoken a number of times about going to the senior prom together. About a month before the prom, Alan broke up with Emma and began dating Salima, whom he subsequently took to the prom. Since that time, Emma has become despondent. She does not go out with her friends, she dropped out of the pep squad, her grades have fallen, and she has lost 10 pounds. She attends classes most of the time, but she spends evenings and weekends in her room alone listening to her music, crying, and sleeping. Her parents are very concerned and contacted the family physician, who has admitted Emma to the psychiatric unit of the local hospital. The admitting psychiatrist has made the diagnosis of Major Depressive Disorder. Emma tells the nurse, "Sometimes I drive around and try to find Alan and Salima. I don't know why he broke up with me. I hate myself! I just want to die!"

Answer the following questions related to Emma:

1. What is the primary nursing diagnosis that is identified for Emma?
2. To determine the seriousness of this problem, what are important nursing assessments that must be made?
3. What medication might the physician order for Emma?
4. What concern has the FDA identified that is associated with this medication?

Communication Exercises

1. Carrie, age 75, is a patient on the psychiatric unit with a diagnosis of Major Depressive Disorder. She says to the nurse, "I never knew my life would end up like this. I've lost my husband, all my friends, and my home."
   What would be an appropriate response by the nurse to this statement by Carrie?
2. "I have spent my whole life taking care of others. Now someone else has to take care of me. I feel so useless." What would be an appropriate response by the nurse to this statement by Carrie?
3. "I don't know why anyone would want to bother taking care of me. I really have nothing left to live for."
   What would be an appropriate response by the nurse to this statement by Carrie?

MOVIE CONNECTIONS

Prozac Nation (Depression) ▪ *The Butcher Boy* (Depression) ▪ *Night, Mother* (Depression) ▪ *The Prince of Tides* (Depression/suicide) ▪ *The Perks of Being a Wallflower* (Depression/suicide) ▪ *The Beaver* (Depression) ▪ *I'm Here, Too* (Depression)

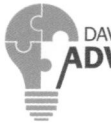

Go to **Davis Advantage** to complete your learning: strengthen understanding, apply your knowledge, and prepare for the Next Gen NCLEX®.

References

Abbott, C. C., Gallegos, P., Rediske, N., Lemke, N. T., & Quinn, D. K. (2014). A review of longitudinal electroconvulsive therapy: Neuroimaging investigations. *Journal of Geriatric Psychiatry and Neurology, 27*(1), 33–46. PMID 24381234. https://doi.org/10.1177/0891988713516542.

Akincigil, A., Olfson, M., Siegel, M., Zurlo, K. A., Walkup, J. T., & Crystal, S. (2012). Racial and ethnic disparities in depression care in community-dwelling elderly in the United States. *American Journal of Public Health, 102*(2), 319–328. https://doi.org/10.2105/AJPH.2011.300349

Akiskal, H. S. (2017). Mood disorders: Historical introduction and conceptual overview. In B. J. Sadock, V. A. Sadock, & P. Ruiz (Eds.), *Comprehensive textbook of psychiatry* (10th ed., pp. 1599–1603). Wolters Kluwer.

American Psychiatric Association. (2001). *The practice of electroconvulsive therapy: Recommendations for treatment, training, and privileging* (2nd ed.).

American Psychiatric Association. (2022). *Diagnostic and statistical manual of mental disorders* (5th ed., text rev.).

American Psychiatric Nurses Association. (2011). *Position statement: Electroconvulsive therapy.* https://www.apna.org/files/public/ECT_POSITION_STATEMENT.pdf

American Thyroid Association. (2021). *General information/Press room.* https://www.thyroid.org/media-main/pressroom/#:~:text=Prevalence%20and%20Impact%20of%20Thyroid,are%20unaware%20of%20their%20condition.

Amick, H. R., Gartlehner, G., Gaynes, B. N., Forneris, C., Asher, G. N., Morgan, L. C., Coker-Schwimmer, E., Boland, E., Lux, L. J., Gaylord, S., Bann, C., Pierl, C. B., & Lohr, K. N. (2015). Comparative benefits and harms of second generation antidepressants and cognitive behavioral therapies in initial treatment of major depressive disorder: Systematic review and meta-analysis. *British Medical Journal, 351*, h6019. https://doi.org/http://dx.doi.org/10.1136/bmj.h6019

Anxiety and Depression Association of America. (2021). *Anxiety and depression in children.* https://adaa.org/find-help/by-demographics/children/anxiety-and-depression

Bauer, A. E., Maegbaek, M. L., Liu, X., Wray, N. R., Sullivan, P. F., Miller, W. C., Meltzer-Brody, S., & Munk-Olsen, T. (2018). Familiality of psychiatric disorders and risk of postpartum psychiatric episodes: A population-based cohort study. *American Journal of Psychiatry, 175*(8), 783–791. https://doi.org/10.1176/appi.ajp.2018.17111184

Berlim, M. T., McGirr, A., Van den Eynde, F., Fleck, M. P., & Giacobbe P. (2014). Effectiveness and acceptability of deep brain stimulation (DBS) of the subgenual cingulate cortex for treatment-resistant depression: A systematic review and exploratory meta-analysis. *Journal of Affective Disorders, 159*, 31–38. https://doi.org/10.1016/j.jad.2014.02.016

Boland, R., & Verduin, M. L. (2022). *Kaplan & Sadock's synopsis of psychiatry* (P. Ruiz, Ed.). (12th ed.). Wolters Kluwer.

Budhwani, H., Hearld, K. R., & Chavez-Yenter, D. (2015). Depression in racial and ethnic minorities: The impact of nativity and discrimination. *Journal of Racial and Ethnic Health Disparities, 2*(1), 34–42.

Burnett, T. (2021). Premenstrual dysphoric disorder: Different from PMS? *Mayo Clinic.* http://www.mayoclinic.org/diseases-conditions/premenstrual-syndrome/expert-answers/pmdd/faq-20058315

Canuso, C. M., Singh, J. B., Fedgchin, M., Alphs, L., Lane, R., Lim, P., Pinter C., Hough, D. Sanacora, G., Husseini, M., & Drevets, W. C. (2018). Efficacy and safety of intranasal esketamine for the rapid reduction of symptoms of depression and suicidality in patients at imminent risk for suicide: Results of a double-blind, randomized, placebo-controlled study. *The American Journal of Psychiatry, 175*(7), 620–630. https://doi.org/10.1176/appi.ajp.2018.17060720

Centers for Disease Control and Prevention. (2021a). *Depression is not a normal part of growing older.* https://www.cdc.gov/aging/depression/

Centers for Disease Control and Prevention. (2021b). *FastStats: Depression.* https://www.cdc.gov/nchs/fastats/depression.htm

Chang, S. C., Wang, W., Pan, A., Jones, R. N., Kawachi, I., & Okereki, O. (2016). Racial variation in depression risk factors and symptom trajectories among older women. *American Journal of Geriatric Psychiatry, 24*(11), 1051–1062. https://doi.org/10.1016/j.jagp.2016.07.008

Cobb, B. S., Coryell, W. H., Cavanough, J., Keller, M., Solomon, D., Endicott, J., & Fiedorowicz, J. G. (2014). Seasonal variation of depressive symptoms in unipolar major depressive disorder. *Comprehensive Psychiatry, 55*(8), 1891–1899. https://doi.org/10.1016/j.comppsych.2014.07.021

Conejero, I., Olié, E., Courtet, P., & Calati, R. (2018). Suicide in older adults: Current perspectives. *Clinical Interventions in Aging, 13*, 691–699. https://doi.org/10.2147/CIA.S130670

Cotterell, D. (2010). Pathogenesis and management of seasonal affective disorder. *Progress in Neurology and Psychiatry, 14*(5), 18–25. https://doi.org/10.1002/pnp.173

Cunningham, J. E. A., Stamp, J. A., & Shapiro, C. M. (2019). Sleep and major depressive disorder: a review of non-pharmacological chronotherapeutic treatments for unipolar depression. *Sleep Medicine, 61*, 6–18. https://doi.org/10.1016/j.sleep.2019.04.012

Davis, A. K., Barrett, F. S., May, D. G., Cosimano, M. P., Sepeda, N. D., Johnson, M. W., Finan, P. H., & Griffiths, R. R. (2020). Effects of psilocybin-assisted therapy on major depressive disorder: A randomized clinical trial. *JAMA Psychiatry, 78*(5), 1–9. https://doi.org/10.1001/jamapsychiatry.2020.3285

Depping, M. S., Nolte, H. M., Hirjak, D., & Thoman, P. A. (2016). Cerebellar volume change in response to electroconvulsive therapy in patients with major depression. *Progress in Neuropsychopharmacology and Biological Psychiatry, 73*, 31–35. https://doi.org/10.1016/j.pnpbp.2016.09.007

Fetterman, T. C., & Ying, P. (2011). Informed consent and electroconvulsive therapy. *Journal of the American Psychiatric Nurses Association, 17*(3), 219–222. https://doi.org/10.1177/1078390311408604

Food and Drug Administration. (2019a). *Zulresso (brexanolone): Highlights of prescribing information.* https://www.accessdata.fda.gov/drugsatfda_docs/label/2019/211371lbl.pdf

Food and Drug Administration. (2019b). *FDA approves new nasal spray medication for treatment-resistant depression; available only at a certified doctor's office or clinic* [Press release]. https://www.fda.gov/news-events/press-announcements/fda-approves-new-nasal-spray-medication-treatment-resistant-depression-available-only-certified

Gautam, M., Tripathi, A., Deshmukh, D., & Gaur, M. (2020). Cognitive behavioral therapy for depression. *Indian Journal of Psychiatry, 62*(Suppl 2), S223–S229. https://doi.org/10.4103/psychiatry.IndianJPsychiatry_772_19

Gaynes, B. N., Lloyd, S. W., Lux, L., Gartlehner, G., Hansen, R. A., Brode, S., Jonas, D. E., Swinson Evans, T., Viswanathan, M., & Lohr, K. N. (2014). Repetitive transcranial magnetic stimulation for treatment-resistant depression. *Journal of Clinical Psychiatry, 75*(5), 477–489.

Geduldig, E. T., & Kellner, C. H. (2016). Electroconvulsive therapy in the elderly: New findings in geriatric depression. *Current Psychiatry Reports, 18*, 40. https://doi.org/10.1007/s11920-016-0674-5

George, M. S., Taylor, J. J., & Short, E. B. (2013). The expanding evidence base for rTMS treatment of depression. *Current Opinion in Psychiatry, 26*(1), 13–18.

Gerhard, T., Stroup, T. S., Correll, C. U., Setoguchi, S., Strom, B. L., Huang, C., Tan, Z., Crystal, S., & Olfson, M. (2020). Mortality risk of antipsychotic augmentation for adult depression. *PLoS ONE, 15*(9), e0239206. https://journals.plos.org/plosone/article?id=10.1371/journal.pone.0239206

Grosse Holtforth, M., Krieger, T., Zimmermann, J., Altenstein-Yamanaka, D., Dörig, N., Meisch, L., & Hayes, A. M. (2019). A randomized-controlled trial of cognitive-behavioral therapy for depression with integrated techniques from emotion-focused and exposure therapies. *Psychotherapy Research. 29*(1), 30–44. https://doi.org/10.1080/10503307.2017.1397796.

Hasin, D. S., Sarvet, A. L., Meyers, J. L., Saha, T. D., Ruan, W. J., Stohl, M., & Grant, B. F. (2018). Epidemiology of adult DSM-5 major depressive disorder and its specifiers in the United States. *JAMA Psychiatry, 75*(4), 336–346. https://doi.org/10.1001/jamapsychiatry.2017.4602

Herdman, T. H., Kamitsuru, S., & Lopes, C. T. (Eds.). (2021). *NANDA-I, Inc. nursing diagnoses: Definitions and classification, 2021–2023.* Thieme.

Holt-Lundstat, J., Robles, T. F., & Sbarra, D. A. (2017). Advancing social connection as a public health priority in the United States. *American Psychologist, 72*(6), 517–530. https://doi.org/10.1037/amp0000103

Holoyda, B. (2021). The rebirth of psychedelic psychiatry. *Current Psychiatry, 20*(1), 13–19.

Jiang, X., Asmaro, R., O'Sullivan, D. O., Budnik, E., & Schnatz, P. F. (2016, October 5–8). *Depression may be one of the strongest risk factors for coronary artery disease in women aged <65 years: A 10-year prospective longitudinal study* [Abstract S-17]. Presented at the NAMS 2016 Annual Meeting, Orlando, FL, United States.

Kauffman, K., Davey, C. H., Dolata, J., Figueroa, M., Gunzler, D., Huml, A. Pencak, J., Sajatovic, M., & Sehgal, A. R. (2021). Changes in self-reported depressive symptoms among adults in the United States From 2005 to 2016. *Journal of the American Psychiatric Nurses Association, 27*(2), 148–155.

Kelsoe, J. R., & Greenwood, T. A. (2017). Mood disorders: Genetics. In B. J. Sadock, V. A. Sadock, & P. Ruiz (Eds.), *Comprehensive textbook of psychiatry* (10 ed., pp. 1619–1630). Wolters Kluwer.

Kubala, J. (2021). 11 herbs, vitamins, and supplements to help fight depression. *Healthline.* https://www.healthline.com/health/depression/herbs-vitamins-supplements

Kurlansik, S. L., & Ibay, A. D. (2013). Seasonal affective disorder. *Indian Journal of Clinical Practice, 24*(7), 607–610.

Lam, R. W., Levitt, A. J., Levitan, R. D., Michelak, E., Morehouse, R., Rammasubbu, R., & Tam, E. M. (2015). Efficacy of bright light treatment, fluoxetine, and the combination in patients with non-seasonal major depressive disorder: A randomized clinical trial. *JAMA Psychiatry, 73*(1), 56–63. https://doi.org/10.1001/jamapsychiatry.2015.2235

Lapate, R. C., Van Reekum, C. M., Schaefer, S. M., Greischar, L. L., Norris, C. J., Bachhuber, D., & Davidson, R. J. (2014). Prolonged marital stress is associated with short-lived responses to positive stimuli. *Psychophysiology, 51*(6), 499–509. https://doi.org/10.1111/psyp.12203

LaPierre, T. A. (2004, August 14). *An investigation of the role of age and life stage in the moderation and mediation of the effect of marital status on depression.* Paper presented at the annual meeting of the American Sociological Association, San Francisco, CA, United States. http://www.allacademic.com/meta/p109917_index.html

Lee, K. C. (2015). Using pharmacogenomics to aid antidepressant prescribing. *Psychiatry Advisor.* http://www.psychiatryadvisor.com/mood-disorders/using-pharmacogenomics-to-aid-antidepressant-prescribing/article/394244/2

Lipp, M., Pasternak, A., & Ward, K. (2020). Impact of the *MTHFR C677T* variant on depression. *Current Psychiatry, 19*(10), 41–53.

Liu, H., Elliott, S., & Umberson, D. J. (2010). Marriage in young adulthood. In J. E. Grant & M. N. Potenza (Eds.), *Young adult mental health* (pp. 169–180). Oxford University Press.

Lyden, H., Espinoza, R. T., Pirnia, T., Clark, K., Joshi, S. H., Leaver, A. M., Woods, R. P., & Narr, K. L. (2014). Electroconvulsive therapy mediates neuroplasticity of white matter microstructure in major depression. *Translational Psychiatry, 4*(4), e380. https://doi.org/10.1038/tp.2014.21

Magnezi, R., Aminov, E., Shmuel, D., Dreifuss, M., & Dannon, P. (2016). Comparison between neurostimulation techniques repetitive transcranial magnetic stimulation vs electroconvulsive therapy for the treatment of resistant depression: Patient preference and cost-effectiveness. *Patient Preference and Adherence, 10*, 1481–1487. https://doi.org/10.2147/PPA.S105654

Mankad, M. V. (2019). Electroconvulsive therapy. *Medscape.* http://emedicine.medscape.com/article/1525957-overview#a1

Marcussen K. (2005). Explaining differences in mental health between married and cohabiting individuals. *Social Psychology Quarterly, 68*, 239–257.

Mårtensson, B., Pettersson, A., Berglund, L., & Ekselius, L. (2015). Bright white light therapy in depression: A critical review of the evidence. *Journal of Affective Disorders, 182*, 1–7. https://doi.org/10.1016/j.jad.2015.04.013.

Mayo Clinic. (2019). *Antidepressants for children and teens.* http://www.mayoclinic.org/diseases-conditions/teen-depression/in-depth/antidepressants/art-20047502

Mayo Clinic. (2021). *Electroconvulsive therapy.* https://www.mayoclinic.org/tests-procedures/electroconvulsive-therapy/about/pac-20393894

McClintock, S. M., & Husain, M. M. (2011). Electroconvulsive therapy does not damage the brain. *Journal of the American Psychiatric Nurses Association, 17*(3), 212–213. https://doi.org/10.1177/1078390311407667

McMahon, B., Andersen, S. B., Madsen, M. K., Hjordt, L. V., Hageman, I., Dam, H., Svarer, C., Cunha-Bang, S., Baaré, W., Madsen, J., Hasholt, L., Holst, K., Frokjaer, V. G., & Knudsen, G. M. (2016). Seasonal difference in brain serotonin transporter binding predicts symptom severity in patients with seasonal affective disorder. *Brain, 139*(Pt. 5), 1605–1614. https://doi.org/10.1093/brain/aww043

Merikangas, K. R., & Rihmer, Z. (2017). Mood disorders: Epidemiology. In B. J. Sadock, V. A. Sadock, & P. Ruiz (Eds.), *Comprehensive textbook of psychiatry* (10th ed., pp. 1614–1619). Wolters Kluwer.

Miller, A. H. (2018). Five things to know about inflammation and depression. *Psychiatric Times.* http://www.psychiatrictimes.com/special-reports/five-things-know-about-inflammation-and-depression/page/0/1

National Center for Health Statistics. (2021). *Faststats: Adolescent health.* https://www.cdc.gov/nchs/fastats/adolescent-health.htm

National Institute of Mental Health. (n.d.). *Postpartum depression facts.* https://www.nimh.nih.gov/health/publications/postpartum-depression-facts/index.shtml

National Institute of Mental Health. (2018). *Depression.* https://www.nimh.nih.gov/health/topics/depression/index.shtml

Natsuaki, M. N., Shaw, D. S., Neiderhiser, J. M., Ganiban, J., Gordon, H. T., Reiss, D., & Leve, L. D. (2014). Raised by depressed parents: Is it an environmental risk? *Clinical Child and Family Psychology Review, 17*(4), 357–367. https://doi.org/10.1007/s10567-014-0169-z

Okereke, O., Reynolds, C., Mischoulon, D., Chang, G., Vyas, C. M., Cook, N., Weinberg, A., Bubes, V., Copeland, T., Friedenberg, G., Lee, M., Buring, J., & Manson, J. E. (2020). Effect of long-term vitamin D3 supplementation vs placebo on risk of depression or clinically relevant depressive symptoms and on change in mood scores: A randomized clinical trial. *JAMA, 324*(5), 471–480. https://doi.org/10.1001/jama.2020.10224

Pirnia, T., Josh, S. H., Leaver, A., & Narr, K. (2016). Electroconvulsive therapy and structural neuroplasticity in neocortical, limbic and paralimbic cortex. *Translational Psychiatry, 6*(6). https://doi.org/10.1038/tp.2016.102

Prudic, J., & Duan, Y. (2017). Electroconvulsive therapy. In B. J. Sadock, V. A. Sadock, & P. Ruiz (Eds.), *Comprehensive textbook of psychiatry* (10th ed., pp. 3280–3298). Wolters Kluwer.

Pulia, K., Vaidya, P., Jayaram, G., Hayat, M. J., & Reti, I. M. (2013). ECT treatment outcomes following performance improvement changes. *Journal of Psychosocial Nursing and Mental Health Services, 51*(11), 20–25. https://doi.org/10.3928/02793695-20130628-02

Raposelli, D. (2015). Is TMS cost effective? *Psychiatric Times.* http://www.psychiatrictimes.com/major-depressive-disorder/tms-cost-effective

Ridley, M., Rao, G., Schilbach, F., & Patel, V. (2020). Poverty, depression, and anxiety: Causal evidence and mechanisms. *Science, 370*(6522). https://doi.org/10.1126/science.aay0214

Rodriguez, T. (2015). Using bright light therapy beyond seasonal affective disorder. *Psychiatry Advisor.* http://www.psychiatryadvisor.com/mood-disorders/depression-mood-winter-season-light-sad-antidepressant/article/457643

Rohan, K. J., Mahon, J. N., Evans, M., Ho, S-Y., Meyerhoff, J., Postolache, T. T., & Vacek, P. M. (2016). Outcomes one and two winters following cognitive-behavioral therapy or light therapy for seasonal affective disorder. *American Journal of Psychiatry, 173*, 244–251.

Sartorius, A., Boehringer, A., Demirakca, J., & Ende, G. (2015). Electroconvulsive therapy increases temporal gray matter volume and cortical thickness. *European Neuropsychopharmacology, 26*(3), 506–517. https://doi.org/10.1016/j.euroneuro.2015.12.036

Sathyanarayana, T. S., Asha, M. R., Ramsh, B. M., & Rao, K. S. (2008). Understanding nutrition, depression, and mental illness. *Indian Journal of Psychiatry, 50*(2), 77–82. https://doi.org/10.4103/0019-5545.42391

Sharma, M. S., Ang-Rabeanes, M., Selek, S., Gajwani, P., & Soares, J. C. (2018). Neuromodulatory options for treatment-resistant depression. *Current Psychiatry, 17*(3), 26–37.

Semkovska, M., & McLoughlin, D. M. (2010). Objective cognitive performance associated with electroconvulsive therapy for depression: a systematic review and meta-analysis. *Biological Psychiatry, 68*(6), 568–577. https://doi.org/10.1016/j.biopsych.2010.06.009

Shin, Y. C., Jung, C. H., Kim, H. J., Kim, E. J., &, Lim, S. W. (2016). The associations among vitamin D deficiency, C-reactive protein, and depressive symptoms. *Journal of Psychosomatic Research, 90*, 98–104. https://doi.org/10.1016/j.jpsychores.2016.10.001

Sikkens, D., Riemersma-Van der Lek, R. F., Meesters, Y., Schoevers, R. A., & Haarman, B. C. M. (2019). Combined sleep deprivation and light therapy: Clinical treatment outcomes in patients with complex unipolar and bipolar depression. *Journal of Affective Disorders, 246*, 727–730. https://doi.org/10.1016/j.jad.2018.12.117

Slezak, M. (2021). Studying depression at a molecular level. *Psychiatric Times.* https://www.psychiatrictimes.com/view/studying-depression-molecular-level

Substance Abuse and Mental Health Services Administration. (2020). *Key substance use and mental health indicators in the United States: Results from the 2019 National Survey on Drug Use and Health* (HHS Publication No. PEP20-07-01-001, NSDUH Series H-55). https://www.samhsa.gov/data/

Teo, A. R., Choi, H., & Valenstein, M. (2013). Social relationships and depression: Ten-year follow-up from a nationally representative study. *PloS ONE, 8*(4), e62396. https://doi.org/10.1371/journal.pone.0062396

Uecker, J. E. (2012). Marriage and mental health among young adults. *Journal of Health and Social Behavior, 53*(1), 67–83. https://doi.org/10.1177/0022146511419206

Wagner, K. D., & Brent, D. A. (2017). Mood disorders in children and adolescents: Depressive disorders and suicide. In B. J. Sadock, V. A. Sadock, & P. Ruiz (Eds.), *Comprehensive textbook of psychiatry* (10th ed., pp. 3674–3685). Wolters Kluwer.

Winthorst, W., Post, W., Meesters, Y., Penninx, B., & Nolen, W. A. (2011). Seasonality in depressive and anxiety symptoms among primary care patients and in patients with depressive and anxiety disorders; results from the Netherlands Study of Depression and Anxiety. *BMC Psychiatry, 11*(1), 1–18. https://doi.org/10.1186/1471-244X-11-198

Classical References

Beck, A. T., Rush, A. J., Shaw, B. F., & Emery, G. (1979). *Cognitive theory of depression.* Guilford Press.

Freud, S. (1957). Mourning and melancholia. In *Standard edition of the complete psychological works of Freud* (Vol. XIV). Hogarth Press.

Hamilton, M. (1960). A rating scale for depression. *Journal of Neurology, Neurosurgery, & Psychiatry, 23*, 56–62.

Seligman, M. E. P. (1973). Fall into helplessness. *Psychology Today, 7*, 43–48.

Bipolar and Related Disorders 17

CHAPTER OUTLINE

Objectives
Introduction
Historical Perspective
Epidemiology
Types of Bipolar Disorders
Predisposing Factors
Developmental Implications
Application of the Nursing Process to Bipolar Disorder (Mania)
Treatment Modalities
Summary and Key Points
Review Questions
Clinical Judgment Questions
Implications for Evidence-Based Practice
Test Your Clinical Reasoning and Clinical Judgment Skills
Communication Exercises
Movie Connections

CORE CONCEPTS

Mood and Affect: Mania
Professional Behavior: Nursing process in the care of patients with bipolar and related disorders
Safety
Clinical Judgment

KEY TERMS

acute mania
bipolar disorder
cyclothymic disorder
delirious mania
flight of ideas
hypomania
mania
pressured speech

OBJECTIVES

After reading this chapter, the student will be able to:

1. Recount historical perspectives of bipolar disorder.
2. Discuss epidemiological statistics related to bipolar disorder.
3. Describe various types of bipolar disorders.
4. Identify predisposing factors in the development of bipolar disorder.
5. Discuss implications of bipolar disorder related to developmental stage.
6. Identify symptomatology associated with bipolar disorder and use this information in patient assessment.
7. Formulate nursing diagnoses and goals of care for patients experiencing a manic episode.
8. Identify topics for patient and family teaching relevant to bipolar disorder.
9. Describe appropriate nursing interventions for patients experiencing a manic episode.
10. Describe relevant criteria for evaluating nursing care of patients experiencing a manic episode.
11. Discuss various modalities relevant to treatment of bipolar disorder.

Introduction

Mood is defined in Chapter 16, "Depressive Disorders," as a pervasive and sustained emotion that may have a major influence on a person's perception of the world. Examples of mood include depression, joy, elation, anger, and anxiety. *Affect* is described as the external, observable emotional reaction associated with an experience.

Chapter 16 focuses on the consequences of maladaptive grieving as it is manifested by depressive disorders. This chapter addresses mood disorders as they are manifested by cycles of mania and depression—called **bipolar disorder.** A historical perspective and epidemiology related to bipolar disorder are presented. Predisposing factors that have been implicated in the etiology of bipolar disorder provide a framework for studying the dynamics of the disorder.

The implications of bipolar disorder relevant to children and adolescents are discussed. An explanation of the symptomatology is presented as background knowledge for assessing the client with bipolar disorder. Nursing care is described in the context of the six steps of the nursing process. Various medical treatment modalities are explored.

CORE CONCEPT

Mania

Mania is an alteration in mood that may be expressed by feelings of elation, inflated self-esteem, grandiosity, hyperactivity, agitation, racing thoughts, and accelerated speech. Mania can occur as part of the psychiatric disorder bipolar disorder, as part of some other medical conditions, or in response to some substances.

Historical Perspective

Documentation of the symptoms associated with bipolar disorder dates back to about the second century in ancient Greece. Aretaeus of Cappadocia, a Greek physician, is credited with associating these extremes of mood as part of the same illness. He described patients who could at times laugh and play all night and day but at other times appeared "torpid, dull, and sorrowful (Burton, 2017). His view that these mood swings were part of the same illness did not gain acceptance until much later.

In early writings, mania was categorized with all forms of "severe madness." In 1025, the Persian physician Avicenna wrote *The Canon of Medicine* in which he described mania as "bestial madness characterized by rapid onset and remission, with agitation and irritability." The modern concept of manic-depressive illness began to emerge in the 19th century. In 1854, Jules Baillarger presented information to the French Imperial Academy of Medicine in which he used the term *dual-form insanity* to describe the illness. In the same year, Jean-Pierre Falret described the same disorder, which he termed *circular insanity* (Burton, 2017). Falret also noted that this disorder appeared to have genetic underpinnings, a belief that is adhered to today (Krans, 2019).

Contemporary thinking has been shaped a great deal by the works of Emil Kraepelin, who first coined the term *manic-depressive* in 1913. He added that this disorder was characterized by acute episodes followed by relatively symptom-free periods. In 1980, the American Psychiatric Association (APA) adopted the term *bipolar disorder* as the diagnostic category for manic-depressive illness in the *Diagnostic and Statistical Manual of Mental Disorders* (3rd ed.; *DSM-III*). This term identified a period of mood elevation and excitation as a defining characteristic that distinguishes it from other mood and psychotic disorders. The term *mania* was replaced in the diagnostic label because the description of people as "maniacs" was considered stigmatizing (Krans, 2019). The term *mania*, however, is still currently used to describe an abnormal mood state of elation with symptoms that include agitation, insomnia, grandiose delusions, racing thoughts, boundless energy, and increased libido among others.

Epidemiology

Bipolar disorder affects approximately 4.4% of American adults, and 82.9% of these cases are considered severe (National Institute of Mental Health [NIMH], 2017). In terms of sex, bipolar disorder roughly equally affects both men and women. The average age of onset for bipolar disorder is 25 years, and following the first manic episode, the disorder tends to be recurrent. Bipolar disorder is associated with increased mortality in general and particularly with death by suicide (Merikangas & Rihmer, 2017).

Unlike depressive disorders, bipolar disorder appears to occur more frequently among the higher socioeconomic classes with an overrepresentation among socially active, creative individuals (Merikangas & Rihmer, 2017). Bipolar disorder is the sixth-leading cause of disability in the middle-aged group, but for those who respond to lithium treatment (about 33% of those treated with lithium), bipolar disorder may be completely treatable with no further episodes. Unfortunately, many individuals go for years without an accurate diagnosis or treatment, and for some the consequences can be devastating.

Types of Bipolar Disorders

A bipolar disorder is characterized by mood swings from profound depression to extreme euphoria (mania) with intervening periods of normalcy. Delusions or hallucinations may or may not be a part of the clinical picture, and onset of symptoms may reflect a seasonal pattern.

During a manic episode, the mood is elevated, expansive, or irritable. The disturbance is sufficiently severe to cause marked impairment in occupational functioning or in usual social activities or relationships with others or to require hospitalization to prevent harm to self or others. Motor activity is excessive and frenzied. Psychotic features may be present. The *Diagnostic and Statistical Manual of Mental Disorders, Fifth Edition, Text Revision* (*DSM-5-TR*) (APA, 2022) diagnostic criteria for a manic episode are presented in Box 17–1.

A somewhat milder degree of this clinical symptom picture is called **hypomania.** In hypomania the symptoms are less intense, and they are not severe enough to cause marked impairment in social or occupational functioning or to require hospitalization. Hypomania does not include psychotic features. The *DSM-5-TR* diagnostic criteria for a hypomanic episode are presented in Box 17–2.

The diagnostic picture for depression associated with bipolar disorder is similar to that described for major depressive disorder, with one major distinction: the client must have a history of one or more manic episodes. When the presentation includes symptoms associated with both depression and mania, the diagnosis is further specified as *with mixed features.*

Bipolar I Disorder

A diagnosis of bipolar I disorder is given to an individual who is experiencing a manic episode or who has a history of one or more manic episodes. The client may also have experienced episodes of depression. This diagnosis is further specified by the current or most recent behavioral episode experienced. For example, the specifier might be *single manic episode* (to describe individuals having a first episode of mania) or *current* (or most recent) *episode manic, hypomanic, mixed,* or *depressed* (to describe individuals who have had recurrent mood episodes). Psychotic or catatonic features may also be noted. Although the length of manic episodes (and depressive episodes) is variable, when an individual

BOX 17–1 Diagnostic Criteria for a Manic Episode

A. A distinct period of abnormally and persistently elevated, expansive, or irritable mood and abnormally and persistently increased goal-directed activity or energy, lasting at least 1 week and present most of the day, nearly every day (or any duration if hospitalization is necessary).

B. During the period of mood disturbance and increased energy or activity, three (or more) of the following symptoms (four if the mood is only irritable) are present to a significant degree and represent a noticeable change from usual behavior:
   1. Inflated self-esteem or grandiosity
   2. Decreased need for sleep (e.g., feels rested after only 3 hours of sleep)
   3. More talkative than usual or pressure to keep talking
   4. Flight of ideas or subjective experience that thoughts are racing
   5. Distractibility (i.e., attention too easily drawn to unimportant or irrelevant external stimuli), as reported or observed
   6. Increase in goal-directed activity (either socially, at work or school, or sexually) or psychomotor agitation (i.e., purposeless non-goal-directed activity)
   7. Excessive involvement in activities that have a high potential for painful consequences (e.g., engaging in unrestrained buying sprees, sexual indiscretions, or foolish business investments)

C. The mood disturbance is sufficiently severe to cause marked impairment in social or occupational functioning or to necessitate hospitalization to prevent harm to self or others, or there are psychotic features.

D. The episode is not attributable to the physiological effects of a substance (e.g., a drug of abuse, a medication, or other treatment) or to another medical condition.

NOTE: A full manic episode that emerges during antidepressant treatment (e.g., medication, electroconvulsive therapy) but persists at a fully syndromal level beyond the physiological effect of that treatment is sufficient evidence for a manic episode and, therefore, a bipolar I diagnosis.

Reprinted with permission from American Psychiatric Association. (2022). *Diagnostic and statistical manual of mental disorders, fifth edition, text revision.*

BOX 17–2 Diagnostic Criteria for a Hypomanic Episode

A. A distinct period of abnormally and persistently elevated, expansive, or irritable mood and abnormally and persistently increased activity or energy, lasting at least 4 consecutive days and present most of the day, nearly every day.
B. During the period of mood disturbance and increased energy and activity, three (or more) of the following symptoms (four if the mood is only irritable) have persisted, represent a noticeable change from usual behavior, and have been present to a significant degree:
   1. Inflated self-esteem or grandiosity
   2. Decreased need for sleep (e.g., feels rested after only 3 hours of sleep)
   3. More talkative than usual or pressure to keep talking
   4. Flight of ideas or subjective experience that thoughts are racing
   5. Distractibility (i.e., attention too easily drawn to unimportant or irrelevant external stimuli), as reported or observed
   6. Increase in goal-directed activity (either socially, at work or school, or sexually) or psychomotor agitation
   7. Excessive involvement in pleasurable activities that have a high potential for painful consequences (e.g., engaging in unrestrained buying sprees, sexual indiscretions, or foolish business investments)
C. The episode is associated with an unequivocal change in functioning that is uncharacteristic of the individual when not symptomatic.
D. The disturbance in mood and the change in functioning are observable by others.
E. The episode is not severe enough to cause marked impairment in social or occupational functioning or to necessitate hospitalization. If there are psychotic features, the episode is, by definition, manic.
F. The episode is not attributable to the physiological effects of a substance (e.g., a drug of abuse, a medication, or other treatment).

NOTE: A full hypomanic episode that emerges during antidepressant treatment (medication, electroconvulsive therapy) but persists at a fully syndromal level beyond the physiological effect of that treatment is sufficient evidence for a hypomanic episode diagnosis. However, caution is indicated so that one or two symptoms (particularly increased irritability, edginess or agitation following antidepressant use) are not taken as sufficient for diagnosis of a hypomanic episode, nor necessarily indicative of a bipolar diathesis.

Reprinted with permission from American Psychiatric Association. (2022). *Diagnostic and statistical manual of mental disorders, fifth edition, text revision.*

has more than four manic and depressive episodes in a year, they are referred to as having *rapid cycling* bipolar disorder.

Bipolar II Disorder

The bipolar II disorder diagnostic category is characterized by recurrent bouts of major depression with episodic occurrence of hypomania. The individual who is assigned this diagnosis may present with symptoms (or history) of depression or hypomania. The client has never experienced a full manic episode, and the hypomanic episode is "not severe enough to cause marked impairment in social or occupational functioning or to necessitate hospitalization" (APA, 2022, p. 151). The diagnosis may specify whether the current or most recent episode is hypomanic, depressed, or with mixed features.

Cyclothymic Disorder

The essential feature of **cyclothymic disorder** is a chronic mood disturbance of at least 2 years' duration, involving numerous periods of elevated mood (hypomanic symptoms) that do not meet the criteria for a hypomanic episode and numerous periods of depressed mood of insufficient severity or duration to meet the criteria for major depressive episode. The individual is never without the symptoms for more than 2 months. The *DSM-5-TR* criteria for cyclothymic disorder are presented in Box 17–3.

Substance/Medication-Induced Bipolar Disorder

The disturbance of mood associated with this disorder is considered to be the direct result of physiological effects of a substance (e.g., ingestion of or withdrawal from a drug of abuse or a medication). The mood disturbance may involve elevated, expansive, or irritable mood with inflated self-esteem, decreased need for sleep, and distractibility. The disorder causes clinically significant distress or impairment in social, occupational, or other important areas of functioning.

Mood disturbances are associated with *intoxication* from substances such as alcohol, amphetamines, cocaine, hallucinogens, inhalants, opioids, phencyclidine, sedatives, hypnotics, and anxiolytics. Symptoms can also occur during *withdrawal* from substances such as alcohol, amphetamines, cocaine, sedatives, hypnotics, and anxiolytics.

BOX 17–3 Diagnostic Criteria for Cyclothymic Disorder

A. For at least 2 years (at least 1 year in children and adolescents) there have been numerous periods with hypomanic symptoms that do not meet criteria for hypomanic episode and numerous periods with depressive symptoms that do not meet the criteria for a major depressive episode.
B. During the above 2-year period (1 year in children and adolescents), Criterion A symptoms have been present for at least half the time, and the individual has not been without the symptoms for more than 2 months at a time.
C. Criteria for a major depressive, manic, or hypomanic episode have never been met.
D. The symptoms in Criterion A are not better explained by schizoaffective disorder, schizophrenia, schizophreniform disorder, delusional disorder, or other specified or unspecified schizophrenia spectrum and other psychotic disorder.
E. The symptoms are not attributable to the physiological effects of a substance (e.g., a drug of abuse, a medication) or another medical condition (e.g., hyperthyroidism).
F. The symptoms cause clinically significant distress or impairment in social, occupational, or other important areas of functioning.

Specify if:
With anxious distress

Reprinted with permission from American Psychiatric Association. (2022). *Diagnostic and statistical manual of mental disorders, fifth edition, text revision.*

Many medications have been known to evoke mood symptoms. Classifications include anesthetics, analgesics, anticholinergics, anticonvulsants, antihypertensives, antiparkinsonian agents, antiulcer agents, cardiac medications, oral contraceptives, psychotropic medications, muscle relaxants, steroids, and sulfonamides. Some specific examples are included in the discussion of predisposing factors associated with bipolar disorders.

Bipolar Disorder Due to Another Medical Condition

This disorder is characterized by an abnormally and persistently elevated, expansive, or irritable mood and excessive activity or energy that is judged to be the direct physiological consequence of another medical condition (APA, 2022). The mood disturbance causes clinically significant distress or impairment in social, occupational, or other important areas of functioning. Types of medical conditions that are associated with bipolar symptoms include thyroid disorders, stroke, traumatic brain injury, multiple sclerosis, systemic lupus erythematosus, AIDS, and others.

Predisposing Factors

The exact etiology of bipolar disorder has yet to be determined. Scientific evidence supports a chemical imbalance in the brain, although the cause of the imbalance remains unclear. Theories that consider a combination of hereditary factors and environmental triggers (stressful life events) appear to hold the most credibility.

Biological Theories

Genetics

Research suggests that bipolar disorder strongly reflects an underlying genetic vulnerability. Evidence from family, twin, and adoption studies exists to support this observation. A large study that looked at genetic variations associated with five major mental illnesses, found that schizophrenia and bipolar disorders had about 15% of genetic variations in common (NIMH, 2013).

Twin Studies

Twin studies have indicated a concordance rate for bipolar disorder among monozygotic twins at 60% to 80% compared to 10% to 20% in dizygotic twins. Because monozygotic twins have identical genes and dizygotic twins share only approximately half their genes, this is strong evidence that genes play a major role in the etiology. However, because identical twins do not always develop the illness, other factors must also be involved. It is likely that many different genes as well as environmental factors are involved, although researchers do not yet know how these factors interact to cause bipolar disorder.

Family Studies

Although the pattern of inheritance for bipolar disorder is not completely understood, the risk is greatest among first-degree relatives (MedlinePlus, 2021). Boland and Verduin (2022) report that a family history of bipolar disorder conveys a higher risk for mood disorders in general and a threefold increase in the rate of bipolar disorder; first degree relatives have a 10-fold risk of developing the disorder. This increased risk is also present in children born to parents with bipolar disorder who were adopted at birth and reared by adoptive parents without evidence of the disorder.

Other Genetic Studies

Soreff (2019) states:

> Bipolar disorder, especially bipolar type I disorder, has a major genetic component, with the involvement of the *ANK3, CACNA1C,* and *CLOCK* genes. The evidence indicating a genetic role in bipolar disorder takes several forms. . . . Gene expression studies also demonstrate that persons with bipolar disorder, major depression, and schizophrenia share similar decreases in the expression of oligodendrocyte-myelin-related genes and abnormalities of white matter in various brain regions.

The *ANK3* protein is located on the first part of the axon and is involved in making the determination of whether a neuron will fire. Studies have shown that lithium carbonate, the most common medication used to prevent manic episodes, reduces expression of *ANK3* (Leussis et al., 2013). The *CACNA1C* protein regulates the influx and outflow of calcium from the cells and is the site of action of the calcium channel blockers sometimes used in the treatment in bipolar disorder. The *CLOCK* gene is associated with circadian rhythm regulation, and sleep-wake cycles are known to be significantly disrupted in patients with bipolar disorder.

Research looking specifically at factors associated with lithium's effectiveness identified "a number of candidate genes related to neurotransmitters, intracellular signaling, neuroprotection, circadian rhythms, and other pathogenic mechanisms of bipolar disorder [that] were found to be associated with lithium's prophylactic response" (Rybakowski, 2014, p. 353). Evidence from another study, which looked at common gene sets that demonstrated altered expression in patients with schizophrenia, bipolar disorder, and depression Darby and colleagues found that ribosomal genes were overexpressed, and those involved with neuronal connections such as gamma-aminobutyric acid (GABA) signaling were underexpressed (Darby et al., 2016).

The researchers suggest that this finding may lead the way to RNA processing and protein synthesis as targets for therapeutic intervention. Ongoing genetic research will continue to shed light on the genetic influences in the development of bipolar disorder and the genetic factors that affect treatment response.

Biochemical Influences

Biogenic Amines

Early studies have associated symptoms of mania with a functional excess of norepinephrine and dopamine. The neurotransmitter serotonin is believed to remain low in both depression and mania. However, the exact mechanisms and biochemical influences are complex and not yet completely understood. For example, even though serotonin is believed to be low in both depression and manic states, selective serotonin reuptake inhibitors (SSRIs) have been shown to sometimes trigger manic episodes and rapid cycling of mood swings in clients with bipolar disorders. Likely, multiple factors influence serotonin's role in this illness. Acetylcholine is another neurotransmitter believed to be related to symptoms in bipolar disorder. Excessive levels of glutamate, an excitatory neurotransmitter, have been associated with bipolar disorder. Many of the mood stabilizers used to treat bipolar disorder inhibit the actions of glutamate. The primary support for neurotransmitter hypotheses has been the effects that neuroleptic drugs have on the levels of these biogenic amines and the resulting reduction in symptoms of the disorder. Although several neurotransmitters have been implicated in influencing symptoms, the cause of bipolar disorder remains unknown.

Physiological Influences

Neuroanatomical Factors

Neuroanatomical changes have been correlated with dysfunction in the prefrontal cortex, basal ganglia, temporal and frontal lobes of the forebrain, and parts of the limbic system, including the amygdala, thalamus, and striatum. The different symptoms in bipolar disorder may be correlated to those specific areas of dysfunction or may be evidence of downregulation of specific circuits in response to abnormal activity in other circuits (Boland & Verduin, 2022). Akiskal (2017) adds that circadian disturbances seen in both depression and manic episodes can be conceptualized as dysfunction in the limbic system. Although causality of bipolar disorder cannot yet be defined as solely a neuroanatomical disorder, it is clear that mood disorders, including bipolar disorder, involve pathology in the brain.

Medication Side Effects

Certain medications used to treat somatic illnesses have been known to trigger a manic response. The most common of these are the steroids frequently used to treat chronic illnesses such as multiple sclerosis and systemic lupus erythematosus (SLE). Some clients whose first episode of mania occurred during steroid therapy have reported spontaneous recurrence of manic symptoms years later. Amphetamines, antidepressants, and high doses of anticonvulsants and narcotics also have the potential for initiating a manic episode.

Psychosocial Theories

Interest in psychosocial theories has declined in recent years with the focus of research on genetic and biochemical predisposing factors. Consequently, conditions such as schizophrenia and bipolar disorder are more often viewed as diseases of the brain with biological etiologies. However, several studies have confirmed a link between childhood trauma (emotional, physical, and sexual abuse) and the development of bipolar disorder (Aas et al., 2016; Janiri et al., 2015; Quidé et al., 2021; Watson et al., 2013). Aas and associates (2016) identify that childhood trauma interacts with genes along several pathways. These genetic changes may be linked not only to an increased risk for bipolar disorder but also to earlier onset, more severe symptoms, substance abuse, and suicide risk. Research efforts continue to focus on this apparent interaction of genetics and psychosocial stressors More research is needed to translate these connections into practical applications for treatment or prevention.

The Transactional Model of Stress and Adaptation

Bipolar disorder most likely results from an interaction among genetic, biological, and psychosocial determinants. The transactional model takes into consideration these various etiological influences as well as those associated with past experiences, existing conditions, and the individual's perception of the event.

Developmental Implications

The lifetime prevalence of adolescent bipolar disorders is estimated to be about 1% and in younger children the incidence is very rare, but children and adolescents are often difficult to diagnose. In the past decade, diagnosis of bipolar I disorder in youth has rapidly increased, prompting researchers to look more closely at factors contributing to this trend. More recent studies have shown that in 50% to 66% of diagnoses, bipolar disorder actually began before age 18, and as many as 14% had an onset before 12 years of age (Chang & DelBello, 2018).

A connection is thought to exist between attention deficit-hyperactivity disorder (ADHD) and the development of bipolar disorder in youth. A recent study found that a diagnosis of ADHD conferred a 10-fold increase in the risk for later development of bipolar disorder compared to children without ADHD (Meier et al., 2018). ADHD is the most common comorbidity in children and adolescents with bipolar disorder. Studies report anywhere from 9% to 94% comorbidity of the two conditions, and there is overlap in both genetics and symptoms (particularly inattention, distractibility, and impulsivity) (Chang & DelBello, 2018). Osser (2021) notes that when ADHD and bipolar disorder are comorbid, the course of the disease is more severe than either diagnosis alone, and there is an increased risk of suicide attempts.

For youth who manifest with a host of atypical symptoms, including nondiscrete mood episodes, chronic irritability, and temper tantrums, the *DSM-5-TR* includes a distinct diagnosis, *disruptive mood dysregulation disorder.* Since then, a longitudinal study of children with nonepisodic irritability found that although these children had higher risk for anxiety and depression, they were not typically at higher risk for developing bipolar disorder (Stringaris et al., 2010). Because family studies show a familial risk for bipolar disorder, whenever a child is exhibiting mood-related symptoms (including depression) and there is a family history of bipolar disorders, the possibility for a developing bipolar disorder should be carefully evaluated. True bipolar disorder in adolescents, as with adults, is considered a chronic illness (much like diabetes) and medication treatment is typically lifelong.

Treatment Strategies

Psychopharmacology

Medications approved by the U.S. Food and Drug Administration (FDA) for treatment of acute mania in children and adolescents include lithium, risperidone, aripiprazole, quetiapine, olanzapine, and asenapine. Only two medications are approved for the treatment of bipolar depression: olanzapine/fluoxetine combination drugs and lurasidone. Chang and DelBello (2018) note that because medication treatment, particularly for bipolar depression in children and adolescents, is controversial, nonpharmacological interventions, including mood charting, managing stress and sleep cycles, maintaining healthy diet and exercise, and avoiding alcohol and drugs, should be considered as well in this population. Nurses can play a primary role in offering such education and interventions.

Because ADHD has been identified as the most common comorbid condition in children and adolescents with bipolar disorder and stimulants can exacerbate mania, it is suggested that medication for ADHD be initiated only after bipolar symptoms have been controlled with a mood-stabilizing agent (Jain & Jain, 2014). Nonstimulant medications indicated for ADHD (e.g., atomoxetine, bupropion, the tricyclic antidepressants) may also induce switches to mania or hypomania. Bipolar disorder in children and adolescents appears to be a chronic condition with a high risk of relapse. Maintenance therapy incorporates the same medications used to treat acute symptoms, although few research studies exist that deal with long-term medication maintenance of bipolar disorder in children.

Family Interventions

Although pharmacological treatment is acknowledged as the primary method of stabilizing acute symptoms, a combination of medications with psychosocial interventions has been recognized as serving an important role in preventing relapses and improving adjustment. Treatment adherence must be emphasized as an essential component of relapse prevention.

Family dynamics and attitudes can influence the outcome of a client's recovery. Interventions with family members must include education that promotes understanding that at least some of the client's negative behaviors are attributable to an illness that must be managed and are not deliberate or under the client's control.

Family-focused treatment (FFT) is an evidence-based intervention for reducing relapses and increasing medication adherence in clients with bipolar disorder (Miklowitz & Chung, 2016). Miklowitz and Chung also found that clients involved in FFT who demonstrated a high risk for developing bipolar disorder (those with depressive symptoms and a first-degree relative with bipolar disorder) recovered more quickly than those who were provided only educational sessions. FFT includes psychoeducation about bipolar disorder (i.e., symptoms, early recognition, etiology, treatment, self-management), communication training, and problem-solving skills training. Teaching the client and family about early warning signs and management strategies provides the client with a needed support system and the family with tools and resources to provide that support.

Application of the Nursing Process to Bipolar Disorder (Mania)

Background Assessment Data

Symptoms of manic states can be described according to three levels of severity: hypomania, acute mania, and delirious mania. Symptoms of mood, cognition and perception, and activity and behavior are presented for each stage.

Hypomania

Hypomania is characterized by a persistent elevated, expansive, or irritable mood with increased activity and energy that is not sufficiently severe enough to cause marked impairment in social or occupational functioning or to require hospitalization (APA, 2022).

Mood

The mood of a person with hypomania is cheerful and expansive; however, there is an underlying irritability that surfaces rapidly when the person's wishes and desires go unfulfilled. The nature of the hypomanic person is very volatile and fluctuating (see Box 17–2 for diagnostic criteria for a hypomanic episode).

Cognition and Perception

Perceptions of the self are exalted—the individual has ideas of great worth and ability. Thinking is flighty with a rapid flow of ideas. Perception of the environment is heightened, but the individual is so easily distracted by irrelevant stimuli that goal-directed activities may be difficult.

Activity and Behavior

Hypomanic individuals exhibit increased motor activity. They are perceived as being very extroverted and sociable, and, consequently, they attract numerous acquaintances. However, they lack the depth of personality and warmth to formulate close friendships. They talk and laugh a great deal, usually very loudly and often inappropriately. Increased libido is common. Some individuals experience anorexia and weight loss. The exalted self-perception leads some hypomanic individuals to engage in inappropriate behaviors, such as phoning the president of the United States or running up debt on a credit card without concern for having the resources to pay.

Acute Mania

Symptoms of **acute mania** may be a progression in intensification of those experienced in hypomania, or they may be manifested directly. Most individuals experience marked impairment in functioning and require hospitalization (see Box 17–1 for diagnostic criteria for a manic episode).

Mood

Acute mania is characterized by euphoria and elation. The person appears to be on a continuous "high." However, the mood is always subject to frequent variation, easily changing to irritability and anger or even to sadness and crying.

Cognition and Perception

Cognition and perception become fragmented and often psychotic in acute mania. Accelerated thinking proceeds to racing thoughts, overconnection of ideas, and **flight of ideas** (rapidly changing focus of ideas with only superficial connections), may be manifested by a continuous flow of accelerated, **pressured speech** (loquaciousness) to the point where trying to converse with the individual may be extremely difficult. When flight of ideas is severe, speech may be disorganized and incoherent. Distractibility becomes all pervasive. Attention can be diverted by even the smallest of stimuli. Hallucinations and delusions (usually paranoid and grandiose) are common.

Activity and Behavior

Psychomotor activity is excessive. Sexual interest is increased. There is poor impulse control and low frustration tolerance, and the individual who is normally discreet may become socially and sexually uninhibited. Excessive spending is common. In acute mania, individuals typically have little insight with regard to their behavior and communication. This manifests, at times, as unreliable reporting of events and denial of problems when confronted by friends or family, both of which may be interpreted as lying. Energy seems inexhaustible, and the need for sleep is diminished. Individuals may go for many days without sleep and still not feel tired. Hygiene and grooming may be neglected. Dress may be disorganized, flamboyant, or bizarre, and the use of excessive makeup or jewelry is common.

Delirious Mania

Delirious mania is a serious form of the disorder characterized by severe clouding of consciousness and an intensification of the symptoms associated with acute mania. This condition has become relatively rare since the availability of antipsychotic medication.

Mood

The mood of delirious patients is very labile. They may exhibit feelings of despair, quickly converting to unrestrained merriment and ecstasy or becoming irritable or totally indifferent to the environment. Panic anxiety may be evident.

Cognition and Perception

Cognition and perception are characterized by a clouding of consciousness with accompanying confusion, disorientation, and sometimes stupor. Other common manifestations include religiosity, delusions of grandeur or persecution, and auditory or visual hallucinations. The individual is extremely distractible and incoherent.

Activity and Behavior

Psychomotor activity is frenzied and characterized by agitated, purposeless movements. The safety of the individual is at stake unless this activity is curtailed. Exhaustion, injury to self or others, and eventually death could occur without intervention.

Diagnosis and Outcome Identification

Using information collected during the assessment, the nurse completes the patient database from which the selection of appropriate nursing diagnoses is determined. Table 17–1 presents a list of patient behaviors and the NANDA International (NANDA-I) nursing diagnoses (Herdman et al., 2021) that correspond to those behaviors, which may be used in planning care for the patient experiencing a manic episode.

Outcome Criteria

The following criteria may be used for measuring outcomes in the care of the patient experiencing a manic episode. The patient:

- Exhibits no evidence of physical injury.
- Has not harmed self or others.
- Is no longer exhibiting signs of physical agitation.
- Eats a well-balanced diet with snacks to prevent weight loss and maintain nutritional status.
- Verbalizes an accurate interpretation of the environment.
- Verbalizes that hallucinations have ceased and demonstrates no outward behavior indicating hallucinations.
- Accepts responsibility for own behaviors.
- Does not manipulate others for gratification of own needs.
- Interacts appropriately with others.
- Is able to fall asleep within 30 minutes of retiring.
- Is able to sleep 6 to 8 hours per night without medication.

Planning and Implementation

Table 17–2 provides a plan of care for the patient experiencing a manic episode. Selected nursing diagnoses are presented, along with outcome criteria, appropriate nursing interventions, and rationales for each.

TABLE 17–1 Assigning Nursing Diagnoses to Behaviors Commonly Exhibited by Individuals Experiencing a Manic Episode

BEHAVIORS	NURSING DIAGNOSES
Extreme hyperactivity; increased agitation and lack of control over purposeless and potentially injurious movements	Risk for injury
Manic excitement, delusional thinking, hallucinations, impulsivity	Risk for violence: Self-directed or other-directed
Loss of weight, amenorrhea, refusal or inability to sit still long enough to eat	Imbalanced nutrition: Less than body requirements
Delusions of grandeur and persecution; inaccurate interpretation of the environment	Disturbed thought processes
Auditory and visual hallucinations; disorientation	Disturbed sensory-perception*
Inability to develop satisfying relationships, manipulation of others for own desires, use of unsuccessful social interaction behaviors	Impaired social interaction
Difficulty falling asleep, sleeping only short periods	Insomnia

*This diagnosis was resigned from the NANDA-I list of approved diagnoses. It is used in this instance because it is most compatible with the identified behaviors.

Table 17–2 | CARE PLAN FOR THE PATIENT EXPERIENCING A MANIC EPISODE

NURSING DIAGNOSIS: RISK FOR INJURY

RELATED TO: Extreme hyperactivity

EVIDENCED BY: Increased agitation and lack of control over purposeless and potentially injurious movements

OUTCOME CRITERIA	NURSING INTERVENTIONS	RATIONALE
Short-Term Goal ■ Patient will no longer exhibit potentially injurious movements after 24 hours, with administration of tranquilizing medication. **Long-Term Goal** ■ Patient will not experience injury.	1. Reduce environmental stimuli. Assign private room with simple decor on quiet unit if possible. Keep lighting and noise level low.	1. Patients are extremely distractible and responses to even the slightest stimuli are exaggerated. A milieu unit may be too stimulating.
	2. Remove hazardous objects and substances (including smoking materials).	2. Rationality is impaired, and the patient may harm self inadvertently.
	3. Stay with the patient who is hyperactive and agitated.	3. Nurse's presence may offer support and provide feeling of security for the patient.
	4. Provide structured schedule of activities that includes established rest periods throughout the day. Limit group activities.	4. A structured schedule and one-to-one activities provide a feeling of security for the patient.
	5. Provide physical activities.	5. Physical activities may help relieve tension and excessive energy.
	6. Administer tranquilizing medication as ordered by physician.	6. Antipsychotics are common and are very effective for providing rapid relief from symptoms of hyperactivity.

Table 17–2 | CARE PLAN FOR THE PATIENT EXPERIENCING A MANIC EPISODE—cont'd

NURSING DIAGNOSIS: RISK FOR VIOLENCE: SELF-DIRECTED OR OTHER-DIRECTED

RELATED TO: Manic excitement, delusional thinking, hallucinations

OUTCOME CRITERIA	NURSING INTERVENTIONS	RATIONALE
Short-Term Goal ■ Patient's agitation will be maintained at a manageable level with the administration of tranquilizing medication during the first week of treatment (decreasing risk of violence to self or others).	1. Maintain low level of stimuli in the patient's environment (low lighting, few people, simple décor, low noise level).	1. Anxiety level rises in a stimulating environment. A suspicious, agitated patient may perceive others and the environment threatening.
	2. Assess for concomitant substance use issues.	2. There is a high incidence of comorbid substance use disorders in patients with bipolar disorder and these can increase risk for harm to self or others. Also, the use of other mood-altering chemicals makes evaluation of pharmacotherapy more difficult.
Long-Term Goal ■ Patient will not harm self or others.	3. Observe the patient's behavior frequently. Do this while carrying out routine activities so as to avoid creating suspiciousness in the individual.	3. Close observation is important to identify the need for redirection or limit setting and to protect patient safety.
	4. Remove all sharp objects, glass or mirrored items, belts, ties, and smoking materials from patient's environment.	4. Dangerous objects are removed to minimize risks that the patient (in an agitated, hyperactive state) may use them to harm self or others.
	5. Intervene at the first signs of increased anxiety, agitation, or verbal or behavioral aggression using empathic responses such as "You seem anxious" or "How can I help?"	5. Validation of the patient's feelings conveys an attitude of caring and collaboration and facilitates establishing trust. Because the patient is highly distractible, providing a distraction can also aid in diffusing anxiety and agitation.
	6. Maintain and convey a calm attitude. Respond matter-of-factly to verbal hostility.	6. Maintaining a calm attitude facilitates de-escalation of the patient's anxiety and agitation.
	7. As anxiety increases, offer some alternatives: to participate in a physical activity (e.g., walking or other physical exercise), talking about the situation, taking some antianxiety medication.	7. Offering alternatives empowers the patient to have a sense of control over the situation.
	8. Have sufficient staff available to safely redirect the patient if it becomes necessary.	8. This provides physical security for staff and patients.
	9. If the patient is not calmed by "talking down" or by medication, use of mechanical restraints may be necessary.	9. Patients should be offered the "least restrictive alternative" to maintain safety. Restraints should be used only as a last resort, after all other interventions have been unsuccessful, and the patient is imminently at risk of harm to self or others.

Continued

Table 17–2 | CARE PLAN FOR THE PATIENT EXPERIENCING A MANIC EPISODE—cont'd

OUTCOME CRITERIA	NURSING INTERVENTIONS	RATIONALE
	10. If restraint is deemed necessary, ensure that sufficient staff is available to assist. Follow protocol established by the institution.	10. Patient safety is a nursing priority.
	11. Observe the patient in restraints continuously and assess patient at least every 15 minutes to ensure that circulation to extremities is not compromised (check temperature, color, pulses); to assist the patient with needs related to nutrition, hydration, and elimination; and to position the patient so that comfort is facilitated and aspiration can be prevented.	11. This intervention ensures that needs for circulation, nutrition, hydration, and elimination are met. Patient safety is a nursing priority.
	12. As agitation decreases, assess the patient's readiness for restraint removal or reduction. Remove restraints gradually, one at a time while assessing the patient's response.	12. Gradual removal of restraints minimizes potential for injury to the patient and staff.

NURSING DIAGNOSIS: IMBALANCED NUTRITION: LESS THAN BODY REQUIREMENTS

RELATED TO: Refusal or inability to sit still long enough to eat

EVIDENCED BY: Weight loss, amenorrhea

OUTCOME CRITERIA	NURSING INTERVENTIONS	RATIONALE
Short-Term Goal ■ Patient will consume sufficient finger foods and between-meal snacks to meet recommended daily allowances of nutrients.	1. Provide high-protein, high-calorie, nutritious finger foods and drinks that can be consumed "on the run."	1. The patient may have difficulty sitting or concentrating long enough to complete a sit-down meal.
	2. Have juice and snacks available on the unit at all times.	2. Nutritious intake must compensate for increased caloric requirement due to hyperactivity.
Long-Term Goal ■ Patient will exhibit no signs or symptoms of malnutrition.	3. Maintain accurate record of intake, output, calorie count, and weight. Monitor daily laboratory values.	3. These are important nutritional assessment data.
	4. Determine the patient's likes and dislikes and collaborate with dietitian to plan meals.	4. Collaboration with the patient on meal planning increases the likelihood of meeting nutrition goals.
	5. Supplement diet with vitamins and minerals.	5. Improvement of nutritional status.
	6. Walk or sit with the patient while the patient is eating.	6. The nurse's presence offers support and encouragement for the patient to eat food that will maintain physical wellness.

Table 17–2 | CARE PLAN FOR THE PATIENT EXPERIENCING A MANIC EPISODE—cont'd

NURSING DIAGNOSIS: IMPAIRED SOCIAL INTERACTION

RELATED TO: Delusional thought processes (grandeur and/or persecution); underdeveloped ego and low self-esteem

EVIDENCED BY: Inability to develop satisfying relationships and manipulation of others for own desires

OUTCOME CRITERIA	NURSING INTERVENTIONS	RATIONALE
Short-Term Goal ■ Patient will verbalize which interaction behaviors are appropriate and which are inappropriate within 1 week. **Long-Term Goal** ■ Patient will demonstrate use of appropriate interaction skills as evidenced by lack of, or marked decrease in, manipulation of others to fulfill own desires.	1. Recognize the purpose that manipulative behaviors serve for the patient: to reduce feelings of insecurity by increasing feelings of power and control.	1. Understanding the motivation behind the manipulation may facilitate acceptance of the individual and the behavior.
	2. Set limits on manipulative behaviors. Explain to the patient what is expected and what the consequences are if the limits are violated. Terms of the limitations must be agreed on by all staff who will be working with the patient.	2. When the patient is unable to establish own limits, this must be done for the patient. Unless administration of consequences for violation of limits is consistent, manipulative behavior will not be eliminated.
	3. Do not argue, bargain, or try to reason with the patient. Merely state the limits and expectations. Confront the patient as soon as possible when interactions with others are manipulative or exploitative. Follow through with established consequences for unacceptable behavior.	3. Because the patient may be vulnerable to impulsive, reckless, or pleasure-seeking behavior without considering consequences, the patient should receive immediate feedback when behavior is unacceptable. Consistency in enforcing the consequences is essential if positive outcomes are to be achieved. Inconsistency creates confusion and encourages testing of limits.
	4. Provide positive reinforcement for nonmanipulative behaviors. Explore feelings and help the patient seek more appropriate ways of dealing with them.	4. Positive reinforcement enhances self-esteem and promotes repetition of desirable behaviors.
	5. Help the patient recognize and accept the consequences of their own behaviors and refrain from attributing them to others.	5. The patient must accept responsibility for their own behaviors before adaptive change can occur.
	6. Help the patient identify positive aspects about self, recognize accomplishments, and feel good about them.	6. As self-esteem is increased, patient will feel less need to manipulate others for their own gratification.

Concept Care Mapping

The concept map care plan (see Chapter 6, "The Nursing Process in Psychiatric Mental Health Nursing") is a diagrammatic teaching and learning strategy that allows visualization of interrelationships between medical diagnoses, nursing diagnoses, assessment data, and treatments. An example of a concept map care plan for a patient experiencing a manic episode is presented in Figure 17–1.

Patient and Family Education

The role of patient teacher is important in the psychiatric area, as it is in all areas of nursing. A list of topics for patient and family education relevant to bipolar disorder is presented in Box 17–4.

Evaluation of Care for the Patient Experiencing a Manic Episode

In the final step of the nursing process, a reassessment is conducted to determine if the nursing

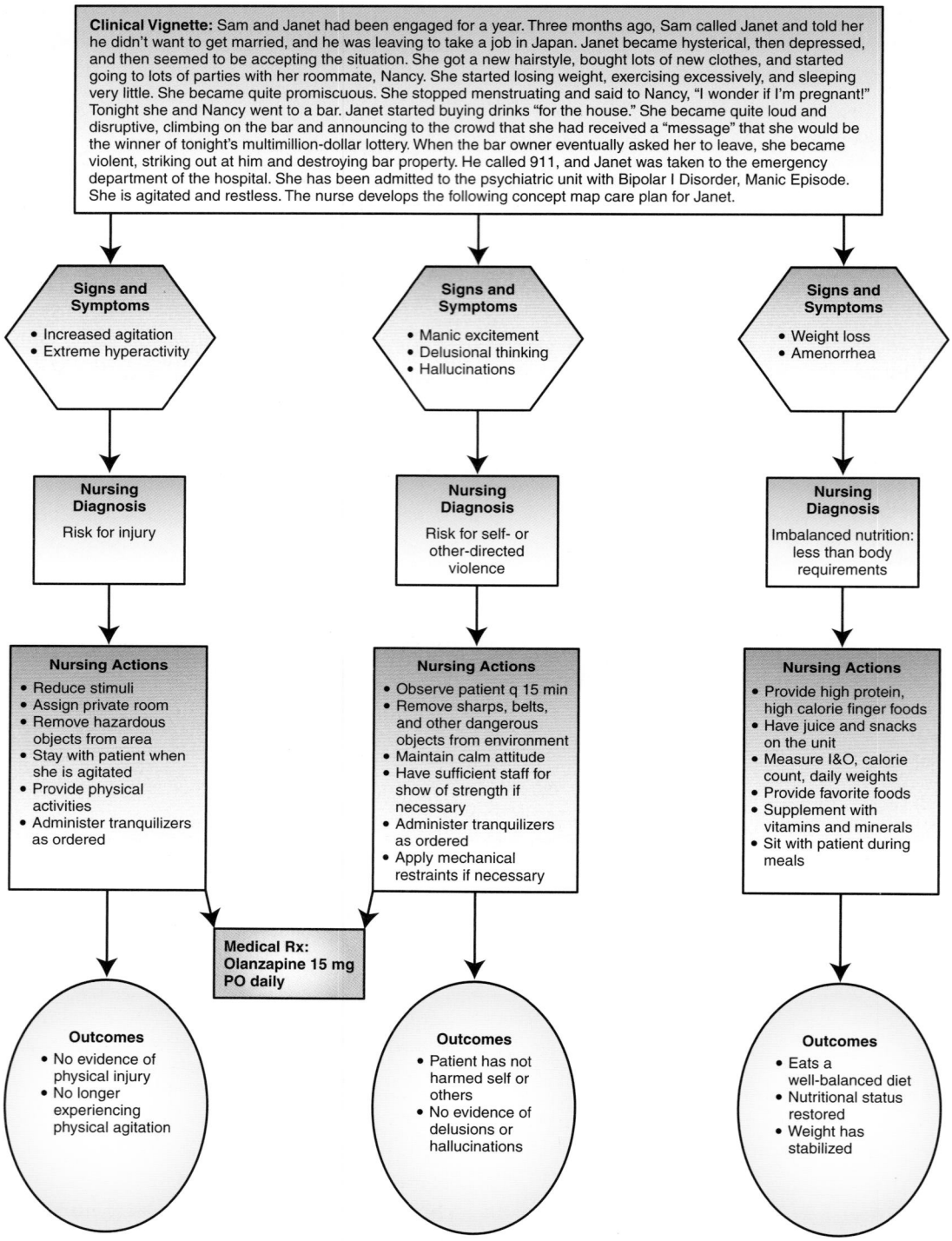

FIGURE 17–1 Concept map care plan for a patient with bipolar disorder, manic episode.

BOX 17–4 Topics for Patient and Family Education Related to Bipolar Disorder

NATURE OF THE ILLNESS

1. Causes of bipolar disorder
2. Cyclic nature of the illness
3. Symptoms of depression
4. Symptoms of mania

MANAGEMENT OF THE ILLNESS

1. Medication management
   a. Lithium
   b. Others
      1) Carbamazepine
      2) Valproic acid
      3) Clonazepam
      4) Verapamil
      5) Lamotrigine
      6) Gabapentin
      7) Topiramate
      8) Oxcarbazepine
      9) Olanzapine
      10) Risperidone
      11) Chlorpromazine
      12) Aripiprazole
      13) Quetiapine
      14) Ziprasidone
      15) Asenapine
   c. Side effects
   d. Symptoms of lithium toxicity
   e. Importance of regular blood tests
   f. Adverse effects
   g. Importance of not stopping medication, even when feeling well
2. Assertive techniques
3. Anger management

SUPPORT SERVICES

1. Crisis hotline
2. Support groups
3. Individual psychotherapy
4. Legal and/or financial assistance

actions have been successful in achieving the objectives of care. Evaluation of the nursing actions for the patient experiencing a manic episode may be facilitated by gathering information using the following types of questions.

- Has the individual avoided personal injury?
- Has violence to the patient and others been prevented?
- Has agitation subsided?
- Have nutritional status and weight been stabilized? Is the patient able to select foods to maintain adequate nutrition?
- Have delusions and hallucinations ceased? Is the patient able to interpret the environment correctly?
- Is the patient able to make decisions about self-care? Has hygiene and grooming improved?
- Is behavior socially acceptable? Is the patient able to interact with others in a satisfactory manner? Has the patient stopped manipulating others to fulfill own desires?
- Is the patient able to sleep 6 to 8 hours per night and awaken feeling rested?
- Does the patient understand the importance of maintenance medication therapy and understand that symptoms may return if medication is discontinued?
- Can the patient taking lithium verbalize early signs of lithium toxicity? Does the patient understand the necessity for monthly blood level checks?

Treatment Modalities

Individual Psychotherapy

In a review of the evidence on psychotherapy for clients with bipolar disorder, Swartz and Swanson (2014) conclude that bipolar-specific psychotherapies in conjunction with medication treatment have better outcomes than medication alone. Evidence supports the benefits of psychoeducation, cognitive behavior therapy, FFT, interpersonal and social rhythm therapy (IPSRT), and integrated care management (Strakowski, 2016).

IPSRT is a type of therapy specifically designed for patients with bipolar disorder. Developed by Frank (2005), the focus of this therapy is helping clients to regulate their social rhythms or daily activities such as the sleep–wake cycle and exercise routines that may otherwise disrupt underlying biological rhythms and contribute to mood disturbances. In combination with this strategy, IPSRT also engages principles of interpersonal therapy to help clients address interpersonal problems.

Group Therapy

Once an acute phase of the illness has passed, groups can provide an atmosphere in which individuals may discuss issues in their lives that cause, maintain, or arise out of having a serious affective disorder. Both group psychoeducation and group cognitive behavior therapy have demonstrated benefits for this population (Swartz & Swanson, 2014). The element of peer support may provide a feeling of security because troublesome or embarrassing issues are discussed and resolved. Some groups have other specific purposes, such as helping to monitor medication-related issues or serving as an avenue for promoting education related to the affective disorder and its treatment.

Support groups help members gain a sense of perspective on their condition and tangibly encourage them to link up with others who have common problems. A sense of hope is conveyed when individuals are able to see that they are not alone or unique in experiencing affective illness.

Self-help groups offer another avenue of support for the individual with bipolar disorder. These groups are usually peer led and are not meant to substitute for or compete with professional therapy. They offer supplementary support that frequently enhances compliance with the medical regimen. Examples of self-help groups are the Depression and Bipolar Support Alliance (DBSA) and the Child and Adolescent Bipolar Foundation; these organizations put individuals in touch with their local support groups. Although self-help groups are not psychotherapy groups, they do provide important adjunctive support experiences, which often have therapeutic benefit for participants.

Family Therapy

The ultimate objectives in working with families of clients with mood disorders are to resolve the symptoms and initiate or restore adaptive family functioning. Boland and Verduin (2022) suggest that efficacious family therapy may include education about the disorder, relapse preventions plans that are agreed upon by the whole family, and communication and problem-solving skills training.

Family functioning and marital relationships are often disrupted in clients with bipolar disorder, especially when symptoms are contributing to disloyalty in the marriage and to financial problems related to the client's excessive spending behaviors. Whether intervention occurs in the form of family education, support, formal therapy, or a combination of these approaches, it is clear that families need to be involved in treatment whenever possible.

Cognitive Behavior Therapy

In cognitive behavior therapy, the individual is taught to control thought distortions that are considered to be a factor in the development and maintenance of mood disorders. In the cognitive model, depression is characterized by a triad of negative distortions related to expectations of the environment, self, and future. The environment and activities within it are viewed as unsatisfying, the self is unrealistically devalued, and the future is perceived as hopeless. In the same model, mania is characterized by exaggeratedly positive cognitions and perceptions. The individual perceives the self as highly valued and powerful. Life is experienced with overstated self-assurance and the future is viewed with unrealistic optimism.

The general goals in cognitive behavior therapy are to obtain symptom relief as quickly as possible, assist the client in identifying dysfunctional patterns of thinking and behaving, and guide the client to evidence and logic that effectively test the validity of the dysfunctional thinking. Therapy focuses on changing "automatic thoughts" that occur spontaneously and contribute to the distorted affect. Examples of automatic thoughts in bipolar mania include the following:

- ***Personalizing:*** "I'm the only reason my husband is a successful businessman."
- ***All or nothing:*** "Everything I do is great."
- ***Mind reading:*** "She thinks I'm wonderful."
- ***Discounting negatives:*** "None of those mistakes are really important."

The client is asked to describe evidence that both supports and disputes the automatic thought. The logic underlying the inferences is then reviewed with the client. Another technique involves evaluating what would most likely happen if the client's automatic thoughts were true. Implications of the consequences are then discussed.

Clients should not become discouraged if one technique seems not to be working. No single technique works with all clients. Clients should be reassured that any of a number of techniques may be used, and both the therapist and client may explore these possibilities.

The Recovery Model

Research provides support for recovery as an obtainable objective for individuals with bipolar disorder. See "Real, People, Real Stories" to learn more about Bridget's recovery journey. Conceptual models of recovery from mental illness are presented in Chapter 10, "The Recovery Model." The recovery model has been used primarily in caring for individuals with serious mental illness, such as schizophrenia and bipolar disorder. However, concepts have utility for all individuals experiencing emotional conditions with which they require assistance and who have a desire to take control and manage their lives more independently.

Real People, Real Stories: Bridget's Story

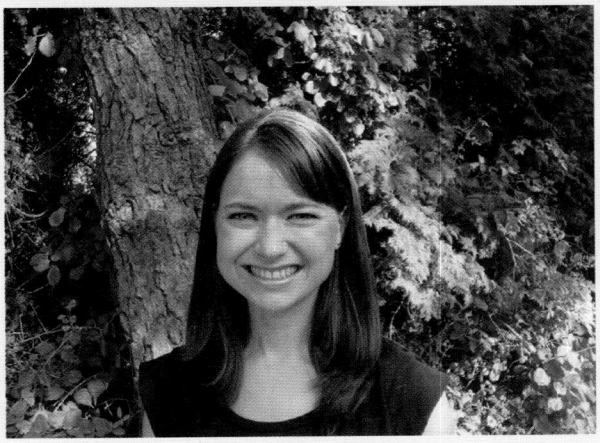

Bridget is a PhD, advanced practice registered nurse with bipolar disorder. Her story highlights the progression of her illness, her insights about illness management, and her courageous efforts to advocate for herself and others.

Karyn: I really appreciate you sharing your insights with other health-care professionals. So tell me about your history with bipolar disorder.

Bridget: I was diagnosed with depression at the age of 13, was on medication for that, and was stable until about 24 years of age. At that time I was working on night shift as a labor and delivery nurse. I remember having a very stressful night and some ethical disagreements with some others and I couldn't sleep for a couple of nights. It threw me into a manic episode. I took melatonin and Nyquil and had a bad reaction. I was having visual hallucinations of interconnecting lights. I have heard other people say that Nyquil can trigger that.

Karyn: I have also read of accounts of people having hallucinations in reaction to dextromethorphan. What happened next?

Bridget: I didn't sleep for days. It was acute and recognizable; very uncomfortable and very scary. I was too sick to return to work and still very upset about ongoing disagreements about patient care issues so when I returned to work it was at a different hospital that rotated shifts. Rotating working the night and day shift worked better for my health. I would work 2 weeks of the night shift and then rotate to working 4 weeks of the day shift. Although not as ideal as working straight day shifts, this month of day shifts allowed me to catch up and stabilize my sleep.

I got accepted into a midwifery program and between the stresses of work, moving, and school, I had a second episode; first manic then depressive. I was concerned that I would have to drop out of school because I couldn't manage graduate school classes along with my recovery. In addition, I read about the importance of regulating sleep patterns in managing this illness and a midwife's schedule requires very irregular sleep patterns. Babies are not born nine to five. However, I couldn't drop out or even go part-time or else I would lose my health insurance. My professors really helped me work out arrangements and accommodations so I could remain a student and keep my insurance and continue working on my degree in midwifery.

The next couple years I was stable but it was frightening; I never knew how well I would recover from episodes. I had a counselor tell me I might have to cut back my expectations for my life. I went to support groups and felt like they brought me down more; there was a lot of complaining and one person told me I would probably only be able to work part-time. I had different expectations for what I wanted to do.

Karyn: How long does an acute episode typically last?

Bridget: The manic episodes seem to be sudden in onset then it "gets dark" and then it's a slow return. The worst episode has been for 2 months but I would say full recovery takes around 9 months to 1 year. After that I'm able to get back into the swing of things.

Karyn: What do you mean when you say it "gets dark"?

Bridget: It's very frightening. There is a sense of loss of control. I lose weight quickly and people think I'm anorexic but it's just that my metabolism gets really fast. Not being able to sleep adds to the traumatization. Then there's the depression and suicidal thoughts. That's when it gets really dark. But I was stable for a 2-to-3-year period before I had a third episode. That was the worst one. I was going through another stressful period but some of it was positive stress; graduating from school, in a new relationship, accepted to a prestigious program for doctoral nursing study, and I was going through some medication changes. It seemed like any treatment was just "putting a bottle cap on a tidal wave." I was hospitalized three times, was having symptoms of psychosis, and it took about a year to get back on track. It's been 6 years since that last episode.

Karyn: What do you think has been most helpful in moving toward this recovery?

Bridget: Having a supportive family. My family has knowledge and history with mental illnesses and that has been a blessing. In my family, recovery is the expectation and chronic illness is the exception. Also, I have long-term friends that stuck with me and never gave up on me; even my doctor said I have amazing friends.

The medications are important even though I have a love-hate relationship with them. The only time I refused medication it was because I thought I was having a bad reaction, but people thought I was just not recognizing

Continued

Real People, Real Stories: Bridget's Story—cont'd

I was sick. It's still a blurry line . . . the judgments were snap . . . in fairness, I was a lot to handle . . . but it was scary. I was being told I had to take something I felt was hurting me so I was uncooperative. Now I recognize they were well-intentioned people doing the best they could.

Also I found work I love; as a childbirth educator. I got married and that has been a stabilizing factor. The medications seem to be working. I had been taking Trileptal but I stopped taking that so I wouldn't have to worry about its effects when I got pregnant, and my workplace has been accommodating.

Karyn: Accommodating?

Bridget: Well, I had been in circumstances prior to my current job; like once I was shoved by a coworker and I threw milk at her. The coworker maintained they were justified. In another circumstance when a coworker found out I had bipolar disorder she told my supervisor I should not be able to work there. I was very scared and felt like I had to become a strong advocate for myself. The truth is my illness requires little accommodation most of the time. When I am well, I am very well and a fairly high-functioning person. I get sick fairly infrequently and when I do, I just need some time to recover, just like any other illness. It does help to have understanding and compassion from my superiors. When I've been able to garner support from them, I've been able to pursue recovery and my life goals.

There was a journal editor and a mentor I connected with after grad school that was so encouraging in terms of me pursuing my PhD. At the time, I had so much shame and guilt about having bipolar disorder, but she extended compassion to me that I wasn't even able to extend to myself. She saw and encouraged me to work to my full potential.

Karyn: What are the most important things that you want nurses to know about providing care for patients with bipolar disorder, particularly in an acute manic episode?

Bridget: Number One: Better listening is key. Even if the patient does not seem to be making sense, there most likely is a kernel of truth in what they are saying. Be patient. Listen and look for that kernel of truth. I remember trying to talk to my psychiatrist about wanting lithium but we never got to discuss that because he was yelling at me that I was being uncooperative with the hospital treatment plan. I signed out AMA [against medical advice] because . . . it felt safer. That's a whole other story.

Number Two: A little compassion goes a long way. Patients can tell right away who is there to help them and who is just there for the paycheck.

Number Three: Look patients in the eye and call them by their name. Many people, when they are in an acute episode of illness, feel very lost and confused; talking to them directly and personally is really grounding. It helps people reclaim their dignity.

Remember, being sick is hard: whether it's cancer or diabetes or bipolar disorder. It takes a lot to manage. Trust that people are truly doing the best that they can with the resources they are given. The mental health system can be very difficult to navigate, especially when someone is acutely ill. It makes it hard to get stabilized and get better. The more you can treat people with dignity, respect their requests when possible, listen, and offer compassion, the better they will do.

In bipolar disorder, recovery is a continuous process. Individuals with bipolar disorder identify goals based on personal values or on what they define as giving meaning and purpose to life. The clinician and client work together to develop a treatment plan that is in alignment with the goals set forth by the client. In the recovery process, the individual may continue to experience symptoms but collaborates with the clinician to develop a management strategy. Management strategies include the following:

- Developing self-awareness
- Becoming an expert on the disorder
- Taking medications regularly
- Avoiding drugs and alcohol
- Recognizing earliest symptoms
- Developing a plan for emergencies
- Identifying and reducing sources of stress
- Knowing when to seek help
- Developing a personal support system

Throughout the ongoing process of recovery, individuals actively work on the strategies they have identified to support their mental health and physical well-being. The clinician serves as a support person.

Although there is no cure for bipolar disorder, there are effective treatments and interventions. Recovery is possible when the client is empowered and actively engaged in a multifaceted illness management approach.

Electroconvulsive Therapy

Episodes of acute mania are occasionally treated with electroconvulsive therapy (ECT), particularly when the client does not tolerate or fails to respond to lithium or other drug treatment or when life is threatened by dangerous behavior or exhaustion (see Chapter 16, "Depressive Disorders," for more information on ECT).

One recent study (McGirr et al., 2021) explored the use of intermittent transcranial magnetic stimulation (which has been used for the treatment of major depression) for patients with acute bipolar depression. However, the study was terminated when they found it to be ineffective, and in some cases, to increase risk for triggering a hypomanic episode.

Psychopharmacology With Mood-Stabilizing Agents

For many years, the drug of choice for treatment and management of bipolar mania was lithium carbonate. However, in recent years, a number of investigators and clinicians have achieved satisfactory results with several other medications, including anticonvulsant drugs, which have a mood-stabilizing effect either alone or in combination with lithium. (See Chapter 4, "Psychopharmacology," for a detailed discussion of indications, actions, contraindications, and other safety issues related to mood-stabilizing agents.)

Both lithium and mood stabilizers demonstrate effectiveness in managing bipolar depression. Three mood stabilizer products are currently approved by the FDA for that purpose: the combination of olanzapine and fluoxetine, quetiapine, and lurasidone (Strakowski, 2016). Antidepressants have shown little evidence of effectiveness in treating bipolar depression as an adjunct to mood stabilizers. Additionally, Strakowski identifies that antidepressants carry as high as a 40% risk of potentially triggering a switch from depression to mania in individuals with bipolar disorder.

Clients who respond to lithium can virtually be symptom free over the long term. Because only about 33% of people treated with lithium respond positively (Rybakowski, 2014), the availability of other pharmacological treatments is important in the management of this illness. Because bipolar disorder is a chronic, episodic illness, most people will remain on medication throughout their lives. See Table 17–3 for a list of commonly used medications in the treatment of bipolar disorder. Lithium, like other medications, has side effects. Most notably its therapeutic range (0.6–1.2 mEq/L) can have toxic side effects and is potentially fatal when exceeded.

Calcium channel blockers, a class of medications used to treat hypertension and cardiac arrhythmias, have been used off-label as a treatment for bipolar disorder based on evidence (D'Onofrio et al., 2017) that calcium signaling dysfunction occurs in bipolar disorder (lithium carbonate has also been shown to down-regulate Ca^{2+}activity). To date, though, use of calcium channel blockers has not become an established or common therapeutic treatment approach.

Patient and Family Education for Lithium

The patient should:

- Take medication on a regular basis, even when feeling well. Discontinuation can result in return of symptoms.
- Not drive or operate dangerous machinery until lithium levels are stabilized. Drowsiness and dizziness can occur.
- Maintain adequate dietary sodium intake. The client should eat a variety of healthy foods and avoid "junk" foods. The patient should drink six to eight large glasses of water each day and avoid excessive use of beverages containing caffeine (coffee, tea, colas), which promote increased urine output.
- Notify the physician if vomiting or diarrhea occurs. These symptoms can result in sodium loss and an increased risk of lithium toxicity.
- Maintain appropriate diet. Include adequate sodium and other nutrients while decreasing number of calories to minimize risks of weight gain.
- Be aware of risks of becoming pregnant while receiving lithium therapy. Notify the physician as soon as possible if pregnancy is suspected or planned.
- Be aware of side effects and symptoms associated with toxicity. Notify the physician if any of the following symptoms occur: persistent nausea and vomiting, severe diarrhea, ataxia, blurred vision, tinnitus, excessive output of urine, increasing tremors, or mental confusion.
- Refer to written materials furnished by health-care providers while receiving self-administered maintenance therapy. Keep appointments for outpatient follow-up; have serum lithium level checked every 1 to 2 months or as advised by physician.
- Carry a card identifying all medications being taken.

Patient and Family Education for Anticonvulsant Mood Stabilizers

The patient should:

- Refrain from discontinuing the drug abruptly. Physician will administer orders for tapering the drug when therapy is to be discontinued.

Text continued on page 468

TABLE 17–3 **Selected Mood-Stabilizing Agents**

CLASSIFICATION: GENERIC (TRADE)	HALF-LIFE/INDICATIONS	MECHANISM OF ACTION	CONTRAINDICATIONS/ PRECAUTIONS	DAILY ADULT DOSAGE RANGE/ THERAPEUTIC PLASMA RANGE
ANTIMANIC				
Lithium carbonate (Eskalith, Lithobid)	24 hr/ ■ Prevention and treatment of manic episodes of bipolar disorder. *Unlabeled uses:* ■ Neutropenia ■ Cluster headaches (prophylaxis) ■ Alcohol dependence ■ Bulimia ■ Postpartum affective psychosis ■ Corticosteroid-induced psychosis	Not fully understood but may modulate the effects of various neurotransmitters, such as norepinephrine, serotonin, dopamine, glutamate, and gamma-aminobutyric acid (GABA), that are thought to play a role in the symptomatology of bipolar disorder (may take 1–3 weeks for symptoms to subside).	Hypersensitivity. Cardiac or renal disease, dehydration; sodium depletion; brain damage; pregnancy and lactation. Caution with thyroid disorders, diabetes, urinary retention, history of seizures, and with elderly.	Acute mania: 1,800–2,400 mg Maintenance: 900–1,200 mg/ Therapeutic range: 0.6–1.2 mEq/L
ANTICONVULSANTS				
Carbamazepine (Tegretol)	25–65 hr (initial); 12–17 hr (repeated doses) ■ Epilepsy ■ Trigeminal neuralgia *Unlabeled uses:* ■ Bipolar disorder ■ Resistant schizophrenia ■ Management of alcohol withdrawal ■ Restless legs syndrome ■ Postherpetic neuralgia	Action in the treatment of bipolar disorder is unclear.	Hypersensitivity. With monoamine oxidase inhibitors (MAOIs), lactation. Caution with elderly; liver, renal, cardiac disease; pregnancy.	200–1,600 mg/ 4–12 mcg/mL
Clonazepam (Klonopin)	18–60 hr/ ■ Petit mal, akinetic, and myoclonic seizures ■ Panic disorder *Unlabeled uses:* ■ Acute manic episodes ■ Uncontrolled leg movements during sleep ■ Neuralgias	Action in the treatment of bipolar disorder is unclear.	Hypersensitivity, glaucoma, liver disease, lactation. Caution in elderly, liver and renal disease, pregnancy.	0.5–20 mg/ 20–80 mg/mL
Valproic acid (Depakene; Depakote)	5–20 hr/ ■ Epilepsy ■ Manic episodes ■ Migraine prophylaxis ■ Adjunct therapy in schizophrenia	Action in the treatment of bipolar disorder is unclear.	Hypersensitivity; liver disease. Caution in elderly, renal and cardiac diseases, pregnancy, and lactation.	5–60 mg/kg/ 50–150 mcg/mL

Lamotrigine (Lamictal)	~33 hr/ ■ Epilepsy *Unlabeled use:* ■ Bipolar disorder	Action in the treatment of bipolar disorder is unclear.	Hypersensitivity. Caution in renal and hepatic insufficiency, pregnancy, lactation, and children <16 y.o.	100–200 mg/ Not established
Gabapentin (Neurontin)	5–7 hr/ ■ Epilepsy ■ Postherpetic neuralgia *Unlabeled uses:* ■ Bipolar disorder ■ Migraine prophylaxis ■ Neuropathic pain ■ Tremors associated with multiple sclerosis	Action in the treatment of bipolar disorder is unclear.	Hypersensitivity and children <3 yr. Caution in renal insufficiency, pregnancy, lactation, children, and the elderly.	900–1,800 mg/ Not established
Topiramate (Topamax)	21 hr/ ■ Epilepsy ■ Migraine prophylaxis *Unlabeled uses:* ■ Bipolar disorder ■ Cluster headaches ■ Bulimia ■ Binge eating disorder ■ Weight loss in obesity	Action in the treatment of bipolar disorder is unclear.	Hypersensitivity. Caution in renal and hepatic impairment, pregnancy, lactation, children, and the elderly.	50–400 mg/ Not established
Oxcarbazepine (Trileptal)	2–9 hr/ ■ Epilepsy *Unlabeled uses:* ■ Bipolar disorder ■ Diabetic neuropathy ■ Neuralgia	Action in the treatment of bipolar disorder is unclear.	Hypersensitivity. Caution in renal and hepatic impairment, pregnancy, lactation, children, and the elderly.	600–2,400 mg/ Not established

Continued

TABLE 17-3 **Selected Mood-Stabilizing Agents–cont'd**

CLASSIFICATION: GENERIC (TRADE)	HALF-LIFE/INDICATIONS	MECHANISM OF ACTION	CONTRAINDICATIONS/ PRECAUTIONS	DAILY ADULT DOSAGE RANGE/ THERAPEUTIC PLASMA RANGE
ANTIPSYCHOTICS		**ALL ANTIPSYCHOTICS**	**ALL ANTIPSYCHOTICS**	
Olanzapine (Zyprexa)	21–54 hr/ ■ Schizophrenia ■ Acute manic episodes ■ Management of bipolar disorder ■ Agitation associated with schizophrenia or mania *Unlabeled uses:* ■ Obsessive-compulsive disorder (OCD)	Efficacy in schizophrenia is achieved through a combination of dopamine and serotonin type 2 (5-HT_2) antagonism. Mechanism of action in the treatment of mania is unknown.	Hypersensitivity, children, lactation. Caution with hepatic or cardiovascular disease, history of seizures, comatose or other central nervous system (CNS) depression, prostatic hypertrophy, narrow-angle glaucoma, diabetes or risk factors for diabetes, pregnancy, elderly and debilitated patients, history of suicide attempts.	10–20 mg/ Not established
Olanzapine and fluoxetine (Symbyax)	(see individual drugs) ■ For the treatment of depressive episodes associated with bipolar disorder	Action may be mediated via effects on dopamine and serotonin (5-HT_{2A}) receptor antagonism.		6/25–12/50 mg/ Not established
Aripiprazole (Abilify)	50–80 hr/ ■ Bipolar mania ■ Schizophrenia			10–30 mg/ Not established
Lurasidone (Latuda)	18 hr/ ■ Depressive episodes in bipolar I disorder ■ Schizophrenia			20–120 mg/ Not established
Chlorpromazine	24 hr/ ■ Bipolar mania ■ Schizophrenia ■ Emesis/hiccoughs ■ Acute intermittent porphyria ■ Preoperative apprehension *Unlabeled uses:* ■ Migraine headaches			75–400 mg/ Not established

Quetiapine (Seroquel)	6 hr/ ■ Schizophrenia ■ Acute manic episodes	100–800 mg/ Not established
Risperidone (Risperdal)	3–20 hr/ ■ Bipolar mania ■ Schizophrenia *Unlabeled uses:* ■ Severe behavioral problems in children ■ Behavioral problems associated with autism ■ Obsessive-compulsive disorder	1–6 mg/ Not established
Ziprasidone (Geodon)	7 hr (oral)/ ■ Bipolar mania ■ Schizophrenia ■ Acute agitation in schizophrenia	40–160 mg/ Not established
Asenapine (Saphris)	24 hr/ ■ Schizophrenia ■ Bipolar mania	10–20 mg/ Not established

- Report the following symptoms to the physician immediately: skin rash, unusual bleeding, spontaneous bruising, sore throat, fever, malaise, dark urine, and yellow skin or eyes.
- Not drive or operate dangerous machinery until reaction to the medication has been established.
- Avoid consuming alcoholic beverages and nonprescription medications without approval from physician.
- Carry a card at all times identifying the name of medications being taken.

CLINICAL PEARL The FDA requires that all antiepileptic (anticonvulsant) drugs carry a warning label indicating that use of the drugs increases risk for suicidal thoughts and behaviors. Patients being treated with these medications should be monitored for the emergence or worsening of depression, suicidal thoughts or behavior, or any unusual changes in mood or behavior.

Patient and Family Education for Calcium Channel Blocker

The patient should:

- Take medication with meals if gastrointestinal upset occurs.
- Use caution when driving or when operating dangerous machinery. Dizziness, drowsiness, and blurred vision can occur.
- Refrain from discontinuing the drug abruptly. To do so may precipitate cardiovascular problems. Physician will administer orders for tapering the drug when therapy is to be discontinued.
- Report occurrence of any of the following symptoms to physician immediately: irregular heartbeat, shortness of breath, swelling of the hands and feet, pronounced dizziness, chest pain, profound mood swings, or severe and persistent headache.
- Rise slowly from a sitting or lying position to prevent a sudden drop in blood pressure.
- Avoid taking other medications (including over-the-counter medications) without physician's approval.
- Carry a card at all times describing medications being taken.

Patient and Family Education for Antipsychotics

The patient should:

- Use caution when driving or operating dangerous machinery. Drowsiness and dizziness can occur.
- Refrain from discontinuing the drug abruptly after long-term use. To do so might produce withdrawal symptoms, such as nausea, vomiting, dizziness, gastritis, headache, tachycardia, insomnia, and tremulousness. Physician will administer orders for tapering the drug when therapy is to be discontinued.
- Use sunblock lotion and wear protective clothing when spending time outdoors. Skin is more susceptible to sunburn, which can occur in as little as 30 minutes.
- Report the occurrence of any of the following symptoms to the physician immediately: sore throat, fever, malaise, unusual bleeding, easy bruising, persistent nausea and vomiting, severe headache, rapid heart rate, difficulty urinating, muscle twitching, tremors, darkly colored urine, excessive urination, excessive thirst, excessive hunger, weakness, pale stools, yellow skin or eyes, muscular incoordination, or skin rash.
- Rise slowly from a sitting or lying position to prevent a sudden drop in blood pressure.
- Take frequent sips of water, chew sugarless gum, or suck on hard candy, if dry mouth is a problem. Good oral care (frequent brushing, flossing) is very important.
- Consult the physician regarding smoking while on antipsychotic therapy. Smoking increases the metabolism of these drugs, requiring an adjustment in dosage to achieve a therapeutic effect.
- Dress warmly in cold weather and avoid extended exposure to very high or low temperatures. Body temperature is harder to maintain with this medication.
- Avoid drinking alcohol while on antipsychotic therapy. These drugs potentiate each other's effects.
- Avoid taking other medications (including over-the-counter products) without the physician's approval. Many medications contain substances that interact with antipsychotic medications in a way that may be harmful.
- Be aware of possible risks of taking antipsychotics during pregnancy. Antipsychotics are thought to readily cross the placental barrier; if so, a fetus could experience adverse effects of the drug. Inform the physician immediately if pregnancy occurs, is suspected, or is planned.
- Be aware of side effects of antipsychotic medications. Refer to written materials furnished by health-care providers for safe self-administration.
- Continue to take the medication, even if feeling well and feeling as though it is not needed. Symptoms may return if medication is discontinued.
- Carry a card or other identification at all times describing medications being taken.

CASE STUDY AND SAMPLE CARE PLAN

NURSING HISTORY AND ASSESSMENT

Candace, age 32, recently moved to New York City from Omaha, Nebraska, where she had been working as a television reporter. She felt that Omaha had become "too boring" and wanted to experience big city life. Candace has a history of bipolar I disorder and has been maintained on lithium since she was 23 years old. Since she arrived in New York, she has run out of her medication and has not found a doctor to have her prescription renewed. She has been staying in an inexpensive apartment, using her savings to live on. She has been seeking employment in her chosen line of work, but it has been 2 months now, and she has been unable to find a job. Candace is becoming anxious because her savings are becoming depleted. She has lost weight and has trouble sleeping.

Today, after two failed interviews, Candace went to a bar and began drinking. She ordered several rounds of drinks for everyone in the bar and told the bartender to "put it on my tab." The bartender called the police when Candace refused to pay her tab and became loud and belligerent. He said she began shouting that she knew the mayor, and he was going to help her find a job, and if they didn't leave her alone, she would tell the mayor how they were treating her. She took out her cell phone and said she was calling the mayor. When others in the room began laughing at her, she began cursing and saying that they would be sorry one day that they laughed at her. When the police arrived, Candace was resistant and had to be physically restrained. The police took Candace to the emergency department of the community hospital, where she was admitted with a diagnosis of Bipolar I Disorder, current episode manic. The psychiatrist ordered olanzapine 10 mg IM STAT, olanzapine 10 mg PO qd, lithium carbonate 600 mg PO bid, and vitamin supplement daily. He ordered a lithium level to be drawn prior to first dose of lithium.

NURSING DIAGNOSES AND OUTCOME IDENTIFICATION

From the assessment data, the admitting nurse develops the following nursing diagnoses for Candace:

1. **Risk for self- or other-directed violence** related to manic hyperactivity, delusional thinking, impulsivity
   a. **Short-Term Goal:** Agitation and hyperactivity will be maintained at manageable level with the administration of tranquilizing medication.
   b. **Long-Term Goal:** Candace will not harm self or others during hospitalization.
2. **Imbalanced nutrition: Less than body requirements** related to lack of appetite and excessive physical agitation, evidenced by loss of weight
   a. **Short-Term Goal:** Candace will consume sufficient finger foods and between-meal snacks to meet recommended daily allowances of nutrients.
   b. **Long-Term Goal:** Candace will begin to regain weight and exhibit no signs or symptoms of malnutrition.

PLANNING AND IMPLEMENTATION

RISK FOR SELF- OR OTHER-DIRECTED VIOLENCE

The following nursing interventions have been identified for Candace:

1. Place Candace in a private room near the nurse's station. Observe her behavior frequently.
2. Remove all dangerous objects from her environment.
3. Plan some physical activities for Candace (e.g., treadmill, punching bag) and regular rest periods during the day.
4. Administer tranquilizing medication as ordered by physician.
5. Monitor lithium levels three times during first week of therapy. Monitor for signs and symptoms of toxicity (e.g., ataxia, blurred vision, severe diarrhea, persistent nausea and vomiting, tinnitus).
6. Ensure that sufficient staff is available to intervene should Candace become agitated and aggressive.

IMBALANCED NUTRITION: LESS THAN BODY REQUIREMENTS

The following nursing interventions have been identified for Candace:

1. Consult dietitian to determine appropriate diet for Candace to restore nutrition and increase weight. Ensure that her diet includes foods that she particularly likes.
2. Ensure that Candace has access to finger foods and between-meal snacks if she cannot or will not sit still to eat from a meal tray.
3. Maintain an accurate record of intake, output, and calorie count.
4. Obtain daily weights.
5. Administer vitamin supplement, as ordered by physician.
6. Sit with Candace during mealtime.

EVALUATION

The outcome criteria identified for Candace have been met. She has not harmed herself or others in any way. She is able to verbalize names of resources outside the hospital from whom she may request help if needed. With help from the social worker, she has applied for unemployment assistance and will begin receiving help within 2 weeks. She has gained 3 pounds in the hospital, and she verbalizes understanding of the importance of maintaining good nutrition. She is taking her medication regularly and has a follow-up appointment with the psychiatric nurse practitioner who will see Candace biweekly and ensure that Candace is adherent with medication and laboratory requirements. Candace verbalizes understanding of the importance of taking her medication on a continuous basis. She has a hopeful but realistic attitude about finding work in New York City and states that she will give herself a deadline, after which she plans to return to her home in Omaha, where she may be near family and friends.

Summary and Key Points

- Bipolar disorder is manifested by mood swings from profound depression to extreme elation or irritable mood, euphoria, and increased activity or energy.
- Genetic influences have been strongly implicated in the development of bipolar disorder. Various other physiological factors, such as biochemical and electrolyte alterations, as well as cerebral structural changes, have also been implicated. Side effects of certain medications may also induce symptoms of mania. No single theory can explain the etiology of bipolar disorder, and it is likely that the illness is caused by a combination of factors.
- Symptoms of mania may be identified by the three different levels of severity: hypomania, acute mania, and delirious mania.
- The symptoms of bipolar disorder may occur in children and adolescents as well as in adults.
- Treatment of bipolar disorders includes individual therapy, group and family therapy, cognitive therapy, electroconvulsive therapy, and psychopharmacology. For the majority of clients, the most effective treatment appears to be a combination of psychotropic medication and psychosocial therapy.
- Some clinicians choose a course of therapy based on a model of recovery similar to that used for many years to treat addiction. The basic premise of a recovery model is empowerment; it allows clients primary control over decisions about their own care and enables a person with a mental health problem to live a meaningful life in a community of choice while striving to achieve full potential.
- For many years, the pharmacological treatment of choice for bipolar mania was lithium carbonate. A number of other medications are now being used with satisfactory results, including anticonvulsants and antipsychotics.
- There is a narrow margin between the therapeutic and toxic levels of lithium. Serum lithium levels must be monitored regularly while the client is on maintenance therapy. The therapeutic range for lithium is 0.6 to 1.2 mEq/L.

Review Questions

Select the answer that is most appropriate for each of the following questions:

1. Which technique is used to promote adequate nutritional intake for a client in an acute manic episode who is not eating?
   a. Sit with the client during meals to reinforce the importance of eating everything on the tray.
   b. Have family members bring food from home so the client will have only favorite foods.
   c. Provide high-calorie, nutritious finger foods and snacks that can be eaten "on the run."
   d. Restrict the client to their room until they begin to gain weight.
2. A client who has been prescribed lithium carbonate for bipolar I disorder asks the nurse what is a normal range for lithium blood levels. Which is the most accurate response?
   a. 0.6 to 1.2 mEq/L
   b. 0.1 to 5 mEq/L
   c. Above 1.2 mEq/L
   d. 6 to 12 mEq/L
3. Although historically lithium has been the medication of choice for mania, several others have been used with good results. Which medication is used in the treatment of bipolar disorder? (Select all that apply.)
   a. Olanzapine (Zyprexa)
   b. Oxycodone (Oxycontin)
   c. Carbamazepine (Tegretol)
   d. Gabapentin (Neurontin)
   e. Tranylcypromine (Parnate)

4. A client who is experiencing a manic episode is admitted to the psychiatric unit after being brought to the emergency department by a family member. The client yells, "I need to get out of here because the interplanetary council has elected me president of the universe." This is an example of:
   a. A delusion of grandeur
   b. A delusion of persecution
   c. Auditory hallucinations
   d. Lithium toxicity
5. Which is the most common comorbid condition in children with bipolar disorder?
   a. Schizophrenia
   b. Substance disorders
   c. Oppositional defiant disorder
   d. Attention deficit-hyperactivity disorder
6. A nurse is educating a client about lithium therapy and is explaining signs and symptoms of lithium toxicity. Which findings should the nurse instruct the client to be on the alert for?
   a. Fever, sore throat, malaise
   b. Tinnitus, severe diarrhea, ataxia
   c. Occipital headache, palpitations, chest pain
   d. Skin rash, marked rise in blood pressure, bradycardia

Clinical Judgment Questions

7. A client is brought to the emergency department by a family member who reports that the client stopped taking mood stabilizer medication a few months ago and is now agitated, pacing, demanding, and speaking very loudly. The client's family member reports that they eat very little, is losing weight, and almost never sleeps. What is the *priority* nursing diagnosis?
   a. Imbalanced nutrition: Less than body requirements related to not eating
   b. Risk for injury related to hyperactivity
   c. Disturbed sleep pattern related to agitation
   d. Ineffective coping related to denial of depression
8. A female client, who is experiencing a manic episode, enters the milieu area dressed in a provocative and physically revealing outfit. Which is the most appropriate intervention by the nurse?
   a. Tell her, in front of the other clients, that she cannot dress like a whore while she is in the hospital.
   b. Do nothing and allow her to learn from the responses of her peers.
   c. Quietly walk with her back to her room and help her change into something more appropriate.
   d. Explain to her that if she wears this outfit, she must remain in her room.
9. The nurse is providing medication education to a client on lithium. Which is an important point to include? (Select all that apply.)
   a. Significant reductions in sodium intake increase the risk for lithium toxicity.
   b. Weight loss is a common side effect of lithium.
   c. Serum lithium levels will need to be checked at regular intervals throughout treatment.
   d. Lithium therapy should be continued even during periods when the client feels well.

Continued

10. A client admitted to the inpatient psychiatric unit with bipolar disorder tells the nurse, "I need to sit in on change-of-shift report because I have been appointed director of this unit." Which action by the nurse demonstrates the best clinical judgment at this point?
    a. Invite the client to sit in on the change-of-shift report, but do not share any confidential client information.
    b. Instruct the client that this is not permitted and redirect the client to other unit activities that are available.
    c. Tell the client that they are delusional but that these symptoms will go away with medication.
    d. Place the client in seclusion for protection of self and others.

IMPLICATIONS FOR EVIDENCE-BASED PRACTICE

Zimmerman, M., Balling, C., Dalrymple, K., & Chelminski, I. (2019). Screening for borderline personality disorder in psychiatric outpatients with major depressive disorder and bipolar disorder. *Journal of Clinical Psychiatry, 80*(1), 18m12257. https://doi.org/10.4088/JCP.18m12257

DESCRIPTION OF THE STUDY: Bipolar disorder is often confused with borderline personality disorder because of several mood symptoms that appear to overlap between the two disorders. In addition, borderline personality disorder and bipolar disorder are sometimes comorbid conditions. Noting that borderline personality disorder is a serious illness and frequently underdiagnosed, the researchers used a semi-structured *DSM*-criteria interview to attempt to differentiate borderline personality disorder from bipolar disorder and from major depressive disorder (n = 3,764).

RESULTS OF THE STUDY: The researchers' findings supported that screening for affective instability was highly predictive of borderline personality disorder (greater than 90% sensitivity) in patients with major depressive disorder, bipolar disorder, and other diagnoses.

IMPLICATIONS FOR NURSING PRACTICE: Affective instability, one of the *DSM-5-TR* criteria for diagnosing borderline personality disorder, is related to "a marked reactivity of mood (e.g., intense episodic dysphoria, irritability, or anxiety usually lasting a few hours and rarely more than a few days") (APA, 2022, p. 753). This is unlike the mood swings from depression to elation that are seen in bipolar disorder in that the mood changes in in borderline personality disorder are rapid, shorter lived, difficult to regulate, and often triggered by interpersonal events in the environment. Nurses should recognize the potential for confusion between symptoms of bipolar disorder and borderline personality disorder and consider screening for evidence of affective instability to determine whether a treatment plan for borderline personality disorder, in addition to bipolar disorder is appropriate. This may be accomplished by incorporating established screening tools such as the Affective Lability Scale or the Affective Intensity Scale and through semi-structured interview questions.

TEST YOUR CLINICAL REASONING AND CLINICAL JUDGMENT SKILLS

Allie, age 29, had been working in the typing pool of a large corporation for 6 years. Her immediate supervisor recently retired, and Alice was promoted to supervisor in charge of 20 people in the department. Allie was flattered by the promotion but anxious about the additional responsibility of the position. Shortly after the promotion, she overheard two of her former coworkers saying, "Why in the world did they choose her? She's not the best one for the job. I know *I* certainly won't be able to respect her as a boss!" Hearing these comments added to Allie's anxiety and self-doubt.

Shortly after Allie began her new duties, her friends and coworkers noticed a change. She had a great deal of energy and worked long hours on her job. She began to speak very loudly and rapidly. Her roommate noticed that Allie slept very little yet seldom appeared tired. Every night, she would go out to bars and dances. Sometimes she brought men she had just met home to the apartment, something she had never done before. She bought lots of clothes and makeup and had her hair restyled in a more youthful look. She failed to pay her share of the rent and bills but came home with a brand-new convertible. She lost her temper and screamed at her roommate, "Mind your own business!" when asked to pay her share.

TEST YOUR CLINICAL REASONING AND CLINICAL JUDGMENT SKILLS—cont'd

Allie became irritable at work, and several of her subordinates reported her behavior to the corporate manager. When the manager confronted Allie about her behavior, she lost control, shouting, cursing, and striking out at anyone and anything that happened to be within her reach. The security officers restrained her and took her to the emergency department of the hospital, where she was admitted to the psychiatric unit. She had no previous history of psychiatric illness.

The psychiatrist assigned a diagnosis of Bipolar I Disorder and wrote orders for olanzapine (Zyprexa) 10 mg IM STAT, olanzapine 15 mg PO daily, and lithium carbonate 600 mg qid.

Answer the following questions related to Allie:

1. What are the most important considerations with which the nurse who is taking care of Allie should be concerned?
2. Why was Allie given the diagnosis of Bipolar I Disorder?
3. The doctor should order a lithium level drawn after 4 to 6 days. For what symptoms should the nurse be on the alert?
4. Why did the physician order olanzapine in addition to the lithium carbonate?

Communication Exercises

1. Kyle, a newly admitted patient, diagnosed with bipolar disorder states to the nurse, "I was looking at the sky, blue is the color of my eyes, too. I went to Florida on a plane."
   How might the nurse respond to this patient's statement?
2. Darcy, who is in a manic phase of bipolar disorder is jumping from chair to chair in the patient lounge during visiting hours, loudly proclaiming to the visitors that she is a famous gymnast. She begins doing somersaults, nearly tripping a visitor.
   How might the nurse respond to the patient at this point?

MOVIE CONNECTIONS

Lust for Life ▪ *Call Me Anna* ▪ *Blue Sky* ▪ *A Woman Under the Influence* (bipolar disorder and substance use disorder) ▪ *Mr. Jones* ▪ *Frances* ▪ *The Whole Wide World* ▪ *Pollock* (bipolar disorder and substance use disorder) ▪ *Silver Linings Playbook* ▪ *No Letting Go* ▪ *A Light Beneath Their Feet* ▪ *Touched With Fire*

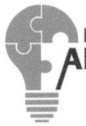

Go to **Davis Advantage** to complete your learning: strengthen understanding, apply your knowledge, and prepare for the Next Gen NCLEX®.

References

Aas, M., Henry, C., Andreassen, O. A. Bellivier, F., Melle, I., & Etain, B. (2016). The role of childhood trauma in bipolar disorders. *International Journal of Bipolar Disorders, 4*(2), 1–10. https://doi.org/10.1186/s40345-015-0042-0

Akiskal, H. S. (2017). Mood disorders: Historical introduction and conceptual overview. In B. J. Sadock, V. A. Sadock, & P. Ruiz (Eds.), *Comprehensive textbook of psychiatry* (10th ed., pp. 1599–1603). Wolters Kluwer.

American Psychiatric Association. (2013). *Diagnostic and statistical manual of mental disorders* (5th ed.).

Boland, R., & Verduin, M. L. (2022). *Kaplan & Sadock's synopsis of psychiatry* (P. Ruiz, Ed.). (12th ed.). Wolters Kluwer.

Burton, N. (2017). A short history of bipolar disorder. *Psychology Today.* https://www.psychologytoday.com/blog/hide-and-seek/201206/short-history-bipolar-disorder

Chang, K. D., & DelBello, M. P. (2018). *Strategies for diagnosis in children and adolescents with bipolar spectrum disorders.* http://www.bipolarkidscme.org/

Darby, M. M., Yolken, R. H., & Sabunciyan, S. (2016). Consistently altered expression of gene sets in postmortem brains of individuals with major psychiatric disorders. *Translational Psychiatry, 6*(9), e890. https://doi.org/10.1038/tp.2016.173

D'Onofrio, S., Mahaffey, S., & Garcia-Rill, E. (2017). Role of calcium channels in bipolar disorder. *Current Psychopharmacology, 6*(2), 122–135. https://doi.org/10.2174/2211556006666171024141949

Frank, E. (2005). *Treating bipolar disorder: A clinician's guide to interpersonal and social rhythm therapy.* Guilford Press.

Herdman, T. H., Kamitsuru, S., & Lopes, C. T. (Eds.). (2021). *NANDA-I, Inc. nursing diagnoses: Definitions and classification, 2021–2023.* Thieme.

Jain, R., & Jain, S. (2014). *Facing the diagnostic challenge of comorbid bipolar disorder and ADHD.* https://www.psychiatryadvisor.com/home/topics/adhd/facing-the-diagnostic-challenge-of-comorbid-bipolar-disorder-and-adhd/

Janiri, D., Sani, G., Danese, E., Simonetti, A., Ambrosi, E., Angeletti, G., Erbuto, D., Caltagirone, C., Girardi, P., & Spalletta, G. (2015). Childhood traumatic experiences of patients with bipolar disorder type I and type II. *Journal of Affective Disorders, 175*(8), 92–97. https://doi.org/10.1016/j.jad.2014.12.055.

Krans, B. (2019). *The history of bipolar disorder.* http://www.healthline.com/health/bipolar-disorder/history-bipolar#1

Leussis, M. P., Berry-Scott, E. M., Saito, M., Jhuang, H., Haan, G., Alkan, O., Luce, C. J., Madison, J. M., Sklar, P., Serre, T., Root, D. E., & Petryshen, T. L. (2013). The *ANK3* bipolar disorder gene regulates psychiatric-related behaviors that are modulated by lithium and stress. *Biological Psychiatry, 73*(7), 683–696. https://doi.org/10.1016/j.biopsych.2012.10.016

McGirr, A., Vila-Rodriguez, F., Cole, J., Torres, I. J., Arumugham, S. S., Keramatian, K., Saraf, G., Lam, R. W., Chakrabarty, T., & Yatham, L. N. (2021). Efficacy of active vs sham intermittent theta burst transcranial magnetic stimulation for patients with bipolar depression: A randomized clinical trial. *JAMA Network Open, 4*(3), e210963. https://doi.org/10.1001/jamanetworkopen.2021.0963

MedlinePlus. (2021). Bipolar disorder. *MedlinePlus.* https://medlineplus.gov/genetics/condition/bipolar-disorder/#inheritance

Meier, S. M., Pavlova, B., Dalsgaard, S., Nordentoft, M., Mors, O., Mortensen, P. B., & Uher, R. (2018). Attention-deficit hyperactivity disorder and anxiety disorders as precursors of bipolar disorder onset in adulthood. *British Journal of Psychiatry, 3*(3), 555–560. https://doi.org/10.1192/bjp.2018.111

Merikangas, K. R., & Rihmer, Z. (2017). Mood disorders: Epidemiology. In B. J. Sadock, V. A. Sadock, & P. Ruiz (Eds.), *Comprehensive textbook of psychiatry* (10th ed., pp.1614–1619). Wolters Kluwer.

Miklowitz, D. J., & Chung, B. (2016). Family-focused therapy for bipolar disorder: Reflections on 30 years of research. *Family Process, 55*(3), 483–499. https://doi.org/10.1111/famp.12237

National Institute of Mental Health. (2013). *New data reveal the extent of genetic overlap between major mental disorders: Schizophrenia, bipolar disorder share the most common genetic variation* [Press release]. http://www.nimh.nih.gov/news/science-news/2013/new-data-reveal-extent-of-genetic-overlap-between-major-mental-disorders.shtml

National Institute of Mental Health. (2017). *Bipolar disorder.* https://www.nimh.nih.gov/health/statistics/bipolar-disorder.shtml

Osser, D. (2021). ADHD in patients with bipolar disorder: Genetics, diagnosis, and treatment. *Psychiatric Times, 38*(1). https://www.psychiatrictimes.com/view/adhd-bipolar-genetics-diagnosis-treatment

Quidé, Y., Tozzi, L., Corcoran, M., Cannon, D. M., & Dauvermann, M. R. (2020). The impact of childhood trauma on developing bipolar disorder: Current understanding and ensuring continued progress. *Neuropsychiatric Disease and Treatment, 16*, 3095–3115. https://doi.org/10.2147/NDT.S285540

Rybakowski, J. (2014). Factors associated with lithium efficacy in bipolar disorder. *Harvard Review of Psychiatry, 22*(6), 353–357. https://doi.org/10.1097/HRP.0000000000000006

Soreff, S. (2019). Bipolar disorder. *Medscape.* https://emedicine.medscape.com/article/286342-overview#a4

Strakowski, S. (2016). A guide to treating unipolar and bipolar depression. *Medscape.* http://www.medscape.com/viewarticle/871539#vp_6

Stringaris, A., Baroni, A., Haimm, C., Brotman, M., Lowe, C. H., Myers, F., Rustgi, E., Wheeler, W., Kayser, R., Towbin, K., & Leibenluft, E. (2010). Pediatric bipolar disorder versus severe mood dysregulation: Risk for manic episodes on follow-up. *Journal of the American Academy of Child and Adolescent Psychiatry, 49*(4), 397–405.

Swartz, H., & Swanson, J. (2014). Psychotherapy for bipolar disorder in adults: A review of the evidence. *American Psychiatric Publishing, 12*(3), 251–266. https://doi.org/10.1176/appi.focus.12.3.251

Watson, S., Gallagher, P., Dougall, D., Porter, R., Moncrieff, J., Ferrier, I. N., & Young, A. H. (2013). Childhood trauma in bipolar disorder. *Australian and New Zealand Journal of Psychiatry, 48*(6), 564–570. https://doi.org/10.1177/0004867413516681

Zimmerman, M., Balling, C., Dalrymple, K., & Chelminski, I. (2019). Screening for borderline personality disorder in psychiatric outpatients with major depressive disorder and bipolar disorder. *Journal of Clinical Psychiatry, 80*(1), 18m12257. https://doi.org/10.4088/JCP.18m12257

Anxiety, Obsessive-Compulsive, and Related Disorders

18

CHAPTER OUTLINE

Objectives
Introduction
Historical Perspectives
Epidemiology
How Much Is Too Much?
Application of the Nursing Process
Treatment Modalities
Summary and Key Points
Review Questions
Clinical Judgment Questions
Implications for Evidence-Based Practice
Test Your Clinical Reasoning and Clinical Judgment Skills
Communication Exercises
Movie Connections

CORE CONCEPTS

Stress and Coping: Anxiety
Mood and Affect
Professional Behavior: Nursing process in the care of patients with anxiety, obsessive-compulsive, and related behaviors
Safety
Clinical Judgment

KEY TERMS

agoraphobia
anxiety
body dysmorphic disorder
compulsions
fear
generalized anxiety disorder
habit reversal training
hoarding disorder
implosion therapy (flooding)
obsessions
obsessive-compulsive disorder
panic disorder
phobia
social anxiety disorder (SAD)
specific phobia
stress
systematic desensitization
trichotillomania

OBJECTIVES

After reading this chapter, the student will be able to:

1. Differentiate among the terms *stress, anxiety*, and *fear*.
2. Discuss historical aspects and epidemiological statistics related to anxiety, obsessive-compulsive, and related disorders.
3. Differentiate between normal anxiety and clinically significant anxiety.
4. Describe various types of anxiety, obsessive-compulsive, and related disorders and identify symptomatology associated with each. Incorporate this information in patient assessment.
5. Identify predisposing factors in the development of anxiety, obsessive-compulsive, and related disorders.
6. Formulate nursing diagnoses and outcome criteria for patients with anxiety, obsessive-compulsive, and related disorders.
7. Describe appropriate nursing interventions for behaviors associated with anxiety, obsessive-compulsive, and related disorders.
8. Identify topics for patient and family teaching relevant to anxiety, obsessive-compulsive, and related disorders.
9. Evaluate nursing care of patients with anxiety, obsessive-compulsive, and related disorders.
10. Discuss various modalities relevant to treatment of anxiety, obsessive-compulsive, and related disorders.

Introduction

Prince Harry, of the British Royal Family, shared in an interview about his incapacitating panic attacks following the death of his mother, Princess Diana (Sykes, 2017). In the interview he described these attacks as follows:

> "In my case, every single time I was in any room with loads of people, which is quite often, I was just pouring with sweat, my heart beating—boom, boom, boom, boom—literally, just like a washing machine. I was like, 'Oh my God, get me out of here now. Oh, hang on, I can't get out of here, I have got to just hide it.'"

He reports having struggled with these attacks for several years before recognizing he needed professional help and learned that the panic attacks were linked to unresolved grief over the death of his mother more than a decade earlier. His story highlights not only the impact that anxiety disorders can have on one's functioning but also that treatment can be successful and improve one's quality of life.

CORE CONCEPT

Anxiety

Anxiety is a feeling of discomfort, apprehension, or dread related to anticipation of danger, the source of which is often nonspecific or unknown. Anxiety is considered a disorder (or pathology) when fears and anxieties are excessive (in a cultural context) and there are associated behavioral disturbances such as interference with social and occupational functioning (American Psychiatric Association [APA], 2022).

Individuals face anxiety on a daily basis. Anxiety, which provides the motivation for achievement, is a necessary force for survival. The term *anxiety* is often used interchangeably with the word *stress*; however, they are not the same. **Stress** or, more properly, a *stressor*, is an external pressure that is brought to bear on the individual. Anxiety is the subjective emotional response to that stressor. (See Chapter 1, "Mental Health and Mental Illness," for an overview of anxiety as a psychological response to stress.)

Anxiety may be distinguished from *fear* in that the former is an internal emotional process, whereas fear is an emotion related to a cognitive sense of danger. In other words, **fear** involves the intellectual appraisal of a stimulus perceived to be threatening; anxiety is an emotional response of internal tension and worry that may be diffuse and not directly related to an external cause.

This chapter focuses on disorders that are characterized by exaggerated and often disabling anxiety reactions. Historical aspects and epidemiological statistics are presented. Predisposing factors that have been implicated in the etiology of the disorders provide a framework for studying the dynamics of phobias, obsessive-compulsive disorders, generalized anxiety disorder, panic disorder, and other anxiety disorders. Various theories of causation are presented, although it is most likely that a combination of factors contribute to the etiology of these disorders. The neurobiology of anxiety disorders is presented in Figure 18–1.

An explanation of the symptomatology is presented as background knowledge for assessing the client with an anxiety or obsessive-compulsive disorder. Nursing care is described in the context of the nursing process. Various treatment modalities are explored.

Historical Perspectives

Individuals have experienced anxiety throughout the ages. Yet anxiety, like fear, was not clearly defined or isolated as a separate entity by psychiatrists or psychologists until the 19th and 20th centuries. In fact, what we now know as anxiety was once solely identified by its physiological symptoms, focusing largely on the cardiovascular system.

Freud first introduced the term *anxiety neurosis* in 1895. Freud described this syndrome as 'anxiety neurosis' because he believed all the various manifestations were related to the chief symptom of anxiety (Freud, 1959). Although Freud attempted to negate the previous concept of the problem as strictly physical, it was some time before physicians of internal medicine were ready to accept the psychological implications for the symptoms. It was not until World War II that the psychological dimensions of various functional heart conditions were recognized.

For many years, anxiety disorders were viewed as purely psychological or purely biological in nature. Researchers have begun to focus on the interrelatedness of mind and body, and anxiety disorders provide an excellent example of this complex relationship. It is likely that various factors, including genetic, developmental, environmental, and psychological, play a role in the etiology of anxiety disorders.

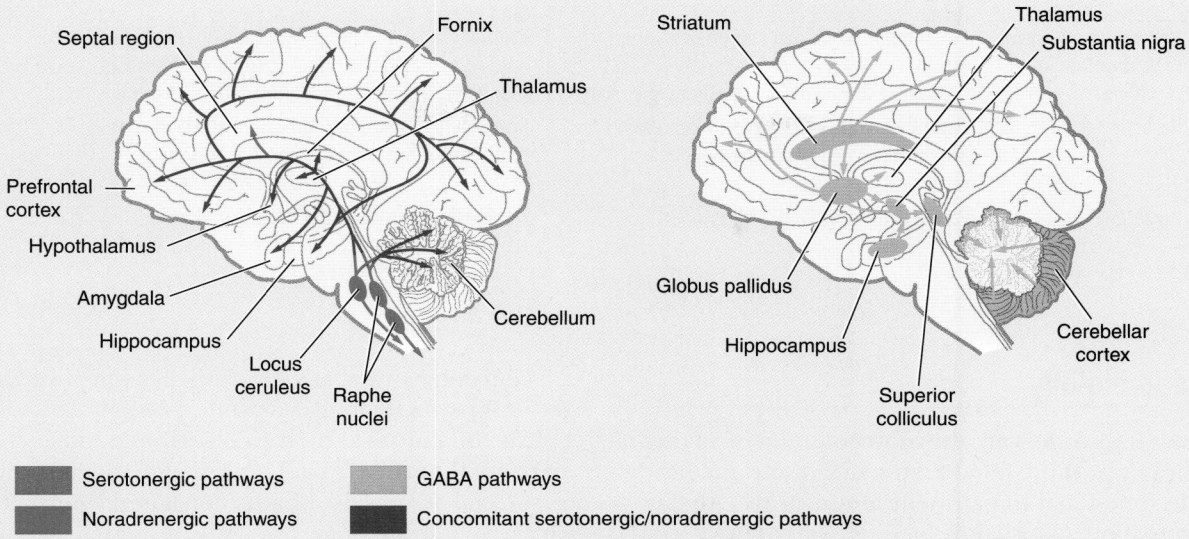

FIGURE 18–1 Neurobiology of anxiety disorders.

NEUROTRANSMITTERS

Although other neurotransmitters have also been implicated in the pathophysiology of anxiety disorders, disturbances in serotonin, norepinephrine, and gamma-aminobutyric acid (GABA) appear to be most significant.

Cell bodies of origin for the serotonin pathways lie within the raphe nuclei located in the brainstem. Serotonin is thought to be decreased in anxiety disorders (based on the efficacy of selective serotonin reuptake inhibitors [SSRIs] in the treatment of anxiety disorders), but some studies suggest that serotonin may have a modulating effect in response to intense emotions in general. Cell bodies for norepinephrine originate in the locus ceruleus. Norepinephrine is thought to be increased in anxiety disorders. GABA is the major inhibitory neurotransmitter in the brain. It is involved in the reduction and slowing of cellular activity. It is synthesized from glutamic acid, with vitamin B_6 as a cofactor. It is found in almost every region of the brain. GABA is thought to be decreased in anxiety disorders (allowing for increased cellular excitability).

AREAS OF THE BRAIN AFFECTED

Areas of the brain affected by anxiety disorders and the symptoms that they mediate include the following:

- ***Amygdala:*** Fear, which is particularly important in panic and phobic disorders
- ***Hippocampus:*** Associated with memory related to fear responses
- ***Locus ceruleus:*** Arousal
- ***Brainstem:*** Respiratory activation, heart rate
- ***Hypothalamus:*** Activation of stress response
- ***Frontal cortex:*** Cognitive interpretations
- ***Thalamus:*** Integration of sensory stimuli
- ***Basal ganglia:*** Tremor

Anxiolytic Agents	Action	Side Effects
Benzodiazepines	Increases the affinity of the $GABA_A$ receptor for GABA	Sedation, dizziness, weakness, ataxia, decreased motor performance, dependence, withdrawal
SSRIs	Block reuptake of serotonin into the presynaptic nerve terminal, increasing synaptic concentration of serotonin	Nausea, diarrhea, headache, insomnia, somnolence, sexual dysfunction
SNRIs	Inhibit reuptake of neuronal serotonin and norepinephrine; mild reuptake of dopamine	Headache, dry mouth, nausea, somnolence, dizziness, insomnia, asthenia, constipation, diarrhea

Continued

Anxiolytic Agents	Action	Side Effects
Noradrenergic agents (e.g., propranolol, clonidine)	Propranolol: blocks beta adrenergic receptor activity Clonidine: stimulates alpha-adrenergic receptors	Propranolol: bradycardia, hypotension, weakness, fatigue, impotence, gastrointestinal upset, bronchospasm Clonidine: Dry mouth, sedation, fatigue, hypotension
Barbiturates	Central nervous system (CNS) depression; also produces effects in the hepatic and cardiovascular systems	Somnolence, agitation, confusion, ataxia, dizziness, bradycardia, hypotension, constipation
Buspirone	Partial agonist of 5-HT_{1A} receptor	Dizziness, drowsiness, dry mouth, headache, nervousness, nausea, insomnia

Epidemiology

Anxiety disorders are the most common of all mental illnesses in the United States and result in considerable functional impairment and distress (Anxiety & Depression Association of America [ADAA], 2021). Statistics vary widely, but most agree that anxiety disorders are more common in women than in men by at least two to one. Prevalence rates (ADAA, 2021) for anxiety disorders within the general population are identified as follows:

- Specific phobias: 8.7%
- Social anxiety disorder: 6.8%
- Post-traumatic stress disorder: 3.5%
- Generalized anxiety disorder: 3.1%
- Panic disorder: 2.7%
- Obsessive-compulsive disorder: 1%

The lifetime prevalence for any anxiety disorder is estimated at 31.1% for adults and 31.9% for adolescents 13 to 18 years of age (National Institute of Mental Health [NIMH], 2017). Common comorbidities include another anxiety disorder, depression, and substance abuse. Vulnerability to comorbidities includes parental psychiatric history, childhood trauma, and negative life events, but regardless of the contributing factors, comorbidities are associated with poorer outcomes, higher health-care utilization, and greater impairment in functioning. In general, studies support a moderate genetic vulnerability, and gene-environment studies support the influence of early developmental trauma and stressful life events in anxiety disorders (Gottschalk & Domschke, 2017).

How Much Is Too Much?

Anxiety is usually considered a normal reaction to a realistic danger or threat to biological integrity or self-concept. Normal anxiety dissipates when the danger or threat is no longer present.

It is difficult to draw a precise line between normal and abnormal anxiety. Normalcy is determined by societal standards; what is considered normal in Chicago, Illinois, may not be considered as such in Cairo, Egypt. There may even be regional differences within a country or cultural differences within a region. So what criteria can be used to determine whether an individual's anxious response is normal? Anxiety can be considered abnormal or pathological if:

1. *It is out of proportion to the situation that is creating it.*

EXAMPLE

Mr. Z witnessed a serious automobile accident two months ago when he was out driving in his car, and since that time refuses to drive even to the grocery store a few miles from his house. He has been relying on others to pick up groceries for him and bring them to his home.

2. *The anxiety interferes with social, occupational, or other important areas of functioning.*

EXAMPLE

Jenna has become increasingly uncomfortable being in social situations based on fears that she will be embarrassed or ridiculed. Her friends have given up inviting her to go out and her boyfriend recently broke up with her related to his complaints that she never wants to go anywhere with his friends.

It is clear that when anxiety becomes excessive and persistent, humans respond in a variety of ways that are likely a complex interaction of genetic vulnerability, biochemical influences, and environmental factors. Various manifestations of pathological anxiety are discussed in the following section.

Application of the Nursing Process

Background Assessment Data

CORE CONCEPT

Panic

A sudden, overwhelming feeling of terror or impending doom. This most severe form of emotional anxiety is usually accompanied by behavioral, cognitive, and physiological signs and symptoms considered extremely intense and frightening.

Panic Disorder

Panic disorder is characterized by recurrent *panic attacks*, the onset of which is unpredictable. Panic attacks are manifested by intense apprehension, fear, or terror, often associated with feelings of impending doom (clients often fear they are dying) and accompanied by intense physical discomfort. The physical sensations can be so intense that individuals experiencing a panic attack believe they are having a heart attack or other critical illness. The symptoms come on suddenly and unexpectedly; that is, they do not occur immediately before or on exposure to a situation that usually causes anxiety (as in specific phobia). They are not triggered by situations in which the person is the focus of others' attention (as in social anxiety disorder [SAD]). The role of organic factors in the etiology has been ruled out.

The *Diagnostic and Statistical Manual of Mental Disorders, Fifth Edition, Text Revision* (*DSM-5-TR*; APA, 2022) states that at least four of the following symptoms must be present to identify the presence of a panic attack:

- Palpitations, pounding heart, or accelerated heart rate
- Sweating
- Trembling or shaking
- Sensations of shortness of breath or smothering
- Feelings of choking
- Chest pain or discomfort
- Nausea or abdominal distress
- Feeling dizzy, unsteady, lightheaded, or faint
- Chills or heat sensations
- Paresthesias (numbness or tingling sensations)
- Derealization (feelings of unreality) or depersonalization (feelings of being detached from oneself)
- Fear of losing control or going crazy
- Fear of dying

Attacks usually last minutes or, more rarely, they can last for hours. The individual often experiences varying degrees of nervousness and apprehension between attacks. Symptoms of depression are common.

The average age of onset of panic disorder is the late 20s. Frequency and severity of the panic attacks vary widely. Some individuals may have attacks of moderate severity weekly; others may have less severe or limited-symptom attacks several times a week. Still others may experience panic attacks that are separated by weeks or months. The disorder may last for a few weeks or months or for a number of years. Sometimes the individual experiences periods of remission and exacerbation. Limited-symptom attacks ("fearful spells" that do not meet criteria for panic attacks) may be a risk factor for later panic attacks and panic disorder. Genetic vulnerability, tendency toward negative emotions, history of trauma, respiratory disturbances such as asthma, and smoking have also been identified as risk factors (APA, 2022).

Generalized Anxiety Disorder

Generalized anxiety disorder (GAD) is characterized by persistent, unrealistic, and excessive anxiety and worry, which have occurred more days than not for at least 6 months and cannot be attributed to specific organic factors, such as caffeine intoxication or hyperthyroidism. The anxiety and worry are associated with three or more of the following symptoms: "restless or feeling keyed up or on edge, being easily fatigued, difficulty concentrating or mind going blank, irritability, muscle tension, and sleep disturbance" (APA, 2022, p. 250).

These symptoms are like those often associated with anxiety in the general population but, unlike the typical experience of anxiety, the symptoms in GAD are intense enough to cause clinically significant impairment in social, occupational, or other important areas of functioning. The individual often avoids activities or events that may result in negative outcomes or spends considerable time and effort preparing for such activities. Anxiety and worry often result in procrastination in behavior or decision making, and the individual repeatedly seeks reassurance from others.

The disorder may begin in childhood or adolescence, but onset is more common after age 20. Depressive symptoms are common, and numerous somatic complaints may also be a part of the clinical picture. GAD tends to be chronic, with frequent stress-related exacerbations and fluctuations in the course of the illness.

Theories of Etiology Related to Panic and Generalized Anxiety Disorders

Psychodynamic Theory

The psychodynamic view focuses on the inability of the ego to intervene when conflict occurs between the id and the superego, producing anxiety. For various reasons (unsatisfactory parent-child relationship, conditional love, or provisional gratification), ego development is delayed. When developmental defects in ego functions compromise the capacity to modulate anxiety, the individual resorts to unconscious mechanisms to resolve the conflict. Use of defense mechanisms rather than coping and management skills results in maladaptive responses to anxiety.

Cognitive Theory

The main thesis of the cognitive view is that faulty, distorted, or counterproductive thinking patterns accompany or precede maladaptive behaviors and emotional disorders. A disturbance in this central mechanism of cognition causes a consequent disturbance in feeling and behavior. Because of distorted thinking, anxiety is maintained by erroneous or dysfunctional appraisal of a situation. There is a loss of ability to reason regarding the problem, whether it is physical or interpersonal. The individual feels vulnerable in a given situation, and the distorted thinking results in an irrational appraisal, fostering a negative outcome.

Biological Aspects

Research investigations into the psychobiological correlation of panic disorder and GAD have implicated a number of possibilities.

- ***Genetics:*** Genetic studies have identified variations in specific genes that may be associated with anxiety disorders (including panic disorder and obsessive-compulsive disorder), and some studies suggest that genetic variations may affect the sensitivity of emotional processing centers in the brain (Ressler & Smoller, 2016). Twin studies identify a 30% to 40% risk of heritability. But as Ressler and Smoller point out, genetic findings are indicative of risk rather than determinants of illness, and many current genetic studies reveal that environmental factors in interaction with genes have more of an impact on risk than genetic influences alone (Gottschalk & Domschke, 2017).
- ***Neuroanatomical:*** Structural brain imaging studies in patients with panic disorder have implicated pathological involvement in the temporal lobes, particularly the hippocampus and the amygdala (Boland & Verduin, 2022). Dysfunctions in the limbic system (often referred to as "the emotional brain") and the frontal cerebral cortex have also been noted in clients with anxiety disorders.
- ***Biochemical:*** Abnormal elevations of blood lactate have been noted in clients with panic disorder. Likewise, infusion of sodium lactate in clients with anxiety neuroses produces symptoms of panic disorder. Studies have suggested that people with panic disorders may be more sensitive to hypercapnia (which increases lactate levels), and carbon dioxide (CO_2) challenge tests have supported this sensitivity (Amaral et al., 2013). Additionally, studies of various medications and treatments such as cognitive behavior therapy (CBT) have demonstrated decreased sensitivity to CO_2 inhalation after treatment, suggesting a relationship between lactate levels and anxiety reduction.
- ***Neurochemical:*** Strong evidence exists for the involvement of the neurotransmitter norepinephrine in the etiology of panic disorder. Norepinephrine is known to mediate arousal and cause hyperarousal and anxiety. This fact has been demonstrated by a notable increase in anxiety following the administration of drugs that increase the synaptic availability of norepinephrine, such as yohimbine. The neurotransmitters serotonin and gamma-aminobutyric acid (GABA) are thought to be decreased in anxiety disorders. These hypotheses are related to the efficacy of benzodiazepines, which enhance the activity of GABA and the efficacy of selective serotonin reuptake inhibitors (SSRIs), which enhance the activity of serotonin. Similarly, deep-breathing exercises have been shown to elevate thalamic GABA levels through stimulation of vagal nerve pathways with a subsequent reduction in heart rate and improvement in emotional regulation and stress responses (Gerbard & Brown, 2016).

CORE CONCEPT

Phobia

A **phobia** is an irrational fear of a specific object or situation resulting in an intense aversion toward the feared stimulus. Exposure to the feared object or situation is typically accompanied by intense anxiety or panic attacks.

Phobias

Two common phobia disorders include agoraphobia and SAD (formerly called social phobia). The estimated lifetime prevalence of agoraphobia among U.S. adults is 1.3%, and approximately 40% of those cases are considered severe (NIMH, 2017). Social anxiety disorder is more common, with an estimated lifetime prevalence of 12.1% (NIMH, 2017). A specific phobia, in which a person has an exaggerated fear response to a specific object or situation, is estimated to affect 12.5 % of the U.S. adult population (NIMH, 2017).

Agoraphobia

The Greek translation of the word *agoraphobia* is "fear of the marketplace." **Agoraphobia** is the fear of being in open shops and markets, but more specifically, it is the fear of being vulnerable and unable to get help or escape the setting (Kimmel & Roy-Burn, 2017) should panic symptoms occur. It is possible that the individual may have experienced symptoms in the past and is preoccupied with fears of their recurrence. The *DSM-5-TR* diagnostic criteria for agoraphobia are presented in Box 18–1.

The onset of symptoms most commonly occurs in one's 20s and 30s and persists for many years. It is diagnosed more commonly in women than in men. Impairment can be severe. In extreme cases, the individual is unable to leave home without being accompanied by a friend or relative. If this is not possible, the person may become totally confined to home.

Social Anxiety Disorder (SAD)

Social anxiety disorder (SAD) is an excessive fear of situations in which a person might do something embarrassing or be evaluated negatively by others. The individual has extreme concerns about being exposed to possible scrutiny by others and fears social or performance situations in which embarrassment may occur (APA, 2022). In some instances, the fear may be quite defined, such as the fear of speaking or eating in a public place, fear of using a public restroom, or fear of writing in the presence of others. In other cases, the social phobia may involve general social situations, such as making comments or answering questions in a manner that would provoke laughter on the part of others. Exposure to the phobic situation usually results in feelings of panic anxiety with sweating, tachycardia, and dyspnea.

Onset of symptoms of this disorder often begins in late childhood or early adolescence and runs a chronic, sometimes lifelong, course. It appears to be more common in women than in men (Kimmel & Roy-Burn, 2017). Impairment interferes with social or occupational functioning and causes marked distress. The *DSM-5-TR* diagnostic criteria for SAD are presented in Box 18–2.

BOX 18–1 Diagnostic Criteria for Agoraphobia

A. Marked fear or anxiety about two (or more) of the following five situations:
   1. Using public transportation (e.g., automobiles, buses, trains, ships, planes)
   2. Being in open spaces (e.g., parking lots, marketplaces, bridges)
   3. Being in enclosed places (e.g., shops, theaters, cinemas)
   4. Standing in line or being in a crowd
   5. Being outside of the home alone

B. The individual fears these situations because of thoughts that escape might be difficult or help might not be available in the event of panic-like symptoms or other incapacitating or embarrassing symptoms (e.g., fear of falling in the elderly, fear of incontinence).

C. The agoraphobic situations almost always provoke fear or anxiety.

D. The agoraphobic situations are actively avoided, require the presence of a companion, or are endured with intense fear or anxiety.

E. The fear or anxiety is out of proportion to the actual danger posed by the agoraphobic situations and to the sociocultural context.

F. The fear, anxiety, or avoidance is persistent, typically lasting 6 months or more.

G. The fear, anxiety, or avoidance causes clinically significant distress or impairment in social, occupational, or other important areas of functioning.

H. If another medical condition (e.g., inflammatory bowel disease, Parkinson's disease) is present, the fear, anxiety, or avoidance is clearly excessive.

I. The fear, anxiety, or avoidance is not better explained by the symptoms of another mental disorder—for example, the symptoms are not confined to specific phobia, situational type; do not involve only social situations (as in social anxiety disorder); and are not related exclusively to obsessions (as in obsessive-compulsive disorder), perceived defects or flaws in physical appearance (as in body dysmorphic disorder), reminders of traumatic events (as in posttraumatic stress disorder), or fear of separation (as in separation anxiety disorder).

Reprinted with permission from American Psychiatric Association. (2022). *Diagnostic and statistical manual of mental disorders, fifth edition, text revision.*

Specific Phobia

Specific phobia is identified by fear of specific objects or situations that could conceivably cause harm (e.g., snakes, heights), but the person's reaction to them is excessive and irrational.

Specific phobias are often identified when other anxiety disorders have become a focus of clinical attention. Treatment is generally aimed at the primary diagnosis because it usually produces the greatest

BOX 18–2 Diagnostic Criteria for Social Anxiety Disorder (Social Phobia)

A. Marked fear or anxiety about one or more social situations in which the individual is exposed to possible scrutiny by others. Examples include social interactions (e.g., having a conversation, meeting unfamiliar people), being observed (e.g., eating or drinking), and performing in front of others (e.g., giving a speech). **NOTE:** In children, the anxiety must occur in peer settings and not just during interactions with adults.
B. The individual fears that he or she will act in a way or show anxiety symptoms that will be negatively evaluated (i.e., will be humiliating or embarrassing; will lead to rejection or offend others).
C. The social situations almost always provoke fear or anxiety. **NOTE:** In children, the fear or anxiety may be expressed by crying, tantrums, freezing, clinging, shrinking, or failing to speak in social situations.
D. The social situations are avoided or are endured with intense fear or anxiety.
E. The fear or anxiety is out of proportion to the actual threat posed by the social situation and to the sociocultural context.
F. The fear, anxiety, or avoidance is persistent, typically lasting 6 months or more.
G. The fear, anxiety, or avoidance causes clinically significant distress or impairment in social, occupation, or other important areas of functioning.
H. The fear, anxiety, or avoidance is not attributable to the physiological effects of a substance (e.g., a drug of abuse, a medication) or another medical condition.
I. The fear, anxiety, or avoidance is not better explained by the symptoms of another mental disorder, such as panic disorder, body dysmorphic disorder, or autism spectrum disorder.
J. If another medical condition (e.g., Parkinson's disease, obesity, disfigurement from burns or injury) is present, the fear, anxiety, or avoidance is clearly unrelated or is excessive.

Specify if:
Performance only: If the fear is restricted to speaking or performing in public

Reprinted with permission from American Psychiatric Association. (2022). *Diagnostic and statistical manual of mental disorders, fifth edition, text revision.*

distress and interferes with functioning more so than does a specific phobia. A diagnosis of specific phobia is made only when the irrational fear restricts the individual's activities and interferes with daily living.

The phobic person may be no more (or less) anxious than anyone else until exposed to the phobic object or situation. Exposure to the phobic stimulus produces overwhelming symptoms of panic, including palpitations, sweating, dizziness, and difficulty breathing. These symptoms may occur in response to the individual's merely *thinking* about the phobic stimulus. Invariably, the person recognizes that the fear is excessive or unreasonable but feels powerless to change. Phobias may begin at almost any age. Those that begin in childhood often disappear without treatment, but those that begin or persist into adulthood usually require assistance with therapy. The disorder is diagnosed more often in women than in men.

Even though the disorder is relatively common among the general population, people seldom seek treatment unless the phobia interferes with ability to function. The individual who has a fear of snakes but who lives on the 23rd floor of an urban, high-rise apartment building is not likely to be bothered by the phobia unless they decide to move to an area where snakes are prevalent. On the other hand, a fear of elevators may very well interfere with this individual's daily functioning.

Specific phobias have been classified according to the phobic stimulus. A list of some of the identified phobias appears in Table 18–1. This list is by no means all-inclusive. People can become phobic about almost any object or situation, and anyone with a little knowledge of Greek or Latin can produce a phobia classification, thereby making possibilities for the list almost infinite.

Theories of Etiology Related to Phobias

The cause of phobias is unknown. However, various theories exist that may offer insight into the etiology.

Psychoanalytic Theory

Modern-day psychoanalysts believe that unconscious fears may be expressed in a symbolic manner as phobias. For example, a female child who was sexually abused by an adult male family friend when he was taking her for a ride in his boat grew up with an intense, irrational fear of all water vessels. Psychoanalytic theory postulates that fear of the man was repressed and displaced onto boats. Boats became an unconscious symbol for the feared person but one that the young girl viewed as safer because her fear of boats prevented her from having to confront the real fear.

Learning Theory

Classic conditioning in the case of phobias may be explained as follows: a stressful stimulus produces an "unconditioned" response of fear. When the stressful stimulus is repeatedly paired with a harmless object,

TABLE 18–1 Classifications of Selected Specific Phobias

CLASSIFICATION	FEAR
Acrophobia	Height
Ailurophobia	Cats
Agoraphobia	Situations or places where escape may be difficult or the person feels trapped
Algophobia	Pain
Anthophobia	Flowers
Anthropophobia	People
Aquaphobia	Water
Arachnophobia	Spiders
Astraphobia	Lightning
Belonephobia	Needles
Brontophobia	Thunder
Claustrophobia	Closed spaces
Cynophobia	Dogs
Dementophobia	Insanity
Equinophobia	Horses
Gamophobia	Marriage
Herpetophobia	Lizards, reptiles
Homophobia	Homosexuality
Murophobia	Mice
Mysophobia	Dirt, germs, contamination
Numerophobia	Numbers
Nyctophobia	Darkness
Ochophobia	Riding in a car
Ophidiophobia	Snakes
Pyrophobia	Fire
Scoleciphobia	Worms
Siderodromophobia	Railroads or train travel
Taphophobia	Being buried alive
Thanatophobia	Death
Trichophobia	Hair
Triskaidekaphobia	The number 13
Xenophobia	Strangers
Zoophobia	Animals

eventually the harmless object alone produces a "conditioned" response: fear. This conditioning becomes a phobia when the individual consciously avoids the harmless object to escape fear.

Some learning theorists hold that fears are conditioned responses and thus are learned by imposing rewards for certain behaviors. In the instance of phobias, when individuals avoid a phobic object, they escape fear, which is indeed a powerful reward.

Phobias also may be acquired by direct learning or imitation (modeling; e.g., a parent who exhibits fear toward an object will provide a model for the child, who may also develop a phobia of the same object).

Cognitive Theory

Cognitive theorists espouse that anxiety is the product of faulty cognitions or anxiety-inducing self-instructions. Two types of faulty thinking have been investigated: negative self-statements and irrational beliefs. Cognitive theorists believe that some individuals engage in negative and irrational thinking that produces anxiety reactions. The individual begins to seek out avoidance behaviors to prevent the anxiety reactions, and phobias result.

Related to the cognitive theory is the involvement of locus of control. Johnson and Sarason (1978) suggested that individuals with internal locus of control and those with external locus of control might respond differently to life change. These researchers proposed that locus of control orientation may be an important variable in the development of phobias. Individuals with an external control orientation experiencing anxiety attacks in a stressful period are likely to mislabel the anxiety and attribute it to external sources (e.g., crowded areas) or to a disease (e.g., heart attack). They may perceive the experienced anxiety as being outside of their control. Figure 18–2 depicts a graphic model of the relationship between locus of control and the development of phobias.

Biological Aspects

- ***Neuroanatomical:*** Specific areas in the prefrontal cortex and the amygdala play a role in storing and recalling information about threatening or potentially deadly events. Similar future events can trigger those memories, after which the amygdala triggers release of fight-or-flight hormones and the individual experiences heightened stress and fear as though the original threat was happening again (Brazier, 2020). Other researchers (Dias & Ressler, 2014) have found that parental traumatic exposure creates genetic "memories" that are passed down to subsequent generations via parental

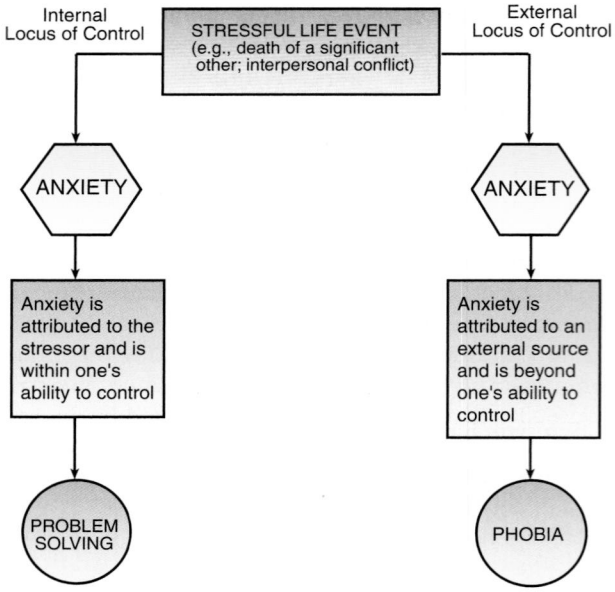

FIGURE 18–2 Locus of control as a variable in the etiology of phobias.

gametes, which are then expressed as phobias in their offspring. Kimmel and Roy-Burn (2017) note that although there may be a genetic vulnerability to phobias, environmental factors such as trauma play a more central role.

- ***Temperament:*** Children experience fears as a part of normal development. Most infants are afraid of loud noises. Common fears of toddlers and preschoolers include strangers, animals, darkness, and being separated from parents or attachment figures. School-age children commonly experience fear of death and anxiety about school achievement. Fears of social rejection and sexual anxieties are common among adolescents.

Innate fears represent a part of the overall characteristics or tendencies with which one is born that influences response throughout life to specific situations. Innate fears usually do not reach phobic intensity but may have the capacity for such development if reinforced by events in later life. For example, a 4-year-old girl is afraid of dogs. By age 5, however, she has overcome her fear and plays with her own dog and the neighbors' dogs without fear. Then, when she is 19, she is bitten by a stray dog and develops a phobia of dogs.

Life Experiences

Certain early experiences may set the stage for phobic reactions later in life. Some researchers believe that phobias, particularly specific phobias, are symbolic of original anxiety-producing objects or situations that have been repressed. Examples include the following:

- A child who is punished by being locked in a closet develops a phobia of elevators or other closed places.
- A child who falls down a flight of stairs develops a phobia of high places.
- A young adult who, as a child, survived a plane crash in which both parents were killed has a phobia of airplanes.

Anxiety Disorder Due to Another Medical Condition and Substance/Medication-Induced Anxiety Disorder

The symptoms associated with these disorders are judged to be the direct physiological consequence of another medical condition or due to the direct physiological effects of substance intoxication or withdrawal or exposure to a medication. Several medical conditions have been associated with the development of anxiety symptoms. Some of these include cardiac conditions, such as myocardial infarction, congestive heart failure, and mitral valve prolapse; endocrine conditions, such as hypoglycemia, hypo- or hyperthyroidism, and pheochromocytoma; respiratory conditions, such as chronic obstructive pulmonary disease and hyperventilation; and neurological conditions, such as complex partial seizures, neoplasms, and encephalitis.

Nursing care of patients with this disorder must take into consideration the underlying cause of the anxiety. Holistic nursing care is essential to ensure that the patient's physiological and psychosocial needs are met. Nursing actions appropriate for the specific medical condition must be considered.

The diagnosis of substance-induced anxiety disorder is made only if the anxiety symptoms are in excess of those usually associated with the intoxication or withdrawal syndrome and warrant independent clinical attention. Evidence of intoxication or withdrawal must be available from history, physical examination, or laboratory findings to substantiate the diagnosis. Substance-induced anxiety disorder may be associated with use of the following substances: alcohol, amphetamines, cocaine, hallucinogens, inhalants, opioids, sedatives, hypnotics, anxiolytics, caffeine, cannabis, or other substances (APA, 2022). Nursing care of the patient with substance-induced anxiety disorder must take into consideration the nature of the substance and the context in which the symptoms occur—that is, intoxication or withdrawal.

CORE CONCEPT

Obsessions

Intrusive thoughts that are recurrent and stressful. Although they are recognized by the individual as irrational, they continue to be repetitive and cannot be ignored.

CORE CONCEPT

Compulsions

Repetitive ritualistic behaviors or mental acts that the individual feels driven to perform according to rigidly applied rules and which are intended to reduce the anxiety associated with obsessive thoughts (APA, 2022).

Obsessive-Compulsive Disorder

The manifestations of **obsessive-compulsive disorder** (OCD) include the presence of **obsessions** (repetitive intrusive thoughts) or compulsions, or both, the severity of which is significant enough to cause distress or impairment in social, occupational, or other important areas of functioning (APA, 2022). With **compulsions** the individual recognizes that the behavior is excessive or unreasonable but, because of the feeling of relief from discomfort that it promotes, is compelled to continue the act. Common compulsions include hand washing, ordering, checking, praying, counting, and repeating words silently.

The disorder is equally common among men and women. It may begin in childhood but more often begins in adolescence or early adulthood. The course is usually chronic and may be complicated by depression or substance abuse. The *DSM-5-TR* diagnostic criteria for OCD are presented in Box 18–3.

Body Dysmorphic Disorder

Body dysmorphic disorder is characterized by the exaggerated belief that the body is deformed or

BOX 18–3 Diagnostic Criteria for Obsessive-Compulsive Disorder

A. Presence of obsessions, compulsions, or both:

Obsessions are defined by (1) and (2)

1. Recurrent and persistent thoughts, urges, or images that are experienced, at some time during the disturbance, as intrusive and unwanted, and that in most individuals cause marked anxiety or distress.
2. The individual attempts to ignore or suppress such thoughts, urges, or images, or to neutralize them with some other thought or action (i.e., by performing a compulsion).

Compulsions are defined by (1) and (2):

1. Repetitive behaviors (e.g., hand washing, ordering, checking) or mental acts (e.g., praying, counting, repeating words silently) that the person feels driven to perform in response to an obsession or according to rules that must be applied rigidly.
2. The behaviors or mental acts are aimed at preventing or reducing anxiety or distress, or preventing some dreaded event or situation; however, these behaviors or mental acts either are not connected in a realistic way with what they are designed to neutralize or prevent or are clearly excessive. **NOTE:** Young children may not be able to articulate the aims of these behaviors or mental acts.

B. The obsessions or compulsions are time consuming (e.g., take more than 1 hour a day) or cause clinically significant distress or impairment in social, occupational, or other important areas of functioning.

C. The obsessive-compulsive symptoms are not attributable to the direct physiological effects of a substance (e.g., a drug of abuse, a medication) or another medical condition.

D. The disturbance is not better explained by the symptoms of another mental disorder (e.g., excessive worries, as in generalized anxiety disorder; preoccupation with appearance, as in body dysmorphic disorder; difficulty discarding or parting with possessions, as in hoarding disorder; hair pulling, as in trichotillomania [hair-pulling disorder]; skin picking, as in excoriation [skin-picking] disorder; stereotypies, as in stereotypic movement disorder; ritualized eating behavior, as in eating disorders; preoccupation with substances or gambling, as in substance-related and addictive disorders; preoccupation with having an illness, as in illness anxiety disorder; sexual urges or fantasies, as in paraphilic disorders; impulses, as in disruptive, impulse-control, and conduct disorders; guilty ruminations, as in major depressive disorder; thought insertion or delusional preoccupations, as in schizophrenia spectrum and other psychotic disorders; or repetitive patterns of behavior, as in autism spectrum disorder).

Specify if:
With good or fair insight
With poor insight
With absent insight/delusional beliefs

Specify if:
Tic-related

Reprinted with permission from American Psychiatric Association. (2022). *Diagnostic and statistical manual of mental disorders, fifth edition, text revision.*

defective in some specific way. The most common complaints involve flaws of the face or head, such as wrinkles or scars, the shape of the nose, excessive facial hair, and facial asymmetry, that are slight or not observable by others (Stein & Lochner, 2017). However, any body part can be the focus of distorted beliefs including the ears, eyes, lips, teeth, stomach, genitalia, or body weight. In some instances, a true defect is present, but the significance of the defect is unrealistically exaggerated, and the person's concern is grossly excessive. These beliefs are differentiated from delusions in that the individual with body dysmorphic disorder is aware that the beliefs are exaggerated. In some cases, though, people with body dysmorphic disorder also develop psychotic disorders.

People with body dysmorphic disorder often have other comorbid mental disorders. The most frequent comorbidity is depression, with a lifetime prevalence rate of 75%; other less common comorbidities include OCD, panic attacks, and substance use disorders (Boland & Verduin, 2022). Social and occupational impairment may occur because of the excessive anxiety experienced by individuals in relation to the imagined defect. Medical histories of clients may reflect numerous visits to plastic surgeons and dermatologists in an unrelenting drive to correct the imagined defect, and they may undergo unnecessary surgical procedures toward this effort. The *DSM-5-TR* diagnostic criteria for body dysmorphic disorder are presented in Box 18–4.

Trichotillomania (Hair-Pulling Disorder)

The *DSM-5-TR* defines **trichotillomania** (hair-pulling disorder) as the recurrent pulling out of one's hair that results in hair loss (APA, 2022). The impulse is preceded by an increasing sense of tension and results in a sense of release or gratification from pulling out the hair. The most common sites for hair pulling are the scalp, eyebrows, and eyelashes but may occur in any area of the body on which hair grows. The areas of hair loss are often found on the opposite side of the body from the dominant hand. Pain is seldom reported to accompany the hair pulling, although tingling and pruritus in the area are not uncommon. Comorbid psychiatric disorders are common with hair-pulling disorder. The most common are mood and other anxiety disorders (Stein & Lochner, 2017).

Some children under 6 years of age have been reported to have mild symptoms of hair-pulling disorder, usually in response to a significant loss or other anxiety-producing event (Koblenzer, 2017). More significant trichotillomania typically begins in adolescence or early adulthood with a variable course. It may be accompanied by nail biting, head banging, scratching, biting, or other acts of self-mutilation. Because the repetitive behavior of hair-pulling is intended to decrease anxiety, it may be considered within the spectrum of obsessive-compulsive disorders, This phenomenon occurs more often in women than in men, and prevalence estimates vary widely from 1% to 13.4% (Koblenzer, 2017).

Hoarding Disorder

The *DSM-5-TR* defines the essential feature of **hoarding disorder** as "persistent difficulties discarding or parting with possessions, regardless of their actual value" (APA, 2022, p. 277). Additionally, the diagnosis may be specified as "*with excessive acquisition*," which identifies the excessive need for continual acquiring of items (either by buying them or by other means).

BOX 18–4 Diagnostic Criteria for Body Dysmorphic Disorder

A. Preoccupation with one or more perceived defects or flaws in physical appearance that are not observable or appear slight to others.

B. At some point during the course of the disorder, the individual has performed repetitive behaviors (e.g., mirror checking, excessive grooming, skin picking, reassurance seeking) or mental acts (e.g., comparing their appearance with that of others) in response to the appearance concerns.

C. The preoccupation causes clinically significant distress or impairment in social, occupational, or other important areas of functioning.

D. The appearance preoccupation is not better explained by concerns with body fat or weight in an individual whose symptoms meet diagnostic criteria for an eating disorder.

Specify if:
With muscle dysmorphia

Specify if:
With good or fair insight
With poor insight
With absent insight/delusional beliefs

Reprinted with permission from American Psychiatric Association. (2022). *Diagnostic and statistical manual of mental disorders, fifth edition, text revision.*

In previous editions of the *DSM*, hoarding was considered a symptom of OCD. However, it is currently (in the *DSM-5-TR*) identified as a distinct disorder.

Individuals with this disorder collect items until virtually all surfaces within the home are covered. There may be only narrow pathways, winding through stacks of clutter, in which to walk. Some individuals also hoard food and animals, keeping dozens or hundreds of pets, often in unsanitary conditions (Mayo Clinic, 2021).

Community surveys estimate the prevalence of clinically significant hoarding in the United States and Europe to range from 1.5% to 6% (APA, 2022). More men than women are diagnosed with the disorder, and it is almost three times more prevalent in older adults (older than age 65) than in younger adults (ages 30–40) (APA, 2022). The symptoms, regardless of when they begin, appear to become more severe with each decade of life. Associated symptoms include perfectionism, indecisiveness, anxiety, depression, distractibility, and difficulty planning and organizing tasks (APA, 2022; Symonds & Janney, 2013). In addition to OCD, hoarding is associated with comorbid generalized anxiety disorder and major depressive disorder (Boland & Verduin, 2022). Research has shown that hoarding disorder runs in families, and there may be a genetic vulnerability (Dozier & Ayers, 2017).

Treatment of hoarding disorder has been met with mixed results. It is often difficult to convince individuals with the disorder that they are actually ill. Change is slow, and the relapse rate is high; when possessions are taken away, they are often quickly replaced to provide emotional comfort (Mayo Clinic, 2021). Psychoeducation about the disorder is almost always the initial intervention, and primary treatment is CBT. Psychopharmacology with SSRIs may be added, particularly when there is evidence of comorbid anxiety or depression. Family and friends may misinterpret hoarding behavior as laziness or uncleanliness. Psychoeducation that includes the patient's identified support system assists the patient in a recovery plan. Some experts (Meyers, 2016) have identified unresolved grief issues and trauma associated with exacerbations of hoarding behavior, which may provide another avenue for psychological intervention.

Theories of Etiology in Obsessive-Compulsive and Related Disorders

Psychoanalytic Theory

Psychoanalytic theorists propose that individuals with OCD have underdeveloped egos (for any of a variety of reasons: unsatisfactory parent-child relationship, conditional love, or provisional gratification). The psychoanalytical concept views clients with OCD as having regressed to earlier developmental stages of the infantile superego—the harsh, exacting, punitive characteristics that now reappear as part of the psychopathology. Regression and use of defense mechanisms (isolation, undoing, displacement, reaction formation) produce the clinical symptoms of obsessions and compulsions.

Learning Theory

Learning theorists explain obsessive-compulsive behavior as a conditioned response to a traumatic event. The traumatic event produces anxiety and discomfort, and the individual learns to prevent the anxiety and discomfort by avoiding the situation with which they are associated. This type of learning is called *passive avoidance* (staying away from the source). When passive avoidance is not possible, the individual learns to engage in behaviors that provide relief from the anxiety and discomfort associated with the traumatic situation. This type of learning is called *active avoidance* and describes the behavior pattern of the individual with OCD.

According to this classic conditioning interpretation, a traumatic event should mark the beginning of the obsessive-compulsive behaviors. However, in a significant number of cases, the onset of the behavior is gradual, and the clients relate the onset of their problems to life stress in general rather than to one or more traumatic events.

Psychosocial Influences

The onset of trichotillomania can be related to stressful situations in more than one-quarter of cases. Additional factors that have been implicated include disturbances in the mother-child relationship, fear of abandonment, and recent object loss. Trichotillomania has at times been connected to childhood trauma, but Woods (as cited by Kaplan, 2012) indicates that only 5% of patients with trichotillomania also meet diagnostic criteria for post-traumatic stress disorder (PTSD). Hoarding disorder has been associated with unmanaged stress following the sudden loss of a loved one, divorce, or other significant life stressors (Mayo Clinic, 2021).

Biological Aspects

- ***Genetics:*** Twin studies and family studies support a genetic susceptibility for OCD, especially in childhood onset OCD (Stein & Lochner, 2017). Trichotillomania has commonly been associated with OCDs among first-degree relatives, leading researchers to conclude that the disorder has a possible hereditary or familial predisposition. Structural abnormalities in various areas of the brain, as well as alterations in the serotonin and endogenous opioid systems, have also been noted.

Genetics also may play a role in the development of hoarding disorder. Family and twin studies indicate that approximately 50% of individuals who hoard report having a relative who also hoards (APA, 2022).

- ***Neuroanatomy:*** Recent findings suggest that neurobiological disturbances may play a role in the pathogenesis and maintenance of OCD. Abnormalities in various regions of the brain have been implicated in the neurobiology of OCD. Neuroimaging and neurocognitive assessment have identified impairment in motor inhibition responses (the ability to stop an action once initiated) in patients with OCD and trichotillomania (Kaplan, 2012). In individuals with hoarding disorder, neuroimaging studies have indicated blunted activity in the cingulate cortex (particularly the insula), the area of the brain that connects the emotional part of the brain with the parts that control higher-level thinking and insular and anterior cingulate cortex overengagement during possession-related choices (Stevens et al., 2020).
- ***Biochemical Factors:*** Dopaminergic, serotonergic, and glutamate systems have all been implicated in the etiology of obsessive-compulsive behaviors. Drugs that have been used successfully in alleviating the symptoms of OCD include clomipramine (a tricyclic antidepressant) and SSRIs, which are believed to block the neuronal reuptake of serotonin, thereby potentiating serotonergic activity in the central nervous system (see Figure 18–1). The serotonergic system may also be a factor in the etiology of body dysmorphic disorder. This relationship between OCD and serotonin levels is suggested by the high incidence of comorbidity with major mood disorder and anxiety disorder and the positive responsiveness of the condition to the serotonin-specific drugs.

  Genome studies have implicated glutamatergic function in OCD, but more research is needed (Stein & Lochner, 2017).

Assessment Scales

A number of assessment rating scales are available for measuring severity of anxiety symptoms. Some are meant to be clinician administered, whereas others may be self-administered. Examples of self-rating scales include the Beck Anxiety Inventory and the Zung Self-Rated Anxiety Scale. One of the most widely used clinician-administered scales is the Hamilton Anxiety Rating Scale (HAM-A), which is used in both clinical and research settings. The scale consists of 14 items and measures both psychic and somatic anxiety symptoms (psychological distress and physical complaints associated with anxiety). The HAM-A scale is presented in Box 18–5.

Diagnosis and Outcome Identification

Nursing diagnoses are formulated from the data gathered during the assessment phase and with background knowledge regarding predisposing factors to the disorder. Table 18–2 presents a list of patient behaviors and the NANDA International (NANDA-I) nursing diagnoses (Herdman et al., 2021) that correspond to those behaviors, which may be used in planning care for patients with anxiety, obsessive-compulsive, and related disorders.

Outcome Criteria

The following criteria may be used for measurement of outcomes in the care of the patient with anxiety disorders. The patient:

- Is able to recognize signs of escalating anxiety and intervene before reaching panic level *(panic and generalized anxiety disorders).*
- Is able to maintain anxiety at manageable level and make independent decisions about life situation *(panic and generalized anxiety disorders).*
- Functions adaptively in the presence of the phobic object or situation without experiencing panic anxiety *(phobic disorder).*
- Verbalizes a plan of action for responding in the presence of the phobic object or situation without developing panic anxiety *(phobic disorder).*
- Is able to maintain anxiety at a manageable level without resorting to the use of ritualistic behavior *(OCD).*
- Demonstrates adaptive coping strategies for dealing with anxiety instead of ritualistic behaviors *(OCD).*
- Verbalizes a realistic perception of personal appearance and expresses feelings that reflect a positive body image *(body dysmorphic disorder).*
- Verbalizes and demonstrates more adaptive strategies for coping with stressful situations *(trichotillomania).*

BOX 18–5 Hamilton Anxiety Rating Scale (HAM-A)

Below are descriptions of symptoms commonly associated with anxiety. Assign the client the rating between 0 and 4 (for each of the 14 items) that best describes the extent to which he/she has these symptoms.
0 = Not present, 1 = Mild, 2 = Moderate, 3 = Severe, 4 = Very severe

1. **Anxious mood** _____ Worries, anticipation of the worst, fearful anticipation, irritability	8. **Somatic (sensory)** _____ Tinnitus, blurred vision, hot/cold flushes, feelings of weakness, tingling sensation
2. **Tension** _____ Feelings of tension, fatigability, startle response, moved to tears easily, trembling, feelings of restlessness, inability to relax	9. **Cardiovascular symptoms** _____ Tachycardia, palpitations, pain in chest, throbbing of vessels, feeling faint
3. **Fears** _____ Of dark, of strangers, of being left alone, of animals, of traffic, of crowds	10. **Respiratory symptoms** _____ Pressure or constriction in chest, choking feelings, sighing, dyspnea
4. **Insomnia** _____ Difficulty in falling asleep, broken sleep, unsatisfying sleep and fatigue on waking, dreams, nightmares, night terrors	11. **Gastrointestinal symptoms** _____ Difficulty swallowing, flatulence, abdominal pain and fullness, burning sensations, nausea/vomiting, borborygmi, diarrhea, constipation, weight loss
5. **Intellectual** _____ Difficulty in concentration, poor memory	12. **Genitourinary symptoms** _____ Urinary frequency, urinary urgency, amenorrhea, menorrhagia, loss of libido, premature ejaculation, impotence
6. **Depressed mood** _____ Loss of interest, lack of pleasure in hobbies, depression, early waking, diurnal swing	13. **Autonomic symptoms** _____ Dry mouth, flushing, pallor, tendency to sweat, giddiness, tension headache
7. **Somatic (muscular)** _____ Pains and aches, twitching, stiffness, myoclonic jerks, grinding of teeth, unsteady voice, increased muscular tone	14. **Behavior at interview** _____ Fidgeting, restlessness or pacing, tremor of hands, furrowed brow, strained face, sighing or rapid respiration, facial pallor, swallowing, clearing throat
Client's Total Score _____	

SCORING
14 – 17 = Mild Anxiety
18 – 24 = Moderate Anxiety
25 – 30 = Severe Anxiety

Source: Hamilton (1959). The HAM-A is in the public domain.

Planning and Implementation

Table 18–3 provides a plan of care for the patient with anxiety, obsessive-compulsive, and related disorders. Nursing diagnoses are presented, along with outcome criteria, appropriate nursing interventions, and rationales for each.

Concept Care Mapping

The concept map care plan (see Chapter 6) is a diagrammatic teaching and learning strategy that allows visualization of interrelationships between medical diagnoses, nursing diagnoses, assessment data, and treatments. An example of a concept map care plan for the patient with an anxiety disorder is presented in Figure 18–3.

Patient and Family Education

The role of patient-teacher is important in the psychiatric area, as it is in all areas of nursing. A list of topics for patient and family education relevant to anxiety disorders is presented in Box 18–6.

Text continued on page 495

TABLE 18–2 Assigning Nursing Diagnoses to Behaviors Commonly Associated With Anxiety, Obsessive-Compulsive, and Related Disorders

BEHAVIORS	NURSING DIAGNOSES
Palpitations, trembling, sweating, chest pain, shortness of breath, fear of going crazy, fear of dying (panic disorder); excessive worry, difficulty concentrating, sleep disturbance (generalized anxiety disorder)	**Anxiety (severe/panic)**
Verbal expressions of having no control over life situation; nonparticipation in decision making related to own care or life situation; expressions of doubt regarding role performance (panic and generalized anxiety disorders)	**Powerlessness**
Behavior directed toward avoidance of a feared object or situation (phobic disorder)	**Fear**
Stays at home alone, afraid to venture out alone (agoraphobia)	**Social isolation**
Ritualistic behavior, obsessive thoughts, inability to meet basic needs; severe level of anxiety (obsessive-compulsive disorder)	**Ineffective coping**
Inability to fulfill usual patterns of responsibility because of need to perform rituals (obsessive-compulsive disorder)	**Ineffective role performance**
Preoccupation with imagined defect; verbalizations that are out of proportion to any actual physical abnormality that may exist; numerous visits to plastic surgeons or dermatologists seeking relief (body dysmorphic disorder)	**Disturbed body image**
Repetitive and impulsive pulling out of one's hair (trichotillomania)	**Ineffective impulse control**

Table 18–3 | CARE PLAN FOR THE PATIENT WITH ANXIETY, OBSESSIVE-COMPULSIVE, AND RELATED DISORDERS

NURSING DIAGNOSIS: PANIC ANXIETY

RELATED TO: Real or perceived threat to biological integrity or self-concept

EVIDENCED BY: Any or all of the physical symptoms identified by the *DSM-5-TR*

OUTCOME CRITERIA	NURSING INTERVENTIONS	RATIONALE
Short-Term Goal ■ The patient will verbalize ways to intervene in escalating anxiety within 1 week. **Long-Term Goal** ■ By time of discharge from treatment, the patient will be able to recognize symptoms of onset of anxiety and intervene before reaching panic level.	1. Stay with the patient and offer reassurance of safety and security. Do not leave the patient in panic anxiety alone.	1. The patient may fear for their life. Presence of a trusted individual provides a feeling of security and assurance of personal safety.
	2. Maintain a calm, nonthreatening, matter-of-fact approach.	2. Anxiety is contagious and may be transferred from staff to patient or vice versa. Patient's sense of security is promoted in the presence of a calm staff person.
	3. Use simple words and brief messages, spoken calmly and clearly, to explain hospital experiences.	3. In an intensely anxious situation, the patient is unable to comprehend anything but the most elemental communication.

Table 18–3 | CARE PLAN FOR THE PATIENT WITH ANXIETY, OBSESSIVE-COMPULSIVE, AND RELATED DISORDERS—cont'd

OUTCOME CRITERIA	NURSING INTERVENTIONS	RATIONALE
	4. Hyperventilation may occur during periods of extreme anxiety. Hyperventilation causes the amount of carbon dioxide (CO_2) in the blood to decrease, possibly resulting in lightheadedness, rapid heart rate, shortness of breath, numbness or tingling in the hands or feet, and syncope. If hyperventilation occurs, assist the patient to breathe into a small paper bag held over the mouth and nose. Six to 12 natural breaths should be taken, alternating with short periods of diaphragmatic breathing.	4. Hyperventilation may result in injury to the patient, and patient safety is a nursing priority. The technique here should not be used with patients who have coronary or respiratory disorders, such as coronary artery disease, asthma, or chronic obstructive pulmonary disease.
	5. Keep immediate surroundings low in stimuli (dim lighting, few people, simple decor).	5. A stimulating environment may increase level of anxiety.
	6. Administer tranquilizing medication, as ordered by physician. Assess for effectiveness and for side effects.	6. Antianxiety medication provides relief from the immobilizing effects of anxiety.
	7. When level of anxiety has been reduced, explore possible reasons for occurrence.	7. Recognition of precipitating factor(s) is the first step in teaching the patient to interrupt escalation of anxiety.
	8. Teach signs and symptoms of escalating anxiety and ways to interrupt its progression (relaxation techniques, such as deep-breathing exercises and meditation, or physical exercise, such as brisk walks and jogging).	8. Relaxation techniques result in a physiological response opposite that of the anxiety response. Physical activities discharge excess energy in a healthful manner.

NURSING DIAGNOSIS: FEAR

RELATED TO: Causing embarrassment to self in front of others, being in a place from which one is unable to escape, or a specific stimulus

EVIDENCED BY: Behavior directed toward avoidance of the feared object or situation

OUTCOME CRITERIA	NURSING INTERVENTIONS	RATIONALE
Short-Term Goal ■ Patient will discuss the phobic object or situation with the health-care provider within (time specified).	1. Reassure the patient that they are safe.	1. At the panic level of anxiety, the patient may fear for their life.
	2. Explore the patient's perception of the threat to physical integrity or threat to self-concept.	2. It is important to understand the patient's perception of the phobic object or situation to assist with the desensitization process.

Continued

Table 18–3 | CARE PLAN FOR THE PATIENT WITH ANXIETY, OBSESSIVE-COMPULSIVE, AND RELATED DISORDERS—cont'd

OUTCOME CRITERIA	NURSING INTERVENTIONS	RATIONALE
Long-Term Goal ■ By time of discharge from treatment, patient will be able to function in presence of phobic object or situation without experiencing panic anxiety.	3. Discuss reality of the situation with the patient to recognize aspects that can be changed and those that cannot.	3. The patient must accept the reality of the situation (aspects that cannot change) before the work of reducing the fear can progress.
	4. Include the patient in making decisions related to selection of alternative coping strategies (e.g., patient may choose either to avoid the phobic stimulus or to attempt to eliminate the fear associated with it).	4. Allowing the patient choices provides a measure of control and serves to increase feelings of self-worth.
	5. If the patient elects to work on elimination of the fear, techniques of desensitization or implosion therapy may be employed. (See explanation of these techniques under "Treatment Modalities" at the end of this chapter.)	5. Fear is decreased as the physical and psychological sensations diminish in response to repeated exposure to the phobic stimulus under nonthreatening conditions.
	6. Encourage the patient to explore underlying feelings that may be contributing to irrational fears and to face them rather than suppress them.	6. Exploring underlying feelings may help the patient to confront unresolved conflicts and develop more adaptive coping abilities.

NURSING DIAGNOSIS: INEFFECTIVE COPING

RELATED TO: Underdeveloped ego, punitive superego; avoidance learning; possible biochemical changes

EVIDENCED BY: Ritualistic behavior or obsessive thoughts

OUTCOME CRITERIA	NURSING INTERVENTIONS	RATIONALE
Short-Term Goal ■ Within 1 week, the patient will decrease participation in ritualistic behavior by half.	1. Work with the patient to determine types of situations that increase anxiety and result in ritualistic behaviors.	1. Recognition of precipitating factors is the first step in teaching the patient to interrupt the escalating anxiety.
Long-Term Goal ■ By time of discharge from treatment, patient will demonstrate ability to cope effectively without resorting to obsessive-compulsive behaviors.	2. In the beginning of treatment, allow plenty of time for rituals. Do not be judgmental or verbalize disapproval of the behavior.	2. To deny the patient this activity may precipitate panic anxiety. Conversely, indulging the patient's need for ritualistic behavior initially decreases anxiety and promotes the ability to learn alternative coping strategies. Learning is best accomplished when the patient's anxiety is at a mild level.

Table 18–3 | CARE PLAN FOR THE PATIENT WITH ANXIETY, OBSESSIVE-COMPULSIVE, AND RELATED DISORDERS—cont'd

OUTCOME CRITERIA	NURSING INTERVENTIONS	RATIONALE
	3. Support the patient's efforts to explore the meaning and purpose of the behavior.	3. The patient may be unaware of the relationship between emotional problems and compulsive behaviors. Recognition is important before change can occur.
	4. Provide structured schedule of activities for the patient, including adequate time for completion of rituals.	4. Structure provides a feeling of security for the anxious patient.
	5. Gradually begin to limit amount of time allotted for ritualistic behavior as the patient becomes more involved in other activities.	5. Anxiety is minimized when the patient is able to replace ritualistic behaviors with more adaptive ones.
	6. Give positive reinforcement for nonritualistic behaviors.	6. Positive reinforcement enhances self-esteem and encourages repetition of desired behaviors.
	7. Help the patient learn ways of interrupting obsessive thoughts and ritualistic behavior with techniques such as thought stopping, relaxation, and physical exercise.	7. Knowledge and practice of coping techniques that are more adaptive will help the patient change and let go of maladaptive responses to anxiety.

NURSING DIAGNOSIS: DISTURBED BODY IMAGE

RELATED TO: Repressed severe anxiety

EVIDENCED BY: Preoccupation with imagined defect; verbalizations that are out of proportion to any actual physical abnormality that may exist; and numerous visits to plastic surgeons or dermatologists seeking relief

OUTCOME CRITERIA	NURSING INTERVENTIONS	RATIONALE
Short-Term Goal ■ Patient will verbalize understanding that changes in bodily structure or function are exaggerated out of proportion to the change that actually exists. (Time frame for this goal must be determined according to individual patient's situation.) **Long-Term Goal** ■ Patient will verbalize perception of own body that is realistic to actual structure or function by time of discharge from treatment.	1. Assess the patient's perception of body image. Keep in mind that this image is real to the patient.	1. Assessment information is necessary in developing an accurate plan of care. Denial of the patient's feelings impedes the development of a trusting, therapeutic relationship.
	2. Help the patient to see that their body image is distorted or that it is out of proportion in relation to the significance of an actual physical anomaly.	2. Recognition that a misperception exists is necessary before the patient can accept reality and reduce the significance of the imagined defect.
	3. Encourage verbalization of fears and anxieties associated with identified stressful life situations. Discuss alternative adaptive coping strategies.	3. Verbalization of feelings with a trusted individual may help the patient come to terms with unresolved issues. Knowledge of alternative coping strategies may help the patient respond to stress more adaptively in the future.

Continued

Table 18–3 | CARE PLAN FOR THE PATIENT WITH ANXIETY, OBSESSIVE-COMPULSIVE, AND RELATED DISORDERS—cont'd

OUTCOME CRITERIA	NURSING INTERVENTIONS	RATIONALE
	4. Involve the patient in activities that reinforce a positive sense of self not based on appearance.	4. When the patient is able to develop self-satisfaction based on accomplishments and unconditional acceptance, significance of the imagined defect or minor physical anomaly will diminish.
	5. Make referrals to support groups of individuals with similar histories (e.g., Adult Children of Alcoholics [ACoA], Victims of Incest, Survivors of Suicide [SOS], Adults Abused as Children).	5. Having a support group of understanding, empathic peers can help the patient accept the reality of the situation, correct distorted perceptions, and make adaptive life changes.

NURSING DIAGNOSIS: INEFFECTIVE IMPULSE CONTROL

RELATED TO: Possible genetic or biochemical factors; poor parent-child relationship; history of child abuse or neglect

EVIDENCED BY: Recurrent pulling out of the hair in response to stressful situations

OUTCOME CRITERIA	NURSING INTERVENTIONS	RATIONALE
Short-Term Goal ■ Patient will verbalize adaptive ways to cope with stress by means other than pulling out own hair (time dimension to be individually determined).	1. Support the patient in efforts to stop hair pulling. Help the patient understand that it is possible to discontinue the behavior.	1. Patients realize that the behavior is maladaptive but feels helpless to stop. Support from the nurse builds trust.
	2. Ensure that a nonjudgmental attitude is conveyed, and criticism of the behavior is avoided.	2. An attitude of acceptance promotes feelings of dignity and self-worth.
Long-Term Goal ■ Patient will be able to demonstrate adaptive coping strategies in response to stress and a discontinuation of pulling out own hair (time dimension to be individually determined).	3. Assist the patient with habit reversal training (HRT). Three components of HRT include the following: a. Awareness training. Help the patient become aware of times when the hair pulling most often occurs (e.g., client learns to recognize urges, thoughts, or sensations that precede the behavior; the therapist points out to the patient each time the behavior occurs).	3. HRT has been shown to be an effective tool in treatment of hair-pulling disorder. a. This helps the patient identify situations in which the behavior occurs or is most likely to occur. Awareness gives the patient a feeling of increased self-control.
	b. Competing response training. In this step, the patient learns to substitute another response to the urge to pull their hair. For example, when a patient experiences a hair-pulling urge, suggest that the individual ball up his/her hands into fists, tightening arm muscles, and "locking" his/her arms so as to make hair pulling impossible at that moment.	b. Substituting an incompatible behavior may help to extinguish the undesirable behavior.

Table 18–3 | CARE PLAN FOR THE PATIENT WITH ANXIETY, OBSESSIVE-COMPULSIVE, AND RELATED DISORDERS—cont'd

OUTCOME CRITERIA	NURSING INTERVENTIONS	RATIONALE
	c. Social support. Encourage family members to participate in the therapy process and to offer positive feedback for attempts at habit reversal.	c. Positive feedback enhances self-esteem and increases patient's desire to continue with the therapy. It also provides cues for family members to use in their attempts to help the patient in treatment.
	4. Once the patient has become aware of hair-pulling times, suggest that patient hold something (a ball, paperweight, or other item) in their hand at times when hair pulling is anticipated.	4. This would help to prevent behaviors occurring without the patient being aware that they are happening.
	5. Practice stress management techniques: deep breathing, meditation, stretching, physical exercise, listening to soft music.	5. Hair pulling is thought to occur at times of increased anxiety.
	6. Offer support and encouragement when setbacks occur. Help the patient to understand the importance of not quitting when it seems that change is not happening as quickly as they would like.	6. Although some people see a decrease in the behavior within a few days, most will take several months to notice the greatest change.

Evaluation

In the final step of the nursing process, a reassessment is conducted in order to determine whether the nursing actions have been successful in achieving the objectives of care. Evaluation of the nursing actions for the patient with an anxiety, OCD, or related disorder may be facilitated by asking, can the patient:

- Recognize signs and symptoms of escalating anxiety?
- Use skills learned to interrupt the escalating anxiety before it reaches the panic level?
- Demonstrate the most appropriate activities that can be used to maintain anxiety at a manageable level (e.g., relaxation techniques, physical exercise)?
- Maintain anxiety at a manageable level without medication?
- Verbalize a long-term plan for preventing panic anxiety in the face of a stressful situation?
- Discuss the phobic object or situation without becoming anxious?
- Function in the presence of the phobic object or situation without experiencing panic anxiety?
- Refrain from performing rituals when anxiety level rises?
- Demonstrate substitute behaviors to maintain anxiety at a manageable level?
- Recognize the relationship between escalating anxiety and the dependence on ritualistic behaviors for relief?
- Refrain from hair pulling? (for patients with trichotillomania)
- Successfully substitute a more adaptive behavior when urges to pull hair occur? (for patients with trichotillomania)
- Verbalize a realistic perception and satisfactory acceptance of personal appearance? (for patients with body dysmorphic disorder)

Treatment Modalities

Individual Psychotherapy

Most clients experience a marked decrease in anxiety when given the opportunity to discuss their difficulties with a concerned and sympathetic therapist.

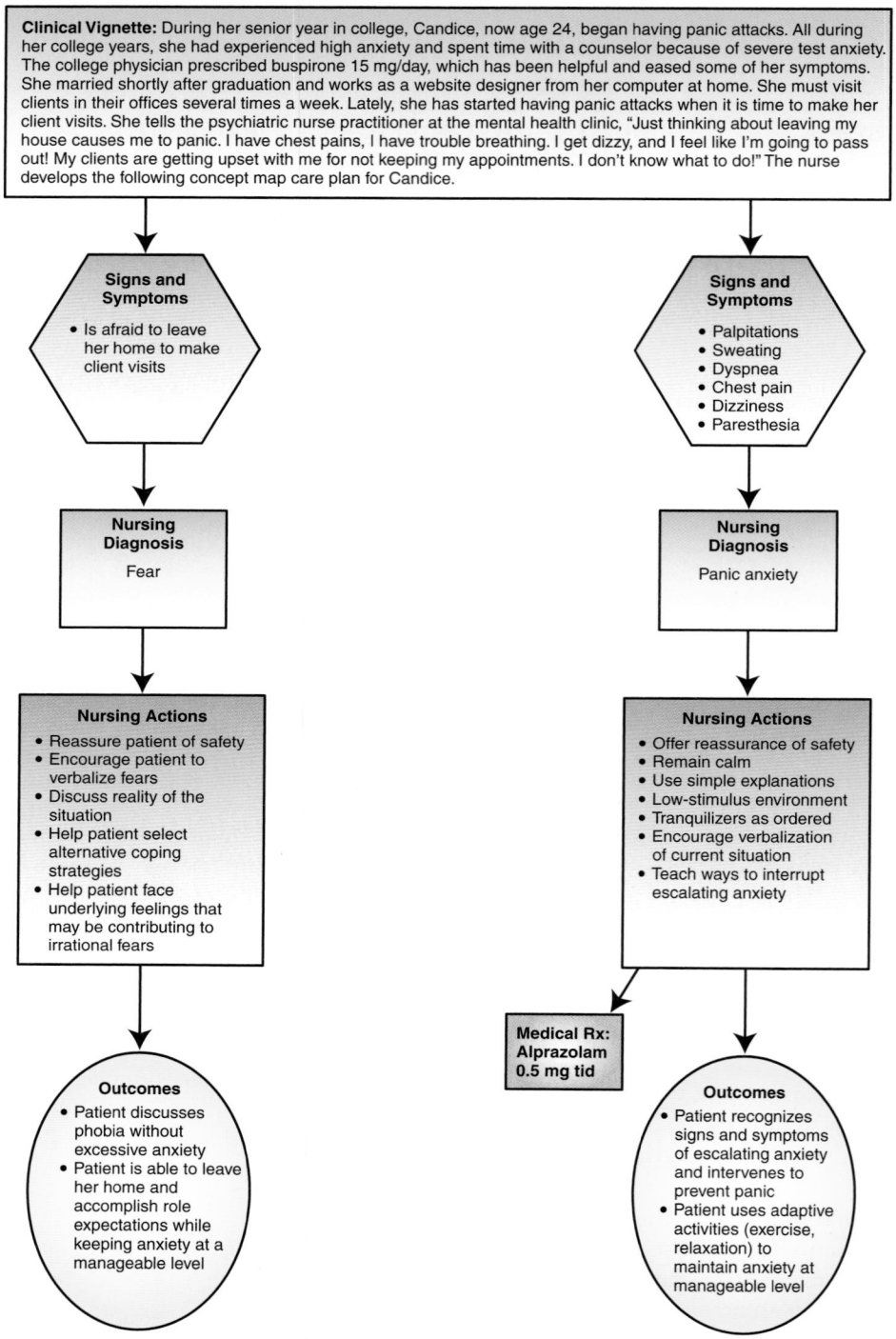

FIGURE 18–3 Concept map care plan for a patient with agoraphobia.

BOX 18–6 Topics for Patient and Family Education Related to Anxiety, OCD, and Related Disorders

NATURE OF THE ILLNESS

1. What is anxiety?
2. To what might it be related?
3. What is OCD?
4. What is body dysmorphic disorder?
5. What is trichotillomania?
6. Symptoms of anxiety disorders.

MANAGEMENT OF THE ILLNESS

1. Medication Management:
   - Possible adverse effects
   - Length of time to take effect
   - What to expect from the medication
   - a. For panic disorder and generalized anxiety disorder
     - 1) Benzodiazepines
     - 2) Buspirone (BuSpar)
     - 3) Tricyclics
     - 4) SSRIs
     - 5) SNRIs
     - 6) Propranolol
     - 7) Clonidine
   - b. For phobic disorders
     - 1) Benzodiazepines
     - 2) Tricyclics
     - 3) Propranolol
     - 4) SSRIs
   - c. For OCD
     - 1) SSRIs
     - 2) Clomipramine
   - d. For body dysmorphic disorder
     - 1) Clomipramine
     - 2) Fluoxetine
   - e. For hair-pulling disorder (trichotillomania)
     - 1) Chlorpromazine
     - 2) Amitriptyline
     - 3) Lithium carbonate
     - 4) SSRIs/pimozide
     - 5) Olanzapine
2. Stress management:
   - a. Teach ways to interrupt escalating anxiety
     - 1) Relaxation techniques
       - (a) Progressive muscle relaxation
       - (b) Imagery
       - (c) Music
       - (d) Meditation
       - (e) Yoga
       - (f) Physical exercise

SUPPORT SERVICES

1. Crisis hotline
2. Support groups
3. Individual psychotherapy

Supportive psychotherapy is designed to help clients identify their personal strengths and explore adaptive coping mechanisms. Insight-oriented psychotherapy, which is rooted in Freudian psychology, is designed to help clients identify, explore, and resolve internal psychological conflicts that are contributing to anxiety.

The psychotherapist also can use logical and rational explanations to increase the client's understanding about various situations that create anxiety. Psychoeducational information may also be presented in individual psychotherapy.

Cognitive Behavior Therapy (CBT)

The cognitive model relates how individuals respond in stressful situations to their subjective cognitive appraisal of the event. Anxiety is experienced when an individual's cognitive appraisal signifies danger with which they are unable to cope. Impaired cognition can contribute to anxiety and related disorders when appraisals are chronically negative. Automatic negative appraisals provoke self-doubts, negative evaluations, and negative predictions. Anxiety is maintained by this dysfunctional appraisal of a situation.

Cognitive behavior therapy strives to assist the individual in reducing anxiety responses by altering cognitive distortions. Anxiety is described as resulting from exaggerated, *automatic* thinking.

Cognitive behavior therapy for anxiety is brief and time limited, usually lasting from 5 to 20 sessions. Brief therapy discourages the client's dependency on the therapist, which is prevalent in anxiety disorders, and encourages the client's self-sufficiency.

A sound therapeutic relationship is a necessary condition for effective CBT. For the therapeutic process to occur, the client must be able to talk openly about fears and feelings. A major component of treatment consists of encouraging the client to face frightening situations in order to view them realistically, and talking about them is one way of achieving this goal. Treatment is a collaborative effort between client and therapist.

Rather than offering suggestions and explanations, the therapist uses questions to encourage the client to correct anxiety-producing thoughts. The client is encouraged to become aware of the thoughts, examine them for cognitive distortions, substitute more balanced thoughts, and eventually develop new patterns of thinking.

Cognitive behavior therapy is structured and orderly, which is important for the client with an anxiety or related disorder who is often confused and lacks self-assurance. The focus is on solving current problems. Together, the client and therapist work to identify and correct maladaptive thoughts and behaviors that maintain a problem and block its solution.

Cognitive behavior therapy is based on education. The premise is that anxiety develops because of learned, inappropriate ways of thinking about and responding to life experiences. The belief is that with practice, individuals can learn more effective ways of responding to these experiences through cognitive reframing. Homework assignments, a central feature of cognitive therapy, provide an experimental, problem-solving approach to overcoming long-held anxieties. Through fulfillment of these personal "experiments," the effectiveness of specific strategies and techniques is determined.

Behavior Therapy

Behavior modification has been used to treat trichotillomania. Various techniques have been used, including covert desensitization and **habit reversal training** (HRT). These may include a system of positive and negative reinforcements in an effort to modify the hair-pulling behaviors. With HRT, in an attempt to extinguish the unwanted behavior, the individual learns to become more aware of the hair pulling, identifies times of occurrence, and substitutes a more adaptive coping strategy. (See interventions listed under the nursing diagnosis "Ineffective Impulse Control.")

Other forms of behavior therapy include systematic desensitization and implosion therapy (flooding). They are commonly used to treat clients with phobic disorders and to modify the stereotyped behavior of clients with OCD. They have also been shown to be effective in a variety of other anxiety-producing situations.

Systematic Desensitization

In **systematic desensitization,** the client is gradually exposed to the phobic stimulus, in either a real or an imagined situation. The concept was introduced by Joseph Wolpe in 1958 and is based on behavioral conditioning principles. Emphasis is placed on reciprocal inhibition or counterconditioning.

Reciprocal inhibition is described as the restriction of anxiety prior to the effort of reducing avoidance behavior. The rationale behind this concept is that because relaxation is antagonistic to anxiety, individuals cannot be anxious and relaxed at the same time.

Systematic desensitization with reciprocal inhibition involves two main elements:

1. Training in relaxation techniques
2. Progressive exposure to a hierarchy of fear stimuli while in the relaxed state

The individual is instructed to use relaxation techniques that they find most effective (e.g., progressive relaxation, mental imagery, tense and relax, meditation). When the individual has mastered the relaxation technique, exposure to the phobic stimulus is initiated. The client is asked to present a hierarchal list of situations involving the phobic stimulus in order from most disturbing to least disturbing. While in a state of maximum relaxation, the client may be asked to imagine the phobic stimulus. Initial exposure is focused on a concept of the phobic stimulus that produces the least amount of fear or anxiety. In subsequent sessions, the individual is gradually exposed to stimuli that are more fearful. Sessions may be executed in fantasy, in real-life *(in vivo)* situations, or sometimes in a combination of both. Following is a case study describing systematic desensitization.

CASE STUDY

SYSTEMATIC DESENSITIZATION

Carlos was afraid to ride on elevators. He had been known to climb 24 flights of stairs in an office building to avoid riding the elevator. Carlos's office had plans to move the company to a high-rise building soon with offices on the 32nd floor. Carlos sought assistance from a therapist for help to treat this fear. He was taught to achieve a sense of calmness and well-being by using a combination of mental imagery and progressive relaxation techniques. In the relaxed state, Carlos was initially instructed to imagine the entry level of his office building with a clear image of the bank of elevators. In subsequent sessions, and always in the relaxed state, Carlos progressed to images of walking onto an elevator, having the elevator door close after he had entered, riding the elevator to the 32nd floor, and emerging from the elevator once the doors were opened. The progression included being accompanied in the activities by the therapist and eventually accomplishing them alone.

Therapy for Carlos also included in vivo sessions in which he was exposed to the phobic stimulus in real-life situations (always after achieving a state of relaxation). This technique, combining imagined and in vivo procedures, proved successful for Carlos, and his employment in the high-rise complex was no longer in jeopardy because of his fear of elevators.

Implosion Therapy (Flooding)

Implosion therapy, or **flooding,** is a therapeutic process in which clients, for a prolonged period, must imagine situations or participate in real-life situations they find extremely frightening.

In implosion therapy, the therapist "floods" the client with information concerning situations that trigger the client's anxiety by describing anxiety-provoking situations in vivid detail. The more anxiety is provoked, the more expedient the therapeutic endeavor. The same theme is continued for as long as it arouses anxiety. The therapy concludes when a topic no longer elicits inappropriate anxiety on the part of the client.

Other Nonpharmacological Treatments for Anxiety

Many treatment modalities are available that may be used alone or in combination with medication to treat anxiety. Examples include deep-breathing exercises, progressive muscle relaxation, imagery, mindfulness meditation, and exercise. (See Chapter 7, "Psychosocial Interventions and Spiritual Care," for further discussion of these topics.)

Psychopharmacology

Antianxiety Agents

Antianxiety drugs are also called *anxiolytics* and historically were referred to as *minor tranquilizers.* Antianxiety agents are used in the treatment of anxiety disorders, anxiety symptoms, acute alcohol withdrawal, skeletal muscle spasms, convulsive disorders, status epilepticus, and preoperative sedation. Their use and efficacy for periods greater than 4 months have not been evaluated.

Benzodiazepines have been the traditional medication used for the treatment of acute anxiety states. By reducing anxiety, they allow learning and adaptation to take place. However, because they also have the potential for dependence, they are typically a short-term intervention. In addition, they pose certain risks for some patients, including those who are pregnant; the elderly; those who have current or past substance use disorders; current users of prescribed opioids (risk of respiratory depression and death); and patients with chronic obstructive pulmonary disease (Weber & Duchemin, 2018). Buspirone and SSRIs have demonstrated efficacy in treating anxiety disorders as well and have the added benefit of not being addictive chemicals. (See Chapter 4, "Psychopharmacology," for a detailed description of contraindications, precautions, and other safety issues for these medications.)

Several drugs can be used off-label to treat anxiety, including atypical antipsychotics; mirtazapine (a tetracyclic antidepressant); gabapentin or pregabalin (analgesic and mood stabilizer that also carries a risk for dependence); antihistamines such as diphenhydramine; and other anticonvulsants such as lamotrigine and topiramate (Weber & Duchemin, 2018). Selected antianxiety agents are presented in Table 18–4.

Medications for Specific Disorders

For Panic and Generalized Anxiety Disorders

Anxiolytics

Benzodiazepines have been used with success in the treatment of GAD. They can be prescribed on an as-needed basis when the client is feeling particularly anxious. Alprazolam, lorazepam, and clonazepam have been particularly effective in the treatment of panic disorder. The major risks with benzodiazepine therapy are physical dependence and tolerance, which may encourage abuse. Because withdrawal symptoms can be life threatening, clients must be warned against abrupt discontinuation of the drug and should be tapered off the medication at the end of therapy. Because of this addiction potential, their use as first-line treatment has been surpassed in favor by SSRIs, serotonin and norepinephrine reuptake inhibitors (SNRIs), and buspirone.

The antianxiety agent buspirone is effective for the treatment of GAD (Boland & Verduin, 2022). One disadvantage of buspirone is its lag period (similar to antidepressants) in alleviating symptoms. However, the benefit of lack of physical dependence and tolerance with buspirone may make it the drug of choice in the treatment of GAD.

Antidepressants

Several antidepressants are effective as major antianxiety agents. The tricyclics clomipramine and imipramine have been used with success in clients experiencing panic disorder. However, since the advent of SSRIs, the tricyclics are less widely used because of their tendency to produce severe side effects at the high doses required to relieve symptoms of panic disorder.

The SSRIs have been effective in the treatment of panic disorder. Paroxetine, fluoxetine, and sertraline have been approved by the U.S. Food and Drug Administration (FDA) for this purpose. Venlafaxine, an SNRI, is also FDA approved for the treatment of panic disorder. Clients with panic disorder appear to be sensitive to treatment with antidepressants, so doses are typically lower initially and titrated slowly.

TABLE 18–4 **Antianxiety Agents**

CLASSIFICATION: GENERIC (TRADE) NAME	HALF-LIFE (HR)	DAILY ADULT DOSAGE RANGE (MG)	COMMON SIDE EFFECTS OF ANTIANXIETY AGENTS
ANTIHISTAMINES			
Hydroxyzine (Vistaril)	(3)	100–400	■ Drowsiness, confusion, lethargy. ■ Tolerance; physical and psychological dependence (does not apply to buspirone or hydroxyzine). Client should be tapered off long-term use. ■ Potentiates the effects of other CNS depressants. Client should not take alcohol or other CNS depressants with the medication. ■ May aggravate symptoms of depression. ■ Orthostatic hypotension. Client should rise slowly from lying or sitting position. ■ Paradoxical excitement. If symptoms opposite of desired effect occur, notify physician immediately. ■ Dry mouth. ■ Nausea and vomiting. May be taken with food or milk. ■ Blood dyscrasias. Symptoms of sore throat, fever, malaise, easy bruising, or unusual bleeding should be reported to the physician immediately. ■ Delayed onset (with buspirone). Lag time of 10 to 14 days for anxiety symptoms to diminish with buspirone. Buspirone is not recommended for prn administration.
BENZODIAZEPINES			
Alprazolam (Xanax, Niravam)	(6.3–26.9)	0.75–4	
Chlordiazepoxide (Librium)	(5–30)	15–100	
Clonazepam (Klonopin)	(18–50)	1.5–20	
Clorazepate (Tranxene)	(40–50)	15–60	
Diazepam (Valium, Diastat)	(20–80)	4–40	
Lorazepam (Ativan)	(10–20)	2–6	
Oxazepam (Serax)	(5–20)	30–120	
Midazolam (Versed)*	(1.8–6.4) (by mouth)	5	
CARBAMATE DERIVATIVE			
Meprobamate (Miltown, Equanil)	(6–17)	400–1,600	
AZASPIRODECANEDION			
Buspirone (BuSpar)	(14)	15–60	

*Primarily used for preoperative sedation, antianxiety, and conscious sedation.

SSRIs and SNRIs are considered first-line treatments for GAD. The FDA has approved paroxetine (Paxil), escitalopram (Lexapro), duloxetine (Cymbalta), and extended-release venlafaxine (Effexor XR) in the treatment of GAD. Atypical antidepressants such as nefazodone (Serzone) and mirtazapine (Remeron), although not FDA approved for anxiety disorder treatment, have also been identified as beneficial (Bhatt, 2019).

Antihypertensive Agents

Several studies have called attention to the effectiveness of beta blockers (e.g., propranolol) and alpha$_2$-receptor agonists (e.g., clonidine) in the amelioration of anxiety symptoms (Bhatt, 2019). Propranolol has potent effects on the somatic manifestations of anxiety (e.g., palpitations, tremors) with less dramatic effects on the psychic component of anxiety. It appears to be most effective in the treatment of acute situational anxiety (e.g., performance anxiety, test anxiety), but it is not the first-line drug of choice in the treatment of panic disorder and GAD. Propranolol also demonstrated effectiveness in reducing hyperarousal states for up to 1 week after patients with PTSD experienced a flashback (Bhatt, 2019).

Clonidine is effective in blocking the acute anxiety effects in conditions such as opioid and nicotine withdrawal. However, it has had limited usefulness in the long-term treatment of panic and generalized anxiety disorders, particularly because of the development of tolerance to its antianxiety effects.

Anticonvulsants

Pregabalin (Lyrica), which is a GABA derivative, may have benefits in treating anxiety disorders, but it is a Schedule V controlled substance and therefore may pose a risk for dependence or drug diversion.

For Phobic Disorders

Anxiolytics

The benzodiazepines have been successful in the treatment of SAD. They are well tolerated and have a rapid onset of action. However, because of their potential for abuse and dependence, they are not considered first-line choice of treatment.

Antidepressants

In recent years, SSRIs have become the first-line treatment of choice for SAD, and paroxetine and sertraline have been FDA approved for this purpose. Several other SSRIs and SNRIs have been used off-label to treat SAD, including fluoxetine, escitalopram, fluvoxamine, duloxetine, and venlafaxine (Garakani et al., 2020). Specific phobias are generally not treated with medication unless panic attacks accompany the phobia.

Antihypertensive Agents

The beta blockers propranolol and atenolol have been tried with success in clients experiencing anticipatory performance anxiety or "stage fright." This type of phobic response produces symptoms such as sweaty palms, racing pulse, trembling hands, dry mouth, labored breathing, nausea, and memory loss. The beta blockers appear to be quite effective in reducing these symptoms in some individuals.

Novel Treatments

Controlled trials for novel treatments including neuropeptides, glutamatergic agents (such as ketamine and D-cycloserine), and cannabinoids (including cannabidiol) primarily in GAD or SAD, have largely been negative, with only some promise for kava and PH94B (an inhaled neurosteroid) (Garakani et al., 2020).

For Obsessive-Compulsive Disorder

Antidepressants

The SSRIs fluoxetine, paroxetine, sertraline, and fluvoxamine have been approved by the FDA for the treatment of OCD. Doses in excess of what is effective for treating depression may be required for OCD. Common side effects include sleep disturbances, headache, and restlessness. These effects are often transient and are less troublesome than those of the tricyclics.

The tricyclic antidepressant clomipramine was the first drug approved by the FDA in the treatment of OCD. Clomipramine is more selective for serotonin reuptake than any of the other tricyclics. Its efficacy in the treatment of OCD is well established, although adverse effects, such as those associated with all the tricyclics, may make it less desirable than the SSRIs.

For Body Dysmorphic Disorder

Antidepressants

SSRIs are effective in treating body dysmorphic disorder but the effective doses are higher than those used to treat depression and the duration of treatment is longer (Boland & Verduin, 2022).

For Trichotillomania

No medications have demonstrated consistent benefits for clients with trichotillomania, but SSRIs have yielded moderate results for some clients with this condition (Elston, 2019).

CASE STUDY AND SAMPLE CARE PLAN

NURSING HISTORY AND ASSESSMENT

Stephanie is a 34-year-old mother of a 7-year-old girl named April. Stephanie's husband, Chris, brought her to the emergency department when she began complaining of chest pain and shortness of breath. Diagnostic testing ruled out cardiac problems, and Stephanie was referred for psychiatric evaluation.

Chris was present at the admission interview. He explained to the nurse that Stephanie has become increasingly "nervous and high strung" over the past few years. Four years ago, April, then 3 years old, was attending nursery school 2 days a week. April came down with a severe case of influenza that developed into pneumonia. She was hospitalized, and her prognosis was questionable for a short while, although she eventually made a complete recovery. Since that time, however, Stephanie has been extremely anxious about her family's health. She is fastidious about housekeeping and scrubs her floors three times a week. She launders the bedclothes daily and uses bleach on all the countertops and door handles several times a day. She washes the woodwork twice a week. She washes her hands incessantly, and they are red and noticeably chapped. Chris explained that Stephanie becomes very upset if she is not able to perform all of her cleaning "chores" according to her self-assigned schedule. This afternoon, April came home from school with a note from the teacher saying that a child in April's class had been diagnosed with a case of meningitis. Chris told the nurse, "Stephanie just lost it. She got all upset and started crying and had trouble breathing. Then she got those pains in her chest. That's when I brought her to the hospital." Stephanie is admitted to the psychiatric unit with a diagnosis of obsessive-compulsive disorder. The physician orders alprazolam 0.5 mg tid and paroxetine 20 mg every morning.

The night nurse finds her up at 2 a.m. scrubbing the shower with a hand towel. She refuses to sleep in the bed, stating that it must certainly be contaminated. When the day nurse makes morning rounds, she finds Stephanie in the bathroom washing her hands.

NURSING DIAGNOSES AND OUTCOME IDENTIFICATION

From the assessment data, the nurse develops the following nursing diagnoses for Stephanie:

1. **Panic anxiety** related to perceived threat to biological integrity evidenced by chest pain and shortness of breath
   a. **Short-Term Goal:** Stephanie will be able to relax with effects of medication.
   b. **Long-Term Goal:** Stephanie will be able to maintain anxiety at manageable level.
2. **Ineffective coping** related to panic anxiety and weak ego strength evidenced by compulsive cleaning and washing hands
   a. **Short-Term Goal:** Stephanie will reduce amount of time performing rituals within 3 days.
   b. **Long-Term Goal:** Stephanie will demonstrate ability to cope effectively without resorting to ritualistic behavior.

PLANNING AND IMPLEMENTATION

PANIC ANXIETY

The following nursing interventions have been identified for Stephanie:

1. Stay with Stephanie and reassure her that she is safe and that she is not going to die.
2. Maintain a calm, nonthreatening manner.
3. Speak very clearly, calmly, and use simple words and messages to communicate with Stephanie.
4. Keep the lights low and the noise level down as much as possible, and allow as few people in her environment as is necessary.
5. Administer the alprazolam and paroxetine as ordered by the physician. Monitor for effectiveness and side effects.
6. After several days, when the anxiety has subsided, discuss with her the reasons that precipitated this attack.
7. Teach her the signs that indicate her anxiety level is rising.
8. Teach strategies that Stephanie may employ to interrupt the escalation of the anxiety. She could choose which is best for her: relaxation exercises, physical exercise, meditation.

INEFFECTIVE COPING

The following nursing interventions have been identified for Stephanie:

1. Initially, allow Stephanie all the time she needs to wash her hands, straighten up her room, change her own sheets, and so on. To deny her these rituals would result in panic anxiety.
2. Initiate discussions with Stephanie about her behavior. She ultimately must come to understand that these rituals are her way of keeping her anxiety under control.
3. Within a couple of days, begin to limit the amount of time Stephanie may spend on her rituals. Assign her to groups and activities that take up her time and distract her from her obsessions.
4. Explore with Stephanie the types of situations that cause her anxiety to rise. Help her to correlate these times of increased anxiety to initiation of the ritualistic behavior.

CASE STUDY AND SAMPLE CARE PLAN—cont'd

5. Help her with problem-solving and with making decisions about more adaptive ways to respond to situations that cause her anxiety to rise.
6. Explore her fears surrounding the health of her daughter. Help her to recognize which fears are legitimate and which are irrational.
7. Discuss possible activities in which she may participate that may distract from obsessions about contamination. Make suggestions and encourage her to follow through. Examples may include enrollment in classes at the local community college, volunteer work at the local hospital, or part-time employment.
8. Explain to her that she will likely be discharged from the hospital with a prescription for paroxetine. Teach her about the medication, how it should be taken, possible side effects, and what to report to the physician.
9. Suggest that she may benefit from attendance in an anxiety disorder support group. If she is interested, help locate one that would be convenient and appropriate for her.

EVALUATION

The outcome criteria for Stephanie have been met. She has remained calm during her hospital stay with the use of the medication. The use of ritualistic behavior in the hospital setting diminished rapidly. She has discussed situations that she knows cause her anxiety to rise. She has learned relaxation exercises and practices them daily. Stephanie plans to start jogging and has the phone number for an anxiety support group that she plans to call. She says that she hopes the support group will help her maintain rationality about her daughter's health. She knows about paroxetine and plans to take it every morning.

Summary and Key Points

- Anxiety is a necessary force for survival and has been experienced by humanity throughout the ages.
- Anxiety was first described as a physiological disorder and identified by its physical symptoms, particularly cardiac symptoms. The psychological implications for the symptoms were not recognized until the early 1900s.
- Anxiety is considered a normal reaction to a realistic danger or threat to biological integrity or self-concept.
- The normality of the anxiety experienced in response to a stressor is defined by societal and cultural standards.
- Anxiety disorders are more common in women than in men by at least two to one.
- Studies of familial patterns suggest a moderate genetic vulnerability to anxiety disorders.
- The *DSM-5-TR* identifies several broad categories of anxiety and related disorders. They include panic and generalized anxiety disorders, phobic disorders, and obsessive-compulsive (OCD) and related disorders, such as body dysmorphic disorder and trichotillomania. Anxiety disorders may also be the result of other medical conditions and intoxication or withdrawal from substances.
- Panic disorder is characterized by recurrent panic attacks, manifested by intense apprehension, fear, and physical discomfort and the onset of which is unpredictable.
- Generalized anxiety disorder (GAD) is characterized by chronic, unrealistic, and excessive anxiety and worry.
- Social anxiety disorder (SAD) is an excessive fear of situations in which a person might do something embarrassing or be evaluated negatively by others.
- Specific phobia is a marked, persistent, and excessive or unreasonable fear when in the presence of, or when anticipating an encounter with, a specific object or situation.
- Agoraphobia is a fear of being in places or situations from which escape might be difficult or in which help might not be available in the event that the person becomes anxious.
- OCD involves recurrent obsessions or compulsions that are severe enough to interfere with social and occupational functioning.
- Body dysmorphic disorder is an exaggerated belief that the body is deformed or defective in some specific way.
- Trichotillomania (also known as hair-pulling disorder) is a disorder of impulse characterized by the recurrent pulling out of one's own hair that results in noticeable hair loss.
- Hoarding disorder is defined by the persistent difficulty of discarding or parting with possessions, regardless of their actual value.

- A number of elements, including genetic vulnerability, psychosocial factors, biological influences, and learning experiences contribute to the development of these disorders.
- Treatment of anxiety and related disorders includes individual psychotherapy, cognitive behavior therapy, behavior therapy (including implosion therapy, systematic desensitization, and habit reversal training [HRT]), and psychopharmacology.
- Nurses can help patients manage anxiety and related disorders through education, psychosocial interventions (such as relaxation exercises) and facilitating increased self-awareness in relation to their illness.
- Intervention focuses on assisting patients to learn techniques with which they may interrupt the escalation of anxiety before it reaches unmanageable proportions and to replace maladaptive behavior patterns with new, more adaptive coping skills.

Review Questions

Select the answer that is most appropriate for each of the following questions:

1. A client has been diagnosed with agoraphobia. Which behavior would be most characteristic of this disorder?
   a. The client experiences panic anxiety in the presence of snakes.
   b. The client refuses to fly in an airplane.
   c. The client fears public ridicule.
   d. The client stays at home for fear of being in a place from which they cannot escape.
2. Which of the following is the most appropriate therapy for a client with agoraphobia?
   a. 10 mg Valium qid
   b. Group therapy with other people with agoraphobia
   c. Facing fears in gradual step progression
   d. Hypnosis
3. With implosion therapy, a client with phobic anxiety would be:
   a. Taught relaxation exercises
   b. Subjected to graded intensities of the fear
   c. Instructed to stop the therapeutic session as soon as anxiety is experienced
   d. Presented with intense exposure to a variety of stimuli associated with the phobic object or situation
4. A client with OCD spends many hours each day washing their hands. Which is the most likely reason for washing hands so much?
   a. Relieve anxiety
   b. Reduce the probability of infection
   c. Reduce delusions
   d. Increase his self-concept
5. A client is receiving habit-reversal therapy. Which element would be included in this therapy? (Select all that apply.)
   a. Awareness training
   b. Competing response training
   c. Social support
   d. Hypnotherapy
   e. Aversive therapy

Clinical Judgment Questions

6. The *initial* care plan for a client with OCD who washes their hands obsessively would include which nursing intervention?
   a. Keep the client's bathroom locked so they cannot wash their hands all the time.
   b. Structure the client's schedule so that they have plenty of time for washing their hands.
   c. Place the client in isolation until they promise to stop washing their hands so much.
   d. Explain the client's behavior to them because they are probably unaware that it is maladaptive.

7. A client with OCD says to the nurse, "I've been here four days now, and I'm feeling better. I feel comfortable on this unit, and I'm not ill at ease with the staff or other clients anymore." In light of this change, which nursing intervention is most appropriate?
   a. Give attention to the ritualistic behaviors each time they occur and point out their inappropriateness.
   b. Ignore the ritualistic behaviors, and they will be eliminated for lack of reinforcement.
   c. Set limits on the amount of time the client may engage in the ritualistic behavior.
   d. Continue to allow the client time to carry out the ritualistic behavior.
8. A new client at the mental health clinic has been diagnosed with body dysmorphic disorder. Which nursing intervention is the priority?
   a. Support the client's efforts to seek corrective surgery.
   b. Recommend the client see the physician for treatment with antipsychotic medication.
   c. Encourage the client to describe reasons for seeking treatment.
   d. Reinforce to the client that their body is perfectly normal.
9. A client who is experiencing a panic attack has just arrived at the emergency department. Which is the *priority* nursing intervention for this client?
   a. Stay with the client and reassure them of their safety.
   b. Administer a dose of diazepam.
   c. Leave the client alone in a quiet room to calm down.
   d. Encourage the client to talk about what triggered the attack.
10. A client diagnosed with generalized anxiety disorder has been prescribed buspirone 15 mg daily. The client says to the nurse, "Why do I have to take this every day? My friend's doctor ordered Xanax for her, and she only takes it when she is feeling anxious." Which response by the nurse would be appropriate?
    a. "Xanax is not effective for generalized anxiety disorder."
    b. "Buspirone must be taken daily in order to be effective."
    c. "I will ask the doctor about changing your dose of buspirone to prn so that you don't have to take it every day."
    d. "Your friend really should be taking the Xanax every day."

IMPLICATIONS FOR EVIDENCE-BASED PRACTICE

Teismann, T., Lukaschek, K., Hiller, T. S. Breitbart, J., Brettschneider, C., Schumacher, U., Margraf, J., Gensichen, J., & the Jena Paradies Study Group. (2018). Suicidal ideation in primary care patients suffering from panic disorder with or without agoraphobia. *BMC Psychiatry, 18*, 305. https://doi.org/10.1186/s12888-018-1894-5

DESCRIPTION OF THE STUDY: Recognizing that suicide ideation is common among individuals with panic disorder, the researchers investigated primary care patients with panic disorder (n = 296) to better understand the rates and risk factors for suicide ideation.

RESULTS OF THE STUDY: Suicidal ideation was experienced by 25% of the respondents. In a logistic regression analysis, depression diagnosis and depression severity emerged as significant risk factors for suicidal ideation. Anxiety measures were not associated with suicidal ideation.

IMPLICATIONS FOR NURSING PRACTICE: Suicide is a major health problem in the United States, and the increase in incidence has prompted researchers to explore variables that are most associated with suicide risk. The findings in this study highlight the importance of assessing for symptoms of depression and suicidal ideation in individuals with anxiety disorders. (See Chapter 11, "Suicide Prevention," for a more thorough discussion of current assessment tools and interventions associated with risks for suicide.) Current research on the topic of suicide is rapidly expanding the evidence base related to this health concern, and nurses in any practice setting need to remain informed of the latest research to improve safety and quality care for this population.

TEST YOUR CLINICAL REASONING AND CLINICAL JUDGMENT SKILLS

Sarah, age 25, was taken to the emergency department by her friends. They were at a dinner party when Sarah suddenly clasped her chest and started having difficulty breathing. She complained of nausea and was perspiring profusely. She had calmed down some by the time they reached the hospital. She denied any pain, and electrocardiogram and laboratory results were unremarkable.

Sarah told the admitting nurse that she had a history of these "attacks." She began having them in her sophomore year of college. She knew her parents had expectations that she should follow in their footsteps and become an attorney. They also expected her to earn grades that would promote acceptance by an Ivy League university. Sarah experienced her first attack when she made a B in English during her third semester of college. Since that time, she has experienced these symptoms sporadically, often in conjunction with her perception of the need to excel. She graduated with top honors from Harvard.

Last week, Sarah was promoted within her law firm. She was assigned her first solo case of representing a couple whose baby had died at birth and who were suing the physician for malpractice. She has experienced these panic symptoms daily for the past week, stating, "I feel like I'm going crazy!"

Sarah is transferred to the psychiatric unit. The psychiatrist diagnoses Panic Disorder.

Answer the following questions related to Sarah:

1. What would be the priority nursing diagnosis for Sarah?
2. What is the priority nursing intervention with Sarah?
3. What medical treatment might you expect the physician to prescribe?

Communication Exercises

1. John, who was just admitted to the psychiatric unit with panic disorder, approaches the nurse with complaints of numbness in his fingers and shortness of breath.
   What would be some appropriate responses by the nurse?
2. After attending a group that discussed irrational thinking patterns, John asks the nurse, "How does this cognitive behavior therapy work?"
   What would be some appropriate responses to John's question?

MOVIE CONNECTIONS

As Good As It Gets (OCD) ▪ *The Aviator* (OCD) ▪ *What About Bob?* (Phobias) ▪ *Copycat* (Agoraphobia) ▪ *Analyze This* (Panic disorder) ▪ *Vertigo* (Specific phobia) ▪ *Dirty, Filthy Love* (Trichotillomania and other anxiety disorders) ▪ *Sparrow's Dance* (Agoraphobia)

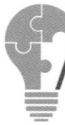

Go to **Davis Advantage** to complete your learning: strengthen understanding, apply your knowledge, and prepare for the Next Gen NCLEX®.

References

Amaral, J. M., Spadaro, P. T., Pereira, V. M., Oliveira e Silva, A. C., & Nardi, A. E. (2013). The carbon dioxide challenge test in panic disorder: A systematic review of preclinical and clinical research. *Revista Brasileira de Psiquiatria, 35*(3), 318–331. https://doi.org/10.1590/1516-4446-2012-1045

American Psychiatric Association. (2013). *Diagnostic and statistical manual of mental disorders* (5th ed.).

Anxiety & Depression Association of America. (2021). *Understand anxiety and depression.* https://adaa.org/understanding-anxiety

Bhatt, N. (2019). Anxiety disorders. *Medscape.* http://emedicine.medscape.com/article/286227-overview#a2

Boland, R., & Verduin, M. L. (2022). *Kaplan & Sadock's synopsis of psychiatry* (P. Ruiz, Ed.). (12th ed.). Wolters Kluwer.

Brazier, Y. (2020). Everything you need to know about phobias. *Medical News Today.* https://www.medicalnewstoday.com/articles/249347

Dias, B. G., & Ressler, K. J. (2014). Parental olfactory experience influences behavior and neural structure in subsequent generations. *Nature Neuroscience, 17,* 86–96. https://doi.org/10.1038/nn.3594

Dozier, M. E., & Ayers, C. R. (2017). The etiology of hoarding disorder: A review. *Psychopathology, 50*(5), 291–296. https://doi.org/10.1159/000479235

Elston, D. M. (2019). Trichotillomania. *Medscape.* http://emedicine.medscape.com/article/1071854-overview#a3

Garakani, A., Murrough, J. W., Freire, R. C., Thom, R. P., Larkin, K., Buono, F. D., & Iosifescu, D. V. (2020). Pharmacotherapy of anxiety disorders: Current and emerging treatment options. *Frontiers in Psychiatry, 11,* 595584. https://doi.org/10.3389/fpsyt.2020.595584

Gerbard, P. L., & Brown, R. P. (2016). Neurobiology and neurophysiology of breath practices in psychiatric care. *Psychiatric Times.* http://www.psychiatrictimes.com/specialreports/neurobiology-and-neurophysiology-breath-practices-psychiatric-care

Gottschalk, M. G., & Domschke, K. (2017). Genetics of generalized anxiety disorder and related traits. *Dialogues in Clinical Neuroscience, 19*(2), 159–168. https://doi.org/10.31887/DCNS.2017.19.2/kdomschke

Herdman, T. H., Kamitsuru, S., & Lopes, C. T. (Eds.). (2021). *NANDA-I, Inc. nursing diagnoses: Definitions and classification, 2021–2023.* Thieme.

Kaplan, K. (2012). Update on trichotillomania. *Psychiatric Times.* https://www.psychiatrictimes.com/view/update-trichotillomania

Kimmel, R. J., & Roy-Burn, P. (2017). Clinical features of the anxiety disorders. In B. J. Sadock, V. A. Sadock, & P. Ruiz (Eds.), *Comprehensive textbook of psychiatry* (10th ed., pp. 1723–1730). Wolters Kluwer.

Koblenzer, C. (2017). Trichotillomania. *PsychiatryAdvisor.* https://www.psychiatryadvisor.com/home/decision-support-in-medicine/dermatology/trichotillomania/

Mayo Clinic. (2021). *Hoarding.* http://www.mayoclinic.com/health/hoarding/DS00966

Meyers, L. (2016). *Help for those who hoard.* https://ct.counseling.org/tag/hoarding/

National Institute of Mental Health. (2017). *Statistics.* https://www.nimh.nih.gov/health/statistics/index.shtml

Ressler, K., & Smoller, J. (2016). *The genetics of anxiety disorders.* https://www.adaa.org/resources-professionals/podcasts/genetics-anxiety-disorders

Stein, D. J., & Lochner, C. (2017). Obsessive-compulsive and related disorders. In B. J. Sadock, V. A. Sadock, & P. Ruiz (Eds.), *Comprehensive textbook of psychiatry* (10th ed., pp. 1785–1798). Wolters Kluwer.

Stevens, M. C., Levy, H. C., Hallion, L. S., Wootton, B. M., & Tolin, D. F. (2020). Functional neuroimaging test of an emerging neurobiological model of hoarding disorder. *Biological Psychiatry: Cognitive Neuroscience and Neuroimaging, 5*(1), 68–75. https://doi.org/10.1016/j.bpsc.2019.08.010

Sykes, T. (2017). Prince Harry on his panic attacks: "We're all mental." *The Daily Beast.* https://www.thedailybeast.com/prince-harry-on-panic-attacks-were-all-mental

Symonds, A., & Janney, R. (2013). Shining a light on hoarding disorder. *Nursing2013, 43*(10), 22–28.

Weber, S. R., & Duchemin, A. M. (2018). Benzodiazepines: Sensible prescribing in light of the risks. *Current Psychiatry, 17*(2), 23–27.

Classical References

Freud, S. (1959). On the grounds for detaching a particular syndrome from neurasthenia under the description "anxiety neurosis." In *Standard edition of the complete psychological works of Freud* (Vol. III). Hogarth Press.

Hamilton, M. (1959). The assessment of anxiety states by rating. *British Journal of Medical Psychology, 32,* 50–55.

Johnson, J. H., & Sarason, I. B. (1978). Life stress, depression and anxiety: Internal-external control as moderator variable. *Journal of Psychosomatic Research, 22*(3), 205–208.

19 Trauma- and Stressor-Related Disorders

CORE CONCEPTS

Stress and Coping: Trauma

Professional Behavior: Nursing process in the care of patients with trauma- and stressor-related disorders

Safety

Clinical Judgment

CHAPTER OUTLINE

Objectives

Introduction

Historical Perspectives and Epidemiology

Application of the Nursing Process—Trauma-Related Disorders

Application of the Nursing Process—Stressor-Related Disorders

Treatment Modalities

Summary and Key Points

Review Questions

Clinical Judgment Questions

Test Your Clinical Reasoning and Clinical Judgment Skills

Movie Connections

KEY TERMS

acute stress disorder

adjustment disorder

post-traumatic stress disorder

prolonged grief disorder

trauma-informed care

OBJECTIVES

After reading this chapter, the student will be able to:

1. Discuss historical perspectives and the epidemiology of trauma- and stressor-related disorders.
2. Describe various types of trauma- and stressor-related disorders and identify symptomatology associated with each; use this information in client assessment.
3. Identify predisposing factors in the development of trauma- and stressor-related disorders.
4. Formulate nursing diagnoses and goals of care for patients with trauma- and stressor-related disorders.
5. Describe the concepts and principles associated with trauma-informed care.
6. Describe appropriate nursing interventions for behaviors associated with trauma- and stressor-related disorders.
7. Evaluate the nursing care of patients with trauma- and stressor-related disorders.
8. Discuss various modalities relevant to treatment of trauma- and stressor-related disorders.

Introduction

In 2011, a massive earthquake and tsunami claimed the lives of thousands and destroyed communities in eastern Japan. Yuri Sato, a public health nurse charged with helping survivors, shares her courageous experience (Frances, 2015):

> As public health nurses, our immediate task was to treat the injured and sick; collect and dispense medicines; and respond to the desperate conditions of the townspeople. We launched and managed an aid station and a welfare evacuation site for those in need of urgent nursing care; established countermeasures against infectious disorders; and arranged for emergency food supplies and sanitation. . . . With the entire town disaster-stricken, I was overcome with a sense of doubt and anxiety. Questions continually spun around in my mind: "What is mental health care when all of us have suffered so greatly?"

> But with everyone in mourning, we were single-mindedly focused on not losing any more lives to suicide or accident. . . . People continued to be unable to accept the deaths of family members, relatives and friends—and the fact that so many were still missing. I often heard "I should have died," "Why did I survive?" or "I want my time to come soon." I also felt this way, but had too much work to do to linger on my own losses and feelings about them.

Disasters such as the Japan earthquake and tsunami of 2011 test the very fiber of our human spirit and sense of emotional well-being. The events recounted by Yuri Sato were painfully traumatic. For some, the stress associated with such traumas continues to cause enduring, significant distress and interference with their ability to function, leading to conditions called *trauma- and stressor-related disorders.*

In the Diagnostic and Statistical Manual of Mental Disorders, Fifth Edition, Text Revision *(DSM-5-TR),* post-traumatic stress disorder (PTSD), acute stress disorder, adjustment disorder, and prolonged grief disorder are included in the chapter "Trauma- and Stressor-Related Disorders" (American Psychiatric Association [APA], 2022). Two additional disorders (reactive attachment disorder and disinhibited social engagement disorder) are also included in that chapter and are identified as childhood disorders associated with absence of adequate caregiving during childhood (social neglect). This classification "reflects increased recognition of trauma as a precipitant, emphasizing common etiology over common phenomenology" (Friedman et al., 2011, p. 737).

Chapter 19 focuses on disorders that occur following exposure to an identifiable stressor or to an extreme traumatic event. Epidemiological statistics are presented, and predisposing factors associated with the etiology of these disorders are discussed. Concepts and principles of trauma-informed care are discussed. An explanation of the symptomatology is presented as background knowledge for assessing clients with trauma- and stressor-related disorders. Nursing care is described in the context of the nursing process. Various treatment modalities are explored.

Historical Perspectives and Epidemiology

The concept of a post-trauma response has been referred to as *shell shock, battle fatigue, accident neurosis,* and *post-traumatic neurosis.* Reports of symptoms and syndromes with features resembling post-traumatic stress disorder (PTSD) have existed in writing throughout the centuries. In the early part of the 20th century, traumatic neurosis was viewed as the ego's inability to master the degree of disorganization brought about by a traumatic experience. Very little was written about "post-traumatic neurosis" between 1950 and 1970. This absence was followed in the 1970s and 1980s with expansive research and writing on the subject. Many of the papers written during this time were about Vietnam War veterans. Although the renewed interest in PTSD was linked to the psychological casualties of war, it is well recognized that any experience of significant trauma may be associated with the development of this disorder.

The diagnostic category of PTSD did not appear until the third edition of the *Diagnostic and Statistical Manual of Mental Disorders* (3rd ed.; *DSM-III*) in 1980, after a need was indicated by increasing numbers of problems identified in Vietnam veterans and victims of multiple disasters. The *DSM-5-TR* (APA, 2022) describes the trauma that precedes PTSD as an event that is either directly experienced, witnessed, occurring in a close family member or close friend, or involving repeated exposure to aversive details about a traumatic event. Examples of such events include (but are not limited to) threatened or actual sexual violence, exposure to war, threatened or actual physical attack, torture, natural or man-made disasters, and severe motor vehicle accidents.

About 60% of men and 50% of women are exposed to a traumatic event in their lifetime (Department of Veterans Affairs, 2019). Women are more likely to experience sexual assault and childhood sexual abuse, whereas men are more likely to experience accidents, physical assaults, combat, or proximity to death or injury. Although the exposure to trauma is high, the National Center for PTSD reports that fewer than 10% of trauma victims develop PTSD (Department of Veterans Affairs, 2019). The disorder appears to be more common in women than in men.

Historically, as previously stated, individuals who experienced stress reactions that followed exposure to an extreme traumatic event were given the diagnosis of PTSD. Accordingly, stress reactions from "less extreme" events (e.g., divorce, failure, rejection) were characterized as adjustment disorders rather than PTSD (Friedman, 1996). Currently, the definition of an adjustment disorder is broader in spectrum and may involve single, multiple, recurrent, or continuous stressors. It is primarily differentiated from PTSD and acute stress disorders by the time of onset and duration of symptoms (APA, 2022).

A number of studies have indicated that adjustment disorders are quite common, although prevalence statistics vary from 3% to 50% depending on the population being studied (Frank, 2016). The *DSM-5-TR*

(APA, 2022) reports that, in hospital psychiatric consultation services, adjustment disorder has often been the most common diagnosis; frequently reaching 50%.

Studies have found that adjustment disorders are more commonly diagnosed in women than in men (Gradus et al., 2014). Examples of situations that result in adjustment disorders include giving birth to a stillborn child, enduring a stressful experience such as a major life change, being a victim of bullying or harassment, or being incarcerated (Katzman & Geppert, 2017).

Application of the Nursing Process—Trauma-Related Disorders

CORE CONCEPT

Trauma

An extremely distressing experience that causes severe emotional shock and may have long-lasting psychological effects.

Trauma-Informed Care

Experts highlight the importance of trauma-informed care as essential to improving the quality of care for clients both in and outside of behavioral health-care settings (Hopper et al., 2010; Substance Abuse and Mental Health Services Administration [SAMHSA], 2019). Trauma-informed care generally describes a philosophical approach that values awareness and understanding of trauma when assessing, planning, and implementing care. SAMHSA (2019) advances the following principles (4Rs) in defining this approach.

Trauma-informed care:

- Realizes the widespread impact of trauma and various paths for recovery.
- Recognizes the signs and symptoms of trauma in clients, families, staff, and all those involved with the system.
- Responds by fully integrating knowledge about trauma in policies, procedures, and practices.
- Seeks to actively resist retraumatization.

Hopper and associates (2010) discuss applying this approach with the homeless population (many of whom are people with severe mental illness). The authors describe the many traumatic experiences that culminate in homelessness and the often co-occurring illnesses such as depression, substance abuse, and severe mental illness. To ignore the significance of trauma or to provide uninformed care leaves this population vulnerable to revictimization and "further complicates their service needs" (p. 81). These authors advance the following definition of trauma-informed care:

> Trauma-informed care is a strength-based framework that is grounded in understanding of and responsiveness to the impact of trauma that emphasizes physical, psychological, and emotional safety for both providers and survivors to rebuild a sense of control and empowerment. (p. 82)

Inherent in this definition is the importance of health-care providers also being aware of the impact of trauma on themselves because it may impact their effectiveness in providing care to clients.

Interventions that are considered trauma-informed highlight the importance of respect for the client, collaboration and connection, providing information about the links between trauma and other health concerns, instilling hope, and empowering the trauma survivor to guide and direct the recovery plan (the essence of patient-centered care).

Childhood trauma, including physical, emotional, and sexual abuse, is identified as significant in the development of behavioral problems, eating disorders, some personality disorders, depression, and substance abuse. Health-care providers, if they do not fully understand the impact of previous trauma on the client's current health concerns, may unwittingly retraumatize clients. Interventions such as seclusion and restraint, which are designed to protect the client's safety when they are at imminent risk of harm to themselves or others, may be retraumatizing to a client with a history of trauma. Much attention has been given to the importance of trauma-informed care in behavioral health-care settings because of the recognition that trauma history may be associated with other mental illnesses. However, nurses in every practice setting must incorporate this approach in assessment and care provision because trauma history can impact any patient's response to care. See the "Real People, Real Stories" feature in Chapter 25, "Survivors of Abuse or Neglect," for Diana's perspective on how previous traumas affect her response in general health-care settings.

Background Assessment Data

Post-Traumatic Stress Disorder

Post-traumatic stress disorder (PTSD) is described as a multisymptom response triggered by an extremely traumatic event. These symptoms are not related to common experiences such as uncomplicated bereavement, marital conflict, or chronic illness but are associated with events that would be markedly distressing to almost anyone. The individual may experience or witness the trauma alone or in the presence of others.

Characteristic symptoms include reexperiencing the traumatic event, a sustained high level of anxiety or arousal, or a general numbing of responsiveness. Intrusive recollections, sleep disturbances, or nightmares of the event are common. Some individuals may be unable to remember certain aspects of the trauma.

Symptoms of depression are common with this disorder and may be severe enough to warrant a diagnosis of a depressive disorder in addition to PTSD. In the case of a life-threatening trauma shared with others, survivors often describe painful guilt feelings about surviving when others lost their lives. They may also express trauma and guilt feelings about the things they had to do to survive. Substance abuse, anger and aggressive behavior, and relationship problems are common. The full symptom picture must be present for more than 1 month and cause significant interference with social, occupational, and other areas of functioning. The disorder can occur at any age. Symptoms may begin within the first 3 months after the trauma, or there may be a delay of several months or even years. The *DSM-5-TR* diagnostic criteria for PTSD are presented in Box 19–1.

Acute Stress Disorder

The *DSM-5-TR* describes another disorder that is similar to PTSD called **acute stress disorder.** There are similarities between the two disorders in terms of precipitating traumatic events and symptomatology, but in acute stress disorder, the symptoms are time limited, up to 1 month following the trauma. By definition, if the symptoms last longer than 1 month, the diagnosis is PTSD. The *DSM-5-TR* diagnostic criteria for acute stress disorder are presented in Box 19–2.

Predisposing Factors Related to Trauma-Related Disorders

Psychosocial Aspects

The psychosocial model seeks to explain why certain persons exposed to massive trauma develop trauma-related disorders and others do not. Variables include characteristics that relate to (1) the traumatic experience, (2) the individual, and (3) the recovery environment.

The Traumatic Experience

Specific characteristics relating to the trauma have been identified as crucial elements in the determination of an individual's long-term response to stress. They include the following:

- Severity and duration of the stressor
- Extent of anticipatory preparation for the event
- Exposure to death
- Numbers affected by life threat
- Amount of control over recurrence
- Location where the trauma was experienced (e.g., familiar surroundings, at home, in a foreign country)

The Individual

The variables that follow are considered important in determining an individual's response to trauma include the following:

- Degree of ego strength
- Effectiveness of coping resources
- Presence of pre-existing psychopathology
- Outcomes of previous experiences with stress or trauma
- Behavioral tendencies (temperament)
- Current psychosocial developmental stage
- Demographic factors (e.g., age, socioeconomic status, education)

The Recovery Environment

It has been suggested that the quality of the environment in which the individual attempts to work through the traumatic experience is correlated with the outcome. Environmental variables include the following:

- Availability of social supports
- The cohesiveness and protectiveness of family and friends
- The attitudes of society regarding the experience
- Cultural and subcultural influences

In a longitudinal study of Vietnam veterans, it was shown that the best predictors of war-related PTSD were "African-American race, lower education level, negative homecoming reception, lower current social support, and greater past-year stress" in the recovery environment (Steenkamp et al., 2017, p. 711). Further, it was found that that these factors can predict PTSD symptom severity and symptom change up to 40 years post-deployment.

Learning Theory

Learning theorists view negative reinforcement as behavior that leads to a reduction in an aversive experience, thereby reinforcing and resulting in repetition of the behavior. The avoidance behaviors and psychic numbing in response to a trauma are

BOX 19–1 Diagnostic Criteria for Post-traumatic Stress Disorder

NOTE: The following criteria apply to adults, adolescents, and children older than 6 years.

A. Exposure to actual or threatened death, serious injury, or sexual violence, in one (or more) of the following ways:
   1. Directly experiencing the traumatic event(s).
   2. Witnessing, in person, the event(s) as it occurred to others.
   3. Learning that the traumatic event(s) occurred to a close family member or close friend. In cases of actual or threatened death of a family member or friend, the event(s) must have been violent or accidental.
   4. Experiencing repeated or extreme exposure to aversive details of the traumatic event(s) (e.g., first responders collecting human remains; police officers repeatedly exposed to details of child abuse). **NOTE:** Criterion A4 does not apply to exposure through electronic media, television, movies, or pictures unless this exposure is work related.

B. Presence of one (or more) of the following intrusion symptoms associated with the traumatic event(s), beginning after the traumatic event(s) occurred:
   1. Recurrent, involuntary, and intrusive distressing memories of the traumatic event(s). **NOTE:** In children older than 6 years, repetitive play may occur in which themes or aspects of the traumatic event(s) are expressed.
   2. Recurrent distressing dreams in which the content and/or effect of the dream is related to the traumatic event(s). **NOTE:** In children, there may be frightening dreams without recognizable content.
   3. Dissociative reactions (e.g., flashbacks) in which the individual feels or acts as if the traumatic event(s) were recurring. (Such reactions may occur on a continuum, with the most extreme expression being a complete loss of awareness of present surroundings.) **NOTE:** In children, trauma-specific reenactment may occur in play.
   4. Intense or prolonged psychological distress at exposure to internal or external cues that symbolize or resemble an aspect of the traumatic event(s).
   5. Marked physiological reactions to internal or external cues that symbolize or resemble an aspect of the traumatic event(s).

C. Persistent avoidance of stimuli associated with the traumatic event(s) beginning after the traumatic event(s) occurred, as evidenced by one or both of the following:
   1. Avoidance of or efforts to avoid distressing memories, thoughts, or feelings about or closely associated with the traumatic event(s).
   2. Avoidance of or efforts to avoid external reminders (people, places, conversations, activities, objects, situations) that arouse distressing memories, thoughts, or feelings about or closely associated with the traumatic event(s).

D. Negative alterations in cognitions and mood associated with the traumatic event(s), beginning or worsening after the traumatic event(s) occurred, as evidenced by two or more of the following:
   1. Inability to remember an important aspect of the traumatic event(s) (typically due to dissociative amnesia and not to other factors such as head injury, alcohol, or drugs).
   2. Persistent and exaggerated negative beliefs or expectations about oneself, others, or the world (e.g., "I am bad," "No one can be trusted," "The world is completely dangerous," "My whole nervous system is permanently ruined").
   3. Persistent, distorted cognitions about the cause or consequences of the traumatic event(s) that lead the individual to blame themselves or others.
   4. Persistent negative emotional state (e.g., fear, horror, anger, guilt, or shame).
   5. Markedly diminished interest or participation in significant activities.
   6. Feelings of detachment or estrangement from others.
   7. Persistent inability to experience positive emotions (e.g., inability to experience happiness, satisfaction, or loving feelings).

E. Marked alterations in arousal and reactivity associated with the traumatic event(s), beginning or worsening after the traumatic event(s) occurred, as evidenced by two or more of the following:
   1. Irritable behavior and angry outbursts (with little or no provocation) typically expressed as verbal or physical aggression toward people or objects.
   2. Reckless or self-destructive behavior.
   3. Hypervigilance.
   4. Exaggerated startle response.
   5. Problems with concentration.
   6. Sleep disturbance (e.g., difficulty falling or staying asleep or restless sleep).

F. Duration of the disturbance (Criteria B, C, D, and E) is more than 1 month.

G. The disturbance causes clinically significant distress or impairment in social, occupation, or other important areas of functioning.

H. The disturbance is not attributable to the physiological effects of a substance (e.g., medication, alcohol) or another medical condition.

Specify whether:

With dissociative symptoms (depersonalization or derealization)

With delayed expression (full diagnostic criteria not met until at least 6 months after the event)

Reprinted with permission from American Psychiatric Association (APA). (2022). Diagnostic and statistical manual of mental disorders, fifth edition, text revision.

BOX 19–2 Diagnostic Criteria for Acute Stress Disorder

A. Exposure to actual or threatened death, serious injury, or sexual violation, in one (or more) of the following ways:
   1. Directly experiencing the traumatic event(s).
   2. Witnessing, in person, the event(s) as it occurred to others.
   3. Learning that the event(s) occurred to a close family member or close friend. **NOTE:** In cases of actual or threatened death of a family member or friend, the event(s) must have been violent or accidental.
   4. Experiencing repeated or extreme exposure to aversive details of the traumatic event(s) (e.g., first responders collecting human remains, police officers repeatedly exposed to details of child abuse). **NOTE:** This does not apply to exposure through electronic media, television, movies, or pictures, unless this exposure is work related.

B. Presence of nine (or more) of the following symptoms from any of the five categories of intrusion, negative mood, dissociation, avoidance, and arousal, beginning or worsening after the traumatic event(s) occurred:

INTRUSION SYMPTOMS

1. Recurrent, involuntary, and intrusive distressing memories of the traumatic event(s). **NOTE:** In children, repetitive play may occur in which themes or aspects of the traumatic event(s) are expressed.
2. Recurrent distressing dreams in which the content and/or affect of the dream are related to the event(s). **NOTE:** In children, there may be frightening dreams without recognizable content.
3. Dissociative reactions (e.g., flashbacks) in which the individual feels or acts as if the traumatic event(s) were recurring. (Such reactions may occur on a continuum, with the most extreme expression being a complete loss of awareness of present surroundings.) **NOTE:** In children, trauma-specific reenactment may occur in play.
4. Intense or prolonged psychological distress or marked physiological reactions in response to internal or external cues that symbolize or resemble an aspect of the traumatic event(s).

NEGATIVE MOOD

5. Persistent inability to experience positive emotions (e.g., inability to experience happiness, satisfaction, or loving feelings).

DISSOCIATIVE SYMPTOMS

6. An altered sense of the reality of one's surroundings or oneself (e.g., seeing oneself from another's perspective, being in a daze, time slowing).
7. Inability to remember an important aspect of the traumatic event(s) (typically due to dissociative amnesia and not to other factors such as head injury, alcohol, or drugs).

AVOIDANCE SYMPTOMS

8. Efforts to avoid distressing memories, thoughts, or feelings about or closely associated with the traumatic event(s).
9. Efforts to avoid external reminders (people, places, conversations, activities, objects, situations) that arouse distressing memories, thoughts, or feelings about or closely associated with the traumatic event(s).

AROUSAL SYMPTOMS

10. Sleep disturbance (e.g., difficulty falling or staying asleep, or restless sleep).
11. Irritable behavior and angry outbursts (with little or no provocation), typically expressed as verbal or physical aggression toward people or objects.
12. Hypervigilance.
13. Problems with concentration.
14. Exaggerated startle response.

C. Duration of the disturbance (symptoms in Criteria B) is 3 days to 1 month after trauma exposure. **NOTE:** Symptoms typically begin immediately after the trauma, but persistence for at least 3 days and up to a month is needed to meet disorder criteria.

D. The disturbance causes clinically significant distress or impairment in social, occupational, or other important areas of functioning.

E. The disturbance is not attributable to the direct physiological effects of a substance (e.g., medication or alcohol) or another medical condition (e.g., mild traumatic brain injury), and is not better explained by brief psychotic disorder.

Reprinted with permission from American Psychiatric Association (APA). (2022). Diagnostic and statistical manual of mental disorders, fifth edition, text revision.

mediated by negative reinforcement (behaviors that decrease the emotional pain of the trauma). Behavioral disturbances, such as anger and aggression and drug and alcohol abuse, are the behavioral patterns that are reinforced by their capacity to reduce objectionable feelings.

Cognitive Theory

These models take into consideration the cognitive appraisal of an event and focus on assumptions that an individual makes about the world. Epstein's classic theory (1991) outlines three fundamental beliefs that most people construct within a personal theory of reality:

1. The world is benevolent and a source of joy.
2. The world is meaningful and controllable.
3. The self is worthy (e.g., lovable, good, and competent).

Park and associates' (2012) research added support to the cognitive theory in their finding that the extent to which an individual's appraisal of an event violates their beliefs about themselves and the world damages their beliefs and is strongly related to the development and maintenance of PTSD over time.

As life situations occur, some disequilibrium is to be expected until accommodation for the change has been made and it has become assimilated into one's personal theory of reality. An individual is vulnerable to trauma-related disorders when fundamental beliefs are invalidated by a trauma that cannot be comprehended and a sense of helplessness and hopelessness prevails. One's appraisal of the environment can be drastically altered.

Biological Aspects

Exposure to trauma has been associated with hyperarousal of the sympathetic nervous system, excessive amygdala activity, and decreased hippocampus volume, all of which are neurobiological reactions to heightened stress. Dysfunctions in the hypothalamic-pituitary-adrenal (HPA) axis, either from chronic stress or exposure to an extreme stressor, have been linked to many psychiatric illnesses including PTSD, depression, Alzheimer's disease, and substance use disorders and to medical conditions such as inflammatory disorders and cardiovascular disease (Valentino & Van Bockstaele, 2015). These links are evident in the comorbidity or increased risk for developing one or more of the above-mentioned disorders. For example, a recent meta-analysis (Günak et al., 2020) found that PTSD is associated with a significant risk for all causes of dementia. Substance use disorders and depression are commonly diagnosed comorbidities with PTSD.

In addition, neuroendocrine abnormalities, including corticotropin releasing hormone, norepinephrine, serotonin, glutamate, thyroid, and endogenous opioids (among others), have been associated with stress responses and PTSD. Valentino and Van Bockstaele (2015) identify that the activation of endogenous opioids both reduces stress and mimics the stress response depending on which opioid receptors are activated. Studies have shown that opioids administered shortly after exposure to a trauma reduced the incidence of PTSD, suggesting a protective effect. Chronic activation, however, may sensitize neurons in a way that increases vulnerability to stress-induced relapse. Lanius (2013) discusses the effects of repeated activation of opioid receptors, including the effect of increasing one's addiction potential to other drugs or even to the learned experience of relief when traumatic stress is reexperienced. He identifies that opiate antagonists such as naltrexone have demonstrated effectiveness in treatment.

Other biological systems have also been implicated in the symptomatology of PTSD. Norepinephrine, dopamine, and benzodiazepine receptors (on gamma-aminobutyric acid [GABA] receptors) are some of the neurotransmitters believed to be dysregulated in individuals with PTSD. Lower concentrations of neuropeptide Y (NPY), an anxiolytic peptide, have been shown to increase susceptibility to PTSD in combat veterans and catechol-o-methyltransferase (COMT) gene variants have been linked to deficits in stress responses and emotional resilience (Togay & El-Mallakh, 2020). Whether these factors are suggestive of vulnerability to PTSD or are changes that result from the brain's efforts to process trauma remains unclear. As with other disorders, it is likely that a complex dynamic of biological, social, and psychological factors is involved.

A large-scale genome study (Stein et al., 2021) of over 250,000 veterans identified specific genes associated with PTSD and related mood symptoms of anxiety and depression. Their research supports a biological and, specifically, genetic influence in the development of this disorder. Further, their finding that genetically regulated gene expression occurs in several cortical and subcortical regions of the brain may have implications for future research into potential drug treatments.

Diagnosis and Outcome Identification

Nursing diagnoses are formulated from the data gathered during the assessment phase and with background knowledge regarding predisposing factors to the disorder. Following are some common NANDA-I nursing diagnoses (Herdman et al., 2021) for patients with trauma-related disorders:

- Post-trauma syndrome related to distressing events considered to be outside the range of usual human experience evidenced by flashbacks, intrusive recollections, nightmares, psychological numbness related to the event, dissociation, or amnesia
- Maladaptive grieving related to loss of perceived sense of security before the trauma or other actual or perceived losses incurred during or after the event evidenced by irritability and explosiveness, self-destructiveness, substance abuse, verbalization of survival guilt, or guilt about behavior required for survival

Outcome Criteria

The following criteria may be used for measurement of outcomes in the care of the patient with a trauma-related disorder. The patient:

- Can acknowledge the traumatic event and the impact it has had on their life.

- Is experiencing fewer flashbacks, intrusive recollections, and nightmares than on admission (or at the beginning of therapy).
- Can demonstrate adaptive coping strategies (e.g., relaxation techniques, mental imagery, music, art).
- Can concentrate and has made realistic goals for the future.
- Includes significant others in the recovery process and willingly accepts their support.
- Verbalizes no ideas or intent of self-harm.
- Has worked through feelings of survivor's guilt.
- Gets enough sleep to avoid risk of injury.
- Verbalizes community resources from which to seek assistance in times of stress.
- Attends support group of individuals who have recovered or are recovering from similar traumatic experiences.
- Verbalizes desire to put the trauma in the past and progress with life.

Planning and Implementation

Table 19–1 provides a care plan for patients with a trauma-related disorder. NANDA International (NANDA-I) (Herdman et al., 2021) nursing diagnoses are presented, along with outcome criteria, appropriate nursing interventions, and rationales for each.

See the feature "Real People, Real Stories" in Chapter 28, "Military Families," to learn more about Sean's post-military experience with PTSD and the importance of compassionate nursing care in his recovery.

Patient and Family Education

The role of patient teacher is important in the psychiatric area, as it is in all areas of nursing. A list of topics for patient and family education relevant to trauma- and stressor-related disorders is presented in Box 19-3.

Table 19–1 | CARE PLAN FOR THE PATIENT WITH A TRAUMA-RELATED DISORDER

NURSING DIAGNOSIS: POST-TRAUMA SYNDROME

RELATED TO: Distressing event considered to be outside the range of usual human experience

EVIDENCED BY: Flashbacks, intrusive recollections, nightmares, psychological numbness related to the event, dissociation, or amnesia

OUTCOME CRITERIA	NURSING INTERVENTIONS	RATIONALE
Short-Term Goals ■ Patient will begin a healthy grief resolution, initiating the process of psychological healing (within time frame specific to individual). Patient will demonstrate ability to deal with emotional reactions in an individually appropriate manner.	1. a. Assign the same staff as often as possible. b. Use a nonthreatening, matter-of-fact but friendly approach. c. Respect the patient's wishes regarding interaction with individuals of opposite gender at this time (especially important if the trauma was rape). d. Be consistent; keep all promises; convey acceptance; spend time with the patient.	1. A post-trauma patient may be suspicious of others in their environment. All of these interventions serve to facilitate a trusting relationship.
Long-Term Goal ■ Patient will integrate the traumatic experience into their persona, renew significant relationships, and establish meaningful goals for the future.	2. Stay with the patient during periods of flashbacks and nightmares. Offer reassurance of safety and security and that these symptoms are not uncommon following a trauma of the magnitude they have experienced.	2. Presence of a trusted individual may calm fears for personal safety and reassure patients that they are not "in danger."
	3. Obtain accurate history from significant others about the trauma and the patient's specific response.	3. Various types of traumas elicit different responses (e.g., human-engendered traumas often generate a greater degree of humiliation and guilt in victims than trauma associated with natural disasters).

Continued

Table 19–1 | CARE PLAN FOR THE PATIENT WITH A TRAUMA-RELATED DISORDER—cont'd

OUTCOME CRITERIA	NURSING INTERVENTIONS	RATIONALE
	4. Encourage the patient to talk about the trauma at their own pace. Provide a non-threatening, private environment, and include a significant other if the patient wishes. Acknowledge and validate patient's feelings as they are expressed.	4. This debriefing process is the first step in the progression toward resolution.
	5. Discuss coping strategies used in response to the trauma as well as those used during stressful situations in the past. Determine those that have been most helpful and discuss alternative strategies for the future. Include available support systems, including religious and cultural influences. Identify maladaptive coping strategies (e.g., substance use, psychosomatic responses) and practice more adaptive coping strategies for possible future post-trauma responses.	5. Resolution of the post-trauma response is largely dependent on the effectiveness of the coping strategies employed.
	6. Assist the individual to comprehend the trauma if possible. Discuss feelings of vulnerability and the individual's "place" in the world following the trauma.	6. Post-trauma response is largely a function of the shattering of basic beliefs the survivor holds about self and world. Assimilation of the event into one's persona requires that some degree of meaning associated with the event be incorporated into the basic beliefs, which will affect how the individual eventually comes to reappraise self and world (Epstein, 1991).

NURSING DIAGNOSIS: MALADAPTIVE GRIEVING

RELATED TO: Loss of sense of self as perceived prior to the trauma or other actual/perceived losses incurred during/following the event

EVIDENCED BY: Irritability and explosiveness, self-destructiveness, substance abuse, verbalization of survival guilt or guilt about behavior required for survival

OUTCOME CRITERIA	NURSING INTERVENTIONS	RATIONALE
Short-Term Goal ■ Patient will verbalize feelings (guilt, anger, self-blame, hopelessness) associated with the trauma.	1. Acknowledge feelings of guilt or self-blame that the patient may express.	1. Guilt at having survived a trauma in which others died is common. Patients need to discuss these feelings and recognize that they are not responsible for what happened but must take responsibility for their own recovery.

Table 19–1 | CARE PLAN FOR THE PATIENT WITH A TRAUMA-RELATED DISORDER—cont'd

OUTCOME CRITERIA	NURSING INTERVENTIONS	RATIONALE
Long-Term Goal ■ Patient will demonstrate progress in dealing with stages of grief and will verbalize a sense of optimism and hope for the future.	2. Assess stage of grief in which the patient is fixed. Discuss normalcy of feelings and behaviors related to stages of grief.	2. Knowledge of grief stages facilitates patients' understanding of their feelings. Guilt may be generated if the patient believes it is unacceptable to have these feelings. Knowing these are part of the normal grief response can provide a sense of relief.
	3. Assess impact of the trauma on the patient's ability to resume regular activities of daily living (ADLs). Consider employment, marital relationship, and sleep patterns.	3. Following a trauma, individuals are at high risk for physical injury because of disrupted concentration and problem-solving abilities and lack of sufficient sleep. Isolation and avoidance behaviors may interfere with interpersonal relatedness.
	4. Assess for self-destructive ideas and behavior.	4. The trauma may result in feelings of hopelessness and worthlessness, leading to high risk for suicide.
	5. Assess for maladaptive coping strategies, such as substance abuse.	5. These behaviors interfere with and delay the recovery process.
	6. Identify available community resources from which the individual may seek assistance if problems with maladaptive grieving persist.	6. Support groups for victims of various types of traumas exist within most communities. The presence of support systems in the recovery environment has been identified as a major predictor in the successful recovery from trauma.

Evaluation

Reassessment is conducted in order to determine whether the nursing actions have been successful in achieving the objectives of care. Evaluation of the nursing actions for the patient with a trauma-related disorder may be facilitated by gathering information using the following types of questions:

Can the patient:

- Discuss the traumatic event without experiencing panic anxiety?
- Voluntarily discuss the traumatic event?
- Discuss changes that have occurred in life because of the traumatic event?
- Verbalize that flashbacks have decreased in intensity or frequency?
- Sleep without medication?
- Verbalize that nightmares have subsided?
- Identify new adaptive coping strategies for assistance with recovery?
- Demonstrate successful use of these new coping strategies in times of stress?
- Verbalize stages of grief and the normal behaviors associated with each?
- Recognize their own position in the grieving process?
- Verbalize that feelings of guilt have decreased in intensity or subsided?
- Maintain satisfactory relationships with significant others?
- Look to the future with optimism?
- Verbalize intent to attend a regular support group for victims of similar traumatic experiences?
- Identify a plan of action for dealing with symptoms if they return?

BOX 19–3 Topics for Patient and Family Education Related to Trauma- and Stressor-Related Disorders

NATURE OF PTSD AND STRESSOR-RELATED DISORDERS

- Definitions of trauma and stressor-related disorders
- Long-term effects of trauma on physical and mental health
- Common comorbidities such as depression, anxiety, and substance use disorders

MANAGEMENT OF PTSD

- Medication management options; SSRIs, anxiolytics, ketamine
- Psychotherapies; trauma-focused psychotherapy, CBT, DBT, Prolonged exposure therapy, eye movement desensitization therapy
- Community resources; trauma-focused support groups, meditation groups

CBT, cognitive behavior therapy; DBT, dialectical behavior therapy; SSRIs, selective serotonin reuptake inhibitors.

Application of the Nursing Process—Stressor-Related Disorders

CORE CONCEPT

Stress

A state of disequilibrium and tension that occurs when there is disharmony between demands occurring within an individual's internal or external environment and their ability to cope with those demands.

Background Assessment Data

An **adjustment disorder** is characterized by a maladaptive reaction to an identifiable stressor or stressors that results in the development of clinically significant emotional or behavioral symptoms (APA, 2022). The response occurs within 3 months after onset of the stressor and has persisted for no longer than 6 months after the stressor or its consequences have ended.

The individual shows impairment in social and occupational functioning or exhibits symptoms that are in excess of an expected reaction to the stressor. The symptoms are expected to remit soon after the stressor is relieved, or if the stressor persists, when a new level of adaptation is achieved.

The stressor itself can be almost anything, but an individual's response to any particular stressor cannot be predicted. If an individual is highly predisposed or vulnerable to maladaptive response, a severe form of the disorder may follow what most people would consider only a mild or moderate stressor. On the other hand, a less vulnerable individual may develop only a mild form of the disorder in response to what others might consider a severe stressor.

In the latest edition of the *Diagnostic and Statistical Manual of Mental Disorders* (*DSM-5-TR*, APA, 2022) a distinct syndrome, prolonged grief disorder, was added. Although symptoms of bereavement (beyond normal bereavement) may occur in adjustment disorders, **prolonged grief disorder** is diagnosed when the stressor is specifically the death of a person who was close to the bereaved individual and clinically significant distress or impairment in functioning endures beyond a year of the associated death.

A number of clinical presentations are associated with adjustment disorders. The following categories, identified by the *DSM-5-TR* (APA, 2022), are distinguished by the predominant features of the maladaptive response.

Adjustment Disorder With Depressed Mood

This category is the most commonly diagnosed adjustment disorder. The clinical presentation is one of predominant mood disturbance, although it is less pronounced than that of major depressive disorder (MDD). The symptoms, such as depressed mood, tearfulness, and feelings of hopelessness, exceed what is an expected or normative response to an identified stressor.

Adjustment Disorder With Anxiety

This category denotes a maladaptive response to a stressor in which the predominant manifestation is anxiety. For example, the symptoms may reveal nervousness, worry, and jitteriness. The clinician must differentiate this diagnosis from those of anxiety disorders.

Adjustment Disorder With Mixed Anxiety and Depressed Mood

The predominant features of this category include disturbances in mood (depression, feelings of hopelessness and sadness) and manifestations of anxiety (nervousness, worry, jitteriness) that are more intense than what would be expected or considered to be a normative response to an identified stressor.

Adjustment Disorder With Disturbance of Conduct

This category is characterized by conduct in which there is violation of the rights of others or of major age-appropriate societal norms and rules. Examples include truancy, vandalism, reckless driving, fighting, and defaulting on legal responsibilities. Differential diagnosis must be made from conduct disorder or antisocial personality disorder.

Adjustment Disorder With Mixed Disturbance of Emotions and Conduct

The predominant features of this category include emotional disturbances (e.g., anxiety or depression) as well as disturbances of conduct in which there is violation of the rights of others or of major age-appropriate societal norms and rules (e.g., truancy, vandalism, fighting).

Adjustment Disorder Unspecified

This subtype is used when the maladaptive reaction is not consistent with any of the other categories. The individual may have physical complaints, withdraw from relationships, or exhibit impaired work or academic performance but without significant disturbance in emotions or conduct.

Predisposing Factors to Adjustment Disorders

Biological Aspects

Chronic disorders, such as neurocognitive or intellectual developmental disorders, are thought to impair the ability of an individual to adapt to stress, causing increased vulnerability to an adjustment disorder. Genetic factors also may influence individual risks for maladaptive response to stress.

Psychosocial Theories

Some proponents of psychoanalytic theory view an adjustment disorder as a maladaptive response to stress that is caused by early childhood trauma, increased dependency, and retarded ego development. Other psychoanalysts give considerable weight to the constitutional factors or birth characteristics that contribute to the manner in which individuals respond to stress. In many instances, an adjustment disorder is precipitated by a specific meaningful stressor having found a point of vulnerability in an individual of otherwise adequate ego strength.

Some studies relate a predisposition to an adjustment disorder to factors such as developmental stage, timing of the stressor, and available support systems. When a stressor occurs, and the individual does not have the developmental maturity, available support systems, or adequate coping strategies to adapt, normal functioning is disrupted, resulting in psychological or somatic symptoms. The disorder also may be related to a maladaptive grieving process. The individual may remain in the denial or anger stage with inadequate defense mechanisms to complete the grieving process.

Transactional Model of Stress and Adaptation

Why are some individuals able to confront stressful situations adaptively and even gain strength from the experience, whereas others not only fail to cope adaptively but may even encounter psychopathological dysfunction? The transactional model of stress and adaptation takes into consideration the interaction between the individual and the environment.

The type of stressor that one experiences may influence one's adaptation. Sudden-shock stressors occur without warning, and continuous stressors are those that an individual is exposed to over an extended period. Although many studies have been directed to individuals' responses to sudden-shock stressors, it has been found that continuous stressors are more commonly cited than sudden-shock stressors as precipitants to maladaptive functioning.

Both situational and intrapersonal factors most likely contribute to an individual's stress response. Situational factors include personal and general economic conditions; occupational and recreational opportunities; and the availability of social supports such as family, friends, neighbors, and cultural or religious support groups.

Pre-existing personality and behavioral traits may also predispose an individual to an adjustment disorder and other stress-related disorders. Studies have found that personality traits (including rigidity, perfectionism, cautiousness, and slow adaptation to change) are related to the development of emotional disorders (Lynch, 2018). Other factors that might influence one's ability to adjust to life changes include social skills, coping strategies, the presence of psychiatric illness, and level of intelligence.

Diagnosis and Outcome Identification

Nursing diagnoses are formulated from the data gathered during the assessment phase and with background knowledge regarding predisposing factors to the disorder. Nursing diagnoses that may be used for the patient with an adjustment disorder include the following:

- Maladaptive grieving related to real or perceived loss of anything of value to the individual, evidenced by interference with life functioning, developmental regression, or somatic complaints
- Risk-prone health behavior related to change in health status requiring modification in lifestyle (e.g., chronic illness, physical disability), as evidenced by inability to problem solve or set realistic goals for the future (appropriate diagnosis for the person with an adjustment disorder if the precipitating stressor was a change in health status)
- Anxiety (moderate to severe) related to situational and/or maturational crisis as evidenced by restlessness, increased helplessness, and diminished productivity

Outcome Criteria

The following criteria may be used for measurement of outcomes in the care of the patient with an adjustment disorder. The patient:

- Verbalizes acceptable behaviors associated with each stage of the grief process.
- Demonstrates a reinvestment in the environment.
- Accomplishes activities of daily living independently.
- Demonstrates ability for adequate occupational and social functioning.
- Verbalizes awareness of change in health status and the effect it will have on lifestyle.
- Solves problems and sets realistic goals for the future.
- Demonstrates ability to cope effectively with change in lifestyle.

Planning and Implementation

Table 19–2 provides a care plan for a patient with an adjustment disorder. NANDA-I nursing diagnoses (Herdman et al., 2021) are presented, along with outcome criteria, appropriate nursing interventions, and rationales for each.

Evaluation

Reassessment is conducted to determine whether the nursing actions have been successful in achieving the objectives of care. Evaluation of the nursing actions for the patient with an adjustment disorder may be facilitated by gathering information using the following types of questions:

Does the patient:

- Verbalize understanding of the grief process and their position in the process?
- Recognize the adaptive and maladaptive behaviors associated with the grief response?
- Demonstrate evidence of progression along the grief response?
- Accomplish activities of daily living independently?
- Demonstrate the ability to perform occupational and social activities adequately?
- Discuss the change in health status and modification of lifestyle it will affect?
- Demonstrate acceptance of the modification?
- Participate in decision making and problem-solving for the future?

Table 19–2 | CARE PLAN FOR THE PATIENT WITH AN ADJUSTMENT DISORDER

NURSING DIAGNOSIS: MALADAPTIVE GRIEVING

RELATED TO: Death of a significant other; lack of social support; emotional instability

EVIDENCED BY: Decreased ability to function in life roles; inappropriate anger; persistent emotional distress; self-blame

OUTCOME CRITERIA	NURSING INTERVENTIONS	RATIONALE
Short-Term Goal ■ By end of 1 week, patient will express anger toward lost entity. **Long-Term Goal** ■ Patient will be able to verbalize behaviors associated with the normal stages of grief and identify own position in grief process, while progressing at own pace toward resolution.	1. Determine the stage of grief in which the patient is fixed. Identify behaviors associated with this stage.	1. Accurate baseline assessment data are necessary to plan effective care for the grieving patient.
	2. Develop a trusting relationship with the patient. Show empathy and caring. Be honest and keep all promises.	2. Trust is the basis for a therapeutic relationship.
	3. Convey an accepting attitude so that the patient is not afraid to express feelings openly.	3. An accepting attitude conveys nonjudgment and enhances trust.
	4. Allow the patient to express anger. Do not become defensive if the initial expression of anger is displaced on the nurse or therapist. Help the patient explore angry feelings so that they may be directed toward the intended object or person.	4. Verbalization of feelings in a nonthreatening environment may help the patient come to terms with unresolved issues.
	5. Assist the patient to discharge pent-up anger through participation in large motor activities (e.g., brisk walks, jogging, physical exercises, volleyball, exercise bike).	5. Physical exercise provides a safe and effective method for discharging pent-up tension.

Table 19–2 | CARE PLAN FOR THE PATIENT WITH AN ADJUSTMENT DISORDER—cont'd

OUTCOME CRITERIA	NURSING INTERVENTIONS	RATIONALE
	6. Explain to the patient the normal stages of grief and the behaviors associated with each stage. Help the patient to understand that feelings such as guilt and anger toward the lost entity/concept are natural and acceptable during the grief process.	6. Knowledge of the acceptability of the feelings associated with normal grieving may help to relieve some of the guilt that these responses generate.
	7. Encourage the patient to review their perception of the loss or change. With support and sensitivity, point out the reality of the situation in areas where misrepresentations are expressed.	7. The patient must give up an idealized perception and be able to accept both positive and negative aspects about the painful life change before the grief process is complete.
	8. Communicate to the patient that crying is acceptable. The use of touch is therapeutic and appropriate with most patients.	8. Knowledge of cultural influences specific to the patient is important before employing this technique. Touch is considered inappropriate in some cultures.
	9. Help the patient to solve problems as attempts are made to determine methods for more adaptive coping with the stressor. Provide positive feedback for strategies identified and decisions made.	9. Positive reinforcement enhances self-esteem and encourages repetition of desirable behaviors.
	10. Encourage the patient to reach out for spiritual support during this time in whatever form is desirable. Assess the patient's spiritual needs and assist as necessary in the fulfillment of those needs.	10. For some individuals, spiritual support can enhance successful adaptation to painful life experiences.

NURSING DIAGNOSIS: RISK-PRONE HEALTH BEHAVIOR

RELATED TO: Inadequate coping strategies; inadequate social support; low self-efficacy

EVIDENCED BY: Demonstrates nonacceptance of health status change

OUTCOME CRITERIA	NURSING INTERVENTIONS	RATIONALE
Short-Term Goals ■ Patient and primary nurse will discuss the kinds of lifestyle changes that will occur because of the change in health status. With the help of the primary nurse, the patient will formulate a plan of action for incorporating those changes into their lifestyle.	1. Encourage the patient to talk about their lifestyle prior to the change in health status. Discuss coping mechanisms that were used at stressful times in the past.	1. It is important to identify the patient's strengths so that they may be used to facilitate adaptation to the change or loss that has occurred.
	2. Encourage the patient to discuss the change or loss and particularly to express anger associated with it.	2. Anger is a normal stage in the grieving process and, if not released in an appropriate manner, may be turned inward on the self, leading to pathological depression.

Continued

Table 19–2 | CARE PLAN FOR THE PATIENT WITH AN ADJUSTMENT DISORDER—cont'd

OUTCOME CRITERIA	NURSING INTERVENTIONS	RATIONALE
■ Patient will demonstrate movement toward independence, considering the change in health status.	3. Encourage the patient to express fears associated with the change or loss or alteration in lifestyle that it has created.	3. Change often creates a feeling of disequilibrium, and the individual may respond with fears that are irrational or unfounded. The patient may benefit from feedback that corrects misperceptions about how life will be with the change in health status.
Long-Term Goal ■ Patient will demonstrate competence to function independently to optimal ability, considering the change in health status, by the time of discharge from treatment.	4. Provide assistance with activities of daily living as required but encourage independence to the limit that the patient's ability will allow. Give positive feedback for activities accomplished independently.	4. Independent accomplishments and positive feedback enhance self-esteem and encourage repetition of desired behaviors. Successes also provide hope that adaptive functioning is possible and decrease feelings of powerlessness.
	5. Help the patient with decision making regarding incorporation of the change or loss into their lifestyle. Identify problems the change or loss is likely to create. Discuss alternative solutions, weighing potential benefits and consequences of each alternative. Support the patient's decision in the selection of an alternative.	5. The great amount of anxiety that usually accompanies a major life change often interferes with an individual's ability to solve problems and to make appropriate decisions. The patient may need assistance with this process in an effort to progress toward successful adaptation.
	6. Use role-play to practice stressful situations that might occur in relation to the health status change.	6. Role-playing decreases anxiety and provides a feeling of security by providing the patient with a plan of action for responding in an appropriate manner when a stressful situation occurs.
	7. Ensure that the patient and family are fully knowledgeable regarding the physiology of the change in health status and understand the necessity of such knowledge for optimal wellness. Encourage them to ask questions and provide printed material explaining the change to which they may refer.	7. Having knowledge about the health status and knowing what to expect regarding the change or loss decreases anxiety and enhances the capacity for wellness.
	8. Ensure that the patient can identify resources within the community from which to seek assistance in adapting to the change in health status. Examples include self-help and support groups and public health nurses, counselors, or social worker. Encourage the patient to keep follow-up appointments with their physician or to call the physician's office prior to the follow-up date if problems or concerns arise.	8. Support services provide a feeling of security that one is not alone and provide a means to prevent decompensation when stress becomes intolerable.

- Set realistic goals for the future?
- Demonstrate new adaptive coping strategies for dealing with the change in lifestyle?
- Verbalize available resources for support or assistance should it be necessary?

Treatment Modalities

Trauma-Related Disorders

Cognitive Behavior Therapy

Cognitive behavior therapy for PTSD and acute stress disorder strives to help the individual recognize and modify trauma-related thoughts and beliefs. The individual learns to modify the relationships between thoughts and feelings and to identify and challenge inaccurate or extreme automatic negative thoughts. The goal is to replace these negative thoughts with more accurate and less distressing thoughts and to cope more effectively with feelings such as anger, guilt, and fear. The individual is assisted to modify the appraisal of self and the world as it has been affected by the trauma and to regain hope and optimism about safety, trust, power and control, esteem, and intimacy. Stress inoculation therapy (SIT) is a type of cognitive behavior therapy (CBT) that focuses on learning new ways of coping with stressful events through education and practicing alternative responses like meditation, deep breathing, and other relaxation exercises. Recent research (Bohus et al., 2020) supported the effectiveness of dialectical behavior therapy DBT (a therapy with several features common to CBT) in patients with complex PTSD associated with severe childhood abuse.

Prolonged Exposure Therapy

Prolonged exposure therapy is a type of behavioral therapy somewhat similar to implosion therapy or flooding (see Chapter 18, "Anxiety, Obsessive-Compulsive, and Related Disorders," for a discussion of implosion therapy). It can be conducted in an imagined or real (in vivo) situation. In the imagined situation, the individual is exposed to repeated and prolonged mental recounting of the traumatic experience within a therapy setting. In vivo exposure involves systematic confrontation outside of therapy and within safe limits to trauma-related stimuli that are feared and avoided. This intense emotional processing of the traumatic event serves to neutralize the memories so that they no longer result in anxious arousal or escape and avoidance behaviors. Prolonged exposure therapy has four main parts: (1) education about the treatment, (2) breath retraining for relaxation, (3) imagined exposure through repeated discussion about the trauma with a therapist, and (4) exposure to real-world situations related to the trauma.

Group and Family Therapy

Group therapy has been strongly advocated for clients with PTSD and has proved especially effective with military veterans and survivors of catastrophic disasters (Boland & Verduin, 2022). The importance of being able to share their experiences with empathetic fellow veterans, to talk about problems in social adaptation, and to discuss options for managing their aggression toward others has been emphasized. Some PTSD groups are informal and leaderless, such as self-help or support groups, and some are led by experienced group therapists who may have had some firsthand experience with the trauma. Some groups involve family members, thereby recognizing that the symptoms of PTSD may also severely affect them. For example, family members of military veterans sometimes develop PTSD as a result of exposure to their loved one's symptoms of PTSD (see Chapter 28, "Military Families," for further discussion of this topic).

Eye Movement Desensitization and Reprocessing

Eye movement desensitization and reprocessing (EMDR) is a type of psychotherapy that was developed in 1989 by psychologist Francine Shapiro. It "has evolved from a simple technique into an integrative psychotherapy approach with a theoretical model that emphasizes the brain's information processing system and memories of disturbing experiences as the basis of pathology" (Shapiro, 2007, p. 3). EMDR has been shown to be an effective therapy for clients with PTSD and other trauma-related disorders (Maxfield & Hyer, 2002; Rothbaum et al., 2005; Valiente-Gómez et al., 2017). It has been used experimentally in the treatment of other disorders, including depression, an adjustment disorder, phobias, addictions, generalized anxiety disorder, and panic disorder. Clinical practice guidelines from both the American Psychiatric Association and the Department of Veterans Affairs support the effectiveness of EMDR for PTSD (WebMD, 2021) and the World Health Organization (2013) supports the use of CBT and EMDR as advanced treatments for patients with PTSD.

The exact biological mechanisms by which EMDR achieves its therapeutic effects are unknown. Some studies have indicated that eye movements cause a decrease in imagery vividness and distress as well as an increase in memory access. The process involves rapid eye movements while processing painful emotions. The EMDR International Association (2021a) clarifies that therapy is not focused on talking in detail about the distressing issue or trying to change associated emotions, thoughts and behaviors; instead, the process allows the brain to resolve unprocessed traumatic memories and "resume its natural healing process." While concentrating on a particular emotion or physical sensation surrounding the traumatic event, the client is asked to focus eye movements on the therapist's fingers as the therapist moves them from left to right and back again. Although some individuals report rapid results with this therapy, research has indicated that from 5 to 12 sessions are required to achieve lasting treatment effects. Special precautions may be needed when using EMDR in clients with neurological impairments (e.g., seizure disorders), severe dissociative disorders, or unstable substance abuse and those who are suicidal or experiencing psychosis (UPMC, Center for Integrative Medicine, 2021).

The treatment encompasses an eight-phase process:

- ***Phase 1: History and treatment planning.*** The therapist takes a thorough history and develops a treatment plan. The problem for which the client is seeking treatment and current symptoms are discussed. However, clients are not required to discuss the traumatic event in detail, unless they choose to do so. Instead, emphasis is placed on the emotions and physical sensations surrounding the traumatic event.
- ***Phase 2: Preparation.*** The therapist teaches the client certain self-care techniques (e.g., relaxation techniques) for dealing with emotional disturbances that may arise during or between sessions. Self-care is an important component of EMDR. It is important for the client to develop a sense of trust in the therapist during this phase.
- ***Phase 3: Assessment.*** The therapist asks the client to identify a specific scene or picture from the target event identified in phase 1 that best represents the memory. The client is then directed to express a negative self-belief associated with the memory (e.g., "I am bad" or "I'm in danger"). The next step is to identify a self-statement that the client would *rather* believe (e.g., "I am good" or "I'm safe now"). When the self-statements have been identified, the client is asked to rate the validity of each of the statements on the Validity of Cognition (VOC) scale from "completely false" (a score of 1) to "completely true" (a score of 7). In this phase, the client is also asked to rank the disturbing emotions on the 0 to 10 Subjective Units of Disturbance (SUD) scale (with 0 meaning the disturbance is not disturbing at all and 10 meaning it is the worst feeling ever had).
- ***Phase 4: Desensitization.*** The client gives attention to the negative beliefs and disturbing emotions associated with the traumatic event while focusing vision on the back-and-forth motion of the therapist's fingers. All personal feelings and physical reactions experienced during this time are noted. Following each set of rapid eye movements, the therapist reassesses the level of disturbance associated with the feelings, images, and beliefs. This desensitization process continues until the distress level (as measured by the SUD scale) is reduced to 0 or 1.
- ***Phase 5: Installation.*** The client gives attention to the positive belief that has been identified to replace the negative belief associated with the trauma. This is accomplished while simultaneously visually tracking the therapist's fingers. Following each set of rapid eye movements, the client is asked to rate the positive belief on the VOC scale. The goal is to strengthen the positive belief or self-statement until it is accepted as completely true (a score of 7 on the VOC scale).
- ***Phase 6: Body scan.*** When the positive cognition has been strengthened, the therapist asks the client to concentrate on any lingering physical sensations. While focusing on the traumatic event, the client is asked to identify any areas of the body where residual tension is experienced. Because positive self-beliefs must be believed on more than just an intellectual level, phase 6 is not complete until the client is able to think about or discuss the traumatic event (or the feelings associated with it) without experiencing bodily tension.
- ***Phase 7: Closure.*** Closure ensures that the client leaves each session feeling better than the client felt at the beginning. If the processing that took place during the session is not complete, the therapist will direct the client through a variety of self-calming relaxation techniques to help them regain emotional equilibrium. The client is briefed about what to expect between sessions. Until processing of the trauma is complete, disturbing images, thoughts, and emotions may arise between therapy sessions. The therapist instructs the client to

record these experiences in a journal so that they may be used as targets for processing in future therapy sessions.

- ***Phase 8: Reevaluation.*** Reevaluation begins each new therapy session. The therapist assesses whether the positive changes have been maintained, determines whether previous target areas need reprocessing, and identifies any new target areas that need attention.

Clients often feel relief quite rapidly with EMDR. However, to achieve lasting results, it is important that each of the eight phases be completed. Treatment is not complete until "EMDR therapy has focused on the past memories that are contributing to the problem, the present situations that are disturbing, and what skills the client may need for the future" (EMDR International Association, 2021b).

Digital Therapeutics

In 2020, the U.S. Food and Drug Administration (FDA) approved a prescription Apple Watch application designed to improve sleep quality in adults with PTSD-related nightmares (FDA, 2020). The watch's sensors detect heart rate abnormalities that might be related to nightmares and then it vibrates, reportedly to interrupt the dream without disturbing sleep. It is currently undergoing additional trials but may be available with a physician's recommendation.

Psychopharmacology

Trauma-focused psychotherapy is considered the first-line treatment for PTSD (Jeffreys, 2021); however, many medications have demonstrated benefits as well.

Antidepressants

Specific selective serotonin reuptake inhibitors (SSRIs) are considered the first-line pharmacological choice for PTSD because of their efficacy, tolerability, and safety ratings. Paroxetine and sertraline have been approved by the FDA for this purpose. Additionally, fluoxetine and the serotonin-norepinephrine reuptake inhibitor (SNRI) venlafaxine (although not FDA-approved for PTSD) have demonstrated effectiveness (Jeffreys, 2021). The tricyclic antidepressants amitriptyline (Elavil) and imipramine (Tofranil) have been supported by several well-controlled studies and may be an alternative if the client is not responding to an SSRI. The monoamine oxidase inhibitor phenelzine has also demonstrated efficacy in the treatment of PTSD.

Anxiolytics

Alprazolam (a benzodiazepine) has been prescribed for clients with PTSD for its antidepressant and antipanic effects despite the absence of controlled studies demonstrating their efficacy for this condition. Jeffreys (2021) recommends against using benzodiazepines in PTSD based on a meta-analysis finding that they worsened patients' PTSD symptoms. In addition, their addictive properties make them less desirable than some of the other medications in the treatment of post-trauma patients.

Buspirone, which has serotonergic properties similar to those of SSRIs, may be useful for treating anxiety in PTSD, and these drugs also have less addiction potential than benzodiazepines. Animal studies (Malikowska-Racia et al., 2020) support its benefit in treating clients with PTSD but more controlled trials with this drug are needed.

Antihypertensives

The beta-blocker propranolol and alpha$_2$-receptor agonist clonidine have been successful in alleviating some of the symptoms associated with PTSD. Some clinical trials have reported reduction in symptoms, such as nightmares and angry outbursts. Although beta blockers are known to reduce hyperarousal states and may decrease aggression, Jeffreys (2021) reports that current evidence is insufficient to support their routine use in PTSD treatment.

Other Medications

Ketamine, an anesthetic agent that has demonstrated benefits in treatment of depression and obsessive-compulsive disorder was found in clinical trials (Feder et al., 2021) to benefit some patients with PTSD. It modulates glutaminergic activity at *N*-methyl-D-aspartate (NMDA) receptors and serotonergic activity at 5-HT$_1$ receptors and is thought to disrupt the fear associated with trauma. Currently, ketamine is not FDA approved for this use but is prescribed as an off-label use. It is administered intravenously at subanesthetic doses and usually involves a series of treatments. Jeffreys (2021) cautions that its effects are short term and there is potential for addiction. MDMA (3,4-methylenedioxymethamphetamine) is also in clinical trials for the treatment of PTSD and early findings suggest that MDMA-assisted psychotherapy may be beneficial in helping reduce fear and facilitate processing of traumatic memories (Mitchell et al., 2021).

The endocannabinoid system may be another avenue for treatment, since decreased levels of endogenous cannabinoids have been found in PTSD patients (Jeffreys, 2021). Although direct stimulation of this pathway has demonstrated negative effects on PTSD and potential for addiction, indirect stimulation of this pathway might provide some additional treatment options. Early trials with fatty acid amide hydrolase (FAAH) inhibitors, which block the breakdown of endocannabinoids, showed promise in helping participants to develop fear-extinction memories (Mayo et al., 2019). More research is needed to confirm these benefits.

The alpha$_1$ antagonist prazosin (Minipress) has been studied for its potential benefit in reducing nightmares and enhancing normal dreaming patterns in clients with PTSD. However, Veterans Health Administration clinical practice guidelines now recommend against its use for clients with PTSD based on a large trial that found no difference between prazosin and placebo (Jeffreys, 2021). Low-dose glucocorticoids have been studied for possible benefit in decreasing recall of traumatic memories; other actions of glucocorticoids that may affect response to PTSD symptoms include potentiating glutamate at NMDA receptors and interactions with noradrenergic systems (Jeffreys, 2021), but more research is needed.

Adjustment Disorders

Various treatments are used for clients with adjustment disorders. The primary focus of intervention is to maximize the potential for adaptation.

Individual Psychotherapy

Individual psychotherapy is the most common treatment for adjustment disorders. Individual psychotherapy allows the client to examine the stressor that is causing the problem, possibly assign personal meaning to the stressor, and confront unresolved issues that may be exacerbating this crisis. Treatment works to remove these blocks to adaptation so that normal developmental progression can resume. Techniques are used to clarify links between the current stressor and past experiences and to assist with the development of more adaptive coping strategies.

Family Therapy

The focus of treatment is shifted from the individual to the system of relationships in which the individual is involved. The maladaptive response of the identified client is viewed as symptomatic of a dysfunctional family system. All family members are included in the therapy, and treatment serves to improve the functioning within the family network. Emphasis is placed on communication, family rules, and interaction patterns among the family members.

Behavior Therapy

The goal of behavior therapy is to replace ineffective response patterns with more adaptive ones. The situations that promote ineffective responses are identified, and carefully designed reinforcement schedules, along with role-modeling and coaching, are used to alter the maladaptive response patterns. This type of treatment is very effective when implemented in an inpatient setting where the client's behavior and its consequences may be more readily controlled.

Self-Help Groups

Group experiences, with or without a professional facilitator, provide an arena in which members may consider and compare their responses with those of individuals with similar life experiences. Members benefit from learning that they are not alone in their painful experiences. Hope is derived from knowing that others have survived and even grown from similar experiences. Members of the group exchange advice, share coping strategies, and provide support and encouragement for each other.

Crisis Intervention

In crisis intervention, the therapist or other intervener becomes a part of the individual's life situation. Because of increased anxiety, the individual with an adjustment disorder is unable to problem solve so requires guidance and support from another to help mobilize the resources needed to resolve the crisis. Crisis intervention is short term and relies heavily on orderly problem-solving techniques and structured activities that are focused on change. The ultimate goal of crisis intervention in the treatment of adjustment disorders is to resolve the immediate crisis, restore adaptive functioning, and promote personal growth.

Psychopharmacology

Adjustment disorders are not commonly treated with medications because (1) their effect may be temporary and only mask the real problem, interfering with the possibility of finding a more permanent solution, and (2) some psychoactive drugs carry the potential for physiological and psychological dependence.

When the client with an adjustment disorder has symptoms of anxiety or depression, the physician may prescribe antianxiety or antidepressant medication. These medications are considered only adjuncts to psychotherapy and should not be given as the primary therapy. In these instances, they are given to alleviate symptoms so that the individual may more effectively cope while attempting to adapt to the stressful situation.

CASE STUDY AND SAMPLE CARE PLAN

NURSING HISTORY AND ASSESSMENT

Marissa, age 22, was born in a small town in Oklahoma. She has lived there her whole life, even living at home while she attended a nearby college to earn a baccalaureate degree in education. She is an only child, and her parents were in their 40s when she was born. She was engaged throughout her college years to her high school sweetheart, Dave, who graduated 6 months ago from the state university with a degree in aeronautical engineering. Upon his graduation, he accepted a position with NASA at Kennedy Space Center in Florida. Marissa and Dave were married 5 months ago and moved to a small apartment in Cape Canaveral, where Dave began his work with NASA. The plan was for Marissa to seek employment upon their arrival, but she has been unable to move ahead with those plans. She stays in their apartment most days, talking on the phone to her parents and crying about how much she misses them and her home in Oklahoma. Marissa has met very few people and has no desire to do so. She sleeps a lot and has lost weight. She has been having severe headaches. Her husband is very concerned about her and made an appointment for her with a private physician. Following a complete and unremarkable physical examination, the physician referred Marissa to the mental health clinic where she was admitted to the day treatment center with a diagnosis of adjustment disorder with depressed mood.

NURSING DIAGNOSES AND OUTCOME IDENTIFICATION

From the assessment data, the nurse develops the following nursing diagnoses for Marissa:

1. **Maladaptive grieving** related to feelings of loss associated with leaving her parents and her lifetime home
   a. **Short-Term Goal:** Within 1 week, Marissa will express anger about the loss associated with her move.
   b. **Long-Term Goal:** Marissa will be able to verbalize behaviors associated with the normal stages of grief and identify her own position in the grief process, while progressing at her own pace toward resolution.
2. **Relocation stress syndrome** related to moving away from parents and familiar environment in which she had spent her whole life
   a. **Short-Term Goal:** Within 1 week, Marissa will verbalize at least one positive aspect regarding relocation to her new environment.
   b. **Long-Term Goal:** Within 1 month, Marissa will demonstrate positive adaptation to her new environment as evidenced by involvement in activities, expression of satisfaction with new acquaintances, and elimination of previously evident physical and psychological symptoms associated with the relocation.

PLANNING AND IMPLEMENTATION

MALADAPTIVE GRIEVING

The following nursing interventions have been identified for Marissa:

1. Determine the stage of grief in which Marissa is fixed. Identify behaviors associated with this stage.
2. Develop a trusting relationship with Marissa. Show empathy and caring. Be honest and keep all promises.
3. Convey an accepting attitude so that Marissa is not afraid to express her feelings openly.
4. Allow Marissa to express her anger. Do not become defensive if the initial expression of anger is displaced on nurse or therapist. Help Marissa explore angry feelings so that they may be directed toward the intended object or situation.
5. Help Marissa discharge pent-up anger through participation in large motor activities (e.g., brisk walks, jogging, physical exercises, or activity of her choice).
6. Explain to Marissa the normal stages of grief and the behaviors associated with each stage. Help her to understand that these feelings are normal and acceptable during a grief process.
7. Encourage Marissa to review her personal perception of the move. With support and sensitivity, point out the reality of the situation in areas where misrepresentations are expressed.
8. Help Marissa solve problems as she attempts to determine methods for more adaptive coping with the life change. Provide positive feedback for strategies identified and decisions made.
9. Encourage Marissa to reach out for spiritual support during this time in whatever form is desirable to her. Assess her spiritual needs and assist as necessary in the fulfillment of those needs.

Continued

CASE STUDY AND SAMPLE CARE PLAN—cont'd

RELOCATION STRESS SYNDROME

The following nursing interventions have been identified for Marissa:

1. Encourage Marissa to discuss feelings (concerns, fears, anger) regarding this relocation.
2. Encourage Marissa to discuss how the change will affect her life. Ensure that Marissa is involved in decision making and problem-solving regarding the move.
3. Help Marissa identify positive aspects about the move.
4. Help Marissa identify resources within the new community from which assistance with various types of services may be obtained.
5. Identify groups within the community that specialize in helping individuals adapt to relocation. Examples include Newcomers' Club, Welcome Wagon International, and school and church organizations.
6. Refer Marissa to a support group (e.g., Depression and Bipolar Support Alliance [DBSA]).

EVALUATION

The outcome criteria for Marissa have been met. She is no longer having headaches, and she has regained some of her weight. She has joined a chapter of DBSA and has made some new acquaintances. She has applied to become a substitute teacher in the local school district, and she and Dave have joined the local Methodist church, where they have started to socialize with several couples their age. They have also adopted Molly, a 2-year-old mutt from the local shelter, who showers Marissa with love and keeps her company when no one else is around. They take daily walks together. Marissa still talks to her parents on the phone daily, but she no longer has feelings of despair about living so far away from them. Her parents provide encouragement and give her positive feedback for achieving a satisfactory adaptation to her new environment. They are planning a visit to see Marissa and Dave in the near future.

Summary and Key Points

- Post-traumatic stress disorder (PTSD) is the development of characteristic symptoms following exposure to an extreme traumatic stressor involving a personal threat to physical integrity or to the integrity of others. Symptoms may begin within the first 3 months after the trauma, or there may be a delay of several months or even years.
- The symptoms of PTSD are associated with events that would be markedly distressing to almost anyone and include reexperiencing the trauma, a sustained high level of anxiety or arousal, or a general numbing of responsiveness.
- A disorder that is similar in terms of precipitating traumatic events and symptomatology to PTSD is called acute stress disorder. In acute stress disorder, the symptoms are time limited, up to 1 month following the trauma. If the symptoms last longer than 1 month, the diagnosis would be PTSD.
- Predisposing factors to trauma-related disorders include psychosocial, learning, cognitive, and biological influences.
- Adjustment disorders are relatively common. Some studies indicate that they are the most commonly ascribed psychiatric diagnoses.
- Clinical symptoms associated with adjustment disorders include inability to function socially or occupationally in response to an identifiable stressor.
- An adjustment disorder is distinguished by the predominant features of the maladaptive response. These include depression, anxiety, mixed anxiety and depression, disturbance of conduct, and mixed disturbance of emotions and conduct.
- Of the two types of stressors discussed (sudden shock and continuous), more individuals respond with maladaptive behaviors to long-term, continuous stressors.
- Treatment modalities for PTSD include cognitive behavior therapy, dialectical behavior therapy, prolonged exposure therapy, group and family therapy, EMDR, digital therapeutics, and psychopharmacology.
- Treatment modalities for adjustment disorders include individual psychotherapy, family therapy, behavior therapy, self-help groups, crisis intervention, and medications to treat anxiety or depression.
- Nursing care of individuals with trauma- and stressor-related disorders is accomplished using the steps of the nursing process.
- Trauma-informed care identifies and considers the impact of previous trauma when developing a care plan for clients in any setting because this client is vulnerable to retraumatization.

Review Questions

Select the answer that is most appropriate for each of the following questions:

1. A client, who is a veteran of the war in Iraq, is diagnosed with PTSD. The client, John, says to the nurse, "I can't figure out why God took my buddy instead of me." From this statement, the nurse assesses which of the following in John?
   a. Repressed anger
   b. Survivor's guilt
   c. Intrusive thoughts
   d. Spiritual distress
2. Which treatment regimen would most appropriately be ordered for a client with PTSD?
   a. Paroxetine and group therapy
   b. Diazepam and implosion therapy
   c. Alprazolam and behavior therapy
   d. Carbamazepine and cognitive therapy
3. Which finding may be influential in the predisposition to PTSD?
   a. Resilient personality traits
   b. Ketamine deficiency
   c. History of dementia
   d. Severity of the stressor and availability of support systems
4. Which statement is true regarding the diagnosis of an adjustment disorder?
   a. The client will require long-term psychotherapy to achieve relief.
   b. The client likely inherited a genetic tendency for the disorder.
   c. Symptoms will likely remit once the client has accepted the changes that precipitated difficulties with adjustment.
   d. Adjustment disorders are not typically related to an identified stressor.
5. The physician orders sertraline (Zoloft) for a client who is hospitalized with an adjustment disorder with depressed mood. Which benefit is intended?
   a. Increase energy and elevate mood
   b. Stimulate the central nervous system
   c. Prevent psychotic symptoms
   d. Produce a calming effect
6. Trauma-informed care is a philosophical approach that includes which principles? (Select all that apply.)
   a. Nurses need to be aware of the potential for trauma in any client and provide care that minimizes the risk of revictimization or retraumatization.
   b. Medications need to be given before any other interventions are considered.
   c. Trauma-informed care highlights the importance of providing care that protects the physical, psychological, and emotional safety of the client.
   d. Trauma-informed care is based on the principle that traumas are not correlated with depression or increased risk for suicide.

Clinical Judgment Questions

7. A client experiences a nightmare during their first night in the hospital. The client explains to the nurse that they were dreaming about gunfire all around and people being killed. Which is the nurse's most appropriate *initial* intervention?
   a. Administer alprazolam as ordered prn for anxiety.
   b. Call the physician and report the incident.
   c. Stay with the client and reassure them of their safety.
   d. Have the client listen to a tape of relaxation exercises.

Continued

8. A client who recently divorced after 10 years of marriage is admitted to the hospital with a diagnosis of adjustment disorder with depressed mood. The client acknowledges difficulty adjusting to an independent lifestyle and having thoughts of taking an overdose of acetaminophen. Which is the priority nursing diagnosis for this client?
   a. Risk-prone health behavior
   b. Maladaptive grieving
   c. Ineffective communication
   d. Risk for suicidal behavior
9. A client, who is depressed following the breakup of a very stormy marriage, says to the nurse, "I feel so bad. I thought I would feel better once I left, but I feel worse!" Which is the *best* response by the nurse?
   a. "Cheer up. You have a lot to be happy about."
   b. "You are grieving the loss of your marriage. It's natural for you to feel bad."
   c. "Try not to dwell on how you feel. If you don't think about it, you'll feel better."
   d. "You did the right thing. Knowing that should make you feel better."
10. A client, age 16, has recently been diagnosed with diabetes mellitus. The client must watch their diet and take an oral hypoglycemic medication daily. The client has become very depressed, and the client's mother reports that they refuse to change their diet and often skips their medication. The client has been hospitalized for stabilization of their blood glucose level. The psychiatric nurse practitioner has been called in as a consultant. Which nursing diagnosis by the psychiatric nurse would be a priority for the client at this time?
    a. Anxiety related to hospitalization evidenced by nonadherence
    b. Low self-esteem related to feeling different from their peers evidenced by social isolation
    c. Risk for suicide related to new diagnosis of diabetes mellitus as evidenced by reports of depression
    d. Risk-prone health behavior related to denial of seriousness of their illness evidenced by refusal to follow diet and take medication

TEST YOUR CLINICAL REASONING AND CLINICAL JUDGMENT SKILLS

Alicia, age 48, underwent a mastectomy of the right breast after her mammogram revealed a lump that proved to be malignant when biopsied. Since her surgery 6 weeks ago, Alicia has refused to see any of her friends. She stays in her bedroom, speaks to her husband only when he speaks first, is having difficulty sleeping, and eats very little. She refuses to look at the mastectomy scar and has refused to see the Reach to Recovery representative who has tried several times to help fit her with a prosthesis. Her husband is very worried about her and spoke to the family doctor, who recommended a psychiatrist. Alicia has been admitted to the psychiatric unit with a diagnosis of adjustment disorder with depressed mood.

Answer the following questions about Alicia:

1. What would be the primary nursing diagnosis for Alicia?
2. Describe a short-term goal and a long-term goal for Alicia.
3. Discuss a priority nursing intervention in working with Alicia.

MOVIE CONNECTIONS

The Deer Hunter (PTSD) ▪ *Hell and Back Again* (PTSD) ▪ *Jackknife* (PTSD) ▪ *Brothers* (PTSD) ▪ *The War at Home* (PTSD) ▪ *Fearless* (PTSD) ▪ *The Fisher King* (PTSD) ▪ *The Changeover* (PTSD and comorbid mental health issues) ▪ *The Perks of Being a Wallflower* (PTSD) ▪ *A Private War* (PTSD)

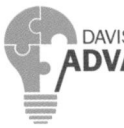

Go to **Davis Advantage** to complete your learning: strengthen understanding, apply your knowledge, and prepare for the Next Gen NCLEX®.

References

American Psychiatric Association. (2000). *Diagnostic and statistical manual of mental disorders* (4th ed., text rev.).

American Psychiatric Association. (2022). *Diagnostic and statistical manual of mental disorders* (5th ed., text rev.).

Bohus, M., Kleindiens, N., Hahn, C., Müller-Engelmann, M., Ludäscher, P., Steil, R., Fydrich, T., Kuehner, C., Resick, P. A., Stiglmayr, C., Schmahl, C., & Priebe, K. (2020). Dialectical behavior therapy for posttraumatic stress disorder (DBT-PTSD) compared with cognitive processing therapy (CPT) in complex presentations of PTSD in women survivors of childhood abuse: A randomized clinical trial. *JAMA Psychiatry, 77*(12), 1235–1245. https://doi.org/10.1001/jamapsychiatry.2020.2148

Boland, R., & Verduin, M. L. (2022). *Kaplan & Sadock's synopsis of psychiatry* (P. Ruiz, Ed.). (12th ed.). Wolters Kluwer.

Department of Veterans Affairs. (2019). *How common is PTSD in adults?* https://www.ptsd.va.gov/understand/common/common_adults.asp

EMDR International Association. (2021a). *About EMDR therapy.* https://www.emdria.org/about-emdr-therapy/

EMDR International Association. (2021b). *Experiencing EMDR therapy.* https://www.emdria.org/about-emdr-therapy/experiencing-emdr-therapy/

Feder, A., Costi, S., Rutter, S. B., Collins, A. B., Govindarajulu, U., Jha, M. K., Horn, S. R., Kautz, M., Corniquel, M., Collins, K. A., Bevilacqua, L., Glasgow, A. M., Brallier, J., Pietrzak, R. H., Murrough, J. W., & Charney, D. S. (2021). A randomized controlled trial of repeated ketamine administration for chronic posttraumatic stress disorder. *American Journal of Psychiatry, 178*(2), 193–202. https://doi.org/10.1176/appi.ajp.2020.20050596

Frances, A. (2015). "We should live"—Surviving after catastrophic death. *Psychiatric Times.* http://www.psychiatrictimes.com/major-depressive-disorder/we-should-live-surviving-after-catastrophic-death

Frank, J. B. (2016). Adjustment disorders. *Medscape.* https://emedicine.medscape.com/article/2192631-overview#a5

Friedman, M. J., Resick, P. A., Bryant, R. A., Strain, J., Horowitz, M., & Spiegel, D. (2011). Classification of trauma and stressor-related disorders in DSM-5. *Depression and Anxiety, 28*(9), 737–749.

Gradus, J. L., Bozi, I., Antonsen, S., Svensson, E., Lash, T.L., Resick, P. A., & Hansen, J. G. (2014). Severe stress and adjustment disorder diagnoses in the population of Denmark. *Journal of Traumatic Stress, 27*(3), 370–374. https://doi.org/10.1002/jts.21926

Günak, M., Billings, J., Carratu, E., Marchant, N., Favarato, G., & Orgeta, V. (2020). Post-traumatic stress disorder as a risk factor for dementia: Systematic review and meta-analysis. *The British Journal of Psychiatry, 217*(5), 600–608. https://doi.org/10.1192/bjp.2020.150

Herdman, T. H., Kamitsuru, S., & Lopes, C. T. (Eds.). (2021). *NANDA-I, Inc. nursing diagnoses: Definitions and classification, 2021–2023.* Thieme.

Hopper, E. K., Bassuk, E. L., & Olivet, J. (2010). Shelter from the storm: Trauma-informed care in homelessness services settings. *Open Health Services and Policy Journal, 3*, 80–100.

Jeffreys, M. (2021). *Clinician's guide to medications for PTSD.* https://www.ptsd.va.gov/professional/treat/txessentials/clinician_guide_meds.asp

Katzman, J. W., & Geppert, C. M. (2017). Adjustment disorders. In B. J. Sadock, V. A. Sadock, & P. Ruiz (Eds.), *Comprehensive textbook of psychiatry* (10th ed., pp. 2116–2125). Wolters Kluwer.

Lanius, U. (2013). *Neurobiology and treatment of traumatic dissociation.* http://www.isst-d.org/downloads/AnnualConference/2013/Baltimore2013handout.pdf

Lynch, T. R. (2018). *Radically open dialectical behavior therapy: Theory and practice for treating disorders of overcontrol.* Context Press.

Malikowska-Racia, N., Popik, P., & Salat, K. (2020). Behavioral effects of buspirone in a mouse model of posttraumatic stress disorder. *Behavioural Brain Research, 381.* https://doi.org/10.1016/j.bbr.2019.112380

Maxfield, L., & Hyer, L. (2002). The relationship between efficacy and methodology in studies investigating EMDR treatment of PTSD. *Journal of Clinical Psychology, 58*(1), 23–41.

Mayo, L. M., Asratian, A., Linde, J., Moreno, M., Haataja, R., Hammar, V., Augier, G., Hill, M. N., & Heilig, M. (2019). Elevated anandamide, enhanced recall of fear extinction, and attenuated stress responses following inhibition of fatty acid amide hydrolase: A randomized, controlled experimental medicine trial. *Biological Psychiatry, 87*(6), 538–547. https://doi.org/10.1016/j.biopsych.2019.07.034

Mitchell, J. M., Bogenschutz, M., Lilienstein, A., Harrison, C., Kleiman, S., Parker-Guilbert, K., Ot'alora, G. M., Garas, W., Paleos, C., Gorman, I., Nicholas, C., Mithoefer, M., Carlin, S., Poulter, B., Mithoefer, A., Quevedo, S., Wells, G., Klaire, S. S., van der Kolk, B., Tzarfaty, K., Amiaz, R., . . . Doblin, R. (2021). MDMA-assisted therapy for severe PTSD: A randomized, double-blind, placebo-controlled phase 3 study. *Nature Medicine, 27*(6), 1025–1033. https://doi.org/10.1038/s41591-021-01336-3

Park, C. L., Mills, M. A., & Edmondson, D. (2012). PTSD as meaning violation: Testing a cognitive worldview perspective. *Psychological Trauma: Theory, Research, Practice and Policy, 4*(1), 66–73. https://doi.org/10.1037/a0018792

Rothbaum, B. O., Astin, M. C., & Marsteller, F. (2005). Prolonged exposure versus and reprocessing (EMDR) for PTSD rape victims. *Journal of Traumatic Stress, 18*(6), 607–616.

Shapiro, F. (2007). EMDR and case conceptualization from an adaptive information processing perspective. In F. Shapiro, F. W. Kaslow, & L. Maxfield (Eds.), *Handbook of EMDR and family therapy processes,* (pp. 3–34). John Wiley & Sons.

Steenkamp, M. M., Schlenger, W. E., Corry, N., Henn-Haase C., Qian, M., Li, M., Horesh, D., Karstoft, K.I., Williams, C., Ho, C. L., Shalev, A., Kulka, R., & Marmar, C. (2017). Predictors of PTSD 40 years after combat: Findings from the National Vietnam Veterans longitudinal study. *Depression and Anxiety, 34*(8), 711–722. https://doi.org/10.1002/da.22628

Stein, M. B., Levey, D. F., Cheng, Z., Wendt, F. R., Harrington, K., Pathak, G. A., Cho, K., Quaden, R., Radhakrishnan, K., Girgenti, M. J., Ho, Y. A., Posner, D., Aslan, M., Duman, R. S., Zhao, H., Department of Veterans Affairs Cooperative Studies Program (no. 575B); VA Million Veteran Program, Polimanti, R., Concato, J., & Gelernter J. (2021). Genome-wide association analyses of post-traumatic stress disorder and its symptom subdomains in the Million Veteran Program. *Nature Genetics, 53*(2), 174–184. https://doi.org/10.1038/s41588-020-00767-

Substance Abuse and Mental Health Services Administration. (2019). *Trauma and violence.* https://www.samhsa.gov/trauma-violence

Togay, B., & El-Mallakh, R. S. (2020). Posttraumatic stress disorder: From pathophysiology to pharmacology. *Current Psychiatry, 19*(5), 33–37.

UPMC, Center for Integrative Medicine. (2021). *Eye movement desensitization and reprocessing.* http://www.upmc.com/Services/integrative-medicine/services/Pages/eye-movement.aspx

U.S. Food and Drug Administration. (2020). *FDA permits marketing of new device designed to reduce sleep disturbance related to nightmares in certain adults* [Press release]. https://www.fda.gov/news-events/press-announcements/fda-permits-marketing-new-device-designed-reduce-sleep-disturbance-related-nightmares-certain-adults

Valentino, R. J., & Van Bockstaele, E. (2015). Endogenous opioids: The downside to opposing stress. *Neurobiology of Stress, 1,* 23–32. https://doi.org//10.1016/j.ynstr.2014.09.006

Valiente-Gómez, A., Moreno-Alcázar, A., Treen, D., Cedrón, C., Colom, F., Pérez, V., & Amann, B. L. (2017). EMDR beyond PTSD: A systematic literature review. *Frontiers in Psychiatry, 8.* https://doi.org/10.3389/fpsyg.2017.01668

WebMD. (2021). *EMDR: Eye movement desensitization and reprocessing.* https://www.webmd.com/mental-health/emdr-what-is-it

World Health Organization. (2013). *WHO releases guidance on mental health care after trauma* [Press release]. https://www.who.int/mediacentre/news/releases/2013/trauma_mental_health_20130806/en/

Classical References

Epstein, S. (1991). Beliefs and symptoms in maladaptive resolutions of the traumatic neurosis. In D. Ozer, J. M. Healy, Jr., & A. J. Stewart (Eds.), *Perspectives on personality* (Vol. 3). Jessica Kingsley.

Friedman, M. J. (1996). PTSD diagnosis and treatment for mental health clinicians. *Community Mental Health Journal, 32*(2), 173–189.

Somatic Symptom and Dissociative Disorders 20

CHAPTER OUTLINE

Objectives
Introduction
Historical Perspectives
Epidemiology
Application of the Nursing Process
Treatment Modalities
Summary and Key Points
Review Questions
Clinical Judgment Questions
Implications for Evidence-Based Practice
Test Your Clinical Reasoning and Clinical Judgment Skills
Movie Connections

KEY TERMS

abreaction
anosmia
aphonia
depersonalization
derealization
factitious disorders
fugue
generalized amnesia
integration
localized amnesia
primary gain
pseudocyesis
secondary gain
selective amnesia
somatization
tertiary gain

OBJECTIVES

After reading this chapter, the student will be able to:

1. Discuss historical perspectives and epidemiology related to somatic symptom and dissociative disorders.
2. Describe various types of somatic symptom and dissociative disorders and identify symptomatology associated with each; use this information in patient assessment.
3. Identify predisposing factors in the development of somatic symptom and dissociative disorders.
4. Formulate nursing diagnoses and goals of care for patients with somatic symptom and dissociative disorders.
5. Describe appropriate nursing interventions for behaviors associated with somatic symptom and dissociative disorders.
6. Evaluate the nursing care of patients with somatic symptom and dissociative disorders.
7. Discuss various modalities relevant to treatment of somatic symptom and dissociative disorders.

CORE CONCEPTS

Stress and Coping: Amnesia, dissociation, and somatic symptoms
Professional Behavior: Nursing process in the care of patients with somatic symptom and dissociative disorders
Safety
Clinical Judgment

Introduction

Disorders with primarily somatic symptoms are characterized by physical symptoms, suggesting medical disease, but without demonstrable organic pathology. For this reason, most clients with a somatic symptom or related disorder are seen in primary care and hospital settings rather than in mental health-care settings. It is important to note that in cases in which modern medicine cannot determine the existence of pathophysiology to explain a client's symptoms, the lack of pathophysiology is not sufficient to diagnose the client with a mental illness. Somatic symptoms and related disorders are classified as mental disorders, according to the *Diagnostic and Statistical Manual of Mental Disorders, Fifth Edition, Text Revision* (American Psychiatric Association [APA], 2022), when the excessive focus on somatic symptoms is beyond any medical explanation *and* when somatic symptoms cause significant distress and impairment in the client's functioning.

The *DSM-5-TR* identifies a specific disorder called *somatic symptom disorder* and several related disorders, including *illness anxiety disorder, conversion disorder, factitious disorders, psychological factors affecting other medical conditions,* and others (APA, 2022). Their common focus is distress and impairment secondary to somatic symptoms, as described previously. The prevalence of somatic symptom disorder in primary care settings is estimated to be as high as 11%, and prevalence of hypochondriasis (no longer a diagnostic category in the *DSM-5-TR* but similar to *illness anxiety disorder*) is estimated to be 1.3% to 10% (APA, 2022). Studies have estimated the incidence of conversion symptoms (somatic symptoms that can't be medically explained) among patients in general hospital settings to be as high as 20% to 25%, with 5% meeting the full criteria for a conversion disorder (Ali et al., 2015). The wide variation in estimates, depending on the population being studied, highlights the difficulties associated with consensus in diagnosing and reporting these conditions.

Dissociative disorders are defined by a disruption in psychobiological functions that would otherwise be integrated aspects of experience and cognition including memory, identity, consciousness, perception, behavior, emotion, body representation, and motor control (Lowenstein et al., 2017). Dissociative responses occur when anxiety becomes overwhelming and the personality becomes disorganized. Defense mechanisms that normally govern consciousness, identity, and memory break down, and behavior occurs with little or no participation on the part of the conscious personality. Types of dissociative disorders described by the *DSM-5-TR* include *depersonalization-derealization disorder, dissociative amnesia, dissociative identity disorder (DID), and others.*

This chapter focuses on disorders characterized by severe anxiety that has been repressed and is being expressed in the form of physical symptoms, fear of illness, and dissociative behaviors. Historical perspectives and epidemiology are presented. Predisposing factors that have been implicated in the etiology of these responses provide a framework for studying the dynamics of somatic symptom and dissociative disorders. An explanation of the symptomatology of these disorders is presented as background knowledge for assessing the patient, and nursing care is described in the context of the nursing process. Additional treatment modalities are explored.

Historical Perspectives

Historically, somatic symptom disorders were identified as *hysterical neuroses.* The concept of hysteria is at least 4,000 years old and probably originated in Egypt. The name has been in use since the time of Hippocrates. In its original use, hysteria was referred to as a condition of emotional excitability that affected psychological, sensory, vasomotor, and visceral functions.

Over the years, symptoms of hysterical neuroses have been associated with witchcraft, demonology, and sorcery; dysfunction of the nervous system; and unexpressed emotions. They have also historically been viewed as primarily an affliction of women. Critics have argued that the depiction of women as prone to hysteria is not only sexist but also has interfered, at times, with women receiving adequate medical evaluation for symptoms.

Somatic symptom disorders are thought to occur in response to repressed severe anxiety. Freud (1962) observed that, under hypnosis, clients with hysterical neurosis could recall memories and emotional experiences that would relieve their symptoms. This observation led to his proposal that unexpressed emotion can be "converted" into physical symptoms.

CORE CONCEPT

Dissociation

An unconscious defense mechanism in which there is separation of normally related mental processes such as identity, memory, and cognition from affect; the detachment of ideas and memories from events or experiences.

Freud (1962) viewed dissociation as a type of repression: an active defense mechanism used to remove threatening or unacceptable mental contents from conscious awareness. He described ego-splitting (division of identity) as a defense mechanism in the management of incompatible mental contents. Although the study of dissociative processes dates to the 19th century, scientists know remarkably little about the phenomena. Questions remain unanswered: Are dissociative disorders psychopathological processes or ego-protective devices? Are dissociative processes under voluntary control, or are they a totally unconscious effort? In either case, they may serve to reduce a person's awareness and anxiety associated with events that are perceived as extremely stressful.

While symptoms such as dissociation are an unconscious defense mechanism, some individuals consciously fabricate symptoms. The syndrome of fabricating symptoms for emotional gain was first described by Richard Asher in 1951. He described a pattern of behavior in which individuals fabricated or embellished their histories and signs and symptoms of illness. He termed this condition *Munchausen syndrome* after Baron Friedrich Hieronymus Freiherr von Munchhausen, a German cavalry officer and nobleman who was known for his fabricated stories and fanciful exaggerations about himself (Asher, 1951). Currently, the *DSM-5-TR* describes these syndromes as **factitious disorders.** These include *factitious disorders imposed on self* or, when someone deceptively induces injury or illness in another person, *factitious disorder imposed on another.*

Epidemiology

The prevalence of somatic symptom disorder in the general population is estimated to be 5% to 7% (Yates, 2019). Although historically this disorder was thought to be more prevalent in women, the *DSM-5-TR* (APA, 2022) suggests that the higher reported prevalence of this disorder in women may be related to the fact that females tend to report somatic symptoms more often than males.

Lifetime prevalence rates of conversion disorder vary widely. Statistics within the general population range from 5% to 30% (Ali, 2015). The disorder occurs more frequently in women than in men and more frequently in adolescents and young adults than in other age-groups.

The prevalence of illness anxiety disorder, which along with somatic symptom disorder replaces hypochondriasis in the *DSM-5-TR*, is especially difficult to establish. The best estimate is based on data about the prevalence of hypochondriasis, which is identified at between 1.3% and 10% (APA, 2022). Some people who were previously diagnosed with hypochondriasis might better meet diagnostic criteria for somatic symptom disorder under this new classification. There are similarities in these two disorders, but the distinguishing feature between illness anxiety disorder and somatic symptom disorder is that in somatic symptom disorder the primary symptom is significant somatic sensations, and in illness anxiety disorder there are few to no somatic symptoms but anxiety or fear about having or acquiring an illness is a primary concern. Kahn (2018) notes that preoccupation with illness is not uncommon since 10% to 20% of people who are healthy and 45% of people without a major psychiatric disorder have intermittent unfounded worries about illness. More research is needed to better understand the epidemiology for each of these disorders.

Hypochondriasis was relabeled as illness anxiety disorder, at least in part, to eliminate myths and stigmas associated with the former diagnosis (Dimsdale, 2020). Illness anxiety disorder is equally common among men and women, and onset most commonly occurs in early adulthood. Data on the prevalence of factitious disorder are limited, so the frequency of the disorder is unknown. Estimates based on samples of hospital patients identify that about 1% meet criteria for factitious disorder (APA, 2022). Factitious disorder imposed on another is most often perpetrated by mothers against infants, and it accounts for less than 0.04% of reported cases of child abuse in the United States each year (Boland & Verduin, 2022).

Dissociative syndromes, although often portrayed in fictional media, are statistically quite rare. However, when they do occur, they may present very dramatic clinical pictures of severe disturbance in normal personality functioning. Dissociative amnesia occurs most frequently under conditions of war or during natural disasters. In recent years, there has been an increase in the number of reported cases, possibly attributed to increased awareness of the phenomenon and identification of cases that were previously undiagnosed. It appears to be equally common in men and women. Dissociative amnesia can occur at any age but is difficult to diagnose in children because it is easily confused with inattention or oppositional behavior.

Estimates of the prevalence of dissociative identity disorder (DID), previously called *multiple personality disorder*, also vary. In early childhood the ratio of female to male DID cases is 1 to 1 but increases steadily to approximately 8 to 1 by late adolescence (Boland & Verduin, 2022). Onset likely occurs in childhood, although manifestations of the disorder may not be recognized until late adolescence or early adulthood.

The prevalence of severe episodes of depersonalization-derealization disorder is unknown. Single brief episodes may occur in as many as 50% of all adults, particularly when under severe psychosocial stress; when sleep deprived; during travel to unfamiliar places; or when intoxicated with hallucinogens, marijuana, or alcohol. Symptoms usually begin in adolescence or early adulthood. The disorder is chronic with periods of remission and exacerbation. The incidence of depersonalization-derealization disorder is high under conditions of sustained traumatization, such as in military combat or prisoner-of-war camps. It has also been reported in many individuals who endure near-death experiences.

Application of the Nursing Process

Background Assessment Data for Somatic Symptom Disorders

Somatic Symptom Disorder

Somatic symptom disorder is a syndrome of multiple somatic symptoms that cannot be explained medically and that are associated with psychosocial distress and long-term seeking of assistance from health-care professionals. Symptoms may be vague, dramatized, or exaggerated in their presentation, and an excessive amount of time and energy is devoted to worry and concern about the symptoms. Individuals with somatic symptom disorder are so convinced that their symptoms are related to organic pathology that they adamantly reject, and are often irritated by, any implication that stress or psychosocial factors play any role in their condition. One study (van den Houte et al., 2017 as cited by Dimsdale, 2017) found that participants who had difficulty identifying feelings (a component of the personality trait *alexithymia*, which is characterized by marked dysfunction in emotional awareness and social attachment), reported more somatic symptoms than healthy controls. Their findings suggest that alexithymia may be an important construct in the development of somatic symptom disorders. The disorder is chronic, with symptoms beginning before age 30. Anxiety and depression are frequent comorbidities, and, consequently, the disorder is associated with an increased risk for suicide attempts (Yates, 2019).

Somatic symptom disorder usually runs a fluctuating course with periods of remission and exacerbation. Clients often receive medical care from several physicians, sometimes concurrently, leading to the possibility of dangerous combinations of treatments. They tend to seek relief through overmedicating with prescribed analgesics or antianxiety agents. Drug abuse and dependence are common complications of somatic symptom disorder. The *DSM-5-TR* diagnostic criteria for somatic symptom disorder are presented in Box 20–1.

Illness Anxiety Disorder

Illness anxiety disorder may be defined as an unrealistic or inaccurate interpretation of physical symptoms or sensations, leading to preoccupation and fear of having a serious disease. The fear becomes disabling

BOX 20–1 Diagnostic Criteria for Somatic Symptom Disorder

A. One or more somatic symptoms that are distressing or result in significant disruption in daily life.
B. Excessive thoughts, feelings, or behaviors related to the somatic symptoms or associated health concerns as manifested by at least one of the following:
   1. Disproportionate and persistent thoughts about the seriousness of one's symptoms.
   2. Persistently high level of anxiety about health or symptoms.
   3. Excessive time and energy devoted to these symptoms or health concerns.
C. Although any one symptom may not be continuously present, the state of being symptomatic is persistent (typically more than 6 months).

Specify if:

With predominant pain (the somatic symptoms predominantly involve pain)

Persistent (a persistent course is characterized by severe symptoms, marked impairment, and long duration [more than 6 months])

Specify current severity:

Mild (only one of the symptoms specified in Criterion B is fulfilled)

Moderate (two or more of the symptoms specified in Criterion B are fulfilled)

Severe (two or more of the symptoms specified in Criterion B are fulfilled, plus there are multiple somatic complaints [or one very severe somatic symptom])

Reprinted with permission from American Psychiatric Association. (2022). Diagnostic and statistical manual of mental disorders, fifth edition, text revision.

and persists despite appropriate medical evaluation and reassurance that no organic pathology can be detected. Symptoms may be minimal or absent, but the individual is highly anxious about and suspicious of the presence of an undiagnosed, serious medical illness (APA, 2022).

Individuals with illness anxiety disorder are extremely conscious of bodily sensations and changes and may become convinced that a rapid heart rate indicates they have heart disease or that a small sore is skin cancer. They are profoundly preoccupied with their bodies and are totally aware of even the slightest change in feeling or sensation. Their response to these small changes, however, is usually unrealistic and exaggerated.

Some individuals with illness anxiety disorder have a long history of "doctor shopping" and are convinced that they are not receiving the proper care.

Collaboration and ongoing communication with other clinicians are essential to "minimize inconsistent or conflicting messages and potentially reduce splitting" (Joshi, 2020, p. 54) in the care of patients with an illness anxiety disorder. *Teamwork and collaboration* form one of the six essential competencies identified by the Institute of Medicine (now the National Academy of Medicine) (2003) and adopted as a Quality and Safety Education for Nurses (QSEN) competency (QSEN Institute, 2020) for improving quality in health-care education and practice.

Others avoid seeking medical assistance because to do so would increase their anxiety to intolerable levels. Psychiatric comorbidities are common, including generalized anxiety disorder, depression, somatization disorder, and panic disorder; in addition, patients with illness anxiety disorder are three times more likely to have a concurrent personality disorder (Soreff, 2018). Preoccupation with the fear of serious disease may interfere with social or occupational functioning. Some individuals are able to function appropriately on the job, however, while limiting their physical complaints to nonwork time.

Individuals with illness anxiety disorder are so apprehensive and fearful that they become alarmed at the slightest intimation of serious illness. Even reading about a disease or hearing that someone they know has been diagnosed with an illness precipitates alarm on their part. Both somatic symptom disorder and illness anxiety disorder have features similar to the now removed hypochondriasis, but the *DSM-5-TR* identifies two separate disorders to distinguish between individuals who are primarily preoccupied with perceived physical symptoms (somatic symptom disorder) and those who are primarily focused on fear of illness in general (illness anxiety disorder). The *DSM-5-TR* diagnostic criteria for illness anxiety disorder are presented in Box 20–2.

Functional Neurological Symptom Disorder (Conversion Disorder)

Functional neurological symptom disorder (previously called conversion disorder) is a loss of or change in body function that cannot be explained by any known medical disorder or pathophysiological mechanism. Although there is a psychological component involved in the initiation, exacerbation, or perpetuation of the symptom, it may or may not be obvious or easily identifiable.

Conversion symptoms affect voluntary motor or sensory functioning suggestive of neurological disease. Examples include paralysis, **aphonia** (inability to produce voice), seizures, coordination disturbance, difficulty swallowing, urinary retention,

BOX 20–2 Diagnostic Criteria for Illness Anxiety Disorder

A. Preoccupation with having or acquiring a serious illness.
B. Somatic symptoms are not present or, if present, are only mild in intensity. If another medical condition is present or there is a high risk for developing a medical condition (e.g., strong family history is present), the preoccupation is clearly excessive or disproportionate.
C. There is a high level of anxiety about health, and the individual is easily alarmed about personal health status.
D. The individual performs excessive health-related behaviors (e.g., repeatedly checks his or her body for signs of illness) or exhibits maladaptive avoidance (e.g., avoids doctors' appointments and hospitals).
E. Illness preoccupation has been present for at least 6 months, but the specific illness that is feared may change over that period of time.
F. The illness-related preoccupation is not better explained by another mental disorder, such as somatic symptom disorder, panic disorder, generalized anxiety disorder, body dysmorphic disorder, obsessive-compulsive disorder, or delusional disorder, somatic type.

Specify whether:

Care-seeking type: Medical care, including physician visits or undergoing tests and procedures, is frequently used.

Care-avoidant type: Medical care is rarely used.

Reprinted with permission from American Psychiatric Association. (2022). Diagnostic and statistical manual of mental disorders, fifth edition, text revision.

akinesia, blindness, deafness, double vision, **anosmia** (inability to perceive smell), loss of pain sensation, and hallucinations. Abnormal limb shaking with impaired or loss of consciousness that resembles epileptic seizures is another type of conversion disorder symptom that is referred to as *psychogenic* or *nonepileptic seizures*. **Pseudocyesis** (false pregnancy) is a conversion symptom and may represent a strong desire to be pregnant.

The *DSM-5-TR* clarifies that although the diagnosis [of functional neurological symptom disorder] requires that the symptom is not explained by neurological disease, it should not be made simply because results from investigations are normal or because the symptom is 'bizarre.' "The diagnosis rests on clinical findings showing clear evidence of incompatibility with recognized neurological disease" (APA, 2022, p. 361). For example, a client who appears to be having a seizure but has a normal electroencephalogram, whose eyes are closed and resist opening, and who has no urinary incontinence may be diagnosed with conversion disorder. It is likely that multiple factors play a role in the etiology.

Although not diagnostic of a functional neurological symptom disorder, an associated symptom is the client's apparent indifference to symptoms that seem very serious to others. This feature is termed *la belle indifference*. Most symptoms of conversion disorder resolve within a few weeks. About 20% of individuals with the diagnosis have a relapse within 1 year. The *DSM-5-TR* states that the prognosis is better when the symptoms are of short duration, when the client accepts the diagnosis, when there is absence of comorbid physical disease, and when the client has no identified maladaptive personality traits (APA, 2022). The *DSM-5-TR* diagnostic criteria for conversion disorder are presented in Box 20–3.

BOX 20–3 Diagnostic Criteria for Functional Neurological Symptom Disorder (Conversion Disorder)

A. One or more symptoms of altered voluntary motor or sensory function.
B. Clinical findings provide evidence of incompatibility between the symptom and recognized neurological or medical conditions.
C. The symptom or deficit is not better explained by another medical or mental disorder.
D. The symptom or deficit causes clinically significant distress or impairment in social, occupational, or other important areas of functioning or warrants medical evaluation.

Specify symptom type:
With weakness or paralysis
With abnormal movement
With swallowing symptoms
With speech symptom
With attacks or seizures
With anesthesia or sensory loss
With special sensory symptom
With mixed symptoms

Specify if:
Acute episode
Persistent

Specify if:
With psychological stressor
Without psychological stressor

Reprinted with permission from American Psychiatric Association. (2022). Diagnostic and statistical manual of mental disorders, fifth edition, text revision.

Psychological Factors Affecting Other Medical Conditions

Psychological factors play a role in virtually any medical condition. However, in this disorder, it is evident that psychological or behavioral factors are clearly implicated in the development, exacerbation, or delayed recovery from a medical condition.

Factitious Disorder

Factitious disorder involves conscious, intentional feigning of physical or psychological symptoms. Individuals with factitious disorder pretend to be ill in order to receive emotional care and support commonly associated with the role of "patient." Even though the behaviors are deliberate and intentional, there may be an associated compulsive element that diminishes personal control. Individuals with this disorder characteristically become skilled at presenting their "symptoms" so well that they successfully gain admission to hospitals and treatment centers. To accomplish this, they may aggravate existing symptoms, induce new ones, or even inflict painful injuries on themselves. The disorder has also been identified as Munchausen syndrome, and symptoms may be psychological or physical, or a combination of both.

Factitious disorder imposed on another (previously called *factitious disorder by proxy*) describes a condition in which physical or psychological symptoms are falsified or induced in another person. Diagnosis of factitious disorder can be very difficult because individuals become very inventive in their quest to produce symptoms. "The most common cause of factitious disorder imposed on another involves a mother who deceives medical personnel into believing her child is ill" (Boland & Verduin, 2022, p. 457). This may be accomplished by lying about the child's medical history, manipulating data such as by contaminating laboratory samples, and inducing illness or injury in their child through use of substances or other physical assaults.

Predisposing Factors Associated With Somatic Symptom and Related Disorders

Genetic

Escobar and Dimsdale (2017) report that somatic symptom and related disorders should be conceptualized as a complex interaction of genetic vulnerabilities; history of trauma; learning; and environmental, psychological, and behavioral influences. Although the specific genetic vulnerabilities are not well understood the authors report that there is no evidence of familial aggregation in somatic symptom disorder.

Biochemical

Although biochemical factors of somatic symptom disorder are not clearly understood, decreased levels of serotonin and endorphins may play a role in the sensation of pain.

Neuroanatomical

Magnetic resonance imaging (MRI) studies of patients with a variety of somatoform disorders found that these patients had volume reductions in the hypothalamus, left fusiform gyrus, right cuneus, left inferior frontal gyrus, left posterior cingulate, and right amygdala (Delvecchio et al., 2019). The authors conclude that these findings suggest selective impairments in specific cortico-limbic regions associated with two overlapping circuits, the neuromatrix of pain and the emotion regulation system.

Psychodynamic

Psychodynamic theorists view illness anxiety disorder as an ego defense mechanism. Physical complaints are seen as the expression of low self-esteem and feelings of worthlessness because it is easier to feel that something is wrong with the body than to feel that something is wrong with the self. Another psychodynamic view of illness anxiety disorder (as well as somatic symptom disorder, predominantly pain) is related to a defense against guilt. The individual views the self as "bad" because of real or imagined past misconduct and views physical suffering as the deserved punishment required for atonement. This view has also been related to individuals with factitious disorder.

The psychodynamic theory of conversion disorder proposes that emotions associated with a traumatic event that the individual cannot express because of moral or ethical unacceptability are "converted" into physical symptoms. The unacceptable emotions are repressed and converted to a somatic symptom that is symbolic in some way of the original emotional trauma.

Another view suggests that individuals with factitious disorders were victims of child abuse or neglect. Frequent childhood hospitalizations provided a reprieve from the traumatic home situation and a supportive, caring environment that was absent in the child's family. This theory proposes that in adulthood, the individual with factitious disorder is attempting to recapture the only positive support known to them by seeking out the environment in which it was received as a child. Regarding factitious disorder imposed on another, Boland and Verduin (2022) have stated, "One apparent purpose of the behavior is for the caretaker to assume the sick role indirectly; another is to be relieved of the caretaking role by having the child hospitalized" (p. 457).

Escobar and Dimsdale (2017) report that up to two-thirds of patients in primary care settings complain of symptoms for which no disease entity can be identified and up to two-thirds of those patients meet criteria for a major psychiatric disorder. The authors suggest that this finding reinforces the belief that individuals with psychiatric disorders more typically present with physical rather than psychological complaints in primary care settings.

Family Dynamics

This view suggests that in families who have difficulty resolving conflicts, a child's illness creates a shift in focus from the unresolved conflicts to the child's illness. This provides a reprieve from the instability posed by issues that the family cannot confront openly, and the child in turn receives positive reinforcement for the illness. **Somatization,** a focus on physical symptoms, becomes reinforced as a way to shift the focus away from family issues and discord.

Learning Theory

Somatic complaints are often reinforced when the sick role relieves the individual from the need to deal with a stressful situation, whether it be within society or within the family. The sick person learns that there are emotional gains conferred by staying in the sick role. For example, they may be able to avoid stressful obligations, postpone unwelcome challenges, or be excused from troublesome duties

(primary gain). They may become the prominent focus of attention because of the illness **(secondary gain)** or being in the sick role relieves conflict within the family as concern is shifted to the ill person and away from the real issue **(tertiary gain).** These types of positive reinforcement virtually guarantee repetition of the response.

Past experience with serious or life-threatening physical illness, either personal or that of close family members, can predispose an individual to illness anxiety disorder. Once an individual has experienced a threat to biological integrity, that person may develop a fear of recurrence. The fear of recurring illness generates an exaggerated response to minor physical changes, leading to excessive anxiety and health concerns.

Background Assessment Data for Dissociative Disorders

Dissociative Amnesia

CORE CONCEPT

Amnesia

Partial or total loss of memory. Memory loss may be temporary or permanent.

Amnesia may be caused by a host of medical conditions, including stroke, encephalitis, degenerative brain diseases (such as Alzheimer's disease), chronic alcohol abuse, brain tumors, seizures, and some medications. Dissociative amnesia stems from extreme emotional or physical trauma and is described in the *DSM-5-TR* as an inability to recall important personal information, usually of a traumatic or stressful nature, that is too extensive to be explained by ordinary forgetfulness and is not due to the direct effects of substance use or a neurological or other medical condition (APA, 2022). The *DSM-5-TR* states that the most common types of dissociative amnesia are localized, selective, or generalized. Localized and selective amnesia are related to a specific stressful event that has occurred. For example, the individual with **localized amnesia** is unable to recall all incidents associated with a stressful event. It may be broader than just a single event, however, such as being unable to remember months or years of child abuse (APA, 2022). In **selective amnesia,** the individual can recall only certain incidents associated with a stressful event for a specific period after the event. In **generalized amnesia,** the individual has amnesia for both identity and total life history.

The individual with amnesia usually appears alert and may give no indication to observers that anything is wrong, although some clients may present with alterations in consciousness, with conversion symptoms, or in trance states. Clients with amnesia are often brought to general hospital emergency departments by police who have found them wandering confusedly around the streets.

The onset of an amnestic episode usually follows severe psychosocial stress. Termination is typically abrupt and followed by complete recovery. Recurrences are unusual. A specific subtype of dissociative amnesia is *dissociative fugue.* Dissociative **fugue** is characterized by a sudden, unexpected travel away from the customary place of daily activities or by bewildered wandering with the inability to recall some or all of one's past. An individual in a fugue state may not be able to recall personal identity and sometimes assumes a new identity. The *DSM-5-TR* diagnostic criteria for dissociative amnesia are presented in Box 20–4.

BOX 20–4 Diagnostic Criteria for Dissociative Amnesia

A. An inability to recall important autobiographical information, usually of a traumatic or stressful nature, that is inconsistent with ordinary forgetting. **NOTE:** Dissociative amnesia most often consists of localized or selective amnesia for a specific event or events; or generalized amnesia for identity and life history.
B. The symptoms cause clinically significant distress or impairment in social, occupational, or other important areas of functioning.
C. The disturbance is not attributable to the physiological effects of a substance (e.g., alcohol or other drug of abuse, a medication) or a neurological or other medical condition (e.g., partial complex seizures, transient global amnesia, sequelae of a closed head injury/traumatic brain injury, other neurological condition).
D. The disturbance is not better explained by dissociative identity disorder, posttraumatic stress disorder, acute stress disorder, somatic symptom disorder, or major or mild neurocognitive disorder.

Specify if:

With dissociative fugue (Apparently purposeful travel or bewildered wandering that is associated with amnesia for identity or for other important **autobiographical** information.)

Reprinted with permission from American Psychiatric Association. (2022). Diagnostic and statistical manual of mental disorders, fifth edition, text revision.

Dissociative Identity Disorder

Dissociative identity disorder (DID) was formerly called *multiple personality disorder*. This disorder is characterized by the existence of two or more personality states in a single individual. These different personality states are sometimes referred to as *alter identities* or just *alters*. Only one of the personalities is evident at any given moment, and one of them is dominant most of the time over the course of the disorder. Each personality is unique and composed of a complex set of memories, behavior patterns, and social relationships that surface at different times. Transition from one personality state to another may be sudden or gradual and is sometimes quite dramatic. Boland and Verduin (2022) state, "Patients often describe a profound sense of concretized internal division or personified internal conflicts between parts of themselves. . . . [T]hese parts may have proper names or be designated by their predominant affect or function, for example, 'the angry one' or 'the wife'" (p. 443).

DID has been a controversial disorder that gained attention after the 1976 movie *Sybil* portrayed the presumed true story of a woman who reported having 16 different personalities. Diagnosis of this disorder increased significantly in the years following the movie, and in 1980, the APA formally recognized the disorder as a psychiatric illness (Haberman, 2014). Since then, critics have reported that both the patient "Sybil" and her psychiatrist acknowledged her case as largely fabrication. Dr. David Speigel, a psychiatrist who was involved in promoting the APA's adoption of DID as the preferred term for this condition, is quoted in Haberman's review (2014) as saying "[the term] multiple personality carries with it the implication that they really have more than one personality. The problem is fragmentation of identity, not that you really are 12 people . . . that you have not more than one but less than one personality."

Although questions persist about whether this disorder has been overdiagnosed, there are certainly individuals who present with this condition of fragmented identity, and most have been victims of severe childhood physical and sexual abuse. It is not uncommon for clients with DID to also manifest with symptoms of other dissociative disorders, such as amnesia, fugue states, depersonalization, and derealization (Boland & Verduin, 2022). Generally, there is amnesia for the events that took place when another personality was being manifested, and clients report "gaps" in autobiographical histories, "lost time" or "blackouts." They may "wake up" in unfamiliar situations with no idea of where they are, how they got there, or the identities of the people around them. They may be accused of lying when they deny remembering or being responsible for events or actions.

DID is not always incapacitating. Some individuals with DID maintain responsible positions, complete graduate degrees, and are successful spouses and parents before diagnosis and while in treatment. Before they are diagnosed with DID, many individuals are misdiagnosed with depression, borderline and antisocial personality disorders, schizophrenia, epilepsy, or bipolar disorder. The *DSM-5-TR* diagnostic criteria for DID are presented in Box 20–5.

Depersonalization-Derealization Disorder

Depersonalization-derealization disorder is characterized by a temporary change in the quality of self-awareness, which often takes the form of feelings of unreality, changes in body image, feelings of detachment from the environment, or a sense of observing oneself from outside the body. For example, a soldier in recalling an experience in combat describes that

BOX 20–5 Diagnostic Criteria for Dissociative Identity Disorder

A. Disruption of identity characterized by two or more distinct personality states, which may be described in some cultures as an experience of possession. The disruption in identity involves marked discontinuity in sense of self and sense of agency, accompanied by related alterations in affect, behavior, consciousness, memory, perception, cognition, and/or sensory-motor functioning. These signs and symptoms may be observed by others or reported by the individual.
B. Recurrent gaps in the recall of everyday events, important personal information, and/or traumatic events that are inconsistent with ordinary forgetting.
C. The symptoms cause clinically significant distress or impairment in social, occupational, or other important areas of functioning.
D. The disturbance is not a normal part of a broadly accepted cultural or religious practice. **NOTE:** In children, the symptoms are not better explained by imaginary playmates or other fantasy play.
E. The symptoms are not attributable to the physiological effects of a substance (e.g., blackouts or chaotic behavior during alcohol intoxication) or another medical condition (e.g., complex partial seizures).

Reprinted with permission from American Psychiatric Association. (2022). Diagnostic and statistical manual of mental disorders, fifth edition, text revision.

he saw himself observing himself from a distance and wondered what he would do if *he* were in that situation. **Depersonalization** (a disturbance in the perception of oneself) is differentiated from **derealization,** which describes an alteration in the perception of the external environment. Both of these phenomena also occur in a variety of psychiatric illnesses, such as schizophrenia, depression, anxiety states, and neurocognitive disorders. As previously stated, the symptoms of depersonalization and derealization are very common. It is estimated that approximately 50% of all adults have experienced transient episodes of the symptoms. They are also identified as the third most common reported psychiatric symptoms after depression and anxiety (Boland & Verduin, 2022). Diagnosis of the disorder is made only if the symptoms cause significant distress or impairment in functioning.

The *DSM-5-TR* describes this disorder as the persistence or recurrence of episodes of depersonalization or derealization, or both (APA, 2022). There may be a mechanical or dreamlike feeling or a belief that the body's physical characteristics have changed. If derealization is present, objects in the environment are perceived as altered in size or shape. Other people in the environment may seem automated or mechanical.

These distorted perceptions are experienced as disturbing and often accompanied by anxiety, depression, fear of going insane, obsessive thoughts, somatic complaints, and an alteration in the subjective sense of time. The *DSM-5-TR* diagnostic criteria for depersonalization-derealization disorder are presented in Box 20–6.

BOX 20–6 Diagnostic Criteria for Depersonalization-Derealization Disorder

A. The presence of persistent or recurrent depersonalization, derealization, or both:
   1. **Depersonalization:** Experiences of unreality, detachment, or being an outside observer with respect to one's thoughts, feelings, sensations, body, or actions (e.g., perceptual alterations, distorted sense of time, unreal or absent self, emotional and/or physical numbing).
   2. **Derealization:** Experiences of unreality or detachment with respect to surroundings (e.g., individuals or objects are experienced as unreal, dreamlike, foggy, lifeless, or visually distorted).
B. During the depersonalization or derealization experiences, reality testing remains intact.
C. The symptoms cause clinically significant distress or impairment in social, occupational, or other important areas of functioning.
D. The disturbance is not attributable to the physiological effects of a substance (e.g., a drug of abuse, medication) or another medical condition (e.g., seizures).
E. The disturbance is not better explained by another mental disorder, such as schizophrenia, panic disorder, major depressive disorder, acute stress disorder, post-traumatic stress disorder, or another dissociative disorder.

Reprinted with permission from American Psychiatric Association. (2022). Diagnostic and statistical manual of mental disorders, fifth edition, text revision.

Predisposing Factors Associated With Dissociative Disorders

Genetics

The overwhelming majority of adults with DID (85% to 97%) have a history of physical and sexual abuse, and although genetic factors may illuminate the interaction of the individual with environmental stress current research does not show evidence of a significant genetic contribution (Şar et al., 2017).

Neurobiological

Şar and associates (2017) report that there are both structural and functional neuroimaging findings that demonstrate differences between patients with DID and nonclinical populations. Areas of the brain that have been associated with memory include the hippocampus, amygdala, fornix, mammillary bodies, thalamus, and frontal cortex. One study found that hippocampal volume was significantly smaller in individuals with DID and it was correlated to a higher severity of childhood trauma and dissociative symptoms (Chalavi et al., 2015).

Various studies have implicated the *N*-methyl-D-aspartate (NMDA) glutamate receptor, neuropeptide Y, norepinephrine, serotonin, and the opioid system in depersonalization (Boland & Verduin, 2022). Dissociative experiences have been reported in patients with temporal lobe epilepsy and severe migraine headaches (Özdemir et al., 2016). Electroencephalographic abnormalities have been observed in some clients with DID.

Psychodynamic Theory

Freud (1962) believed that dissociative behaviors occurred when individuals repressed distressing mental contents from conscious awareness. He believed that the unconscious was a dynamic entity in which repressed mental contents were stored and unavailable to conscious recall. Current psychodynamic explanations of dissociation are based on Freud's concepts. The repression of mental contents is believed to protect the client from extreme emotional pain triggered by either disturbing external circumstances or anxiety-provoking internal urges and feelings. In the case of depersonalization and derealization, the pain and anxiety are expressed as feelings of unreality or detachment from the environment of the painful situation.

Psychological Trauma

Several studies support the etiology of dissociative disorders as a response to traumatic experiences that overwhelm the individual's capacity to cope by any means other than dissociation (Chavali et al., 2015; Irwin, 1999; Muller, 2014). In DID, these experiences are most often physical, sexual, or psychological abuse by a parent or significant other in the child's life. The most widely accepted explanation for DID is that it begins as a survival strategy that serves to help children cope with the severe sexual, physical, or psychological abuse and evolves into a fragmented identity as the victim struggles to integrate conflicting aspects of their personality into a cohesive whole. Dissociative amnesia is frequently related to acute and extreme trauma but may also develop in the clinical presentation of DID. Dissociative amnesia is also often noted in response to combat trauma during wartimes.

Diagnosis and Outcome Identification

Nursing diagnoses are formulated from the data gathered during the assessment phase and with background knowledge regarding predisposing factors to the disorder. Table 20–1 presents a list of patient behaviors and the NANDA-I nursing diagnoses (Herdman et al., 2021) that correspond to those behaviors, which may be used in planning care for patients with somatic symptom and dissociative disorders.

TABLE 20–1 Assigning Nursing Diagnoses to Behaviors Commonly Associated With Somatic Symptom and Dissociative Disorders

BEHAVIORS	NURSING DIAGNOSES
Verbalization of numerous physical complaints in the absence of any pathophysiological evidence; focus on the self and physical symptoms (somatic symptom disorder)	Ineffective coping; chronic pain
History of "doctor shopping" for evidence of organic pathology to substantiate physical symptoms; statements such as, "I don't know why the doctor put me on the psychiatric unit. I have a physical problem" (somatic symptom disorder)	Deficient knowledge (psychological causes for physical symptoms)
Preoccupation with and unrealistic interpretation of bodily signs and sensations (illness anxiety disorder)	Fear (of having a serious disease)
Loss or alteration in physical functioning without evidence of organic pathology (conversion disorder) Alteration in the perception or experience of the self or the environment (depersonalization-derealization disorder)	Disturbed sensory perception*
Need for assistance to carry out self-care activities such as eating, dressing, maintaining hygiene, and toileting due to alteration in physical functioning (conversion disorder)	Self-care deficit
History of numerous exacerbations of physical illness; inappropriate or exaggerated behaviors; denial of emotional problems (psychological factors affecting other medical conditions)	Deficient knowledge (psychological factors affecting medical condition); denial
Loss of memory (dissociative amnesia)	Impaired memory
Verbalizations of frustration over lack of control and dependence on others (dissociative amnesia)	Powerlessness
Unresolved grief; depression; self-blame associated with childhood abuse (dissociative identity disorder)	Risk for suicidal behavior
Presence of more than one personality within the individual (dissociative identity disorder)	Disturbed personality identity
Feigning of physical or psychological symptoms to gain attention (factitious disorder)	Ineffective coping

*This diagnosis has been resigned from the NANDA-I list of approved diagnoses. It is used in this instance because it is most compatible with the identified behaviors.

Outcome Criteria

The following criteria may be used for measurement of outcomes in the care of the patient with somatic symptom and dissociative disorders. The patient:

- Effectively uses adaptive coping strategies during stressful situations without resorting to physical symptoms (*somatic symptom disorder*).
- Interprets bodily sensations rationally, verbalizes understanding of the significance the irrational fear held for them, and has decreased the number and frequency of physical complaints (*illness anxiety disorder and somatic symptom disorder*).
- Is free of physical disability and verbalizes understanding of the possible correlation between the loss of or alteration in function and extreme emotional stress (*conversion disorder*).
- Recalls events associated with a traumatic or stressful situation (*dissociative amnesia*).
- Verbalizes the extreme anxiety that precipitated the dissociation (*depersonalization-derealization disorder*).
- Demonstrates more adaptive coping strategies to avert dissociative behaviors in the face of severe anxiety (*depersonalization-derealization disorder*).
- Verbalizes understanding of the existence of multiple personality states and the purposes they serve (*dissociative identity disorder*).
- Maintains a sense of reality during stressful situations (*depersonalization-derealization disorder*).

Planning and Implementation

Tables 20–2 and 20–3 provide plans of care for patients with somatic symptom disorders and dissociative disorders. NANDA-I nursing diagnoses (Herdman et al., 2021) are presented along with outcome criteria, appropriate nursing interventions, and rationales for each.

Concept Care Mapping

The concept map care plan is a diagrammatic teaching and learning strategy that allows visualization of interrelationships between medical diagnoses, nursing diagnoses, assessment data, and treatments. Examples of concept map care plans for patients with somatic symptom and dissociative disorders are presented in Figures 20–1 and 20–2.

Text continued on page 552

Table 20–2 | CARE PLAN FOR THE PATIENT WITH A SOMATIC SYMPTOM DISORDER

NURSING DIAGNOSIS: INEFFECTIVE COPING/CHRONIC PAIN

RELATED TO: Repressed anxiety and unmet dependency needs

EVIDENCED BY: Verbalization of numerous physical complaints in the absence of any pathophysiological evidence; total focus on the self and physical symptoms

OUTCOME CRITERIA	NURSING INTERVENTIONS	RATIONALE
Short-Term Goal ■ Within (specified time), patient will verbalize understanding of correlation between physical symptoms and psychological problems. **Long-Term Goal** ■ By time of discharge from treatment, patient will demonstrate ability to cope with stress by means other than preoccupation with physical symptoms.	1. Monitor physician's ongoing assessments, laboratory reports, and other data to maintain assurance that possibility of organic pathology is clearly ruled out. Review findings with the patient.	1. Accurate medical assessment is vital for the provision of adequate and appropriate care. Honest explanation may help the patient understand psychological implications.
	2. Recognize and accept that the physical complaint is real to the patient, even though no organic etiology can be identified.	2. Denial of the patient's feelings is nontherapeutic and interferes with establishment of a trusting relationship.
	3. Provide pain medication as prescribed by physician.	3. Patient comfort and safety are nursing priorities.
	4. Identify gains that the physical symptoms are providing: increased dependency, attention, distraction from other problems.	4. Identification of underlying motivation is important in assisting the patient with problem resolution.
	5. Initially, fulfill the patient's most urgent dependency needs, but gradually withdraw attention to physical symptoms. Minimize time given in response to physical complaints.	5. Anxiety and maladaptive behaviors will increase if dependency needs are ignored initially. Gradual lack of positive reinforcement will discourage repetition of maladaptive behaviors.

Table 20–2 | CARE PLAN FOR THE PATIENT WITH A SOMATIC SYMPTOM DISORDER—cont'd

OUTCOME CRITERIA	NURSING INTERVENTIONS	RATIONALE
	6. Encourage the patient to verbalize fears and anxieties. Explain that attention will be withdrawn if rumination about physical complaints begins. Follow through.	6. The possibility of organic pathology must always be considered. Failure to do so could jeopardize patient safety.
	7. Discuss possible alternative coping strategies the patient may use in response to stress (e.g., relaxation exercises; physical activities; assertiveness skills). Give positive reinforcement for use of these alternatives.	7. Without consistency of limit setting, change will not occur.
	8. Help the patient identify ways to achieve recognition from others without resorting to physical symptoms.	8. Patients may need help with problem-solving. Positive reinforcement encourages repetition. Positive recognition from others enhances self-esteem and minimizes the need for attention through maladaptive behaviors.

NURSING DIAGNOSIS: FEAR (OF HAVING A SERIOUS DISEASE)

RELATED TO: Past experience with life-threatening illness of self or significant others

EVIDENCED BY: Preoccupation with and unrealistic interpretation of bodily signs and sensations

OUTCOME CRITERIA	NURSING INTERVENTIONS	RATIONALE
Short-Term Goal ■ Patient will verbalize that fears associated with bodily sensations are irrational (within time limit deemed appropriate for specific individual). **Long-Term Goal** ■ Patient will interpret bodily sensations correctly.	1. Monitor physician's ongoing assessments and laboratory reports.	1. Organic pathology must be clearly ruled out.
	2. Assess and refer all new physical complaints to physician. Acknowledge these complaints and that they are genuinely experienced perceptions.	2. To ignore all physical complaints could place the patient's safety in jeopardy. Acknowledging the patient's experience provides validation and promotes trust.
	3. Assess the function that the patient's excessive concern is fulfilling (e.g., unfulfilled needs for dependency, nurturing, caring, attention, or control). Educate the patient that their perceptions could be symptoms of anxiety.	3. This information may provide insight into reasons for maladaptive behavior and provide direction for planning patient care.
	4. Identify times during which preoccupation with physical symptoms is worse. Determine extent of correlation of physical complaints with times of increased anxiety.	4. Patients may be unaware of the psychosocial implications of the physical complaints. Knowledge of the relationship is the first step in the process for creating change.
	5. Convey empathy. Let the patient know that you understand how a specific symptom may conjure up fears of previous life-threatening illness.	5. Unconditional acceptance and empathy promote a therapeutic nurse/patient relationship.

Continued

Table 20–2 | CARE PLAN FOR THE PATIENT WITH A SOMATIC SYMPTOM DISORDER—cont'd

OUTCOME CRITERIA	NURSING INTERVENTIONS	RATIONALE
	6. Initially provide the patient a limited amount of time (e.g., 10 minutes each hour) to discuss physical concerns.	6. Because this has been the patient's primary method of coping for so long, complete prohibition of this activity would likely raise the patient's anxiety level significantly, further exacerbating the behavior.
	7. Help the patient determine what techniques may be most useful to implement when fear and anxiety are exacerbated (e.g., relaxation techniques, mental imagery, thought-stopping techniques, physical exercise).	7. All of these techniques are effective to reduce anxiety and may assist the patient in the transition from focusing on fear of physical illness to the discussion of honest feelings.
	8. Gradually increase the limit on amount of time spent each hour in discussing physical concerns. If the patient violates the limits, withdraw attention.	8. Lack of positive reinforcement may help to extinguish maladaptive behavior.
	9. Facilitate discussion of feelings associated with fear of serious illness and avoid reassuring patients they are medically healthy (Joshi, 2020).	9. Verbalization of feelings in a nonthreatening environment facilitates expression and resolution of disturbing emotional issues. When the patient can express feelings directly, there is less need to express them through physical symptoms. Reassurance of being medically healthy quickly fades and may worsen anxiety (Joshi, 2020).
	10. Role-play the patient's plan for dealing with the fear the next time it assumes control and before anxiety becomes disabling.	10. Anxiety and fears are minimized when the patient has achieved a degree of comfort through practicing a plan for dealing with stressful situations in the future.

NURSING DIAGNOSIS: DISTURBED SENSORY PERCEPTION

RELATED TO: Repressed severe anxiety

EVIDENCED BY: Loss or alteration in physical functioning, without evidence of organic pathology

OUTCOME CRITERIA	NURSING INTERVENTIONS	RATIONALE
Short-Term Goal ■ Patient will verbalize understanding of emotional problems as a contributing factor to the alteration in physical functioning (within time limit appropriate for specific individual).	1. Monitor physician's ongoing assessments, laboratory reports, and other data to ensure that possibility of organic pathology is clearly ruled out.	1. Failure to do so may jeopardize patient safety.
	2. Identify primary or secondary gains that the physical symptom may be providing (e.g., increased dependency, attention, protection from experiencing a stressful event).	2. Primary and secondary gains are often etiological factors and may be used to assist in problem resolution.

Table 20–2 | CARE PLAN FOR THE PATIENT WITH A SOMATIC SYMPTOM DISORDER—cont'd

OUTCOME CRITERIA	NURSING INTERVENTIONS	RATIONALE
Long-Term Goal ■ Patient will demonstrate recovery of lost or altered function.	3. Do not focus on the disability and encourage the patient to be as independent as possible. Intervene only when the patient requires assistance.	3. Positive reinforcement would encourage continual use of the maladaptive response for secondary gains, such as dependency.
	4. Maintain nonjudgmental attitude when providing assistance to the patient. The physical symptom is not within the patient's conscious control and is very real to them.	4. A judgmental attitude interferes with the nurse's ability to establish trust and provide therapeutic care for the patient.
	5. Identify the expectation and importance of the patient attending therapeutic activities. Withdraw attention if the patient continues to focus on physical limitations as a reason to avoid participation.	5. Somatization may be used to avoid addressing issues. Clarifying expectations facilitates follow-through. Lack of reinforcement may help to extinguish the maladaptive response.
	6. Encourage the patient to verbalize fears and anxieties. Help identify physical symptoms as a coping mechanism that is used in times of extreme stress.	6. Patients with conversion disorder are usually unaware of the psychological implications of their illness.
	7. Help the patient identify coping mechanisms to be used when faced with stressful situations, rather than retreating from reality with a physical disability.	7. Educating and engaging the patient in identifying alternative coping strategies help diminish the need for maladaptive responses.
	8. Give positive reinforcement for identification or demonstration of alternative, more adaptive coping strategies.	8. Positive reinforcement enhances self-esteem and encourages repetition of desirable behaviors.

NURSING DIAGNOSIS: DEFICIENT KNOWLEDGE

RELATED TO: Psychological factors affecting medical condition

EVIDENCED BY: Statements such as, "I don't know why the doctor thinks this could be psychological. I have a physical problem."

OUTCOME CRITERIA	NURSING INTERVENTIONS	RATIONALE
Short-Term Goal ■ Patient will cooperate with plan for teaching provided by primary nurse.	1. Assess level of knowledge regarding effects of psychological problems on the body.	1. An adequate database is necessary for the development of an effective teaching plan.
	2. Assess level of anxiety and readiness to learn.	2. Learning does not occur beyond the moderate level of anxiety.
Long-Term Goal ■ By time of discharge from treatment, patient will be able to verbalize psychological factors affecting their physical condition.	3. Discuss physical examinations and laboratory tests that have been conducted. Explain purpose and results of each.	3. Fear of the unknown may contribute to elevated level of anxiety. The patient has the right to know about and accept or refuse any medical treatment.
	4. Explore feelings and fears. Go slowly. These feelings may have been suppressed or repressed for so long that their disclosure may be a very painful experience. Be supportive.	4. Expression of feelings in the presence of a trusted individual and in a nonthreatening environment may encourage the individual to confront unresolved issues.

Continued

Table 20–2 | CARE PLAN FOR THE PATIENT WITH A SOMATIC SYMPTOM DISORDER—cont'd

OUTCOME CRITERIA	NURSING INTERVENTIONS	RATIONALE
	5. Have the patient keep a diary of appearance, duration, and intensity of physical symptoms. A separate record of situations that the patient finds especially stressful should also be kept.	5. Comparison of these records may provide objective data from which to observe the relationship between physical symptoms and stress.
	6. Help the patient identify needs that are being met through the sick role. Together, formulate more adaptive means for fulfilling these needs. Practice by role-playing.	6. Repetition through practice serves to reduce discomfort in the actual situation.
	7. Provide instruction in assertiveness techniques, especially the ability to recognize the differences among passive, assertive, and aggressive behaviors and the importance of respecting the rights of others while protecting one's own basic rights.	7. These skills will preserve the patient's self-esteem while also improving their ability to form satisfactory interpersonal relationships.
	8. Discuss adaptive methods of stress management, such as relaxation techniques, physical exercise, meditation, breathing exercises, and autogenics (a relaxation technique using focused attention to enable an individual to induce relaxation in themselves).	8. Use of these adaptive techniques may decrease appearance of physical symptoms in response to stress.

Table 20–3 | CARE PLAN FOR THE PATIENT WITH A DISSOCIATIVE DISORDER

NURSING DIAGNOSIS: IMPAIRED MEMORY

RELATED TO: Severe psychological stress and repression of anxiety

EVIDENCED BY: Loss of memory

OUTCOME CRITERIA	NURSING INTERVENTIONS	RATIONALE
Short-Term Goal ■ Patient will verbalize understanding that loss of memory is related to a stressful situation and begin discussing the stressful situation with nurse or therapist.	1. Obtain as much information as possible about the patient from family and significant others if possible. Consider likes, dislikes, important people, activities, music, and pets.	1. A comprehensive baseline assessment is important for the development of an effective plan of care.
	2. Do not flood the patient with data regarding their past life.	2. Individuals who are exposed to painful information from which the amnesia is providing protection may decompensate even further into a psychotic state.
	3. Instead, expose the patient to stimuli that represent pleasant experiences from the past, such as smells associated with enjoyable activities, beloved pets, and music known to have been pleasurable to the patient. As memory begins to return, engage the patient in activities that may provide additional stimulation.	3. Recall may occur during activities that simulate life experiences.

Table 20–3 | CARE PLAN FOR THE PATIENT WITH A DISSOCIATIVE DISORDER—cont'd

OUTCOME CRITERIA	NURSING INTERVENTIONS	RATIONALE
Long-Term Goal ■ Patient will recover deficits in memory and develop more adaptive coping mechanisms to deal with stressful situations.	4. Encourage the patient to discuss situations that have been especially stressful and to explore the feelings associated with those times. 5. Identify specific conflicts that remain unresolved and assist the patient to identify possible solutions. Provide instruction regarding more adaptive ways to respond to anxiety.	4. Verbalization of feelings in a nonthreatening environment may help the patient come to terms with unresolved issues that may be contributing to the dissociative process. 5. Unless these underlying conflicts are resolved, any improvement in coping behaviors must be viewed as only temporary.

NURSING DIAGNOSIS: DISTURBED PERSONAL IDENTITY

RELATED TO: Childhood trauma/abuse

EVIDENCED BY: The presence of more than one personality within the individual

OUTCOME CRITERIA	NURSING INTERVENTIONS	RATIONALE
Short-Term Goals ■ Patient will verbalize understanding about the existence of multiple identities within the self. ■ Patient will be able to recognize stressful situations that precipitate transition from one identity to another. **Long-Term Goals** ■ Patient will verbalize understanding of the reason for existence of each personality and the role each plays for the individual. ■ Patient will enter into and cooperate with long-term therapy, the ultimate goal being integration into one personality.	1. The nurse must develop a trusting relationship with the patient regardless of which identities are being manifested. 2. Help the patient understand the existence of the subpersonalities and the need each serves in the personal identity of the individual. 3. Help the patient identify stressful situations that precipitate transition from one identity to another. Carefully observe and record these transitions. 4. Use nursing interventions necessary to deal with maladaptive behaviors associated with individual subpersonalities. For example, if one identity is suicidal, precautions must be taken to guard against the patient's self-harm. If another identity has a tendency toward physical hostility, precautions must be taken to protect others. **NOTE:** It may be possible to seek assistance from one of the identities. For example, the patient's strong-willed identity may be able to help control the behaviors of a "suicidal" identity.	1. Trust is the basis of a therapeutic relationship. Each of the identities views itself as a separate entity and must initially be treated as such. 2. Patients may initially be unaware of the dissociative response. Knowledge of the needs each identity fulfills is the first step in the integration process. 3. Identification of stressors is required to assist the patient in responding more adaptively and to eliminate the need for transition to other identities. 4. The safety of the patient and others is a nursing priority.

Continued

Table 20–3 | CARE PLAN FOR THE PATIENT WITH A DISSOCIATIVE DISORDER—cont'd

OUTCOME CRITERIA	NURSING INTERVENTIONS	RATIONALE
	5. Help the patient recognize that intervention is intended to promote an integrated, unified identity within the individual.	5. Because subpersonalities function as separate entities, the idea of total elimination generates fear and defensiveness.
	6. Provide support during disclosure of painful experiences and reassurance when the patient becomes discouraged with lengthy treatment.	6. Positive reinforcement may encourage repetition of desirable behaviors.

NURSING DIAGNOSIS: DISTURBED SENSORY PERCEPTION (VISUAL/KINESTHETIC)

RELATED TO: Severe psychological stress and repression of anxiety

EVIDENCED BY: Alteration in the perception or experience of the self or the environment

OUTCOME CRITERIA	NURSING INTERVENTIONS	RATIONALE
Short-Term Goal ■ Patient will verbalize adaptive ways of coping with stress. **Long-Term Goal** ■ Patient will demonstrate the ability to perceive stimuli correctly and maintain a sense of reality during stressful situations.	1. Provide support and encouragement during times of depersonalization.	1. Patients manifesting these symptoms may express fear and anxiety at experiencing such behaviors. They do not understand the response and may express a fear of going insane. Support and encouragement from a trusted individual provide a feeling of security when fears and anxieties are manifested.
	2. Explain the depersonalization behaviors and the purpose they usually serve for the patient.	2. This knowledge may help to minimize fears and anxieties associated with their occurrence.
	3. Explain the relationship between severe anxiety and depersonalization behaviors. Help relate these behaviors to times of severe psychological stress that the patient has experienced.	3. The patient may be unaware that the occurrence of depersonalization behaviors is related to severe anxiety. Knowledge of this relationship is the first step in the process of behavioral change.
	4. Explore past experiences and possibly repressed painful situations, such as trauma or abuse, *as the patient demonstrates readiness*.	4. Prompting patients to recall traumatic events and experiences before they are ready can be retraumatizing, and premature recounting of traumatic experiences may predispose individuals to dissociative disorders.
	5. Discuss these painful experiences with the patient and encourage them to deal with the feelings associated with these situations. Work to resolve the conflicts these repressed feelings have nurtured.	5. Conflict resolution will serve to decrease the need for the dissociative response to anxiety.
	6. Discuss ways the patient may more adaptively respond to stress and use role-play to practice using these new methods.	6. Role-play helps to prepare the patient to face stressful situations by using these new behaviors when they occur in real life.

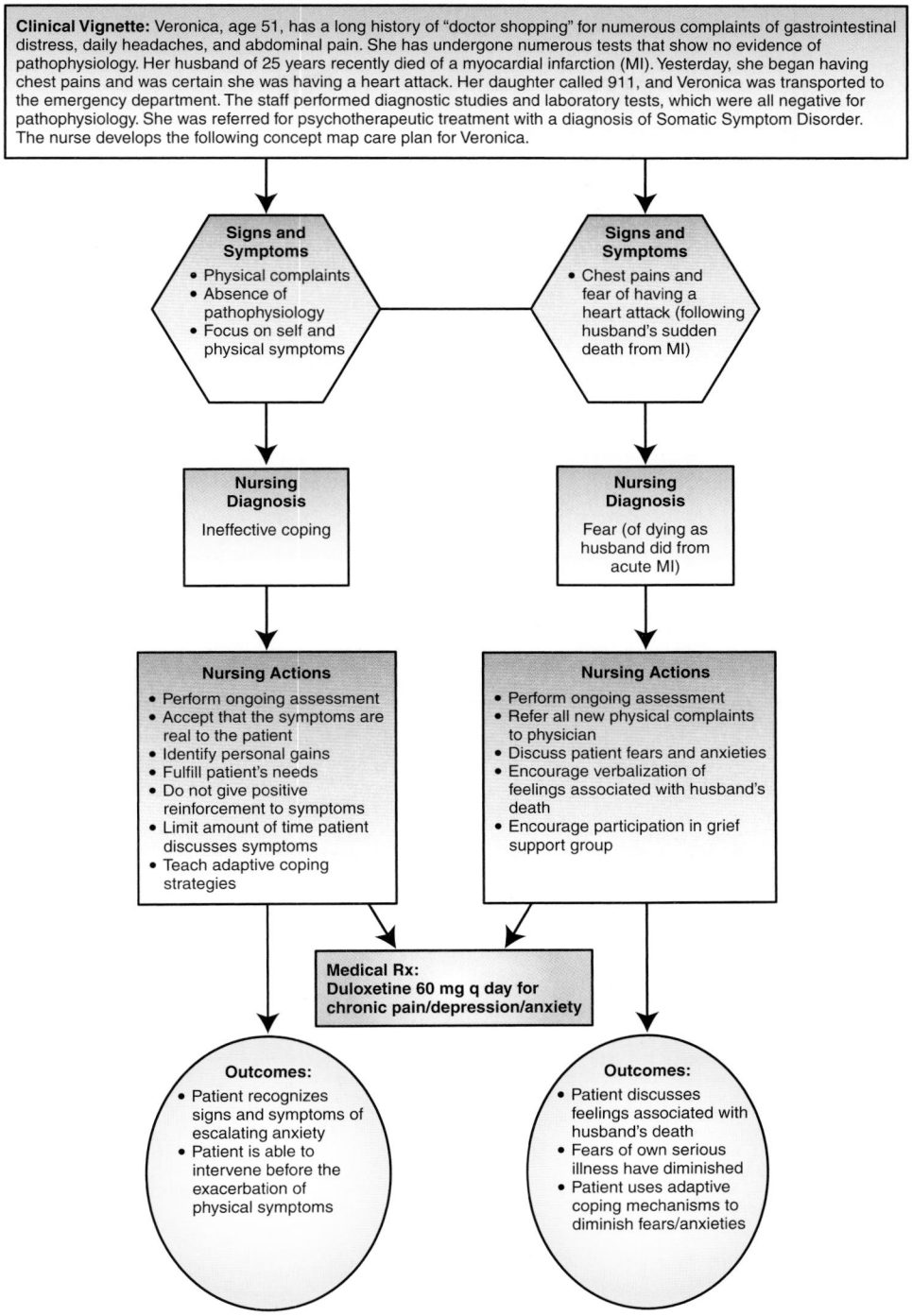

FIGURE 20–1 Concept map care plan for a patient with somatic symptom disorder.

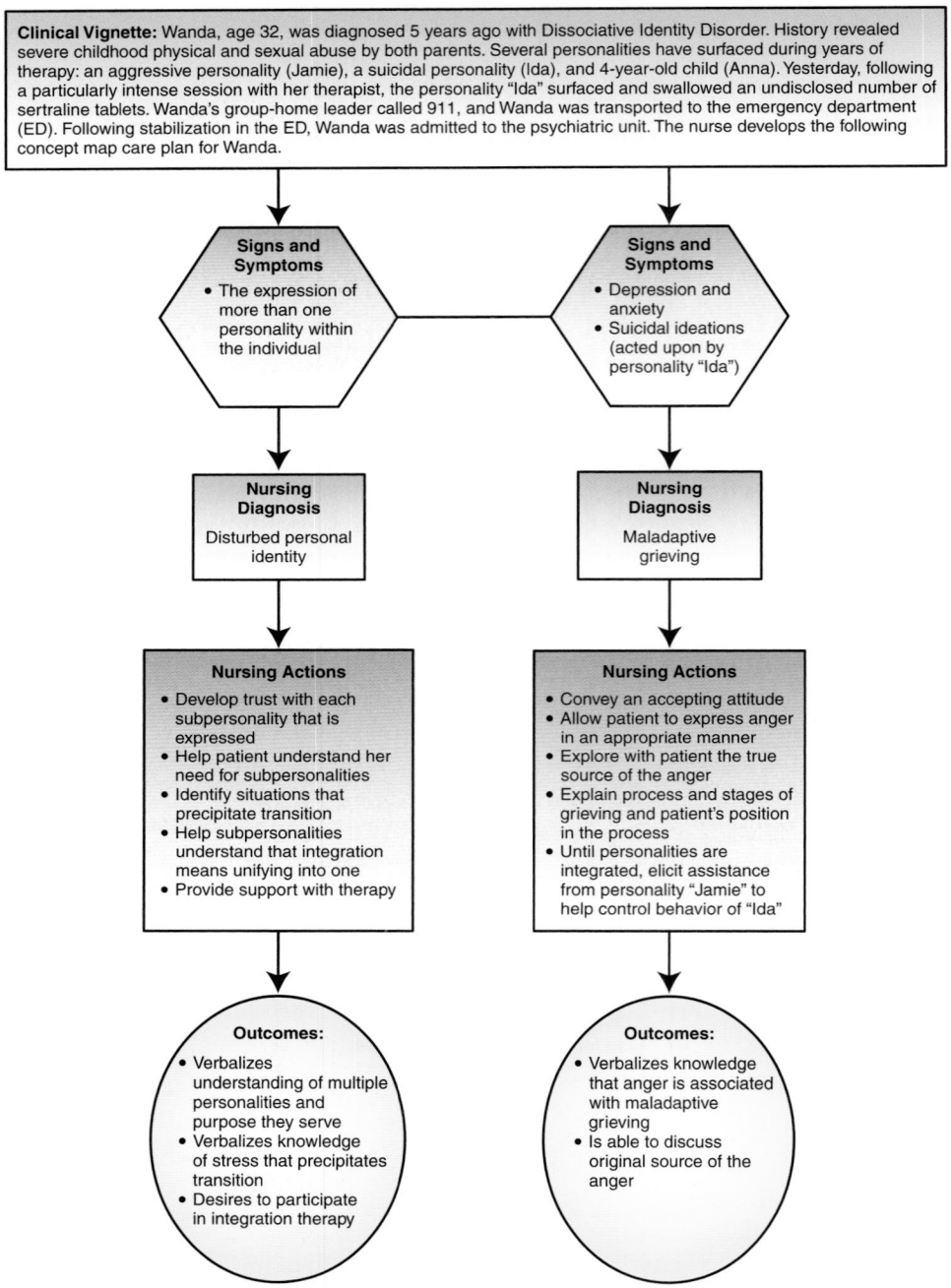

FIGURE 20–2 Concept map care plan for a patient with dissociative identity disorder.

Patient and Family Education

The role of patient teacher is important in the psychiatric area, as it is in all areas of nursing. For patients with dissociative disorders, the patient and family need to be educated about various treatment options that are focused on trauma treatment. Family therapy may be recommended and is often crucial for long-term stabilization (Boland & Verduin, 2022). For patients with somatic symptom disorders, it is important to educate about the benefits of CBT but Boland and Verduin (2022) note that patients may respond better to recommendations for exercise, yoga, meditation, and massage since some may not be open to psychological explanations for their symptoms.

Evaluation

Reassessment is conducted to determine whether the nursing actions have been successful in achieving the objectives of care. Evaluation of the nursing actions for the patient with a somatic symptom disorder may be facilitated by gathering information using the following types of questions:

Does the patient:

- Recognize signs and symptoms of escalating anxiety?
- Intervene with adaptive coping strategies to interrupt the escalating anxiety before physical symptoms are exacerbated?
- Verbalize an understanding of the correlation between physical symptoms and times of escalating anxiety?
- Have a plan for dealing with increased stress to prevent exacerbation of physical symptoms?
- Demonstrate a decrease in ruminations about physical symptoms?
- Express that fears of serious illness have diminished?
- Demonstrate full recovery from previous loss or alteration of physical functioning?

Evaluation of the nursing actions for the patient with a dissociative disorder may be facilitated by gathering information using the following types of questions:

Does the patient:

- Recall memories accurately?
- Connect occurrence of psychological stress to loss of memory?
- Discuss fears and anxieties with members of the staff in an effort toward resolution?
- Discuss the presence of various identities within the self?
- Verbalize situations that precipitate transition from one identity to another?
- Maintain a sense of reality during stressful situations?
- Verbalize a correlation between stressful situations and the onset of depersonalization behaviors?
- Demonstrate more adaptive coping strategies for dealing with stress without resorting to dissociation?

Treatment Modalities

Somatic Symptom Disorders

Individual Psychotherapy

The goal of psychotherapy is to help clients develop healthy and adaptive behaviors and to encourage them to move beyond their somatization and manage their lives more effectively. The focus is on personal and social difficulties that the client is experiencing in daily life as well as the achievement of practical solutions for these difficulties.

Treatment is initiated with a complete physical examination to rule out organic pathology. Clients may be more amenable to psychotherapeutic treatment, particularly stress management, when it is conducted in a medical setting. Regular noninvasive medical assessments are recommended to reassure clients that their concerns are being heard (Yates, 2019). In addition, regular assessment may limit health-care seeking behavior and provide an ongoing opportunity for education and stress management.

Group Psychotherapy

Group therapy may be helpful for somatic symptom disorders because it provides a setting where clients can share their experiences of illness, can learn to verbalize thoughts and feelings, and can be confronted by group members and leaders when they reject responsibility for maladaptive behaviors. It has been reported to be the treatment of choice for both somatic symptom disorder and illness anxiety disorder, in part because it provides the social support and anxiety reduction that these clients need.

Cognitive Behavior Therapy (CBT) and Psychoeducation

Escobar and Dimsdale (2017) report that several studies support cognitive behavior therapy (CBT) as an effective strategy for reducing symptoms in clients with somatic diseases. Evidence supports that CBT is particularly effective in reducing depressive symptoms in clients with somatic disorders (Yates, 2019). Psychoeducation includes teaching patients that their symptoms may be related to or exacerbated by stress and anxiety. This teaching should be done in the context of a trusting relationship between the health-care provider and the client because the client may resist the suggestion that physical symptoms could have a psychological foundation. Psychoeducation for family members and other support systems focuses on teaching these individuals to reward the client's autonomy, self-sufficiency, and independence while being careful not to reinforce passivity and dependence associated with the sick role. This process becomes more difficult when the client is very regressed and the sick role is well established. In conversion disorder, symptoms usually abate spontaneously, but behavior therapy may be beneficial.

Psychopharmacology

While studies have shown CBT to have the highest efficacy in patients with somatic symptom and related disorders, antidepressants (and particularly first generation tricyclics) have demonstrated benefit for pain syndromes (Boland & Verduin, 2022). Anxiety may be treated in the short term with antianxiety agents, but long-term use should be avoided because of the potential for physical dependence. Benzodiazepines should be used cautiously in patients with dissociative disorders since they can also exacerbate dissociation (Gentile et al., 2014). In the treatment of conversion disorders, parenteral amobarbital or lorazepam may be helpful in revealing historical information related to trauma.

Dissociative Amnesia

Many cases of dissociative amnesia resolve spontaneously when the individual is removed from the stressful situation. For more refractory conditions, intravenous administration of amobarbital is useful in the retrieval of lost memories. Most clinicians recommend supportive psychotherapy as well to reinforce adjustment to the psychological impact of the retrieved memories and the emotions associated with them.

In some instances, psychotherapy is used as the primary treatment. Techniques of persuasion and free or directed association are used to help the client remember. In other cases, hypnosis may be required to mobilize the memories. Hypnosis is sometimes facilitated by pharmacological agents, such as sodium amobarbital. Once the memories have been obtained through hypnosis, supportive psychotherapy, group psychotherapy, and cognitive behavior therapy may be employed to help the client integrate the memories into their conscious state. CBT has an added benefit that when clients begin to correct cognitive distortions about the associated trauma, they may develop better recall of details about traumatic events (Boland & Verduin, 2022).

Dissociative Identity Disorder

The goal of therapy for the client with DID is to optimize the client's function and potential. The achievement of **integration** (a blending of all the personality states into one) is usually considered desirable, but some clients choose not to pursue this lengthy therapeutic regimen. In these cases, resolution, or a smooth collaboration among the subpersonalities, may be all that is realistic.

Intensive, long-term psychotherapy with the DID client is directed toward uncovering the underlying psychological conflicts, helping them gain insight into these conflicts, and striving to synthesize the various identities into one integrated personality. The therapist who engages in psychotherapy with this client must be skilled in various approaches, including insight-oriented psychotherapy, CBT, and especially trauma-informed and post-traumatic stress disorder (PTSD) treatment approaches. Clients are assisted to recall past traumas in detail. They must mentally reexperience the abuse that caused their illness. This process, called **abreaction,** or "remembering with feeling," is so painful that clients may actually cry, scream, and feel the pain that they felt at the time of the abuse.

During therapy, each personality state is actively explored and encouraged to become aware of the others across previously amnestic barriers. Traumatic memories associated with the different personality manifestations, especially those related to childhood abuse, are examined. The course of treatment is often difficult and anxiety provoking to client and therapist alike, especially when aggressive or suicidal personalities are in the dominant role. In these instances, brief periods of hospitalization may be necessary as an interim supportive measure. Escobar and Dimsdale (2017) identify that the standard of care for clients with DID (and dissociative amnesia) is a three-phase process: (1) stabilization in which the focus is on safety and symptom control, (2) an intensive focus on trauma issues, and (3) reintegration of the personality and a moving away from a framework of traumatization and victimization.

When integration is achieved, individuals are able to integrate all the feelings, experiences, memories, skills, and talents that were previously in the command of the various identities. They learn how to function effectively without the necessity for creating separate identities to cope with life. This is possible only after years of intense psychotherapy, and even then, recovery is often incomplete.

Depersonalization-Derealization Disorder

Information about the treatment of depersonalization-derealization disorder is sparse and inconclusive. Various psychiatric medications have been tried, both singly and in combination: antidepressants, mood stabilizers, anticonvulsants, and antipsychotics. Results have been sporadic at best. If other psychiatric disorders, such as schizophrenia, are evident, they too may be treated pharmacologically. For clients with evident intrapsychic conflict, analytically oriented insight psychotherapy may be useful. Some clients with depersonalization-derealization disorder have benefited from hypnotherapy or CBT.

CASE STUDY AND SAMPLE CARE PLAN

NURSING HISTORY AND ASSESSMENT

Jake is a 54-year-old client of the psychiatric outpatient department of the VA Medical Center. At age 42, Jake was diagnosed with colon cancer and underwent a colon resection. Since that time, he has had regular follow-up examinations with no recurrence of the cancer and no residual effects. He did not require follow-up chemotherapy or radiation therapy. For 10 years, Jake has had yearly physical and laboratory examinations. He regularly complains to his family physician of mild abdominal pain, sensations of "fullness," "bowel rumblings," and what he calls a "firm mass," which he says he can sometimes feel in his lower left quadrant. The physician has performed x-rays of the entire gastrointestinal (GI) tract, an esophagoscopy, gastroscopy, and colonoscopy. All results were negative for organic pathology. Rather than being relieved, Jake appears to be resentful and disappointed that the physician has not been able to reveal a pathological problem. Jake's job is in jeopardy because of excessive use of sick leave. The family physician has referred Jake for psychiatric evaluation. Jake was admitted as an outpatient with the diagnosis of Illness Anxiety Disorder. He has been assigned to Lisa, a psychiatric nurse practitioner.

In her assessment, Lisa learns that Jake has lived most of his adult life in isolation. He was never close to his parents, who worked and seldom had time for Jake or his sister. Jake told Lisa, "My parents really didn't care about me. They were too busy taking care of the farm. Dad wanted me to take over the farm, but I was never interested. I liked working on cars and went to vocational school to learn how to be a mechanic. I thought they would be proud of me, but they never cared. I think they only had kids so they would have some help on the farm. When I left home, they really didn't care if they ever saw me again." He has never been married nor had a really serious relationship. "Women don't like me much. I spend most of my time alone. I guess I don't really like people, and they don't really like me."

NURSING DIAGNOSES AND OUTCOME IDENTIFICATION

From the assessment data, the nurse develops the following nursing diagnoses for Jake:

1. **Fear** (of cancer recurrence) related to history of colon cancer evidenced by numerous complaints of the GI tract and insistence that something is wrong despite objective tests that rule out pathophysiology
   a. **Short-Term Goal:** Jake will verbalize that fears associated with bodily sensations are irrational.
   b. **Long-Term Goal:** Jake interprets bodily sensations correctly.
2. **Chronic low self-esteem** related to unfulfilled childhood needs for nurturing and caring evidenced by transformation of internalized anger into physical complaints and hostility toward others
   a. **Short-Term Goal:** Within 2 weeks, Jake will verbalize aspects about self that he likes.
   b. **Long-Term Goal:** By discharge from treatment, Jake will demonstrate acceptance of self as a person of worth, as evidenced by setting realistic goals, limiting physical complaints and hostility toward others, and verbalizing positive prospects for the future.

PLANNING AND IMPLEMENTATION

FEAR (OF CANCER RECURRENCE)

The following nursing interventions have been identified for Jake.

1. Monitor the physician's ongoing assessments and laboratory reports to ensure that pathology is clearly ruled out.
2. Refer any new physical complaints to the physician.
3. Assess what function these physical complaints are fulfilling for Jake. Is it a way for him to get attention that he can't get in any other way?
4. Show empathy for Jake's feelings. Let him know that it is understood how GI symptoms may bring about fears of the colon cancer recurring.
5. Encourage Jake to talk about his fears of cancer recurrence. What feelings did he have when it was first diagnosed? How did he deal with those feelings? What are his fears at this time?
6. Have Jake keep a diary of the appearance of the symptoms. In a separate diary, have Jake keep a record of situations that create stress for him. Compare these two records. Correlate whether symptoms appear at times of increased anxiety.
7. Help Jake determine what techniques may be useful for him to implement when fear and anxiety are exacerbated (e.g., relaxation techniques, mental imagery, thought-stopping techniques, physical exercise).
8. Offer positive feedback when Jake responds to stressful situations with coping strategies other than physical complaints.

CHRONIC LOW SELF-ESTEEM

The following nursing interventions have been identified for Jake.

1. Convey acceptance and unconditional positive regard and remain nonjudgmental at all times.
2. Encourage Jake to participate in decision making regarding his care as well as in life situations.

Continued

CASE STUDY AND SAMPLE CARE PLAN—cont'd

3. Help Jake to recognize and focus on strengths and accomplishments. Minimize attention given to past (real or perceived) failures.
4. Encourage Jake to talk about feelings related to his unsatisfactory relationship with his parents.
5. Discuss things in his life that Jake would like to change. Help him determine what *can* be changed and what changes are not realistic.
6. Encourage participation in group activities and in therapy groups that offer simple methods of achievement. Give recognition and positive feedback for actual accomplishments.
7. Teach assertiveness techniques and effective communication techniques.
8. Offer positive feedback for appropriate social interactions with others. Role-play with Jake situations that he finds particularly stressful. Help him to understand that ruminations about himself and his health may cause others to reject him socially.
9. Help Jake to set realistic goals for his future.

EVALUATION

Some of the outcome criteria for Jake have been met, and some are ongoing. He has come to realize that the fears about his "symptoms" are not rational. He understands that the physician has performed adequate diagnostic procedures to rule out illness. He still has fears of cancer occurrence and discusses these fears with the nurse practitioner on a weekly basis. He has kept his symptoms/stressful situations diary and has correlated the appearance of some of the symptoms to times of increased anxiety. Jake has started running and tries to use this exercise as a strategy to keep the anxiety from escalating out of proportion and bringing on new physical symptoms. He continues to discuss feelings associated with his childhood, and the nurse has helped him see that he has had numerous accomplishments in his life even though they were not recognized by his parents or others. He has joined a support group for depressed persons and states that he "has made a few friends." Jake has made a long-term goal of joining a church with the hope of meeting new people. He is missing fewer workdays because of illness, and his job is no longer in jeopardy.

Summary and Key Points

- Somatic symptom and related disorders and dissociative disorders are associated with anxiety that occurs at the severe level. The anxiety is repressed and manifested in the form of symptoms and behaviors associated with these disorders.
- Somatic symptom and related disorders affect about 5% to 7% of the general population. Types of somatic disorders include somatic symptom disorder, illness anxiety disorder, conversion disorder, psychological factors affecting other medical conditions, factitious disorder, and other specified or unspecified somatic symptom and related disorders.
- Somatic symptom disorder is manifested by physical symptoms that may be vague, dramatized, or exaggerated in their presentation. No evidence of organic pathology can be identified.
- Illness anxiety disorder is an unrealistic preoccupation with fear of having a serious illness. This disorder may follow a personal experience or the experience of a close family member with serious or life-threatening illness.
- The individual with conversion disorder experiences a loss of or alteration in bodily functioning, unsubstantiated by medical or pathophysiological explanation. Psychological factors may be evident by the primary or secondary gains that the individual achieves from experiencing the physiological manifestation.
- With the diagnosis of psychological factors affecting medical condition, psychological or behavioral factors have been implicated in the development, exacerbation, or delayed recovery from a medical condition.
- In factitious disorder, the individual falsifies physical or psychological signs or symptoms or induces injury on the self or another person in order to receive attention from medical personnel.
- A dissociative response has been described as a defense mechanism to protect the ego in the face of overwhelming anxiety.
- Dissociative responses result in an alteration in the normally integrative functions of identity, memory, or consciousness.
- Classification of dissociative disorders includes dissociative amnesia, dissociative identity disorder

(DID), depersonalization-derealization disorder, and other specified or unspecified dissociative disorders.

- The individual with dissociative amnesia is unable to recall important personal information that is too extensive to be explained by ordinary forgetfulness.
- The prominent feature of DID is the existence of two or more personality states within a single individual. An individual may have many personality states, each of which serves a purpose for that individual of enduring painful stimuli that the person's identity is too fragmented to integrate as one whole personality.
- Depersonalization-derealization disorder is characterized by an alteration in the perception of oneself and/or the environment. Depersonalization is described as a feeling of unreality or detachment from one's body. Derealization is an experience of unreality or detachment with respect to one's surroundings.
- Individuals with somatic symptom and dissociative disorders often receive health care initially in settings other than psychiatry.
- Nurses can assist patients with these disorders by helping them to understand the role of anxiety in symptom development and identify and establish new, more adaptive cognitive and behavior patterns.
- History of child abuse and other traumas is not uncommon in clients with these disorders. Nurses should provide trauma-informed care and be aware of resources for referral to specialists in trauma care and post-traumatic stress disorder (PTSD) treatment.

Review Questions

Select the answer that is most appropriate for each of the following questions:

1. Which symptom profiles would you expect when assessing a client with somatic symptom disorder?
   a. Multiple somatic symptoms in several body systems
   b. Fear of having a serious disease
   c. Loss or alteration in sensorimotor functioning
   d. Belief that their body is deformed or defective in some way
2. Which ego defense mechanism describes the underlying psychodynamics of somatic symptom disorder?
   a. Denial of depression
   b. Repression of anxiety
   c. Suppression of grief
   d. Displacement of anger
3. Nursing care for a client with somatic symptom disorder should focus on helping the client to achieve which goal?
   a. Eliminate stressors.
   b. Discontinue focusing on numerous physical complaints.
   c. Take medication only as prescribed.
   d. Learn more adaptive coping strategies.
4. A client diagnosed with somatic symptom disorder, states, "My doctor thinks I should see a psychiatrist. I can't imagine why he would make such a suggestion." What is the most common basis for the client's statement?
   a. Lack of trust in the physician
   b. Lack of understanding about the correlation of symptoms and stress
   c. Lack of understanding about the role of a psychiatrist
   d. Lack of financial resources

Continued

5. What is the ultimate goal of therapy for a client with DID?
   a. Integration of the identities into one cohesive personality
   b. The ability to switch from one identity to another voluntarily
   c. The ability to select one personality as the dominant self the dominant self
   d. Recognition that the various identities exist
6. The ultimate goal of therapy for a client with DID is most likely achieved through which intervention?
   a. Crisis intervention and directed association
   b. Psychotherapy and hypnosis
   c. Psychoanalysis and free association
   d. Insight psychotherapy and dextroamphetamines
7. Which manifestations would be consistent with the diagnosis of illness anxiety disorder?
   a. Complains of a multitude of incapacitating physical symptoms
   b. Presents with pseudoseizures or pseudocyesis
   c. Takes substances to induce vomiting in order to convince the nurse that of the need for treatment
   d. Expresses persistent fears of having life-threatening disease

Clinical Judgment Questions

8. A client diagnosed with somatic symptom disorder tells the nurse about a pain in their side. The client says they have not experienced it before. Which is the most appropriate response by the nurse?
   a. "I don't want to hear about another physical complaint. You know they are all in your head. It's time for group therapy now."
   b. "Let's sit down here together, and you can tell me about this new pain you are experiencing. You'll just have to miss group therapy today."
   c. "I will report this pain to your physician. In the meantime, group therapy starts in 5 minutes."
   d. "I will call your physician and see if he will order a new pain medication for your side. The one you have now doesn't seem to provide relief. Why don't you get some rest for now?"
9. A client with a history of childhood physical and sexual abuse was diagnosed with dissociative identity disorder (DID) 6 years ago and has been admitted to the psychiatric unit following a suicide attempt. What is the primary nursing diagnosis for this client?
   a. Disturbed personal identity related to childhood abuse
   b. Disturbed sensory perception related to repressed anxiety
   c. Impaired memory related to disturbed thought processes
   d. Risk for suicide related to unresolved grief
10. In establishing trust with a client diagnosed with dissociative identity disorder, the nurse should use which intervention?
   a. Tell the client that their personality states are related to severe childhood trauma and ask them to elaborate.
   b. Listen nonjudgmentally and respond empathetically when the client transitions to different personality states.
   c. Ignore communication that appears to be that of another personality.
   d. Explain to the client that they must remain in their primary identity state while communicating with the nurse.
   e. All of the above.

IMPLICATIONS FOR EVIDENCE-BASED PRACTICE

Lebel, S., Mutsaers, B., Tomei, C., Leclair, C. S., Jones, G., Petricone-Westwood, D., Rutkowski, N., Ta, V., Trudel, G., Laflamme, S. Z., Lavigne, A-A., & Dinkel, A. (2020). Health anxiety and illness-related fears across diverse chronic illnesses: A systematic review on conceptualization, measurement, prevalence, course, and correlates. *PLoS ONE, 15*(7), e0234124. https://doi.org/10.1371/journal.pone.0234124

DESCRIPTION OF THE STUDY: The authors, noting that health-related fears are common among patients with chronic illnesses, conducted a systematic review of 401 articles to investigate the conceptual, theoretical, measurement overlap, and differences between distinct perspectives on management of illness-related fears in various chronic illnesses and to clarify the prevalence, course, and correlates of these fears.

RESULTS OF THE STUDY: The review found that, across different conceptualizations of illness anxiety, there were three commonalities: a high level of clinically significant levels of fear, a stable course over time, and a deleterious impact on the quality of life. While there appeared to be applicability of *DSM-5-TR* disorders to the experience of fear in patients with chronic illnesses, only a minority of the reviewed articles employed a psychiatric perspective. The authors recommend conceptualizing health anxiety (HA) on a continuum from mild and transient to severe. They further identify the need to conceptualize HA as having affective, cognitive, behavioral, and perceptual features.

IMPLICATIONS FOR NURSING PRACTICE: The setting, patient population, and perspectives of different healthcare professionals can all be influential in how nurses respond to the needs of a patient with illness anxiety. The authors' research underscores the importance of systematic review to clarify and unify conceptualizations with the goal of assuring that, across settings and across populations of patients with chronic illnesses, illness anxiety is recognized as not only a significant concern but also one that affects an individual's mood, cognition, behavior, and perceptions. Nurses in any practice setting should be attentive to assessing for the severity of illness or health anxiety and consider interventions that address mood, cognitive, perceptual, and behavioral symptoms.

TEST YOUR CLINICAL REASONING AND CLINICAL JUDGMENT SKILLS

Tom was admitted to the psychiatric unit from the emergency department of a general hospital in the Midwest. The owner of a local bar called the police when Tom suddenly seemed to "lose control. He just went ballistic." The police reported that Tom did not know where he was or how he got there. He kept saying, "My name is John Brown, and I live in Philadelphia." When the police ran an identity check on Tom, they found that he was indeed John Brown from Philadelphia, and his wife had reported him missing a month ago. Mrs. Brown explained that about 12 months before his disappearance, her husband, who was a shop foreman at a large manufacturing plant, had been having considerable difficulty at work. He had been passed over for a promotion, and his supervisor had been very critical of his work. Several of his staff had left the company for other jobs, and without enough help, Tom had been unable to meet shop deadlines. Work stress made him very difficult to live with at home. Previously an easygoing, extroverted individual, he became withdrawn and extremely critical of his wife and children. Immediately preceding his disappearance, he had had a violent argument with his 18-year-old son, who called Tom a "loser." His son stormed out of the house to stay with some friends. It was the day after this argument that Tom disappeared. The psychiatrist assigns a diagnosis of Dissociative Amnesia, with dissociative fugue.

Answer the following questions related to Tom:

1. Describe the *priority* nursing intervention with Tom as he is admitted to the psychiatric unit.
2. What approach should be taken to help Tom with his problem?
3. What is the long-term goal of therapy for Tom?

MOVIE CONNECTIONS

Bandits (Illness anxiety disorder) ▪ *Hanna and Her Sisters* (Illness anxiety disorder) ▪ *Send Me No Flowers* (Illness anxiety disorder) ▪ *Dead Again* (Amnesia) ▪ *Mirage* (Amnesia) ▪ *Suddenly Last Summer* (Amnesia) ▪ *Sybil* (DID) ▪ *The Three Faces of Eve* (DID) ▪ *Identity* (DID)

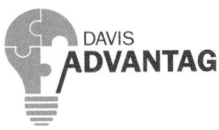

Go to **Davis Advantage** to complete your learning: strengthen understanding, apply your knowledge, and prepare for the Next Gen NCLEX®.

References

Ali, S., Jabeen, S., Pate, R. J., Shahid, M., Chinala, S., Nathani, M., & Shah, R. (2015). Conversion disorder—mind versus body: A review. *Innovations in Clinical Neuroscience, 12*(5-6), 27–33.

American Psychiatric Association. (2022). *Diagnostic and statistical manual of mental disorders* (5th ed., text rev.).

Boland, R., & Verduin, M. L. (2022). *Kaplan & Sadock's synopsis of psychiatry* (P. Ruiz, Ed.). (12th ed.). Wolters Kluwer.

Chalavi, S., Vissia, E. M., Giesen, M. E., Nijenhuis, E. R. S., Draijer, N., Cole, J. H., Dazzan, P., Pariante, C. M., Madsen, S. K., Rajagopalan, P., Thompson, P. M., Toga, A. W., Veltman, D. J. & Reinders, A. T. (2015). Abnormal hippocampal morphology in dissociative identity disorder and post-traumatic stress disorder correlates with childhood trauma and dissociative symptoms. *Human Brain Mapping, 36*, 1692–1704.

Delvecchio, G., Rossetti, M. G., Caletti, E., Arighi, A., Galimberti, D., Basilico, P., Mercurio, M., Paoli, R., Cinnante, C., Triulzi, F., Altamura, A. C., Scarpini, E., & Brambilla, P. (2019). The neuroanatomy of somatoform disorders: A magnetic resonance imaging study. *Psychosomatics, 60*(3), 278–288. https://doi.org/10.1016/j.psym.2018.07.005

Dimsdale J. E. (2017). Research on somatization and somatic symptom disorders: Ars longa, vita brevis. *Psychosomatic Medicine, 79*(9), 971–973. https://doi.org/10.1097/PSY.0000000000000533

Dimsdale, J. (2020). Illness anxiety disorder. In *Merck manual: Professional version.* http://www.merckmanuals.com/professional/psychiatric-disorders/somatic-symptom-and-related-disorders/illness-anxiety-disorder

Escobar, J. I., & Dimsdale, J. E. (2017). Somatic symptom and related disorders. In B. J. Sadock, V. A. Sadock, & P. Ruiz (Eds.), *Comprehensive textbook of psychiatry* (10th ed., pp. 1827–1845). Wolters Kluwer.

Gentile, J. P., Snyder, M., & Marie Gillig, P. (2014). Stress and trauma: Psychotherapy and pharmacotherapy for depersonalization/derealization disorder. *Innovations in Clinical Neuroscience, 11*(7-8), 37–41.

Haberman, C. (2014, November 24). Debate persists over diagnosing mental disorders, long after "Sybil." *New York Times.* http://www.nytimes.com/2014/11/24/us/debate-persists-over-diagnosing-mental-health-disorders-long-after-sybil.html?_r=0

Herdman, T. H., Kamitsuru, S., Lopes, C. T. (Eds.). (2021). *NANDA-I Inc. nursing diagnoses: Definitions and classification, 2021–2023.* Thieme.

Institute of Medicine. (2003). *Health professions education: A bridge to quality.* National Academies Press.

Joshi, K. G. (2020). Strategies for treating patients with health anxiety. *Current Psychiatry, 19*(4), 54–60.

Kahn, D. (2018). Illness anxiety disorder (formerly hypochondriasis). *Medscape.* https://emedicine.medscape.com/article/290955-overview#a6

Lebel, S., Mutsaers, B., Tomei, C., Leclair, C. S., Jones, G., Petricone-Westwood, D., Rutkowski, N., Ta, V., Trudel, G., Laflamme, S. Z., Lavigne, A-A., & Dinkel, A. (2020). Health anxiety and illness-related fears across diverse chronic illnesses: A systematic review on conceptualization, measurement, prevalence, course, and correlates. *PLoS ONE 15*(7), e0234124. https://doi.org/10.1371/journal.pone.0234124

Lowenstein, R. J., Frewen, P., & Lewis-Fernandez, R. (2017). Dissociative disorders. In B. J. Sadock, V. A. Sadock, & P. Ruiz (Eds.), *Comprehensive textbook of psychiatry* (10th ed., pp. 1866–1952). Wolters Kluwer.

Muller, M. (2014). Fragmented child: Disorganized attachment and dissociation. *Psychology Today.* https://www.psychologytoday.com/us/blog/talking-about-trauma/201406/fragmented-child-disorganized-attachment-and-dissociation

Özdemir, O., Cilingir, V., Özdemir, P. G., Milanlioglu, A., Hamamci, M., & Yilmaz, E. (2016). Dissociative experiences in patients with epilepsy. *Arquivos de Neuro-Psiquiatria, 74*(3), 189–194. https://doi.org/10.1590/0004-282X20160045

QSEN Institute. (2020). *Competencies.* http://qsen.org/competencies/

Şar, V., Dorahy, M. J., & Krüger, C. (2017). Revisiting the etiological aspects of dissociative identity disorder: A biopsychosocial perspective. *Psychology Research and Behavior management, 10*, 137–146. https://doi.org/10.2147/PRBM.S113743

Soreff, S. (2018). Fast five quiz: Are you prepared to treat patients with illness anxiety disorder? *Medscape.* https://reference.medscape.com/viewarticle/895692_2

Van den Houte, M., Bogaerts, K., Van Diest, I., De, J., Persoons, P., Van Oudenhove, L., & Van den Bergh, O. (2017). Inducing somatic symptoms in functional syndrome patients: Effects of manipulating state negative affect. *Psychosomatic Medicine, 79*(9), 1000–1007. https://doi.org/10.1097/PSY.0000000000000527

Yates, W. (2019). Somatic symptom disorders. *Medscape.* http://emedicine.medscape.com/article/294908-overview

Classical References

Asher, R. (1951). Munchausen's syndrome. *Lancet, 257*(6650), 339–341.

Freud, S. (1962). The neuro-psychoses of defense. In *Standard edition of the complete psychological works of Freud* (Vol. III). Hogarth Press.

Irwin, H. J. (1999). Pathological and nonpathological dissociation: the relevance of childhood trauma. *The Journal of Psychology, 133*(2), 157–164.

Eating Disorders 21

CHAPTER OUTLINE

Objectives
Introduction
Epidemiology
Application of the Nursing Process
Treatment Modalities
Summary and Key Points
Review Questions
Clinical Judgment Questions
Implications for Evidence-Based Practice
Test Your Clinical Reasoning and Clinical Judgment Skills
Communication Exercises
Movie Connections

CORE CONCEPTS

Stress and Coping
Maladaptive Behaviors: Anorexia; bulimia
Self-Image
Professionalism: Nursing process in the care of patients with an eating disorder
Clinical Judgment

KEY TERMS

amenorrhea
anorexia nervosa (AN)
binging
binge eating disorder (BED)
bulimia nervosa (BN)
emaciated
lanugo
obesity
purging

OBJECTIVES

After reading this chapter, the student will be able to:

1. Identify and differentiate among several eating disorders.
2. Discuss the epidemiology of eating disorders.
3. Describe symptomatology associated with anorexia nervosa, bulimia nervosa, and binge eating disorder, and use the information in patient assessment.
4. Identify predisposing factors in the development of eating disorders.
5. Formulate nursing diagnoses and outcomes of care for patients with eating disorders.
6. Describe appropriate interventions for behaviors associated with eating disorders.
7. Identify topics for patient and family teaching relevant to eating disorders.
8. Evaluate the nursing care of patients with eating disorders.
9. Discuss various modalities relevant to treatment of eating disorders.

Introduction

Nutrition is required to sustain life, and most individuals acquire nutrients from eating food; however, nutrition and life sustenance are not the only reasons most people eat food. In an affluent culture, life sustenance may not even be a consideration. It is sometimes difficult to remember that many people in this affluent American culture, as well as all over the world, are starving from lack of food.

The hypothalamus contains the appetite regulation center in the brain. This complex neural system regulates the body's ability to recognize when it is hungry and when it has been sated. Some studies have shown evidence of serotonin and dopamine dysfunction in individuals with eating disorders (Riva, 2016). These neurotransmitters both play a role in regulating eating behavior in the hypothalamus.

Society and culture also have a great deal of influence on eating behaviors. Eating is a social activity; seldom does an event of any social significance occur without the presence of food. Yet, society and culture also influence how people (and in particular, women) must look. History reveals a regularity of fluctuation in what society has considered desirable in the human female body. Archives and historical paintings from the 16th and 17th centuries reveal that plump, full-figured women were considered fashionable and desirable. In the Victorian era, beauty was characterized by a slender, wan appearance that continued through the flapper era of the 1920s. During the Depression era and World War II, the full-bodied woman was again admired, only to be superseded in the late 1960s by the image of the super-thin model propagated by the media, which remains the ideal of today. As it has been said, "A woman can't be too rich or too thin." Eating disorders, as we know them, can refute this concept.

This chapter explores the disorders associated with undereating and overeating. Because psychological and behavioral factors play a potential role in the presentation of these disorders, they fall well within the realm of psychiatry and psychiatric nursing. Epidemiological statistics are presented along with factors that have been implicated in the etiology of anorexia nervosa, bulimia nervosa, and binge eating disorder. An explanation of the symptomatology is presented as background knowledge for assessing the patient with an eating disorder. Nursing care is described in the context of the nursing process. Various treatment modalities are explored.

Epidemiology

The prevalence of anorexia nervosa has increased since the mid-20th century both in the United States and in Western Europe. Epidemiological studies have found that across all ages and genders, the lifetime prevalence for an episode of anorexia nervosa is 2.4% to 4.3% (Call et al., 2017). Once thought to be rare among males, more recent data (Woolridge & Lemberg, 2016) identify that men account for 25% of those with anorexia and bulimia and 36% of those with binge eating disorders. The authors also note that for the first time, the incidence in males may be increasing at a more rapid rate than in females. See "Real People, Real Stories" for more about Vic's experience with an eating disorder.

Social interests may also play a role in the prevalence of eating disorders. Ballet, modeling, wrestling, and other sports that focus on weight restriction may lead to preoccupation with one's body and increase the risk for anorexia nervosa. Anorexia nervosa was once believed to be more prevalent in the higher socioeconomic classes, but evidence is lacking to support this hypothesis.

Bulimia nervosa has a lifetime prevalence of 2% among women (Call et al., 2017). Onset of bulimia nervosa occurs in late adolescence or early adulthood and is more common in women than men.

Binge eating disorder (BED) is defined in the *Diagnostic and Statistical Manual of Mental Disorders, Fifth Edition, Text Revision* (*DSM-5-TR*; American Psychiatric Association [APA], 2022) as recurrent episodes of eating significantly more than most people would eat in a similar period under similar circumstances, and these episodes occur at least once a week for 3 months. It is the most common eating disorder and affects women almost twice as often as men (Boland & Verduin, 2022). Its prevalence is estimated at 2.8% of the U.S. population (National Institute of Mental Health [NIMH], 2017). Weight gain and obesity are major health risks associated with this disorder and rates of BED are particularly high in obese and overweight individuals (Boland & Verduin, 2022).

Obesity has been defined as a body mass index (BMI) (weight/height^2) of 30 or greater. In the United States, the prevalence of obesity is 42.4% (Centers for Disease Control and Prevention [CDC], 2021). This percentage is higher among non-Hispanic black (49.6%) and Hispanic (44.8%) populations (CDC, 2021). The association between socioeconomics and obesity is complex, but one finding is a lower prevalence of obesity in both men and women from the highest income groups (CDC, 2021). Interestingly, the *DSM-5-TR* does not include obesity as a mental health disorder with the rationale that "a range of genetic, physiological, behavioral, and environmental factors that vary across individuals contributes to the development of obesity; thus obesity is not considered a mental disorder" (APA, 2022, p. 371). The *DSM-5-TR* also notes, however, that there are several mental disorders in which obesity is a significant problem (at least in part related to side effects of psychotropic medications) and that obesity may be a risk factor for the development of illnesses such as depression. BED, which *is* identified as a mental illness, carries a high risk for weight gain and obesity.

Real People, Real Stories: Living With an Eating Disorder

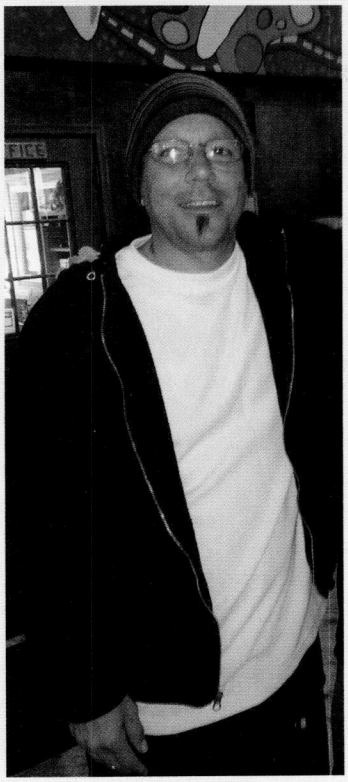

(Following is an excerpt of our conversation.)

Karyn: First of all, I appreciate your willingness to share your story.

Vic: I want to talk about this because there is such a stigma associated with being a guy and having an eating disorder. And it's hard for guys to find a support group of people who really "get it."

Karyn: What has your experience been with encountering stigma?

Vic: Well, my weight has sometimes been really high and sometimes very low. I fluctuate between anorexia and bulimia. So when my weight is really low, people have presumed I have AIDS. And in general, because eating disorders are presumed to be a female disorder, people have assumed I was gay. In high school, I was very heavy and the guys on the football team teased me a lot. I talked to my girlfriend at the time, and she suggested I try purging. I was using food and alcohol for comfort, but then I had to purge. I started working out a lot, and when I started getting compliments on my appearance, I began binging and purging every day and drinking alcohol. It was a stress relief for a while, but then it just wasn't working anymore and I still hated my appearance. To this day, there's not one thing I like about my appearance even though my physician is happy with my current weight. I was hiding it from my family for some time: wearing baggy clothes and two sets of clothes so people wouldn't see my flaws. The behaviors are very isolating. When I tried to talk to my dad he just told me to be a man . . . but there was a lot of physical and emotional abuse from him, so I didn't get support there.

Karyn: Where have you found support?

Vic: My mom and my fiancée are my biggest supports, but it's a struggle to find support with other guys who have eating disorders, and I feel like they would really understand. I tried to start a support group on Facebook, and no one responded. I have an individual counselor who knows a lot about eating disorders, and I have a family practice physician, and they are both helpful. It's just not the same as having the support of others who are having the same experiences that you are.

Karyn: Have you ever been engaged in group treatment specifically for eating disorders?

Vic: I tried, at one point, but most insurances don't cover eating disorder treatment, or the treatment program doesn't take insurance. I went into treatment in 2009 for alcohol rehabilitation, and they didn't address the eating disorder. In fact, they kind of force you to eat and tell you that you'll probably gain weight as you go through rehab, so the bulimia kicked in again for me because I didn't want to get fat like the other people in recovery. But I've been sober since 2009, and I take Vivitrol injections (to manage alcohol dependence) once a month; it blocks the pleasure centers.

Karyn: And has that been effective?

Vic: Oh yes, definitely. And my AA buddies are very supportive, but they don't see food as a similar issue to alcohol, so they don't really see a need to discuss that. Plus, you can't abstain from food like you can from alcohol. And society itself can be a trigger: television, all the messages that you need to be a certain way, picnics, going out to eat, grocery stores, talking about food, et cetera. And I think I have an element of "people pleasing" in my personality, so I'm always worried about what other people are thinking about me.

Karyn: It's not uncommon for people with eating disorders to also have depression and sometimes have suicide thoughts. Have you ever been in that place?

Vic: Yeah, once last year I took an overdose of pills with some alcohol, but I called some friends and they got me in to get help.

Karyn: Do you still have times when you have those thoughts?

Continued

Real People, Real Stories: Living With an Eating Disorder—cont'd

Vic: No. I'm doing really well right now. I still dabble from time to time with "the behavior" [Vic described this as his term for binging/purging or calorie restriction, stating that sometimes using the words can be a trigger for him], but not like before when I was taking up to 20 laxatives a day and my whole day was preoccupied with planning "the behaviors." I'm working in a setting that treats dual diagnosis clients, and I am hopeful that there may be opportunities to establish peer support groups for men with eating disorders, much like what exists in AA for alcohol recovery. As a guy, you just can't go to a group that is all women and talk about this stuff, especially what's going on with your body. And I don't want to be accused of "thirteen-steppin'."

Karyn: "Thirteen steppin'"?

Vic: Yeah, that's the "thirteenth step" in the twelve-step program. It's the guys that go to AA meetings to pick up girls who are in recovery because they know they are more vulnerable when they're trying to stay sober. [Chuckles]

Karyn: [Chuckles] I didn't know that was a thing. But I understand what you're saying about the difficulty of finding support with other men who understand and are willing to acknowledge their eating disorder. I hope the peer support group works out, and in the meantime, I'm glad to hear that you are accessing resources to support your own health.

Application of the Nursing Process

Background Assessment Data

CORE CONCEPT

Anorexia

Prolonged loss of appetite.

CORE CONCEPT

Body Image

A subjective concept of one's physical appearance based on the personal perceptions of self and the reactions of others.

Anorexia Nervosa (AN)

Anorexia nervosa (AN) is characterized by a morbid fear of obesity. Symptoms include gross distortion of body image, preoccupation with food, and refusal to eat, leading to extremely low body weight. The term *anorexia* is actually a misnomer. It was initially believed that individuals with anorexia nervosa did not experience sensations of hunger. However, research indicates that they do suffer from pangs of hunger, and it is only with food intake of less than 200 calories per day that hunger sensations actually cease.

The distortion in body image is manifested by the individual's perception of being "fat" when the person is obviously underweight or even **emaciated** (excessively thin). Weight loss is usually accomplished by reduction in food intake and often extensive exercising. Self-induced vomiting and the abuse of laxatives or diuretics may occur. The *DSM-5-TR* further specifies that some individuals with AN lose weight exclusively by restricting intake while others have binging and purging episodes.

Weight loss is excessive, with some individuals presenting for health-care services weighing less than 85% of expected weight. Despite a weight that is "less than minimally expected" or "less than minimally normal," behaviors to interfere with weight gain persist (Toulany & Katzman, 2021). Other symptoms include hypothermia, bradycardia, hypotension with orthostatic changes, peripheral edema, **lanugo** (fine, neonatal-like hair growth), and a variety of metabolic changes. In women **amenorrhea** (absence of menstruation) usually follows weight loss, but sometimes it happens early in the disorder, even before severe weight loss has occurred. Associated symptoms include cold intolerance, dizziness, chest pain, abdominal bloating, pain or discomfort, constipation, weakness, decreased concentration, and poor memory (Toulany & Katzman, 2021).

Individuals with AN may be obsessed with food. For example, they may hoard or conceal food, talk about food and recipes at great length, or prepare elaborate meals for others, only to restrict themselves to a limited amount of low-calorie food intake. Compulsive behaviors, such as hand washing, may also be present.

Age at onset is usually early to late adolescence, and psychosexual development is often delayed. Feelings of depression and anxiety or irritability often accompany the disorder. Depression is strongly correlated with eating disorders, some of which may be secondary to malnutrition. However, even in those who have recovered from AN, there is a higher incidence of depression, anxiety, and obsessive thinking than in the general population (Uniacke & Broft, 2016). Box 21–1 outlines the *DSM-5-TR* diagnostic criteria for anorexia nervosa.

CORE CONCEPT

Bulimia

Excessive, insatiable appetite.

Bulimia Nervosa (BN)

Bulimia nervosa (BN) is an episodic, uncontrolled, compulsive, rapid ingestion of large quantities of food over a short period **(binging),** followed by inappropriate compensatory behaviors to rid the body of the excess calories. The food consumed during a binge often has a high caloric content, a sweet taste, and a soft or smooth texture that can be eaten rapidly, sometimes even without being chewed, although sometimes bulky foods are preferred without regard for taste (Boland & Verduin, 2022). The binging episodes often occur in secret and are usually terminated by abdominal discomfort, sleep, social interruption, or self-induced vomiting. Although the eating binges may bring pleasure while they are occurring, self-degradation and depressed mood commonly follow.

To rid the body of the excessive calories, the individual engages in **purging** behaviors (self-induced vomiting or the misuse of laxatives, diuretics, or enemas) or other inappropriate compensatory behaviors, such as fasting or excessive exercise. There is a persistent, excessive concern with personal appearance, particularly regarding how the individual believes others perceive them. Weight fluctuations are common because of the alternating binges and fasts. However, most individuals with BN are within a normal weight range—some slightly underweight, some slightly overweight.

Excessive vomiting and laxative or diuretic abuse may lead to problems with dehydration and electrolyte imbalance. Gastric acid in the vomitus also contributes to the erosion of tooth enamel. In rare instances, the individual may experience tears in the gastric or esophageal mucosa. Some individuals develop calluses on the dorsal surface of their hands, typically on knuckles, secondary to long-term, repeated self-induced vomiting. This feature is called *Russell's sign* after the British psychiatrist who first described it. It cannot be a reliable diagnostic symptom, however, because many individuals with purging behavior have developed skill in inducing vomiting at will, without using their hands.

BOX 21–1 Diagnostic Criteria for Anorexia Nervosa

A. Restriction of energy intake relative to requirements leading to a significantly low body weight in the context of age, sex, developmental trajectory, and physical health. Significantly low weight is defined as a weight that is less than minimally normal, or, for children and adolescents, less than that minimally expected.

B. Intense fear of gaining weight or becoming fat, or persistent behavior that interferes with weight gain, even though at a significantly low weight.

C. Disturbance in the way in which one's body weight or shape is experienced, undue influence of body weight or shape on self-evaluation, or persistent lack of recognition of the seriousness of the current low body weight.

Specify whether:

Restricting Type: During the last 3 months, the individual has not engaged in recurrent episodes of binge eating or purging behavior (i.e., self-induced vomiting or the misuse of laxatives, diuretics, or enemas). This subtype describes presentations in which weight loss is accomplished primarily through dieting, fasting, and/or excessive exercise.

Binge-Eating/Purging Type: During the last 3 months, the individual has engaged in recurrent episodes of binge eating or purging behavior (i.e., self-induced vomiting or the misuse of laxatives, diuretics, or enemas).

Specify if:

In partial remission

In full remission

Specify current severity:

Mild: BMI >17 kg/m^2

Moderate: BMI 16–16.99 kg/m^2

Severe: BMI 15–15.99 kg/m^2

Extreme: BMI <15 kg/m^2

Reprinted with permission from American Psychiatric Association (APA) (2022). Diagnostic and statistical manual of mental disorders, fifth edition, text revision (DSM-5-TR).

Common comorbidities include mood disorders, anxiety disorders, or substance abuse, most frequently involving central nervous system (CNS) stimulants or alcohol. Research has shown that about one-third of those with AN cross over to BN (Eddy et al., 2008) and patients with BN and a history of previous lifetime AN had worse decision-making ability, worse general and specific functioning, decreased bone density, more antecedents of lifetime suicide attempts, more dietary restraint, and more frequent use of laxatives (Strumila et al., 2020). The *DSM-5-TR* diagnostic criteria for BN are presented in Box 21–2.

Binge Eating Disorder (BED)

Individuals with BED have episodes of binge eating that may be similar to those with bulimia nervosa. However, one differential feature in BED is the absence of compensatory purging. As a result, clients with BED are at risk for substantial weight gain. The episodes of eating are referred to as binges when they occur over a discrete period, usually defined as less than 2 hours (APA, 2022). Food consumption is not only rapid but also often continues to the point that the individual feels uncomfortably full. Interpersonal stressors, low self-esteem, and boredom are identified as possible triggers. Typically, clients describe their eating as out of control (an important diagnostic clinical symptom) and, after an episode, report accompanying guilt and depression. As many as 50% of individuals with BED have a history of depression (WebMD, 2021). Another difference between bulimia nervosa and BED is that rates of improvement are consistently higher among individuals with BED than among those with bulimia nervosa (APA, 2022). The *DSM-5-TR* diagnostic criteria for BED are presented in Box 21–3.

Predisposing Factors and Theories of Etiology Associated With AN, BN, and BED

Biological Influences

Genetics

A hereditary predisposition to eating disorders has been hypothesized on the basis of family histories and an apparent association with other disorders for which the likelihood of genetic influences exists. Twin studies identify higher concordance rates in monozygotic than in dizygotic twins for AN and BN (Boland & Verduin, 2022). AN is more common among sisters and mothers of those with the disorder than among the general population, but social factors, such as modeling and mimicking, may influence these relationships. Family studies find that a history of AN confers up to 11 times the risk for family members (Call et al., 2017), and those with a

BOX 21–2 Diagnostic Criteria for Bulimia Nervosa

A. Recurrent episodes of binge eating. An episode of binge eating is characterized by both of the following:
   1. Eating, in a discrete period of time (e.g., within any 2-hour period) an amount of food that is definitely larger than most individuals would eat during a similar period of time and under similar circumstances.
   2. A sense of lack of control over eating during the episode (e.g., a feeling that one cannot stop eating or control what or how much one is eating).

B. Recurrent inappropriate compensatory behaviors in order to prevent weight gain, such as self-induced vomiting; misuse of laxatives, diuretics, or other medications; fasting; or excessive exercise.

C. The binge eating and inappropriate compensatory behaviors both occur, on average, at least once a week for 3 months.

D. Self-evaluation is unduly influenced by body shape and weight.

E. The disturbance does not occur exclusively during episodes of anorexia nervosa.

Specify if:

In partial remission

In full remission

Specify current severity:

Mild: An average of 1–3 episodes of inappropriate compensatory behaviors per week.

Moderate: An average of 4–7 episodes of inappropriate compensatory behaviors per week.

Severe: An average of 8–13 episodes of inappropriate compensatory behaviors per week.

Extreme: An average of 14 or more episodes of inappropriate compensatory behaviors per week.

Reprinted with permission from American Psychiatric Association (APA) (2022). Diagnostic and statistical manual of mental disorders, fifth edition, text revision (DSM-5-TR).

BOX 21–3 Diagnostic Criteria for Binge Eating Disorder

A. Recurrent episodes of binge eating. An episode of binge eating is characterized by both of the following:
   1. Eating, in a discrete period of time (e.g., within any 2-hour period), an amount of food that is definitely larger than what most people would eat in a similar period of time under similar circumstances
   2. A sense of lack of control over eating during the episode (e.g., a feeling that one cannot stop eating or control what or how much one is eating)

B. The binge-eating episodes are associated with 3 (or more) of the following:
   1. Eating much more rapidly than normal
   2. Eating until feeling uncomfortably full
   3. Eating large amounts of food when not feeling physically hungry
   4. Eating alone because of feeling embarrassed by how much one is eating
   5. Feeling disgusted with oneself, depressed, or very guilty after overeating

C. Marked distress regarding binge eating is present.

D. The binge eating occurs, on average, at least once a week for 3 months.

E. The binge eating is not associated with the recurrent use of inappropriate compensatory behavior as in bulimia nervosa and does not occur exclusively during the course of bulimia nervosa or anorexia nervosa.

Specify if:
In partial remission
In full remission

Specify current severity:
Mild: 1–3 binge-eating episodes per week
Moderate: 4–7 binge-eating episodes per week
Severe: 8–13 binge-eating episodes per week
Extreme: 14 or more binge-eating episodes per week

Reprinted with permission from American Psychiatric Association (APA) (2022). Diagnostic and statistical manual of mental disorders, fifth edition, text revision (DSM-5-TR).

family history of BN, mood disorders, substance use disorders, or obesity are at greater risk for developing bulimia.

Neurobiological Influences

Neurochemical influences in BN and AN may be associated with the neurotransmitters serotonin, dopamine, and norepinephrine. Neurobiological changes that occur in starvation, including depression and obsessional thinking, may contribute to maintaining the illness (Call et al., 2017). Selective serotonin reuptake inhibitors (SSRIs) (particularly fluoxetine) have demonstrated effectiveness in treating patients with BN but not those with AN (WebMD, 2020). However, SSRIs may be used to treat depression that often accompanies AN. Individuals with BED have manifested several neurobiological disturbances, including delayed gastric emptying, enlarged stomach capacity, and decreased secretion of cholecystokinin (CCK), which is a hormone responsible for signaling satiety (Call et al., 2017). Endogenous opioid peptides appear to play a role in individuals with AN and may be associated with the addictive components of the disorder and with denial of hunger (Hasan & Hasan, 2011). Some individuals with AN have been shown to gain weight when given naloxone, an opioid antagonist. Questions still remain as to whether neurochemical changes are causal or are an outcome of the body's reaction to changes in nutrition and mood.

The etiology of BED is unknown. Brain imaging studies of people with BED reveal increased activity in the orbitofrontal cortex, which is associated with reward and pleasure responses such as those seen in response to substances of abuse (Balodis et al., 2015). These studies support the hypothesis that BED may be an illness of addiction.

Psychodynamic Influences

Psychodynamic theories suggest that the development of an eating disorder is rooted in an unfulfilled sense of separation-individuation. When events occur that threaten the vulnerable ego, feelings of lack of control over one's body (self) emerge. Behaviors associated with food and eating serve to provide feelings of control over one's life.

Family Influences

Historically, parents of individuals with eating disorders have often been presumed to be overcontrolling and perfectionistic, which is then misconstrued as causing pathology in their children. This theory has been problematic, at least in part, because not all siblings in the same family develop eating disorders. There is no sufficient evidence to support these claims, and, in fact, they may have contributed to a resistance to seeking health care based on parents' fear that they will be judged as the cause of the problem. The American Academy for Eating Disorders published a position statement (2009) that includes the following:

> The AED stands firmly against any model of eating disorders in which family influences are seen as the primary cause of eating disorders, condemns statements that blame families for their child's illness, and recommends that families be included in the treatment of younger patients, unless this is clearly ill-advised on clinical grounds.

Conflicts certainly arise in a family when a child is starving, but it has become clear that family members need to be involved in treatment rather than shunned or blamed, and family-based approaches, such as the Maudsley approach (see later in this chapter), are supported by clinical evidence (Reinicke, 2017).

Body Mass Index

Assessment for the presence of an eating disorder requires an understanding of the measurements for BMI. The following formula is used to determine an individual's BMI:

$$\text{Body mass index} = \frac{\text{Weight (kg)}}{\text{Height (m)}^2}$$

The BMI range for normal weight is 20 to 24.9. Studies by the National Center for Health Statistics indicate that *overweight* is defined as a BMI of 25 to 29.9 (based on U.S. Dietary Guidelines for Americans). Based on World Health Organization criteria, *obesity* is defined as a BMI of 30 or greater. These guidelines, which were released by the National Heart, Lung, and Blood Institute in July 1998, markedly increased the number of Americans considered to be overweight. The average American woman has a BMI of 26, and fashion models typically have a BMI of 18. Anorexia nervosa is characterized by a BMI of 17 or lower. In extreme anorexia nervosa, the BMI may be less than 15. Table 21–1 presents an example of some BMIs based on weight (in pounds) and height (in inches).

Diagnosis and Outcome Identification

Nursing diagnoses are formulated from the data gathered during the assessment phase and with background knowledge regarding predisposing factors to the disorder. Table 21–2 presents a list of patient behaviors and the NANDA-International (NANDA-I) nursing diagnoses (Herdman et al., 2021) that correspond to those behaviors, which may be used in planning care for patients with eating disorders.

Outcome Criteria

The following criteria may be used for measurement of outcomes in the care of the patient with eating disorders. The patient:

- Has achieved and maintained an expected BMI for age with consideration for body build, weight history, and any physiological disturbances.
- Has vital signs, blood pressure, and laboratory serum studies within normal limits.
- Verbalizes importance of adequate nutrition.
- Verbalizes knowledge regarding consequences of fluid loss caused by self-induced vomiting (or laxative/diuretic abuse) and importance of adequate fluid intake (AN, BN).
- Verbalizes events that precipitate anxiety and demonstrates techniques for its reduction.
- Verbalizes ways to may gain more control of the environment and thereby reduce feelings of powerlessness.
- Expresses less preoccupation with own appearance (AN, BN).
- Demonstrates ability to take control of own life without resorting to maladaptive eating behaviors (AN, BN, BED).
- Establishes a healthy pattern of eating for weight control, and weight loss toward a desired goal is progressing (BED).
- Verbalizes plans for maintenance of weight control and relapse prevention (BED).

Planning and Implementation

In most instances, individuals with eating disorders are treated on an outpatient basis, but in some cases hospitalization becomes necessary. Reasons for hospitalization include the following:

- ***Malnutrition:*** Individuals 20% below expected weight for height require inpatient treatment; those 30% below expected weight for height are recommended for long-term intensive hospital treatment (2 to 6 months) (Boland & Verduin, 2022)
- ***Dehydration:*** Assessment includes thirst, orthostatic hypotension, tachycardia, elevated sodium levels, and other symptoms
- ***Severe electrolyte imbalance:*** Potassium levels below 3 mmol/L; phosphate levels below 3 mg/dL; magnesium levels below 1.4 mEq/L
- ***Cardiac arrhythmias:*** ST segment and T wave changes usually related to electrolyte imbalances
- ***Severe bradycardia:*** Below 50 beats per minute
- ***Hypothermia:*** Body temperature below 96.8°F

TABLE 21–1 **Body Mass Index (BMI) Chart**

BMI	19	20	21	22	23	24	25	26	27	28	29	30	31	32	33	34	35	36	37	38	39	40
HEIGHT (INCHES)	BODY WEIGHT (POUNDS)																					
58	91	96	100	105	110	115	119	124	129	134	138	143	148	153	158	162	167	172	177	181	186	191
59	94	99	104	109	114	119	124	128	133	138	143	148	153	158	163	168	173	178	183	188	193	198
60	97	102	107	112	118	123	128	133	138	143	148	153	158	163	168	174	179	184	189	194	199	204
61	100	106	111	116	122	127	132	137	143	148	153	158	164	169	174	180	185	190	195	201	206	211
62	104	109	115	120	126	131	136	142	147	153	158	164	169	175	180	186	191	196	202	207	213	218
63	107	113	118	124	130	135	141	146	152	158	163	169	175	180	186	191	197	203	208	214	220	225
64	110	116	122	128	134	140	145	151	157	163	169	174	180	186	192	197	204	209	215	221	227	232
65	114	120	126	132	138	144	150	156	162	168	174	180	186	192	198	204	210	216	222	228	234	240
66	118	124	130	136	142	148	155	161	167	173	179	186	192	198	204	210	216	223	229	235	241	247
67	121	127	134	140	146	153	159	166	172	178	185	191	198	204	211	217	223	230	236	242	249	255
68	125	131	138	144	151	158	164	171	177	184	190	197	203	210	216	223	230	236	243	249	256	262
69	128	135	142	149	155	162	169	176	182	189	196	203	209	216	223	230	236	243	250	257	263	270
70	132	139	146	153	160	167	174	181	188	195	202	209	216	222	229	236	243	250	257	264	271	278
71	136	143	150	157	165	172	179	186	193	200	208	215	222	229	236	243	250	257	265	272	279	286
72	140	147	154	162	169	177	184	191	199	206	213	221	228	235	242	250	258	265	272	279	287	294
73	144	151	159	166	174	182	189	197	204	212	219	227	235	242	250	257	265	272	280	288	295	302
74	148	155	163	171	179	186	194	202	210	218	225	233	241	249	256	264	272	280	287	295	303	311
75	152	160	168	176	184	192	200	208	216	224	232	240	248	256	264	272	279	287	295	303	311	319
76	156	164	172	180	189	197	205	213	221	230	238	246	254	263	271	279	287	295	304	312	320	328

Source: National Heart, Lung, and Blood Institute. (n.d.).

TABLE 21–2 Assigning Nursing Diagnoses to Behaviors Commonly Associated With Eating Disorders

BEHAVIORS	NURSING DIAGNOSES
Refusal to eat; abuse of laxatives, diuretics, and/or diet pills; loss of 15% of expected body weight; pale conjunctiva and mucous membranes; poor muscle tone; amenorrhea; poor skin turgor; electrolyte imbalances; hypothermia; bradycardia; hypotension; cardiac irregularities; edema	**Imbalanced nutrition: Less than body requirements**
Decreased fluid intake; abnormal fluid loss caused by self-induced vomiting; excessive use of laxatives, enemas, or diuretics; electrolyte imbalance; decreased urine output; increased urine concentration; elevated hematocrit; decreased blood pressure; increased pulse rate; dry skin; decreased skin turgor; weakness	**Deficient fluid volume**
Minimizes symptoms; unable to admit impact of disease on life pattern; does not perceive personal relevance of symptoms; does not perceive personal relevance of danger	**Denial**
Compulsive eating; excessive intake in relation to metabolic needs; sedentary lifestyle; weight 20% over ideal for height and frame; BMI of 30 or more; reports the perception that eating is out of control	**Obesity**
Distorted body image; views self as fat, even in the presence of normal body weight or severe emaciation; denies that problem with low body weight exists; difficulty accepting positive reinforcement; self-destructive behavior (self-induced vomiting, abuse of laxatives or diuretics, refusal to eat); preoccupation with appearance and how others perceive it (anorexia nervosa, bulimia nervosa) Verbalization of negative feelings about their looks and the desire to lose weight (obesity) Lack of eye contact; depressed mood (all)	**Disturbed body image/Low self-esteem**
Increased tension; increased helplessness; overexcited; apprehensive; fearful; restlessness; poor eye contact; increased difficulty taking oral nourishment; inability to learn	**Anxiety (moderate to severe)**

- ***Hypotension:*** A pattern of low blood pressure or orthostatic hypotension (20 mm Hg or greater drop in systolic blood pressure with positional changes and pulse rate increase by 20 or more beats per minute)
- ***Suicidal ideation*** (see Chapter 11, "Suicide Prevention," for an in-depth discussion of suicide risk assessment)

In addition to the physical assessment parameters listed previously, when an eating disorder is suspected, a general assessment includes asking patients about their eating patterns and body image, their dieting patterns, whether they feel driven to be thin, exercise patterns, and any use of substances including diet pills, laxatives, or diuretics. Assess where the patient is getting information about weight loss, eating behaviors, and calorie restriction methods; several Web sites are established that teach others how to starve themselves and avoid detection. Although the individual may not be forthcoming with this information, asking the parents about their child's use of Internet resources may reveal the need for close monitoring and restrictions on Internet use. Evidence of calluses on the dorsum of the hands, parotid enlargement, mouth ulcers, dental caries, and edema may also be assessment findings in the patient with purging behaviors.

Individuals with AN should be carefully assessed for infections since studies have found an increased risk of morbidity and mortality from infectious diseases in this population (DeSarbo & DeSarbo, 2020). Factors that can complicate this assessment include delayed fever response in patients with AN. Further similar changes in laboratory values (lower lymphocyte counts; elevated inflammatory cytokines and leukocyte counts; significantly decreased T-cell counts) occur in both AN and infectious disease processes like COVID-19, which could delay diagnosis and treatment (DeSarbo & DeSarbo, 2020).

Tables 21–3 and 21–4 provide plans of care for patients with eating disorders. NANDA-I nursing diagnoses (Herdman et al., 2021) are presented, along with outcome criteria, appropriate nursing interventions, and rationales.

Text continued on page 576

Table 21–3 | CARE PLAN FOR PATIENT WITH EATING DISORDERS: ANOREXIA NERVOSA AND BULIMIA NERVOSA

NURSING DIAGNOSES: IMBALANCED NUTRITION: LESS THAN BODY REQUIREMENTS/DEFICIENT FLUID VOLUME (RISK FOR OR ACTUAL)

RELATED TO: Refusal to eat/drink; self-induced vomiting; abuse of laxatives/diuretics

EVIDENCED BY: Loss of weight; poor muscle tone and skin turgor; lanugo; bradycardia; hypotension; cardiac arrhythmias; pale, dry mucous membranes

OUTCOME CRITERIA	NURSING INTERVENTIONS	RATIONALE
Short-Term Goals ■ Patient will gain x pounds per week (amount to be established by the interdisciplinary team including the patient, nurse, and dietitian). ■ Patient will drink x mL of fluid each hour during waking hours. **Long-Term Goal** ■ By time of discharge from treatment, patient will exhibit no signs or symptoms of malnutrition or dehydration.	1. For the patient who is emaciated and is unable or unwilling to maintain an adequate oral intake, the physician may order a liquid diet to be administered via nasogastric tube. Nursing care of the individual receiving tube feedings should be administered according to established hospital procedures.	1. Without adequate nutrition, a life-threatening situation exists.
	2. For the patient who is able and willing to consume an oral diet, collaborate with the dietitian to determine the appropriate amount of calories and fluids required to provide adequate nutrition and realistic weight gain.	2. Adequate calories are required to allow a weight gain of 2–3 pounds per week.
	3. Monitor laboratory values for phosphate, potassium, calcium, and magnesium while nutrition is being restored.	3. **Refeeding syndrome** (a series of negative intracellular shifts associated with aggressive renourishment in a malnourished patient) poses a risk for hypophosphatemia, hypokalemia, hypocalcemia, and hypomagnesemia. Cardiovascular collapse, arrhythmias, altered mental status, and death can occur in untreated refeeding syndrome. Electrolyte supplementation may be indicated (Toulany & Katzman, 2021).
	4. Explain to the patient that privileges and restrictions will be based on compliance with treatment and direct weight gain. Minimize the focus on food and eating.	4. The real issues have little to do with food or eating patterns. Focus on the control issues that have precipitated these behaviors.
	5. Weigh the patient daily, immediately upon arising and following first voiding. Always use the same scale, if possible. Keep strict record of intake and output. Assess skin turgor and integrity regularly. Assess moistness and color of oral mucous membranes.	5. These assessments are important measurements of nutritional status and provide guidelines for treatment.

Continued

Table 21–3 | CARE PLAN FOR PATIENT WITH EATING DISORDERS: ANOREXIA NERVOSA AND BULIMIA NERVOSA—cont'd

OUTCOME CRITERIA	NURSING INTERVENTIONS	RATIONALE
	6. Stay with the patient during established time for meals (usually 30 min) and for at least 1 hour following meals.	6. Lengthy mealtimes put excessive focus on food and eating and provide the patient with attention and reinforcement. The hour following meals may be used to discard food stashed from tray or to engage in self-induced vomiting.
	7. If weight loss occurs, enforce restrictions.	7. Restrictions and limits must be established and carried out consistently to avoid power struggles, to encourage patient compliance with therapy, and to ensure patient safety.
	8. Ensure that the patient and family understand that if nutritional status deteriorates, tube feedings will be initiated. This is implemented in a matter-of-fact, nonpunitive way.	8. This intervention is carried out for the patient's safety and protection from a life-threatening condition.
	9. Encourage the patient to explore and identify the true feelings and fears that contribute to maladaptive eating behaviors.	9. Emotional issues must be resolved if these maladaptive responses are to be eliminated.

NURSING DIAGNOSIS: DENIAL

RELATED TO: Ineffective coping mechanisms, anxiety, fear of losing control

EVIDENCED BY: Inability to admit the impact of maladaptive eating behaviors on life pattern

OUTCOME CRITERIA	NURSING INTERVENTIONS	RATIONALE
Short-Term Goal ■ Patient will verbalize understanding of the correlation between emotional issues and maladaptive eating behaviors (within time deemed appropriate for individual patient).	1. Establish a trusting relationship with the patient by being honest, accepting, and available, and by keeping all promises. Convey unconditional positive regard.	1. Trust and unconditional acceptance promote dignity and self-worth and provide a strong foundation for a therapeutic relationship.
Long-Term Goal ■ By time of discharge from treatment, patient will demonstrate the ability to discontinue use of maladaptive eating behaviors and to cope with emotional issues in a more adaptive manner.	2. Acknowledge the patient's anger at feelings of loss of control brought about by the established eating regimen associated with the program of behavior modification.	2. Anger is a normal human response and should be expressed in an appropriate manner. Feelings that are not expressed remain unresolved and add an additional component to an already serious situation.

Table 21–3 | CARE PLAN FOR PATIENT WITH EATING DISORDERS: ANOREXIA NERVOSA AND BULIMIA NERVOSA—cont'd

OUTCOME CRITERIA	NURSING INTERVENTIONS	RATIONALE
	3. Avoid arguing or bargaining with the patient who is resistant to treatment. State matter-of-factly which behaviors are unacceptable and how privileges will be restricted for noncompliance.	3. The person who is denying a problem and who also has a weak ego will use manipulation to achieve control. Consistency and firmness by staff will decrease use of these behaviors.
	4. Encourage the patient to verbalize feelings regarding their role within the family and issues related to dependence/independence, the intense need for achievement, and sexuality. Help the patient recognize how maladaptive eating behaviors may be related to these emotional issues. Discuss ways to gain control over these problematic areas of life without resorting to maladaptive eating behaviors.	4. When the patient feels control over major life issues, the need to gain control through maladaptive eating behaviors will diminish.

NURSING DIAGNOSIS: DISTURBED BODY IMAGE/LOW SELF-ESTEEM

RELATED TO: Ineffective coping, history of trauma, guilt or shame

EVIDENCED BY: Distorted body image, difficulty accepting positive reinforcement, depressed mood and self-deprecating thoughts

OUTCOME CRITERIA	NURSING INTERVENTIONS	RATIONALE
Short-Term Goal ■ Patient will verbally acknowledge misperception of body image as "fat" within specified time (depending on severity and chronicity of condition). **Long-Term Goal** ■ By time of discharge from treatment, patient will demonstrate an increase in self-esteem as manifested by verbalizing positive aspects of self and exhibiting less preoccupation with own appearance as a more realistic body image is developed.	1. Help the patient to develop a realistic perception of body image and relationship with food. Compare specific measurement of the patient's body with the patient's perceived calculations.	1. There may be a large discrepancy between actual body size and the patient's perception of their body size. The patient needs to recognize that the misperception of body image is unhealthy and that maintaining control through maladaptive eating behaviors is dangerous—even life threatening.
	2. Promote feelings of control within the environment through participation and independent decision making. Through positive feedback, help the patient learn to accept self as is, including weaknesses as well as strengths.	2. Patients must come to understand that they are capable, autonomous individuals who can perform outside the family unit and who are not expected to be perfect. Sense of control must be achieved in other ways besides dieting and weight loss.

Continued

Table 21–3 | CARE PLAN FOR PATIENT WITH EATING DISORDERS: ANOREXIA NERVOSA AND BULIMIA NERVOSA—cont'd

OUTCOME CRITERIA	NURSING INTERVENTIONS	RATIONALE
	3. Help the patient realize that perfection is unrealistic and explore this need.	3. As the patient begins to feel better about self, identifies positive self-attributes, and develops the ability to accept certain personal inadequacies, the need for unrealistic achievement should diminish.
	4. Assess the patient for history of trauma and other adverse childhood life events.	4. Assessing for trauma history is foundational to pursuing trauma-informed care.

Table 21–4 | CARE PLAN FOR THE PATIENT WITH A BINGE EATING DISORDER: OBESITY

NURSING DIAGNOSIS: IMBALANCED NUTRITION: MORE THAN BODY REQUIREMENTS

RELATED TO: Compulsive overeating

EVIDENCED BY: Weight of more than 20% over expected body weight for age and height; BMI >30

OUTCOME CRITERIA	NURSING INTERVENTIONS	RATIONALE
Short-Term Goal ■ Patient will identify desired weight loss plan. **Long-Term Goal** ■ Patient will demonstrate a change in eating patterns that results in the patient's desired weight loss.	1. Encourage the patient to keep a diary of food intake.	1. A food diary provides the opportunity for the patient to gain a realistic picture of the amount of food ingested and provides a database on which to tailor the dietary program.
	2. Discuss feelings and emotions associated with eating.	2. This helps to identify when the patient is eating to satisfy an emotional need rather than a physiological one.
	3. With input from the patient, formulate an eating plan that includes food from the required food groups with emphasis on low-fat intake. It is helpful to keep the plan as similar to the patient's usual eating pattern as possible.	3. Diet for the patient with BED must focus on establishing healthy eating patterns and eliminating binging behaviors; weight loss is a secondary outcome (O'Melia, 2014). Patients are more likely to stay on the eating plan if they participate in its creation and it deviates as little as possible from usual types of foods.
	4. Identify realistic incremental goals for weekly weight loss.	4. Reasonable weight loss (1–2 pounds per week) results in more lasting effects. Excessive, rapid weight loss may result in fatigue and irritability and ultimately lead to failure in meeting goals for weight loss. Motivation is more easily sustained by meeting "stair-step" goals.

Table 21–4 | CARE PLAN FOR THE PATIENT WITH A BINGE EATING DISORDER: OBESITY—cont'd

OUTCOME CRITERIA	NURSING INTERVENTIONS	RATIONALE
	5. Plan a progressive exercise program tailored to individual goals and choice.	5. Exercise may enhance weight loss by burning calories and reducing appetite, increasing energy, toning muscles, and enhancing sense of well-being and accomplishment. Walking is an excellent choice for overweight individuals.
	6. Discuss the probability of reaching plateaus when weight remains stable for extended periods.	6. The patient should know that this is likely to happen as changes in metabolism occur. Plateaus cause frustration, and patient may need additional support during these times to remain on the weight loss program.
	7. Provide instruction about medications to assist with weight loss if ordered by physician.	7. Appetite-suppressant drugs and others that have weight loss as a side effect may be helpful to someone who is severely overweight. They should be used for this purpose for only a short period while the individual attempts to adjust to the new pattern of eating.

NURSING DIAGNOSIS: DISTURBED BODY IMAGE/LOW SELF-ESTEEM

RELATED TO: Dissatisfaction with appearance, trauma history

EVIDENCED BY: Verbalization of negative feelings about their looks and desire to lose weight

OUTCOME CRITERIA	NURSING INTERVENTIONS	RATIONALE
Short-Term Goal ■ Patient will begin to accept self, based on self-attributes rather than on appearance. **Long-Term Goal** ■ Patient will pursue loss of weight as desired.	1. Assess the patient's feelings and attitudes about being obese.	1. Obesity and compulsive eating behaviors may have deep-rooted psychological implications, such as compensation for lack of love and nurturing or a defense against intimacy.
	2. Assess for history of trauma and adverse childhood life events.	2. Assessing for trauma history is foundational to providing trauma-informed care.
	3. Ensure that the patient has privacy during self-care activities.	3. The obese individual may be sensitive or self-conscious about their body.
	4. Have the patient recall coping patterns related to food in family of origin and explore how these may affect current situation.	4. Parents are role models for their children. Maladaptive eating behaviors may be learned within the family system and are supported through positive reinforcement. Food may be substituted by the parent for affection and love, and eating is associated with a feeling of satisfaction, becoming the primary defense.

Continued

Table 21–4 | CARE PLAN FOR THE PATIENT WITH A BINGE EATING DISORDER: OBESITY—cont'd

OUTCOME CRITERIA	NURSING INTERVENTIONS	RATIONALE
	5. Determine the patient's motivation for weight loss and set goals.	5. The individual may harbor repressed feelings of hostility, which may be expressed inward on the self. Because of a poor self-concept, the person often has difficulty with relationships. When the motivation is to lose weight for someone else, successful weight loss is less likely to occur.
	6. Help the patient identify positive self-attributes. Focus on strengths and past accomplishments unrelated to physical appearance.	6. It is important that self-esteem not be tied solely to size of the body. The patient needs to recognize that obesity need not interfere with positive feelings regarding self-concept and self-worth.
	7. Refer the patient to support or therapy group.	7. Support groups can provide companionship, increase motivation, decrease loneliness and social ostracism, and give practical solutions to common problems. CBT has demonstrated effectiveness in treating eating disorders. Group therapy can be helpful in dealing with underlying psychological concerns.

Concept Care Mapping

The concept map care plan is a diagrammatic teaching and learning strategy that allows visualization of interrelationships between medical diagnoses, nursing diagnoses, assessment data, and treatments. Examples of concept map care plans for patients with eating disorders are presented in Figures 21–1 and 21–2.

Patient and Family Education

The role of patient teacher is important in the psychiatric area, as it is in all areas of nursing. It is essential to include the family in education and treatment unless there are overriding issues against it. A list of topics for patient and family education relevant to eating disorders is presented in Box 21–4.

Evaluation

Evaluation of the patient with an eating disorder requires a reassessment of the behaviors for which the patient sought treatment. Behavioral change will be required on the part of both the patient and family members. The following types of questions may provide assistance in gathering data required for evaluating whether the nursing interventions have been effective in achieving the goals of therapy.

For the Patient With AN or BN

Has the patient:

- Steadily gained 2 to 3 pounds per week to at least 80% of expected body weight for age and size?
- Demonstrated no signs or symptoms of malnutrition and dehydration?
- Consistently consumed adequate calories as determined by the dietitian?
- Attempted to stash food from the tray to discard later?
- Attempted to self-induce vomiting?
- Admitted that a problem exists and that eating behaviors are maladaptive?

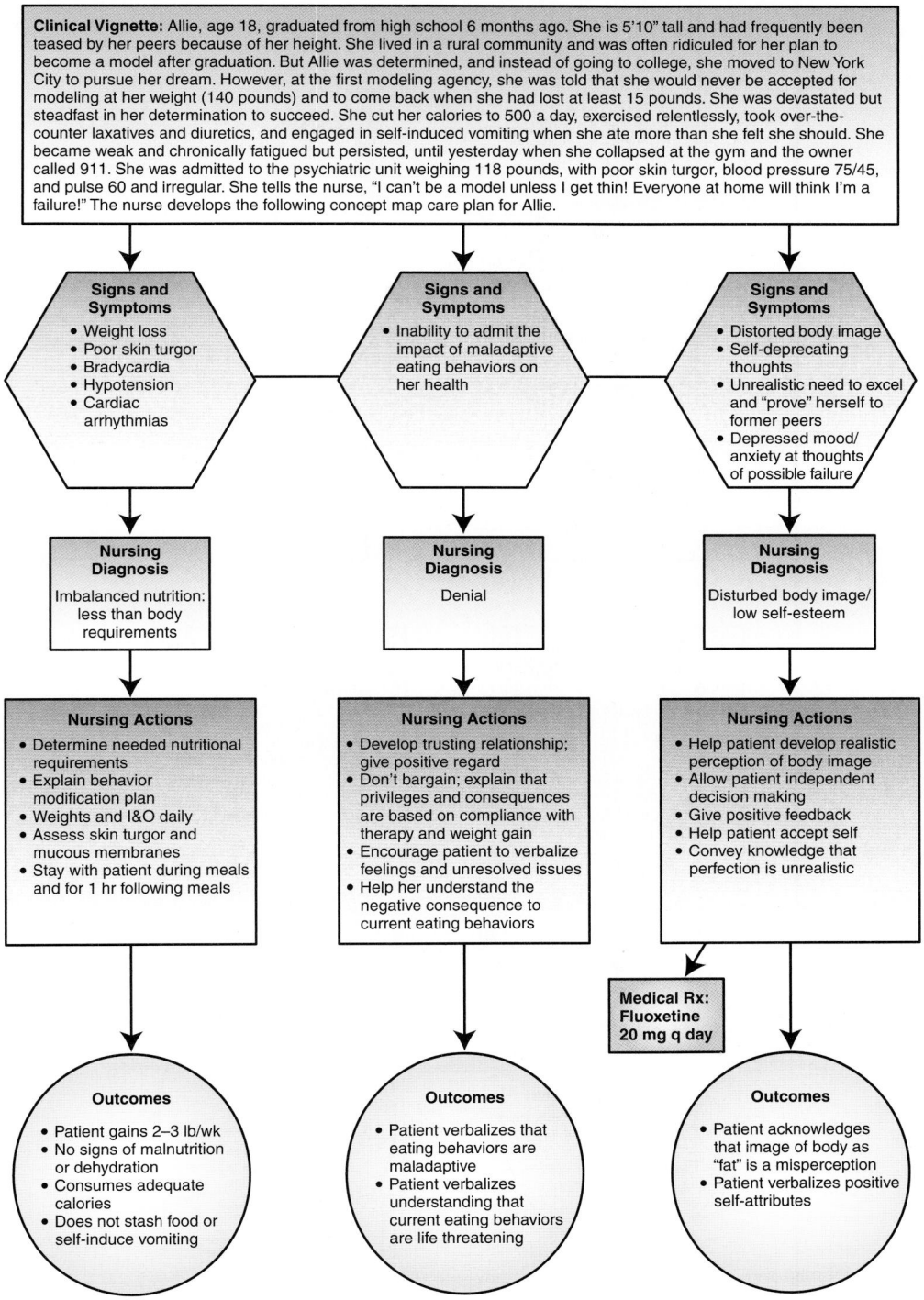

FIGURE 21–1 Concept map care plan for a patient with anorexia nervosa.

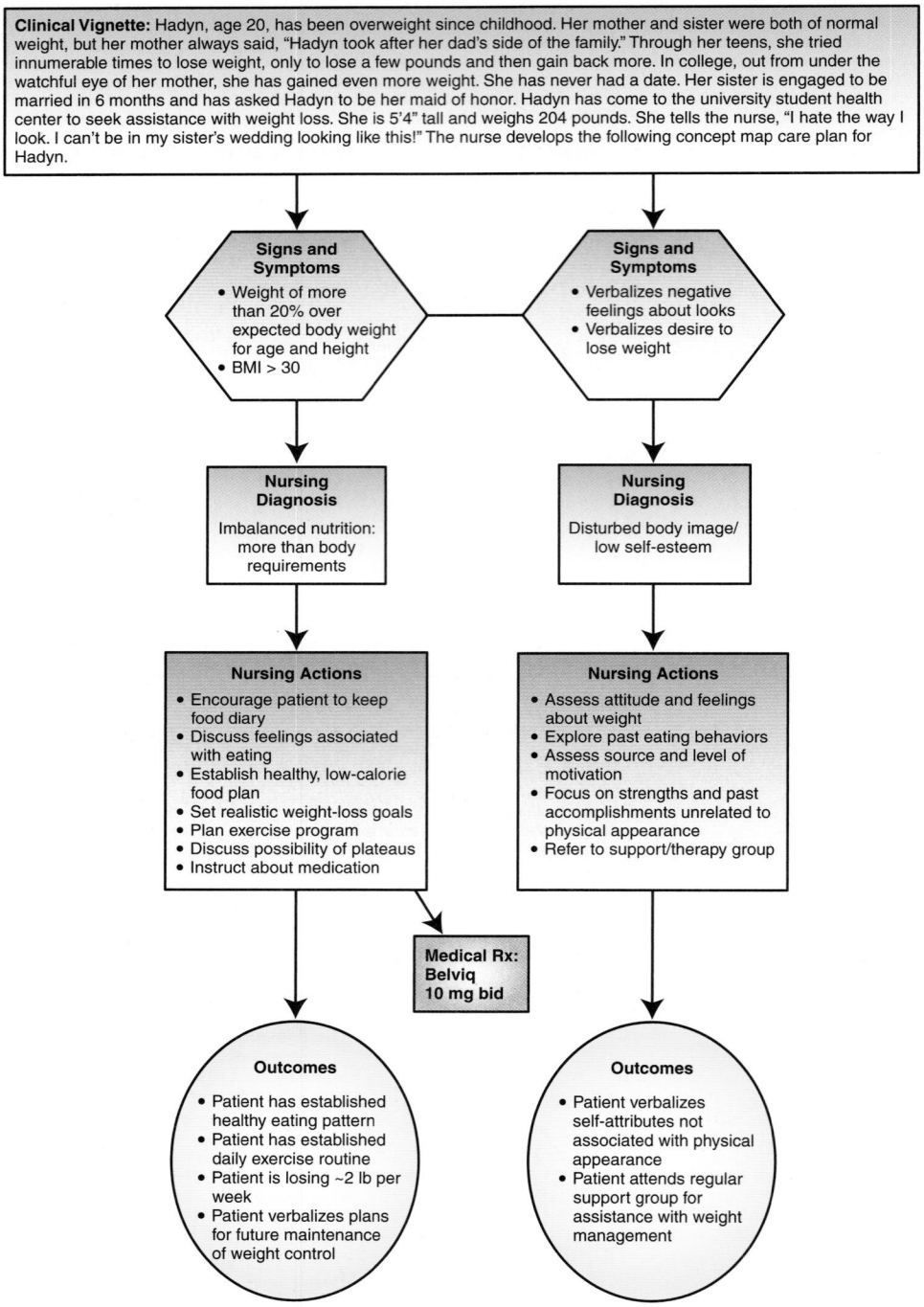

FIGURE 21–2 Concept map care plan for a patient with obesity.

BOX 21–4 Topics for Patient and Family Education Related to Eating Disorders

NATURE OF THE ILLNESS

1. Symptoms of anorexia nervosa
2. Symptoms of bulimia nervosa
3. Symptoms of BED
4. What constitutes obesity
5. Causes of eating disorders
6. Effects of the illness or condition on the body
7. Behaviors that may reinforce unhealthy responses, such as television and social media, peer focus on clothing sizes, eating, and weight. Internet sources have become a means for sharing information among people with anorexia about how the individual can distract parents and health-care providers from recognizing the extent of weight loss. Family members can learn more about some of these behaviors to look out for and may want to monitor their child's use of Internet and social media resources

MANAGEMENT OF THE ILLNESS

1. Principles of nutrition (foods for maintenance of wellness)
2. Ways patient may feel in control of life (aside from eating)
3. Importance of expressing fears and feelings, rather than holding them inside
4. Alternative coping strategies (to maladaptive eating behaviors)
5. For the obese patient:
   a. How to plan a reduced-calorie, nutritious diet
   b. How to read food content labels
   c. How to establish a realistic weight loss plan
   d. How to establish a planned program of physical activity
6. Correct administration of prescribed medications
7. Indication for and side effects of prescribed medications
8. Relaxation techniques
9. Problem-solving skills
10. Discuss the Maudsley approach for treatment of anorexia nervosa as an evidence-based option for family involvement in the recovery program

SUPPORT SERVICES

1. Weight Watchers International (WW)
   www.weightwatchers.com
2. Overeaters Anonymous
   oa.org
3. National Association of Anorexia Nervosa and Associated Disorders (ANAD)
   (888) 375-7767(helpline)
   www.anad.org
4. National Eating Disorders Association (NEDA)
   (800) 931-2237 (helpline)
   www.nationaleatingdisorders.org
5. National Association for Males with Eating Disorders
   (In 2019, this organization merged with NEDA)
   https://www.nationaleatingdisorders.org

- Discontinued maladaptive behaviors to manipulate calorie restriction?
- Discussed feelings related to family roles, sexuality, dependence/independence, and the need for achievement?
- Verbalized understanding of how the use of maladaptive eating behaviors was an effort to achieve a feeling of some control over life events?
- Acknowledged that perception of body image as "fat" is incorrect?

For the Patient With BED and Associated Obesity

Has the patient:

- Shown a steady weight loss since starting the new eating plan?
- Verbalized a relapse prevention plan to avoid triggers and abstain from binging?
- Verbalized positive self-attributes not associated with body size or appearance?

For the Patient With AN, BN, or BED and Associated Obesity

Has the patient:

- Been able to develop a more realistic perception of body image?
- Acknowledged that past self-expectations may have been unrealistic?
- Verbalized improvement in self-acceptance?
- Developed adaptive coping strategies to deal with stress without resorting to maladaptive eating behaviors?

Treatment Modalities

The immediate aim of treatment in eating disorders is to restore and stabilize the patient's nutritional status. Complications of emaciation, dehydration, and electrolyte imbalance can lead to death. Once the physical condition is no longer life threatening, other treatment modalities may be initiated. Electrolytes should be monitored for the first week after initiation of nutritional rehabilitation and refeeding because the greatest risk for refeeding syndrome (a series of negative intracellular shifts associated with aggressive renourishment in a malnourished patient) occurs during this time (Toulany & Katzman, 2021).

Behavior Modification

Efforts to change the maladaptive eating behaviors of clients with AN and BN have become widely accepted treatment approaches. Traditional behavior modification programs are designed to allow the client a degree of autonomy that promotes a sense of control over the treatment process based on the belief that control issues are central dynamics in this disorder. The client has input into the care plan and can clearly see what the treatment choices are. The client has control over eating, over the amount of exercise pursued, and even over whether or not to induce vomiting. Goals of therapy, along with the responsibilities for achieving each goal, are agreed on by the client and staff.

Staff and the client also agree on a system of rewards and privileges that can be earned by the client, who is given ultimate control. The client has a choice of whether or not to abide by the contract—a choice of whether or not to gain weight and whether or not to earn the desired privilege.

This method of treatment gives a great deal of autonomy to the client. It must be understood, however, that these behavior modification techniques are helpful for weight restoration only. Concomitant individual and/or family psychotherapy are required to prevent or reduce further morbidity. Cognitive behavior therapy (CBT) and dialectical behavior therapy (DBT) have demonstrated benefits in clients with AN, BN, and BED (Call et al., 2017; O'Melia, 2014). By confronting irrational thinking patterns and associated feelings, CBT and DBT strive to eliminate the emotional components associated with unhealthy eating patterns.

Family Treatment: The Maudsley Approach

The Maudsley approach is an evidence-based, family-centered program for the treatment of adolescents with AN that modifies the traditional concept of the adolescent being in control of their calorie intake (Le Grange et al., 2016; Lock et al., 2010). This approach actively involves the family in each step of the process. Available evidence supports the use of family-based treatment as the first line of outpatient psychological treatment for adolescents with AN (Toulany & Katzman, 2021). Evidence also supports family-based programs in the treatment of BN (Rienecke et al., 2017). In some of the first controlled studies of this method, 90% of the clients showed improvement compared to 36% of those in individual therapies (Le Grange, 2005).

The treatment program is conducted as an intensive outpatient program, and it involves three phases. Phase I is focused on weight restoration, and in this phase, treatment is designed to encourage parental control of eating, and control is returned to the adolescent after the child demonstrates the readiness and ability to establish control in healthier ways. Parents often need a lot of support during this phase because they typically encounter frequent power struggles with their child. When the child accepts parental demands for increased food intake and demonstrates steady weight gain, and when there is a change in the mood of the family (i.e., relief at having taken charge of the eating disorder; both the adolescent and the parents identify reduced anxiety), phase II is ready to begin (Le Grange & Lock, n.d.). In this phase, control of maintaining weight gain is returned to the adolescent. Once the teen demonstrates the ability to maintain above 95% of ideal weight, the shift to phase III focuses on assisting the adolescent to develop a healthy self-identity. This phase includes incorporating CBT and DBT skills, which have also demonstrated effectiveness in treating this condition.

Individual Therapy

Although individual psychotherapy is not the therapy of choice for eating disorders, it may be an adjunct to a comprehensive, multifaceted treatment approach when underlying comorbid psychological problems are contributing to the maladaptive behaviors. In supportive psychotherapy, the therapist encourages the client to explore unresolved conflicts and to recognize the maladaptive eating behaviors as defense mechanisms used to ease the emotional pain. The goals are to resolve the personal issues and establish more adaptive coping strategies for dealing with stressful situations.

Psychopharmacology

Medication research has not yet identified a medication that results in definitive improvement in the core symptoms of AN (Boland & Verduin, 2022). As mentioned previously, SSRIs (particularly fluoxetine) have demonstrated effectiveness in treating bulimia but not anorexia (WebMD, 2020). SSRIs may be beneficial in the treatment of comorbid depression, but they also carry a black box warning about risk of increasing suicide ideation in adolescents. The anticholinergic side effects of tricyclic antidepressants, including orthostatic hypotension, may be problematic for patients who are already at risk for these symptoms. It is important to recognize that depression and other mood and cognitive symptoms can be a sign of malnutrition and starvation. When nutrition is restored, those symptoms often improve.

Antidepressants, and particularly fluoxetine, have been found to be useful in the treatment of BN (Call et al., 2017) and appear to have benefits for patients with and without depressive symptoms. It is possible that fluoxetine, an SSRI, may decrease the craving for carbohydrates, thereby decreasing the incidence of binge eating, which is often associated with consumption of large amounts of carbohydrates. A dosage of 60 mg to 80 mg/day (triple the usual antidepressant dosage) may be required. Other SSRIs, tricyclic antidepressants (particularly amitriptyline and desipramine), trazodone, and monoamine oxidase inhibitors may also be helpful (Boland & Verduin, 2022).

High-dose SSRIs have demonstrated some effectiveness in promoting weight loss for those with BED, but the weight loss was temporary (Boland & Verduin, 2022). Remember, too, that weight gain is a secondary symptom of BED. An effective medication needs to also manage the symptom of binging. Two medications, topiramate and lisdexamfetamine (a dopamine-norepinephrine reuptake inhibitor, originally used in the treatment of attention deficit-hyperactivity disorder) have demonstrated benefits in reducing both incidents of binge eating and weight gain (Balodis et al., 2015). Currently, lisdexamfetamine (Vyvanse) has been approved by the U.S. Food and Drug Administration (FDA) specifically for short-term treatment of BED. Most studies reveal that medication in combination with CBT is more beneficial than medication alone (Boland & Verduin, 2022).

CASE STUDY AND SAMPLE CARE PLAN

NURSING HISTORY AND ASSESSMENT

When Katie fainted in history class, she was taken to the university health center by her roommate, Ashley. Ashley told the nurse that Katie had been taking a lot of over-the-counter laxatives and diuretics. She also said that Katie often self-induced vomiting when she felt that she had eaten too much. After an initial physical assessment, the nurse in the university health center referred Katie to the mental health clinic.

At the mental health clinic, Katie weighed 110 pounds and measured 5 feet 6 inches tall. She admitted to the psychiatric nurse that she tried to keep her weight down by dieting but sometimes she got so hungry that she would overeat, and then she felt the need to self-induce vomiting to get rid of the calories. "I really don't like doing it, but lots of the girls do. In fact, that is where I got the idea. I always thought I was too fat in high school, but the competition wasn't so great there. Here all the girls are so pretty . . . and so thin! It's the only way I can keep my weight down!"

Katie also admitted that she hoards food in her dorm room and that she eats when she is feeling particularly anxious and depressed (often during the night). She admitted to having eaten several bags of potato chips and whole packages of cookies in a single sitting. She sometimes drives to the local hamburger stand in the middle of the night, orders several hamburgers, fries, and milkshakes, and consumes them as she sits in her car alone. She stated that she feels so much better while she is eating these foods but then feels panicky after they have been consumed. That is when she self-induces vomiting. "Then I feel more depressed, and the only thing that helps is eating! I feel so out of control!"

NURSING DIAGNOSES AND OUTCOME IDENTIFICATION

From the assessment data, the nurse develops the following nursing diagnosis for Katie:

1. **Ineffective coping** related to feelings of helplessness, low self-esteem, and lack of control in life situation
   a. **Short-Term Goal:** Katie will identify and discuss fears and anxieties with the nurse.
   b. **Long-Term Goal:** Katie will identify adaptive coping strategies that can be realistically incorporated into her lifestyle, thereby eliminating binging and purging in response to anxiety.

Continued

CASE STUDY AND SAMPLE CARE PLAN—cont'd

PLANNING AND IMPLEMENTATION

INEFFECTIVE COPING

The following nursing interventions have been identified for Katie:

1. Establish a trusting relationship with Katie. Be honest and accepting. Show unconditional positive regard.
2. Help Katie identify the situations that produce anxiety and discuss how she coped with these situations before she began binging and purging.
3. Help Katie identify the emotions that precipitate binging (e.g., fear, boredom, anger, loneliness).
4. Once these high-risk situations have been identified, help her identify alternative behaviors, such as exercise, a hobby, or a warm bath.
5. Encourage Katie to express feelings that have been suppressed because they were considered unacceptable. Help her identify healthier ways to express those feelings.
6. Use role-play with Katie to deal with feelings and experiment with new behaviors.
7. Explore the dynamics of Katie's family and encourage family involvement for support with Katie's consent.
8. Teach the concepts of good nutrition and the importance of healthy eating patterns in overall wellness.
9. Consult with the physician about a prescription for fluoxetine for Katie.
10. Help Katie find a support group for individuals with eating disorders. Encourage regular attendance in this group.

EVALUATION

The outcome criteria for Katie have been met. She discussed with the nurse the feelings that triggered binging episodes and the situations that precipitated those feelings. She has joined a support group of individuals with eating disorders and now has a "buddy" whom she may call (even in the middle of the night) when she is feeling like binging. She has started riding her bicycle regularly and goes to the fitness center when she is feeling especially anxious. Katie still sees the mental health nurse weekly and continues to discuss her fears and anxieties. The urges to binge at stressful times have not disappeared completely. However, they have decreased in frequency, and Katie is now able to choose more adaptive strategies for dealing with stress.

Summary and Key Points

- The incidence of eating disorders has continued to increase since the middle of the 20th century.
- Individuals with anorexia nervosa (AN), a disorder that is characterized by a morbid fear of obesity and a gross distortion of body image, literally can starve themselves to death.
- Individuals with AN believe they are fat even when emaciated. The disorder is commonly accompanied by depression and anxiety.
- Bulimia nervosa (BN) is an eating disorder characterized by the consumption of large amounts of food, usually in a short period and often in secret.
- With BN, tension is relieved and pleasure is felt during the time of the binge, but feelings of guilt and depression follow soon after the binge.
- Individuals with BN purge themselves of the excessive intake with self-induced vomiting or the misuse of laxatives, diuretics, or enemas. They also at risk for mood and anxiety disorders.
- Binge eating disorder (BED) is characterized by the consumption of huge amounts of food by an individual who feels a lack of control over the eating behavior. BED differs from BN in that the individual does not engage in behaviors to rid the body of the excess calories.
- Compulsive eating can result in obesity, which is defined by the National Institutes of Health as a BMI of 30 or more.
- Obesity predisposes the individual to many health concerns, and at the morbid level (a BMI of 40), weight alone can contribute to increases in morbidity and mortality.
- Predisposing factors to eating disorders include genetics, physiological factors, family dynamics, and environmental and lifestyle factors.
- Treatment modalities for eating disorders may include behavior modification, individual psychotherapy, cognitive behavior therapy (CBT), dialectical behavior therapy (DBT), family treatment (such as the Maudsley approach), and psychopharmacology to treat symptoms of mood or anxiety disorders.

Review Questions

Select the answer that is most appropriate for each of the following questions:

1. Some obese individuals take amphetamines to suppress appetite and help them lose weight. Which is an adverse effect associated with use of amphetamines that makes this practice undesirable?
   a. Bradycardia
   b. Amenorrhea
   c. Tolerance
   d. Convulsions
2. The Maudsley approach to treatment of adolescents with anorexia nervosa advances which fundamental concept?
   a. Family should be actively involved in each phase of treatment.
   b. Parents should be prohibited from involvement in helping their child eat more because there are often control issues.
   c. Adolescents need to work on developing healthy self-identities before they can begin to gain weight.
   d. Individual psychotherapy is the most effective treatment for adolescents with anorexia nervosa.
3. A client has sought help for their concern that they are binge eating, and the client believes it has "gotten out of control." The client asks the nurse what can be done to help them. Which is the most accurate response?
   a. "There are no recognized treatments for binge eating disorder."
   b. "Some medications and psychological treatments that have demonstrated effectiveness in reducing binge eating behaviors."
   c. "The primary problem is obesity. I can help you set up a calorie-restricted diet."
   d. "Medications can help with weight loss, but there are no medications effective for reducing binge eating."
4. Which physical manifestations would you expect to assess in a client with anorexia nervosa?
   a. Tachycardia, hypertension, hyperthermia
   b. Bradycardia, hypertension, hyperthermia
   c. Bradycardia, hypotension, hypothermia
   d. Tachycardia, hypotension, hypothermia
5. Which medication has been used with some success in clients with bulimia nervosa?
   a. Lorcaserin (Belviq)
   b. Diazepam (Valium)
   c. Fluoxetine (Prozac)
   d. Carbamazepine (Tegretol)
6. A client is hospitalized on the psychiatric unit with a history and current diagnosis of bulimia nervosa. Which symptoms would be congruent with this client's diagnosis?
   a. Binging, purging, obesity, hyperkalemia
   b. Binging, purging, normal weight, hypokalemia
   c. Binging, laxative abuse, amenorrhea, severe weight loss
   d. Binging, purging, severe weight loss, hyperkalemia

Continued

Clinical Judgment Questions

7. A 14-year-old client has just been admitted to the psychiatric unit for anorexia nervosa. They are emaciated and refuses to eat. What is the primary nursing diagnosis for this client?
   a. Complicated grieving
   b. Imbalanced nutrition: Less than body requirements
   c. Interrupted family processes
   d. Anxiety (severe)
8. The nurse is caring for a client who has been hospitalized with anorexia nervosa and is severely malnourished. The client continues to refuse to eat. What is the most appropriate response by the nurse?
   a. "You know that if you don't eat, you will die."
   b. "If you continue to refuse to take food orally, you will be fed through a nasogastric tube."
   c. "You might as well leave if you are not going to follow your therapy regimen."
   d. "You don't have to eat if you don't want to. It is your choice."
9. A hospitalized client with bulimia nervosa has stopped vomiting in the hospital and tells the nurse they are afraid they're going to gain weight. Which is the most appropriate response by the nurse?
   a. "Don't worry. The dietitian will ensure you don't get too many calories in your diet."
   b. "Don't worry about your weight. We are going to work on other problems while you are in the hospital."
   c. "I understand that you are concerned about your weight, and we will talk about the importance of good nutrition; but for now, I want you to tell me about your recent invitation to join the National Honor Society. That's quite an accomplishment."
   d. "You are not fat, and the staff will ensure that you do not gain weight while you are in the hospital, because we know that is important to you."
10. A client presents in the emergency department with complaints of suicidal ideation. The following data is collected by the nurse. Which assessment findings suggest that bulimia nervosa might be a health problem? (Select all that apply.)
   a. Parotid glands appear enlarged.
   b. Teeth have a "moth eaten" pattern of tooth decay.
   c. Client reports taking laxatives daily.
   d. Client's weight is within the expected range.

IMPLICATIONS FOR EVIDENCE-BASED PRACTICE

Bakalar, J. L., Barmine, M., Druskin, L., Olsen, C. H., Quinlan, J., Sbrocco, T., & Tanofsky-Kraff, M. (2018). Childhood adverse life events, disordered eating, and body mass index in US military service members. *International Journal of Eating Disorders, 51*(11). https://doi.org/10.1002/eat.22851

DESCRIPTION OF THE STUDY: The authors, noting a high prevalence of overweight and obesity and a high prevalence of childhood adverse life events among U.S. military personnel, conducted an online survey (N = 179) of active-duty military personnel to explore the associations between these two phenomena.

RESULTS OF THE STUDY: Multiple indices of childhood adverse life events (both traumatic and subjective impact) were positively associated with a higher body mass index and were mediated by disordered eating.

IMPLICATIONS FOR NURSING PRACTICE: This study underscores the importance of trauma assessment and trauma-informed care for military personnel. Additionally, as the authors note, because there have been consistent links demonstrated between childhood adverse life events and eating disorders in the general population, assessment of trauma history should also be conducted for any client presenting with an eating disorder.

TEST YOUR CLINICAL REASONING AND CLINICAL JUDGMENT SKILLS

Janice, a high school sophomore, wanted desperately to become a cheerleader. She practiced endlessly before tryouts, but she was not selected. A week later, her boyfriend, Roy, broke up with her to date another girl. Janice, who was 5 feet 3 inches tall and weighed 110 pounds, decided it was because she was too fat. She began to exercise at every possible moment. She skipped meals and tried to keep her daily consumption to no more than 300 calories. She lost a great deal of weight but became very weak. She felt cold all the time and wore sweaters in the warm weather. Janice collapsed during her physical education class at school and was rushed to the emergency department. On admission, she weighed 90 pounds. She was emaciated and anemic. The physician admitted her with a diagnosis of Anorexia Nervosa.

Answer the following questions about Janice:

1. What will be the *primary* consideration in Janice's care?
2. How will treatment be directed toward helping her gain weight?
3. How will the nurse know if Janice is using self-induced vomiting to rid herself of food consumed at meals?

Communication Exercises

1. Helena was admitted to the psychiatric unit with a diagnosis of severe anorexia nervosa. After completing a meal, she asks the nurse to be excused so she can use the restroom.
   How would the nurse respond to Helena's request?
2. John has been seeking counseling for a binge eating disorder. When the nurse is weighing him, John states, "I hate myself. I should never have let myself get like this. I'm completely out of control."
   What would be the most empathic response by the nurse?

MOVIE CONNECTIONS

The Best Little Girl in the World (AN) ▪ *Kate's Secret* (BN) ▪ *For the Love of Nancy* (AN) ▪ *Super Size Me* (Obesity). *To the Bone* (AN) ▪ *Sharing the Secret* (BN) ▪ *Life Is Sweet* (BN)

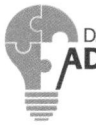

Go to **Davis Advantage** to complete your learning: strengthen understanding, apply your knowledge, and prepare for the Next Gen NCLEX®.

References

American Academy for Eating Disorders. (2009). *Position statement: The role of the family in eating disorders.* https://www.aedweb.org/advocate/press-releases/role-of-the-family

American Psychiatric Association. (2022). *Diagnostic and statistical manual of mental disorders* (5th ed., text rev.).

Bakalar, J. L., Barmine, M., Druskin, L., Olsen, C. H., Quinlan, J., Sbrocco, T., & Tanofsky-Kraff, M. (2018). Childhood adverse life events, disordered eating, and body mass index in US military service members. *International Journal of Eating Disorders, 51*(11). https://doi.org/10.1002/eat.22851

Balodis, I. M., Grilo, C. M., & Potenza, M. N. (2015). Neurobiological underpinnings of obesity and addiction: A focus on binge eating disorder and implications for treatment. *Psychiatric Times.* http://www.psychiatrictimes.com/cme/neurobiological-underpinnings-obesity-and-addiction-focus-binge-eating-disorder-and-implications/page/0/2#sthash.D9vZ5Ijs.dpuf

Boland, R., & Verduin, M. L. (2022). *Kaplan & Sadock's synopsis of psychiatry* (P. Ruiz, Ed.). (12th ed.). Wolters Kluwer.

Call, C. C., Attia, E., & Walsh, B. T. (2017). Feeding and eating disorders. In B. J. Sadock, V. A. Sadock, & P. Ruiz (Eds.), *Comprehensive textbook of psychiatry* (10th ed., pp. 2065–2082). Wolters Kluwer.

Centers for Disease Control and Prevention. (2021). *Overweight and obesity.* http://www.cdc.gov/obesity/adult/index.html

DeSarbo, J. R., & DeSarbo, L. (2020). Anorexia nervosa and COVID-19. *Current Psychiatry, 19*(8), 23–27.

Eddy, K. T., Dorer, D. J., Franko, D. L., Tahilani, K., & Thompson-Brenner, H. (2008). Diagnostic crossover in anorexia nervosa and bulimia nervosa: Implications for DSM-V. *American Journal of Psychiatry.* https://doi.org/10.1176/appi.ajp.2007.07060951

Hasan, T. F., & Hasan, H. (2011). Anorexia nervosa: A unified neurological perspective. *International Journal of Medical Sciences, 8*(8), 679–703. https://doi.org/10.7150/ijms.8.679

Herdman, T. H., Kamitsuru, S., & Lopes, C. T. (Eds.). (2021). *NANDA-I Inc. nursing diagnoses: Definitions and classification, 2021–2023.* Thieme.

Le Grange, D. (2005). The Maudsley family-based treatment for adolescent anorexia nervosa. *World Psychiatry, 4*(3), 142–146.

Le Grange, D., & Lock, J. (n.d.). *Family-based treatment of adolescent anorexia nervosa: The Maudsley approach.* http://www.maudsleyparents.org/whatismaudsley.html

Le Grange, D., Hughes, E. K., Court, A., Yeo, M., Crosby, R. D., & Sawyer, S.M. (2016). Randomized clinical trial of parent-focused treatment and family-based treatment for adolescent anorexia nervosa. *Journal of the American Academy of Child and Adolescent Psychiatry, 55*(8), 683–692. https://doi.org/10.1016/j.jaac.2016.05.007

Lock, J., Le Grange, D., Agras, W. S., Moye, A., Bryson, S. W., & Jo, B. (2010). Randomized clinical trial comparing family-based treatment with adolescent-focused individual therapy for adolescents with anorexia nervosa. *Archives of General Psychiatry, 67*(10), 1025–1032. https://doi.org/10.1001/archgenpsychiatry.2010.128

National Heart, Lung, and Blood Institute. (1998). *Clinical guidelines on the identification, evaluation, and treatment of overweight and obesity in adults: Body mass index tables.* http://www.nhlbi.nih.gov/guidelines/obesity/bmi_tbl.htm

National Institute of Mental Health. (2017). *Eating disorders.* https://www.nimh.nih.gov/health/statistics/eating-disorders#part_155059

O'Melia, A. M. (2014). Binge eating disorder. *Current Psychiatry, 13*(4). http://www.currentpsychiatry.com/specialty-focus/eating-disorders/article/binge-eating-disorder/1e566fd65698cb7b06e0d2b355284392.html

Rienecke, R. D. (2017). Family-based treatment of eating disorders in adolescents: Current insights. *Adolescent Health, Medicine and Therapeutics, 8,* 69–79. https://doi.org/10.2147/AHMT.S115775

Riva, G. (2016). Neurobiology of anorexia nervosa: Serotonin dysfunctions link self-starvation with body image disturbances through an impaired body memory. *Frontiers in Human Neuroscience, 24.* https://doi.org/10.3389/fnhum.2016.00600

Strumila, R., Nobile, B., Maimoun, L., Jaussent, I., Seneque, M., Thiebaut, S., Iceta, S., Dupuis-Maurin, K., Lefebvre, P., Courtet, P., Renard, E., & Guillaume, S. (2020). The implications of previous history of anorexia nervosa in patients with current bulimia nervosa: Alterations in daily functioning, decision-making, and bone status. *European Eating Disorders Review, 28*(1), 34–45.

Toulany, A., & Katzman, D. K. (2021). Restrictive anorexia nervosa. *Psychiatric Advisor.* https://www.psychiatryadvisor.com/home/decision-support-in-medicine/pediatrics/restrictive-anorexia-nervosa/

Uniacke, B., & Broft, A. (2016). The interplay of mood disorders and eating disorders. *Psychiatric Times, 33*(5). http://www.psychiatrictimes.com/special-reports/interplay-mood-disorders-and-eating-disorders

WebMD. (2020). *When do doctors prescribe antidepressants for anorexia?* https://www.webmd.com/mental-health/eating-disorders/anorexia-nervosa/antidepressants-eating-disorders

WebMD. (2021). *Symptoms of binge eating disorder.* https://www.webmd.com/mental-health/eating-disorders/binge-eating-disorder/binge-eating-symptoms#2

Woolridge, T., & Lemberg, R. (2016). Macho, bravado, and eating disorders in men: Special issues in diagnosis and treatment. *Psychiatric Times, 33*(5). http://www.psychiatrictimes.com/special-reports/macho-bravado-and-eating-disorders-men-special-issues-diagnosis-and-treatment

22 Personality Disorders

CHAPTER OUTLINE

Objectives
Introduction
Historical Perspectives
Types of Personality Disorders
Application of the Nursing Process: Borderline Personality Disorder
Application of the Nursing Process: Antisocial Personality Disorder
Treatment Modalities
Summary and Key Points
Review Questions
Clinical Judgment Questions
Implications for Evidence-Based Practice
Test Your Clinical Reasoning and Clinical Judgment Skills
Communication Exercises
Movie Connections

CORE CONCEPTS

Maladaptive Behavior
Stress and Coping
Professionalism: Nursing process in the care of patients with personality disorders
Safety
Clinical Judgment

KEY TERMS

antisocial personality disorder
avoidant personality disorder
borderline personality disorder (BPD)
dependent personality disorder
histrionic personality disorder
narcissistic personality disorder
object constancy
obsessive-compulsive personality disorder
paranoid personality disorder
personality
schizoid personality disorder
schizotypal personality disorder
splitting

OBJECTIVES

After reading this chapter, the student will be able to:

1. Define *personality*.
2. Compare stages of personality development according to Sullivan, Erikson, and Mahler.
3. Identify various types of personality disorders.
4. Discuss history and epidemiology related to various personality disorders.
5. Describe symptomatology associated with borderline personality disorder (BPD) and antisocial personality disorder and use these data in patient assessment.
6. Identify predisposing factors for BPD and antisocial personality disorder.
7. Formulate nursing diagnoses and goals of care for patients with BPD and antisocial personality disorder.
8. Describe appropriate nursing interventions for behaviors associated with BPD and antisocial personality disorder.
9. Evaluate nursing care of patients with BPD and antisocial personality disorder.
10. Discuss various modalities relevant to treatment of personality disorders.

Introduction

CORE CONCEPT

Personality

Personality is the totality of emotional and behavioral characteristics that are particular to a specific person and that remain somewhat stable and predictable over time.

The word *personality* is derived from the Greek term *persona.* It was originally used to describe the theatrical mask worn by some dramatic actors at the time. Over the years, it lost its connotation of pretense and illusion and came to represent the person behind the mask—the "real" person.

Personality *traits* may be defined as characteristics with which an individual is born or that develop early in life. They influence the way the individual perceives and relates to the environment and are quite stable over time. Personality *disorders* occur when these traits deviate markedly from the expectations of the individual's culture, become pervasive and inflexible, contribute to maladaptive patterns of behavior or impairment in functioning, and lead to distress (American Psychiatric Association [APA], 2022). The most common symptoms occurring in personality disorders are impairment in interpersonal relationship functions (41%) and dysfunctions in cognition (30%), affect (18%), and impulse control (6%) (Bornstein et al., 2014). In specific types of personality disorders, such as paranoid and schizotypal personality disorders, cognitive symptoms may appear more prominently; in other types, such as borderline personality and antisocial personality disorders, interpersonal dysfunctions may predominate (Bornstein et al., 2014). Virtually all individuals exhibit some behaviors associated with the various personality disorders from time to time. As previously stated, it is only when significant functional impairment occurs in response to these personality characteristics that the individual is thought to have a personality disorder.

Personality development occurs in response to a number of biological and psychological influences. These variables include (but are not limited to) heredity, temperament, experiential learning, and social interaction. Recent research on the psychobiology of human personality conducted through person-centered, functional brain imaging has broadened our understanding of healthy personality development and the factors that contribute to individual differences (Cloninger & Svrakic, 2017). For example, functional brain imaging and person-centered analysis have confirmed a model for human temperaments and character traits that is consistent among people from various cultures (Cloninger & Svrakic, 2017). These advances provide a firmer foundation for treatment of personality disorders based on a thorough assessment that includes laboratory findings, mental status, and clinical history.

A number of theorists have attempted to provide information about the psychological aspects of personality development. Most suggest that it occurs in an orderly, stepwise fashion. These stages overlap, however, as maturation occurs at different rates in different individuals. The theories of Sullivan (1953), Erikson (1963), and Mahler (Mahler et al., 1975) are presented at length in Chapter 29, "Concepts of Personality Development." The stages of personality development according to these three theorists are compared in Table 22–1. The nurse should understand "normal" personality development before learning about what is considered maladaptive.

Individuals with a primary diagnosis of a personality disorder are not often treated in acute care settings. However, many clients with other psychiatric and medical diagnoses manifest symptoms of personality disorders. Nurses are likely to encounter clients with these personality characteristics in all healthcare settings.

Nurses working in psychiatric settings are likely to encounter clients with borderline and antisocial personality characteristics. The behavior of clients with borderline personality disorder (BPD) is unstable, and hospitalization is often required as a result of attempts at self-injury, persistent suicide risk, substance abuse and dependence, or a combination of these behaviors. The client with antisocial personality disorder may enter psychiatric care as a result of judicially ordered evaluation. Psychiatric intervention may be an alternative to imprisonment for antisocial behavior if the intervention is deemed potentially helpful.

Historical and epidemiological aspects of personality disorders are discussed in this chapter. Predisposing factors that have been implicated in the etiology of personality disorders are presented, and symptomatology is explained to provide background knowledge for assessing clients with personality disorders. Nursing care of patients with BPD or antisocial personality disorder is presented in the context of the nursing process. Various medical treatment modalities for personality disorders are also explored.

TABLE 22–1 Comparison of Personality Development—Sullivan, Erikson, and Mahler

MAJOR DEVELOPMENTAL TASKS AND DESIGNATED AGES

SULLIVAN	ERIKSON	MAHLER
Birth to 18 months: Relief from anxiety through oral gratification of needs.	Birth to 18 months: To develop a basic trust in the mothering figure and be able to generalize it to others.	Birth to 1 month: Fulfillment of basic needs for survival and comfort.
18 months to 6 years: Learning to experience a delay in personal gratification without undue anxiety.	18 months to 3 years: To gain some self-control and independence within the environment.	1 to 5 months: Developing awareness of external source of need fulfillment.
6 to 9 years: Learning to form satisfactory peer relationships.	3 to 6 years: To develop a sense of purpose and the ability to initiate and direct own activities.	5 to 10 months: Commencement of a primary recognition of separateness from the mothering figure.
9 to 12 years: Learning to form satisfactory relationships with persons of the same gender; the initiation of feelings of affection for another person.	6 to 12 years: To achieve a sense of self-confidence by learning, competing, performing successfully, and receiving recognition from significant others, peers, and acquaintances.	10 to 16 months: Increased independence through locomotor functioning; increased sense of separateness of self.
12 to 14 years: Learning to form satisfactory relationships with persons of the opposite gender; developing a sense of identity.	12 to 20 years: To integrate the tasks mastered in the previous stages into a secure sense of self.	16 to 24 months: Acute awareness of separateness of self; learning to seek "emotional refueling" from mothering figure to maintain feeling of security.
14 to 21 years: Establishing self-identity; experiences satisfying relationships; working to develop a lasting, intimate opposite-gender relationship.	20 to 30 years: To form an intense, lasting relationship or a commitment to another person, a cause, an institution, or a creative effort.	24 to 36 months: Sense of separateness established; on the way to object constancy: able to internalize a sustained image of loved object/person when it is out of sight; resolution of separation anxiety.
	30 to 65 years: To achieve the life goals established for oneself, while also considering the welfare of future generations.	
	65 years to death: To review one's life and derive meaning from both positive and negative events, while achieving a positive sense of self-worth. In late, older adulthood (80 years and beyond) an additional stage of development, *transcendence*, refers to a period in which one develops a broader sense of one's meaning and spirituality that transcends oneself.	

Historical Perspectives

In the 4th century BC, Hippocrates concluded that all disease stemmed from an excess of or imbalance among four bodily humors: yellow bile, black bile, blood, and phlegm. Hippocrates identified four fundamental personality styles that he concluded stemmed from excesses in the four humors: the irritable and hostile choleric (yellow bile); the pessimistic melancholic (black bile); the overly optimistic and extraverted sanguine (blood); and the apathetic phlegmatic (phlegm).

In 1801 the medical profession first recognized that personality disorders, apart from psychosis, were cause for special concern with the realization that an individual can behave irrationally even when the powers of intellect are intact. Nineteenth-century psychiatrists embraced the term *moral insanity*, the concept of which defines what we know today as personality disorders.

Historically, individuals with personality disorders have been labeled as "bad" or "immoral" and as deviants in the range of normal personality dimensions. The events and sequences that result in pathology of the personality are complicated and difficult to unravel. Continued study is needed to facilitate understanding of this complex behavioral phenomenon.

A major difficulty for psychiatrists has been the establishment of a classification of personality disorders. Ten specific types of personality disorders are identified in the *Diagnostic and Statistical Manual of Mental Disorders, Fifth Edition, Text Revision* (*DSM-5-TR*; APA, 2022). Looking toward the future, the APA has proposed a different and complex diagnostic system to identify impairments in personality functioning specifically related to the dimensions of *self* and *interpersonal relations* and to personality *trait domains* and *facets*. This diagnostic system is very specific and addresses symptoms that may differ not only among personality disorders but also among individuals with the same personality disorder. This trait-specific diagnostic methodology is described in the *DSM-5-TR* as an alternative approach to diagnosis of personality disorder and is recommended for further study.

The current diagnostic system classifies the personality disorders into three clusters according to description of personality traits:

1. ***Cluster A:*** Behaviors described as odd or eccentric
   a. Paranoid personality disorder
   b. Schizoid personality disorder
   c. Schizotypal personality disorder
2. ***Cluster B:*** Behaviors described as dramatic, emotional, or erratic
   a. Antisocial personality disorder
   b. Borderline personality disorder
   c. Histrionic personality disorder
   d. Narcissistic personality disorder
3. ***Cluster C:*** Behaviors described as anxious or fearful
   a. Avoidant personality disorder
   b. Dependent personality disorder
   c. Obsessive-compulsive personality disorder

Types of Personality Disorders

Paranoid Personality Disorder

Definition and Epidemiology

Paranoid personality disorder is defined as a pattern of pervasive mistrust and suspicion of others and misinterpretation of others' motives as malevolent (APA, 2022). This pattern begins by early adulthood and remains present in a variety of contexts. Prevalence has been estimated at 1% to 4% of the general population. Symptoms are generally mild but interfere with occupational and social functioning (Cloninger & Svrakic, 2017). The disorder is more commonly diagnosed in men than in women.

Clinical Picture

Individuals with paranoid personality disorder are constantly on guard, hypervigilant, and ready for any real or imagined threat. They appear tense and irritable. They have developed a hard exterior and become insensitive to the feelings of others. They avoid interactions with other people lest they are forced to relinquish some of their own power. They most often feel that other people will take advantage of them, and perceived slights, injuries, or insults become long-held grudges.

They are overly sensitive and tend to misinterpret even minute cues within the environment, magnifying and distorting them into thoughts of trickery and deception. Because they trust no one, they are constantly "testing" the honesty of others. Their intimidating manner provokes exasperation and anger in almost everyone with whom they come in contact.

Individuals with paranoid personality disorder maintain their self-esteem by attributing their shortcomings to others. They do not accept responsibility for their own behaviors and feelings and project this responsibility onto others. They are envious and hostile toward those who are highly successful and believe that the only reason they are not as successful is because they have been treated unfairly. People who are paranoid are extremely vulnerable and constantly on the defensive. Any real or imagined threat can release hostility and anger that is fueled by animosities from the past. The desire for reprisal and vindication is so intense that a perceived loss of control can result in aggression and violence. These outbursts are usually brief, and the paranoid person soon regains external control, rationalizes the behavior, and reconstructs the defenses central to the personality pattern.

Predisposing Factors

Research has indicated a possible hereditary link in paranoid personality disorder. Studies have revealed a higher incidence of paranoid personality disorder among relatives of individuals with schizophrenia and delusional disorder, persecutory type (Boland & Verduin, 2022).

Psychological predisposing factors, as is the case with many personality disorders, include a history of childhood trauma, including neglect. People with paranoid personality disorder may have been subjected to parental antagonism and harassment. They learned to perceive the world as harsh and unkind, a place calling for protective vigilance and mistrust. They entered the world with a "chip-on-the-shoulder" attitude and were met with many rebuffs and rejections from others. Anticipating humiliation and betrayal by others, they learned to defend themselves by attacking first.

Schizoid Personality Disorder

Definition and Epidemiology

Schizoid personality disorder is characterized primarily by a profound defect in the ability to form personal relationships, and individuals with this disorder are often seen by others as eccentric, isolated, aloof, or lonely. These individuals display a lifelong pattern of social withdrawal, and their discomfort with human interaction is apparent. The prevalence of schizoid personality disorder is difficult to determine because, as is the case with many other personality disorders, it may go undiagnosed unless it has been recognized when the individual seeks health care for other reasons. Estimates within the general population vary from 3% to 5%. Significant numbers of people with the disorder are never observed in a clinical setting. Diagnosis of this disorder is more common in men than in women.

Clinical Picture

People with schizoid personality disorder appear cold, aloof, and indifferent to others. They typically have a long-standing history of engaging in primarily solitary activities or engaging more with animals than with people. They prefer to work in isolation and are unsociable, with little need or desire for emotional ties. They are able to invest enormous affective energy in intellectual pursuits. They may appear withdrawn anxious or uneasy in social situations and have difficulty being jovial. Their behavior and conversation exhibit little or no spontaneity and their affect is commonly bland and constricted.

The *DSM-5-TR* identifies schizoid personality disorder as a "pervasive pattern of detachment from social relationships and a restricted range of expression of emotions in interpersonal settings" (APA, 2022, p. 741).

Predisposing Factors

Although the role of heredity in the etiology of schizoid personality disorder is unclear, the feature of introversion appears to be a highly inheritable characteristic. It is more common in individuals with relatives who have schizophrenia or schizotypal personality disorder.

Psychosocially, the development of schizoid personality is probably influenced by early interactional patterns that the person found cold and unsatisfying. The childhoods of these individuals have often been characterized as bleak, cold, and notably lacking in empathy and nurturing. A child brought up in this environment may develop schizoid personality traits if that child possesses a temperamental disposition that is shy, anxious, and introverted.

Schizotypal Personality Disorder

Definition and Epidemiology

Individuals with **schizotypal personality disorder** (although this statement is true and occasionally people with schizotypal personality disorder develop schizophrenia, it might mislead the reader to think that this is the norm) present with behavior that is odd and eccentric but does not decompensate to the level of schizophrenia. Schizotypal personality is marked by symptoms that look more like schizophrenia than do those in schizoid personality, and as such show significant peculiarities in thinking, behavior, and appearance. Schizotypal personality disorder has a prevalence of around 4%. More than one-half of these individuals have had at least one episode of comorbid major depressive disorder (Cloninger & Svrakic, 2017).

Clinical Picture

Individuals with schizotypal personality disorder are aloof and isolated and behave in a bland and apathetic manner. Magical thinking, ideas of reference, illusions, and depersonalization are part of their everyday world. Examples include superstitiousness; belief in clairvoyance, telepathy, or "sixth sense"; and beliefs that "others can feel my feelings."

The speech pattern is sometimes bizarre. People with this disorder often cannot orient their thoughts logically and become lost in personal irrelevancies and in tangential asides that seem vague, digressive, and not pertinent to the topic at hand. This feature of their personality only further alienates them from others.

Individuals with schizotypal personality disorder are distinguished from those with schizophrenia by the absence of psychosis. Under stress, these individuals may decompensate and demonstrate psychotic symptoms, such as delusional thoughts, hallucinations, or bizarre behaviors, but they are usually of brief duration (Boland & Verduin, 2022). They often talk or gesture to themselves, as if "living in their own world." Their affect is bland or inappropriate, such as laughing at their own problems or at a situation that most people would consider sad.

Predisposing Factors

Evidence suggests that schizotypal personality disorder is more common among the first-degree relatives of people with schizophrenia than among the general population and, although a personality disorder, it is also included as one of the schizophrenia spectrum disorders in the *DSM-5-TR* (APA, 2022). Twin studies reveal a higher incidence in monozygotic twins than in dizygotic twins (Boland & Verduin, 2022).

Psychological and environmental factors may also interact with genetic vulnerability in the development of schizotypal personality traits. For children with schizotypal personality disorder, their affective blandness, peculiar behaviors, and discomfort with interpersonal relationships may provoke other children to avoid relationships with them or, worse, to engage in bullying, which reinforces their withdrawal from others. Having failed repeatedly to cope with these adversities, they withdraw and reduce contact with individuals and situations that evoked sadness and humiliation. Their new inner world provides them with a more significant and potentially rewarding existence than the one experienced in reality.

Antisocial Personality Disorder

Definition and Epidemiology

Antisocial personality disorder is a pattern of socially irresponsible, exploitative, and guiltless behavior that reflects a general disregard for the rights of others. These individuals exploit and manipulate others for personal gain and are unconcerned with obeying the law. They have difficulty sustaining consistent employment and developing stable relationships. This personality disorder has been extensively studied and has been included in all editions of the *Diagnostic and Statistical Manual of Mental Disorders*. In the United States, prevalence is estimated to be about 3% in the general population, but in prison populations, the prevalence is 50% or higher (Hatchett, 2015). It is more common in men than in women and in the lower socioeconomic classes, especially among highly mobile inhabitants of impoverished urban areas. The *DSM-5-TR* currently identifies *antisocial personality* and *psychopathy* as synonymous terms, but recent research reveals that these are better understood as distinct disorders (Hatchett, 2015; Thompson et al., 2014). Substance use disorder is commonly identified as a comorbid disorder.

NOTE: The clinical picture, predisposing factors, nursing diagnoses, and interventions for care of clients with antisocial personality disorder are presented later in this chapter.

Borderline Personality Disorder

Definition and Epidemiology

Borderline personality disorder (BPD) is characterized by a pattern of intense and chaotic relationships with affective instability and fluctuating attitudes toward other people. These individuals are impulsive, are directly and indirectly self-destructive, and lack a clear sense of identity. Prevalence of borderline personality is estimated at 1% to 2% of the population, with impairment being frequent, severe, and influencing and characterized by job losses, education interruptions, and marriage breakups (Cloninger & Svrakic, 2017). It is generally estimated to be more common in women than men, and more common in younger persons, suggesting a tendency toward maturation and remission (Boland & Verduin, 2022). Some researchers have estimated female-to-male ratios as high as 4 to 1 (Lubit, 2018).

NOTE: The clinical picture, predisposing factors, nursing diagnoses, and interventions for care of clients with BPD are presented later in this chapter.

Histrionic Personality Disorder

Definition and Epidemiology

Histrionic personality disorder is characterized by colorful, dramatic, and extroverted behavior in excitable, emotional people. They have difficulty maintaining long-lasting relationships, although they require constant affirmation of approval and acceptance from others. This need often gives rise to seductive, flirtatious behavior in efforts to reassure themselves of their attractiveness and to gain approval. The disorder has a prevalence of about 2% and tends to run in families; some researchers have identified a genetic link between histrionic personality disorder, antisocial personality disorder, and alcohol use disorder (Boland & Verduin, 2022).

Clinical Picture

People with histrionic personality disorder tend to be self-dramatizing, attention seeking, overly gregarious, and seductive. They use manipulative and exhibitionistic behaviors in their demands to be the center of attention. People with histrionic personality disorder often demonstrate, to an extreme, what our society tends to foster and admire in its members: to be well liked, successful, popular, extroverted, attractive, and sociable. However, beneath these surface characteristics is a driven quality—an all-consuming need for approval and a desperate striving to be conspicuous and to evoke affection or attract attention at all costs. Failure to evoke the attention and approval they seek often results in feelings of dejection and anxiety.

Individuals with this disorder are highly distractible and flighty by nature. They have difficulty paying attention to detail. They can portray themselves as carefree and sophisticated on the one hand and as inhibited and naive on the other. They tend to be highly suggestible, impressionable, and easily influenced by others. They are strongly dependent.

Interpersonal relationships are fleeting and superficial. Interaction with others may be provocative or sexually inappropriate. The person with histrionic personality disorder, having failed throughout life to develop the richness of inner feelings and lacking resources from which to draw, lacks the ability to provide another with genuinely sustained affection. Somatic complaints are not uncommon in these individuals, and fleeting episodes of psychosis may occur during periods of extreme stress.

The *DSM-5-TR* summarizes histrionic personality disorder as a "pervasive pattern of excessive emotionality and attention-seeking" (APA, 2022, p. 757).

Predisposing Factors

Heredity may be a factor in histrionic personality disorder because the disorder is apparently more common among first-degree biological relatives of people with the disorder than in the general population. Some traits may be inherited, whereas others are related to a combination of genetic predisposition and childhood experiences. At present, however, the exact cause is unknown.

From a psychosocial perspective, learning experiences may contribute to the development of histrionic personality disorder. The child may have learned that positive reinforcement was contingent on the ability to perform approved and admired behaviors.

Narcissistic Personality Disorder

Definition and Epidemiology

Persons with **narcissistic personality disorder** have an exaggerated sense of self-worth. They lack empathy and are hypersensitive to the evaluation of others. They believe that they have the inalienable right to receive special consideration and that their desire is sufficient justification for possessing whatever they seek.

This diagnosis appeared for the first time in the third edition of the *DSM*. However, the concept of narcissism has its roots in the 19th century. It was viewed by early psychoanalysts as a normal phase of psychosexual development. The prevalence of narcissistic personality disorder is estimated at 1% to 6%. It is diagnosed more often in men than in women.

Clinical Picture

Individuals with narcissistic personality disorder appear to lack humility, be overly self-centered, and exploit others to fulfill their own desires. They often do not perceive their behavior as being inappropriate or objectionable. Because they view themselves as "superior" beings, they believe they are entitled to special rights and privileges.

Although often grounded in grandiose distortions of reality, their mood is usually optimistic, relaxed, cheerful, and carefree. This mood can easily change, however, because of their fragile self-esteem. If they do not meet self-expectations, do not receive the positive feedback they expect from others, or draw criticism from others, they may respond with rage, shame, humiliation, or dejection. They may turn inward and fantasize rationalizations that convince them of their continued stature and perfection.

The exploitation of others for self-gratification results in impaired interpersonal relationships. In selecting a mate, narcissistic individuals frequently choose a person who will provide them with the praise and positive feedback that they require and who will not ask much from their partner in return.

The *DSM-5-TR* identifies the various behaviors in narcissistic personality disorder as a "pervasive pattern of grandiosity (in fantasy or behavior), need for admiration, and lack of empathy" (APA, 2022, p. 760).

Predisposing Factors

Although the causes are unknown, psychodynamic theories have suggested that narcissistic personality disorder evolves from a parent-child dynamic of excessive adoration or excessive criticism that is poorly attuned with the child's experience (Mayo Clinic, 2021). Children may then grow to project an image of invulnerability and self-sufficiency that conceals their true sense of emptiness and contributes to their inability to feel deep emotion.

Genetics and environment may both have a role in the development of narcissistic personality disorder. Having an innately oversensitive temperament may be an associated factor. In addition, research has identified a decreased volume of gray matter in areas of the brain responsible for empathy, emotional regulation, compassion, and cognitive functions (Gregory, 2021).

Avoidant Personality Disorder

Definition and Epidemiology

The individual with **avoidant personality disorder** is extremely sensitive to rejection and consequently may lead a very socially withdrawn life. Such individuals are not asocial; in fact, they may have a strong desire for companionship. The extreme shyness and fear of rejection, however, create needs for unusually strong assurances of unconditional acceptance. Prevalence of the disorder in the general population is about 2% to 3%, and it appears to be equally common in men and women.

Clinical Picture

Individuals with this disorder are awkward and uncomfortable in social situations. From a distance, others may perceive them as timid, withdrawn, or perhaps cold and strange. Those who have closer relationships with them, however, soon learn of their sensitivities, touchiness, evasiveness, and mistrustful qualities.

Their speech is usually slow and constrained with frequent hesitations, fragmentary thought sequences, and occasional confused and irrelevant digressions. They are often lonely and express feelings of being unwanted. They view others as critical, betraying, and humiliating. They desire to have close relationships but avoid them because of their fear of being rejected. Depression, anxiety, and anger at oneself for failing to develop social relations are commonly experienced.

The *DSM-5-TR* describes the various manifestations of avoidant personality disorder as a "pervasive pattern of social inhibition, feelings of inadequacy, and hypersensitivity to negative evaluation" (APA, 2022, p. 764).

Predisposing Factors

There is no clear cause of avoidant personality disorder. Contributing factors are most likely a combination of biological, genetic, and psychosocial influences. Some infants who exhibit hyperirritability, crankiness, tension, and withdrawal behaviors may possess a temperamental disposition toward an avoidant pattern later in life. Psychosocial influences may include childhood trauma or neglect leading to fears of abandonment or to viewing the world as a hostile and dangerous place.

Dependent Personality Disorder

Definition and Epidemiology

Dependent personality disorder is characterized by lack of self-confidence and extreme reliance on others, sometimes to the point of intense discomfort with being alone for even a brief period. This mode of behavior is evident in the tendency to allow others to make decisions, to feel helpless when alone, to act submissively, to subordinate needs to others, to tolerate mistreatment by others, to demean oneself to gain acceptance, and to fail to function adequately in situations that require assertive or dominant behavior.

Clinical Picture

Individuals with dependent personality disorder have a notable lack of self-confidence that is often apparent in their posture, voice, and mannerisms. They are typically passive and acquiescent to the desires of others. They are overly generous and thoughtful and underplay their own attractiveness and achievements. They may appear to others to "see the world through rose-colored glasses." But when alone, they may feel pessimistic, discouraged, and dejected, and they hide those feelings from others.

Individuals with dependent personality disorder assume the passive and submissive role in relationships. They are willing to let others make their important decisions. Should the dependent relationship end, they feel fearful and vulnerable because they lack confidence in their ability to care for themselves. They may hastily and indiscriminately attempt to establish another relationship with someone they believe can provide them with the nurturance and guidance they need.

They avoid positions of responsibility and become anxious when forced into them. They have feelings of low self-worth and are easily hurt by criticism and disapproval. They will do almost anything, even if it is unpleasant or demeaning, to earn the acceptance of others.

The *DSM-5-TR* describes the manifestations of dependent personality disorder as a "pervasive and excessive need to be taken care of that leads to submissive and clinging behaviors and fears of separation" (APA, 2022, p. 768).

Predisposing Factors

An infant may be genetically predisposed to a dependent temperament. Twin studies support a genetic vulnerability (Gjerde et al., 2012) but the authors clarify that while about two-thirds of the characteristic traits can be linked to genes, expression of the disorder depends on a complex interplay of both genetic and environmental factors.

Psychosocially, dependency is fostered in infancy when stimulation and nurturance are experienced exclusively from one source. The infant becomes attached to one source to the exclusion of all others. If this exclusive attachment continues as the child grows, the dependency is nurtured. A problem may arise when parents become overprotective and discourage independent behaviors on the part of the child. Parents who make new experiences unnecessarily easy for the child and refuse to allow them to learn by experience encourage their child to give up efforts at achieving autonomy. Dependent behaviors may be subtly rewarded in this environment, and the child may come to fear a loss of love or attachment from the parental figure if independent behaviors are attempted.

Obsessive-Compulsive Personality Disorder

Definition and Epidemiology

Individuals with **obsessive-compulsive personality disorder** are very serious and formal and have difficulty expressing emotions. They are overly disciplined, perfectionistic, and preoccupied with rules. They are inflexible about the way in which things must be done and have a devotion to productivity to the exclusion of personal pleasure. An intense fear of making mistakes leads to difficulty with decision making. The disorder is relatively common and occurs more often in men than in women. Within the family constellation, it appears to be most common in oldest children. Recurrent obsessions and compulsions are absent in this personality disorder, and clients who present with such symptoms are diagnosed with obsessive-compulsive disorder rather than obsessive compulsive *personality* disorder. Prevalence is estimated at anywhere from 2% to 8%.

Clinical Picture

Individuals with obsessive-compulsive personality disorder are inflexible and lack spontaneity. They are meticulous and work diligently and patiently at tasks that require accuracy and discipline. They are especially concerned with matters of organization and efficiency and tend to be rigid and unbending about rules and procedures.

Social behavior tends to be polite and formal. They are very "rank conscious," a characteristic that is reflected in their contrasting behaviors with "superiors" as opposed to "inferiors." They tend to be very solicitous to and ingratiating with authority figures. With subordinates, however, the compulsive person can become quite autocratic and condemnatory, often appearing pompous and self-righteous.

People with obsessive-compulsive personality disorder typify the "bureaucratic personality," the so-called company man. They see themselves as conscientious, loyal, dependable, and responsible and are contemptuous of people whose behavior they consider frivolous and impulsive. Emotional behavior is considered immature and irresponsible.

Although on the surface these individuals appear to be calm and controlled, underneath this exterior lies a great deal of ambivalence, conflict, and hostility. Individuals with this disorder commonly use the defense mechanism of reaction formation. Not daring to expose their true feelings of defiance and anger, they withhold these feelings so strongly that the opposite feelings come forth. The defenses of isolation, intellectualization, rationalization, and undoing are also commonly evident.

The *DSM-5-TR* diagnostic criteria for obsessive-compulsive personality disorder are presented in Box 22–1. These criteria can be compared and contrasted to the diagnostic criteria for obsessive-compulsive disorder presented in Chapter 18, "Anxiety, Obsessive-Compulsive, and Related Disorders."

Predisposing Factors

Genetic vulnerability may be a predisposing factor because some studies have found a familial aggregation of obsessive-compulsive personality disorder (Boland & Verduin, 2022).

The psychoanalytical view posits that the individual with obsessive-compulsive personality disorder was reared in an overly controlled environment with parents who expected their children to live up to their imposed standards of conduct and condemned

BOX 22–1 Diagnostic Criteria for Obsessive-Compulsive Personality Disorder

A pervasive pattern of preoccupation with orderliness, perfectionism, and mental and interpersonal control, at the expense of flexibility, openness, and efficiency, beginning by early adulthood and present in a variety of contexts, as indicated by four (or more) of the following:

1. Is preoccupied with details, rules, lists, order, organization, or schedules to the extent that the major point of the activity is lost
2. Shows perfectionism that interferes with task completion (e.g., is unable to complete a project because his or her own overly strict standards are not met)
3. Is excessively devoted to work and productivity to the exclusion of leisure activities and friendships (not accounted for by obvious economic necessity)
4. Is overconscientious, scrupulous, and inflexible about matters of morality, ethics, or values (not accounted for by cultural or religious identification)
5. Is unable to discard worn-out or worthless objects even when they have no sentimental value
6. Is reluctant to delegate tasks or to work with others unless they submit to exactly his or her way of doing things
7. Adopts a miserly spending style toward both self and others; money is viewed as something to be hoarded for future catastrophes
8. Shows rigidity and stubbornness

Reprinted with permission from American Psychiatric Association. (2022). *Diagnostic and statistical manual of mental disorders, fifth edition, text revision (DSM-5-TR).*

them if they did not. Praise for positive behaviors is bestowed on the child with much less frequency than punishment for undesirable behaviors. In this environment, individuals become experts in learning what they must *not* do to avoid punishment and condemnation rather than what they *can* do to achieve attention and praise. They learn to heed rigid restrictions and rules. Positive achievements are expected, taken for granted, and only occasionally acknowledged by their parents, whose comments and judgments are limited to pointing out transgressions and infractions of rules.

Application of the Nursing Process: Borderline Personality Disorder

Background Assessment Data

Historically, there have been clients who did not classically conform to the standard categories of neuroses or psychoses. The designation "borderline" was introduced to identify clients who seemed to fall on the border between the two categories. Other terminology that has been used in an attempt to identify this disorder includes *ambulatory schizophrenia, pseudoneurotic schizophrenia,* and *emotionally unstable personality.* When the term *borderline* was first proposed for inclusion in the third edition of the *DSM,* some psychiatrists feared that it might be used as a "wastebasket" diagnosis for difficult-to-treat clients. However, a specific set of *DSM-5-TR* criteria, listed in Box 22–2, has been established for diagnosing what has been described as "a consistent and stable course of unstable behavior."

Clinical Picture

Individuals with BPD always seem to be in a state of crisis and have frequent mood swings (although there may also be comorbid bipolar disorder). Their affect is one of extreme intensity, and their behavior reflects frequent changeability within days, hours, or even minutes. They are sometimes described as "thriving on chaos" because their behaviors frequently generate chaos, particularly in interpersonal relationships. Often, these individuals exhibit a single, dominant affective tone, such as depression, which may give way periodically to anxious agitation or inappropriate outbursts of anger.

Chronic Depression

Depression is so common in clients with this disorder that before the inclusion of BPD in the *DSM,* many of these clients were diagnosed with depressive disorder. Depression may be rooted in feelings of abandonment by the mother in early childhood (see "Predisposing Factors" in the section on borderline personality disorder). Underlying the depression is a sense of rage that is sporadically turned inward on the self and externally on the environment. Associated symptoms include uncontrolled anger and chronic feelings of emptiness. The individual is seldom aware of the true source of these feelings until well into long-term therapy.

Bipolar Disorder

Much has been written about the common comorbidity of BPD with bipolar disorder and the overlap of features. There are so many features in common that it has been suggested by some that BPD should be considered a disorder along a bipolar spectrum (Rodriguez, 2017). Predisposing factors common to both illnesses include: shared genetic variants, childhood loss of a parent, early childhood trauma, and dysfunctional family environments (Rodriguez, 2017).

BOX 22–2 Diagnostic Criteria for Borderline Personality Disorder

A pervasive pattern of instability of interpersonal relationships, self-image, and affects, and marked impulsivity beginning by early adulthood and present in a variety of contexts, as indicated by five (or more) of the following:

1. Frantic efforts to avoid real or imagined abandonment (**NOTE:** Do not include suicidal or self-mutilating behavior covered in criterion 5.)
2. A pattern of unstable and intense interpersonal relationships characterized by alternating between extremes of idealization and devaluation
3. Identity disturbance: markedly and persistently unstable self-image or sense of self
4. Impulsivity in at least two areas that are potentially self-damaging (e.g., spending, sex, substance abuse, reckless driving, binge eating) (**NOTE:** Do not include suicidal or self-mutilating behavior covered in criterion 5.)
5. Recurrent suicidal behavior, gestures, or threats, or self-mutilating behavior
6. Affective instability due to marked reactivity of mood (e.g., intense episodic dysphoria, irritability, or anxiety, usually lasting a few hours and only rarely more than a few days)
7. Chronic feelings of emptiness
8. Inappropriate, intense anger or difficulty controlling anger (e.g., frequent displays of temper, constant anger, recurrent physical fights)
9. Transient, stress-related paranoid ideation or severe dissociative symptoms

Reprinted with permission from American Psychiatric Association. (2022). *Diagnostic and statistical manual of mental disorders, fifth edition, text revision (DSM-5-TR).*

Affective instability, moods that shift from depression to irritability or anxiety, are so common (reported in over 90% of patients with BPD) that Zimmerman (2017) notes that if these symptoms are not present, it is likely that BPD can be ruled out.

Inability to Be Alone

Because of this chronic fear of abandonment, clients with BPD have little tolerance for being alone. They prefer a frantic search for companionship, no matter how unsatisfactory, to sitting with feelings of loneliness, emptiness, and boredom (Boland & Verduin, 2022).

Patterns of Interaction

Clinging and Distancing

The client with BPD commonly exhibits a pattern of interaction with others that is characterized by clinging and distancing behaviors. When clients are clinging to another individual, they may exhibit helpless, dependent, or even childlike behaviors. They overidealize a single individual with whom they want to spend all their time, with whom they express a frequent need to talk, or from whom they seek constant reassurance. Impulsive behaviors, even self-mutilation, may result when they cannot be with this chosen individual. Distancing behaviors are characterized by hostility, anger, and devaluation of others, arising from a feeling of discomfort with closeness. Distancing behaviors also occur in response to separations, confrontations, or attempts to limit certain behaviors. Devaluation of others is manifested by discrediting or undermining their strengths and personal significance.

Splitting

Splitting is a primitive ego defense mechanism that is common in people with BPD. It is believed to arise from their lack of achievement of **object constancy** and is manifested by an inability to integrate and accept both positive and negative feelings. In their view, people—including themselves—and life situations are either all good or all bad. For example, a nurse-patient relationship may be perceived to be very intense and overvalued (e.g., "No one else in the world can help me the way you do") until the individual with BPD feels threatened in any way. The reason for feeling threatened could be as simple as a perception that the nurse looked at the individual with a different expression or that the nurse was not immediately available to spend time with the client. Because this individual also struggles with emotional regulation, suddenly the nurse is devalued, valuing is shifted to another nurse, and the idealized image changes from beneficent caregiver to one of hateful and cruel persecutor. These shifting allegiances and valuing/devaluing responses can generate conflict, anger, and frustration in staff members (or in any interpersonal relationships) unless this dynamic is clearly understood and managed appropriately.

Manipulation

In their efforts to prevent the separation they so desperately fear, clients with this disorder become masters of manipulation. Virtually any behavior becomes an acceptable means of achieving the desired result: relief from separation anxiety. Pitting one individual against another is a common ploy to allay these fears of abandonment.

Self-Destructive Behaviors

Repetitive, self-mutilative behaviors are classic manifestations of BPD. About 75% of individuals with

BPD have a history of at least one deliberate act of self-harm, and about 1 in 10 die by suicide (Lubit, 2018). Although these acts can be fatal, most commonly they are manipulative gestures designed to elicit a rescue response from significant others. Suicide attempts are quite common and result from feelings of abandonment following separation from a significant other. The endeavor is often attempted, however, incorporating a measure of "safety" into the plan (e.g., swallowing pills in an area where the person will surely be discovered by others or swallowing pills and making a phone call to report the deed to someone).

Other types of destructive behaviors include cutting, scratching, and burning. Various theories abound regarding why these individuals are able to inflict pain on themselves. One hypothesis suggests that they may have higher levels of endorphins in their bodies than most people, thereby increasing their threshold for pain. Another theory relates to the individual's personal identity disturbance. It proposes that because many of the self-mutilating behaviors take place when individuals are in a state of depersonalization and derealization, they do not initially feel the pain. The mutilation continues until pain is felt in an attempt to counteract the feelings of unreality. Some clients with BPD have reported that "to feel pain is better than to feel nothing." The pain validates their existence.

Impulsivity

Individuals with BPD have poor impulse control. Impulsive behaviors associated with BPD include substance misuse, gambling, promiscuity, reckless driving, and bingeing and purging. These behaviors often occur in response to real or perceived feelings of abandonment.

Predisposing Factors

Biological Influences

BPD, once thought to be an entirely psychodynamic illness, has been the focus of much current research revealing a wealth of information about the neurobiological underpinnings of this illness. Current research clearly shows that BPD evolves through a complex interplay of environmental factors, brain anatomy and function, genetics, and epigenetics (Pier et al., 2016).

- ***Biochemical:*** Clients with BPD have a high incidence of major depressive episodes, and antidepressants have demonstrated benefits in some cases (Boland & Verduin, 2022). This fact and supporting information from brain imaging studies (Lis et al., 2007) have led to the hypothesis that serotonin and/or norepinephrine dysregulation may contribute to the development of BPD. As stated elsewhere, questions remain about whether these dysfunctions contribute to the development of such disorders or whether they are a neurochemical response to intense emotional states.
- ***Genetic:*** An increased prevalence of major depression, antisocial personality disorder, and substance use disorders in first-degree relatives of individuals with borderline personality suggest that there are complex genetic vulnerabilities as well as environmental influences (Boland & Verduin, 2022). Clients with BPD are five times more likely than others to have a first-degree relative with BPD, and many studies have shown personality traits such as impulsivity, affect lability, and neuroticism to be heritable traits (MacIntosh et al., 2015). Epigenetic studies have identified changes to the oxytocin system (related to being a carrier of a specific allele) as associated with negative perceptions of others, increased stress markers, decreased empathy, confidence, and positivity (Pier et al., 2016). In this scenario, prosocial behaviors such as empathy, positivity, and confidence decrease. Treatment with oxytocin has demonstrated some benefits in individuals with BPD. Several studies (Bertsch & Herpertz, 2018; Domes et al., 2019; Schneider et al., 2020) found that intranasal oxytocin strengthened avoidance of interpersonal threat cues, improved empathy, and thus decreased impulsive interpersonal reactions in individuals with BPD, but more research with larger samples is needed.
- ***Neurobiological:*** Magnetic resonance imaging (MRI) studies to assess anatomical and functional activities in the brain have identified several factors associated with BPD. The left amygdala, left hippocampus, and posterior cingulate cortex show heightened activation, and the prefrontal cortex shows decreased activation during the processing of negative emotions (Pier et al., 2016).

Psychosocial Influences

Research about specific types of trauma that predispose one to the development of BPD is inconsistent, but there is strong evidence that a history of childhood trauma is associated with this disorder (MacIntosh et al., 2015). One recent model describes BPD as influenced by a triad of factors that includes childhood trauma, a vulnerable temperament, and a series of triggering events (Cloninger & Svrakic, 2017). Some of the symptoms in BPD are similar to those in post-traumatic stress disorder (PTSD). In fact, some experts have considered BPD a controversial diagnosis because of the many apparent overlaps with PTSD (and bipolar disorder). But as described by MacIntosh and associates (2015), research by Hodges and colleagues (2013) demonstrates that the complexity of symptoms seen in BPD does not fit with general profiles of individuals with PTSD. Ford and Courtois (2014) cite several studies identifying a 30% to 40% comorbidity of PTSD and BPD and indicate that about 85% of those diagnosed with BPD were initially diagnosed with PTSD. In these cases, BPD symptoms persisted after remission of PTSD symptoms. Comorbid substance use disorders may also complicate the differentiation of symptoms and treatment needs. Thorough assessment to identify the multiple psychosocial influences in BPD is clearly essential.

Developmental Factors

According to Mahler's theory of object relations (Mahler et al., 1975), infants pass through six phases from birth to 36 months, when a sense of separateness from the parenting figure is finally established. Between the ages of 16 and 24 months (phase 5, the rapprochement phase), children become acutely aware of their separateness, and because this is frightening, they look to the mother for "emotional refueling" and to maintain a sense of security while at the same time beginning to explore their separateness and independence. (See Table 22–1 for a more detailed outline of Mahler's theory.) According to object relations theorists, the individual with BPD becomes fixed in the rapprochement phase of development. This occurs when the child shows increasing separation and autonomy. The mother, who feels secure in the relationship as long as the child is dependent, begins to feel threatened by the child's increasing independence. The mother may be experiencing her own fears of abandonment. In response to separation behaviors, the mother withdraws the emotional support or "refueling" that is so vitally needed during this phase for the child to feel secure. Instead, the mother rewards clinging, dependent behaviors and punishes independent behaviors by withholding emotional support. With the sense of emotional survival at stake, the child learns to behave in a manner that satisfies the parental wishes. The child develops an internal conflict based on fear of abandonment. The child wants to achieve independence common to this stage of development but fears that the mother will withdraw emotional support as a result. This unresolved fear of abandonment remains with the child into adulthood. Unresolved grief for the nurturing they failed to receive results in internalized rage that manifests itself in the depression so common in people with BPD.

Other research (Mak & Lam, 2013; Pier et al., 2016) looking at attachment issues in childhood suggests that childhood maltreatment, particularly neglect, may be associated with reactive attachment disorder, which results in the development of neurocognitive deficits, particularly temporal limbic dysfunction. The symptoms of BPD with regard to unhealthy attachment in relationships may be related, at least in part, to these neurocognitive deficits rooted in childhood development disruptions.

Diagnosis and Outcome Identification

Nursing diagnoses are formulated from the data gathered during the assessment phase and with background knowledge regarding predisposing factors to the disorder. Table 22–2 presents a list of patient behaviors and the NANDA International (NANDA-I) nursing diagnoses (Herdman et al., 2021) that correspond to these behaviors, which may be used in planning care for patients with BPD.

Outcome Criteria

The following criteria may be used for measurement of outcomes in the care of patients with BPD. The patient:

- Has not harmed self.
- Seeks out staff when desire for self-mutilation is strong.
- Is able to identify true source of anger.
- Expresses anger appropriately.
- Relates to more than one staff member.
- Completes activities of daily living independently.
- Does not manipulate one staff member against the other in order to fulfill own desires.

Planning and Implementation

The patient with BPD is at high risk for being stigmatized, even among health-care professionals (Black et al., 2011; McNee et al., 2014; Quenneville et al., 2020; Weight & Kendal, 2013; Westwood & Baker, 2010). Patient behaviors such as manipulating, lying, and splitting violate the nurse's sense of success in establishing a trusting relationship with this individual and may culminate in negative or distancing behaviors from the nurse. The following guidelines

TABLE 22–2 Assigning Nursing Diagnoses to Behaviors Commonly Associated With Borderline Personality Disorder

BEHAVIORS	NURSING DIAGNOSES
Risk factors: History of self-injurious behavior; history of inability to plan solutions; impulsivity; irresistible urge to damage self; feels threatened with loss of significant relationship	**Risk for self-mutilation**
Risk factors: History of suicide attempts; suicidal ideation; suicidal plan; impulsiveness; childhood abuse; fears of abandonment; internalized rage	**Risk for self-directed violence** **Risk for suicidal behavior**
Risk factors: Body language (e.g., rigid posture, clenching of fists and jaw, hyperactivity, pacing, breathlessness, threatening stances); history of childhood abuse; impulsivity; transient psychotic symptomatology	**Risk for other-directed violence**
Depression; persistent emotional distress; rumination; separation distress; traumatic distress; verbalizes feeling empty; inappropriate expression of anger	**Maladaptive grieving**
Alternating clinging and distancing behaviors; staff splitting; manipulation	**Impaired social interaction**
Feelings of depersonalization and derealization	**Disturbed personal identity**
Transient psychotic symptoms (disorganized thinking; misinterpretation of the environment); increased tension; decreased perceptual field	**Anxiety (severe to panic)**
Dependent on others; excessively seeks reassurance; manipulation of others; inability to tolerate being alone	**Chronic low self-esteem**

are helpful in decreasing negative attitudes and stigmatization of this patient:

- Understand the disorder and the impact of childhood trauma on the dynamics of the patient's behavior to develop an approach of compassion and convey hopefulness that this is a treatable rather than an untreatable condition.
- Recognize that even brief encounters with a patient, during short hospital stays, provide an opportunity to convey connectedness and a sense that the patient is valued. This is particularly important because the patient with BPD is interpersonally hypersensitive, fears abandonment, and has had a history of instability in interpersonal relationships (Helleman et al., 2014).
- Frequently reflect on your feelings in response to patient behavior. For example, self-harming behaviors by the patient frequently generate feelings of anger and frustration in nurses when the behavior seems to be manipulative rather than a sign of true distress. These feelings may culminate in the nurse maintaining distance from the patient (Westwood & Baker, 2010). Indeed, self-harming behaviors may be used as a tool for manipulating others and be a sign of true distress.
- Develop a clear model of communication and intervention among team members for the hospitalized patient with BPD. Consistency in intervention helps to model healthy interpersonal skills for the patient and may minimize successful efforts at splitting staff members. In addition, when health-care team members develop strong communication skills with each other, it provides a foundation for discussing and confronting negative attitudes toward the patient and promotes culture change. For example, McNee and associates (2014) developed a commitment among their team members that they would avoid using phrases such as "acting out" and "attention seeking" because these reinforced a culture of negativity toward the patient.

In Table 22–3, selected nursing diagnoses common to the patient with borderline personality disorder are presented in a plan of care. Outcome criteria, along with appropriate nursing interventions and rationales, are included for each.

Concept Care Mapping

The concept map care plan is a diagrammatic teaching and learning strategy that allows visualization of interrelationships between medical diagnoses, nursing diagnoses, assessment data, and treatments. An example of a concept map care plan for a patient with BPD is presented in Figure 22–1.

Table 22–3 | CARE PLAN FOR THE PATIENT WITH BORDERLINE PERSONALITY DISORDER

NURSING DIAGNOSIS: RISK FOR SELF-INJURY/RISK FOR SELF-DIRECTED OR OTHER-DIRECTED VIOLENCE

RELATED TO: Parental emotional deprivation (unresolved fears of abandonment)

OUTCOME CRITERIA	NURSING INTERVENTIONS	RATIONALE
Short-Term Goals ■ Patient will seek out staff member if feelings of harming self or others emerge. ■ Patient will not harm self or others. **Long-Term Goal** ■ Patient will not harm self or others.	1. Observe the patient's behavior frequently. Do this through routine activities and interactions; avoid appearing watchful and suspicious.	1. Close observation is required so that intervention can occur if required to ensure the patient's (and others') safety.
	2. Encourage the patient to seek out a staff member when the urge for self-injury intensifies.	2. Discussing feelings of self-harm with a trusted individual may provide some relief to the patient. An attitude of acceptance of the patient as a worthwhile individual is conveyed.
	3. If self-mutilation occurs, care for the patient's wounds in a matter-of-fact manner. Do not give positive reinforcement to this behavior by offering sympathy or additional attention.	3. Lack of attention to the maladaptive behavior may decrease repetition of its use.
	4. Encourage the patient to talk about feelings that occurred just before this behavior.	4. To problem-solve the situation with the patient, knowledge of the precipitating factors is important.
	5. Act as a role model for appropriate expression of angry feelings and give positive reinforcement when attempts to conform are made.	5. It is vital that the patient learns to express angry feelings in adaptive ways; suicide and other self-destructive behaviors are often viewed as a result of anger turned inward on the self.
	6. Remove all dangerous objects (sharp items, razors, etc.) from the patient's environment.	6. Patient safety is a nursing priority.
	7. Redirect violent behavior with physical outlets for the patient's anxiety (e.g., exercises, jogging).	7. Physical exercise is a safe and effective way of relieving pent-up tension.
	8. Have sufficient staff available to indicate a show of strength to the patient if it becomes necessary.	8. This conveys to the patient evidence of control over the situation and provides some physical security for patient and staff.
	9. Administer tranquilizing medications as ordered by the physician or obtain an order if necessary. Monitor the patient for effectiveness of the medication, for the appearance of adverse side effects, and to ensure that the patient is not hoarding medication.	9. Tranquilizing medications, such as anxiolytics or antipsychotics, may have a calming effect on the patient and may prevent aggressive behaviors. Close monitoring is important because impulsivity is a common symptom in BPD and may increase risk for an overdose attempt.

Continued

Table 22–3 | CARE PLAN FOR THE PATIENT WITH BORDERLINE PERSONALITY DISORDER–cont'd

OUTCOME CRITERIA	NURSING INTERVENTIONS	RATIONALE
	10. If the patient is not calmed by "talking down" or by medication, use of mechanical restraints may be necessary.	10. The avenue of the "least restrictive alternative" must be selected when planning interventions for a violent patient. Restraints should be used only as a last resort, after all other interventions have been unsuccessful, and the patient is clearly at risk of harm to self or others.
	11. If restraint is deemed necessary, ensure that sufficient staff is available to assist. Follow protocol established by the institution. Provide care with consideration for the patient's trauma history.	11. Restraints should be used only as a last resort, after all other interventions have been unsuccessful and the patient is clearly at imminent risk of harming self or others. The safety and protection of the patient, staff, and other patients is a top priority. Trauma-informed care should always be the foundation for decisions about appropriateness of interventions.
	12. If warranted by high acuity of the situation, staff may need to be assigned on a one-to-one basis.	12. Because of their extreme fear of abandonment, patients with this disorder should not be left alone at a stressful time because it may cause an acute rise in anxiety and agitation levels.
	13. As agitation decreases, assess the patient's readiness for restraint removal or reduction. Remove one restraint at a time while assessing the patient's response.	13. This minimizes the risk of injury to patients and staff.

NURSING DIAGNOSIS: MALADAPTIVE GRIEVING

RELATED TO: Fixation in anger stage of grieving process; fear of abandonment, possible childhood physical or sexual abuse

EVIDENCED BY: Depressed mood, maladaptive expressions of anger

OUTCOME CRITERIA	NURSING INTERVENTIONS	RATIONALE
Short-Term Goal ■ Within 5 days, patient will discuss with nurse or therapist maladaptive patterns of expressing anger.	1. Convey an accepting attitude—one that creates a nonthreatening environment for the patient to express feelings. Be honest and keep all promises.	1. An accepting attitude conveys to the patient that you believe in their worth. Trust is enhanced.
	2. Identify the function that anger, frustration, and rage serve for the patient. Allow expression of these feelings within reason.	2. Verbalization of feelings in a nonthreatening environment may help the patient come to terms with unresolved issues.
	3. Encourage the patient to discharge pent-up anger through participation in large motor activities (e.g., brisk walks, jogging, physical exercises, volleyball, exercise bike).	3. Physical exercise provides a safe and effective method for discharging pent-up tension.

Table 22–3 | CARE PLAN FOR THE PATIENT WITH BORDERLINE PERSONALITY DISORDER–cont'd

OUTCOME CRITERIA	NURSING INTERVENTIONS	RATIONALE
Long-Term Goal ■ By time of discharge from treatment, patient will be able to identify the true source of angry feelings, accept ownership of these feelings, and express them in a socially acceptable manner, in an effort to satisfactorily progress through the grieving process.	4. Explore with the patient the true source of the anger. This is a painful therapy that often leads to regression as the patient deals with the feelings of early abandonment or issues of abuse.	4. Reconciliation of the feelings associated with this stage is necessary before progression through the grieving process can continue.
	5. Because anger may be displaced onto the nurse, caution must be taken to guard against the negative effects of countertransference.	5. Countertransference has the potential to generate an array of negative feelings from the nurse. The existence of negative feelings must be acknowledged, but they must not be allowed to interfere with the therapeutic process.
	6. Explain the behaviors associated with the normal grieving process. Help the patient recognize their position in this process.	6. Knowledge of the acceptability of the feelings associated with normal grieving may help to relieve some of the guilt that these responses generate.
	7. Help the patient understand appropriate ways to express anger. Give positive reinforcement for behaviors used to express anger appropriately. Act as a role model. It is important to let patients know when they have done something that has generated angry feelings in others.	7. Positive reinforcement enhances self-esteem and encourages repetition of desirable behaviors. Role-modeling ways to express anger in an appropriate manner is a powerful learning tool.
	8. Set limits on maladaptive behaviors and explain consequences of violation of those limits. Be supportive, yet consistent and firm in caring for this patient.	8. Patients lack sufficient self-control to limit maladaptive behaviors, so assistance is required. Consistency on the part of all staff members working with this patient is essential for achieving positive outcomes.

NURSING DIAGNOSIS: IMPAIRED SOCIAL INTERACTION

RELATED TO: Extreme fears of abandonment and engulfment

EVIDENCED BY: Alternating clinging and distancing behaviors and staff splitting

OUTCOME CRITERIA	NURSING INTERVENTIONS	RATIONALE
Short-Term Goal ■ Within 5 days, patient will discuss with nurse or therapist behaviors that impede the development of satisfactory interpersonal relationships.	1. Encourage the patient to examine maladaptive behaviors (to recognize that they are occurring).	1. Patients may be unaware of splitting or of clinging and distancing pattern of interaction with others. Recognition must occur before change can occur.
	2. Reinforce that you will be available, without reinforcing dependent behaviors.	2. Knowledge of your availability may provide needed security for the patient.
	3. Rotate staff members who work with the patient in order to avoid their developing dependence on particular individuals.	3. Patients must learn to relate to more than one staff member in an effort to decrease use of splitting and to diminish fears of abandonment.

Continued

Table 22–3 | CARE PLAN FOR THE PATIENT WITH BORDERLINE PERSONALITY DISORDER–cont'd

OUTCOME CRITERIA	NURSING INTERVENTIONS	RATIONALE
Long-Term Goal ■ By time of discharge from treatment, patient will interact appropriately with others in the therapy setting in both social and therapeutic activities (evidencing a discontinuation of splitting and clinging and distancing behaviors).	4. Discuss with the patient and other staff members when it is apparent that the patient is pitting one staff member against another. Do not listen as patient tries to degrade other staff members. Suggest instead that the patient discuss the problem directly with the staff person involved.	4. Splitting is the primary defense mechanism of patients with BPD, and the impressions they have of others as either "good" or "bad" are a manifestation of this defense. These interventions are intended to help the individual understand that staff splitting will not be tolerated, and to work toward diminishing clinging and distancing behaviors.
	5. With the patient, explore feelings that relate to fears of abandonment and engulfment. Help the patient to understand that clinging and distancing behaviors are engendered by these fears.	5. Exploration of feelings with a trusted individual may help the patient come to terms with unresolved issues.
	6. Help the patient explore how these behaviors interfere with satisfactory relationships.	6. Patients may be unaware of how others perceive these behaviors and why they are not acceptable.
	7. Assist the patient to work toward achievement of object constancy. Be available, without promoting dependency.	7. This may help the patient resolve fears of abandonment in the process toward developing the ability to establish satisfactory intimate relationships.
	8. Provide education, support, and referral resources for family members and significant others who may also experience anger and frustration at failed attempts to navigate interpersonal relationships with this individual.	8. Research has found that family members often report feeling excluded and discriminated against by health-care providers (Lawn et al., 2015).

Evaluation

Reassessment is conducted to determine whether the nursing actions have been successful in achieving the objectives of care. Evaluation of the nursing actions for the patient with BPD may be facilitated by gathering information using the following types of questions. Has the patient:

- Been able to seek out staff when feeling the desire for self-harm?
- Avoided self-harm?
- Correlated times of desire for self-harm to times of elevation in level of anxiety?
- Discussed feelings with staff (particularly feelings of depression and anger)?
- Identified the true source toward which the anger is directed?
- Verbalized understanding of the basis for anger?
- Expressed anger appropriately?
- Demonstrated ability to function independently?
- Related to more than one staff member?
- Verbalized the knowledge that the staff members are not abandoning the patient when leaving for the day?
- Separated from the staff in an appropriate manner?
- Demonstrated ability to delay gratification and refrain from manipulating others in order to fulfill own desires?
- Identified resources within the community from whom to seek assistance in times of extreme stress?

Application of the Nursing Process: Antisocial Personality Disorder

Background Assessment Data

In the *DSM-I*, antisocial behavior was categorized as a "sociopathic or psychopathic" reaction that was

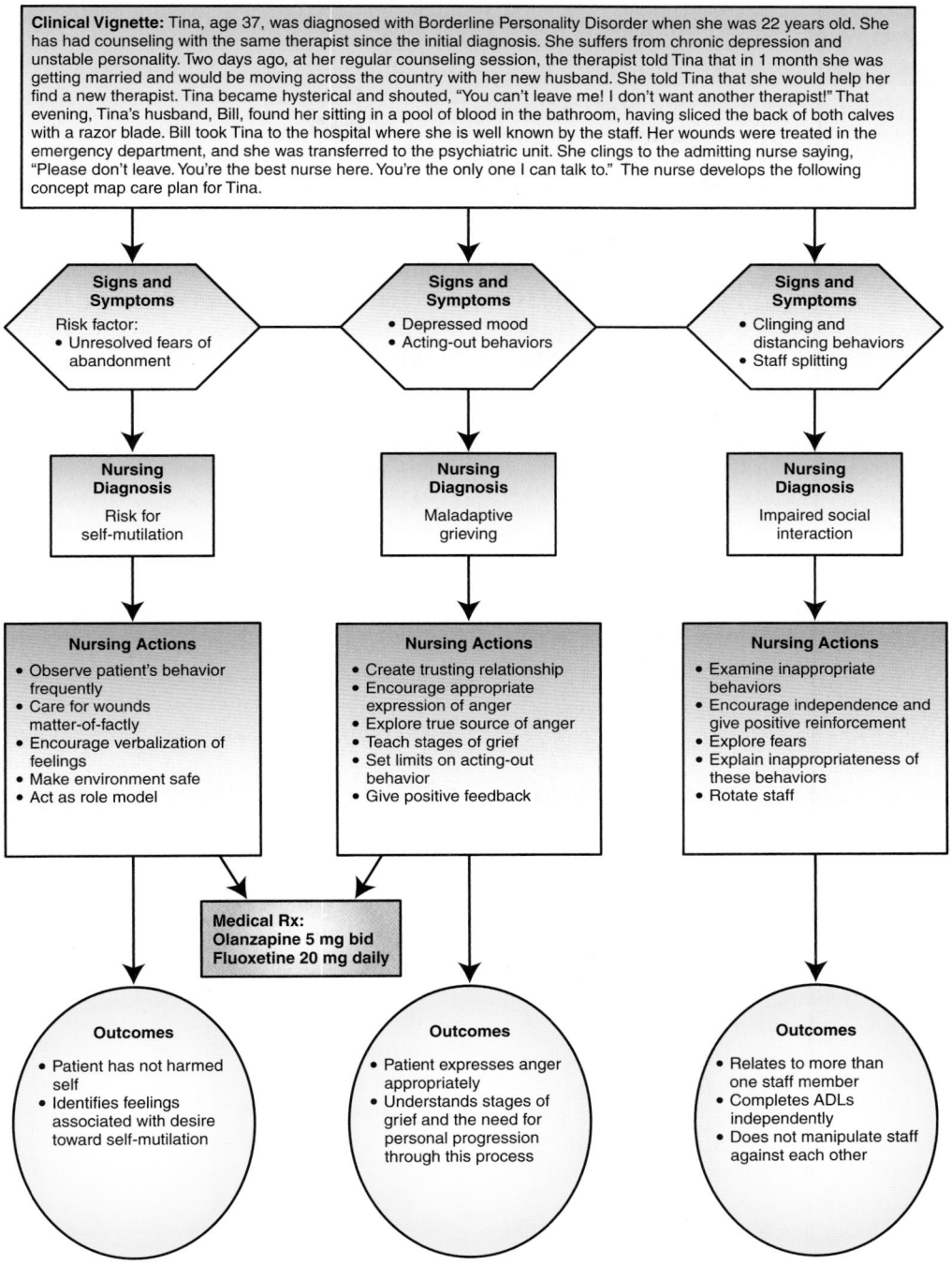

FIGURE 22–1 Concept map care plan for a patient with BPD.

symptomatic of any of several underlying personality disorders. The *DSM-II* represented it as a separate personality type, a distinction that has been retained in subsequent editions. The *DSM-5-TR* diagnostic criteria for antisocial personality disorder are presented in Box 22–3.

Individuals with antisocial personality disorder are seldom seen in most clinical settings, and when they are, it is commonly a way to avoid legal consequences. Sometimes they are admitted to the health-care system by court order for psychological evaluation. Most frequently, however, these individuals may be

BOX 22–3 Diagnostic Criteria for Antisocial Personality Disorder

A. A pervasive pattern of disregard for and violation of the rights of others occurring since age 15 years, as indicated by three (or more) of the following:
   1. Failure to conform to social norms with respect to lawful behaviors as indicated by repeatedly performing acts that are grounds for arrest
   2. Deceitfulness, as indicated by repeated lying, use of aliases, or conning others for personal profit or pleasure
   3. Impulsivity or failure to plan ahead
   4. Irritability and aggressiveness, as indicated by repeated physical fights or assaults
   5. Reckless disregard for safety of self or others
   6. Consistent irresponsibility, as indicated by repeated failure to sustain consistent work behavior or honor financial obligations
   7. Lack of remorse, as indicated by being indifferent to or rationalizing having hurt, mistreated, or stolen from another

B. Individual is at least 18 years.

C. There is evidence of conduct disorder with onset before age 15 years.

D. The occurrence of antisocial behavior is not exclusively during the course of schizophrenia or bipolar disorder.

Reprinted with permission from American Psychiatric Association. (2022). *Diagnostic and statistical manual of mental disorders, fifth edition, text revision (DSM-5-TR).*

encountered in prisons, jails, and rehabilitation services.

Although the *DSM-5-TR* continues to identify antisocial personality disorder as synonymous with psychopathy, recent evidence is beginning to distinguish these as separate entities (Anderson et al., 2014; APA, 2022; Thompson et al., 2014; Verona & Patrick, 2015). Antisocial personality disorder as a distinct entity is characterized by *behaviors* that are reactive to perceived threats, control, and a negative affect; psychopathy is described as *personality traits* that include low fear, low empathy, domination, callous cruelty, and emotional insensitivity (Thompson et al., 2015; Verona & Patrick, 2015). Both disorders include being prone to violence. But the two disorders have different etiologies and potentially different responses to treatment. For the purpose of discussion here, they are identified together as antisocial personality disorder.

Clinical Picture

Antisocial personality disorder is a pattern of socially irresponsible, exploitative, and guiltless behavior that reflects a general disregard for the rights of others. Individuals with this disorder exploit and manipulate others for personal gain and are unconcerned with obeying the law. They have difficulty sustaining consistent employment and in developing stable relationships. They appear cold and callous, often intimidating others with their brusque and belligerent manner. They tend to be argumentative and, at times, cruel and malicious. They lack warmth and compassion and are often suspicious of these qualities in others.

Individuals with antisocial personality have a very low tolerance for frustration, act impulsively, and are unable to delay gratification. They are restless and easily bored, often taking chances and seeking thrills, as if they were immune to danger. Their pattern of impulsivity may be manifested in failure to plan ahead, culminating in sudden job, residence, or relationship changes (APA, 2022).

When things go their way, individuals with this disorder act cheerful, even gracious and charming. Because of their low tolerance for frustration, this pleasant exterior can change very quickly. When what they desire at the moment is challenged, they are likely to become furious and vindictive. Easily provoked to attack, their first inclination is to demean and dominate. They believe that "good guys come in last," and they show contempt for the weak and underprivileged. They exploit others to fulfill their own desires, showing no trace of shame or guilt for their behavior. Individuals with antisocial personalities see themselves as victims, using projection, devaluing, and denial as primary ego defense mechanisms. They do not accept responsibility for the consequences of their behavior. In their own minds, the perception that they are being victimized by others justifies their malicious behavior, lest they be the recipient of unjust persecution and hostility from others. Physical attacks or other acts of aggression are not uncommon.

Satisfying interpersonal relationships are not possible because individuals with antisocial personalities have learned to place their trust only in themselves. They have a philosophy that "it's every man for himself" and that one should stop at nothing to avoid being manipulated by others. They may disregard the safety of themselves and others through reckless sexual activity, substance use, reckless driving, or child neglect (APA, 2022).

One of the most distinctive characteristics of individuals with antisocial personality disorder is their tendency to ignore conventional authority and rules. They act as though established social norms and guidelines for self-discipline and cooperative behavior do not apply to them. They are flagrant in their disrespect for the law and for the rights of others.

Predisposing Factors

Biological Influences

Antisocial personality is more common among first-degree biological relatives of those with the disorder than among the general population. Twin and adoptive studies have implicated the role of genetics in antisocial personality disorder, especially for the personality traits of callousness and unemotional responses, which may be more definitive of psychopathy (Thompson et al., 2014). Interestingly, other antisocial behaviors among twins appear to be environmentally influenced and both biological and adoptive children of parents with antisocial personality disorder are at greater risk for this personality disorder (Cloninger & Svrakic, 2017), suggesting that this is a complex disorder with both genetic and environmental influences. Conduct disorder is more likely to develop into antisocial personality disorder in adulthood when the child is exposed to erratic parenting, neglect, or inconsistent parenting (Boland & Verduin, 2022).

Recent research has suggested that a particular gene, *MAOA*, may be moderated after exposure to violence such as child maltreatment, physical abuse, or sexual abuse (Ouellet-Morin et al., 2016). Mutations in this gene are believed to be associated with the eventual development of differential features of antisocial personality, although the authors note that more research is needed. A recent systematic review (Moore et al., 2019) concluded that the callous-unemotional personality trait (a recognized risk factor for psychopathic traits and antisocial behavior) appears to be substantially influenced by genetic factors, but more research is needed to clarify the exact mechanisms. Nonetheless, it adds support to the evidence that genetics and environment interact in the development of antisocial personality disorder and underscores the influence of childhood trauma.

Characteristics associated with temperament in the newborn may be significant in the predisposition to antisocial personality disorder. Parents who bring their children with behavior disorders to clinics often report that the child displayed temper tantrums from infancy and would become furious when awaiting a bottle or a diaper change. As these children mature, they commonly develop a bullying attitude toward other children. Parents report that they are undaunted by punishment and generally quite unmanageable.

The likelihood of developing antisocial personality disorder is increased if the individual had attention deficit-hyperactivity disorder and conduct disorder as a child that began under the age of 10 (APA, 2022). Brain imaging studies have identified deficits in prefrontal cortex gray matter, which regulates cognitive control and inhibition, altered activity in the amygdala, which is responsible for modulating fearful or threatening stimuli, and inefficient (reduced) whole-brain network connectivity particularly in the frontal regions of the brain (Jiang et al., 2017). Other studies have identified dysregulation of neurotransmitters (dopamine and serotonin), and endocrine abnormalities (testosterone and cortisol) as present in individuals with antisocial personality disorder, and these dysregulations may be related to the symptoms of impulsivity (Thompson et al., 2014). Neuropsychological studies have demonstrated an increased reactivity to environmental irritants and cues that may be triggers for disinhibition (Verona & Patrick, 2015). Slow wave activity changes in EEGs have been associated with antisocial and borderline personality traits (Boland & Verduin, 2022).

Family Dynamics

Antisocial personality disorder frequently arises from a chaotic home environment. Parental deprivation during the first 5 years of life appears to be a critical predisposing factor in the development of antisocial personality disorder. Separation due to parental delinquency appears to be more highly correlated with the disorder than is parental loss from other causes.

Studies have shown that antisocial personality disorder in adulthood is highly associated with physical abuse and neglect, teasing, and lack of parental bonding in childhood (Cloninger & Svrikac, 2017; Kolla et al., 2013; Krastins et al., 2014). Severe physical abuse is particularly correlated to violent offending, triggering the development of a pattern of reactive aggression that is persistent over the lifetime (Kolla et al., 2013). The abuse also contributes to the development of antisocial behavior in that it provides a model for behavior, and it may result in injury to the child's central nervous system, thereby impairing the child's ability to function appropriately. Although a diagnosis of antisocial personality disorder is made only when the client is at least 18 years of age, these behavioral patterns first appear earlier in childhood and adolescence. When they are identified in children and adolescents, the diagnosis is *conduct disorder*, and the common symptoms are bullying, fighting, physical cruelty to animals, destruction of property, and theft, among others (APA, 2022). Evidence of a conduct disorder with onset before the age of 15 is, in fact, one of the diagnostic criteria for antisocial personality disorder. Whether better identification and early intervention might prevent more dangerous behavior in adulthood is yet to be determined through ongoing research.

Diagnosis and Outcome Identification

Nursing diagnoses are formulated from the data gathered during the assessment phase and with background knowledge regarding predisposing factors to the disorder. Table 22–4 presents a list of patient behaviors and the NANDA-I nursing diagnoses (Herdman et al., 2021) that correspond to those behaviors, which may be used in planning care for patients with antisocial personality disorder.

Outcome Criteria

The following criteria may be used for measurement of outcomes in the care of the patient with antisocial personality disorder. The patient:

- Discusses angry feelings with staff and in group sessions.
- Has not harmed self or others.
- Can rechannel hostility into socially acceptable behaviors.
- Follows rules and regulations of the therapy environment.
- Can verbalize which behaviors are not acceptable.
- Shows regard for the rights of others by delaying gratification of own desires when appropriate.
- Does not manipulate others in an attempt to increase feelings of self-worth.
- Verbalizes understanding of knowledge required to maintain basic health needs.

Planning and Implementation

Table 22–5 presents selected nursing diagnoses common to patients with antisocial personality disorder with short- and long-term goals, nursing interventions, and rationales for each.

Concept Care Mapping

The concept map care plan is a diagrammatic teaching and learning strategy that allows visualization of interrelationships between medical diagnoses, nursing diagnoses, assessment data, and treatments. An example of a concept map care plan for a patient with antisocial personality disorder is presented in Figure 22–2.

Evaluation

Reassessment is conducted to determine whether the nursing actions have been successful in achieving the objectives of care. Evaluation of the nursing actions for the patient with antisocial personality

TABLE 22–4 Assigning Nursing Diagnoses to Behaviors Commonly Associated With Antisocial Personality Disorder

BEHAVIORS	NURSING DIAGNOSES
Risk factors: Body language (e.g., rigid posture, clenching of fists and jaw, hyperactivity, pacing, breathlessness, threatening stances); cruelty to animals; rage reactions; history of childhood abuse; history of violence against others; impulsivity; substance abuse; negative role modeling; inability to tolerate frustration	**Risk for other-directed violence**
Disregard for societal norms and laws; absence of guilty feelings; inability to delay gratification; denial of obvious problems; grandiosity; hostile laughter; projection of blame and responsibility; ridicule of others; superior attitude toward others	**Defensive coping**
Manipulation of others to fulfill own desires; inability to form close, personal relationships; frequent lack of success in life events; passive-aggressiveness; overt aggressiveness (hiding feelings of low self-esteem)	**Chronic low-self esteem**
Inability to form a satisfactory, enduring, intimate relationship with another; dysfunctional interaction with others; use of unsuccessful social interaction behaviors	**Impaired social interaction**
Demonstration of inability to take responsibility for meeting basic health practices; history of lack of health-seeking behavior; demonstrated lack of knowledge regarding basic health practices; lack of expressed interest in improving health behaviors	**Ineffective health maintenance**

Table 22–5 | CARE PLAN FOR THE PATIENT WITH ANTISOCIAL PERSONALITY DISORDER

NURSING DIAGNOSIS: RISK FOR OTHER-DIRECTED VIOLENCE
RELATED TO: Unresolved anger

OUTCOME CRITERIA	NURSING INTERVENTIONS	RATIONALE
Short-Term Goals ■ Within 3 days, patient will discuss angry feelings and situations that precipitate hostility. ■ Patient will not harm others.	1. Convey an accepting attitude toward this patient. Feelings of rejection are undoubtedly familiar to the patient. Work on development of trust. Be honest, keep all promises, and convey the message that it is not the individual but the behavior that is unacceptable.	1. An attitude of acceptance promotes feelings of self-worth. Trust is the basis of a therapeutic relationship.
Long-Term Goal ■ Patient will not harm others.	2. Don't misconstrue charm or compliments as indicative of mutual trust. Maintain clear, professional boundaries.	2. Manipulation is characteristic of patients with antisocial personality disorder. Professional boundaries are essential to developing a therapeutic relationship.
	3. Maintain a low level of stimuli in the patient's environment (low lighting, few people, simple decor, low noise level).	3. An overly stimulating environment may increase agitation and promote aggressive behavior.
	4. Observe the patient's behavior frequently. Do this through routine activities and interactions; avoid appearing watchful and suspicious.	4. Close observation is required so that intervention can occur if needed to ensure the patient's (and others') safety.
	5. Remove all dangerous objects from the patient's environment so that patients may not purposefully or inadvertently use them to inflict harm to self or others.	5. Patient safety is a priority.
	6. Help the patient identify the true object of hostility (e.g., "You seem to be upset with . . ."). Encourage the patient to gradually verbalize hostile feelings.	6. Because of weak ego development, the patient may use the defense mechanism of displacement. Helping the patient recognize this in a nonthreatening manner may help reveal unresolved issues so that they may be confronted.
	7. Explore with the patient alternative ways of handling frustration (e.g., large motor skills that channel hostile energy into socially acceptable behavior).	7. Physically demanding activities help to relieve pent-up tension.
	8. The staff should maintain and convey a calm attitude toward the patient.	8. Anxiety is contagious and can be transferred from staff to patient. A calm attitude provides the patient with a feeling of safety and security.
	9. Have sufficient staff available to present a show of strength to the patient if necessary.	9. This conveys to the patient evidence of control over the situation and provides some physical security for the staff.

Continued

Table 22–5 | CARE PLAN FOR THE PATIENT WITH ANTISOCIAL PERSONALITY DISORDER—cont'd

OUTCOME CRITERIA	NURSING INTERVENTIONS	RATIONALE
	10. Administer tranquilizing medications as ordered by the physician or obtain an order if necessary. Monitor the patient for effectiveness of the medication as well as for appearance of adverse side effects.	10. Antianxiety agents (e.g., lorazepam, chlordiazepoxide, oxazepam) produce a calming effect and may help to allay hostile behaviors. (**NOTE:** Medications are not often prescribed for patients with antisocial personality disorder because of these individuals' strong susceptibility to substance use disorders.)
	11. If the patient is not calmed by "talking down" or with medication and becomes an imminent threat to the safety of others, use of mechanical restraints may be necessary. The avenue of the "least restrictive alternative" must be selected when planning interventions for a violent patient.	11. Restraints should be used only as a last resort, after all other interventions have been unsuccessful, and the patient is clearly at risk of harm to self or others.
	12. If restraint is deemed necessary, ensure that sufficient staff is available to assist. Follow protocol established by the institution.	12. Team intervention assures patient and staff safety.
	13. As agitation decreases, assess the patient's readiness for restraint removal or reduction. Remove one restraint at a time while assessing the patient's response.	13. This minimizes the risk of injury to patient and staff.

NURSING DIAGNOSIS: DEFENSIVE COPING
RELATED TO: Disrupted personal relationships, early childhood trauma
EVIDENCED BY: Violating rules, lying, and manipulation

OUTCOME CRITERIA	NURSING INTERVENTIONS	RATIONALE
Short-Term Goals ■ Within 24 hours after admission, patient will verbalize understanding of treatment, setting rules and regulations, and the consequences for violation of them. ■ Patient will verbalize personal responsibility for difficulties experienced in interpersonal relationships within (time period reasonable for patient).	1. At admission, the patient should be made aware of which behaviors are acceptable and which are not. Explain consequences of violation of the limits. A consequence must involve something of value to the patient. All staff must be consistent in enforcing these limits.	1. Because the patient cannot (or will not) impose own limits on maladaptive behaviors, these behaviors must be delineated and enforced by staff.
	2. If consequences are warranted, they should be administered in a matter-of-fact manner immediately following the infraction. Undesirable consequences may help to decrease repetition of these behaviors.	2. Timely response to rule infractions reinforces acceptable versus nonacceptable behavior.
	3. Explanations must be concise, concrete, and clear with little or no capacity for misinterpretation. This involves a step-by-step, "either/or" approach on the unit (either you do [don't do] this, or this will occur).	3. This minimizes the patient's potential to manipulate or rationalize unacceptable behaviour and reinforces that there are consequences for unacceptable behaviors.

Table 22–5 | CARE PLAN FOR THE PATIENT WITH ANTISOCIAL PERSONALITY DISORDER—cont'd

OUTCOME CRITERIA	NURSING INTERVENTIONS	RATIONALE
Long-Term Goals ■ By the time of discharge from treatment, patient will be able to cope more adaptively by delaying gratification of own desires and following rules and regulations of the treatment setting. ■ By the time of discharge from treatment, patient will demonstrate ability to interact with others without becoming defensive, rationalizing behaviors, or manipulating others.	4. Do not attempt to coax or convince the patient to do the "right thing." Do not use the words "You should (or shouldn't) . . ."; instead, use the words "You will be expected to . . ."	4. Communicating in a matter-of-fact manner reduces the potential for misinterpretation about expected behaviors.
	5. Provide positive feedback or reward for acceptable behaviors.	5. Positive reinforcement enhances self-esteem and encourages repetition of desirable behaviors.
	6. In the context of a therapeutic milieu, assist the patient to delay gratification; begin to increase the length of time requirement for acceptable behavior in order to achieve the reward. For example, 2 hours of acceptable behavior may be exchanged for a phone call; 4 hours of acceptable behavior for 2 hours of television; 1 day of acceptable behavior for a recreational therapy bowling activity; 5 days of acceptable behavior for a weekend pass.	6. A milieu unit provides the appropriate environment for the patient with antisocial personality disorder. A community environment with rules and expectations and consequences for unacceptable behaviour sessions emulates the type of societal situation in which the patient must learn to live. Feedback from peers is often more effective than confrontation from an authority figure. The patient learns to follow the rules of the group as a positive step in the progression toward internalizing the rules of society.
	7. Help the patient to gain insight into their own behavior. For example, the patient's thinking may be reflected in statements such as "The owner of this store has so much money, he'll never miss the little bit I take. He has everything, and I have nothing. It's not fair! I deserve to have some of what he has." Patients must come to understand that certain behaviors will not be tolerated within the society and that severe consequences will be imposed on those individuals who refuse to comply.	7. The patient may rationalize to such an extent that they deny that their behavior is inappropriate. Note, though, that patients must want to change behavior before they can be helped. One of the difficulties posed in interventions for personality disorders is that often the behaviors are ego-syntonic—in other words, patients may not perceive these behaviors as requiring change.
	8. Talk about past behaviors with the patient. Discuss which behaviors are acceptable by societal norms and which are not. Help the patient identify ways in which they have exploited others and the benefits versus consequences of previous behavior. Explore the patient's insights into feelings associated with their behavior.	8. This approach conveys caring and concern and promotes the development of insight. Helping the patient to connect behaviors to specific feelings may reduce the need for defensive coping. Promoting self-awareness helps the patient gain insight into their own behavior.
	9. Throughout the relationship with the patient, maintain an attitude of "It is not you but your behavior that is unacceptable."	9. An attitude of acceptance promotes feelings of dignity and self-worth.

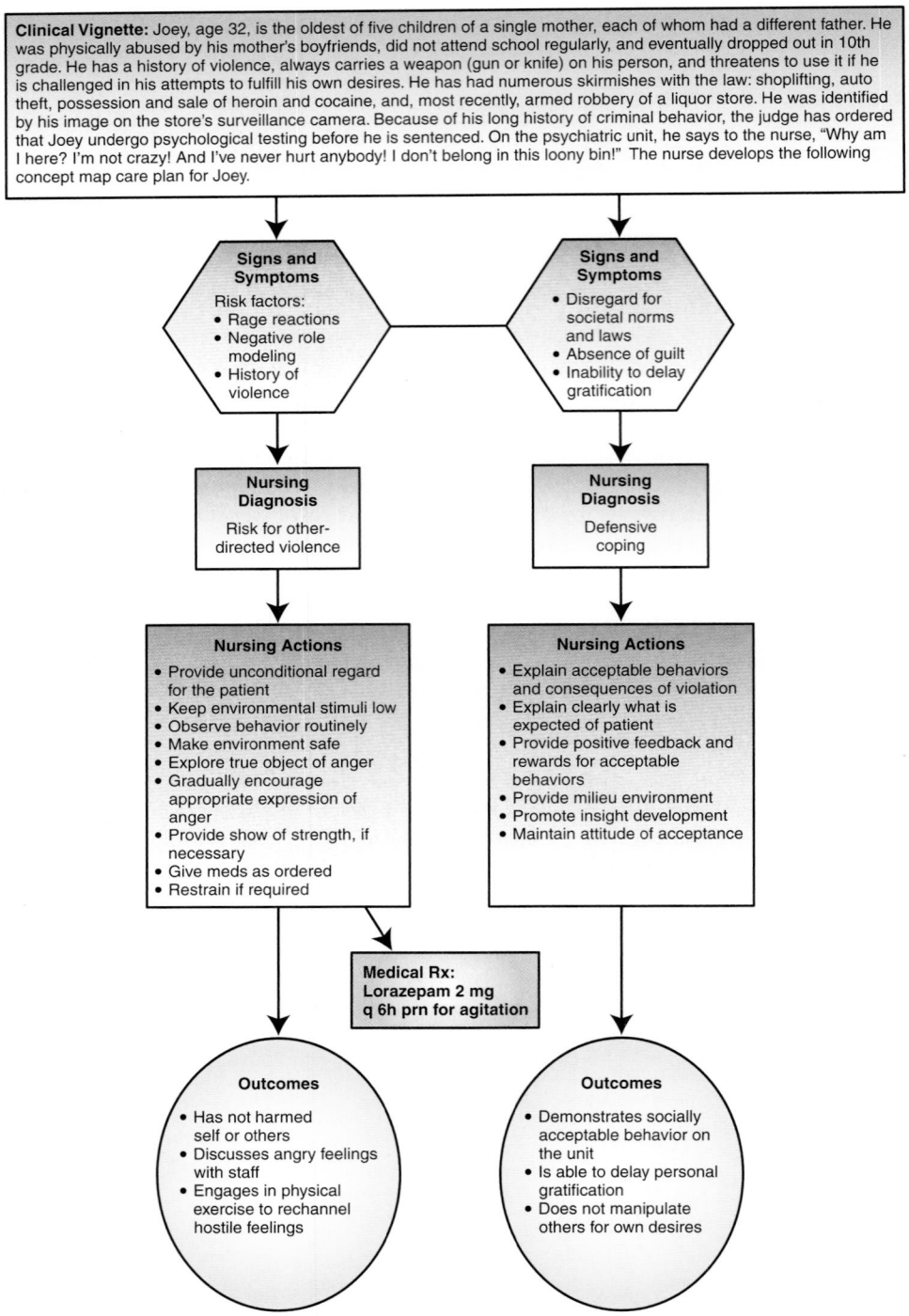

FIGURE 22–2 Concept map care plan for a patient with antisocial personality disorder.

disorder may be facilitated by gathering information using the following types of questions. Has the patient:

- Recognized when anger is getting out of control?
- Sought out staff instead of expressing anger in an inappropriate manner?
- Used other sources for rechanneling anger (e.g., physical activities)?
- Expressed anger without physical aggression or harm to others?
- Followed rules and regulations of the therapeutic milieu with little or no reminding?

- Verbalized which behaviors are appropriate and which are not?
- Expressed a desire to change?
- Demonstrated ability to delay gratifying own desires in deference to those of others when appropriate?
- Refrained from manipulating others to fulfill own desires?
- Fulfilled activities of daily living willingly and independently?
- Verbalized methods of achieving and maintaining optimal wellness?
- Identified community resources from which to seek assistance with daily living and health-care needs when required?

Treatment Modalities

Treatment of individuals with personality disorders is difficult. Personality characteristics are learned very early in life and may be genetically influenced. Many of the symptoms of a personality disorder are viewed by the individual as ego-syntonic, so there may be little motivation to seek treatment or to explore change. It is not surprising, then, that these enduring patterns of behavior may take years to change, if change occurs at all. However, we now understand the personality as a dynamic, adaptive system and, as such, may be modifiable. Cloninger and Svrakic (2017) offer the description of personality as a "multidimensional interaction among temperament, character, and psyche" (p. 2141) and one that can undergo maturation through a complex process of developing awareness of those interactions. Zimmerman (2017) stresses that screening is imperative to appropriate treatment. In particular, BPD is a comorbid condition in 40% of hospitalized psychiatric patients, but it often goes undetected. Although extended inpatient hospitalization for treatment of personality disorders has historically been believed to be associated with adverse events and deterioration, Fowler and associates (2018) found that longer-term stays, of 40 days or more, resulted in significant improvement for patients with BPD. Treatment programs such as these, however, are in short supply. The main treatment modalities for all personality disorders are psychosocial and pharmacological, but most of the available evidence comes from studies of borderline and antisocial personality disorders.

Comorbid conditions are common in most personality disorders, and there is evidence that treating these conditions may have positive outcomes. For example, in a review of the literature, Hatchett (2015) identifies that psychosocial interventions for clients with antisocial personality disorder have lacked both treatment efficacy and clinical utility; however, treatment of comorbid substance use disorder has demonstrated positive outcomes. Furthermore, when the client with antisocial personality disorder has comorbid depression, the individual is more likely to persevere with treatment. This may be related to the fact that symptoms of depression are considered undesirable (not ego-syntonic) and therefore may promote interest in change or improvement. Hatchett notes that this review should not be interpreted as meaning that a client's personality disorder is untreatable. Instead, Hatchett cites Skeem and associates (2011) as saying this client should be identified as "high risk" and requiring intensive treatment to maximize public safety.

While Hatchett (2015) reviewed the literature specifically related to treatment for antisocial personality disorders, other researchers identify in their literature reviews that, for personality disorders in general, there is strong evidence of the effectiveness of psychotherapeutic interventions (Papaioannou et al., 2013; Stoffers et al., 2012), although, again, the bulk of research focuses on borderline and antisocial personality disorders (Bateman et al., 2015).

Other researchers identify that treatment focused on tackling the defense mechanisms associated with each of the personality disorders may be a more effective way to mediate improvement (Perry et al., 2013). For example, therapy focused on exploring the dissociation that is common in patients with BPD or focusing on exploring the defense mechanism of devaluing others, as seen in clients with antisocial personality, may promote overall improvement in symptoms. There is general agreement that all treatment modalities for personality disorders require intensive and longer-term plans of care. Selection of intervention is generally based on the area of greatest dysfunction, such as cognition, affect, behavior, or interpersonal relations. Following is a brief description of various types of therapies and the disorders to which they are customarily suited.

Individual Psychotherapy

Depending on the therapeutic goals, psychotherapy for individuals with personality disorders may be time-limited interpersonal psychotherapy, or it may involve long-term psychoanalytic therapy. Interpersonal psychotherapy may be particularly appropriate because personality disorders largely reflect problems in interpersonal relationship skills.

Long-term psychotherapy attempts to understand and modify the maladjusted behaviors, cognition, and affects of clients with personality disorders that dominate their personal lives and relationships.

Milieu or Group Therapy

This treatment is especially appropriate for individuals with antisocial personality disorder who respond more adaptively to support and feedback from peers. In milieu or group therapy, feedback from peers is more effective than in one-to-one interaction with a therapist.

Group therapy—particularly homogenous supportive groups that emphasize the development of social skills—may be helpful in overcoming social anxiety and developing interpersonal trust and rapport in clients with avoidant personality disorder.

Cognitive Behavior Therapy (CBT)

Behavioral strategies offer reinforcement for positive change. Social skills training and assertiveness training teach alternative ways to deal with frustration. Cognitive strategies help the client recognize and correct distorted and irrational thinking patterns. Davidson and colleagues (2009) found that the addition of cognitive behavior therapy (CBT) to usual treatment for clients with antisocial personality disorders afforded a reduction in both verbal and physical aggression symptoms. There is also some limited evidence that CBT is beneficial for clients with schizotypal personality disorder (Bateman et al., 2015).

Dialectical Behavior Therapy (DBT)

Dialectical behavior therapy (DBT) is a type of psychotherapy that was originally developed by Marsha Linehan, PhD, specifically as a treatment for the chronic self-injurious and parasuicidal behavior of clients with BPD. It is rooted in a belief that the primary problem for these clients is emotional dysregulation (a kind of emotional reactivity to perceived threats), and it has become a well-established treatment for clients with BPD. It is a complex, eclectic treatment that combines the concepts of cognitive, behavioral, and interpersonal therapies with Eastern mindfulness practices.

The four primary modes of treatment in DBT include the following:

1. ***Group skills training:*** These groups focus on teaching skills considered relevant to the particular problems experienced by people with BPD, such as core mindfulness skills, interpersonal effectiveness skills, emotion modulation skills, and distress tolerance skills.
2. ***Individual psychotherapy:*** Dysfunctional behavioral patterns, personal motivation, and skills strengthening are addressed in weekly sessions.
3. ***Telephone contact:*** The therapist is available to the client by telephone, usually on a 24-hour basis, but according to limits set by the therapist. The purpose is to provide appropriate support, to counter abandonment fears, and to reduce episodes of self-harming behaviors.
4. ***Therapist consultation and team meeting:*** Therapists meet regularly to review their work with their clients. These meetings are focused specifically on providing support for each other, keeping the therapists motivated, and providing effective treatment to their clients. DBT has been well studied, and the evidence supports the benefits of this treatment for clients with BPD. O'Connell and Dowling (2014), citing a systematic review of seven studies (Binks et al., 2006), report that:

> Despite the difficulty in treating people with BPD, if the person with BPD is engaged in their treatment plan, there was a reduction in anxiety levels, depression, self-harm, hospital admission, and the use of prescribed medication. (p. 522)

This method of treatment is now being used with other disorders, including substance use disorders, eating disorders, schizophrenia, and PTSD (Boland & Verduin, 2022). Bateman and colleagues (2015) caution, however, that of the many interventions that have been specialized for the treatment of personality disorders, improvement is more often evidenced by symptom reduction; the interventions that have been specialized for the treatment of personality disorders have failed to produce significant improvements in social functioning.

Psychoanalytic Therapies

Two psychoanalytically oriented approaches that have demonstrated benefit in the treatment of BPD include mentalization therapy and transference therapy. Mentalization therapy focuses on assisting the client to improve their ability to reflect on and understand internal states (their own and others) and how those impact behavior so that the client can use mentalization when they are experiencing stressful situations and ultimately improve their ability to relate to others (Yasgur, 2017). Transference therapy seeks to use the transference that occurs in a client-therapist relationship to help the client improve self-perception and relationship skills.

Psychopharmacology

Psychopharmacology may be helpful in some instances. Although these medications have no effect in the direct treatment of the disorder itself, some symptomatic relief can be achieved. Among the cluster A disorders, there has been some limited evidence of the benefits of antipsychotic medication in the treatment of schizotypal personality disorder, but the risk-to-benefit ratio is unclear (Bateman et al., 2015).

For the treatment of BPD, symptom-targeted pharmacotherapy has been identified as an important adjunct. Antipsychotic medications show some benefits in treating cognitive-perceptual symptoms, selective serotonin reuptake inhibitors show some benefit in treating emotional dysregulation, and mood-stabilizing agents have shown some benefit in treating emotional dysregulation and impulsive aggressive symptoms (Bateman et al., 2015). Lithium may be of benefit to the patient with narcissistic personality disorder who has mood swings (Boland & Verduin, 2022).

For antisocial personality disorder, pharmacotherapy is generally not recommended unless it is being used to treat a comorbid condition although anticonvulsants may be of benefit to treat aggressive behavior, especially in the presence of abnormal electroencephalogram (EEG) waveforms (Boland & Verduin, 2022).

Caution must be used when prescribing medications outside the structured setting because of the high risk for substance use disorders in this population. In addition, benzodiazepines should be avoided, particularly in patients with BPD, because of the increased risk for disinhibition, which may increase acting out and self-harm behaviors (Black, 2021).

CASE STUDY AND SAMPLE CARE PLAN

NURSING HISTORY AND ASSESSMENT

Anthony, age 34, has been admitted to the psychiatric unit with a diagnosis of antisocial personality disorder. He was recently arrested and convicted of armed robbery of a convenience store and attempted murder of the store clerk. Due to the actions of the store clerk, who quickly alerted police, and to the store surveillance camera, Anthony was identified and apprehended within hours of the crime. The judge has ordered physical, neurological, and psychiatric evaluations before sentencing Anthony.

Anthony was physically and psychologically abused as a child by his alcoholic father. He was suspended from high school because of failing grades and habitual truancy. He has a long history of arrests, beginning with shoplifting at age 7 and progressing in adolescence to burglary, auto theft, and sexual assault and finally to armed robbery and attempted murder. He was out on probation when he committed his latest crime.

On the psychiatric unit, Anthony is loud, belligerent, and uncooperative. When Julie, his admitting nurse, arrives to work the evening shift on Anthony's second hospital day, he says to her, "I'm so glad you are finally here. You are the best nurse on the unit. I can't talk to anyone but you. These people are nothing but a bunch of jerks around here . . . and that includes staff as well as patients! Maybe you and I could walk down to the coffee shop together later. Are you married? I'd sure like to get to know you better after I get out of this nut house!"

NURSING DIAGNOSES OUTCOME IDENTIFICATION

From the assessment data, the nurse develops the following nursing diagnoses for Anthony:

1. **Risk for other-directed violence** related to history of violence against others and history of childhood abuse
   a. **Short-Term Goals:**
      - Patient will discuss angry feelings and situations that precipitate hostility.
      - Patient will not harm others.
   b. **Long-Term Goal:** Patient will not harm others.
2. **Defensive coping** related to low self-esteem, dysfunctional nuclear family, underdeveloped ego and superego, evidenced by absence of guilt feelings, disregard for societal laws and norms, inability to delay gratification, superior attitude toward others, denial of problems, and projection of blame and responsibility
   a. **Short-Term Goal:** Patient will verbalize understanding of unit rules and regulations and consequences for violation of them.
   b. **Long-Term Goals:**
      - Patient will be able to delay gratification and follow rules and regulations of the unit.
      - Patient will verbalize personal responsibility for own actions and behaviors.

PLANNING AND IMPLEMENTATION

RISK FOR OTHER-DIRECTED VIOLENCE

The following nursing interventions have been identified for Anthony:

1. Develop a trusting relationship with Anthony by conveying an accepting attitude. Ensure that he understands it is not *him* but *his behavior* that is unacceptable.
2. Try to keep excess stimuli out of the environment. Speak to Anthony in a calm, quiet voice.
3. Observe Anthony's behavior regularly. Do so through routine activity so that he doesn't become suspicious and angry about being watched. This is important so that if hostile and aggressive behaviors are observed, intervention may prevent harm to Anthony, staff members, and/or other patients.

Continued

CASE STUDY AND SAMPLE CARE PLAN—cont'd

4. Sit with Anthony and encourage him to talk about his anger and hostile feelings. Help him understand where these feelings originate and who the true target of the hostility is.
5. Help him develop adaptive ways of dealing with frustration, such as exercise and other physical activities.
6. Administer tranquilizing medication, as ordered by the physician.
7. If Anthony should become out of control and mechanical restraints become necessary, ensure that sufficient staff is available to intervene. Do not use restraints as a punishment but only as a protective measure for Anthony and the other patients.

DEFENSIVE COPING

The following nursing interventions have been identified for Anthony:

1. Explain to Anthony which of his behaviors are acceptable on the unit and which are not. Simply state that unacceptable behaviors will not be tolerated.
2. Determine appropriate consequences for violation of these limits (e.g., no TV or movies; no phone calls; time-out room). Ensure that all staff members follow through with these consequences.
3. Recognize that many of these patients use charm and compliments to manipulate others. Explain to Anthony that you will not accept these types of comments from him, and if they continue, impose consequences.
4. Encourage Anthony to talk about his past misdeeds. Try to help him understand how he would feel if someone treated him in the manner that he has treated others.

EVALUATION

The outcome criteria for Anthony has only partially been met. Personality characteristics such as those of Anthony's are deep-rooted and enduring. He is not likely to change. Unless testing reveals a serious medical problem, Anthony will no doubt go to prison for most of the rest of his life. During his time on the psychiatric unit, harm to self and others has been avoided. He has discussed his anger and hostile feelings with Julie and other staff members. He continues to become belligerent when told that he cannot smoke on the unit and must wait for someone to escort him to the smoking area. He yells at the other patients and calls them "nut cases." He refuses to take responsibility for his actions and blames negative behavioral outcomes on others. He has begun a regular exercise program in the fitness room and receives positive feedback from the staff for this attempt to integrate healthier coping strategies.

Summary and Key Points

- Clients with personality disorders present with some of the most challenging symptoms that health-care workers are likely to encounter.
- Personality characteristics are formed very early in life and are difficult to change because they are complex in nature and the individual with personality disorder traits may not recognize the need to change. Some clinicians believe that the therapeutic approach is not to focus on changing the characteristics but rather to focus on decreasing the inflexibility of the maladaptive traits and reduce their interference with everyday functioning and meaningful relationships.
- The concept of a personality disorder has been present throughout the history of medicine. Attempts to establish a classification system for these disorders have been problematic.
- The *DSM-5-TR* identifies 10 individual personality disorders: antisocial, avoidant, borderline, histrionic, dependent, narcissistic, obsessive-compulsive, paranoid, schizoid, and schizotypal.
- Nursing care of the patient with a personality disorder is accomplished using the steps of the nursing process.
- Other treatment modalities include interpersonal psychotherapy, psychoanalytical psychotherapy (including mentalization and transference therapy), milieu or group therapy, cognitive behavior therapy (CBT), dialectical behavior therapy (DBT), and psychopharmacology.
- Individuals with borderline personality disorder (BPD) may enter the health-care system because of their instability and frequent attempts at self-destructive behavior.
- The individual with antisocial personality disorder may become part of the health-care system to avoid legal consequences or because of a court order for psychological evaluation.
- Nurses who work in all types of clinical settings should be familiar with the characteristics associated with personality disorders.
- Nurses working with patients who manifest symptoms of personality disorders, particularly BPD and antisocial personality disorder, must be skilled in clear and consistent communication, effective limit setting, and maintaining professional boundaries. Trauma-informed care is foundational in assessment and intervention.

Review Questions

Select the answer that is most appropriate for each of the following questions:

1. A client diagnosed with BPD manipulates the staff in an effort to fulfill their own desires. All of the following may be examples of manipulative behaviors *except*:
   a. Refusal to stay in room alone, stating, "It's so lonely."
   b. Asking the nurse for cigarettes after 30 minutes, knowing that the assigned nurse has explained the client must wait 1 hour.
   c. Stating to the nurse, "I really like having you for my nurse. You're the best one around here."
   d. Making superficial cuts to their arms after discussing discharge plans with physician.
2. A client on the psychiatric unit has a diagnosis of antisocial personality disorder. Which characteristic is consistent with this diagnosis?
   a. Lack of guilt for wrongdoing
   b. Insight into own behavior
   c. Ability to learn from past experiences
   d. Compliance with authority
3. A nurse on the psychiatric unit documents that the client is using "splitting" behaviors with staff. This should be interpreted to mean that the client is exhibiting what behavior?
   a. Trying to keep the staff away from other clients
   b. Characterizing staff members as either all good or all bad
   c. Having brief psychotic episodes
   d. Manifesting two or more distinct subpersonalities when communicating with staff
4. According to researchers, which is a common theme in the health history of the client with BPD?
   a. Autism
   b. Attention deficit-hyperactivity disorder
   c. Positive and fulfilling interpersonal relationships
   d. Early childhood trauma
5. Which behavioral pattern is characteristic of individuals with narcissistic personality disorder?
   a. Overly self-centered and exploitative of others
   b. Suspicious and mistrustful of others
   c. Rule conscious and disapproving of change
   d. Anxious and socially isolated
6. Which behavioral pattern is characteristic of individuals with schizoid personality disorder?
   a. Belittling themselves and their abilities
   b. A lifelong pattern of social withdrawal
   c. Suspiciousness and mistrust of others
   d. Overreacting inappropriately to minor stimuli

Clinical Judgment Questions

7. A client with a diagnosis of BPD often exhibits alternating clinging and distancing behaviors. Which is the most appropriate nursing intervention for the client with this type of behavior?
   a. Encourage the client to establish trust in one staff person with whom all therapeutic interaction should take place.
   b. Secure a verbal contract from the client to discontinue these behaviors.
   c. Withdraw attention if these behaviors continue.
   d. Rotate staff members who work with the client so that the client will learn to relate to more than one person.

Continued

8. A client diagnosed with antisocial personality disorder approaches the nurse and says "You're so cute, are you married?" Which is the most appropriate response by the nurse?
   a. "I'm married but that's none of your business."
   b. "Let's talk about your love life instead."
   c. "Thank-you so much for the compliment but I'm married."
   d. "Our relationship is strictly professional. It's not appropriate for us to have that kind of discussion."
9. A client with BPD reports to the nurse that they are having abdominal pain and is requesting pain medication. Which action by the nurse is a priority?
   a. Explore alternative pain management strategies
   b. Confront the client about their manipulation to try to get drugs
   c. Assess the client's pain in more detail
   d. Set limits on the client's attempts to cling to the nurse
10. A male client with antisocial personality disorder was found on the bed in a female client's room. When instructed to leave the room, the client states, "I'm sick of you telling me what I can and can't do. If I want to carry on a relationship with one of these ladies, it's my right. I'll do exactly as I please!" Which action by the nurse is a priority at this point?
   a. Reassure the client that he will have plenty of opportunities with women after he is discharged.
   b. Reinforce the rules of the treatment program that all clients are expected to follow.
   c. Escort the client to a seclusion room.
   d. Establish a trusting relationship by telling the client that an exception will be made just this once.

IMPLICATIONS FOR EVIDENCE-BASED PRACTICE

Yen, S., Peters, J. R., Nishar, S., Grilo, C. M., Sanislow, C. A., Shea, M. T., Zanarini, M. C., McGlashan, T. H., Morey, L. C., & Skodol, A. E. (2020). Association of borderline personality disorder criteria with suicide attempts: Findings from the collaborative longitudinal study of personality disorders over 10 years of follow-up. *JAMA Psychiatry, 78*(2), 187–194. https//doi.org/10.1001/jamapsychiatry.2020.3598

DESCRIPTION OF THE STUDY: This longitudinal follow-up study of treatment-seeking individuals (n = 701) with personality disorders sought to identify factors associated with risk for suicide behavior, including suicide attempts. The intent was to identify those risk factors that could inform interventions. Participants were assessed annually using semi-structured diagnostic interviews and a variety of self-report measures for up to 10 years.

RESULTS OF THE STUDY: Of all disorders, BPD emerged as the most robust factor associated with prospectively observed suicide attempt(s) (odds ratio, even after controlling for significant demographic [sex, employment, and education] and clinical [childhood sexual abuse, alcohol use disorder, substance use disorder, and posttraumatic stress disorder] factors. Among BPD criteria, identity disturbance [inconsistency in beliefs, values, and actions]), chronic feelings of emptiness, and frantic efforts to avoid abandonment emerged as significant independent factors associated with suicide attempt(s) over follow-up.

IMPLICATIONS FOR NURSING PRACTICE: BPD has long been identified as a disorder associated with frequent suicidal behavior. Understanding the features that may increase risk for these behaviors can guide the nurse's assessment and interventions directed toward suicide prevention.

TEST YOUR CLINICAL REASONING AND CLINICAL JUDGMENT SKILLS

Dana, age 32, was diagnosed with BPD when she was 26 years old. Her husband took her to the emergency department when he walked into the bathroom and found her cutting her legs with a razor blade. At that time, assessment revealed that Dana had a long history of self-mutilation, which she had carefully hidden from her husband and others. Dana began long-term psychoanalytical psychotherapy on an outpatient basis. Therapy revealed that Dana had been physically and sexually abused as a child by both her mother and her father, both now deceased. She admitted to having chronic depression and her husband related episodes of rage reactions. Dana has been hospitalized on the psychiatric unit for a week because of suicidal ideations. The psychiatrist has ordered that she is allowed to leave the unit on pass to keep a dental appointment that she made a number of weeks ago. She has just returned to the unit and says to her nurse, "I just took 20 Desyrel while I was sitting in my car in the parking lot."

Answer the following questions related to Dana:

1. The nurse is well acquainted with Dana and believes that her suicide attempt is a manipulative gesture. How should the nurse handle this situation?
2. What is the priority nursing diagnosis for Dana?
3. Dana likes to "split" the staff into "good guys" and "bad guys." What is the most important intervention for splitting by a person with BPD?

Communication Exercises

1. Nathan, age 37, has been admitted to the hospital for a psychiatric evaluation after being arrested for armed robbery of a convenience store. He has a history of encounters with law enforcement since early adolescence. He has been diagnosed with antisocial personality disorder. Nathan says to the nurse, "Hey pretty lady! Where have you been all my life?"
   How would the nurse respond appropriately to this statement by Nathan?
2. "I really got a bum rap! I had no intentions of hurting anyone. The gun only had one bullet in it! I just wanted to scare that clerk into giving me a few bucks! Just my bad luck an off-duty cop had to walk in about that time."
   How would the nurse respond appropriately to this statement by Nathan?
3. "You're really cute. Are you married? I'm pretty sure my lawyer can get me out of this rap, and I'll be a free man! Why don't you give me your phone number and I'll call you sometime. We could go out and have some fun!"
   How would the nurse respond appropriately to this statement by Nathan?

MOVIE CONNECTIONS

Taxi Driver (Schizoid personality) ▪ *One Flew Over the Cuckoo's Nest* (Antisocial) ▪ *The Boston Strangler* (Antisocial) ▪ *Just Cause* (Antisocial) ▪ *The Dream Team* (Antisocial) ▪ *Goodfellas* (Antisocial) ▪ *Fatal Attraction* (BPD) ▪ *Play Misty for Me* (BPD) ▪ *Girl, Interrupted* (BPD) ▪ *Gone With the Wind* (Histrionic) ▪ *Wall Street* (Narcissistic) ▪ *The Odd Couple* (Obsessive-compulsive) ▪ *Welcome to Me* (BPD)

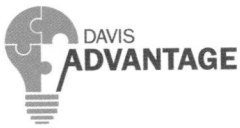

Go to **Davis Advantage** to complete your learning: strengthen understanding, apply your knowledge, and prepare for the Next Gen NCLEX®.

References

American Psychiatric Association. (2022). *Diagnostic and statistical manual of mental disorders* (5th ed., text rev.).

Anderson, J. L., Sellbom, M., Wygant, D. B., Salekin, R. T., & Krueger, R. F. (2014). Examining the association between *DSM-5* section III antisocial personality traits and psychopathy in community and university samples. *Journal of Personality Disorders, 28*(5), 675–697.

Bateman, A. W., Gunderson, J., & Mulder, R. (2015). Treatment of personality disorder. *Lancet, 385*, 735–743.

Bertsch, K., & Herpertz, S. C. (2018). Oxytocin and borderline personality disorder. *Current Topics in Behavioral Neurosciences, 35*, 499–514. https://doi.org/10.1007/7854_2017_26

Binks, C., Fenton, M., McCarthy, L., Lee, T., Adams, C., & Duggan, C. (2006). Psychological therapies for people with BPDs [Review]. *Cochrane Database of Systematic Reviews.* https://doi.org/10.1002/14651858.CD005652

Black, D. (2021). A clinical approach to pharmacotherapy for personality disorders. *Current Psychiatry, 20*(4), 27–32.

Black, D., Pfhol, B., & Blum, M. (2011). Attitudes towards BPD: A survey of 706 mental health clinicians. *CNS Spectrums, 16*(3), 67–74.

Boland, R., & Verduin, M. L. (2022). *Kaplan & Sadock's synopsis of psychiatry* (P. Ruiz, Ed.). (12th ed.). Wolters Kluwer.

Bornstein, R. F., Bianucci, V., Fishman, D. P., & Biars, J. W. (2014). Toward a firmer foundation for *DSM-5.1*: Domains of impairment in *DSM IV/DSM-5* personality disorders. *Journal of Personality Disorders, 28*(2), 212–224.

Cloninger, C. R., & Svrakic, D. M. (2017). Personality disorders. In B. J. Sadock, V. A. Sadock, & P. Ruiz (Eds.), *Comprehensive textbook of psychiatry* (10th ed., pp. 2126–2176). Wolters Kluwer.

Davidson, K. M., Tyrer, P., Tata, P., Cook, D., Gumely, A., Ford, I., Walker, A., Bezlyak, V., Sievewright, H., Robertson, H., & Crawford, M. J. (2009). Cognitive behaviour therapy for violent men with antisocial personality disorder in the community: An exploratory randomized controlled trial. *Psychological Medicine, 39*(4), 569–577. https://doi.org/10.1017/S0033291708004066

Domes, G., Ower, N., von Dawans, B., Spengler, F. B., Ziobek, I., Bohus, M., Matthies, S. Philipsen, A., & Heinrichs, S. (2019). Effects of intranasal oxytocin administration on empathy and approach motivation in women with borderline personality disorder: A randomized controlled trial. *Translational Psychiatry, 9*(328). https://doi.org/10.1038/s41398-019-0658-4

Ford, J. D., & Courtois, C. A. (2014). Complex PTSD, affect dysregulation, and borderline personality disorder. *Borderline Personality Disorder and Emotion Dysregulation, 1*(9), 1–7. https://doi.org/10.1186/2051-6673-1-9

Fowler, J. C., Clapp, J. D., Madan, A., Allen, J. G., Frueh, C., Fonagy, P., & Oldham, J. M. (2018). A naturalistic longitudinal study of extended inpatient treatment for adults with borderline personality disorder: An examination of treatment response, remission and deterioration. *Journal of Affective Disorders, 235*, 323–331. https://doi.org/10.1016/j.jad.2017.12.054

Gjerde, L. C., Czajkowski, N., Røysamb, E., Ørstavik, R. E., Knudsen, G. P., Østby, K., Torgersen, S., Myers, J., Kendler, K. S., & Reichborn-Kjennerud, T. (2012). The heritability of avoidant and dependent personality disorder assessed by personal interview and questionnaire. *Acta Psychiatrica Scandinavica, 126*(6), 448–457. https://doi.org/10.1111/j.1600-0447.2012.01862.x

Gregory, C. (2021). *Narcissistic personality disorder: A guide to signs, diagnosis, and treatment.* https://www.psycom.net/personality-disorders/narcissistic

Hatchett, G. (2015). Treatment guidelines for clients with antisocial personality disorder. *Journal of Mental Health Counseling, 37*(1), 15–27.

Helleman, M., Goossens, P. J., Kaasenbrood, A., & Van Achterberg, T. (2014). Experiences of patients with BPD with the brief admission intervention: A phenomenological study. *International Journal of Mental Health Nursing, 23*, 442–450.

Herdman, T. H., Kamitsuru, S., & Lopes, C. T. (Eds.). (2021). *NANDA-I, Inc. nursing diagnoses: Definitions and classification, 2021–2023.* Thieme.

Hodges, M., Godbout, N., Briere, J., Lanktree, C., Gilbert, A., & Kletzka, N. T. (2013). Cumulative trauma and symptom complexity in children: A path analysis. *Child Abuse and Neglect, 37*, 891–898.

Jiang, W., Shi, F., Liao, J., Liu, H., Wang, T., Shen, C., Shen, H., Hu, D., Wang, W., & Shen, D. (2017). Disrupted functional connectome in antisocial personality disorder. *Brain Imaging and Behavior, 11*(4), 1071–1084. https://doi.org/10.1007/s11682-016-9572-z

Kolla, N. J., Malcolm, C., Attard, S., Arenovich, T., Blackwood, N., & Hodgins, S. (2013). Childhood maltreatment and aggressive behavior in violent offenders with psychopathy. *Canadian Journal of Psychiatry, 58*(8), 487–494.

Krastins, A., Francis, A. J., Field, A. M., & Carr, S. N. (2014). Childhood predictors of adult antisocial personality disorder symptomatology. *Australian Psychologist, 49*, 142–150.

Lawn, S., Diped, B. A., & McMahon, J. (2015). Experience of family carers of people diagnosed with BPD. *Journal of Psychiatric and Mental Health Nursing, 22*, 234–243.

Lis, E., Greenfield, B., Henry, M., Guilé, J. M., & Dougherty, G. (2007). Neuroimaging and genetics of borderline personality disorder: A review. *Journal of Psychiatry & Neuroscience, 32*(3), 162–173.

Lubit, R. H. (2018). BPD. *Medscape.* http://emedicine.medscape.com/article/913575-overview

MacIntosh, H. B., Godbout, N., & Dubash, N. (2015). BPD: Disorder of trauma or personality, a review of the empirical literature. *Canadian Psychology, 56*(2), 227–241.

Mak, A. D., & Lam, L. C. (2013). Neurocognitive profiles of people with borderline personality disorder. *Current Opinion in Psychiatry, 26*(1), 90–96. https://doi.org/10.1097/YCO.0b013e32835b57a9

Mayo Clinic. (2021). *Narcissistic personality disorder.* https://www.mayoclinic.org/diseases-conditions/narcissistic-personality-disorder/symptoms-causes/syc-20366662

McNee, L., Donogue, C., & Coppola, A. M. (2014). A team approach to BPD. *Mental Health Practice, 17*(10), 33–35.

Moore, A. A., Blair, R. J., Hettema, J. M., & Roberson-Nay, R. (2019). The genetic underpinnings of callous-unemotional traits: A systematic research review. *Neuroscience and Biobehavioral Reviews, 100*, 85–97. https://doi.org/10.1016/j.neubiorev.2019.02.018

O'Connell, B., & Dowling, M. (2014). Dialectical behavior therapy (DBT) in the treatment of BPD. *Journal of Psychiatric and Mental Health Nursing, 21*, 518–525.

Ouellet-Morin, I., Côté, S. M., Vitaro, F., Hébert, M., Carbonneau, R., Lacourse, E., & Tremblay, R. E. (2016). Effects of the *MAOA* gene and levels of exposure to violence on antisocial outcomes. *British Journal of Psychiatry, 208*(1), 42–48. https://doi.org/10.1192/bjp.bp.114.162081

Papaioannou, D., Brazier, J., & Parry, G. (2013). How to measure quality of life for cost effectiveness analyses or personality disorders: A systematic review. *Journal of Personality Disorders, 27*(3), 383–401.

Perry, J. C., Presniak, M. D., & Olson, T. R. (2013). Defense mechanisms in schizotypal, borderline, antisocial, and narcissistic personality disorders. *Psychiatry, 76*(1), 32–52.

Pier, K., Marin, L. K., Wilsnack, J., & Goodman, M. (2016). The neurobiology of borderline personality disorder. *Psychiatric Times, 33*(3). http://www.psychiatrictimes.com/borderline-personality/neurobiology-borderline-personality-disorder/page/0/2

Quenneville, A. F., Badouda, D., Nicastro, R., Jermann, F., Favre, S., Kung, A., Euler, S., Perroud, N., & Richard-Lepouriel, H. (2020). Internalized stigmatization in borderline personality disorder and attention deficit hyperactivity disorder in comparison to bipolar disorder. *Journal of Affective Disorders, 262*(1), 317–322. https://doi.org/10.1016/j.jad.2019.10.053

Rodriguez, T. (2017). Bipolar disorder, borderline personality disorder may represent the same disorder. *PsychiatryAdvisor.* http://www.psychiatryadvisor.com/bipolar-disorder/bipolar-disorder-same-as-borderline-personality-disorder/article/712397

Schneider, I., Boll, S., Volman, I. Roelofs, K., Spohn, A., Herpertz, S. C., & Bertch, K. (2020). Oxytocin normalizes approach–avoidance behavior in women with borderline personality disorder. *Frontiers in Psychiatry, 11.* https://doi.org/10.3389/fpsyt.2020.00120

Skeem, J. L., Polaschek, D. L., Patrick, C. J., & Lilienfeld, S. O. (2011). Psychopathic personality: Bridging the gap between scientific evidence and public policy. *Psychological Science in the Public Interest, 12*, 95–162. https://doi.org/10.1177/1529100611426707

Stoffers, J. M., Vollm, B., Rucker, G., Timmer, A., Huband, N., & Lieb, K. (2012). Psychological therapies for people with BPDs [Review]. *Cochrane Database of Systematic Reviews.* https://doi.org/10.1002/14651858.CD005652.pub2

Thompson, D. F., Ramos, C. L., & Willett, J. K. (2014). Psychopathy: Clinical features, developmental basis, and therapeutic challenges. *Journal of Clinical Pharmacology and Therapeutics, 39*, 485–495.

Verona, E., & Patrick, C. J. (2015). Psychobiological aspects of antisocial personality disorder, psychopathy, and violence. *Psychiatric Times*, 1–7. http://www.psychiatrictimes.com

Weight, J., & Kendal, S. (2013). Staff attitudes towards inpatients with BPD. *Mental Health Practice, 17*(3), 35–38.

Westwood, I., & Baker, J. (2010). Attitudes and perceptions of mental health nurses towards BPD clients in acute mental health settings: A review of the literature. *Journal of Psychiatric and Mental Health Nursing, 17*(7), 657–662.

Yasgur, B. S. (2017). Borderline personality disorder: Not just an adult condition. *PsychiatryAdvisor.* https://www.psychiatryadvisor.com/home/topics/child-adolescent-psychiatry/borderline-personality-disorder-not-just-an-adult-condition/

Zimmerman, M. (2017). Improving the recognition of borderline personality disorder. *Current Psychiatry, 16*(10), 13–19.

Classical References

Erikson, E. (1963). *Childhood and society* (2nd ed.). W.W. Norton.

Mahler, M., Pine, F., & Bergman, A. (1975). *The psychological birth of the human infant.* Basic Books.

Sullivan, H. S. (1953). *The interpersonal theory of psychiatry.* W.W. Norton.

UNIT 4

Psychiatric Mental Health Nursing of Special Populations

23 Children and Adolescents

CORE CONCEPTS

Growth and Development
Health Promotion
Maladaptive Behavior
Stress and Coping
Professionalism: Nursing process in the care of patients with selected disorders occurring in children and adolescents

CHAPTER OUTLINE

Objectives
Introduction
Neurodevelopmental Disorders
Disruptive Behavior Disorders
Anxiety Disorders
Treatment Modalities
Summary and Key Points
Review Questions
Clinical Judgment Questions
Implications for Evidence-Based Practice
Test Your Clinical Reasoning and Clinical Judgment Skills
Movie Connections

KEY TERMS

aggression
attention deficit-hyperactivity disorder (ADHD)
autism spectrum disorder (ASD)
clinging
conduct disorder (CD)
echolalia
hyperactivity
impulsivity
intellectual developmental disorder (intellectual disability)
negativism
oppositional defiant disorder (ODD)
palilalia
separation anxiety disorder
Tourette's disorder

OBJECTIVES

After reading this chapter, the student will be able to:

1. Identify psychiatric disorders that most commonly have their onset in infancy, childhood, or adolescence.
2. Discuss predisposing factors implicated in the etiology of intellectual disability, autism spectrum disorder, attention deficit-hyperactivity disorder, conduct disorder, oppositional defiant disorder, Tourette's disorder, and separation anxiety disorder.
3. Identify symptomatology and use the information in the assessment of clients with the aforementioned disorders.
4. Identify nursing diagnoses common to patients with these disorders and select appropriate nursing interventions for each.
5. Discuss relevant criteria for evaluating nursing care of patients with selected infant, childhood, and adolescent psychiatric disorders.
6. Describe treatment modalities relevant to selected disorders of infancy, childhood, and adolescence.

Introduction

This chapter examines various disorders in which the symptoms usually first become evident during infancy, childhood, or adolescence. It is important to note, however, that some of the disorders discussed in this chapter do appear later in life, and that symptoms associated with other disorders, such as major depressive disorder or bipolar disorder, also can appear in childhood or adolescence.

All nurses working with children or adolescents should be knowledgeable about typical stages of growth and development. Chapter 29, "Concepts of Personality Development," discusses this topic, and a summary of personality development theories appears in Chapter 22, "Personality Disorders." The developmental process is one that is fraught with challenges. Behavioral responses are individual and idiosyncratic. They are, indeed, *human* responses.

Whether a child's behavior indicates emotional problems is often difficult to determine. Guidelines for making such a determination should consider appropriateness of the behavior regarding age and cultural norms and whether the behavior interferes with adaptive functioning. This chapter focuses on the nursing process in care of patients with intellectual disability, autism spectrum disorder (ASD), attention deficit-hyperactivity disorder (ADHD), conduct disorder, oppositional defiant disorder (ODD), Tourette's disorder, and separation anxiety disorder. A discussion of treatment modalities is included.

Neurodevelopmental Disorders

Intellectual Developmental Disorder (Intellectual Disability)

Clinical Findings

The *Diagnostic and Statistical Manual of Mental Disorders, Fifth Edition, Text Revision.* (*DSM-5-TR,* American Psychiatric Association [APA], 2022) defines **intellectual developmental disorder (intellectual disability)** as a "disorder with onset during the developmental period that includes both intellectual and adaptive functioning deficits in conceptual, social, and practical domains" (p. 37). The incidence rate in the general population is about 1% (APA, 2022). Onset of intellectual and adaptive deficits occurs during the developmental period. Level of impairment (mild, moderate, severe, or profound) is based on adaptive functioning within the three domains. General intellectual functioning is measured by both clinical assessment and an individual's performance on intelligence quotient (IQ) tests. Adaptive functioning refers to the person's ability to adapt to the requirements of daily living and the expectations of the individual's age and cultural group. According to the *DSM-5-TR* (APA, 2022), a diagnosis of intellectual disability requires the presence of deficits in intellectual (cognitive and learning functions) and adaptive (such as independent functioning, communication, and social) domains that began during the developmental period.

Predisposing Factors

The etiology of intellectual disability may be primarily biological or primarily psychosocial, or a combination of both, or, in some instances, unknown. The common factors, regardless of etiology, are significant impairments in intellectual functions and social adaptation.

Genetic Factors

Genetic factors are implicated as the cause of intellectual disability in approximately 5% of the cases. These factors include inborn errors of metabolism, such as Tay-Sachs disease, phenylketonuria, and hyperglycinemia. Also included are chromosomal disorders such as Down's syndrome and Klinefelter's syndrome and single-gene abnormalities such as fragile X syndrome, tuberous sclerosis, and neurofibromatosis.

Disruptions in Embryonic Development

Conditions affecting early (embryonic) development account for approximately 30% of intellectual disability cases. Damage may occur in response to toxicity associated with maternal ingestion of alcohol or other drugs. Fetal alcohol syndrome is an example, and this disorder has been identified as one of the leading preventable causes of intellectual disability. Maternal illnesses and infections during pregnancy (e.g., rubella, cytomegalovirus) and complications of pregnancy (e.g., pre-eclampsia, uncontrolled maternal diabetes) may also play a role in causing congenital intellectual disability (Boland & Verduin, 2022).

Pregnancy and Perinatal Factors

Approximately 10% of cases of intellectual disability are the result of circumstances that occur during pregnancy (e.g., fetal malnutrition, viral and other infections, and prematurity) or during the birth process. Examples of the latter include trauma to the head incurred during the process of birth, placenta previa or premature separation of the placenta, and prolapse of the umbilical cord.

General Medical Conditions Acquired in Infancy or Childhood

General medical conditions acquired during infancy or childhood account for approximately 5% of cases of intellectual disability. They include infections, such as meningitis and encephalitis; poisonings, such as from insecticides, medications, and lead; and physical trauma, such as head injuries, asphyxiation, and hyperpyrexia. Universal use of the measles vaccine had virtually eliminated measles encephalitis but recent refusal by individuals and communities has increased this risk (Boland & Verduin, 2022).

Sociocultural Factors and Other Mental Disorders

Between 15% and 20% of cases of intellectual disability may be attributed to deprivation of nurturance and social stimulation and to impoverished environments associated with poor prenatal and perinatal care and inadequate nutrition. Additionally, other mental disorders, such as ASD, can result in intellectual disability.

Recognition of the cause and period of inception provides information regarding what to expect in terms of behavior and potential. However, each child is different, and consideration must be given on an individual basis.

Application of the Nursing Process to Intellectual Disability

Background Assessment Data

The degree of severity of intellectual disability may be measured by the client's IQ level and measures of adaptive functioning. Four levels have been delineated: mild, moderate, severe, and profound. The various behavioral manifestations and abilities associated with each of these levels of severity are outlined in Table 23–1.

Nurses should assess and focus on each child's strengths and individual abilities. Knowledge regarding level of independence in the performance of self-care activities is essential to the development of an adequate plan for the provision of nursing care.

Nursing Diagnoses

Selection of appropriate nursing diagnoses for the patient with intellectual disability depends largely

TABLE 23–1 Developmental Characteristics of Intellectual Developmental Disorder by Degree of Severity

LEVEL (IQ)	ABILITY TO PERFORM SELF-CARE ACTIVITIES	COGNITIVE/EDUCATIONAL CAPABILITIES	SOCIAL/COMMUNICATION CAPABILITIES	PSYCHOMOTOR CAPABILITIES
Mild (50–70)	Capable of independent living, with assistance during times of stress.	Capable of academic skills to sixth-grade level. As adult can achieve vocational skills for minimum self-support.	Capable of developing social skills. Functions well in a structured, sheltered setting.	Psychomotor skills usually not affected, although may have some slight problems with coordination.
Moderate (35–49)	Can perform some activities independently. Requires supervision.	Capable of academic skill to second-grade level. As adult may be able to contribute to own support in sheltered workshop.	May experience some limitation in speech communication. Difficulty adhering to social convention may interfere with peer relationships.	Motor development is fair. Vocational capabilities may be limited to unskilled gross motor activities.
Severe (20–34)	May be trained in elementary hygiene skills. Requires complete supervision.	Unable to benefit from academic or vocational training. Benefits from systematic habit training.	Minimal verbal skills. Wants and needs often communicated by acting-out behaviors.	Poor psychomotor development. Able to perform only simple tasks under close supervision.
Profound (below 20)	No capacity for independent functioning. Requires constant aid and supervision.	Unable to benefit from academic or vocational training. May respond to minimal training in self-help if presented in the close context of a one-to-one relationship.	Little, if any, speech development. No capacity for socialization skills.	Lack of ability for both fine and gross motor movements. Requires constant supervision and care. May be associated with other physical disorders.

Sources: Compiled from Boat & Wu (2015) and Boland & Verduin (2022).

on the degree of severity of the condition and the patient's capabilities. Possible nursing diagnoses include the following:

- Risk for injury related to altered physical mobility or aggressive behavior
- Self-care deficit related to altered physical mobility or lack of maturity
- Impaired verbal communication related to developmental alteration
- Impaired social interaction related to speech deficiencies or difficulty adhering to conventional social behavior
- Delayed growth and development related to isolation from significant others, inadequate environmental stimulation, genetic factors
- Anxiety (moderate to severe) related to hospitalization and absence of familiar surroundings
- Defensive coping related to feelings of powerlessness and threat to self-esteem
- Ineffective coping related to inadequate coping skills secondary to developmental delay

Outcome Identification

Outcome criteria include short- and long-term goals. Timelines are individually determined. The following criteria may be used for measurement of outcomes in the care of the patient with intellectual disability. The patient:

- Has experienced no physical harm.
- Has self-care needs fulfilled.
- Interacts with others in a socially appropriate manner.
- Maintains anxiety at a manageable level.
- Is able to accept direction without becoming defensive.
- Demonstrates adaptive coping skills in response to stressful situations.

Planning and Implementation

Table 23–2 provides a plan of care for the child with intellectual disability using selected nursing diagnoses, outcome criteria, and appropriate nursing interventions and rationales.

Although this plan of care is directed toward the individual patient, it is essential that family members or primary caregivers participate in the ongoing care of the patient with intellectual disability. They need to receive information regarding the scope of the condition, realistic expectations and patient potentials, methods for modifying behavior as required, and community resources from which they may seek assistance and support.

Evaluation

Evaluation of care given to the patient with intellectual disability should reflect positive behavioral changes. Evaluation is accomplished by determining whether the goals of care (previously identified) have been met through implementation of the nursing actions selected. The nurse reassesses the plan and makes changes as required. Reassessment data may include information gathered by asking the following questions. Has the patient:

- Remained free from injury?
- Had self-care needs fulfilled? Been able to fulfill some of these needs independently?
- Been able to communicate needs and desires in a way that can be understood?
- Learned to interact appropriately with others?
- Accepted constructive feedback and discontinued inappropriate behavior when regressive behavior surfaces?
- Maintained anxiety at a manageable level?
- Learned new coping skills through behavior modification?
- Demonstrated evidence of increased self-esteem because of the accomplishment of these new skills and adaptive behaviors?

Have primary caregivers:

- Demonstrated understanding of realistic expectations for patient's behavior and methods for attempting to modify unacceptable behaviors?
- Demonstrated awareness of various resources from which they can seek assistance and support within the community?

CORE CONCEPT

Autism Spectrum Disorder

A heterogenous group of neurodevelopmental syndromes characterized by a wide range of social difficulties, communication impairments, and restricted and repetitive behaviors (Boland & Verduin, 2022).

Autism Spectrum Disorder

Clinical Findings

In the *Diagnostic and Statistical Manual of Mental Disorders* (4th ed., text revision; *DSM-IV-TR*; APA, 2000), the autism spectrum disorders were encompassed in a broad spectrum of pervasive development disorders that included autistic disorder, Rett's disorder, childhood disintegrative disorder, pervasive developmental

Table 23–2 | CARE PLAN FOR THE CHILD WITH INTELLECTUAL DISABILITY

NURSING DIAGNOSIS: RISK FOR INJURY

RELATED TO: Altered physical mobility or aggressive behavior

OUTCOME CRITERIA	NURSING INTERVENTIONS	RATIONALE
Short- and Long-Term Goal ■ Patient will not experience injury.	1. Create a safe environment for the patient. 2. Ensure that small items are removed from area where patient will be ambulating and that sharp items are out of reach. 3. Store items that the patient uses frequently within easy reach. 4. Pad side rails and headboard of the patient with history of seizures. 5. Prevent physical aggression and acting-out behaviors by learning to recognize signs that the patient is becoming agitated.	1–5. Patient safety is a nursing priority.

NURSING DIAGNOSIS: SELF-CARE DEFICIT

RELATED TO: Altered physical mobility or lack of maturity

OUTCOME CRITERIA	NURSING INTERVENTIONS	RATIONALE
Short-Term Goal ■ Patient will be able to participate in aspects of self-care. **Long-Term Goal** ■ Patient will have all self-care needs met.	1. Identify aspects of self-care that may be within the patient's capabilities. Work on one aspect of self-care at a time. Provide simple, concrete explanations. Offer positive feedback for efforts.	1. Positive reinforcement enhances self-esteem and encourages repetition of desirable behaviors.
	2. When one aspect of self-care has been mastered to the best of the patient's ability, move on to another. Encourage independence but intervene when the patient is unable to perform.	2. Patient comfort and safety are nursing priorities.

NURSING DIAGNOSIS: IMPAIRED VERBAL COMMUNICATION

RELATED TO: Developmental alteration

OUTCOME CRITERIA	NURSING INTERVENTIONS	RATIONALE
Short-Term Goal ■ Patient will establish trust with caregiver and a means of communication of needs.	1. Maintain consistency of staff assignment over time.	1. Consistency of staff assignments facilitates trust and the ability to understand the patient's actions and communications.
Long-Term Goals ■ Patient's needs are being met through established means of communication. ■ If patient cannot speak or communicate by other means, needs are met by caregiver's anticipation of patient's needs.	2. Anticipate and fulfill the patient's needs until satisfactory communication patterns are established. Learn (from family, if possible) special words the patient uses that are different from the norm. Identify nonverbal gestures or signals that patient may use to convey needs if verbal communication is absent. Practice these communications skills repeatedly.	2. Some children with intellectual disability, particularly at the severe level, can learn only by systematic habit training.

Table 23–2 | CARE PLAN FOR THE CHILD WITH INTELLECTUAL DISABILITY—cont'd

NURSING DIAGNOSIS: IMPAIRED SOCIAL INTERACTION

RELATED TO: Speech deficiencies or difficulty adhering to conventional social behavior

OUTCOME CRITERIA	NURSING INTERVENTIONS	RATIONALE
Short-Term Goal ■ Patient will attempt to interact with others in the presence of trusted caregiver. **Long-Term Goal** ■ Patient will be able to interact with others using behaviors that are socially acceptable and appropriate to developmental level.	1. Remain with the patient during initial interactions with others on the unit. 2. Explain to other patients the meaning behind some of patient's nonverbal gestures and signals. Use simple language to explain to the patient which behaviors are acceptable and which are not. Establish a procedure for behavior modification with rewards for appropriate behaviors and aversive reinforcement for inappropriate behaviors.	1. Presence of a trusted individual provides a feeling of security. 2. Positive, negative, and aversive reinforcements can contribute to desired changes in behavior. These privileges and penalties are individually determined as staff learns the likes and dislikes of the patient.

disorder not otherwise specified, and Asperger's disorder. The *DSM-5-TR* groups these disorders into a single diagnostic category—**autism spectrum disorder (ASD).** The diagnosis is adapted to each individual by clinical specifiers (e.g., level of required support, presence or absence of language impairment, and presence or absence of intellectual impairment) and associated features (e.g., known genetic or other medical conditions or environmental factors, or associated with a neurodevelopmental, mental, or behavior problem) (APA, 2022). ASD includes a wide range of symptoms and levels of severity that affect thinking, feeling, communication, and social relationships. Behavior is often limited and repetitive, but each child is likely to have a unique pattern of behavior and level of severity—from low functioning to high functioning (Mayo Clinic, 2021a).

Epidemiology and Course

The Centers for Disease Control and Prevention (CDC) Autism and Developmental Disabilities Monitoring (ADDM) Network estimates that 1 in 54 children in the United States is identified with ASD, a prevalence that has more than doubled since 2000 (CDC, 2020a). It occurs about four times more often in boys than in girls. Almost half (44%) of individuals with ASD have an average or above average IQ. Onset of the disorder occurs in early childhood, and in most cases, it runs a chronic course with symptoms persisting into adulthood.

Predisposing Factors

Neurological Implications

Imaging studies have revealed a number of alterations in major brain structures of individuals with ASD. Total brain volume, the size of the amygdala, and the size of the striatum are enlarged in about 9% to 16% of children under the age of 4 with ASD and there is evidence of decrease in the size of the amygdala over time (Boland & Verduin, 2022; Kranjac, 2016). Boland and Verduin (2022) identify that this dynamic pattern of change in total brain volume over time lends support for the hypothesis that there are critical periods in the brain's plasticity that, when disrupted, may contribute to the development of ASD. These findings related to brain plasticity also support that early recognition and intervention can be meaningful in improving functional abilities over time. Volkmar and associates (2017) report that the Infant Brain Imaging Study, a national study of developmental changes in at-risk infants, has repeatedly demonstrated abnormal organizational properties in white matter within the first year of life that accentuate over time. In vitro stem cell reprogramming research is beginning to identify the cellular mechanisms responsible for early brain overgrowth and the subsequent disruptions in neural connectivity that may yield valuable information about causes and treatment options (Marchetto et al., 2017).

Genetics

Family and twin studies support that genetic factors play a significant role in the etiology of ASD; about 15% of ASD cases are related to a known genetic mutation, but, in most cases, its expression is related to multiple genes (Boland & Verduin, 2022). Genetic studies have identified genes that confer risk for both autism and schizophrenia, suggesting that these conditions are related (Gilman et al., 2012), but the same genetic variations also appear to confer risk for some other neurodevelopmental disorders as well (Volkmar et al., 2017). Kranjac (2016) reports that rare genetic variants such as copy number variations increase the risk for autism by 20% to 60%. DNA studies have implicated areas on several chromosomes containing genes that may contribute to the development of ASD. Genetic studies have also identified disruptions in serotonin (5-HT), and because 5-HT is important in brain development, it is postulated that changes in 5-HT may be associated with enlargement in the brain (Boland & Verduin, 2022).

Prenatal and Perinatal Influences

Some of the prenatal risk factors that have been associated with development of ASD include advanced parental age, fetal exposure to valproate, gestational diabetes, and maternal gestational bleeding (APA, 2022; Boland & Verduin, 2022). Perinatal influences include low birth weight, obstetrical complications (particularly those associated with neonatal hypoxia), hyperbilirubinemia, congenital malformation, and ABO or Rh factor incompatibilities (Boland & Verduin, 2022). Exposure to environmental toxins, including air pollution and pesticides, showed the strongest links to ASD when it occurred during preconception, gestational, and early childhood stages (Rossignol & Frye, 2016). Volkmar and associates (2017) note that "despite multiple focused investigations, there is no evidence that vaccinations play a role in the environmental liability for ASD" (p. 3576).

Application of the Nursing Process to Autism Spectrum Disorder

Background Assessment Data

The symptomatology presented here is common among children with ASD, but it is important to understand these autism symptoms appear along a spectrum and with varying levels of functionality. Some individuals who meet criteria for ASD may be highly functional and highly intelligent in spite of communication impairments and repetitive or restrictive behaviors. The dramatic increase in prevalence of ASD has led to research focused on differential and common features along the continuum as well as etiological factors. This information is important in creating an accurate plan of care for the patient. Because ASD is a *spectrum* disorder, the symptomatology described here should be understood on a continuum ranging from quite mild to more severe.

- ***Impairment in social interaction:*** Children with ASD have difficulty forming interpersonal relationships with others. They show little interest in people and often do not respond to others' attempts at interaction. As infants, they may have an aversion to affection and physical contact. As toddlers, the attachment to a significant adult may be either absent or manifested as exaggerated adherence behaviors. In childhood, there is a lack of spontaneity manifested in less cooperative play, less imaginative play, and fewer friendships. Those children with milder difficulties may progress to the point of recognizing other children as part of their environment but struggle nonetheless in interpersonal relationships. Social interaction is further impaired by deficits in ability to accurately process others' feelings or affect. Higher functioning children may recognize their difficulty with social skills even though they may desire friendship. In one study (Strunz et al., 2015), the researchers noted that as these relational struggles unfold into adulthood, it is difficult at times to distinguish ASD from personality disorders because there are disruptions in interpersonal relationships within both groups. They found that the differential features in ASD were less extroversion, less openness to experience, increased inhibition, and increased compulsivity than among those with personality disorders.
- ***Impairment in communication and imaginative activity:*** Both verbal and nonverbal skills are affected. In more severe levels of ASD, language may be totally absent or characterized by immature structure or idiosyncratic utterances whose meaning is clear only to those who are familiar with the child's past experiences. Nonverbal communication, such as facial expression or gestures, may be absent or socially inappropriate. Some children with autism spectrum disorder are misdiagnosed as being hearing impaired as a result of their lack of response to sounds, while other children may overreact to sound or other stimuli. In some cases, children with ASD demonstrate special abilities, such as fluent reading skills while still in preschool (Boland & Verduin, 2022). The pattern of play is often restricted and repetitive.

- ***Restricted activities and interests:*** Even minor changes in the environment are often met with resistance or sometimes with agitated irritability. Attachment to, or extreme fascination with, objects that move or spin (e.g., fans) is common. Stereotyped body movements (hand flapping, rocking, whole-body swaying) and verbalizations (repetition of words or phrases) are typical. Diet abnormalities may include eating only a few specific foods or consuming an excessive amount of fluids. Behaviors that are self-injurious, such as head banging or biting the hands or arms, may be evident. Harrop and associates (2014) studied children with ASD compared to children without this disorder and found that all children demonstrated some repetitive behaviors as part of their development of skill mastery, but children with ASD displayed a wider range of repetitive behaviors in many different circumstances.

The *DSM-5-TR* (APA, 2022) diagnostic criteria for ASD are presented in Box 23–1. The criteria specify a range of behaviors, thus addressing the spectrum of symptomatology associated with this diagnosis.

BOX 23–1 Diagnostic Criteria for Autism Spectrum Disorder

A. Persistent deficits in social communication and social interaction across multiple contexts, as manifested by the following, currently or by history (examples are illustrative, not exhaustive):
   1. Deficits in social-emotional reciprocity, ranging, for example, from abnormal social approach and failure of normal back-and-forth conversation; to reduced sharing of interests, emotions, or affect; to failure to initiate or respond to social interactions.
   2. Deficits in nonverbal communicative behaviors used for social interaction, ranging, for example, from poorly integrated verbal and nonverbal communication; to abnormalities in eye contact and body language or deficits in understanding and use of gestures; to a total lack of facial expressions and nonverbal communication.
   3. Deficits in developing, maintaining, and understanding relationships, ranging, for example, from difficulties adjusting behavior to suit various social contexts; to difficulties in sharing imaginative play or in making friends; to absence of interest in peers.

B. Restricted, repetitive patterns of behavior, interests, or activities, as manifested by at least two of the following, currently or by history (examples are illustrative, not exhaustive):
   1. Stereotyped or repetitive motor movements, use of objects, or speech (e.g., simple motor stereotypes lining up toys or flipping objects, echolalia, idiosyncratic phrases).
   2. Insistence on sameness, inflexible adherence to routines, or ritualized patterns of verbal or nonverbal behavior (e.g., extreme distress at small changes, difficulties with transitions, rigid thinking patterns, greeting rituals, need to take same route or eat same food every day).
   3. Highly restricted, fixated interests that are abnormal in intensity or focus (e.g., strong attachment to or preoccupation with unusual objects, excessively circumscribed or perseverative interests).
   4. Hyper- or hypo-reactivity to sensory input or unusual interest in sensory aspects of environment (e.g., apparent indifference to pain/temperature, adverse response to specific sounds or textures, excessive smelling or touching of objects, visual fascination with lights or movement).

C. Symptoms must be present in the early developmental period (but may not become fully manifest until social demands exceed limited capacities, or may be masked by learned strategies in later life).

D. Symptoms cause clinically significant impairment in social, occupational, or other important areas of current functioning.

E. These disturbances are not better explained by intellectual disability (intellectual developmental disorder) or global developmental delay. Intellectual disability and autism spectrum disorder frequently co-occur; to make comorbid diagnoses of autism spectrum disorder and intellectual disability, social communication should be below that expected for general developmental level.

Specify current level of severity based on social communication impairments and restricted, repetitive patterns of behavior:

Requiring very substantial support

Requiring substantial support

Requiring support

Specify if:

With or without accompanying intellectual impairment

With or without accompanying language impairment

Associated with a known medical or genetic condition or environmental factor

Associated with another neurodevelopmental, mental, or behavioral disorder

With catatonia

Reprinted with permission from American Psychiatric Association. (2022). Diagnostic and statistical manual of mental disorders, fifth edition, text revision.

Nursing Diagnoses

Based on data collected during the nursing assessment, possible nursing diagnoses for the patient with ASD include the following:

- Risk for self-mutilation or self-injury related to neurological, cognitive, or social deficits.
- Impaired social interaction related to inability to trust; neurological alterations, evidenced by lack of responsiveness to or interest in people.
- Impaired verbal communication related to withdrawal into self; neurological alterations, evidenced by inability or unwillingness to speak; lack of nonverbal expression.
- Disturbed personal identity related to neurological alterations; delayed developmental stage, evidenced by difficulty separating own physiological and emotional needs and personal boundaries from those of others.

Outcome Identification

Outcome criteria include both short- and long-term goals. Timelines are individually determined. The following criteria may be used for measurement of outcomes in the care of the patient with ASD. The patient:

- Exhibits no evidence of self-harm.
- Interacts appropriately with at least one staff member.
- Demonstrates trust in at least one staff member.
- Is able to communicate in a way that can be understood by at least one staff member.
- Demonstrates behaviors that indicate progress in the separation/individuation process.

Planning and Implementation

Table 23–3 provides a plan of care for the child with ASD, including selected nursing diagnoses, outcome criteria, and appropriate nursing interventions and rationales.

Evaluation

Evaluation of care for the child with ASD reflects whether the nursing actions have been effective in achieving the established goals. The nursing process calls for reassessment of the plan. Questions for gathering reassessment data may include the following. Has the child:

- Been able to establish trust with at least *one* caregiver?
- Remained free from self-mutilation or other self-harm?
- Attempted to interact with others?
- Improved in ability to indicate that attention is being paid?
- Established a means of communicating needs and desires to others? Have all self-care needs been met?
- Demonstrated an awareness of self as separate from others?
- Accepted touch from others and been appropriate in touching others?

Psychopharmacological Intervention for ASD

Behavioral interventions are first line treatments for core symptoms of ASD. Pharmacological interventions are directed toward relief of associated symptoms, such as **aggression, hyperactivity,** self-harm, **impulsivity,** and temper tantrums. There are no medications that treat the core symptoms of ASD. The U.S. Food and Drug Administration (FDA) has approved two medications for the treatment of irritability associated with ASD: risperidone (Risperdal; in children and adolescents 5 to 16 years) and aripiprazole (Abilify; in children and adolescents 6 to 17 years). When administering risperidone, caution must be maintained concerning less common but more serious side effects, including neuroleptic malignant syndrome, tardive dyskinesia, hyperglycemia, and diabetes. A review and meta-analysis (Fallah et al., 2019) concluded that risperidone was more effective than aripiprazole, lurazidone, or placebo in reducing irritability symptoms.

In clinical studies with aripiprazole, the most frequently reported adverse events included sedation, fatigue, weight gain, vomiting, somnolence, and tremor. The most common reasons for discontinuation of aripiprazole were sedation, drooling, tremor, vomiting, and extrapyramidal disorder.

Recent studies and meta-analyses as cited by Kothadia and associates (2021) have identified several other medications for the treatment of ASD associated symptoms: donepezil and a choline supplement improved receptive language skills in children age 5 to 10 years (Gabis et al., 2019); bumetanide improved social communication, interaction and restricted interests in children with moderate to severe ASD (James et al., 2019); and vitamin D with omega-3 long chain polyunsaturated fatty acids (LCPUFA) reduced associated irritability and hyperactivity (Mazahery et al., 2019).

Nonpharmacological Treatments for ASD

Conventional nonpharmacological treatments include behavior and communication therapies, education therapies, and family therapies (Mayo Clinic, 2021a).

These programs may focus on reducing problem behaviors or teaching social and communication skills. Applied behavior analysis (ABA) is referred to as the gold standard behavioral treatment for ASD and it involves tailoring a reward-based motivation program specific to each child's needs (Raypole, 2019). Family therapies involve engaging family members in learning how to interact with their children to promote social interaction skills and manage problem behaviors. Education programs are typically highly structured to facilitate learning and meet the individual needs of the child. Speech therapy,

Table 23–3 | CARE PLAN FOR THE CHILD WITH AUTISM SPECTRUM DISORDER

NURSING DIAGNOSIS: RISK FOR SELF-MUTILATION

RELATED TO: Neurological alterations; history of self-mutilation behaviors; hysterical reactions to changes in the environment

OUTCOME CRITERIA	NURSING INTERVENTIONS	RATIONALE
Short-Term Goal ■ Patient will demonstrate alternative behavior (e.g., initiating interaction between self and nurse) in response to anxiety within specified time. (Length of time required for this objective will depend on severity and chronicity of the disorder.) **Long-Term Goal** ■ Patient will not harm self.	1. Work with the child on a one-to-one basis.	1. One-to-one interaction facilitates trust.
	2. Try to determine whether the self-mutilation behavior occurs in response to increasing anxiety and, if so, to what the anxiety may be attributed.	2. Self-mutilation behaviors may be averted if the cause can be determined and alleviated.
	3. Try to intervene with diversion or replacement activities and offer self to the child as anxiety level starts to rise.	3. Diversion and replacement activities may provide needed feelings of security and substitute for self-mutilation behaviors.
	4. Protect the child when self-mutilative behaviors occur. Devices such as a helmet, padded hand mitts, or arm covers may provide protection when the risk for self-harm exists.	4. Patient safety is a priority nursing intervention.

NURSING DIAGNOSIS: IMPAIRED SOCIAL INTERACTION

RELATED TO: Inability to trust; neurological alterations

EVIDENCED BY: Lack of responsiveness to, or interest in, people

OUTCOME CRITERIA	NURSING INTERVENTIONS	RATIONALE
Short-Term Goal ■ Patient will demonstrate trust in one caregiver within specified time (depending on severity and chronicity of disorder). **Long-Term Goal** ■ Patient will initiate social interactions (physical, verbal, nonverbal) with caregiver by time of discharge from treatment.	1. Assign a limited number of caregivers to the child. Ensure that warmth, acceptance, and availability are conveyed.	1. Warmth, acceptance, and availability, along with consistency of assignment, enhance the establishment and maintenance of a trusting relationship.
	2. Provide child with familiar objects, such as familiar toys or a blanket. Support child's attempts to interact with others.	2. Familiar objects and presence of a trusted individual provide security during times of distress.
	3. Give positive reinforcement for appropriate behaviors with something acceptable to the child (e.g., food, familiar object). Gradually replace with social reinforcement (e.g., touch, smiling, hugging).	3. Positive reinforcement promotes repetition of appropriate behaviors.

Continued

Table 23–3 | CARE PLAN FOR THE CHILD WITH AUTISM SPECTRUM DISORDER—cont'd

NURSING DIAGNOSIS: IMPAIRED VERBAL COMMUNICATION

RELATED TO: Withdrawal into the self; neurological alterations

EVIDENCED BY: Inability or unwillingness to speak; lack of nonverbal expression

OUTCOME CRITERIA	NURSING INTERVENTIONS	RATIONALE
Short-Term Goal ■ Patient will establish trust with one caregiver by specified time (depending on severity and chronicity of disorder). **Long-Term Goal** ■ Patient will establish a means of communicating needs and desires to others.	1. Maintain consistency in assignment of caregivers.	1. Consistency facilitates trust and enhances the caregiver's ability to understand the child's attempts to communicate.
	2. Anticipate and fulfill the child's needs until communication can be established.	2. Anticipating needs helps to minimize frustration while the child is learning communication skills.
	3. Seek clarification and validation.	3. Validation ensures that the intended message has been conveyed.
	4. Give positive reinforcement when the patient establishes means to communicate needs and desires to others.	4. Positive reinforcement increases self-esteem and encourages repetition.

NURSING DIAGNOSIS: DISTURBED PERSONAL IDENTITY

RELATED TO: Neurological alterations; delayed developmental stage

EVIDENCED BY: Difficulty separating own physiological and emotional needs and personal boundaries from those of others

OUTCOME CRITERIA	NURSING INTERVENTIONS	RATIONALE
Short-Term Goal ■ Patient will name own body parts as separate and individual from those of others. **Long-Term Goal** ■ Patient will develop ego identity (evidenced by ability to recognize physical and emotional self as separate from others) by time of discharge from treatment.	1. Assist the child to recognize separateness during self-care activities, such as dressing and feeding.	1. Recognition of body parts during dressing and feeding increases the child's awareness of self as separate from others.
	2. Assist the child in learning to name own body parts. This can be facilitated by the use of mirrors, drawings, and pictures of the child. Encourage appropriate touching of, and being touched by, others.	2. All of these activities may help increase the child's awareness of self as separate from others.

occupational therapy, and physical therapy may also be beneficial. Adjunctive treatments may include art, music, or sensory-based therapies aimed at reducing the child's sensitivity to touch or sound, but while these approaches may support evidence-based treatment approaches, more research is needed to support their efficacy alone (DeBoth & Reynolds, 2017).

CORE CONCEPT

Hyperactivity

Excessive psychomotor activity that may be purposeful or aimless, accompanied by physical movements and verbal utterances that are usually more rapid than normal. Inattention and distractibility are common with hyperactive behavior.

Attention Deficit-Hyperactivity Disorder

Clinical Findings, Epidemiology, and Course

The essential behavior pattern of a child with **attention deficit-hyperactivity disorder (ADHD)** is one of inattention and/or hyperactivity and impulsivity. The most frequently cited characteristics (in order of frequency) are hyperactivity, attention deficit, impulsivity, memory and thinking deficits, specific learning disabilities, and speech and hearing deficits (Boland & Verduin, 2022). Children with ADHD are highly distractible and unable to contain stimuli. Motor activity is excessive, and movements are random and impulsive. Onset of the disorder is difficult to diagnose in children younger than age 4 years because their characteristic behavior is much more variable than that of older children. Frequently, the disorder is not recognized until the child enters school. It is more common in boys (14.6%) than girls (6.9%), and the overall prevalence among school-age children is 10.8% (CDC, 2021a). It is estimated that in 50% to 70% of the cases, ADHD persists into young adulthood and beyond, and unlike other psychiatric disorders that are typically episodic, the adult with ADHD has symptoms that are chronic and unrelenting (McGough, 2017). Without prompt diagnosis and treatment, the child with ADHD is at higher risk for substance abuse and negative consequences associated with risky behavior; the adult is at higher risk for restlessness and functional impairment, occupation difficulties, and disorganization (Mathews-Wilson & Daitch, 2016). See "Real People, Real Stories" to learn more about Myrle's experience as an adult living with ADHD.

Real People, Real Stories: Attention Deficit-Hyperactivity Disorder

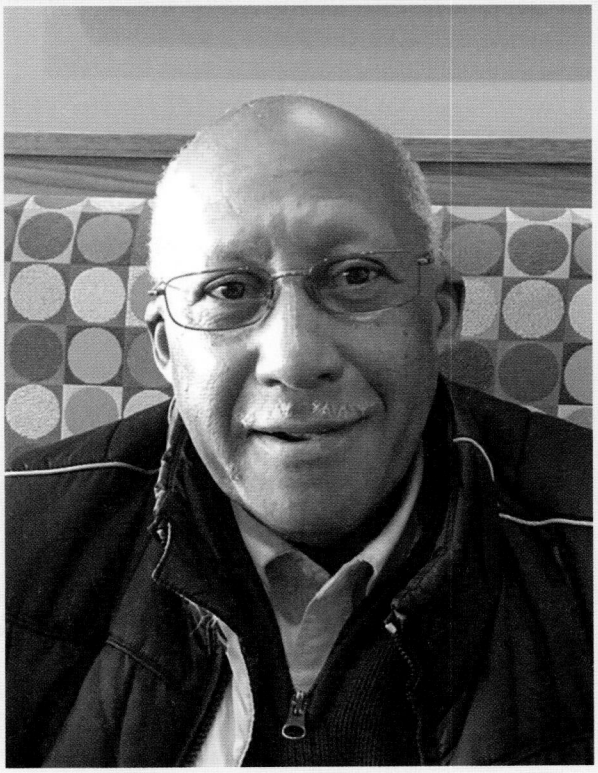

Karyn: When did you first become aware that you had ADHD?

Myrle: I had symptoms as a child but I didn't get diagnosed or treated until I was 50 years old. They put me on Ritalin first and then on Ritalin-XR. When I first started to take it I got very high and very talkative, then after a little while I could focus better and then it wears off.

Karyn: What symptoms do you remember having as a child?

Myrle: I guess I thought of myself as selfish; I was easily distracted, I couldn't handle noise; like the noise at a basketball game was unmanageable and agitating. I was the youngest child but even so, I wanted my way right now. No one else had anything important to say. Later I realized it wasn't that I was so smart but that everyone else seemed to go too slow.

Karyn: How did you get along in school?

Myrle: I didn't have any trouble. I went to school in the country and the classrooms were very small and very quiet so that helped me. When I graduated from high school I went into the military and that was when I really realized I had a problem. I got into fights a lot because the noise and the talking and all the activity really agitated me.

Karyn: Impulsivity is a common symptom in ADHD. Did you experience that?

Myrle: I don't think so. I was pretty forward, outgoing, and I liked to take the lead but I had trouble paying attention. I did become hypersexual as I got older and as an adult, I started smoking pot because it improved my sexual performance and I started drinking alcohol because it helped me sleep. Then those became problems, too. I always wanted to be a lawyer so I went to law school after I got out of the military but I was on probation because I got involved in too many things and

Continued

Real People, Real Stories: Attention Deficit-Hyperactivity Disorder—cont'd

couldn't focus on my studies. I eventually did graduate with a PhD but then I took the bar exam four times and couldn't pass it; sometimes I would get sick and couldn't study; even after I got accommodations when I had less noise and twice the time, I would second-guess myself and change my answers. I had a lot of anxiety. Then I got fired from a job I had at the sewer department and since I had admitted to lying, I was unable to take the bar exam for another five years. I never was able to pass.

I got a job at the Department of Education as a disabilities investigator and I was good at handling these cases. I had cases of people with attention deficit disorders that were being discriminated against. I was very detailed but it took me a lot longer to get things done. I collected a lot of information but I was unable to shorten the process compared to my coworkers. It was there that I had the epiphany that I had a lot of the same symptoms that my clients were describing. In general, I've always had a lot of trouble separating myself from the noise and other distractions.

Karyn: How would you describe your ability to function now that you are being treated with medication?

Myrle: Well, just like I'm doing now, I can go on and on talking about nothing.

(There were several subject changes and refocusings; at times Myrle had difficulty refocusing, stating that he just had to finish one more point.)

Myrle: I'm still very disorganized and sometimes have trouble with attention. The meds help somewhat but I still can't stop talking. My current medical record says I also have OCD, hoarding disorder, and depression. I see a psychiatrist for medications but I still have symptoms. I never feel very confident and I can't seem to get all my ducks in a row. The medication helps me not get quite so agitated as I used to. So I am able to conduct my current role as a minister and I am better able to listen.

Karyn: Yes, I heard you preach a sermon and it sounded like a very focused message.

Myrle: Well, I do better with structured time limits and I let the Spirit take over when I preach. I know this is what I was called to do and I serve a congregation that has a lot of disabilities so I understand their needs because of my own experiences.

Karyn: What is the most important thing that nurses need to know about an adult with ADHD?

Myrle: They need to understand the impact my attention deficit symptoms have on getting my health-care needs met.

I was admitted to a medical unit and was told I needed to stay in a situation that was literally driving me crazy. I was in a room with three patients, nurses were talking outside the door, buzzers and alarms were beeping and they weren't being shut off. The more I asked for help, the more I felt like they weren't listening and then I started to think they were retaliating or doing it deliberately. . . . or maybe I was getting a little paranoid as I was becoming more agitated.

It's really important that nurses listen to me when I'm telling them I can't tolerate the noise and try to reduce the noise as much as possible. I ask for a private room if that's possible. Sometimes I might get pegged as a problem patient because I do get agitated, but a lower stimulation environment could prevent that.

In making the diagnosis of ADHD, the *DSM-5-TR* criteria are further specified according to current clinical presentation. These subtypes include a combined presentation (meeting the criteria for both inattention and hyperactivity/impulsivity), a predominantly inattentive presentation, and a predominantly hyperactive/impulsive presentation.

CORE CONCEPT

Impulsivity

The trait of acting without reflection and without thought to the consequences of the behavior. An abrupt inclination to act (and the inability to resist acting) on certain behavioral urges.

Predisposing Factors

Biological Influences

- ***Genetics:*** A number of studies have revealed supportive evidence of genetic influences in the etiology of ADHD. Twin and family studies showed that the heritability for ADHD exceeds 75% (McGough, 2017). Adoption studies reveal that biological parents of children with ADHD have more psychopathology than the adoptive parents. Studies of genetic evidence for ADHD found copy number variants on a specific region of chromosome 16 (Acosta et al., 2016; Williams et al., 2010). Researchers have also found that these copy number variants overlap with chromosomal regions previously linked to ASD and schizophrenia. Most molecular research has implicated genes that influence the metabolism or action of dopamine (Boland & Verduin, 2022).

- ***Biochemical theory:*** Hypotheses about the impact of neurotransmitters have been based on benefits associated with taking stimulant medications, which are thought to increase the availability of dopamine. Several studies, using single-photon emission computed tomography (SPECT), have now demonstrated increased dopamine transporter-binding densities in the striatal regions (McGough, 2017) (Fig. 23–1). Not surprisingly, researchers have also found a risk of new-onset psychosis in ADHD patients taking amphetamines almost double the risk than for those taking methylphenidate (Griffin & Harari, 2019).
- ***Anatomical changes:*** Brain imaging studies show decreased volume and activity in the prefrontal cortex, anterior cingulated, globus pallidus, caudate, thalamus, and cerebellum (Boland & Verduin, 2022). Several alterations occur in neural connectivity, with evidence of decreased activation in frontoparietal areas and overactivation in visual, dorsal attention, and default networks (McGough, 2017). A recent study by Humphreys and associates (2018) found a correlation between brain volume changes, elevated ADHD symptoms, and the number of childhood stressors. This finding underscores the interaction between genetics and environmental influences and reinforces the need for trauma-informed care.
- ***Prenatal, perinatal, and postnatal factors:*** Early risk factors for the development of ADHD include prenatal tobacco exposure, premature birth, and low birth weight (ADHD Institute, 2021). Froehlich and associates (2009), in a large U.S. study, found that maternal cigarette smoking during pregnancy was *significantly* associated with childhood ADHD. Intrauterine exposure to toxic substances, including alcohol, can produce effects on behavior. Fetal alcohol syndrome includes hyperactivity, impulsivity, and inattention as well as physical anomalies. Maternal infections during pregnancy have also been associated with higher risks for ADHD. Other perinatal and postnatal influences that may contribute to ADHD are low birth weight, trauma, early infancy infections, or other insults to the brain during this period (Boland & Verduin, 2022). Maternal hypertension has also been implicated as a risk factor for both ADHD and ASD (Maher et al., 2018).

Environmental Influences

- ***Environmental lead:*** Studies continue to provide evidence of the adverse effects of elevated serum levels of lead on cognitive and behavioral development in children (Froehlich et al., 2009; Nigg et al., 2010; Rossignol & Frye, 2016). Froehlich and associates (2009) showed a direct link to ADHD. The government has placed tighter restrictions on the substance in recent years, making exposure to toxic levels less prevalent than it once was. However, reports indicate that at least 4 million households in the United States include children who are being exposed to lead and that approximately 500,000 U.S. children ages 1 to 5 have blood lead levels above 5 micrograms per deciliter, the reference level at which the initiation of public health actions is recommended (CDC, 2021b). The ongoing water crisis that was first noted in 2014 in Flint, Michigan, highlighted concerns about lead exposure that continues to be a public health concern in thousands of cities in the U.S (CDC, 2019).
- ***Diet factors:*** The possible link between food dyes and additives such as artificial flavorings, preservatives, and sugar was introduced in the mid-1970s. Studies on these possibilities have failed to confirm a clear link to ADHD. However, a recent large study did find a connection between higher consumption of artificially sweetened soft drinks and increased risk for dementia and stroke, suggesting that some dietary factors have an impact on brain function (Pase et al., 2017).

Psychosocial Influences

Disorganized or chaotic environments or a disruption in family equilibrium may contribute to ADHD in some individuals. Psychosocial risk factors include nonintact or single-parent families, young maternal age at birth of the target child paternal history of antisocial behavior, maternal depression, and lower socioeconomic class (ADHD Institute, 2021).

Application of the Nursing Process to ADHD

Background Assessment Data

A major portion of the hyperactive child's problems relates to difficulties in performing age-appropriate tasks. Children with hyperactivity are highly distractible and have extremely limited attention spans. They often shift from one uncompleted activity to another. Impulsivity, or deficit in inhibitory control, is also common.

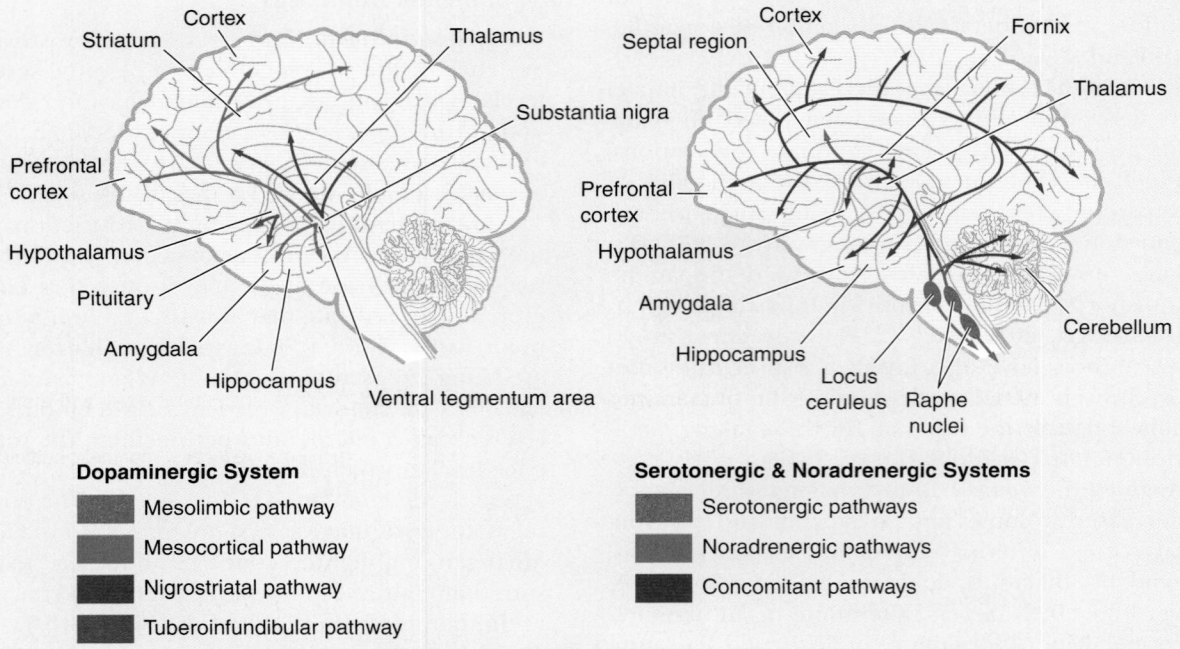

FIGURE 23–1 Neurobiology of attention deficit-hyperactivity disorder.

NEUROTRANSMITTERS

The major neurotransmitters implicated in the pathophysiology of ADHD are dopamine, norepinephrine, and possibly serotonin. Dopamine and norepinephrine appear to be depleted in ADHD. Serotonin in ADHD has been studied less extensively, but recent evidence suggests that it also is reduced in children with ADHD.

NEUROTRANSMITTER FUNCTIONS

- Norepinephrine is thought to play a role in the ability to perform executive functions, such as analysis and reasoning, and in the cognitive alertness essential for processing stimuli and sustaining attention and thought.
- Dopamine is thought to play a role in sensory filtering, memory, concentration, controlling emotions, locomotor activity, and reasoning.
- Deficits in norepinephrine and dopamine have both been implicated in the inattention, impulsiveness, and hyperactivity associated with ADHD.
- Serotonin appears to play a role in ADHD, although possibly less significant than norepinephrine and dopamine. It has been suggested that alterations in serotonin may be related to the disinhibition and impulsivity observed in children with ADHD. It may play a role in mood disorders, particularly depression, which is a common comorbid disorder associated with ADHD.

FUNCTIONAL AREAS OF THE BRAIN AFFECTED

- ***Prefrontal cortex:*** Associated with maintaining attention, organization, and executive function. Also serves to modulate behavior inhibition with serotonin as the predominant central inhibiting neurotransmitter for this function.
- ***Basal ganglia*** (particularly the caudate nucleus and globus pallidus): Involved in the regulation of high-level movements. In association with its connecting circuits to the prefrontal cortex, may also be important in cognition. Interruptions in these circuits may result in inattention or impulsivity.
- ***Hippocampus:*** Plays an important role in learning and memory.
- ***Limbic system*** (the amygdala, hippocampus, mammillary body, hypothalamus, thalamus, fornix, cingulate gyrus, and septum pellucidum): Regulation of emotions. A neurotransmitter deficiency in this area may result in restlessness, inattention, or emotional volatility.
- ***Reticular activating system*** (composed of the reticular formation [located in the brain stem] and its connections): It is the major relay system among the many pathways that enter and leave the brain. It is thought to be the center of arousal and motivation and is crucial for maintaining a state of consciousness.

MEDICATIONS FOR ADHD

CNS Stimulants

- Amphetamines (dextroamphetamine, lisdexamfetamine, methamphetamine, and mixtures): Cause the release of norepinephrine from central noradrenergic neurons. At higher doses, dopamine may be released in the mesolimbic system.
- Methylphenidate and dexmethylphenidate: Block the reuptake of norepinephrine and dopamine into the presynaptic neuron and increase the release of these monoamines into the extraneuronal space.
- Side effects of CNS stimulants include restlessness, insomnia, headache, palpitations, weight loss, suppression of growth in children (with long-term use), increased blood pressure, abdominal pain, anxiety, tolerance, and physical and psychological dependence.

Others

- Atomoxetine: Selectively inhibits the reuptake of norepinephrine by blocking the presynaptic transporter.
  - Side effects include headache, upper abdominal pain, nausea and vomiting, anorexia, cough, dry mouth, constipation, increase in heart rate and blood pressure, and fatigue.
- Bupropion: Inhibits the reuptake of norepinephrine and dopamine into presynaptic neurons.
  - Side effects include headache, dizziness, insomnia or sedation, tachycardia, increased blood pressure, dry mouth, nausea and vomiting, weight gain or loss, seizur es (dose dependent).
- Alpha agonists (clonidine, guanfacine): Stimulate central alpha-adrenoreceptors in the brain, resulting in reduced sympathetic outflow from the CNS.
  - Side effects include palpitations, bradycardia, constipation, dry mouth, and sedation.

Children with ADHD have difficulty forming satisfactory interpersonal relationships. They demonstrate behaviors that inhibit acceptable social interaction. They are disruptive and intrusive in group endeavors. They have difficulty complying with social norms. Some children with ADHD are very aggressive or oppositional, whereas others exhibit more regressive and immature behaviors. Low frustration tolerance and outbursts of temper are common.

Children with ADHD may have boundless energy, exhibiting excessive levels of activity, restlessness, and fidgeting. They have been described as "perpetual motion machines," continuously running, jumping, wiggling, or squirming. They experience a greater-than-average number of accidents, from minor mishaps to more serious incidents that may lead to physical injury or the destruction of property. The *DSM-5-TR* diagnostic criteria for ADHD are presented in Box 23–2.

The prevalence of comorbid psychiatric disorders with ADHD is common, with up to 30% experiencing comorbid depression and 20% experiencing a comorbid anxiety disorder (Sherman & Tarnow, 2013). The APA (2022) reports that in children with ADHD who have symptoms of both inattention and hyperactivity/impulsivity, oppositional defiant disorder co-occurs about 50% of the time. They further identify that most children and adolescents with disruptive mood dysregulation disorder also meet criteria for ADHD. Other comorbidities include conduct disorder, specific learning disorder, anxiety, depression, and intermittent explosive disorder. Boland and Verduin (2022) identify that although bipolar mania and ADHD share many core features, such as distractibility, excessive talking, and hyperactivity, children with bipolar I disorder exhibit symptoms that wax and wane; children with ADHD have more persistent continuous symptoms. They note that bipolar disorder and ADHD can coexist and that when certain features of ADHD occur, they do appear to predict future mania. Sherman and Tarnow (2013) estimate the prevalence of comorbid bipolar disorder and ADHD at around 20%. In addition, ADHD is associated with frontal lobe abnormalities, which supports their finding that 89.4% of children with frontal lobe epilepsy also have comorbid ADHD.

Nursing Diagnoses

Based on the data collected during the nursing assessment, possible nursing diagnoses for the child with ADHD include the following:

- Risk for injury related to impulsive and accident-prone behavior and the inability to perceive self-harm
- Impaired social interaction related to intrusive and immature behavior
- Low self-esteem related to dysfunctional family system and negative feedback
- Noncompliance with task expectations related to low frustration tolerance and short attention span

BOX 23–2 Diagnostic Criteria for Attention Deficit-Hyperactivity Disorder

A. A persistent pattern of inattention and/or hyperactivity-impulsivity that interferes with functioning or development, as characterized by (1) and/or (2):

1. **Inattention:** Six (or more) of the following symptoms have persisted for at least 6 months to a degree that is inconsistent with developmental level and that negatively impacts directly on social and academic/occupational activities. **NOTE:** The symptoms are not solely a manifestation of oppositional behavior, defiance, hostility, or failure to understand tasks or instructions. For older adolescents and adults (age 17 and older), at least five symptoms are required.
   a. Often fails to give close attention to details or makes careless mistakes in schoolwork, at work, or during other activities (e.g., overlooks or misses details, work is inaccurate).
   b. Often has difficulty sustaining attention in tasks or play activities (e.g., has difficulty remaining focused during lectures, conversations, or lengthy reading).
   c. Often does not seem to listen when spoken to directly (e.g., mind seems elsewhere, even in the absence of any obvious distraction).
   d. Often does not follow through on instructions and fails to finish schoolwork, chores, or duties in the workplace (e.g., starts tasks but quickly loses focus and is easily sidetracked).
   e. Often has difficulty organizing tasks and activities (e.g., difficulty managing sequential tasks; difficulty keeping materials and belongings in order; messy, disorganized, work; has poor time management; fails to meet deadlines).
   f. Often avoids, dislikes, or is reluctant to engage in tasks that require sustained mental effort (e.g., schoolwork or homework; for older adolescents and adults, preparing reports, completing forms, reviewing lengthy papers).
   g. Often loses things necessary for tasks or activities (e.g., school materials, pencils, books, tools, wallets, keys, paperwork, eyeglasses, or mobile telephones).
   h. Is often easily distracted by extraneous stimuli (for older adolescents and adults, may include unrelated thoughts).
   i. Is often forgetful in daily activities (e.g., chores, running errands; for older adolescents and adults, returning calls, paying bills, keeping appointments).
2. **Hyperactivity and Impulsivity:** Six (or more) of the following symptoms have persisted for at least 6 months to a degree that is inconsistent with developmental level and that negatively impacts directly on social and academic/occupational activities.

   NOTE: The symptoms are not solely a manifestation of oppositional behavior, defiance, hostility, or a failure to understand tasks or instructions. For older adolescents and adults (age 17 and older), at least five symptoms are required.

   a. Often fidgets with or taps hands or feet or squirms in seat.
   b. Often leaves seat in situations when remaining seated is expected (e.g., leaves his or her place in the classroom, in the office or other workplace, or in other situations that require remaining in place).
   c. Often runs about or climbs in situations where it is inappropriate. (**NOTE:** In adolescents or adults, may be limited to feeling restless.)
   d. Often unable to play or engage in leisure activities quietly.
   e. Is often "on the go," acting as if "driven by a motor" (e.g., is unable to be or uncomfortable being still for extended time, as in restaurants, meetings; may be experienced by others as being restless and difficult to keep up with).
   f. Often talks excessively.
   g. Often blurts out an answer before a question has been completed (e.g., completes people's sentences; cannot wait for turn in conversation).
   h. Often has difficulty waiting his or her turn (e.g., while waiting in line).
   i. Often interrupts or intrudes on others (e.g., butts into conversations, games, or activities; may start using other people's things without asking or receiving permission; for adolescents or adults, may intrude into or take over what others are doing).

B. Several inattentive or hyperactive-impulsive symptoms were present prior to age 12 years.

C. Several inattentive or hyperactive-impulsive symptoms are present in two or more settings (e.g., at home, school, or work; with friends or relatives; in other activities).

D. There is clear evidence that the symptoms interfere with or reduce the quality of social, academic, or occupational functioning.

E. The symptoms do not occur exclusively during the course of schizophrenia or another psychotic disorder and are not better explained by another mental disorder (e.g., mood disorder, anxiety disorder, dissociative disorder, personality disorder, substance intoxication or withdrawal).

Specify whether:

Combined presentation: If both Criterion A1 (inattention) and Criterion A2 (hyperactivity-impulsivity) are met for the past 6 months.

Predominantly inattentive presentation: If Criterion A1 (inattention) is met but Criterion A2 (hyperactivity-impulsivity) is not met for the past 6 months.

Predominantly hyperactive/impulsive presentation: If Criterion A2 (hyperactivity-impulsivity) is met and Criterion A1 (inattention) is not met for the past 6 months.

Specify if:

In partial remission

Specify current severity:

Mild

Moderate

Severe

Reprinted with permission from American Psychiatric Association. (2022). Diagnostic and statistical manual of mental disorders, fifth edition, text revision.

Outcome Identification

Outcome criteria include short- and long-term goals. Timelines are individually determined. The following criteria may be used for measurement of outcomes in the care of the child with ADHD. The patient:

- Experiences no physical harm.
- Interacts with others appropriately.
- Verbalizes positive aspects about self.
- Demonstrates fewer demanding behaviors.
- Cooperates with staff in an effort to complete assigned tasks.

Planning and Implementation

Table 23–4 provides a plan of care for the child with ADHD using nursing diagnoses common to the disorder, outcome criteria, and appropriate nursing interventions and rationales.

Concept Care Mapping

The concept map care plan is a diagrammatic teaching and learning strategy that allows visualization of interrelationships between medical diagnoses, nursing diagnoses, assessment data, and treatments. An example of a concept map care plan for a client with ADHD is presented in Figure 23–2.

Evaluation

Evaluation of the care of a patient with ADHD involves examining patient behaviors following implementation of the nursing actions to determine whether the goals of therapy have been achieved. Collecting data by using the following types of questions may provide appropriate information for evaluation. Has the child:

- Remained free from injury?
- Been able to establish a trusting relationship with the primary caregiver?
- Responded to limits set on unacceptable behaviors?
- Been able to interact appropriately with others?
- Been able to verbalize positive statements about self?
- Been able to complete tasks independently or with a minimum of assistance? Can the child follow through after listening to simple instructions?
- Been able to apply self-control to decrease motor activity?

Psychopharmacological Treatment for ADHD

Medications, and particularly CNS stimulants, are considered first-line treatment for ADHD (Boland & Verduin, 2022). For a list of agents to treat ADHD, see Table 23–5. The mechanism of action is unclear, but because these drugs are known to elevate dopamine and norepinephrine levels, it has been hypothesized that their effectiveness is in response to neurotransmitter dysregulation. They have generally mild side effects, but they are contraindicated in anyone with cardiac problems or risks for cardiac problems. There is a high potential for abuse, tolerance, and dependence. As previously mentioned, there is also an increased risk for new-onset psychosis with amphetamine stimulants, which release about four times as much dopamine as methylphenidate (Griffin & Harari, 2019).

One study (Van den Ban et al., 2014) explored whether use of stimulants had an impact on reducing injuries and hospital admissions for children with ADHD. This study is relevant because these children have a high incidence of injury and hospital admissions related to hyperactivity and impulsivity. About 60% show suboptimal motor performance, which may also increase their risks for injury. The researchers found that children treated with ADHD drugs (mostly stimulants) had a twofold higher risk of injury-related hospital admissions than those not treated with ADHD drugs. They also found that children taking ADHD drugs and psychotropic drugs such as antipsychotics and benzodiazepines had a five times increase risk for injuries and hospital admissions than those who were on ADHD medication alone. The severity of ADHD in children on medication, may, in part, account for these findings, but it is significant that these medications, while mediating other core symptoms of ADHD, may not reduce risks for injury. Amphetamines are a common substance of abuse and demonstrate high risk for dependence, and similar concerns have been identified for clients with ADHD. The recent FDA approval of Adzenys XR-ODT, a flavored chewable amphetamine mixture tablet, has raised concerns that it may increase use or abuse in children and become a gateway drug (Grohol, 2016). See Chapter 4, "Psychopharmacology," for a complete discussion of the medications used in the treatment of ADHD, including safety and education issues.

Nonpharmacological Treatment for ADHD

A recent study using trigeminal nerve stimulation in patients with ADHD demonstrated potential

Table 23–4 | CARE PLAN FOR THE CHILD WITH ATTENTION DEFICIT-HYPERACTIVITY DISORDER

NURSING DIAGNOSIS: RISK FOR INJURY

RELATED TO: Impulsive and accident-prone behavior and the inability to perceive self-harm

OUTCOME CRITERIA	NURSING INTERVENTIONS	RATIONALE
Short- and Long-Term Goal ■ Patient will be free of injury.	1. Ensure that the patient has a safe environment. Remove from immediate area objects on which the patient could injure self as a result of random, hyperactive movements.	1. Objects that are appropriate to the normal living situation can be hazardous to the child whose motor activities are out of control.
	2. Identify deliberate behaviors that put the child at risk for injury. Institute consequences for repetition of this behavior.	2. Behavior can be modified with aversive reinforcement.
	3. Provide adequate supervision and assistance while providing opportunities for physical exercise such as team sports, walking or running, dancing, and others.	3. Patient safety is a nursing priority. Exercise is an important outlet for hyperactivity and may also improve focus.

NURSING DIAGNOSIS: IMPAIRED SOCIAL INTERACTION

RELATED TO: Intrusive and immature behavior

OUTCOME CRITERIA	NURSING INTERVENTIONS	RATIONALE
Short-Term Goal ■ Patient will interact in age-appropriate manner with nurse in one-to-one relationship within 1 week. **Long-Term Goal** ■ Patient will observe limits set on intrusive behavior and will demonstrate ability to interact appropriately with others.	1. Develop a trusting relationship with the child. Convey acceptance of the child separate from the unacceptable behavior.	1. Unconditional acceptance increases feelings of self-worth.
	2. Discuss with the patient those behaviors that are and are not acceptable. Describe in a matter-of-fact manner the consequences of unacceptable behavior. Follow through.	2. Aversive reinforcement can alter undesirable behaviors.
	3. Provide group situations for the patient.	3. Appropriate social behavior is often learned from the positive and negative feedback of peers.

NURSING DIAGNOSIS: LOW SELF-ESTEEM

RELATED TO: Dysfunctional family system and negative feedback

OUTCOME CRITERIA	NURSING INTERVENTIONS	RATIONALE
Short-Term Goal ■ Patient will independently direct own care and activities of daily living within 1 week.	1. Ensure that goals are realistic.	1. Unrealistic goals set patients up for failure, which diminishes self-esteem.
	2. Plan activities that provide opportunities for success.	2. Success enhances self-esteem.
	3. Convey unconditional acceptance and positive regard.	3. Affirmation of the patient as worthwhile human being promotes self-esteem.

Table 23–4 | CARE PLAN FOR THE CHILD WITH ATTENTION DEFICIT-HYPERACTIVITY DISORDER—cont'd

OUTCOME CRITERIA	NURSING INTERVENTIONS	RATIONALE
Long-Term Goal ■ Patient will demonstrate increased feelings of self-worth by verbalizing positive statements about self and exhibiting fewer demanding behaviors.	4. Offer recognition of successful endeavors and positive reinforcement for attempts made. Give immediate positive feedback for acceptable behavior.	4. Positive reinforcement enhances self-esteem and may increase the desired behaviors.

NURSING DIAGNOSIS: NONCOMPLIANCE (WITH TASK EXPECTATIONS)

RELATED TO: Low frustration tolerance and short attention span

OUTCOME CRITERIA	NURSING INTERVENTIONS	RATIONALE
Short-Term Goal ■ Patient will participate in and cooperate during therapeutic activities. **Long-Term Goal** ■ Patient will be able to complete assigned tasks independently or with a minimum of assistance.	1. Provide an environment for task efforts that is as free as possible of distractions.	1. Patient is highly distractible and is unable to perform in the presence of even minimal stimulation.
	2. Provide assistance on a one-to-one basis, beginning with simple, concrete instructions.	2. Patients lack the ability to assimilate information that is complicated or has abstract meaning.
	3. Ask the patient to repeat instructions back.	3. Repetition of the instructions helps to determine the patient's level of comprehension.
	4. Establish goals that allow the patient to complete a part of the task, rewarding completion of each step with a break for physical activity.	4. Short-term goals are not so overwhelming to one with such a short attention span. The positive reinforcement (physical activity) increases self-esteem and provides incentive for the patient to pursue the task to completion.
	5. Gradually decrease the amount of assistance given, while assuring the patient that assistance is still available if deemed necessary.	5. This intervention encourages the patient to perform independently while providing a feeling of security with the presence of a trusted individual.

benefits for improving attention and decreasing both hyperactivity and impulsivity (McGough et al., 2019). The treatment can be administered nightly at home, and after a 4-week trial, study participants showed sustained improvement in lessening both hyperactivity and inattention. Longer-term studies are needed to evaluate outcomes and best practice guidelines.

In a systematic review (Goode et al., 2018), the authors concluded that while numerous nonpharmacological treatments for ADHD have been studied and are widely used (including neurofeedback, cognitive training, cognitive behavioral therapy, child or parent training, dietary omega fatty acid supplementation, and herbal and/or dietary approaches), there are significant gaps in knowledge about their effectiveness.

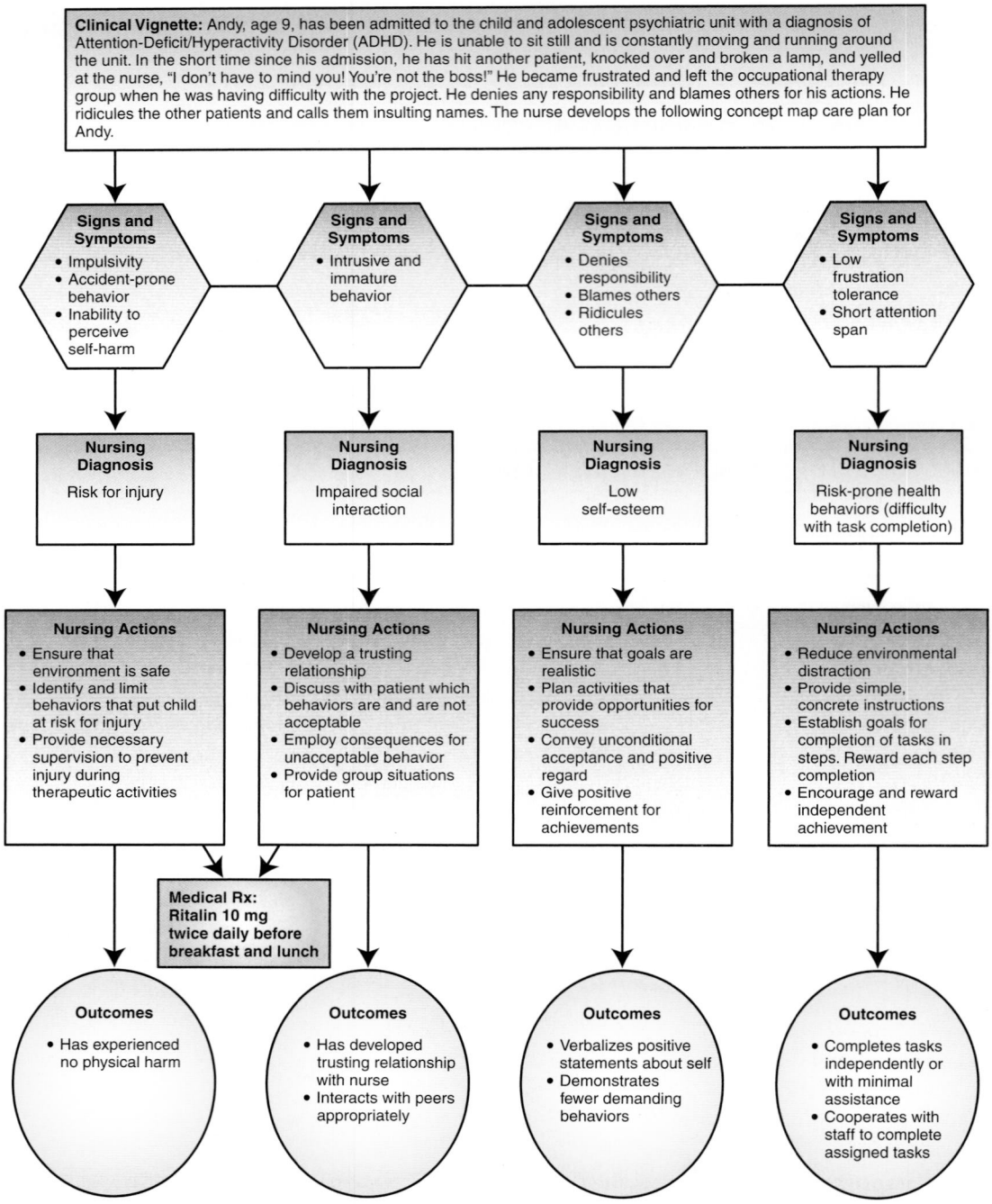

FIGURE 23–2 Concept map care plan for a patient with attention deficit-hyperactivity disorder.

Tourette's Disorder

Clinical Findings, Epidemiology, and Course

Tourette's disorder is characterized by the presence of multiple motor tics and one or more vocal tics, which may appear simultaneously or at different periods during the illness (APA, 2022). The disturbance may cause distress or interfere with social, occupational, or other important areas of functioning. The age at onset of Tourette's disorder can be as early as 2 years, but the disorder occurs most commonly during childhood (around age 6 to

TABLE 23–5 Agents for Attention Deficit-Hyperactivity Disorder

CHEMICAL CLASS	GENERIC (TRADE) NAME	DAILY DOSAGE RANGE (mg)	CONTROLLED CATEGORIES
CNS STIMULANTS			
AMPHETAMINES	Dextroamphetamine sulfate (Dexedrine; Dextrostat)	2.5–40	CII
	Methamphetamine (Desoxyn)	5–25	CII
	Lisdexamfetamine (Vyvanse)	20–70	CII
AMPHETAMINE MIXTURES	Dextroamphetamine/ amphetamine (Adderall; Adderall XR) Adderall XR-ODT	2.5–40 6.3–18.8	CII CII
MISCELLANEOUS	Methylphenidate (Ritalin; Ritalin-SR; Ritalin LA; Methylin; Methylin ER; Metadate ER; Metadate CD; Concerta; Daytrana)	10–60	CII
	Dexmethylphenidate (Focalin) Serdexmethylphenidate and dexmethylphenidate (Azstarys)	5–20 26.1/5.–52.3/10.4	CII CII
ALPHA AGONISTS	Clonidine (Catapres)	0.05–0.3	—
	Guanfacine (Tenex; Intuniv)	1–4	—
MISCELLANEOUS	Atomoxetine (Strattera)	>70 kg: 40–100; <70 kg: 0.5–1.4 (or 100 mg—whichever is less)	—
	Bupropion (Wellbutrin; Wellbutrin SR; Wellbutrin XL)	3 mg/kg (ADHD); 100–300 (depression)	—

7 years). Prevalence of the disorder is estimated at 3 to 9 per 1,000 in school-age children (APA, 2022). The lifetime prevalence is estimated to be about 1% (Boland & Verduin, 2022). It is two to four times more common in boys than in girls. Although the disorder can be lifelong, most people with this condition experience the worst tic symptoms in their early teens with gradual improvement thereafter; some may become symptom free and no longer require medication for tic suppression (National Institutes of Health [NIH], 2021).

Predisposing Factors

Biological Factors

- ***Genetics:*** Various genetic studies, including twin and adoption studies, support a genetic basis for this neurological disorder (Boland & Verduin, 2022). Recent studies suggest that the pattern of inheritance is complex, probably involving several genes influenced by environmental factors (NIH, 2021). In addition, genetic studies suggest that ADHD and obsessive-compulsive disorder are genetically related to Tourette's disorder; as many as 50% of patients with Tourette's disorder also have ADHD, and up to 40% have obsessive-compulsive disorder (Boland & Verduin, 2022; NIH, 2021).
- ***Biochemical factors:*** Abnormalities in levels of dopamine, choline, *N*-acetylaspartate, creatine, myoinositol, and norepinephrine have all been demonstrated in neuroimaging studies, and the effectiveness of antipsychotic medication (particularly haloperidol and fluphenazine) in suppressing tics also supports neurotransmitter involvement in Tourette's disorder (Boland & Verduin, 2022). However, Boland and Verduin add that there is variability in response to antipsychotic medications, and Tourette's disorder has sometimes emerged while a client is being treated with antipsychotics. Although there appear to be several biochemical

influences in this disorder, these interactions are complex and not well understood.

- ***Structural factors:*** Abnormalities in the basal ganglia, frontal lobes, cortex, and circuits that connect these regions have also been implicated in the pathology of this disorder (NIH, 2021). Although many structural influences have been identified, the direct cause is not yet known. It is probably a complex interaction of genetics, biochemistry, and environmental influences.

Environmental Factors

Some studies have shown that environmental influences, such as maternal alcohol use during pregnancy, low birth weight, complications during childbirth, and infection, may be associated with the development of Tourette's disorder (Boland & Verduin, 2022; CDC, 2020b). Further research is needed to confirm these influences.

Application of the Nursing Process to Tourette's Disorder

Background Assessment Data

The motor tics of Tourette's disorder may involve the head, torso, and upper and lower limbs. Initial symptoms may begin with a single motor tic, most commonly eye blinking, or with multiple symptoms. Initially, tics tend to occur in the face and neck and progress downward to the torso and lower limbs over time (Boland & Verduin, 2022). Simple motor tics include movements such as eye blinking, neck jerking, shoulder shrugging, and facial grimacing. The more complex motor tics include squatting, hopping, skipping, tapping, touching behaviors, grooming rituals, echopraxia, and retracing steps. Some tics involve self-harm, such as punching oneself in the face (NIH, 2021).

Vocal tics include various words or sounds such as squeaks, grunts, barks, sniffs, snorts, coughs, and, in rare instances, a complex vocal tic involving the uttering of obscenities. Vocal tics may include repeating certain words or phrases out of context, repeating one's own sounds or words **(palilalia),** or repeating what others say **(echolalia).**

The movements and vocalizations are experienced as compulsive and irresistible, but they can be suppressed for varying lengths of time. Many individuals with Tourette's disorder report a buildup of tension as they attempt to suppress tics to the point where they feel the tic must be expressed against their will. Tics are often worse during periods of stress or excitement and better during periods of calm, focused activity (NIH, 2021). In most cases, tics are diminished during sleep. Neurobehavioral disorders that are common in conjunction with Tourette's disorder (and may be more troublesome than the tics themselves) are inattention, hyperactivity, and impulsivity as are seen in ADHD; and obsessive-compulsive disorder, depression, and anxiety. Many children with Tourette's disorder also manifest difficulty with reading, writing, and arithmetic (NIH, 2021). The *DSM-5-TR* diagnostic criteria for Tourette's disorder require that both motor and vocal tics have been present at some time during the illness and are persistent for more than one year.

Nursing Diagnoses

Based on data collected during the nursing assessment, possible nursing diagnoses for the patient with Tourette's disorder include the following:

- Risk for self-directed or other-directed violence related to low tolerance for frustration
- Impaired social interaction related to impulsiveness, oppositional and aggressive behavior
- Low self-esteem related to embarrassment associated with tic behaviors

Outcome Identification

Outcome criteria include short- and long-term goals. Timelines are individually determined. The following criteria may be used for measurement of outcomes in the care of the patient with Tourette's disorder. The patient:

- Has not harmed self or others.
- Interacts with staff and peers in an appropriate manner.
- Demonstrates self-control by managing tic behavior.
- Follows rules without becoming defensive.
- Verbalizes positive aspects about self.

Planning and Implementation

Table 23–6 provides a plan of care for the child or adolescent with Tourette's disorder using selected nursing diagnoses, outcome criteria, and appropriate nursing interventions and rationales.

Evaluation

Evaluation of care for the child with Tourette's disorder reflects whether or not the nursing actions have been effective in achieving the established goals. The nursing process calls for reassessment of the

Table 23–6 | CARE PLAN FOR THE CHILD OR ADOLESCENT WITH TOURETTE'S DISORDER

NURSING DIAGNOSIS: RISK FOR SELF-DIRECTED OR OTHER-DIRECTED VIOLENCE

RELATED TO: Low tolerance for frustration

OUTCOME CRITERIA	NURSING INTERVENTIONS	RATIONALE
Short-Term Goal ■ Patient will seek out staff or support person at any time if thoughts of harming self or others should occur. **Long-Term Goal** ■ Patient will not harm self or others.	1. Observe the patient's behavior frequently through routine activities and interactions. Become aware of behaviors that indicate a rise in agitation.	1. Stress commonly increases tic behaviors. Recognition of behaviors that precede the onset of aggression may provide the opportunity to intervene before violence occurs.
	2. Monitor for self-destructive behavior and impulses. A staff member may need to stay with the patient to prevent self-mutilation.	2. Patient safety is a nursing priority.
	3. Provide hand coverings and other restraints that prevent the patient from self-mutilative behaviors.	3. For the patient's protection, provide immediate external controls against self-aggressive behaviors.
	4. Redirect violent behavior with physical outlets for frustration.	4. Excess energy is released through physical activities and a feeling of relaxation is induced.

NURSING DIAGNOSIS: IMPAIRED SOCIAL INTERACTION

RELATED TO: Impulsiveness; oppositional and aggressive behavior

OUTCOME CRITERIA	NURSING INTERVENTIONS	RATIONALE
Short-Term Goal ■ Patient will develop a one-to-one relationship with a nurse or support person within 1 week. **Long-Term Goal** ■ Patient will be able to interact with staff and peers using age-appropriate, acceptable behaviors.	1. Develop a trusting relationship with the patient. Convey acceptance of the person separate from the unacceptable behavior.	1. Unconditional acceptance increases feelings of self-worth.
	2. Discuss with the patient which behaviors are and are not acceptable. Describe in matter-of-fact manner the consequences of unacceptable behavior. Follow through.	2. Aversive reinforcement can alter undesirable behaviors.
	3. Provide group situations for the patient.	3. Appropriate social behavior is often learned from the positive and negative feedback of peers.

NURSING DIAGNOSIS: LOW SELF-ESTEEM

RELATED TO: Embarrassment associated with tic behaviors

OUTCOME CRITERIA	NURSING INTERVENTIONS	RATIONALE
Short-Term Goal ■ Patient will verbalize positive aspects about self not associated with tic behaviors.	1. Convey unconditional acceptance and positive regard.	1. Communicating a perception of the patient as a worthwhile human being promotes self-esteem.
	2. Set limits on manipulative behavior. Take precautions not to reinforce manipulative behaviors by providing desired attention. Identify the consequences of manipulation. Administer consequences in a matter-of-fact manner when manipulation occurs.	2. Aversive consequences may work to decrease unacceptable behaviors.

Continued

Table 23–6 | CARE PLAN FOR THE CHILD OR ADOLESCENT WITH TOURETTE'S DISORDER—cont'd

OUTCOME CRITERIA	NURSING INTERVENTIONS	RATIONALE
Long-Term Goal ■ Patient will exhibit increased feeling of self-worth as evidenced by verbal expression of positive aspects about self, past accomplishments, and future prospects.	3. Help the patient understand the use of manipulation to try to increase own self-esteem. Interventions should reflect other actions to accomplish this goal.	3. When the patient feels better about self, the need to manipulate others will diminish.
	4. If the patient chooses to suppress tics in the presence of others, provide a specified "tic time" during which the patient "vents" tics, feelings, and behaviors (alone or with staff).	4. Allows for release of tics and assists in sense of control and management of symptoms.
	5. Ensure that the patient has regular one-to-one time with nursing staff.	5. One-to-one time gives the nurse the opportunity to provide the patient with information about the illness and healthy ways to manage it. Exploring feelings about the illness helps the patient incorporate the illness into a healthy sense of self.

plan. Questions for gathering reassessment data may include the following. Has the patient:

- Refrained from causing harm to self or others during times of increased tension?
- Developed adaptive coping strategies for dealing with frustration to prevent resorting to self-destruction or aggression to others?
- Been able to interact appropriately with staff and peers?
- Been able to suppress tic behaviors when choosing to do so?
- Set a time for "release" of the suppressed tic behaviors?
- Verbalized positive aspects about self, particularly as they relate to the ability to manage the illness?
- Complied with treatment in a nondefensive manner?

Psychopharmacological Intervention for Tourette's Disorder

Systematic review of current evidence supports the efficacy of antipsychotic agents, both typical and atypical agents, and the use of alpha$_2$-adrenergic agonist agents (such as clonidine) in treating tics (Weisman et al., 2013). Medications are reserved for those with significant impairment and unresponsive to psychological therapies. Weisman and associates (2013) note that alpha$_2$ agonists are more efficacious in treating tics among patients with ADHD. Other medications that have demonstrated potential benefits, but need more research, include tetrabenazine, topiramate, and tetrahydrocannabinol. Pharmacotherapy is most effective when it is combined with psychosocial therapy, such as behavioral therapy, individual counseling or psychotherapy, and/or family therapy. Medications that are used in the treatment of Tourette's disorder include antipsychotics, and alpha agonists.

Antipsychotics

The typical antipsychotics, haloperidol (Haldol) and pimozide (Orap), and the atypical antipsychotic aripiprazole have been approved by the FDA for control of tics and vocal utterances associated with Tourette's disorder. These drugs have been widely investigated and have proved to be highly effective in alleviating these symptoms. Conventional antipsychotics are often not the first-line choice of therapy, however, because of their propensity for severe adverse effects, such as extrapyramidal symptoms, neuroleptic malignant syndrome, tardive dyskinesia, and electrocardiographic changes. Haloperidol is not recommended for children younger than 3 years of age, and pimozide should not be administered to children younger than 12 years.

Although not at present approved by the FDA for use in Tourette's disorder, some clinicians prefer to prescribe other atypical antipsychotics, such as risperidone (Risperdal), olanzapine (Zyprexa), or ziprasidone (Geodon), because of their more favorable side effect profiles. Boland and Verduin (2022) identify risperidone as the most well-studied atypical antipsychotic for the treatment of tics and report that there is considerable evidence for its efficacy. These medications have a lower incidence of neurological side effects than the typical antipsychotics, although extrapyramidal symptoms have been observed with risperidone. Metabolic side effects include weight gain and hyperprolactinemia. Ziprasidone has been associated with increased risk of QTc interval prolongation. Hyperglycemia has also been reported in some patients taking atypical antipsychotics.

Alpha Agonists

Clonidine (Catapres) and guanfacine (Tenex, Intuniv) are alpha-adrenergic agonists that are approved for use as antihypertensive agents. The extended-release forms have been approved by the FDA for the treatment of ADHD. Atomoxetine, a selective norepinephrine reuptake inhibitor (SNRI), has also been used, but more research is needed to confirm safety and efficacy in treating children with Tourette's disorder (Boland & Verduin, 2022). These medications may be used for treatment of Tourette's disorder because of their favorable side effect profile and because they are often effective in treating comorbid symptoms of ADHD, anxiety, and insomnia. Common side effects include dry mouth, sedation, headaches, fatigue, and dizziness or postural hypotension.

Guanfacine is longer lasting and less sedating than clonidine; however, its efficacy in reducing tics is controversial (Boland & Verduin, 2022). Alpha agonists should not be prescribed for children and adolescents with pre-existing cardiac or vascular disease. They should not be discontinued abruptly; to do so could result in symptoms of nervousness, agitation, and tremor, as well as a rapid rise in blood pressure.

Nonpharmacological Treatments for Tourette's Disorder

Nonpharmacological treatments for tic disorders include comprehensive behavioral intervention for tics (CBIT), habit reversal training, behavioral therapy, speech therapy, and deep brain or transcranial magnetic stimulation. CBIT is an evidence-based approach that includes habit reversal training and teaches individuals how to recognize and manage environmental factors that trigger or worsen tics. Studies have demonstrated improvement at least 6 months after CBIT (Tourette's Association of America, n.d.), and habit reversal is currently the first-line behavioral treatment for tic disorders (Boland & Verduin, 2022). Individuals with Tourette's syndrome who also have other co-occurring conditions such as social language impairments, learning disabilities, or other communication disorders may benefit from speech and language therapy. Deep brain stimulation is an experimental surgical treatment that involves connecting electrodes to brain centers and implanting a pulse generator to stimulate areas of the brain associated with communication. It is yet to be determined which centers are the best targets for neuromodulation, but it has demonstrated success in some patients. This treatment is an option when all other treatments have been tried and found ineffective.

Disruptive Behavior Disorders

Oppositional Defiant Disorder

Clinical Findings, Epidemiology, and Course

Oppositional defiant disorder (ODD) is characterized by a frequent and persistent pattern of angry mood and defiant behavior that occurs more frequently than is usually observed in individuals of comparable age and developmental level and interferes with social, educational, occupational, or other important areas of functioning (APA, 2022). It must be understood as distinct, pervasive, and more disruptive than the sometimes negativistic and oppositional behavior that is typical in childhood and adolescence. The disorder typically begins by 8 years of age and usually not later than early adolescence. Prevalence estimates range from 1% to 11%, and common comorbid disorders include ADHD, anxiety, major depressive disorder, conduct disorder, and substance use disorders (APA, 2022). It is more prevalent in boys than in girls before puberty, but the rates are more equal after puberty. The *DSM-5-TR* identifies that ODD often precedes conduct disorder, especially in children with onset of conduct disorder prior to 10 years of age (APA, 2022).

Predisposing Factors

Biological Influences

What role, if any, genetics, temperament, or biochemical alterations play in the etiology of ODD is still unclear. Some studies have identified genetic influences in the establishment of a child's temperament, but there is no clear evidence of this connection in ODD. However, having a temperament in which the child has difficulty regulating emotions and has low frustration tolerance is an identified risk factor for ODD (Mayo Clinic, 2021b).

Family Influences

Opposition during various developmental stages is both normal and healthy. Children first exhibit oppositional behaviors at around 10 or 11 months of age, again as toddlers between 18 and 36 months of age, and finally during adolescence. Pathology is considered only when the developmental phase is prolonged or when there is overreaction in the child's environment to the behavior.

Some children exhibit these behaviors in a more intense form than others. Boland and Verduin (2022) report, "Epidemiological studies of negativistic traits in nonclinical populations found such behavior in 16% to 22% of school-age children" (p. 189).

Some parents interpret average or increased level of developmental oppositional behavior as hostility and a deliberate effort on the part of the child to be in control. If power and control are issues for parents, or if they exercise authority for their own needs, a power struggle can be established between the parents and the child that sets the stage for the development of ODD. Lubit (2015) suggested the following pattern of family dynamics:

- There is the combination of a strong-willed child with a reactive and high-energy temperament and parents who are authoritarian rather than authoritative.
- The parents become frustrated with the strong-willed child who does not obey and increase their attempts to enforce authority.
- The child reacts to the excessive parental control with anger and increased self-assertion.

Lubit (2015) stated:

> These patterns develop when parents inadvertently reinforce disruptive and deviant behaviors in a child by giving those behaviors a significant amount of negative attention. At the same time, the parents, who are often exhausted by the struggle to obtain compliance with simple requests, usually fail to provide positive attention; often, the parents have infrequent positive interactions with their children. The pattern of negative interactions evolves quickly as the result of repeated, ineffective, emotionally expressed commands and comments; ineffective harsh punishments; and insufficient attention and modeling of appropriate behaviors.

A childhood history of trauma can be influential in the appearance of ODD behaviors, so it is essential to assess the child for history of abuse, neglect, or other traumas.

Application of the Nursing Process to ODD

Background Assessment Data

ODD is characterized by passive-aggressive behaviors such as stubbornness, procrastination, disobedience, carelessness, **negativism,** testing of limits, resistance to directions, deliberately ignoring the communication of others, and unwillingness to compromise. Other symptoms that may be evident are running away, school avoidance, school underachievement, temper tantrums, fighting, and argumentativeness.

Initially, the oppositional attitude is directed toward the parents, but, in time, relationships with peers and teachers become affected. These impairments in social interaction often lead to depression, anxiety, and additional problematic behavior (Lubit, 2015).

Usually, these children do not see themselves as being oppositional but view the problem as arising from others who they believe are making unreasonable demands on them. These children are often friendless, perceiving human relationships as negative and unsatisfactory. School performance is usually poor because of their refusal to participate and their resistance to external demands.

The *DSM-5-TR* diagnostic criteria for ODD are presented in Box 23–3.

Nursing Diagnoses

Based on the data collected during the nursing assessment, possible nursing diagnoses for the patient with ODD include the following:

- Noncompliance with therapy related to negative temperament, denial of problems, underlying hostility
- Defensive coping related to retarded ego development, low self-esteem, unsatisfactory parent-child relationship
- Low self-esteem related to lack of positive feedback, retarded ego development
- Impaired social interaction related to negative temperament, underlying hostility, manipulation of others

BOX 23–3 Diagnostic Criteria for Oppositional Defiant Disorder

A. A pattern of angry/irritable mood, argumentative/defiant behavior, or vindictiveness lasting at least 6 months as evidenced by at least four symptoms from any of the following categories and exhibited during interaction with at least one individual that is not a sibling.

ANGRY/IRRITABLE MOOD

1. Often loses temper.
2. Is often touchy or easily annoyed.
3. Is often angry and resentful.

ARGUMENTATIVE/DEFIANT BEHAVIOR

1. Often argues with authority figures or, for children and adolescents, with adults.
2. Often actively defies or refuses to comply with requests from authority figures or with rules.
3. Often deliberately annoys others.
4. Often blames others for his or her mistakes or misbehavior.

VINDICTIVENESS

1. Has been spiteful or vindictive at least twice within the past 6 months.

NOTE: The persistence and frequency of these behaviors should be used to distinguish a behavior that is within normal limits from a behavior that is symptomatic. For children younger than 5 years, the behavior should occur on most days for a period of at least 6 months unless otherwise noted (Criterion A8). For individuals 5 years or older, the behavior should occur at least once per week for at least 6 months, unless otherwise noted (Criterion A8). While these frequency criteria provide guidance on a minimal level of frequency to define symptoms, other factors should also be considered, such as whether the frequency and intensity of the behaviors are outside a range that is normative for the individual's developmental level, gender, and culture.

B. The disturbance in behavior is associated with distress in the individual or others in his or her immediate social context (e.g., family, peer group, work colleagues), or it impacts negatively on social, educational, occupational, or other important areas of functioning.

C. The behaviors do not occur exclusively during the course of a psychotic, substance use, depressive, or bipolar disorder. Also, the criteria are not met for disruptive mood dysregulation disorder.

Specify current severity:

Mild: Symptoms are confined to only one setting (e.g., at home, at school, at work, with peers).

Moderate: Some symptoms are present in at least two settings.

Severe: Some symptoms are present in three or more settings.

Reprinted with permission from American Psychiatric Association. (2022). Diagnostic and statistical manual of mental disorders, fifth edition, text revision.

Outcome Identification

Outcome criteria include short- and long-term goals. Timelines are individually determined. The following criteria may be used for measurement of outcomes in the care of the patient with ODD. The patient:

- Complies with treatment by participating in therapies without negativism.
- Accepts responsibility for their part in the problem.
- Takes direction from staff without becoming defensive.
- Does not manipulate other people.
- Verbalizes positive aspects about self.
- Interacts with others in an appropriate manner.

Planning and Implementation

Table 23–7 provides a plan of care for the child with ODD using nursing diagnoses common to the disorder, outcome criteria, and appropriate nursing interventions and rationales.

Evaluation

The evaluation step of the nursing process calls for reassessment of the plan of care to determine whether the nursing actions have been effective in achieving the goals of therapy. The following questions can be used with the child or adolescent with ODD to gather information for the evaluation. Is the patient:

- Cooperating with schedule of therapeutic activities? Is level of participation adequate?
- Manifesting a less negative attitude toward therapy?
- Accepting responsibility for problem behavior?
- Verbalizing the unacceptability of the passive-aggressive behavior?
- Able to identify which behaviors are unacceptable and substitute more adaptive behaviors?
- Able to interact with staff and peers without defending behavior in an angry manner?
- Able to verbalize positive statements about self?

- Manifesting fewer manipulative behaviors?
- Able to make compromises with others when issues of control emerge?
- Expressing anger and hostility appropriately and verbalizing ways of releasing anger adaptively?
- Able to verbalize true feelings instead of allowing them to emerge through use of passive-aggressive behaviors?

Conduct Disorder

Clinical Findings, Epidemiology, and Course

With **conduct disorder (CD),** there is a repetitive and persistent pattern of behavior in which the basic rights of others or major age-appropriate societal norms or rules are violated (APA, 2022). This feature distinguishes it from ODD. Physical aggression

Table 23–7 | CARE PLAN FOR THE CHILD/ADOLESCENT WITH OPPOSITIONAL DEFIANT DISORDER

NURSING DIAGNOSIS: NONCOMPLIANCE WITH THERAPY

RELATED TO: Negative temperament; denial of problems; underlying hostility

OUTCOME CRITERIA	NURSING INTERVENTIONS	RATIONALE
Short-Term Goal ■ Patient will participate in and cooperate during therapeutic activities. **Long-Term Goal** ■ Patient will complete assigned tasks willingly and independently or with a minimum of assistance.	1. Set forth a structured plan of therapeutic activities. Start with minimum expectations and increase as the patient begins to manifest evidence of compliance. 2. Establish a system of rewards for compliance with therapy and consequences for noncompliance. Ensure that the rewards and consequences are concepts of value to the patient. 3. Convey acceptance of the patient separate from the undesirable behaviors being exhibited ("It is not *you* but your *behavior* that is unacceptable").	1. Structure provides security, and one or two activities may not seem as overwhelming as the whole schedule of activities presented at one time. 2. Positive, negative, and aversive reinforcements can contribute to desired changes in behavior. 3. Unconditional acceptance enhances self-worth and may contribute to a decrease in the need for passive-aggression toward others.

NURSING DIAGNOSIS: DEFENSIVE COPING

RELATED TO: Retarded ego development; low self-esteem; unsatisfactory parent-child relationship

OUTCOME CRITERIA	NURSING INTERVENTIONS	RATIONALE
Short-Term Goal ■ Patient will verbalize personal responsibility for difficulties experienced in interpersonal relationships within (time period reasonable for patient). **Long-Term Goal** ■ Patient will accept responsibility for own behaviors and interact with others without becoming defensive.	1. Teach the patient that feelings of inadequacy provoke many defensive behaviors, such as blaming others for problems and the need to "get even." 2. Provide immediate, nonthreatening feedback for passive-aggressive behavior. 3. Help identify situations that provoke defensiveness, and practice through role-play more appropriate responses. 4. Provide immediate positive feedback for acceptable behaviors.	1. Recognition of the problem is the first step toward initiating change. 2. When the patient denies responsibility for problems, the patient is denying the inappropriateness of behavior. 3. Role-playing provides confidence to deal with difficult situations when they actually occur. 4. Positive feedback encourages repetition, and immediacy is significant for these children who respond to immediate gratification.

Table 23–7 | CARE PLAN FOR THE CHILD/ADOLESCENT WITH OPPOSITIONAL DEFIANT DISORDER—cont'd

NURSING DIAGNOSIS: LOW SELF-ESTEEM

RELATED TO: Lack of positive feedback; retarded ego development

OUTCOME CRITERIA	NURSING INTERVENTIONS	RATIONALE
Short-Term Goal ■ Patient will participate in own self-care and discuss with nurse aspects of self about which the patient feels good. **Long-Term Goal** ■ Patient will demonstrate increased feelings of self-worth by verbalizing positive statements about self and exhibiting fewer manipulative behaviors.	1. Ensure that goals are realistic.	1. Unrealistic goals set the patient up for failure, which diminishes self-esteem.
	2. Plan activities that provide opportunities for success.	2. Success enhances self-esteem.
	3. Convey unconditional acceptance and positive regard.	3. Affirmation of the patient as a worthwhile human being promotes positive self-esteem.
	4. Set limits on manipulative behavior. Take precautions not to reinforce manipulative behaviors by providing desired attention. Identify the consequences of manipulation. Administer consequences matter-of-factly when manipulation occurs.	4. Aversive reinforcement may work to decrease unacceptable behaviors.
	5. Help the patient understand the use of this behavior to try to increase own self-esteem. Interventions should reflect other actions to accomplish this goal.	5. When the patient feels better about self, the need to manipulate others will diminish.

NURSING DIAGNOSIS: IMPAIRED SOCIAL INTERACTION

RELATED TO: Negative temperament; underlying hostility; manipulation of others

OUTCOME CRITERIA	NURSING INTERVENTIONS	RATIONALE
Short-Term Goal ■ Patient will interact in age-appropriate manner with nurse in one-to-one relationship within 1 week. **Long-Term Goal** ■ Patient will be able to interact with staff and peers using age-appropriate, acceptable behaviors.	1. Develop a trusting relationship. Convey acceptance of the person separate from the unacceptable behavior and listen to the patient's perceptions about relationships and behaviors.	1. Unconditional acceptance increases feelings of self-worth and may serve to diminish feelings of rejection that have accumulated over a long period.
	2. Explain to the patient about passive-aggressive behavior. Explain how these behaviors are perceived by others. Describe which behaviors are not acceptable, and role-play more adaptive responses. Give positive feedback for acceptable behaviors.	2. Role-playing is a way to practice behaviors that do not come readily to the patient, making it easier when the situation actually occurs. Positive feedback enhances repetition of desirable behaviors.
	3. Provide peer group situations for the patient.	3. Appropriate social behavior is often learned from the positive and negative feedback of peers. Groups also provide an atmosphere for using the behaviors rehearsed in role-play.

is common, and peer relationships are disturbed. This is one of the most frequent reasons that children and adolescents are referred for psychiatric intervention (Boland & Verduin, 2022). Prevalence estimates range from 2% to more than 10%, the prevalence rises from childhood to adolescence, and it is more common in males than females (APA, 2022). There is a higher male predominance among those with the childhood-onset subtype. A number of comorbidities are common with CD, including ADHD, mood disorders, learning disorders, and substance use disorders. The symptoms of ODD are generally considered less severe than those of CD, but ODD may progress to CD and both ODD and CD confer greater risk for antisocial personality disorder in adulthood (Connor, 2017). When the disorder begins in childhood, there is more likely to be a history of ODD and a greater likelihood of antisocial personality disorder in adulthood than if the disorder is diagnosed in adolescence.

CORE CONCEPT

Temperament

Personality characteristics that define an individual's mood and behavioral tendencies. The sum of physical, emotional, and intellectual components that affect or determine a person's actions and reactions.

Predisposing Factors

Biological Influences

- ***Genetics:*** Family, twin, and adoptive studies have revealed a significantly higher number of individuals with CD among those who have family members with the disorder. Although genetic factors appear to be involved in the etiology of CD, little is yet known about the actual mechanisms involved in genetic transmission. A potential role for X-linked monoamine oxidase A gene in the etiology of antisocial behavior suggests the need for more research into its potential role in conduct disorder (Boland & Verduin, 2022). There is some evidence of a distinction between behaviors that appear to be genetic versus environmental risk factors. In a large study of male twins (N = 2,769), researchers attempted to determine the structure of genetic and environmental influences in CD and found that the familial risk to CD is composed of two discrete dimensions of genetic risk: rule breaking (such as truancy) and overt aggression (harming other people) and one dimension of shared environmental risk, reflecting covert delinquency (such as stealing and hurting animals) (Kendler et al., 2013). Studies such as these support a complex dynamic of both genetic and environmental factors in the development of conduct disorder.
- ***Temperament:*** The term *temperament* refers to personality traits that become evident very early in life and may be present at birth. As early as 2 years of age, children who show signs of an irritable temperament, poor compliance, inattentiveness, and impulsivity can begin to show signs of CD at later ages (Bernstein, 2018). Bernstein adds that children with severe temperamental disturbances, including poor attachment, may develop ODD and CD despite adequate parental intervention, but it is more common that these children come from unstable families with frequent changes in residence and economic stress. Evidence suggests a genetic influence in temperament and an association between temperament and behavioral problems later in life.
- ***Neurobiological factors:*** Boland and Verduin (2022) identify three neurobiological findings relevant to CDs. First, neuroimaging studies identify decreased gray matter in limbic structures, bilateral insula (an area of the cortex that plays a role connecting emotional responses to pain), and the left amygdala. Second, studies have found high plasma concentration of serotonin and low levels in cerebrospinal fluid, both of which are correlated with aggression and violence. The third finding is that aggressive children had "significantly greater relative right frontal brain activity at rest than healthy controls" (p. 194).

Psychosocial Influences

Poor academic performance and social maladaptation often lead to affiliations with a deviant peer group. "Considerable research indicates that the deviant peer group provides training in criminal and delinquent behavior including substance abuse" (Bernstein, 2018). In addition, there is some evidence that engaging in risk-taking behaviors can yield reinforcement on a social level (acceptance within a peer group), and as Bernstein cites, "Studies of neural processing show that risk-taking may be associated with reward-related brain activation."

Family Influences

The following factors related to family dynamics have been implicated as contributors in the predisposition to CD and are typically in combination with one another to create a pattern of chaotic disruption in family life (Bernstein, 2018; Boland & Verduin, 2022; Woodward et al., 2019):

- Parental rejection, neglect, or severe physical and verbal aggression
- Inconsistent or harsh punitive discipline
- Parental sociopathy
- Lack of parental supervision
- Frequent changes in residence
- Economic stressors
- Parents with antisocial personality disorder, severe psychopathology, and/or alcohol or other substance dependence
- Marital conflict and divorce (particularly where there is persistence of hostility)

Application of the Nursing Process to Conduct Disorder

Background Assessment Data

The classic characteristic of CD is the use of physical aggression in the violation of the rights of others. The behavior pattern manifests itself in virtually all areas of the child's life (home, school, with peers, and in the community). Stealing, lying, and truancy are common problems. The child lacks feelings of guilt or remorse.

The use of tobacco, liquor, or nonprescribed drugs, as well as the participation in sexual activities, occurs earlier than at the expected age for the peer group. Projection is a common defense mechanism.

Low self-esteem is manifested by a "tough guy" image. Characteristics include poor frustration tolerance, irritability, and frequent temper outbursts. Symptoms of anxiety and depression are not uncommon.

Level of academic achievement may be low in relation to age and IQ. Manifestations associated with ADHD (e.g., attention difficulties, impulsiveness, and hyperactivity) are common in children with CD.

The *DSM-5-TR* diagnostic criteria for CD are presented in Box 23–4.

Nursing Diagnoses

Based on the data collected during the nursing assessment, possible nursing diagnoses for the patient with CD include the following:

- Risk for other-directed violence related to characteristics of temperament, peer rejection, negative parental role models, dysfunctional family dynamics
- Impaired social interaction related to negative parental role models, impaired peer relations leading to inappropriate social behaviors
- Defensive coping related to low self-esteem and dysfunctional family system
- Low self-esteem related to lack of positive feedback and unsatisfactory parent-child relationship

Outcome Identification

Outcome criteria include short- and long-term goals. Timelines are individually determined. The following criteria may be used for measurement of outcomes in the care of the patient with CD. The patient:

- Has not harmed self or others.
- Interacts with others in a socially appropriate manner.
- Accepts direction without becoming defensive.
- Demonstrates evidence of increased self-esteem by discontinuing exploitative and demanding behaviors toward others.

Planning and Implementation

Table 23–8 provides a plan of care for the child with CD using nursing diagnoses common to the disorder, outcome criteria, and appropriate nursing interventions and rationales.

Evaluation

Following the planning and implementation of care, evaluation is made of the behavioral changes in the child with CD. This is accomplished by determining whether the goals of therapy have been achieved. Reassessment, the next step in the nursing process, may be initiated by gathering information using the following questions. Has the patient:

- Been able to manage aggressive impulses?
- Been able to prevent harm to others or others' property?
- Been able to express anger in an appropriate manner?
- Developed more adaptive coping strategies to deal with anger and feelings of aggression?
- Demonstrated the ability to trust others and interact with staff and peers in an appropriate manner?
- Been able to accept responsibility for their own behavior? Is there less blaming of others?
- Been able to accept feedback from others without becoming defensive?
- Been able to verbalize positive statements about self?
- Been able to interact with others without engaging in manipulation?

BOX 23–4 Diagnostic Criteria for Conduct Disorder

A. A repetitive and persistent pattern of behavior in which the basic rights of others or major age-appropriate societal norms or rules are violated, as manifested by the presence of at least three of the following 15 criteria in the past 12 months from any of the categories below, with at least one criterion present in the past 6 months:

AGGRESSION TO PEOPLE AND ANIMALS

1. Often bullies, threatens, or intimidates others.
2. Often initiates physical fights.
3. Has used a weapon that can cause serious physical harm to others (e.g., a bat, brick, broken bottle, knife, gun).
4. Has been physically cruel to people.
5. Has been physically cruel to animals.
6. Has stolen while confronting a victim (e.g., mugging, purse snatching, extortion, armed robbery).
7. Has forced someone into sexual activity.

DESTRUCTION OF PROPERTY

8. Has deliberately engaged in fire setting with the intention of causing serious damage.
9. Has deliberately destroyed others' property (other than by fire setting).

DECEITFULNESS OR THEFT

10. Has broken into someone else's house, building, or car.
11. Often lies to obtain goods or favors or to avoid obligations (i.e., "cons" others).
12. Has stolen items of nontrivial value without confronting a victim (e.g., shoplifting, but without breaking and entering; forgery).

SERIOUS VIOLATIONS OF RULES

13. Often stays out at night despite parental prohibitions, beginning before age 13 years.
14. Has run away from home overnight at least twice while living in parental or parental surrogate home, or once without returning for a lengthy period.
15. Is often truant from school, beginning before age 13 years.

B. The disturbance in behavior causes clinically significant impairment in social, academic, or occupational functioning.

C. If the individual is age 18 years or older, criteria are not met for antisocial personality disorder.

Specify whether:

Childhood-Onset Type: Individuals show at least one symptom characteristic of conduct disorder prior to age 10 years.

Adolescent-Onset Type: Individuals show no symptom characteristic of conduct disorder prior to age 10 years.

Unspecified Onset: Criteria for a diagnosis of conduct disorder are met, but there is not enough information available to determine whether the onset of the first symptom was before or after age 10 years.

Specify if:

With limited prosocial emotions

Specify current severity:

Mild

Moderate

Severe

Reprinted with permission from American Psychiatric Association. (2022). Diagnostic and statistical manual of mental disorders, fifth edition, text revision.

Anxiety Disorders

Separation Anxiety Disorder

Clinical Findings, Epidemiology, and Course

Separation anxiety disorder is characterized by excessive fear or anxiety concerning separation from those to whom the individual is attached (APA, 2022). The anxiety is beyond that which would be expected for the individual's developmental level and interferes with social, academic, occupational, or other areas of functioning. In children, onset may occur any time before age 18 years, but the disorder is most commonly diagnosed around age 5 or 6, when the child goes to school. Diagnosis at this time may be related to the surfacing of symptoms when the child faces new stressors. Typically, schoolteachers and counselors are the first to recognize anxiety and associated behavioral disturbances. Because there is also a high prevalence of separation anxiety disorders (43%) with onset after the age of 18, the *DSM-5* removed the diagnostic criteria that specified this disorder as one that occurs only in children and adolescents. Prevalence estimates for the disorder average about 4%. It is more common in young children than in adolescents and occurs equally between boys and girls (Boland & Verduin, 2022). Over 50% experience remission of symptoms within 10 years of onset, but there are several common comorbidities, including panic disorder, social anxiety disorders, specific phobias, depression, and bipolar disorders (Kimmel & Roy-Byrne, 2017).

Table 23–8 | CARE PLAN FOR CHILD/ADOLESCENT WITH CONDUCT DISORDER

NURSING DIAGNOSIS: RISK FOR OTHER-DIRECTED VIOLENCE

RELATED TO: Characteristics of temperament, peer rejection, negative parental role models, dysfunctional family dynamics

OUTCOME CRITERIA	NURSING INTERVENTIONS	RATIONALE
Short-Term Goal ■ Patient will discuss feelings of anger with nurse or therapist. **Long-Term Goal** ■ Patient will not harm others or others' property.	1. Observe the patient's behavior frequently through routine activities and interactions. Become aware of behaviors that indicate a rise in agitation.	1. Recognition of behaviors that precede the onset of aggression may provide the opportunity to intervene before violence occurs.
	2. Redirect violent behavior with physical outlets for suppressed anger and frustration.	2. Excess energy is released through physical activities, inducing a feeling of relaxation.
	3. Encourage the patient to express anger, and act as a role model for appropriate expression of anger.	3. Discussion of situations that create anger may lead to more effective ways of dealing with them.
	4. Ensure that a sufficient number of staff are available to indicate a show of strength if necessary.	4. This conveys evidence of control over the situation and provides physical security for staff and others.
	5. Administer tranquilizing medication, if ordered, or use mechanical restraints or isolation room only if situation cannot be controlled with less restrictive means.	5. Medications, mechanical restraint, and seclusion are only used if less restrictive measures have been unsuccessful and the patient is an imminent danger to the safety of self or others.

NURSING DIAGNOSIS: IMPAIRED SOCIAL INTERACTION

RELATED TO: Negative parental role models; impaired peer relations leading to inappropriate social behavior

OUTCOME CRITERIA	NURSING INTERVENTIONS	RATIONALE
Short-Term Goal ■ Patient will interact in age-appropriate manner with nurse in one-to-one relationship within 1 week. **Long-Term Goal** ■ Patient will be able to interact with staff and peers using age-appropriate, acceptable behaviors.	1. Develop a trusting relationship. Convey acceptance of the person separate from the unacceptable behavior.	1. Unconditional acceptance promotes feelings of self-worth.
	2. Discuss which behaviors are and are not acceptable. Describe in matter-of-fact manner the consequence of unacceptable behavior. Follow through.	2. Aversive reinforcement can alter or extinguish undesirable behaviors.
	3. Provide group situations for the patient.	3. Appropriate social behavior is often learned from the positive and negative feedback of peers.

NURSING DIAGNOSIS: DEFENSIVE COPING

RELATED TO: Low self-esteem and dysfunctional family system

OUTCOME CRITERIA	NURSING INTERVENTIONS	RATIONALE
Short-Term Goal ■ Patient will verbalize personal responsibility for difficulties experienced in interpersonal relationships within a time period reasonable for patient.	1. Explain to the patient the correlation between feelings of inadequacy and the need for acceptance from others and how these feelings provoke defensive behaviors, such as blaming others for own behaviors.	1. Recognition of the problem is the first step in the change process toward resolution.

Continued

Table 23–8 | CARE PLAN FOR CHILD/ADOLESCENT WITH CONDUCT DISORDER—cont'd

OUTCOME CRITERIA	NURSING INTERVENTIONS	RATIONALE
Long-Term Goal ■ Patient will accept responsibility for own behaviors and interact with others without becoming defensive.	2. Provide immediate, matter-of-fact, nonthreatening feedback for unacceptable behaviors. 3. Help identify situations that provoke defensiveness, and practice through role-play more appropriate responses. 4. Provide immediate positive feedback for acceptable behaviors.	2. Patients may not realize how these behaviors are being perceived by others. 3. Role-playing provides confidence to deal with difficult situations when they actually occur. 4. Positive feedback encourages repetition, and immediacy is significant for these children, who respond to immediate gratification.

NURSING DIAGNOSIS: LOW SELF-ESTEEM

RELATED TO: Lack of positive feedback and unsatisfactory parent/child relationship

OUTCOME CRITERIA	NURSING INTERVENTIONS	RATIONALE
Short-Term Goal ■ Patient will participate in own self-care and discuss with nurse aspects of self about which the patient feels good. **Long-Term Goal** ■ Patient will demonstrate increased feelings of self-worth by verbalizing positive statements about self and exhibiting fewer manipulative behaviors.	1. Ensure that goals are realistic. 2. Plan activities that provide opportunities for success. 3. Convey unconditional acceptance and positive regard. 4. Set limits on manipulative behavior. Take precautions not to reinforce manipulative behaviors by providing desired attention. Identify the consequences of manipulation. Administer consequences matter-of-factly when manipulation occurs. 5. Help the patient understand the use of this behavior in order to try to increase own self-esteem. Interventions should reflect other actions to accomplish this goal.	1. Setting goals that the patient can realistically accomplish promotes self-esteem. 2. Success promotes self-esteem. 3. Communicating that patient is a worthwhile human being promotes positive self-esteem. 4. Aversive consequences may work to decrease unacceptable behaviors. 5. When the patient feels better about self, the need to manipulate others will diminish.

Predisposing Factors

Biological Influences

■ ***Genetics:*** A greater number of children with relatives who manifest anxiety problems develop anxiety disorders themselves than do children with no such family patterns. The results are significant enough to speculate that there is a hereditary influence in the development of separation anxiety disorder, but the mode of genetic transmission has not been determined. Boland and Verduin (2022) state:

> The current consensus on the genetics of anxiety disorders suggests that what is inherited is a general predisposition toward anxiety, with resulting heightened levels of arousability, emotional reactivity, and increased negative affect, all of which increase the risk for the development of separation anxiety disorder [and other anxiety disorders]. (p. 201)

- ***Temperament:*** It is well established that children differ from birth, or shortly thereafter, on a number of temperamental characteristics. While the temperamental traits of behavioral inhibition, excessive shyness, and the tendency to withdraw from unfamiliar situations represent a genetic contribution to development of anxiety disorders later in life, "one third to two thirds of young children with behavioral inhibition do not develop anxiety disorders" (Boland & Verduin, p. 2022). So heritable temperament traits may influence the risk anxiety disorders, but they are not predictive.

Environmental Influences

Studies have shown a relationship between life events and the development of anxiety disorders. Significant changes or losses often coincide with the development of the disorder (Boland & Verduin, 2022). Children of mothers who were stressed during pregnancy also appear to be at greater risk for developing separation anxiety disorder (Dryden-Edwards, 2021).

Family Influences

Various theories expound on the idea that anxiety disorders in children are related to attachment issues with the mother. Three family influences that have demonstrated an increased risk for anxiety disorders in children include parental overprotection, insecure parent-child attachment, and maternal depression (Boland & Verduin, 2022).

Some parents may also transfer their fears and anxieties to their children through role modeling. For example, a parent who becomes significantly fearful and apprehensive when confronted with unfamiliar circumstances, such as a job or residence change, teaches the child that this is an appropriate response.

Application of the Nursing Process to Separation Anxiety Disorder

Background Assessment Data

Onset of this disorder may occur as early as preschool age; it rarely begins as late as adolescence. In most cases, the child has difficulty separating from the mother. Occasionally, the separation reluctance is directed toward the father, siblings, or other significant individual to whom the child is attached. Anticipation of separation may result in tantrums, crying, screaming, complaints of physical problems, and **clinging** behaviors.

Reluctance or refusal to attend school occurs in the majority of these children. Up to 80% of children with school refusal meet criteria for separation anxiety disorder (Dryden-Edwards, 2021). Younger children may "shadow," or follow around the person from whom they are afraid to be separated. During middle childhood or adolescence, they may refuse to sleep away from home (e.g., at a friend's house or at camp). Interpersonal peer relationships are usually not a problem with these children. They are generally well liked by their peers and are reasonably socially skilled.

Worrying is common and relates to the possibility of harm coming to self or to the attachment figure. Younger children may even have nightmares to this effect. Specific phobias are not uncommon (e.g., fear of the dark, ghosts, animals). Depressed mood is frequently present and often precedes the onset of the anxiety symptoms, which commonly occur following a major stressor. The *DSM-5-TR* diagnostic criteria for separation anxiety disorder are presented in Box 23–5.

Nursing Diagnoses

Based on the data collected during the nursing assessment, possible nursing diagnoses for the patient with separation anxiety disorder include the following:

- Anxiety (severe) related to family history, temperament, overattachment to parent, negative role modeling
- Ineffective coping related to unresolved separation conflicts and inadequate coping skills evidenced by numerous somatic complaints
- Impaired social interaction related to reluctance to be away from attachment figure

Outcome Identification

Outcome criteria include short- and long-term goals. Timelines are individually determined. The following criteria may be used for measurement of outcomes in the care of the patient with separation anxiety disorder. The patient:

- Is able to maintain anxiety at manageable level.
- Demonstrates adaptive coping strategies for dealing with anxiety when separation from attachment figure is anticipated.
- Interacts appropriately with others and spends time away from attachment figure to do so.

Planning and Implementation

Table 23–9 provides a plan of care for the child or adolescent with separation anxiety, using nursing diagnoses common to this disorder, outcome criteria, and appropriate nursing interventions and rationales.

BOX 23–5 Diagnostic Criteria for Separation Anxiety Disorder

A. Developmentally inappropriate and excessive fear or anxiety concerning separation from those to whom the individual is attached, as evidenced by at least three of the following:
   1. Recurrent excessive distress when anticipating or experiencing separation from home or major attachment figures.
   2. Persistent and excessive worry about losing major attachment figures or about possible harm to them, such as illness, injury, disasters, or death.
   3. Persistent and excessive worry about experiencing an untoward event (e.g., getting lost, being kidnapped, having an accident, becoming ill) that causes separation from a major attachment figure.
   4. Persistent reluctance or refusal to go out, away from home, to school, to work, or elsewhere because of fear of separation.
   5. Persistent and excessive fear of or reluctance about being alone or without major attachment figures at home or in other settings.
   6. Persistent reluctance or refusal to sleep away from home or to go to sleep without being near a major attachment figure.
   7. Repeated nightmares involving the theme of separation.
   8. Repeated complaints of physical symptoms (e.g., headaches, stomachaches, nausea, vomiting) when separation from major attachment figures occurs or is anticipated.

B. The fear, anxiety, or avoidance is persistent, lasting at least 4 weeks in children and adolescents and typically 6 months or more in adults.

C. The disturbance causes clinically significant distress or impairment in social, academic, occupational, or other important areas of functioning.

D. The disturbance is not better accounted for by another mental disorder, such as refusing to leave home because of excessive resistance to change in autism spectrum disorder; delusions or hallucinations concerning separation in psychotic disorders; refusal to go outside without a trusted companion in agoraphobia; worries about ill health or other harm befalling significant others in generalized anxiety disorder; or concerns about having an illness in illness anxiety disorder.

Reprinted with permission from American Psychiatric Association. (2022). Diagnostic and statistical manual of mental disorders, fifth edition, text revision.

Evaluation

Evaluation of the child or adolescent with separation anxiety disorder requires reassessment of the behaviors for which the family sought treatment. Both the patient and the family members may need to change their behavior. The following types of questions may provide assistance in gathering data required for evaluating whether the nursing interventions have been effective in achieving the goals of therapy. Has the patient:

- Been able to maintain anxiety at a manageable level (i.e., without temper tantrums, screaming, or clinging)?
- Had fewer complaints of physical symptoms?
- Demonstrated the ability to cope in more adaptive ways in the face of escalating anxiety?
- (Parents) Identified more adaptive coping strategies?
- Verbalized an intention to return to school?
- Been able to sleep without nightmares?
- Been able to interact with others away from the attachment figure?

Treatment Modalities

Treatment for neurodevelopmental disorders, disruptive behavior disorders, and anxiety disorders poses many challenges and requires a comprehensive treatment plan that may include individual, group, and family therapies; family education; pharmacotherapy; and psychotherapeutic interventions specifically designed for the unique clinical issues presented in each disorder. The following general therapeutic approaches are described.

Behavior Therapy

Behavior therapy is based on the concepts of classical conditioning and operant conditioning. Behavior therapy is a common and effective treatment with disruptive behavior disorders such as ADHD, ODD, and CD. With this approach, rewards are given for appropriate behaviors and withheld when behaviors are disruptive or otherwise inappropriate. The principle behind behavior therapy is that positive reinforcements encourage repetition of desirable behaviors, and aversive reinforcements (punishments) discourage repetition of undesirable behaviors. Behavior modification techniques—the system of rewards and consequences—can be taught to parents to be used in the home environment. Consistency is an essential component. In the treatment setting, individualized behavior modification programs are designed for each client.

As mentioned previously, ABA is a type of behavior therapy that is considered the gold standard treatment for children with autism (although it is

Table 23–9 | CARE PLAN FOR THE CHILD WITH SEPARATION ANXIETY DISORDER

NURSING DIAGNOSIS: ANXIETY (SEVERE)

RELATED TO: Family history; temperament; overattachment to parent; negative role modeling

OUTCOME CRITERIA	NURSING INTERVENTIONS	RATIONALE
Short-Term Goal ■ Patient will discuss fears of separation with trusted individual. **Long-Term Goal** ■ Patient will maintain anxiety at no higher than moderate level in the face of events that formerly have precipitated panic.	1. Establish an atmosphere of calmness, trust, and genuine positive regard.	1. Trust and unconditional acceptance are necessary for satisfactory nurse-patient relationship. Calmness is important because anxiety is easily transmitted from one person to another.
	2. Assure the patient of safety and security.	2. Symptoms of panic and anxiety are very frightening.
	3. Explore the child's or adolescent's fears of separating from the parents. Explore with the parents possible fears they may have of separation from the child.	3. Some parents may have an underlying fear of separation from the child of which they are unaware and which they are unconsciously transferring to the child.
	4. Help parents and child initiate realistic goals (e.g., child to stay with sitter for 2 hours with minimal anxiety; or child to stay at friend's house without parents until 9 p.m. without experiencing panic or anxiety).	4. Parents may be so frustrated with their child's clinging and demanding behaviors that assistance with problem-solving may be required.
	5. Give, and encourage parents to give, positive reinforcement for desired behaviors.	5. Positive reinforcement encourages repetition of desirable behaviors.

NURSING DIAGNOSIS: INEFFECTIVE COPING

RELATED TO: Unresolved separation conflicts and inadequate coping skills

EVIDENCED BY: Numerous somatic complaints

OUTCOME CRITERIA	NURSING INTERVENTIONS	RATIONALE
Short-Term Goal ■ Patient will verbalize relationship of somatic symptoms to fear of separation. **Long-Term Goal** ■ Patient will demonstrate use of more adaptive coping strategies (than physical symptoms) in response to stressful situations.	1. Encourage the child or adolescent to discuss specific situations in life that produce the most distress and to describe their response to these situations. Include parents in the discussion.	1. The patient and family may be unaware of the correlation between stressful situations and the exacerbation of physical symptoms.
	2. Help the child or adolescent who is perfectionistic to recognize that self-expectations may be unrealistic. Connect times of unmet self-expectations to the exacerbation of physical symptoms.	2. Recognition of maladaptive patterns is the first step in the change process.
	3. Encourage parents and their child to identify more adaptive coping strategies that the child could use in the face of anxiety that feels overwhelming. Practice through role-play.	3. Practice facilitates the use of the desired behavior when the individual is actually faced with the stressful situation.

Continued

Table 23–9 | CARE PLAN FOR THE CHILD WITH SEPARATION ANXIETY DISORDER—cont'd

NURSING DIAGNOSIS: IMPAIRED SOCIAL INTERACTION

RELATED TO: Reluctance to be away from attachment figure

OUTCOME CRITERIA	NURSING INTERVENTIONS	RATIONALE
Short-Term Goal ■ Patient will spend time with staff or other support person, without presence of attachment figure, without excessive anxiety. **Long-Term Goal** ■ Patient will be able to spend time with others (without presence of attachment figure) without excessive anxiety.	1. Develop a trusting relationship.	1. This is the first step in helping the child learn to interact with others.
	2. Attend groups with the child, and support efforts to interact with others. Give positive feedback.	2. Presence of a trusted individual provides security during times of distress. Positive feedback encourages repetition.
	3. Convey to the child the acceptability of their not participating in group in the beginning. Gradually encourage small contributions until the patient is able to participate more fully.	3. Small successes will gradually increase self-confidence and decrease self-consciousness so that patient will feel less anxious in the group situation.
	4. Help the patient set small personal goals (e.g., "Today I will speak to one person I don't know").	4. Simple, realistic goals provide opportunities for success that increase self-confidence and may encourage the patient to attempt more difficult objectives in the future.

used to treat other conditions, too). It begins with a thorough consultation and assessment by an ABA-trained therapist and culminates in the development of a specific, individualized, behavioral treatment plan to teach social and communication skills and reduce problem behaviors such as tantrums or self-injury. ABA relies on caregiver training to assure that parents and other caregivers are reinforcing the treatment plan outside of the formal therapy setting (Raypole, 2019).

Family Therapy

Therapy for children and adolescents must involve the entire family if problems are to be resolved. Parents should be involved in designing and implementing the treatment plan for the child and should be involved in all aspects of the treatment process.

The genogram can be used to identify problem areas between family members. It provides an overall picture of the life of the family over several generations, including roles that various family members play and emotional distance between specific individuals. Areas for change can be easily identified.

The impact of family dynamics on disruptive behavior disorders has been identified. The impact of disruptive behavior on family dynamics cannot be ignored. Family coping can become severely compromised by the chronic stress of dealing with a child with a behavior disorder. It is therefore imperative that the treatment plan for the identified patient be instituted within the context of family-centered care.

Group Therapy

Group therapy provides children and adolescents with the opportunity to interact within an association of their peers. This interaction can be both gratifying and overwhelming, depending on the child.

Group therapy provides a number of benefits. Appropriate social behavior often is learned from the positive and negative feedback of peers. Opportunity is provided to learn to tolerate and accept differences in others, to learn that it is acceptable to disagree, to learn to offer and receive support from others, and to practice these new skills in a safe environment. It provides a way to learn from the experiences of others.

Group therapy with children and adolescents can take several forms. Music therapy groups provide the opportunity to express feelings through; some children may be unable to express themselves in any other way. Art and activity/craft therapy groups allow individual expression through artistic means.

Group play therapy is the treatment of choice for many children between the ages of 3 and 9 years. The Association for Play Therapy (n.d.) states:

> The systematic use of a theoretical model to establish an interpersonal process wherein trained play therapists use the therapeutic powers of play to help clients prevent or resolve psychosocial difficulties and achieve optimal growth and development.

Child play therapy is a way of being with the child that honors their unique developmental level and looks for ways of helping in the "language" of the child—play. Licensed mental health professionals often use play therapy when intervening with children to help them express themselves and resolve problems.

Psychoeducational groups are very beneficial for adolescents. The only drawback to this type of group is that it works best when the group is closed-ended; that is, once the group has been formed, no one is allowed to join until the group has reached its pre-established closure. Members are allowed to propose topics for discussion. The leader serves as teacher much of the time and facilitates discussion of the proposed topic. Members may from time to time be presenters and serve as discussion leaders. Sometimes, psychoeducation groups evolve into traditional therapy discussion groups.

Cognitive behavior therapy (CBT) has demonstrated benefit in the treatment of tic disorders (Tourette's); separation anxiety disorder; and the disruptive behavior disorders including ADHD, ODD, and CD. It has also been identified as beneficial for clients with ASD to treat secondary issues such as depression, anger, anxiety, and social skills deficits (Creed, 2015). Creed notes that because people on the autism spectrum are typically concrete thinkers CBT may be adapted to meet their individual needs and level of functioning.

Psychopharmacology

Several of the disorders presented in this chapter are treated with medications. The appropriate pharmacology is presented following the section in which the disorder is discussed. Medication should never be the sole method of treatment. It is undeniable that medication can and does improve quality of life for families of children and adolescents with these disorders. However, research has indicated that medication alone is not as effective as a combination of medication and psychosocial therapy. The importance of the psychosocial therapies cannot be overstressed. Some clinicians will not prescribe medications for patients unless they also participate in concomitant psychotherapy sessions.

Summary and Key Points

- Intellectual disability is defined by deficits in general intellectual functioning and adaptive functioning.
- Four levels of intellectual disability—mild, moderate, severe, and profound—are associated with various behavioral manifestations and abilities.
- Autism spectrum disorder (ASD) includes a wide variety of symptoms and levels of severity that affect thinking, feeling, communication, and social relationships. Behavior is often limited and repetitive but each child is likely to have a unique pattern of behavior and level of severity form low to high functioning.
- It is generally accepted that ASD is caused by abnormalities in brain structures or functions. Genetic factors are also thought to play a significant role in ASD.
- Children with attention deficit-hyperactivity disorder (ADHD) may exhibit symptoms of inattention or hyperactivity and impulsiveness or a combination of the two.
- Genetics plays a role in the etiology of ADHD. Neurotransmitters that have been implicated include dopamine, norepinephrine, and serotonin. Exposure to tobacco smoke, maternal smoking, and alcohol use during pregnancy have been linked to hyperactive behavior in offspring.
- Central nervous system (CNS) stimulants, alpha agonists, atomoxetine, and bupropion are commonly used to treat ADHD.
- The essential feature of Tourette's disorder is the presence of multiple motor tics and one or more vocal tics.
- Common medications used with Tourette's disorder include haloperidol; pimozide; aripiprazole; clonidine; guanfacine; and atypical antipsychotics such as risperidone. Nonpharmacological interventions include comprehensive behavioral intervention for tics (CBIT), habit reversal training, cognitive behavior therapy (CBT), speech therapy, deep brain stimulation and transcranial magnetic stimulation.
- Oppositional defiant disorder (ODD) is characterized by a pattern of negativistic, defiant,

disobedient, and hostile behavior toward authority figures that occurs more frequently than is usually observed in individuals of comparable age and developmental level.

- Conduct disorder is characterized by a repetitive and persistent pattern of behavior in which the basic rights of others or major age-appropriate societal norms or rules are violated.
- The essential feature of separation anxiety disorder is excessive anxiety concerning separation from the home or from those to whom the person is attached.
- Children with separation anxiety disorder may have temperamental characteristics present at birth that predispose them to the disorder.
- General therapeutic approaches for child and adolescent psychiatric disorders include behavior therapy, family therapy, group therapies (including music, art, crafts, play, and psychoeducation), CBT, and psychopharmacology.

Review Questions

Select the answer that is most appropriate for each of the following questions:

1. Which drug class is most commonly used for management of the child with ADHD?
   a. CNS depressants (e.g., diazepam [Valium])
   b. CNS stimulants (e.g., methylphenidate [Ritalin])
   c. Anticonvulsants (e.g., phenytoin [Dilantin])
   d. Major tranquilizers (e.g., haloperidol [Haldol])
2. The nursing history and assessment of an adolescent with a conduct disorder might reveal all behaviors *except:*
   a. Manipulation of others for fulfillment of own desires
   b. Chronic violation of rules
   c. Feelings of guilt associated with the exploitation of others
   d. Inability to form close peer relationships
3. Certain family dynamics are believed to predispose adolescents to the development of conduct disorder. Which pattern is thought to be a contributing factor?
   a. Parents who are overprotective
   b. Parents who have high expectations for their children
   c. Parents who consistently set limits on their children's behavior
   d. Parents who are alcohol dependent
4. Which statement about oppositional behavior in children is true?
   a. Oppositional behavior in a child over 2 years of age is diagnostic of ODD.
   b. Oppositional behavior at various stages of development is normal and healthy.
   c. Oppositional behavior is genetic.
   d. Oppositional behavior is characterized by limited and repetitive rituals.
5. Which of the following medications is used to treat Tourette's disorder?
   a. Methylphenidate (Ritalin)
   b. Haloperidol (Haldol)
   c. Imipramine (Tofranil)
   d. Phenytoin (Dilantin)

Clinical Judgment Questions

6. A child with ADHD has a nursing diagnosis of impaired social interaction. Which nursing interventions are appropriate for this child? (Select all that apply.)
   a. Socially isolate the child when interactions with others are inappropriate.
   b. Set limits with consequences on inappropriate behaviors.
   c. Provide rewards for appropriate behaviors.
   d. Provide group situations for the child.

7. To help a child with mild to moderate intellectual developmental disorder develop satisfying relationships with others, which nursing intervention is most appropriate?
   a. Interpret the child's behavior for others.
   b. Set limits on behavior that is socially inappropriate.
   c. Allow the child to behave spontaneously without the concept of right or wrong.
   d. Discourage relationships because the child is not capable of forming social relationships.
8. The child with autism spectrum disorder often has difficulty with trust. With this in mind, which nursing action would be most appropriate?
   a. Encourage all staff to hold the child as often as possible, conveying trust through touch.
   b. Assign a different staff member each day so the child will learn that everyone can be trusted.
   c. Assign the same staff person as often as possible to promote feelings of security and trust.
   d. Avoid eye contact because it is extremely uncomfortable for the child and may even discourage trust.
9. Which nursing diagnosis would be considered the priority in planning care for a child with a severe ASD?
   a. Risk for self-mutilation evidenced by banging head against wall
   b. Impaired social interaction evidenced by unresponsiveness to people
   c. Impaired verbal communication evidenced by absence of verbal expression
   d. Disturbed personal identity evidenced by inability to differentiate self from others
10. A client with ODD has been admitted to a residential treatment setting and tells the nurse, "I don't want to be here and you're not in charge of me." Which intervention by the nurse is a priority?
   a. Instruct the client that they will have to follow the rules, or they will be put in seclusion.
   b. Provide information about the structured activities and behavioral expectations in the treatment program.
   c. Give positive feedback to the client for their assertive communication.
   d. Ask the client whether they would rather go to jail.

IMPLICATIONS FOR EVIDENCE-BASED PRACTICE

Lavallee, K., Schuck, K., Blatter-Meunier, J., & Schneider, S. (2019). Transgenerational improvements following child anxiety treatment: An exploratory examination. *PloS ONE, 14*(2), Article e0212667. https://doi.org/10.1371/journal.pone.021266

DESCRIPTION OF THE STUDY: This study was a secondary analysis of a randomized controlled trial to examine the transgenerational relationship between CBT for child separation anxiety disorder and the mental health of parents. One hundred and seven children ages 4 to 14 years with separation anxiety disorder received one of two cognitive behavioral treatment programs. Their parents (N = 189; 101 mothers and 88 fathers) were assessed at baseline and post-treatment for symptoms of separation anxiety, general anxiety, and depression. A comparison group of parents (N = 74; 42 mothers and 32 fathers) of 45 children without separation anxiety disorder, who did not receive any treatment, were also assessed.

RESULTS OF THE STUDY: Maternal symptoms of depression and separation anxiety improved in the child treatment group in comparison to mothers of healthy children. There was no significant improvement in parental pathology levels among fathers of children treated for separation anxiety disorder.

IMPLICATIONS FOR NURSING PRACTICE: This study has implications for nurses who work with children that have separation anxiety disorder. Providing care and intervention for a child always involves working with parents. This study expands the focus of treatment to understanding the benefits not just for the child but also for evaluating the anxiety and depression in parents as well. While the authors acknowledge that more research is needed to better understand the mechanisms, nurses can educate parents about research findings such as these to promote confidence in the treatment process.

TEST YOUR CLINICAL REASONING AND CLINICAL JUDGMENT SKILLS

Jimmy, age 9, has been admitted to the child psychiatric unit with a diagnosis of attention deficit-hyperactivity disorder. He has been unmanageable at school and at home and has had several suspensions from school for continuous disruption of his class. He refuses to sit in his chair or do his work. He yells out in class, interrupts the teacher and the other students, and lately has become physically aggressive when he cannot have his way. Most recently, he was suspended after hitting his teacher when she asked him to return to his seat.

Jimmy's mother describes him as a restless and demanding baby who grew into a restless and demanding toddler. He has never gotten along well with his peers. Even as a small child, he would take his friends' toys away from them or bite them if they tried to hold their own with him. His 5-year-old sister is afraid of him and refuses to be alone with him.

During the nurse's intake assessment, Jimmy paced the room or rocked in his chair. He talked incessantly on a superficial level and jumped from topic to topic. He told the nurse that he did not know why he was there. He acknowledged that he had some problems at school but said that was only because the other kids picked on him and the teacher did not like him. He said he got into trouble at home sometimes but that was because his parents liked his little sister better than they liked him.

The physician has ordered methylphenidate 5 mg twice a day for Jimmy. His response to this order is, "I'm not going to take medicine. I'm not sick!"

Answer the following questions related to Jimmy:

1. What are the pertinent assessment data to be noted by the nurse?
2. What is the primary nursing diagnosis for Jimmy?
3. Aside from patient safety, to what problems would the nurse want to direct intervention with Jimmy?

MOVIE CONNECTIONS

Bill (Intellectual disability) ▪ *Bill, On His Own* (Intellectual disability) ▪ *Sling Blade* (Intellectual disability) ▪ *Forrest Gump* (Intellectual disability) ▪ *Rain Man* (ASD) ▪ *Mercury Rising* (ASD) ▪ *Niagara, Niagara* (Tourette's disorder) ▪ *Toughlove* (Conduct disorder) ▪ *Life, Animated* (ASD) ▪ *The A Word* (ASD) ▪ *Front of the Class* (Tourette's disorder)

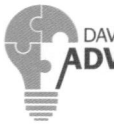

Go to **Davis Advantage** to complete your learning: strengthen understanding, apply your knowledge, and prepare for the Next Gen NCLEX®.

References

Acosta, M. T., Swanson, J., Stehli, A., Molina, B., The MTA Team, Martinez, A. F., Arcos-Burgos, M., & Muenke, M. (2016). *ADGRL3 (LPHN3)* variants are associated with a refined phenotype of ADHD in the MTA study. *Molecular Genetics and Genomic Medicine, 4*(5), 540–547. https://doi.org/10.1002/mgg3.230

ADHD Institute. (2021). *Environmental risk factors.* http://www.adhd-institute.com/burden-of-adhd/aetiology/environmental-risk-factors

American Psychiatric Association. (2000). *Diagnostic and statistical manual of mental disorders* (4th ed., text rev.).

American Psychiatric Association (2022). *Diagnostic and statistical manual of mental disorders* (5th ed., text rev.).

Association for Play Therapy. (n.d.). *Play therapy makes a difference.* http://www.a4pt.org/?page=PTMakesADifference

Bernstein, B. E. (2018). Conduct disorder. *Medscape.* http://emedicine.medscape.com/article/918213-over view#a3

Boat, T. F., & Wu, J. T. (Eds.). (2015). *Mental disorders and disabilities among low-income children.* National Academies Press.

Boland, R., & Verduin, M. L. (2022). *Kaplan & Sadock's synopsis of psychiatry* (P. Ruiz, Ed.). (12th ed.). Wolters Kluwer.

Centers for Disease Control and Prevention. (2019). A renewed commitment to prevent childhood lead exposure in the post-Flint era. https://www.cdc.gov/grand-rounds/pp/2019/20190212-childhood-lead-exposure.html

Centers for Disease Control and Prevention. (2020a). *Autism spectrum disorders. Autism and Developmental Disabilities Monitoring Network.* http://www.cdc.gov/ncbddd/autism/addm.html

Centers for Disease Control and Prevention. (2020b). *Tourette syndrome: Risk factors and causes.* http://www.cdc.gov/ncbddd/tourette/riskfactors.html

Centers for Disease Control and Prevention. (2021a). *FastStats: Attention deficit hyperactivity disorder.* http://www.cdc.gov/nchs/fastats/adhd.htm

Centers for Disease Control and Prevention. (2021b). *Childhood lead poisoning prevention.* http://www.cdc.gov/nceh/lead

Connor, D. (2017). Disruptive behavior disorders in children and adolescents. In B. J. Sadock, V. A. Sadock, & P. Ruiz (Eds.), *Comprehensive textbook of psychiatry* (10th ed., pp. 3605–3621). Wolters Kluwer.

Creed, T. (2015). *An introduction to CBT for people with autism spectrum disorder.* https://beckinstitute.org/an-introduction-to-cbt-for-people-with-an-autism-spectrum-disorder/

DeBoth, K. K., & Reynolds, S. (2017). A systematic review of sensory-based autism subtypes. *Research in Autism Spectrum Disorders, 36,* 44–56. https://doi.org/10.1016/j.rasd.2017.01.005

Dryden-Edwards, R. (2021). *Separation anxiety.* http://www.medicinenet.com/separation_anxiety/page4.htm

Fallah, M. S., Shaikh, M. R., Neupane, B., Rusiecki, D., Bennett, T. A., & Beyene, J. (2019). Atypical antipsychotics for irritability in pediatric autism: A systematic review and network meta-analysis. *Journal of Child and Adolescent Psychopharmacology, 29*(3), 168–180. http://doi.org/10.1089/cap.2018.0115

Froehlich, T. E., Lanphear, B. P., Auinger, P., Hornung, R., Epstein, J. N., Braun, J., & Kahn, R. S. (2009). Association of tobacco and lead exposures with attention-deficit/hyperactivity disorder. *Pediatrics, 124,* 1054–1063. http://www.ncbi.nlm.nih.gov/pmc/articles/PMC2853804/

Gabis, L. V., Ben-Hur, R., Shefer, S., Jokel, A., & Shalom, D. B. (2019). Improvement of language in children with autism with combined donepezil and choline treatment. *Journal of Molecular Neuroscience, 69*(2), 224–234. https://doi.org/10.1007/s12031-019-01351-7.

Gilman, S. R., Chang, J., Xu, B., Bawa, T. S., Gogos, J. A., Karayiorgou, M., & Vitkup, D. (2012). Diverse types of genetic variation converge on functional gene networks involved in schizophrenia. *Nature Neuroscience, 15*(12), 1723–1728. https://doi.org/10.1038/nn.3261

Goode, A. P., Coeytaux, R. R., Maslow, G. R., Davis, N., Hill, S., Namdari, B., Allen LaPointe, N. M., Befus, D., Lallinger, K. R., Bowen, S. E., Kosinski, A., McBroom, A. J., Sanders, G. D., & Kemper, A. R. (2018). Nonpharmacologic treatments for attention-deficit/hyperactivity disorder: A systematic review. *Pediatrics, 141*(6), e20180094. https://doi.org/10.1542/peds.2018-0094

Griffin, M., & Harari, E. (2019). Research sheds light on two types of treatment for ADHD. *Psychiatric Times, 36*(7). https://www.psychiatrictimes.com/adhd/research-sheds-lighttwo-types-treatment-adhd

Grohol, J. (2016). New chewable ADHD medication, Adzenys, has some worried. *PsychCentral.* http://psychcentral.com/news/2016/05/31/new-chewableadhd-medication-adzenys-has-some-worried/104077.html

Harrop, C., McConachie, H., Emsly, R., Leadbitter, K., Green, J., & PACT Consortium. (2014). Restricted and repetitive behaviors in autism spectrum disorders and typical development: Cross sectional and longitudinal comparisons. *Journal of Autism and Developmental Disorders, 44,* 1207–1219. https://doi.org/10.1007/s10803-13-1986-5

Humphreys, K. L., Watts, E. L., Dennis, E. L., King, L. S., Thompson, P. M., & Gotlib, I. H. (2018). Stressful life events, ADHD symptoms, and brain structure in early adolescence. *Journal of Abnormal Child Psychology, 47*(3), 421–432. https://doi.org/10.1007/s10802-018-0443-5

James, B. J., Gales, M. A., & Gales, B. J. (2019). Bumetanide for autism spectrum disorder in children: A review of randomized controlled trials. *Annals of Pharmacotherapy, 53*(5), 537–544.

Kendler, K. S., Aggen, S. H., & Patrick, C. J. (2013). Familial influences on conduct disorder reflect 2 genetic factors and 1 shared environmental factor. *JAMA Psychiatry, 70*(1), 78–86. https://doi.org/10.1001/jamapsychiatry.2013.267

Kimmel, R. J., & Roy-Byrne, P. (2017). Clinical features of anxiety disorders. In B. J. Sadock, V. A. Sadock, & P. Ruiz (Eds.), *Comprehensive textbook of psychiatry* (10th ed., pp. 1723–1730). Wolters Kluwer.

Kothadia, R. J., Krause, M., & Saeed, S. A. (2021). Pharmacologic management of autism spectrum disorder: A review of 7 studies. *Current Psychiatry, 20*(1), 33–38.

Kranjac, D. (2016). In vitro modeling of early brain overgrowth in autism. *PsychiatryAdvisor.* http://www.psychiatryadvisor.com/neurodevelopmental-disorder/modeling-early-brainovergrowth-in-autism/article/508852/

Lavallee, K., Schuck, K., Blatter-Meunier, J., & Schneider, S. (2019). Transgenerational improvements following child anxiety treatment: An exploratory examination. *PloS ONE, 14*(2), Article e0212667. https://doi.org/10.1371/journal.pone.021266

Lubit, R. H. (2015). Oppositional defiant disorder. *Medscape.* http://emedicine.medscape.com/article/918095-overview

Maher, G. M., O'Keeffe, G. W., Kearney, P. M., Kenny, L. C., Dinan, T. G., Mattsson, M., & Khashan, A. S. (2018). Association of hypertensive disorders of pregnancy with risk of neurodevelopmental disorders in offspring: A systematic review and meta-analysis. *JAMA Psychiatry, 75*(8), 809–819. https://doi.org/10.1001/jamapsychiatry.2018.0854

Marchetto, M. C., Belinson, H., Tian, Y., Freitas, B. C., Fu, C., Vadodaria, K. C., Beltrao-Braga, P., Trujillo, C. A., Mendes, A. P. D., Padmanabhan, K., Nunez, Y., Ou, J., Ghosh, H., Wright, R., Brennand, K., Pierce, K., Eichenfield, L., Pramparo, T., Eyler, L., Barnes, C. C., . . . Muotri, A. R. (2017). Altered proliferation and networks in neural cells derived from idiopathic autistic individuals. *Molecular Psychiatry, 22,* 820–835. https://doi.org/10.1038/mp.2016.95

Mathews-Wilson, L., & Daitch, L. (2016). *The psychosocial implications of ADHD in adults.* http://nursing.advanceweb.com/the-psychosocial-implications-of-adhd-in-adults/

Mayo Clinic. (2021a). *Autism spectrum disorder.* https://www.mayoclinic.org/diseases-conditions/autismspectrum-disorder/symptoms-causes/syc-20352928

Mayo Clinic. (2021b). *Oppositional defiant disorder.* http://www.mayoclinic.org/diseases-conditions/oppositional-defiant-disorder/basics/risk-factors/con-20024559

Mazahery, H., Conlon, C. A., Beck, K. L. Mugridge, O., Kruger, M. C., Stonehouse, W., Camargo, C. A. Jr, Meyer, B. J., Jones, B., & von Hurst, P. R. (2019). A randomised controlled trial of vitamin D and omega-3 long chain polyunsaturated fatty acids in the treatment of irritability and hyperactivity among children with autism spectrum disorder. *Journal of Steroid Biochemistry and Molecular Biology, 187,* 9–16. https://doi.org/10.1016/j.jsbmb.2018.10.017

McGough, J. J. (2017). Adult manifestations of attention-deficit/hyperactivity disorder. In B. J. Sadock, V. A. Sadock, & P. Ruiz (Eds.), *Comprehensive textbook of psychiatry* (10th ed., pp. 3598–3604). Philadelphia, PA: Wolters Kluwer.

McGough, J. J., Sturm, A., Cowen, J., Tung, K., Salgari, G. C., Leuchter, A. F., Cook, I. A., Sugar, C. A., & Loo, S. K. (2019). Double-blind, sham-controlled, pilot study of trigeminal nerve stimulation for attention-deficit/hyperactivity disorder. *Journal of the American Academy of Child and Adolescent Psychiatry, 58*(4), 403–411.

National Institutes of Health. (2021). *Tourette's syndrome information page.* https://www.ninds.nih.gov/Disorders/All-Disorders/Tourette-Syndrome-Information-Page

Nigg, J. T., Nikolas, M., Mark Knottnerus, G., Cavanagh, K., & Friderici, K. (2010). Confirmation and extension of association of blood lead with attention-deficit/hyperactivity disorder (ADHD) and ADHD symptom domains at population-typical exposure levels. *Journal of Child Psychology and Psychiatry, 51*(1), 58–65.

Pase, M. P., Himali, J. J., Beiser, A. S., Aparicio, H. J., Satizabal, C. L., Vasan, R. S., Seshadri, S. & Jacques, P. F. (2017). Sugar- and artificially sweetened beverages and the risks of incident stroke and dementia: A prospective cohort study. *Stroke, 48*(5), 1139–1146. https://doi.org/10.1161/STROKEAHA.116.016027

Raypole, C. (2019). *Is applied behavioral analysis (ABA) right for your child?* https://www.healthline.com/health/aba-therapy

Rossignol, D. A., & Frye, R. E. (2016). Environmental toxicants and autism spectrum disorder. *Psychiatric Times.* http://www.psychiatrictimes.com/special-reports/environmentaltoxicants-and-autism-spectrum-disorder

Sherman, J., & Tarnow, J. (2013). What are common comorbidities in ADHD? *Psychiatric Times.* http://www.psychiatrictimes.com/adhd/what-are-common-comorbidities-in-adhd

Strunz, S., Westphal, L., Ritter, K., Heuser, I., Dziobek, I., & Roepke, S. (2015). Personality pathology of adults with autism spectrum disorder without accompanying intellectual impairment in comparison to adults with personality disorders. *Journal of Autism and Developmental Disorders, 45,* 4026–4038. https://doi.org/10.1007/s10803-14-2183-x

Tourette's Association of America. (n.d.). *What is Tourette.* https://tourette.org/about-tourette/overview/what-is-tourette/

Van den Ban, E., Souverein, P., Meijer, W., van Engeland, H., Swaab, H., Egber, T., & Heerdinle, E. (2014). Association between ADHD drug use and injuries among children and adolescents. *European Child and Adolescent Psychiatry, 23,* 95–102. https://doi.org/10.1007/s00787-013-0432-8

Volkmar, F. R., Klin, A., Schultz, R. T., & State, M. W. (2017). Autism spectrum and social communication disorder. In B. J. Sadock, V. A. Sadock, & P. Ruiz (Eds.), *Comprehensive textbook of psychiatry* (10th ed., pp. 3571–3586). Wolters Kluwer.

Weisman, H., Qureshi, I. A., Leckman, J. F., Scahill, L., & Bloch M. H. (2013). Systematic review: Pharmacological treatment of tic disorders—Efficacy of antipsychotic and alpha-2 adrenergic agonist agents. *Neuroscience and Biobehavioral Reviews, 37*(6), 1162–1171. https://doi.org/10.1016/j.neubiorev.2012.09.008

Williams, N. M., Zaharieva, I., Martin, A., Langley, K., Mantripragada, K., Fossdal, R., Stefansson, H., Stefansson, K., Magnusson, P., Gudmundsson, O. O., Gustafsson, O., Holmans, P., Owen, M. J., O'Donovan, M., & Thapar, A. (2010). Rare chromosomal deletions and duplications in attention-deficit hyperactivity disorder: A genome-wide analysis. *Lancet, 376*(9750), 1401–1408.

Woodward, T. J., Ume, U., & Davis, R. (2019). An introduction to oppositional defiant disorder and conduct disorder. *U.S. Pharmacist, 44*(11), 29–32. https://www.uspharmacist.com/article/an-introduction-to-oppositional-defiant-disorder-and-conduct-disorder

The Aging Individual 24

CHAPTER OUTLINE

Objectives
Introduction
How Old Is *Old*?
Epidemiology
Theories of Aging
The Normal Aging Process
Special Concerns of the Older Population
Application of the Nursing Process
Summary and Key Points
Review Questions
Clinical Judgment Questions
Implications for Evidence-Based Practice
Test Your Clinical Reasoning and Clinical Judgment Skills
Movie Connections

CORE CONCEPTS

Health Promotion
Grief and Loss
Clinical Judgment
Professionalism: Nursing process in the care of older adults

KEY TERMS

attachment
bereavement overload
disengagement theory
elder abuse
geriatrics
gerontology
geropsychiatry
long-term memory
Medicaid
Medicare
menopause
osteoporosis
reminiscence therapy
short-term memory
transcendence

OBJECTIVES

After reading this chapter, the student will be able to:

1. Discuss societal perspectives on aging.
2. Describe an epidemiological profile of aging in the United States.
3. Discuss various theories of aging.
4. Describe biological, psychological, sociocultural, and sexual aspects of the normal aging process.
5. Discuss retirement as a special concern to the aging individual.
6. Explain personal and sociological perspectives of long-term care of the aging individual.
7. Describe the problem of elder abuse as it exists in today's society.
8. Discuss the implications of the increasing number of suicides among older adults.
9. Apply the steps of the nursing process to the care of older adults.

Introduction

What is it like to grow old? It is not likely that many people in American culture would state that it is something they want to do. Most would agree, however, that it is "better than the alternative."

Supreme Court Justice Oliver Wendell Holmes, Jr., who retired at the age of 91, is quoted as saying, "Old is fifteen years older than I am." Obviously, being old is relative to the individual experiencing aging, and as the population of older adults continues to grow, our norms about aging will no doubt be reconceptualized. Growing old has not been popular among the youth-oriented American culture. However, with 66 million adults reaching their 65th birthdays by 2030, greater emphasis is being placed on the needs of older adults. The disciplines of **gerontology** (the study of the aging process), **geriatrics** (the branch of clinical medicine specializing in problems of older adults), and **geropsychiatry** (the branch of clinical medicine specializing in psychopathology of the older population) are expanding rapidly in response to this predictable demand.

Growing old in a society that has been obsessed with youth may have a critical impact on the mental health of many people. This situation has serious implications for psychiatric nursing.

What is it like to grow old? Increasing numbers of people will be able to answer this question as the 21st century progresses. Perhaps they will also be asking the question that Roberts (1991) asks: "How did I get here so fast?"

This chapter focuses on physical and psychological changes associated with the aging process as well as on special concerns of older adults, such as retirement, long-term care, elder abuse, polypharmacy, and high suicide rates. The nursing process is presented as the vehicle for delivery of nursing care to older adults.

How Old Is *Old*?

The concept of "old" has changed drastically over the years. Our prehistoric ancestors probably had a life span of 40 years, with the average individual living around 18 years. As civilization developed, mortality rates remained high as a result of periodic famine and frequent malnutrition. Improvement in the standard of living was not truly evident until about the middle of the 17th century. Since that time, ensured food supply, changes in food production, better housing conditions, and more progressive medical and sanitation facilities have contributed to population growth, declining mortality rates, and substantial increases in longevity.

In 1900, the average life expectancy in the United States was 47 years, and only 4% of the population was age 65 or older. In 2018, the average life expectancy at birth was 78.7 years (76.2 years for men and 81.2 years for women) (National Center for Health Statistics [NCHS], 2020).

The U.S. Census Bureau has created a system for classification of older Americans:

- ***Older:*** 55 through 64 years
- ***Elderly:*** 65 through 74 years
- ***Aged:*** 75 through 84 years
- ***Very old:*** 85 years and older

Some gerontologists use a simpler classification system:

- ***Young old:*** 60 through 74 years
- ***Middle old:*** 75 through 84 years
- ***Old old:*** 85 years and older

So how old is *old?* Obviously, the term cannot be defined by a number. Myths and stereotypes of aging have long obscured our understanding of the aged and the process of aging. Ideas that all older individuals are sick, depressed, obsessed with death, senile, and incapable of change affect the way older adults are treated. They even shape the pattern of aging of the people who believe them. They can become self-fulfilling prophecies—people start to believe they should behave in certain ways and therefore act according to those beliefs. Generalized assumptions can be demeaning and interfere with the quality of life for older individuals.

Just as there are many differences in individual adaptation at earlier stages of development, so it is in the aging population. Erikson (1963) suggested that the mentally healthy older person possesses a sense of ego integrity and self-acceptance that will help in adapting to the ambiguities of the future with a sense of security and optimism.

The World Health Organization (WHO, 2017) reports that over 20% of adults over the age of 60 have a mental or neurological disorder and that the keys to mental health in older adulthood are resources to meet their needs, including security and freedom, adequate housing, social support, programs to prevent elder abuse, availability of health and social programs for vulnerable populations such as those who live alone, and community development programs. Everyone, particularly health-care workers, should see aging people as individuals, each with specific needs and abilities, rather than as a stereotypical group. Some individuals may seem old at 40, whereas others may not seem old at 70. Variables such as attitude, mental health, physical health, and degree of independence strongly influence how individuals perceive themselves. Surely, in the final analysis, whether one is considered old must be self-determined.

Epidemiology

The Population

In 1980, Americans 65 years of age or older numbered 25.5 million. By 2018, these numbers had increased to 52.4 million, and this number is expected to double by 2060 to 94.7 million (Administration on Aging [AoA], 2020). The 85 and older population, which numbered 6.5 million in 2019, is expected to more than double by 2040. In 2019 there were 93,927 persons age 100 years or older.

Marital Status

In 2019, of individuals age 65 and older, 69% of men and 47% of women were married (AoA, 2020). Of the women in this age-group, 31% were widowed.

Living Arrangements

About 28% of older adults and 44% of women older than age 75 years live alone (AoA, 2020). Approximately 1.1 million grandparents age 60 years and older were responsible for the basic needs of one or more grandchildren younger than age 18 years living with them in 2018, a trend that continues to grow. A relatively small number (1.2 million) adults older than 65 years lived in nursing homes in 2018. This percentage increases dramatically with age, ranging from 1% for people ages 65 to 74 years to 7% for those ages 85 years and older. See Figure 24–1 for a distribution of living arrangements for people ages 65 years and older.

Economic Status

About 9.7% of persons age 65 or older were below the poverty level in 2018, and when the U.S Census Bureau figures adjusted for regional variations in cost of housing, other benefits, and out-of-pocket expenses for needs such as medical care, the percentage of those living below the poverty level rose to 13.6% (AoA, 2020). Older women had a higher poverty rate than older men, and older Hispanic women living alone had the highest poverty rate.

Of individuals 75 years or older who were living in a house, 76% owned their own homes and 37% spent one-third or more of their income on housing expenses in maintenance and repairs (AoA, 2020). Poor people who have worked all their lives can expect to become poorer in old age, and others will become poor only after becoming old. However, there are a substantial number of affluent and middle-income older persons.

Employment

With the passage of the Age Discrimination in Employment Act in 1967, forced retirement and age discrimination for employees over the age of 40 is now illegal, although there are some exceptions to protections under this law. It is well accepted that involvement in purposeful activity is vital to successful adaptation and perhaps even to survival at any age. Increasing numbers of adults over 65 are remaining active in employment environments. In 2019, 10.7 million Americans (20.2%) age 65 and older were in the labor force (working or actively seeking work), and that number represents a steady increase for women since around the year 2000 (AoA, 2020). The data do not clarify whether this tendency to remain in the labor force during older adulthood is related to the desire to remain active and productive through the labor force or whether it is based in necessity for income.

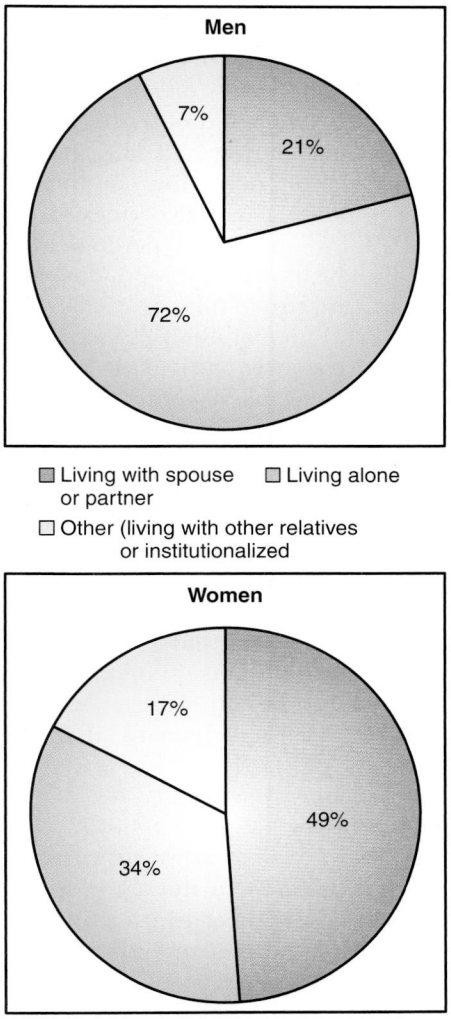

FIGURE 24–1 Living arrangements of noninstutionalized individuals ages 65 and older (AoA 2020).

Health Status

The number of days in which usual activities are restricted because of illness or injury increases with age. Most adults age 65 and older have at least one chronic illness and almost half have two or three. The most commonly occurring conditions among the elderly population are hypertension (67% for men and 79% for women), hyperlipidemia (48%), arthritis (54%), heart disease (28%), diabetes (28%), cancer (19%), and stroke (9%) (AoA, 2020).

Emotional and mental illnesses increase over the life cycle. Depression is particularly prevalent, and suicide is a serious problem among older Americans. Prevalence of major depression is estimated between 1% and 5% for the general population of older adults, but may rise as high as 13.5% for older adults requiring hospitalization or home health care (Centers for Disease Control and Prevention [CDC], 2021). The CDC adds that depression in this age-group is particularly underdiagnosed and undertreated by both health-care providers and older adults themselves, perhaps related to a misperception that this is a normal part of aging or a natural reaction to illnesses. Neurocognitive disorders increase dramatically in old age.

Theories of Aging

Several theories related to the aging process have been described. These theories are grouped into two broad categories: biological and psychosocial.

Biological Theories

Biological theories attempt to explain the physical process of aging, including molecular and cellular changes in the major organ systems and the body's ability to function adequately and resist disease. They also attempt to explain why people age differently and what factors affect longevity and the body's ability to resist disease.

Genetic Theory

According to one genetic theory, aging is an involuntarily inherited process that operates over time to alter cellular or tissue structures. This theory suggests that life span and longevity changes are predetermined. The theory is supported by the finding that there are similar life spans among identical twins and children of parents with a long life span (Rogers et al., 2020).

A second genetic theory identifies aging as a process of genetic mutations that essentially create "errors" in transmission of information, resulting in malfunction of specific proteins. Epigenetics (the study of the ways behavior and environment change how genes are expressed without changes in the DNA sequence) has confirmed some fascinating findings that have implications for aging and illness. First, it was discovered that DNA methylation (the addition of a methyl group to a DNA base) is a mechanism responsible for gene regulation. Genome studies of aging cells and tissues have shown that a variable "DNA methylation drift" creates changes in aging stem cells culminating in reduced stem cell plasticity, stem cell exhaustion, and focal defects that can lead to illnesses such as cancer (Issa, 2014). Issa describes that "aging pathologies in turn accelerate methylation drift by promoting chronic inflammation and uncontrolled proliferation which creates a vicious cycle that may explain why some illnesses increase . . . exponentially . . . with age" (p. 28). It is possible, with ongoing research, that we may discover what aging will look like for an individual and what their disease risks are. If epigenetic drift can be prevented, it may be possible to prevent diseases associated with aging.

Wear-and-Tear Theory

Proponents of this theory believe that the body wears out on a scheduled basis. Because animals have some ability to repair themselves, it would seem that this theory does not fit what we know about biological systems (Rogers et al., 2020). A related theory suggests that free radicals, which are the waste products of metabolism, accumulate and cause damage to important biological structures. Free radicals are molecules with unpaired electrons that exist normally in the body; they also are produced by ionizing radiation, ozone, and chemical toxins. According to this theory, these free radicals cause DNA damage, cross-linkage of collagen, and the accumulation of age pigments.

Environmental Theory

According to this theory, factors in the environment (e.g., industrial carcinogens, sunlight, trauma, and infection) bring about changes in the aging process. Although these factors are known to accelerate aging, the impact of the environment is a secondary rather than a primary factor in aging. Science is only beginning to uncover the many environmental factors that affect aging.

Autoimmune Theory

The autoimmune theory describes an age-related decline in the immune system. As people age, their ability to defend against foreign organisms decreases, resulting in susceptibility to diseases such as cancer and infection. Aging immune cells become unable to distinguish between "self" proteins and foreign proteins and begin to attack the body's own cells. A rise in the body's autoimmune response occurs, leading to the development of autoimmune diseases such as rheumatoid arthritis and allergies to food and environmental agents. This theory, however, is based on clinical rather than experimental evidence (Rogers et al., 2020).

Neuroendocrine Theory

The neuroendocrine theory was first developed in 1954 by Vladimir Dilman, MD. Dilman subsequently worked with another physician, Ward Dean, to update this theory in the early 1990s. The theory suggests that as humans age, the hypothalamus declines in its ability to regulate hormones and becomes less sensitive to them. Consequently, hormone secretion and hormone effectiveness decline. Dilman identified several hypotheses to explain why the hypothalamus becomes less sensitive, including reduced neurotransmitter levels (serotonin in particular), decline in the secretion of pineal gland hormones, reduced glucose utilization and fat accumulation, neuronal lesions caused by chronically elevated cortisol levels secondary to stress, and accumulation of cholesterol in plasma membranes of neurons (Dean, 2021). Some believe that hormone replacements impacted by the hypothalamus may be a future treatment to counter the effects of aging, but more research is needed.

Psychosocial Theories

Psychosocial theories focus on social and psychological changes that accompany advancing age rather than on the biological implications of anatomic deterioration. Several theories have attempted to describe how attitudes and behavior in the early phases of life affect people's reactions during the late phase. This work is called the process of "successful aging."

Personality Theory

In a review of research on personality and aging that studied people between 60 and 80 years of age, Srivastava and Das (2013) identify support for the premise that personality traits are relatively stable but may change somewhat over the long term related to aging and possibly in response to intervention. The personality trait of conscientiousness, for example, when viewed over the course of a lifetime, was found to be relatively stable.

As the population of older adults continues to grow, research has focused not only on what constitutes aging but also more specifically on what constitutes successful aging. Srivastava and Das stress that personality is undeniably influential in successful aging (they note that the term *successful aging* is often used but is controversial to some). Rowe and Kahn (1997) provide the classic paradigm for successful aging, identifying three criteria that must be met: (1) absence of disease, disability, and risk factors; (2) maintenance of physical and mental functioning; and (3) active engagement in life.

What role do personality factors play in these aspects of successful aging? The research of Kern and Friedman (2008) identified the personality trait of conscientiousness as most linked to health-promoting behaviors. Terracciano and colleagues (2010) identified a gene associated with the trait of conscientiousness. They found that this personality trait gene was associated with the same gene that has been linked to some neurodegenerative diseases, including Alzheimer's disease. Several studies have found that the personality trait of conscientiousness is protective against dementia, and the facets of conscientiousness most protective against cognitive impairment are one's sense of personal responsibility, one's belief in one's ability to control own behavior, and one's sense of self as hard working (Sutin et al., 2018). This research suggests that personality may indeed play a significant role in aging and age-related illness. What all of this means for intervention in and possible improvement of the aging process is still unknown. Future research may begin to reveal the intricate interaction between genetic and environmental influences such that personality traits might become alterable to promote healthier, more successful aging.

Developmental Task Theory

In contrast to the personality trait theories of aging, which discuss a largely stable process that continues into old age, developmental task theory holds that there are activities and challenges that one must accomplish at predictable, changing stages in life to achieve successful aging. Erikson (1963) described the primary task of old age as being able to see one's life as having been lived with integrity. In the absence of achieving that sense of having lived well, the older adult is at risk of becoming preoccupied with feelings of regret or despair. As noted previously, the life span was significantly different when Erikson's developmental tasks and stages were first identified, and in the late 1990s, Erikson expanded the concept of **transcendence** as an additional stage that occurs after the stage of integrity versus despair (Erikson & Erikson, 1997). McCarthy and colleagues (2013) identify transcendence as a concept within the spiritual domain, and they cite McCarthy and Bockweg's (2012) definition:

> Transcendence [is] an inherent developmental process, resulting in a shift from a rational, materialistic view to a wider world view characterized by broadened personal boundaries, within interpersonal, intrapersonal, transpersonal, and temporal dimensions resulting in an increased sense of meaning in life, well-being, and life satisfaction. (p. 180)

McCarthy and associates' research (2013) on transcendence supports that transcendence is a significant contributor to successful aging. McCarthy adds that even in the face of chronic illness and functional limitations, individuals can age successfully depending on their ability to cope and adapt while maintaining a sense of connectedness and meaning in life (News Medical, 2014).

Disengagement Theory

Disengagement theory describes the process of withdrawal by older adults from societal roles and responsibilities. According to this theory, this withdrawal process is predictable, systematic, inevitable, and necessary for the proper functioning of a growing society. Older adults were said to be happy when social contacts diminished and responsibilities were assumed by a younger generation. The benefit to the older adult is thought to be in providing time for reflecting on life's accomplishments and for coming to terms with unfulfilled expectations. The benefit to society is thought to be an orderly transfer of power from old to young.

There have been many critics of this theory, and the postulates have been challenged. For many healthy and productive older individuals, the prospect of a slower pace and fewer responsibilities is undesirable.

Activity Theory

In direct opposition to the disengagement theory is the activity theory of aging, which holds that the way to age successfully is to stay active. Boland and Verduin (2022) report that growing evidence supports the importance of remaining socially active for both physical and emotional well-being. Cultural expectations are influential, and as older Americans are identified as reaping the benefits of physical and social activity, cultural expectations begin to shift. Many fitness classes, for example, are now finding a membership of people in their 80s and beyond.

Continuity Theory

This theory, also known as the developmental theory, is a follow-up to the disengagement and activity theories. It emphasizes the individual's previously established coping abilities and personal character traits as a basis for predicting how the person will adjust to the changes of aging. Basic lifestyle characteristics are likely to remain stable in old age, barring physical or other types of complications that necessitate change. A person who has enjoyed the company of others and an active social life will continue to enjoy this lifestyle into old age. One who has preferred solitude and a limited number of activities will probably find satisfaction in a continuation of this lifestyle.

Maintenance of internal continuity is motivated by the need for preservation of self-esteem, ego integrity, cognitive function, and social support. As they age, individuals maintain their self-concept by reinterpreting their current experiences so that old values can take on new meanings in keeping with present circumstances. Internal self-concepts and beliefs are not readily vulnerable to environmental change, and external continuity in skills, activities, roles, and relationship styles can remain remarkably stable into the 70s and beyond.

The Normal Aging Process

Biological Aspects of Aging

Individuals are unique in their physical and psychological aging processes, as influenced by their predisposition or resistance to illness; the effects of their external environment and behaviors; their exposure to trauma, infections, and past diseases; and the health and illness practices they have adopted during their life span. As the individual ages, there is a quantitative loss of cells and changes in many of the enzymatic activities within cells, resulting in a diminished responsiveness to biological demands made on the body. Age-related changes occur at different rates for different individuals, although in actuality, when growth stops, aging begins. This section presents a brief overview of the normal biological changes that occur with the aging process.

Integumentary System

One of the most dramatic changes that occurs in aging is the loss of elastin in the skin. This effect, as well as changes in collagen, causes aged skin to wrinkle and sag. Excessive exposure to sunlight compounds these changes and increases the risk of developing skin cancer.

Fat redistribution results in a loss of the subcutaneous cushion of adipose tissue. Thus, older people lose "insulation," their skin appears thinner, and they are more sensitive to extremes of ambient temperature than are younger people. A diminished supply of blood vessels to the skin results in a slower rate of healing.

Cardiovascular System

The age-related decline in the cardiovascular system is thought to be the major determinant of decreased tolerance for exercise and loss of conditioning and the overall decline in energy reserve. The aging heart is characterized by modest hypertrophy and loss of pacemaker cells, resulting in a decrease in maximal heart rate and diminished cardiac output. This results in a decrease in response to work demands and some diminishment of blood flow to the brain, kidneys, liver, and muscles. Heart rate also slows with time. If arteriosclerosis is present, cardiac function is further compromised.

Respiratory System

Thoracic expansion is diminished by an increase in fibrous tissue and loss of elastin. Pulmonary vital capacity decreases, and the amount of residual air increases. Scattered areas of fibrosis in the alveolar septa interfere with exchange of oxygen and carbon dioxide. These changes are accelerated by the use of cigarettes or other inhaled substances. Cough and laryngeal reflexes are reduced, causing decreased ability to defend the airway. Decreased pulmonary blood flow and diffusion ability result in reduced efficiency in responding to sudden respiratory demands.

Musculoskeletal System

Skeletal aging involving the bones, muscles, ligaments, and tendons probably generates the most frequent limitations on activities of daily living experienced by aging individuals. Loss of muscle mass is significant, although this occurs more slowly in men than in women. Demineralization of the bones occurs at a rate of about 1% per year throughout the life span in both men and women. However, this increases to approximately 10% in women around **menopause,** making them particularly vulnerable to **osteoporosis.**

Individual muscle fibers become thinner and less elastic with age. Muscles become less flexible following disuse. Diminished storage of muscle glycogen results in loss of energy reserve for increased activity. These changes are accelerated by nutritional deficiencies and inactivity.

Gastrointestinal System

In the oral cavity, the teeth show a reduction in dentine production, shrinkage and fibrosis of root pulp, gingival retraction, and loss of bone density in the alveolar ridges. There is some loss of peristalsis in the stomach and intestines, and gastric acid production decreases. Levels of intrinsic factor may also decrease, resulting in vitamin B_{12} malabsorption in some aging individuals. A significant decrease in absorptive surface area of the small intestine may be associated with some decline in nutrient absorption. Motility slowdown of the large intestine, combined with poor dietary habits, dehydration, lack of exercise, and some medications, may give rise to problems with constipation.

A modest decrease in size and weight of the liver results in losses in enzyme activity required to deactivate certain medications by the liver. These age-related changes can influence the metabolism and excretion of these medications. These changes, along with the pharmacokinetics of a drug, must be considered when giving medications to aging individuals.

Endocrine System

A decreased level of thyroid hormones causes a lowered basal metabolic rate. Decreased amounts of adrenocorticotropic hormone may result in less efficient stress response.

Impairments in glucose tolerance are evident in aging individuals. Glucose challenge tests show that insulin levels are equivalent to or slightly higher than those in younger individuals, although peripheral insulin resistance appears to play a significant role in carbohydrate intolerance. The observed glucose clearance abnormalities and insulin resistance in older people may be related to many factors other than biological aging (e.g., obesity, family history of diabetes) and may be influenced substantially by diet or exercise.

Genitourinary System

Age-related declines in renal function occur because of a steady attrition of nephrons and sclerosis within the glomeruli over time. Vascular changes affect blood flow to the kidneys, which results in reduced glomerular filtration and tubular function. Older adults have an increased risk of developing the syndrome of inappropriate antidiuretic hormone secretion, and levels of blood urea nitrogen and creatinine may be elevated slightly. The overall decline in renal functioning has important implications for physicians who prescribe medications for elderly individuals.

In men, enlargement of the prostate gland is common as aging occurs. Symptoms include urgency, difficulty urinating, nocturia, and inability to empty the bladder completely. In addition to changes that may occur as part of the normal aging process, obesity, lack of activity, and erectile dysfunction can also increase the risk (American Urology Association, 2019).

Loss of muscle and sphincter control, as well as the use of some medications, may cause urinary incontinence in women. Not only is this problem a cause of social stigma, but, if left untreated, it also increases the risk of urinary tract infection and local skin irritation. Normal changes in the genitalia are discussed in the section "Sexual Aspects of Aging."

Immune System

Aging results in changes in both cell-mediated and antibody-mediated immune responses. The size of the thymus gland declines continuously from just beyond puberty to about 15% of its original size by age 50. The consequences of these changes include a greater susceptibility to infections and a diminished inflammatory response that results in delayed healing. There is also evidence of an increase in various autoantibodies as a person ages, increasing the risk of autoimmune disorders, such as rheumatoid arthritis (National Institutes of Health [NIH], 2021).

Because of the overall decrease in efficiency of the immune system, the proliferation of abnormal cells is facilitated in older adults. Cancer is the best example of aberrant cells that proliferate due to the ineffectiveness of the immune system.

Nervous System

Brain weight decreases about 11% by age 85 (Galasko, 2017), but the significance of neuron loss as a causal factor is controversial. Neuroimaging studies reveal that brain volume decreases particularly in the frontal, parietal, and hippocampal areas, and that the ventricles become enlarged.

The brain has enormous reserve, and little cerebral function is lost over time, although greater functional decline is noted in the periphery. There appears to be a disproportionately greater loss of cells in the cerebellum, the locus ceruleus, the substantia nigra, and olfactory bulbs, accounting for some of the more characteristic aging behaviors such as mild gait disturbances, sleep disruptions, and decreased smell and taste perception.

Some of the age-related changes within the nervous system may be due to alterations in neurotransmitter release, uptake, turnover, catabolism, or receptor functions (Galasko, 2017). Decreases in dopamine and acetylcholine are of particular interest because of their significance in cognition and mood. Biochemical changes may be responsible for the altered responses of many older persons to stressful events and some biological treatments.

Sensory Systems

Vision

Visual acuity begins to decrease in midlife. Presbyopia (blurred near vision) is the standard marker of aging of the eye. It is caused by a loss of elasticity of the crystalline lens and results in compromised accommodation.

Cataract development is inevitable if the individual lives long enough for the changes to occur. Cataracts occur when the lens of the eye becomes less resilient (due to compression of fibers) and increasingly opaque (as proteins lump together), ultimately resulting in a loss of visual acuity.

The color in the iris may fade, and the pupil may become irregular in shape. A decrease in production of secretions by the lacrimal glands may cause dryness and result in increased irritation and infection. The pupil may become constricted, requiring an increase in the amount of light needed for reading.

Hearing

Hearing changes significantly with the aging process. Gradually over time, the ear loses its sensitivity to discriminate sounds because of damage to the hair cells of the cochlea. The most dramatic decline appears to be in perception of high-frequency sounds.

Age-related hearing loss, called *presbycusis,* is common and affects more than one-half of all adults by age 75 years and most adults over the age of 80 (Blevins, 2021). It is more common in men than it is in women, a fact that may be related to differences in levels of lifetime noise exposure.

Taste and Smell

Beyond 70 years of age, taste sensitivity begins to decline related to atrophy and loss of taste buds (Shock, 2020). Taste discrimination decreases, and bitter taste sensations predominate. Sensitivity to sweet and salty tastes is diminished.

The deterioration of the olfactory bulbs is accompanied by loss of smell acuity. The effect of aging on the sense of smell has not been precisely identified, though, and is difficult to evaluate because so many environmental factors influence sensitivity to smell (Shock, 2020). However, some decreased sensitivity may be related to loss of nerve endings in the nose and less mucus production (MedlinePlus, 2021).

Touch and Pain

Although the primary sensory changes that occur specifically related to aging are in hearing and vision, sensitivity to touch and pain may also decline or change with age related to less blood flow to nerve endings, in the spinal cord, or to the brain (MedlinePlus, 2021). These changes have critical implications for older adults in their potential inability to use sensory warnings to escape serious injury.

Psychological Aspects of Aging

Memory Functioning

Age-related memory deficiencies and slower response times have been extensively reported in the literature. Although **short-term memory** seems to deteriorate with age, perhaps because of poorer sorting strategies, **long-term memory** does not show similar changes. However, in nearly every instance, well-educated, mentally active people do not exhibit the same decline in memory functioning as their age peers who lack similar opportunities to flex their minds. Nevertheless, with few exceptions, the time required for memory scanning is longer for both recent and remote recall among older people. This change can sometimes be attributed to social or health factors (e.g., stress, fatigue, illness), but it can also occur because of certain normal physical changes associated with aging (e.g., decreased blood flow to the brain).

Intellectual Functioning

There appears to be a high degree of regularity in intellectual functioning across the adult age span. Crystallized abilities, or knowledge acquired in the course of the socialization process, tend to remain stable over the adult life span. Fluid abilities, those involved in solving novel problems, tend to decline gradually from young to old adulthood and are thought to be more associated with the integrity of brain function.

Learning Ability

The ability to learn is not diminished by age. Studies, however, have shown that some aspects of learning do change with age. The ordinary slowing of reaction time with age for nearly all tasks or the overarousal of the central nervous system may account for lower performance levels on tests requiring rapid responses. Under conditions that allow for self-pacing by the participant, differences in accuracy of performance diminish. The ability to learn continues throughout life, although it is strongly influenced by interests, activity, motivation, health, and experience. Adjustments need to be made in teaching methodology and time allowed for learning.

Adaptation to the Tasks of Aging

Loss and Grief

Individuals experience losses from the very beginning of life. By the time individuals reach their 60s and 70s, they have experienced numerous losses, and mourning has become a lifelong process. Unfortunately, with the aging process comes a convergence of losses, the timing of which makes it impossible for the aging individual to complete the grief process in response to one loss before another occurs. Because grief is cumulative, this can result in **bereavement overload,** which has been implicated in the predisposition to depression in the elderly.

Attachment to Others

The importance of interpersonal relationships at all stages of the life cycle is widely accepted as key to successful aging. Benefits include decreased sense of loneliness, increased life satisfaction, and support to facilitate coping with stressful changes and events. This need for **attachment** is consistent with the activity theory of aging that correlates the importance of social integration with successful adaptation in later life. Evidence supports that, in addition to psychosocial benefits, social engagement is also correlated with physical and cognitive health in older adulthood (Myhre et al., 2017; Thomas, 2011; Watanabe et al., 2016).

Maintenance of Self-Identity

Maintaining a positive self-concept and identity is important in successful aging. Individuals who tend toward a rigid self-identity and a negative self-concept will no doubt struggle with any changes and adaptations faced in the process of aging. For example, individuals whose identity centers entirely on their job may struggle more with their identity in retirement than those whose identity includes job, family, travel, and so on. Researchers in one study found that maintaining a youthful age identity and positive perceptions and experiences related to aging had a self-enhancing function for self-esteem and identity (Westerhof et al., 2012). The authors compared citizens in the United States with citizens in the Netherlands and found that this self-enhancing function was stronger for Americans than for Netherlanders. Their conclusion was that factors influencing self-identity and self-concept in older age need to be considered within the cultural context.

Dealing With Death

Death anxiety is a universal phenomenon, and attitudes about death are a result of cumulative life experiences (Lehto & Stein, 2009). As more people are living longer there has been a resurgence of interest in research about death anxiety. Lehto and Stein conducted an extensive review of the research to lay a foundation for an emerging understanding of this concept. Kübler-Ross's (1969) pioneering research on attitudes about death and the experience of dying paved the way for discussions of this issue, but as Lehto and Stein (2009) identify in their review of literature, death anxiety is largely denied or repressed. They cite several studies confirming that religious beliefs reduce death anxiety and suggest that such beliefs are beneficial because they provide a context for meaning about life and death. Positive self-esteem mediates death anxiety or at least "assists in preventing overt manifestations of death anxiety" (p. 27). Other researchers found similarly that fear of the dying process among older individuals in care institutions was correlated with low self-esteem, purposelessness, and poor mental health (Missler et al., 2012). These authors also found that, in their sample, death anxiety was more correlated with fears for significant others than fear of the unknown.

Interestingly, death anxiety seems to be the highest during middle age and stabilizes by later adulthood. But as Lehto and Stein (2009) identified, maladaptive consequences of death anxiety include mental illnesses such as depression and anxiety disorders, so assessing and intervening with regard to death anxiety may be beneficial in preventing longer-term consequences. Self-esteem interventions, for example, may be beneficial in preventing depression in older adults secondary to death anxiety. Some research has shown that death education is beneficial in reducing anxiety associated with fear of death (McClatchey & King, 2015). Addressing these issues with middle-aged patients may be in the interest of primary or secondary prevention in the aging process.

Psychiatric Disorders in Later Life

Cognitive disorders, mood disorders, phobias, and alcohol use disorders are among the most common psychiatric illnesses in later life (Boland & Verduin, 2022). Many factors, including medical conditions and medications, may influence symptomatology. One should never assume that psychiatric symptoms are a usual part of aging. A thorough assessment is essential to distinguish the multiple factors that may concurrently influence symptomatology.

Neurocognitive Disorders

Neurocognitive disorders (NCDs) are common causes of psychopathology in older adults and are expected to increase over the next few decades as the population of older adults increases and research on early identification of NCDs improves (Jeste, 2017). About one-half of these disorders are of the Alzheimer's type, which is characterized by an insidious onset and a gradually progressive course of cognitive impairment. No curative treatment is currently available. Symptomatic treatments, including pharmacological interventions, attention to the environment, and family support, can help to maximize the client's level of functioning.

Delirium

Delirium is one of the most common and critical forms of psychopathology in later life. A number of factors have been identified that predispose aging individuals to delirium, including structural brain disease, reduced capacity for homeostatic regulation, impaired vision and hearing, a high prevalence of chronic disease, reduced resistance to acute stress, and age-related changes in the pharmacokinetic and pharmacodynamics of drugs. Delirium needs to be recognized and the underlying condition treated as soon as possible. A high mortality rate is associated with this condition.

Depression

Depressive disorders are the most common affective illnesses occurring after the middle years. The incidence of depression among older adults is influenced by many variables, particularly physical illness and losses. Somatic symptoms such as changes in appetite and complaints of pain are common in the depressed elderly but should always be assessed to rule out other illnesses. Symptomatology often mimics that of NCD, a condition that is referred to as *pseudodementia.* (See Table 13–1, Chapter 13, for a comparison of the symptoms of NCD and pseudodementia.) Suicide is prevalent in older adults, with declining health and decreased economic status being considered important influencing factors. Studies have noted that depression, depression-related suicide, and substance abuse are higher in the baby boomer generation than in those born prior to World War II (Jeste, 2017), although the reasons are unclear. Treatment of depression in the older individual may include psychotropic medications or electroconvulsive therapy. Tricyclic antidepressants pose a risk for orthostatic hypotension and other anticholinergic effects, and selective serotonin reuptake inhibitors (SSRIs) pose a higher risk for hyponatremia in older adults, so risks and benefits of medication use should be carefully reviewed. Cardiac disease in older adults with untreated depression can negatively affect outcome (Celano & Huffman, 2011).

Schizophrenia

Schizophrenia is an illness that typically begins in young adulthood. In most instances, individuals who manifest psychotic disorders early in life show a decline in psychopathology as they age. Late-onset schizophrenia (after age 60) is rare, and when it does occur, it is more common in women and is often characterized by paranoid delusions or hallucinations. Antipsychotic agents may be beneficial for the older adult with schizophrenia but should be used judiciously and at lower than usual doses (Boland & Verduin, 2022).

Anxiety Disorders

Anxiety disorders are the third most common (3.8%) mental disorders in older adults (WHO, 2017). Most anxiety disorders begin in early to middle adulthood, but some appear for the first time after age 60. Because the autonomic nervous system is more fragile in older persons, the response to a major stressor is often quite intense. The presence of physical disability frequently compounds the situation, resulting in a more severe post-traumatic stress response than is commonly observed in younger persons. In older adults, symptoms of anxiety and depression often accompany each other, making it difficult to determine which disorder is dominant.

Anxiety disorders are also associated with cardiac disease in older adults and to adverse cardiovascular outcomes (Celano et al., 2016). There may be physiological (inflammation, autonomic and endothelial dysfunction, platelet aggregation) as well as behavioral mechanisms involved in the link between anxiety and cardiovascular disease, but careful identification and treatment of both conditions is essential.

Substance Use Disorders

It is believed that the incidence of substance abuse and addiction in older adults may have been underdiagnosed, but nationwide attention to the epidemic use and abuse of opioid pain medication has shed light on this problem in the older population.

Older adults use prescription and over-the-counter (OTC) medications at least three times as frequently as the general population (Jeste, 2017) and may have more difficulty tolerating some drugs, particularly some long-acting drugs, sedative hypnotics, and benzodiazepines. For these reasons (and others), older adults are an at-risk population for substance use disorders and should be screened for prescription, OTC, and other substance use to identify an emerging problem. Benzodiazepines used concomitantly with opiate medication have been identified as a potentially fatal combination of drugs.

Many older adults with alcohol dependence have a long-standing history, and consequently many have Wernicke's encephalopathy or Korsakoff syndrome. "The sudden onset of delirium in older adults hospitalized for a medical illness is most often caused by alcohol withdrawal" (Boland & Verduin, 2022, p. 807), so careful evaluation for alcohol use history is important in assessment of this population.

Sleep Disorders

Sleep disorders are very common in older adults. Boland and Verduin (2022) identify that advanced age is the single most important factor related to the increased prevalence of sleep disorders. However, as Rodriguez and associates (2015, p. 431) note, "sleep problems are not an inherent part of the aging process. . . . [T]herefore, a focused evaluation of sleep, specifically sleep apnea and insomnia, and related daytime functioning should be performed in every older adult in whom sleep disturbances are suspected." Contributing factors include medical conditions, medications, age-related changes in circadian rhythms, sleep disordered breathing, and restless leg syndrome. Sedative-hypnotics, along with nonpharmacological approaches, are often used as sleep aids with the elderly. Changes in aging associated with metabolism and elimination must be considered when maintenance medications are administered for chronic insomnia in the aging client.

Sociocultural Aspects of Aging

Old age brings many important socially induced changes, some of which have the potential for negative effect on both the physical and mental well-being of older persons. In American society, *old age* is defined arbitrarily as being 65 years or older because that is the age when most people have been able to retire with full Social Security and other pension benefits. Recent legislation has increased the age beyond 65 years for full Social Security benefits. Currently, the age increases yearly (based on year of birth) until 2027, when the age for full benefits will be 67 years for all individuals.

Older people in virtually all cultures share some basic needs and interests. There is little doubt that most individuals choose to live the most satisfying life possible for as long as possible. They want protection from hazards and release from the weariness of everyday tasks. They want to be treated with the respect and dignity they deserve as individuals who have reached this pinnacle in life; and they want to die with the same respect and dignity.

Historically, the aged have had a special status in society. Even today, in some cultures, the aged are the most powerful, the most engaged, and the most respected members of society. This has not been the case in the modern industrial societies, although trends in the status of the aged differ widely among industrialized countries. For example, the status and integration of the aged in Japan have remained relatively high when compared with other industrialized nations, such as the United States.

Many negative stereotypes influence the perspective on aging in the United States. Ideas that elderly individuals are always tired or sick, slow and forgetful, isolated and lonely, unproductive, and angry determine the way younger individuals relate to the elderly in this society. Increasing disregard for older adults has resulted in a type of segregation, as aging individuals voluntarily seek out or are involuntarily placed in special residences for the aged.

Retirement apartment complexes, assisted living centers, and even entire retirement communities intended solely for individuals over age 50 are becoming increasingly common. Geographic distribution of older populations varies significantly in different states. In 2018, more than half (51%) of those age 65 and older lived in 9 states with the largest numbers in California, Florida, Texas, New York, and Pennsylvania (AoA, 2020). Older adults may be migrating to these areas in an effort to achieve integration with others in their age-group. This phenomenon provides additional corroboration for the activity theory of aging and the importance of attachment to others.

The status of the elderly may improve with time and as their numbers increase with the aging of the baby boomers. As older individuals gain political power and increase in number, the benefits and privileges designed for the elderly will increase.

Sexual Aspects of Aging

Sexuality and the sexual needs of older people are frequently misunderstood, condemned, stereotyped, ridiculed, repressed, and ignored. Americans have grown up in a society that has liberated sexual expression for all other age-groups but still maintains old-fashioned standards for sexual expression by older adults. Negative stereotyped notions include ideas that older people have no sexual interests or desires, that they are sexually undesirable, or that they are too fragile or too ill to engage in sexual activity. Some people even believe that it is disgusting or comical to consider elderly individuals as sexual beings.

These cultural stereotypes undoubtedly play a large part in the misperception that many people hold regarding sexuality of the aged, and they may be reinforced by the common tendency of the young to deny the inevitability of aging. With reasonably good health and an interesting and interested partner, there is no inherent reason that individuals should not enjoy an active sexual life well into late adulthood.

Physical Changes Associated With Sexuality

Many of the changes in sexuality that occur in later years are related to the physical changes that are taking place at that time of life.

Changes in Women

Menopause may begin anytime during the 40s or early 50s. During this time, there is a gradual decline in the functioning of the ovaries and the subsequent production of estrogen, which results in a number of changes. The walls of the vagina become thin and inelastic, the vagina itself shrinks in both width and length, and the amount of vaginal lubrication decreases noticeably. Orgastic uterine contractions may become spastic. All of these changes can result in painful penetration, vaginal burning, pelvic aching, or irritation on urination. In some women, the discomfort may be severe enough to result in an avoidance of intercourse. Paradoxically, these symptoms are more likely to occur with infrequent intercourse of only one time a month or less. Regular and more frequent sexual activity results in a greater capacity for sexual performance (King & Regan, 2013).

Changes in Men

Testosterone production declines gradually over the years, beginning between ages 40 and 60. A major change resulting from this hormone reduction is that erections occur more slowly and require more direct genital stimulation to achieve. There may also be a modest decrease in the firmness of the erection in men older than age 60. The refractory period lengthens with age, increasing the amount of time following orgasm before the man may achieve another erection. The volume of ejaculate gradually decreases, and the force of ejaculation lessens. The testes become somewhat smaller, but most men continue to produce viable sperm well into old age. Prolonged control over ejaculation in middle-aged and elderly men may bring increased sexual satisfaction for both partners. Adverse effects of some medications and circulatory problems may increase risks for erectile dysfunction in older adult men. Vasodilator medications such as sildenafil (Viagra) and tadalafil (Cialis) are treatment options.

Sexual Behavior in the Older Adults

The overall quantity of sexual activity between ages 20 and 40 correlates significantly with frequency patterns of sexual activity during aging (Masters et al., 1995). Although sexual interest and behavior do appear to decline somewhat with age, studies show that significant numbers of elderly men and women have active and satisfying sex lives well into their 80s. According to a University of Michigan national poll (Solway et al., 2018) on sexual behavior and health among adults ages 65 to 80, 40% identified being sexually active. Some statistics from the survey are summarized in Table 24–1. A large, longitudinal study (n = 6021) on sexual health and well-being in older adults within the United Kingdom (Lee et al., 2016)

TABLE 24–1 Sexuality at Midlife and Beyond

	SEX IS AN IMPORTANT PART OF A ROMANTIC RELATIONSHIP AT ANY AGE. (n = 989) PERCENTAGE THAT AGREED OR STRONGLY AGREED	SEX IS IMPORTANT TO MY OVERALL QUALITY OF LIFE. (n = 979) PERCENTAGE THAT AGREED OR STRONGLY AGREED	HOW WOULD YOU DESCRIBE YOUR INTEREST IN SEX? (n = 979) PERCENTAGE THAT WERE EXTREMELY OR STRONGLY INTERESTED	HOW SATISFIED ARE YOU WITH YOUR SEX LIFE? (n = 956) PERCENTAGE THAT WERE EXTREMELY OR VERY SATISFIED
All Respondents	76%	54%	30%	37%
AGE				
65–70	78%	57%	34%	38%
71–75	72%	52%	28%	37%
76–80	77%	50%	19%	36%
GENDER				
Male	84%	70%	50%	31%
Female	69%	40%	12%	43%
RELATIONSHIP STATUS				
Married/Partnered/In a relationship	76%	61%	34%	40%
Not in a relationship	75%	36%	19%	30%
PHYSICAL HEALTH				
Excellent/Very good/Good	77%	56%	32%	40%
Fair/Poor	71%	49%	21%	28%
SEXUALLY ACTIVE				
Yes	92%	83%	52%	49%
No	66%	35%	16%	29%

Source: Solway, E., Clark, S., Singer, D., Kirch, M., & Malani P. (2018). *Let's talk about sex, national poll on healthy aging*. Institute for Healthcare Policy and Innovation, University of Michigan. https://www.healthyagingpoll.org/reports-more/report/lets-talk-about-sex. With permission.

also included the age-group of 80 to >90 years and found that roughly 14% of women and 37% of men reported being sexually active. The information from these surveys clearly indicates that sexual activity can and does continue well past the 70s for healthy, active individuals who have regular opportunities for sexual expression. King and Regan (2013) identify that if an individual has healthy attitudes about sexuality and healthy sexual relationships in younger adulthood, those will probably continue into older adulthood.

Special Concerns of the Older Population

Retirement

Statistics reflect that a larger percentage of Americans are living longer and that many of them are retiring earlier. Reasons often given for the increasing pattern of early retirement include health problems, Social Security and other pension benefits, attractive "early out" packages offered by companies, and long-held plans (e.g., turning a hobby into a money-making situation). Although many Americans are retiring earlier, the Bureau of Labor Statistics notes that the growth rates of older adults continuing to work into their 70s, 80s, and beyond are increasing rapidly. They estimate that in the decade from 2014 to 2024, the growth rate will increase 55% for those 65 to 75 years old and 86% for those 75 and older (Toossi & Torpey, 2017).

It is estimated that about 29% of Americans reenter the workforce after retirement, even though current estimates suggest that there will still be dramatic shortages in the number of needed employees (Sullivan & Ariss, 2018). In the field of nursing, for example, the American Association of Colleges of Nursing (AACN, 2020) predicts that, as more nurses retire, there will be an annual shortage of 175,900 nurses through 2029. Sullivan and Ariss propose that these anticipated shortages, a larger number of retirees, and longer life spans require the development of a new paradigm for examining the role of older adults in the workforce. The authors also cite reasons for older adults not wanting to return to the workforce included ageism, unsupportive work climates, lack of flexibility in the availability of part-time positions, and their own inability to effectively search for employment.

Retirement has both social and economic implications for older individuals. The role is fraught with a great deal of ambiguity and is one that requires many adaptations on the part of those involved.

Social Implications

Retirement is often anticipated as an achievement in principle but met with a great deal of ambiguity when it actually occurs. Our society places a great deal of importance on productivity, making as much money as possible, and doing it at as young an age as possible. These types of values contribute to the ambiguity associated with retirement. Although leisure has been acknowledged as a legitimate reward for workers, leisure during retirement historically has lacked the same social value. Adjustment to this life-cycle event becomes more difficult in the face of societal values that are in direct conflict with the new lifestyle.

American society often identifies individuals by their occupation. This is reflected in the conversation of people who are meeting each other for the first time. Undoubtedly, most people have either asked or been asked at some point in time, "What do you do?" or "Where do you work?" Occupation determines status, and retirement represents a significant change in status. The basic ambiguity of retirement occurs in an individual's or society's definition of this change. Is it undertaken voluntarily or involuntarily? Is it desirable or undesirable? Is one's status made better or worse by the change? It is a major life event that requires planning and realistic expectations of life changes.

Economic Implications

Because retirement is generally associated with a 20% to 40% reduction in personal income, the standard of living after retirement may be adversely affected. Most older adults derive post-retirement income from a combination of Social Security benefits, public and private pensions, and income from savings or investments.

The Social Security Act of 1935 promised assistance with financial security for older adults. Since then, the original legislation has been modified, yet the basic philosophy remains intact. Its effectiveness, however, is now being questioned. Faced with deficits, the program is forced to pay benefits to those currently retired from both the reserve funds and monies being collected at present. There is genuine concern about paying Social Security benefits to future generations, when there may be no reserve funds from which to draw. Because many of the programs that benefit older adults depend on contributions from the younger population, the growing ratio of older Americans to younger people may affect society's ability to supply the goods and services necessary to meet this expanding demand.

Medicare and **Medicaid** were established by the government to provide medical care benefits for older and indigent Americans. The Medicaid program is jointly funded by state and federal governments, and coverage varies significantly from state to state. Medicare covers only a percentage of healthcare costs; therefore, to reduce risk related to out-of-pocket expenditures, many older adults purchase private "Medigap" policies designed to cover charges in excess of those approved by Medicare.

The magnitude of retirement earnings depends almost entirely on preretirement income. The poor will remain poor and the wealthy are unlikely to lower their status during retirement; however, for many in the middle classes, the relatively fixed income sources may be inadequate, possibly forcing them to face financial hardship for the first time in their lives.

Long-Term Care

Long-term care facilities are defined by the level of care they provide. They may be skilled nursing facilities or intermediate care facilities, or a combination of the two. Some institutions provide convalescent care for individuals recovering from acute illness or injury, some provide long-term care for individuals with chronic illness or disabilities, and still others provide both types of assistance.

Most older individuals prefer to remain in their own homes or in the homes of family members for as long as this arrangement can meet their needs without deterioration of family or social patterns. Many older people are placed in institutions as a last resort only after heroic efforts have been made to keep them in their own or a relative's home. The increasing emphasis on home health care has extended the period of independence for aging individuals.

As mentioned previously, fewer than 4% of the population age 65 and older live in nursing homes. The percentage increases dramatically with age, ranging from 1% for persons ages 65 to 74, to 3% for persons ages 75 to 84, to 7% for persons age 85 and older (AoA, 2020). A profile of the "typical" nursing home resident is someone who is about 80 years of age, white, female, widowed, and with multiple chronic health conditions.

Risk Factors for Institutionalization

In determining who in our society will need long-term care, several factors have been identified that appear to place people at risk. Factors that influence the need for long-term care include prevalence of chronic health conditions and disabilities, level of ability to independently provide self-care, presence of mental disorders (particularly NCDs), financial hardships that prohibit exploring other options (such as senior living settings), and lack of a spouse or other support network to provide care or assistance.

Attitudinal Factors

Many people dread the thought of even visiting a nursing home, let alone moving to one or placing a relative in one. Negative perceptions exist of nursing homes as "places to go to die." The media picture and subsequent reputation of nursing homes have not been positive. Stories of substandard care and patient abuse have scarred the industry, making it difficult for those facilities that are clean and well managed and that provide innovative, quality care to their residents to rise above the stigma.

State and national licensing boards perform periodic inspections to ensure that standards set forth by the federal government are being met. These standards address quality of patient care as well as adequacy of the nursing home facility. Yet, many older individuals and their families perceive nursing homes as a place to go to die, and the fact that many of these institutions are poorly equipped, understaffed, and disorganized keeps this societal perception alive. There are, however, many excellent nursing homes that strive to go beyond the minimum federal regulations for Medicaid and Medicare reimbursement. In addition to medical, nursing, rehabilitation, and dental services, social and recreational services are provided to increase the quality of life for residents of nursing homes. These activities include playing cards, bingo, and other games; parties; church activities; books; television; movies; and arts, crafts, and other classes. Some nursing homes provide occupational and professional counseling. These facilities strive to enhance opportunities for improving quality of life and for becoming places to *live* rather than to die.

Elder Abuse

Elder abuse is defined as the psychological, physical, or financial abuse, or intentional or unintentional neglect, of an older adult. Elder abuse occurs within families and inside of institutions such as nursing homes and long-term care facilities (WHO, 2021). Psychological abuse includes yelling, insulting, harsh commands, threats, silence, and social isolation. Physical abuse is described as striking, shoving, beating, or restraint. Financial abuse refers to misuse or theft of finances, property, or material possessions. Neglect implies failure to fulfill the physical needs of an individual who cannot do so independently. Unintentional neglect is inadvertent, whereas intentional neglect is deliberate. In addition, older individuals may be the victims of sexual abuse, which is sexual intimacy between two persons that occurs without the consent of one of the persons involved. Types of elder abuse are summarized in Box 24–1.

Statistics regarding the prevalence of elder abuse are difficult to determine. It is estimated that 1 in 10 older adults in the United States is a victim of abuse (National Council on Aging, 2021). However, one study found that only 45% of victims of violence over age 65 reported those crimes to the police (National Crime Justice Reference Center, 2018). The abuser is often a relative who lives with the elderly person and may be the assigned caregiver. Factors that may contribute to risks for caregiver elder abuse include economic stress, substance abuse, difficulty coping with the caregiver role, and history of criminal behavior (Gillbard & Leggatt-Cook, 2019). Identified risk factors for victims of abuse include being a white female age 70 or older, being mentally or physically impaired, being unable to meet daily self-care needs, and having care needs that exceed the caretaker's ability.

Victims of elder abuse often minimize the abuse or deny that it has occurred. The older person may be unwilling to disclose information because of fear of retaliation, embarrassment about the existence of abuse in the family, protectiveness toward a family member, or unwillingness to institute legal action. Adding to this unwillingness to report is the fact that older adults may be isolated, so their mistreatment is less likely to be noticed by those who might be alert to symptoms of abuse. For these reasons, detection of abuse of older adults is difficult at best.

Factors That Contribute to Abuse

A number of contributing factors have been implicated in the abuse of older individuals who are cared for by family members.

- ***Longer life:*** The 65-and-older age-group has become the fastest-growing segment of the population. Within this segment, the number of persons older than age 75 has increased most rapidly. This trend is expected to continue well into the 21st century. The 75-and-older age-group is the one most likely to be physically or mentally impaired, requiring assistance and care from family members. This group also is the most vulnerable to abuse from caregivers.
- ***Dependency:*** Dependency appears to be the most common precondition in elder abuse. Changes associated with normal aging or induced by chronic illness often result in loss of self-sufficiency

BOX 24–1 Examples of Elder Abuse

PHYSICAL ABUSE
Striking, hitting, beating
Shoving
Bruising
Cutting
Restraining

PSYCHOLOGICAL ABUSE
Yelling
Insulting, name-calling
Harsh commands
Threats
Ignoring, silence, social isolation
Withholding of affection

NEGLECT (INTENTIONAL OR UNINTENTIONAL)
Withholding food and water
Inadequate heating
Unclean clothes and bedding
Lack of needed medication
Lack of eyeglasses, hearing aids, false teeth

FINANCIAL ABUSE OR EXPLOITATION
Misuse of the older person's income by the caregiver
Forcing the older person to sign over financial affairs to another person against their will or without sufficient knowledge about the transaction

SEXUAL ABUSE
Sexual molestation; rape
Any type of sexual contact against the elderly person's will

in older adults, requiring that they become dependent on others for assistance with daily functioning. Long life may also consume finances to the point that the older individual becomes financially dependent on others as well. This type of dependency also increases the older person's vulnerability to abuse.

- ***Stress:*** The stress inherent in the caregiver role is a factor in most abuse cases. Some clinicians believe that elder abuse results from individual or family psychopathology. Others suggest that even psychologically healthy family members can become abusive as the result of the exhaustion and acute stress caused by overwhelming caregiving responsibilities. This is compounded in an age-group that has been dubbed the "sandwich generation"—those individuals who delayed childbearing so that they are now at a point in their lives when they are "sandwiched" between providing care for their children and providing care for their aging parents.
- ***Learned violence:*** Children who have been abused or have witnessed abusive and violent parents are more likely to evolve into abusive adults. In some families, abusive behavior is the normal response to tension or conflict, and this type of behavior can be transmitted from one generation to another. There may be some unresolved family conflicts or retaliation for previous maltreatment that foster and promote abuse of the elderly person.

Identifying Elder Abuse

Because so many older individuals are reluctant to report personal abuse, health-care workers need to be able to detect signs of mistreatment when they are in a position to do so. Box 24–1 lists a number of *types* of elder abuse. The following *manifestations* of the various categories of abuse have been identified:

- ***Psychological and verbal abuse:*** The older adult may appear depressed, withdrawn, more confused, or agitated.
- ***Physical abuse:*** The victim has unexplained bruises, welts, lacerations, burns, puncture wounds, evidence of hair-pulling, skeletal dislocations and fractures, or broken glasses.
- ***Neglect:*** The victim may present with unexplained weight loss, poor hygiene, inappropriate dress, consistent fatigue or listlessness, unattended physical problems or medical needs, or abandonment.
- ***Sexual abuse:*** The patient may present with pain or itching in the genital area; bruising or bleeding in external genitalia, vaginal, or anal areas; unexplained sexually transmitted disease; torn or ripped clothing
- ***Financial abuse:*** There is evidence of disparity between assets and satisfactory living conditions, or the older adult may complain of a sudden lack of sufficient funds for daily living expenses.

Health-care workers often feel intimidated when confronted with cases of elder abuse. In these instances, referral to an individual experienced in management of victims of such abuse may be the most effective approach to evaluation and intervention. Health-care workers are responsible for reporting any suspicions of elder abuse. An investigation is then conducted by regulatory agencies, whose job it is to determine whether the suspicions are corroborated. Every effort must be made to ensure the safety of clients, but it is important to remember that competent older adults have the right to choose their health-care options. As inappropriate as it may seem, some older individuals choose to return to abusive situations. In this instance, provide the patient with names and phone numbers to call for assistance if needed. A follow-up visit by an adult protective services representative should be conducted.

Increased efforts need to be made to ensure that health-care providers have comprehensive training in the detection of and intervention in elder abuse. More research is needed to increase knowledge and understanding of the phenomenon of elder abuse and ultimately to effect more sophisticated strategies for prevention, intervention, and treatment.

Suicide

In 2019, the highest rates of suicide occurred in those age 85 and older (American Foundation for Suicide Prevention [AFSP], 2021). The AFSP also reports that men, and particularly white men (in all age-groups), die by suicide more often than do women. The suicide rate for white men over the age of 65 is five times higher than that of the general population (Boland & Verduin, 2022). Predisposing factors include loneliness, financial problems, physical illness, loss, and depression.

It has been suggested that increased social isolation may be a contributing factor to suicide among older populations. Boland and Verduin (2022) identify that older suicide victims are more likely to be widowed, and the most common precipitants are physical illness and loss.

Many older individuals express symptoms associated with depression that are never recognized as such, particularly somatic symptoms. Any sign of helplessness or hopelessness should prompt an assessment for suicide risk using clear and, often, closed-ended questions to elicit a specific response, such as the following:

- Have you thought of hurting yourself or taking your own life?
- Do you have a plan for hurting yourself?
- Have you ever acted on that plan?
- Have you ever attempted suicide?

Components of intervention with a suicidal older person should include demonstrations of genuine concern, interest, and caring; indications of empathy for their fears and concerns; and help in identifying, clarifying, and formulating a plan of action to manage risks for suicidal behavior. Loneliness and social isolation are often compounding issues and should be addressed as part of collaborative suicide prevention plan.

Application of the Nursing Process

Background Assessment Data

Assessment of the older individual may follow the same framework used for all adults but with consideration of the possible biological, psychological, sociocultural, and sexual changes that occur in the normal aging process described previously in this chapter. In no other area of nursing is it more important for nurses to practice holistic nursing than with older patients. Older adults are likely to have multiple physical problems that contribute to problems in other areas of their lives, and these components cannot be addressed as separate entities. Nursing care of older adults is a multifaceted, challenging process because of the multiple changes occurring at this time in the life cycle and the way in which each change affects every aspect of the individual.

Several considerations are unique to assessment of older populations. Assessment of the older person's thought processes is a primary responsibility. Knowledge about the presence and extent of disorientation or confusion will influence the way in which the nurse approaches care.

Information about sensory capabilities is also extremely important. Because hearing loss is common, the nurse should lower the pitch of the voice when addressing the older person and speak clearly. Looking directly into the face of the older person when talking facilitates communication. Questions that require a declarative sentence in response should be asked; in this way, the nurse is able to assess the client's ability to use words correctly. Visual acuity can be determined by assessing adaptation to the dark, color matching, and the perception of color contrast. Knowledge about these aspects of sensory functioning is essential in the development of an effective care plan.

The nurse should be familiar with the normal physical changes associated with the aging process. Examples of some of these changes include that older clients may have:

- Less effective response to changes in environmental temperature, resulting in hypothermia
- Decreases in oxygen use and the amount of blood pumped by the heart, resulting in cerebral anoxia or hypoxia
- Skeletal muscle wasting and weakness, resulting in difficulty in physical mobility
- Limited cough and laryngeal reflexes, resulting in risk of aspiration
- Demineralization of bones, resulting in spontaneous fracturing
- Decrease in gastrointestinal motility, resulting in constipation
- Decrease in the ability to interpret painful stimuli, resulting in risk of injury

Common psychosocial changes associated with aging include the following:

- Prolonged, maladaptive grief, resulting in depression
- Physical changes, resulting in disturbed body image
- Changes in status, resulting in loss of self-worth

This list is by no means exhaustive. Nurses should consider many other alterations in their assessment of older patients. Knowledge of the older patient's functional capabilities is essential for determining their physiological, psychological, and sociological needs. Age alone does not preclude the occurrence of all these changes. The aging process progresses at a wide range of variance, and each client must be assessed as a unique individual.

Diagnosis and Outcome Identification

Virtually any nursing diagnosis may be applicable to the aging patient, depending on individual needs for assistance. Based on normal changes that occur in older adults, the following nursing diagnoses may be considered.

Physiologically related diagnoses include:

- Risk for trauma related to confusion, disorientation, muscular weakness, spontaneous fractures, falls

- Hypothermia related to loss of adipose tissue under the skin, evidenced by increased sensitivity to cold and body temperature below 98.6°F
- Decreased cardiac output related to decreased myocardial efficiency secondary to age-related changes, evidenced by decreased tolerance for activity and decline in energy reserve
- Ineffective breathing pattern related to increase in fibrous tissue and loss of elasticity in lung tissue, evidenced by dyspnea and activity intolerance
- Risk for aspiration related to diminished cough and laryngeal reflexes
- Impaired physical mobility related to muscular wasting and weakness, evidenced by need for assistance in ambulation
- Imbalanced nutrition, less than body requirements, related to inefficient absorption from gastrointestinal tract, difficulty chewing and swallowing, anorexia, difficulty in feeding self, evidenced by wasting syndrome, anemia, weight loss
- Constipation related to decreased motility; inadequate diet; insufficient activity or exercise, evidenced by decreased bowel sounds; hard, formed stools; or straining at stool
- Stress urinary incontinence related to degenerative changes in pelvic muscles and structural supports associated with increased age, evidenced by reported or observed dribbling with increased abdominal pressure or urinary frequency
- Urinary retention related to prostatic enlargement, evidenced by bladder distention, frequent voiding of small amounts, dribbling, or overflow incontinence
- Disturbed sensory perception related to age-related alterations in sensory transmission, evidenced by decreased visual acuity, hearing loss, diminished sensitivity to taste and smell, or increased touch threshold. (This diagnosis has been retired by NANDA International [NANDA-I] but retained in this text because of its appropriateness to the specific behaviors described.)
- Insomnia related to age-related cognitive decline, decrease in ability to sleep ("sleep decay"), or medications, evidenced by interrupted sleep, early awakening, or falling asleep during the day
- Chronic pain related to degenerative changes in joints, evidenced by verbalization of pain or hesitation to use weight-bearing joints
- Self-care deficit (specify) related to weakness, confusion, or disorientation, evidenced by inability to feed self, maintain hygiene, dress/groom self, or toilet self without assistance
- Risk for impaired skin integrity related to alterations in nutritional state, circulation, sensation, or mobility

Psychosocially related diagnoses include:

- Disturbed thought processes related to age-related changes that result in cerebral anoxia, evidenced by short-term memory loss, confusion, or disorientation
- Maladaptive grieving related to bereavement overload, evidenced by symptoms of depression
- Risk for suicide related to depressed mood and feelings of low self-worth
- Powerlessness related to lifestyle of helplessness and dependency on others, evidenced by depressed mood, apathy, or verbal expressions of having no control or influence over life situation
- Low self-esteem related to loss of preretirement status, evidenced by verbalization of negative feelings about self and life
- Fear related to nursing home placement, evidenced by symptoms of severe anxiety and statements such as "Nursing homes are places to go to die"
- Disturbed body image related to age-related changes in skin, hair, and fat distribution, evidenced by verbalization of negative feelings about body
- Ineffective sexuality pattern related to pain associated with vaginal dryness, evidenced by reported dissatisfaction with decrease in frequency of sexual intercourse
- Sexual dysfunction related to medications (e.g., antihypertensives) evidenced by inability to achieve an erection
- Social isolation related to total dependence on others, evidenced by expression of inadequacy in or absence of significant purpose in life
- Risk for trauma (elder abuse) related to caregiver role strain
- Caregiver role strain related to severity and duration of the care receiver's illness; lack of respite and recreation for the caregiver, evidenced by feelings of stress in relationship with care receiver; feelings of depression and anger; or family conflict around issues of providing care

Outcome Criteria

The following criteria may be used for measurement of outcomes in the care of the older patient. The patient:

- Has not experienced injury.
- Maintains reality orientation consistent with cognitive level of functioning.

- Manages self-care with assistance.
- Expresses positive feelings about self, past accomplishments, and hope for the future.
- Compensates adaptively for diminished sensory perception.

Caregivers:

- Can problem solve effectively regarding care of the elderly patient.
- Demonstrate adaptive coping strategies for dealing with stress of caregiver role.
- Openly express feelings.
- Express desire to join a support group of other caregivers.

Planning and Implementation

In Table 24–2, selected nursing diagnoses are presented for the older patient. Outcome criteria are included along with appropriate nursing interventions and rationale for each.

Reminiscence therapy is especially helpful with older patients. This therapeutic intervention is highlighted in Box 24–2.

Evaluation

Reassessment is conducted to determine whether the nursing actions have been successful in achieving the objectives of care. Evaluation of the nursing actions for the older patient may be facilitated by gathering information using the following types of questions. Has the patient:

- Remained free from injury from falls, burns, or other vulnerabilities?
- Maintained reality orientation for optimal cognitive functioning?
- Distinguished between reality-based and non-reality-based thinking?
- Accomplished self-care activities independently for optimal level of functioning?
- Sought assistance for aspects of self-care that cannot be perform independently?
- Expressed positive feelings about self?
- Reminisced about accomplishments that have occurred in life?
- Expressed some hope for the future?
- Used eyeglasses or a hearing aid, if needed, to compensate for sensory deficits?
- Consistently looked others in the face to facilitate hearing?
- Used helpful aids, such as signs identifying various rooms, to help maintain orientation?

Have the caregivers:

- Verbalized the means to provide a safe environment for the patient?
- Verbalized strategies for reality orientation, if needed?
- Worked through problems and made decisions regarding care of the older patient?
- Included the older family member in the decision-making process, if appropriate?
- Demonstrated adaptive coping strategies for dealing with the strain of long-term caregiving?
- Been open and honest in expression of feelings?
- Verbalized community resources to which they can go for assistance with their caregiving responsibilities?
- Joined a support group?

Summary and Key Points

- Care of the aging individual presents one of the greatest challenges for nursing.
- The growing population of individuals age 65 and older suggests that the trend will progress well into the 21st century.
- A growing number of seniors are living independently in residential communities designed specifically for senior citizens.
- America is a youth-oriented society and, as such, older adults may be at risk for being stigmatized.
- In some cultures, older adults are revered and hold a special place of honor within the society, but in highly industrialized countries such as the United States, status declines with the decrease in productivity and participation in the mainstream of society.
- Individuals experience many changes as they age. Physical changes occur in virtually every body system.
- Psychologically, there may be age-related memory deficiencies, particularly for recent events.
- Intellectual functioning does not decline with age, but length of time required for learning increases.
- Aging individuals experience many losses, potentially leading to bereavement overload. They are vulnerable to depression and to feelings of low self-worth.
- The older population, especially those older than age 85, represents a disproportionately high percentage of individuals who die by suicide.

Text continued on page 694

Table 24–2 | CARE PLAN FOR THE ELDERLY PATIENT

NURSING DIAGNOSIS: RISK FOR PHYSICAL TRAUMA

RELATED TO: Confusion, disorientation, muscular weakness, spontaneous fractures, falls

OUTCOME CRITERIA	NURSING INTERVENTIONS	RATIONALE
Short-Term Goals ■ Patient will call for assistance when ambulating or carrying out other activities. ■ Patient will not experience injury. **Long-Term Goal** ■ Patient will not experience injury.	1. The following measures may be instituted: a. Arrange furniture and other items in the room to accommodate the patient's disabilities. b. Store frequently used items within easy access. c. Keep bed in unelevated position. Pad side rails and headboard if patient has history of seizures. Keep bed rails up when the patient is in bed (if permitted by institutional policy). d. Assign room near nurses' station; observe frequently. e. Assist the patient with ambulation. f. Keep a dim light on at night. g. Frequently orient the patient to place, time, and situation.	1. Patient safety is a priority.

NURSING DIAGNOSIS: DISTURBED THOUGHT PROCESSES

RELATED TO: Age-related changes that result in cerebral anoxia

EVIDENCED BY: Short-term memory loss, confusion, or disorientation

OUTCOME CRITERIA	NURSING INTERVENTIONS	RATIONALE
Short-Term Goal ■ Patient will accept explanations of inaccurate interpretations of the environment within (time to be determined based on patient condition). **Long-Term Goal** ■ Patient will interpret the environment accurately and maintain reality orientation to the best of their cognitive ability.	1. Frequently orient the patient to reality. Use clocks and calendars with large numbers that are easy to read. Notes and large, bold signs may be useful as reminders. Allow the patient to have personal belongings.	1. To help maintain orientation and aid in memory and recognition.
	2. Keep explanations simple. Use face-to-face interaction. Speak slowly, and do not shout.	2. To facilitate comprehension. Shouting may create discomfort and, in some instances, provoke anger.
	3. Discourage rumination of delusional thinking. Talk about real events and real people.	3. Rumination promotes disorientation. Reality orientation increases sense of self-worth and personal dignity.
	4. Monitor for medication side effects.	4. Physiological changes in the elderly can alter the body's response to certain medications. Toxic effects may intensify altered thought processes.

Continued

Table 24–2 | CARE PLAN FOR THE ELDERLY PATIENT—cont'd

NURSING DIAGNOSIS: SELF-CARE DEFICIT (SPECIFY)

RELATED TO: Weakness, disorientation, confusion, or memory deficits

EVIDENCED BY: Inability to fulfill activities of daily living (ADLs)

OUTCOME CRITERIA	NURSING INTERVENTIONS	RATIONALE
Short-Term Goal ■ Patient will participate in ADLs with assistance from caregiver. **Long-Term Goals** ■ Patient will accomplish ADLs to the best of their ability. ■ Unfulfilled needs will be met by caregivers.	1. Provide a simple, structured environment: a. Identify self-care deficits and provide assistance as required. Promote independent actions as able. b. Allow plenty of time for the patient to perform tasks. c. Provide guidance and support for independent actions by talking the patient through the task one step at a time. d. Provide a structured schedule of activities that does not change from day to day. e. ADLs should follow home routine as closely as possible. f. Allow consistency in assignment of daily caregivers.	1. To minimize confusion.

NURSING DIAGNOSIS: CAREGIVER ROLE STRAIN

RELATED TO: Severity and duration of the care receiver's illness; lack of respite and recreation for the caregiver

EVIDENCED BY: Feelings of stress in relationship with care receiver; feelings of depression and anger; family conflict around issues of providing care

OUTCOME CRITERIA	NURSING INTERVENTIONS	RATIONALE
Short-Term Goal ■ Caregivers will verbalize understanding of ways to facilitate the caregiver role. **Long-Term Goal** ■ Caregivers will achieve effective problem-solving skills and develop adaptive coping mechanisms to regain equilibrium.	1. Assess prospective caregivers' ability to anticipate and fulfill the patient's unmet needs. Provide information to assist caregivers with this responsibility. Ensure that caregivers are aware of available community support systems from which they can seek assistance when required. Examples include adult day-care centers, housekeeping and homemaker services, respite care services, or a local chapter of the Alzheimer's Association. This organization sponsors a nationwide 24-hour hotline to provide information and link families who need assistance with nearby chapters and affiliates. The hotline number is 800-272-3900.	1. Caregivers require relief from the pressures and strain of providing 24-hour care for their loved one. Studies have shown that elder abuse arises out of caregiving situations that place overwhelming stress on the caregivers.

Table 24–2 | CARE PLAN FOR THE ELDERLY PATIENT—cont'd

OUTCOME CRITERIA	NURSING INTERVENTIONS	RATIONALE
	2. Encourage caregivers to express feelings, particularly anger.	2. Release of these emotions can serve to prevent psychopathology, such as depression or psychophysiological disorders, from occurring.
	3. Encourage participation in support groups composed of members with similar life situations.	3. Hearing others who are experiencing the same problems discuss ways in which they have coped may help caregivers to adopt more adaptive strategies. Individuals with similar life experiences provide empathy and support for each other.

NURSING DIAGNOSIS: LOW SELF-ESTEEM
RELATED TO: Loss of preretirement status; early stages of cognitive decline
EVIDENCED BY: Verbalization of negative feelings about self and life

OUTCOME CRITERIA	NURSING INTERVENTIONS	RATIONALE
Short-Term Goal ■ Patient will verbalize positive aspects of self and past accomplishments.	1. Encourage the patient to express honest feelings in relation to loss of prior status. Acknowledge pain of loss. Support the patient through the process of grieving.	1. Patient may be fixed in anger stage of grieving process, which is turned inward on the self, resulting in diminished self-esteem.
Long-Term Goal ■ Patient will participate in group activities to experience a feeling of enjoyment and accomplishment (as much as possible).	2. If lapses in memory are occurring, devise methods for assisting the patient with memory deficit. Examples: a. Name sign on door identifying the patient's room. b. Identifying sign on outside of dining room door. c. Identifying sign on outside of restroom door. d. Large clock, with oversized numbers and hands, appropriately placed. e. Large calendar, indicating one day at a time, with month, day, and year in bold print. f. Printed, structured daily schedule, with one copy for the patient and one posted on unit wall. g. "News board" on unit wall where current news of national and local interest may be posted.	2. These aids may assist the patient to function more independently, thereby increasing self-esteem.

Continued

Table 24–2 | CARE PLAN FOR THE ELDERLY PATIENT—cont'd

OUTCOME CRITERIA	NURSING INTERVENTIONS	RATIONALE
	3. Encourage the patient's attempts to communicate. If verbalizations are not understandable, express to the patient what you think they intended to say. It may be necessary to reorient the patient frequently.	3. The ability to communicate effectively with others may enhance self-esteem.
	4. Encourage reminiscence and discussion of life review (see Box 24–2). Sharing picture albums, if possible, is especially good. Also discuss present-day events.	4. Reminiscence and life review help the patient resume progression through the grief process associated with disappointing life events and increase self-esteem as successes are reviewed.
	5. Encourage participation in group activities. May need to accompany the patient at first, so that they feel secure that the group members will be accepting, regardless of limitations in verbal communication.	5. Positive feedback from group members will increase self-esteem.
	6. Encourage the patient to be as independent as possible in self-care activities. Provide written schedule of tasks to be performed. Provide assistance in areas where the patient is unable to perform tasks independently.	6. The ability to perform independently preserves self-esteem.

NURSING DIAGNOSIS: DISTURBED SENSORY PERCEPTION

RELATED TO: Age-related alterations in sensory transmission

EVIDENCED BY: Decreased visual acuity, hearing loss, diminished sensitivity to taste and smell, and increased touch threshold

OUTCOME CRITERIA	NURSING INTERVENTIONS*	RATIONALE
Short-Term Goal ■ Patient will not experience injury due to diminished sensory perception. **Long-Term Goals** ■ Patient will attain optimal level of sensory stimulation. ■ Patient will not experience injury due to diminished sensory perception.	1. The following nursing strategies are indicated: a. Provide meaningful sensory stimulation to all special senses through conversation, touch, music, or pleasant smells. b. Encourage wearing of glasses, hearing aids, prostheses, and other adaptive devices. c. Use bright, contrasting colors in the environment. d. Provide large-print reading materials, such as books, clocks, calendars, and educational materials. e. Maintain room lighting that distinguishes day from night and that is free of shadows and glare.	1. Patient safety is a priority.

Table 24–2 | CARE PLAN FOR THE ELDERLY PATIENT—cont'd

OUTCOME CRITERIA	NURSING INTERVENTIONS*	RATIONALE
	f. Teach the patient to scan the environment to locate objects. g. Help the patient to locate food on plate using "clock" system and describe food if the patient is unable to visualize; assist with feeding as needed. h. Arrange physical environment to maximize functional vision. i. Place personal items and call light within the patient's field of vision. j. Teach the patient to watch the person who is speaking. k. Reinforce wearing of hearing aid; if the patient does not have an aid, may consider a communication device (e.g., amplifier). l. Communicate clearly, distinctly, and slowly, using a low-pitched voice and facing the patient; avoid overarticulation. m. Remove as much unnecessary background noise as possible. n. Do not use slang or extraneous words. o. As speaker, position self at eye level and no farther than 6 feet away. p. Get the patient's attention before speaking. q. Avoid speaking directly into the patient's ear. If the patient does not understand what is being said, rephrase the statement rather than simply repeating it. r. Help the patient select foods from the menu that will ensure discrimination between various tastes and smells. s. Ensure that food has been properly cooled so that the patient with diminished pain threshold is not burned. t. Ensure that bath or shower water is appropriate temperature. u. Use backrubs and massage as therapeutic touch to stimulate sensory receptors.	

*The interventions for this nursing diagnosis were adapted from Rogers-Seidl, F. F. (1997). *Geriatric nursing care plans* (2nd ed). Mosby-Year Book.

BOX 24–2 Reminiscence Therapy and Life Review With Older Adults

Studies have indicated that *reminiscence*, or thinking about the past and reflecting on it, may promote better mental health in old age. *Life review* is related to reminiscence but differs from it in that it is a more guided or directed cognitive process that constructs a history or story in an autobiographical way.

Older individuals who spend time thinking about the past experience an increase in self-esteem and are less likely to suffer depression. Some psychologists believe that life review may help some people adjust to memories of an unhappy past. Others view reminiscence and life review as ways to bolster feelings of well-being, particularly in older people who can no longer remain active.

Reminiscence therapy can take place on a one-to-one basis or in a group setting. In reminiscence groups, older individuals share significant past events with peers. The nurse leader facilitates the discussion of topics that deal with specific life transitions, such as childhood, adolescence, marriage, childbearing, grandparenthood, and retirement. Members share both positive and negative aspects, including personal feelings, about these life-cycle events.

Reminiscence on a one-to-one basis can provide a way for the older individual to work through unresolved issues from the past. Painful issues may be too difficult to discuss in a group setting. As the individual reviews their life process, the nurse can validate feelings and help the older patient to come to terms with painful issues that may have been long suppressed. This process is necessary if the older individual is to maintain (or attain) a sense of positive identity and self-esteem and ultimately achieve the goal of ego integrity, as described by Erikson (1963).

A number of creative measures can be used to facilitate life review with the older individual. Having the patient keep a journal for sharing may be a way to stimulate discussion (as well as provide a permanent record of past events for significant others). Pets, music, and special foods have a way of provoking memories from the patient's past. Photographs of family members and past significant events are an excellent way of guiding the older patient through an autobiographical review.

Care must be taken in the life review to assist clients to work through unresolved issues. Anxiety, guilt, depression, and despair may result if the individual is unable to work through the problems and accept them. Life review can work in a negative way if the individual comes to believe that their life was meaningless. However, it can be a positive experience for the person who can take pride in past accomplishments and feel satisfied with life, resulting in a sense of serenity and inner peace in the older adult.

- Neurocognitive disorders, depression, and anxiety are the most frequent causes of psychopathology in older adults. Anxiety disorders are the second most common. Sleep disorders and substance use disorders are also common.
- The need for sexual expression in the older population is often misunderstood within our society. Although many physical changes occur at this time of life that alter people's sexuality, if they have reasonably good health and a willing partner, sexual activity can continue well past the 70s for most people.
- Retirement has both social and economic implications for older individuals. Society often equates an individual's status with occupation, and loss of employment may result in the need for adjustment in the standard of living because retirement income may be reduced by 20% to 40% of preretirement earnings.
- Less than 4% of the population age 65 and older live in nursing homes, with a higher percentage among those age 85 and older. A profile of the typical nursing home resident is a white woman about 80 years old, widowed, with multiple chronic health conditions. Much stigma is attached to what some still call "rest homes" or "old age homes," and many older adults still equate them with a place to go to die.
- The strain of the caregiver role has become a major dilemma in our society. Elder abuse is sometimes inflicted by caregivers for whom the role has become overwhelming and intolerable. Assistance for family caregivers, who are providing care for their loved ones on a 24-hour basis, is an essential part of the care plan. Home health care, respite care, support groups, and financial assistance are needed to ease the burden of this role strain.
- Caring for older individuals requires a special kind of inner strength and compassion. The poem that follows conveys a vital message for nurses.

What Do You See, Nurse?

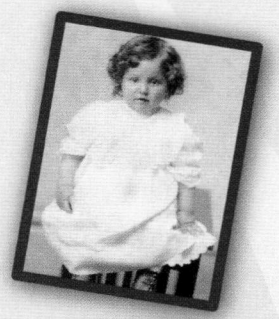

What do you see, nurse, what do you see?
What are you thinking when you look at me?
A crabbed old woman, not very wise.
Uncertain of habit, with faraway eyes.
Who dribbles her food and makes no reply
When you say in a loud voice, "I do wish you'd try."
Who seems not to notice the things that you do
And forever is losing a stocking or shoe.
Who unresisting or not, lets you do as you will
With bathing and feeding, the long day to fill.
Is that what you're thinking, is that what you see?
Then open your eyes, you're not looking at me.
I'll tell you who I am as I sit there so still.
As I move at your bidding, as I eat at your will.
I'm a small child of ten with a father and a mother,
Brothers and sisters who love one another.

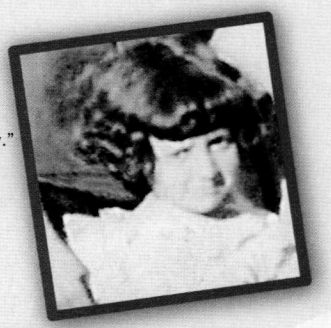

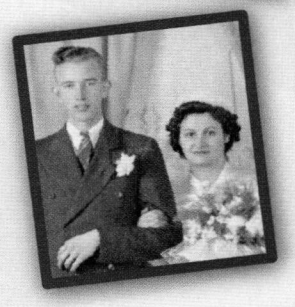

A young girl at sixteen with wings on her feet
Dreaming that soon now a lover she'll meet.
A bride soon at twenty—my heart gives a leap
Remembering the vows that I promised to keep.
At twenty-five, now, I have young of my own
Who need me to build a secure happy home.
A woman of thirty, my young now grow fast
Bound to each other with ties that should last.

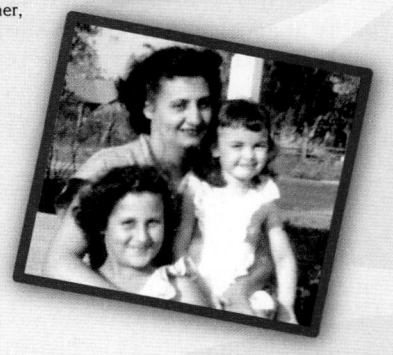

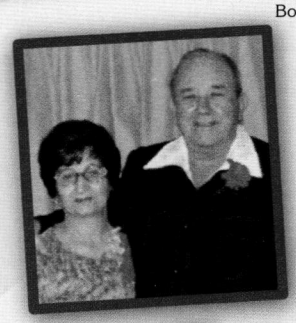

At forty my young will now soon be gone,
But my man stays beside me to see I don't mourn.
At fifty once more babies play round my knee.
Again we know children, my loved one and me.

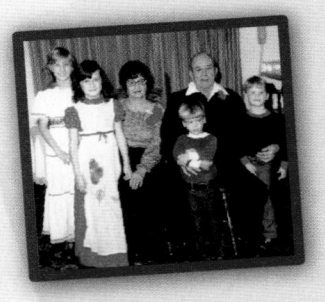

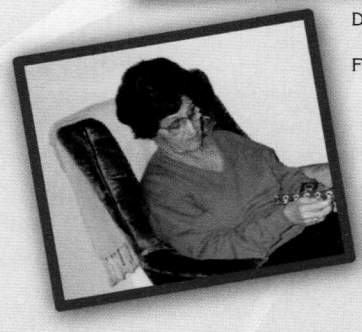

Dark days are upon me, my husband is dead.
I look at the future, I shudder with dread.
For my young are all busy rearing young of their own.
And I think of the years and the love I have known.

I'm an old woman now and nature is cruel.
Tis her jest to make old age look like a fool.
The body it crumbles, grace and vigor depart.
There is now just a stone where I once had a heart.
But inside this old carcass a young girl still dwells.
And now and again my battered heart swells.

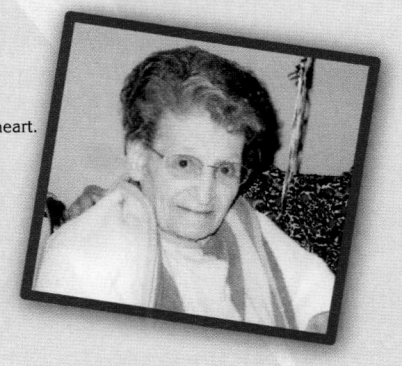

I remember the joys, I remember the pain.
And I'm loving and living life all over again.
I think of the years all too few—gone so fast.
And accept the stark fact that nothing can last.
So open your eyes, nurse, open and see.
Not a crabbed old woman—look closer—SEE ME.

Author Unknown

Review Questions

Select the answer that is most appropriate for each of the following questions:

1. During the admission assessment for a 72-year-old male client the nurse notices an open sore on his arm. When she questions him about it, he says, "I scraped it on the fence two weeks ago. It's smaller than it was." Which of the following is the best interpretation of this finding?
   a. Lower testosterone levels in older adult men results in injury-prone skin.
   b. Confusion is common in older adults, so the client probably doesn't remember how long ago he sustained the injury.
   c. A diminished inflammatory response in older adults increases healing time.
   d. The supply of blood vessels to the skin increases with age and delays healing time.
2. What is the most appropriate way to communicate with an older client who is deaf in their right ear?
   a. Speak loudly into their left ear.
   b. Speak to the client from a position on their left side.
   c. Speak face-to-face in a high-pitched voice.
   d. Speak face-to-face in a low-pitched voice.
3. Which factor is most associated with mental health in older adults?
   a. Pureed foods and warm beverages
   b. Physical activity and socialization
   c. Moderate alcohol and lower calorie intake
   d. Living alone and adhering to antidepressant medications
4. In a group exercise class, Mr. B., a 79-year-old man with major depression, becomes tired and short of breath very quickly. This symptom is most likely due to which cause?
   a. Age-related changes in the cardiovascular system
   b. Anxiety
   c. The effects of pathological depression
   d. Medication the physician has prescribed for depression
5. The developmental task of transcendence suggests that mental health in older adulthood is contingent upon:
   a. Being able to ignore the stigmas associated with being old
   b. Developing the ability to be alone
   c. Transcending physical limitations imposed by age-related changes in the body
   d. Having a sense of meaning in life and a sense of satisfaction

Clinical Judgment Questions

6. A male client, age 79, is admitted to the psychiatric unit for depression. He has lost weight and become socially isolated. His wife died 5 years ago, and his son tells the nurse, "He did very well when Mom died. He didn't even cry." Which is the priority nursing diagnosis?
   a. Maladaptive grieving
   b. Imbalanced nutrition: less than body requirements
   c. Social isolation
   d. Risk for injury
7. A male client, age 79, is admitted to the psychiatric unit for depression. He has lost weight and has become socially isolated. His wife died 5 years ago, and his son tells the nurse, "He did very well when Mom died. He didn't even cry." Which is the priority nursing intervention?
   a. Take blood pressure once each shift.
   b. Ensure that the client attends group activities.
   c. Encourage the client to eat all of the food on his food tray.
   d. Encourage the client to talk about his wife's death.

8. A 75-year-old male client, who is taking a selective serotonin reuptake inhibitor (SSRI) for depression, reports to the nurse that he recently began having erectile dysfunction. Which is the most appropriate action by the nurse?
   a. Set clear boundaries that this is not an appropriate topic to discuss with the nurse.
   b. Instruct the client that this is a potential side effect of his medication and ask whether he would prefer to explore other treatment options.
   c. Educate the client that this is a normal age-related change and cannot be treated.
   d. Reinforce that this is a common symptom of depression and should subside after 4 to 6 weeks of antidepressant treatment.
9. An 80-year-old client says to the nurse, "I'm all alone now. My husband is gone. My best friend is gone. My daughter is busy with her work and family. I might as well just go, too." Which is the best response by the nurse?
   a. "Are you having thoughts of wanting to hurt yourself or take your own life?"
   b. "You have lots to live for, but we need to talk to your daughter about her priorities."
   c. "It's hard getting old."
   d. "Tell me about your family."
10. An older male client with depression says to the nurse, "I don't want to go to that crafts class. I'm too old to learn anything." Which of these is the most appropriate action by the nurse at this point?
   a. Tell the client that groups are mandatory and escort him by the hand.
   b. Pat the client on the shoulder and tell him "We all feel that way sometimes."
   c. Educate the client that people don't typically lose the ability to learn as they age and encourage him to express his thoughts and feelings associated with aging.
   d. Assess the client for suicide risk and warning signs.

IMPLICATIONS FOR EVIDENCE-BASED PRACTICE

Estebsari, F., Dastoorpoor, M., Khalifehkandi, Z. R., Nouri, A., Mostafaei, D., Hosseini, M., Esmaeili, R., & Aghababaeian, H. (2020). The concept of successful aging: A review article. *Current Aging Science, 13*(1), 4–10. https://doi.org/10.2174/1874609812666191023130117

DESCRIPTION OF THE STUDY: The authors sought to review the literature on successful aging to better explain this phenomenon. Twenty-seven articles met the quality criteria for inclusion in this review.

RESULTS OF THE STUDY: Definitions of successful aging covered a range of criteria depending on the article. The authors concluded that "successful aging" does not follow a universal standard and the concept depends on the cultural context of the community. The most common factors influencing successful aging were physical activity level, social interactions, and attitudes of the individual.

IMPLICATIONS FOR NURSING PRACTICE: The authors note that elderly people need information, support, and encouragement to be empowered for successful aging. Nurses can play a key role in providing education about these principles. Discussing with older adults regarding the importance of physical activity and social connection and assisting them to explore their personal attitudes about aging provides a framework for offering support and resources to promote successful aging.

TEST YOUR CLINICAL REASONING AND CLINICAL JUDGMENT SKILLS

Mrs. M, age 76, is seeing her primary physician for her regular 6-month physical examination. Mrs. M's husband died 2 years ago, at which time she sold her home in Kansas and came to live in California with her only child, a daughter. The daughter is married and has three children (one in college and two teenagers at home). The daughter reports that her mother is becoming increasingly withdrawn, stays in her room, and eats very little. She has lost 13 pounds since her last 6-month visit. The primary physician refers Mrs. M to a psychiatrist, who hospitalizes her for evaluation. He diagnoses Mrs. M with Major Depressive Disorder (MDD).

Mrs. M tells the nurse, "I didn't want to leave my home, but my daughter insisted. I would have been all right. I miss my friends and my church. Back home I drove my car everywhere. But there's too much traffic out here. They sold my car, and I have to depend on my daughter or grandkids to take me places. I hate being so dependent! I miss my husband so much. I just sit and think about him and our past life all the time. I don't have any interest in meeting new people. I want to go home!"

Mrs. M admits to having some thoughts of dying, although she denies feeling suicidal. She denies having a plan or means for taking her life. "I really don't want to die, but I just can't see much reason for living. My daughter and her family are so busy with their own lives. They don't need me—or even have time for me!"

Answer the following questions about Mrs. M:

1. What would be the *primary* nursing diagnosis for Mrs. M?
2. Formulate a short-term goal for Mrs. M.
3. From the assessment data, identify the major problem that may be a long-term focus of care for Mrs. M.

MOVIE CONNECTIONS

The Hiding Place (loss and grief, transcendence) ▪ *On Golden Pond* (dementia) ▪ *To Dance With the White Dog* (loss and grief) ▪ *5 Flights Up* (aging, resilience) ▪ *Still Alice* (Alzheimer's disease) ▪ *The Second Best Exotic Marigold Hotel* (aging, resilience) ▪ *A Man Called Ove* (depression, suicidal behavior) ▪ *The Truth* (aging) ▪ *Tea With the Dames* (reminiscence)

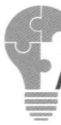

Go to **Davis Advantage** to complete your learning: strengthen understanding, apply your knowledge, and prepare for the Next Gen NCLEX®.

References

Administration on Aging. (2020). *2019 Profile of older Americans.* https://acl.gov/sites/default/files/Aging%20and%20Disability%20in%20America/2019ProfileOlderAmericans508.pdf

American Association of Colleges of Nursing. (2020). The future of the nursing workforce in the United States: Data, trends and implications. http://www.aacnnursing.org/News-Information/Nursing-Shortage-Resources

American Foundation for Suicide Prevention. (2021). *Suicide statistics.* https://afsp.org/suicide-statistics/

American Urology Association. (2019). *Benign prostatic hypertrophy.* https://www.urologyhealth.org/urologic-conditions/benign-prostatic-hyperplasia-(bph)

Blevins, N. H. (2021). *Presbycusis.* http://www.uptodate.com/contents/presbycusis

Boland, R., & Verduin, M. L. (2022). *Kaplan & Sadock's synopsis of psychiatry* (P. Ruiz, Ed.). (12th ed.). Wolters Kluwer.

Celano, C. M., & Huffman, J. C. (2011). Depression and cardiac disease: A review. *Cardiology in Review, 19,* 130–142.

Celano, C. M., Daunis, D. J., Lokko, H. N., Campbell, K. A., & Huffman, J. C. (2016). Anxiety disorders and cardiovascular disease. *Current Psychiatry Reports, 18*(11), 101. https://doi.org/10.1007/s11920-016-0739-5

Centers for Disease Control and Prevention. (2021). *Depression is not a normal part of growing older.* https://www.cdc.gov/aging/depression/

Dean, W. (2021). *Neuroendocrine theory of aging: Chapter 1.* http://warddeanmd.com/articles/neuroendocrine-theory-of-aging-chapter-1

Gillbard, A., & Leggatt-Cook, C. (2019). *Elder Abuse Prevention Unit: Year in review 2018–2019.* https://www.researchgate.net/publication/347515852_Year_in_Review_2018-19?channel=doi&linkId=5fe016a8299bf140882f8b5c&showFulltext=true

Galasko, D. R. (2017). The aging brain. In B. J. Sadock, V. A. Sadock, & P. Ruiz (Eds.), *Comprehensive textbook of psychiatry* (10th ed., pp. 3986–3995). Wolters Kluwer.

Issa, J. P. (2014). Aging and epigenetic drift: A vicious cycle. *Journal of Clinical Investigation, 124*(1), 24–29.

Jeste, D. V. (2017). Introduction to geriatric psychiatry. In B. J. Sadock, V. A. Sadock, & P. Ruiz (Eds.), *Comprehensive textbook of psychiatry* (10th ed., pp. 3947–3955). Wolters Kluwer.

Kern, M. L., & Friedman, H. S. (2008). Do conscientious individuals live longer? A quantitative review. *Health Psychology, 27*(5), 505–512. https://doi.org/10.1037/0278-6133.27.5.505

King, B. M., & Regan, P. (2013). *Human sexuality today* (8th ed.). Pearson Prentice Hall.

Lee, D. M., Nazroo, J., O'Connor, D. B., Blake, M., & Pendleton, N. (2016). Sexual health and well-being among older men and women in England: Findings from the English longitudinal study of ageing. *Archives of Sexual Behavior, 45*(1), 133–144. https://doi.org/10.1007/s10508-014-0465-1

Lehto, R. H., & Stein, K. I. (2009). Death anxiety: An analysis of an evolving concept. *Research and Theory for Nursing Practice, 23*(1), 23–41.

McCarthy, V. L., & Bockweg, M. (2012). The role of transcendence in a holistic view of successful aging: A concept analysis and model of transcendence in maturation and aging. *Journal of Holistic Nursing, 31*(2), 84–92. https://doi.org/10.1177/0898010112463492

McCarthy, V. L., Ling, J., & Carini, R. M. (2013). The role of self-transcendence: A missing variable in the pursuit of successful aging? *Research in Gerontological Nursing, 6*(3), 178–186.

McClatchey, I. S., & King, S. (2015). The impact of death education on fear of death and death Anxiety among human services students. *Omega (Westport), 71*(4), 343–361.

MedlinePlus. (2021). Aging changes in the senses. *Medical encyclopedia.* https://medlineplus.gov/ency/article/004013.htm

Missler M., Stroebe, M., Geurtsen, L., Mastenbroek, M., Chmoun, S., & van der Houwen, K. (2012). Exploring death anxiety among elderly people: A literature review and empirical investigation. *Omega (Westport), 64*(4), 357–379.

Myhre, J. W., Mehl, M. R., & Glisky, E. L. (2017). Cognitive benefits of online social networking for healthy older adults. *The Journals of Gerontology: Series B, 72*(5), 752–760. https://doi.org/10.1093/geronb/gbw025

National Center for Health Statistics. (2020). *Mortality in the United States: 2018.* https://www.cdc.gov/nchs/products/databriefs/db355.htm

National Crime Justice Reference Center. (2018). *Elder victimization fact sheet.* https://ovc.ojp.gov/sites/g/files/xyckuh226/files/ncvrw2018/info_flyers/fact_sheets/2018NCVRW_OlderAdults_508_QC.pdf

National Council on Aging. (2021). *Elder abuse facts.* https://www.ncoa.org/public-policy-action/elder-justice/elder-abuse-facts/

National Institutes of Health. (2021). *Aging changes in immunity.* https://www.nlm.nih.gov/medlineplus/ency/article/004008.htm

News Medical. (2014). *Transcendence is the best predictor of positive aging, study show.* https://www.news-medical.net/news/20140521/Transcendence-is-the-best-predictor-of-positive-aging-shows-study.aspx

Rodriguez, J. C., Dzierzewski, J. M., & Alessi, C. A. (2015). Sleep problems in the elderly. *Medical Clinics of North America, 99*(2), 431–439. https://doi.org/10.1016/j.mcna.2014.11.013

Rogers, K., Simic, P., & Guarente, L. P. (2020). *Aging: Life process.* http://www.britannica.com/science/aging-life-process

Shock, N. W. (2020). *Human aging: Physiology and sociology.* http://www.britannica.com/science/human-aging

Solway, E., Clark, S., Singer, D., Kirch, M., & Malani P. (2018). *Let's talk about sex, national poll on healthy aging.* Institute for Healthcare Policy and Innovation, University of Michigan.

Srivastava, S., & Das, R. C. (2013). Personality pathways of successful ageing. *Industrial Psychiatry Journal, 22*(1), 1–3. https://doi.org/10.4103/0972-6748.123584

Sullivan, S., & Ariss, A. A. (2018). Employment after retirement: A review and framework for future research. *Journal of Management, 45*(1), 262–284. https://doi.org/10.1177/0149206318810411

Sutin, A. R., Stephan, Y., & Terracciano, A. (2018). Facets of conscientiousness and risk of dementia. *Psychological Medicine, 48,* 974–982. https://doi.org/10.1017/S0033291717002306

Terracciano, A., Sanna, S., Uda, M., Deiana, B., Usala, G., Busonero, F., Maschio, A., Scally, M., Patriciu, N., Chen, W-M., Distel, M. A., Slagboom, E. P., Boomsma, D. I., Villafuerte, S., Śliwerska, E., Burmeister, M., Amin, N., Janssens, A. C. J. W., van Duijn, C. M., . . . Costa, P. T. (2010). Genome-wide association scan for five major dimensions of personality. *Molecular Psychiatry, 15*(6), 647656. https://doi.org/10.1038/mp.2008.113

Thomas, P. A. (2011). Trajectories of social engagement and limitations in late life. *Journal of Health and Social Behavior, 52*(4), 430–443. https://doi.org/10.1177/0022146511411922

Toossi, M., & Torpey, E. (2017). *Older workers: Labor force trends and career options.* https://www.bls.gov/careeroutlook/2017/article/older-workers.htm

Watanabe, K., Tanaka, E., Watanabe, T., Chen, W., Wu, B., Ito, S., Okumura, R., & Anme, T. (2016). Association between social relationships and cognitive function among the elderly. *Public Health Research, 6*(2), 59–63. https://doi.org/10.5923/j.phr.20160602.05

Westerhof, G. J., Whitbourne, S. K., & Freeman, J. P. (2012). The aging self in a cultural context: The relation of conceptions of aging to identity processes and self-esteem in the United States and the Netherlands. *Journals of Gerontology. Series B, Psychological Sciences and Social Sciences. 67*(1), 52–60. https://doi.org/10.1093/geronb/gbr075

World Health Organization. (2017). *Mental health of older adults.* https://www.who.int/en/news-room/fact-sheets/detail/mental-health-of-older-adults

World Health Organization. (2021). *Elder abuse.* https://www.who.int/news-room/fact-sheets/detail/elder-abuse

Classical References

Dilman, V. (1954). *Data regarding the origin of climacteric and the role of age-associated "perestroika" in the elevation of blood pressure, blood cholesterol levels, and body weight* [Unpublished master's thesis]. Leningrad.

Erikson, E. H. (1963). *Childhood and society* (2nd ed.). W. W. Norton.

Erikson, E. H., & Erikson, J. M. (1997). *The life cycle completed: Extended version with new chapters on the ninth stage of development.* W. W. Norton.

Kübler-Ross, E. (1969). *On death and dying.* Macmillan.

Masters, W. H., Johnson, V. E., & Kolodny, R. C. (1995). *Human sexuality* (5th ed.). Addison-Wesley Longman.

Roberts, C. M. (1991). *How did I get here so fast?* Warner Books.

Rogers-Seidl, F. F. (1997). *Geriatric nursing care plans* (2nd ed.). Mosby-Year Book.

Rowe, J. W., & Kahn, R. L. (1997). Successful aging. *Gerontology, 37*(4), 433–440.

25 Survivors of Abuse or Neglect

CORE CONCEPTS

Stress and Coping

Safety

Professionalism: Nursing process in the care of survivors of abuse or neglect

Clinical Judgment

CHAPTER OUTLINE

Objectives
Introduction
Predisposing Factors
Application of the Nursing Process
Treatment Modalities
Summary and Key Points
Review Questions
Clinical Judgment Questions
Implications for Evidence-Based Practice
Test Your Clinical Reasoning and Clinical Judgment Skills
Communication Exercises
Movie Connections

KEY TERMS

abuse
acquaintance rape
adverse childhood experiences (ACEs)
child abuse
child sexual abuse
compounded rape reaction
controlled response pattern
cycle of battering
date rape
emotional abuse
emotional neglect
expressed response pattern
forensic nursing
incest
intimate partner violence
marital rape
physical neglect
rape-trauma syndrome
safe houses or shelters
sexual assault
sexual exploitation of a child
silent rape reaction
statutory rape
trauma-informed care
retraumatization

OBJECTIVES

After reading this chapter, the student will be able to:

1. Describe epidemiological statistics associated with intimate partner violence, child abuse, and sexual assault.
2. Discuss characteristics of victims and victimizers.
3. Identify predisposing factors to abusive behaviors.
4. Describe physical and psychological effects on the survivors of intimate partner violence, child abuse, and sexual assault.
5. Identify nursing diagnoses, goals of care, and appropriate nursing interventions for care of survivors of intimate partner violence, child abuse, and sexual assault.
6. Evaluate nursing care of survivors of intimate partner violence, child abuse, and sexual assault.
7. Define the terms *forensic* and *forensic nursing*.
8. Discuss various modalities relevant to treatment of survivors of abuse.

Introduction

CORE CONCEPT

Abuse

The maltreatment of one person by another.

Abuse is a significant and frightening public health problem. The National Intimate Partner and Sexual Violence Survey (NISVS) (D'Inverno et al., 2019) found that during their lifetime, 1 in 4 women and 1 in 10 men experienced contact sexual violence, physical violence, and/or stalking by an intimate partner and reported at least one form of intimate partner violence (IPV). Commonly experienced IPV-related issues, reported by both women and men, included concern for safety, being fearful, injury, post-traumatic stress disorder (PTSD) symptoms, and needing help from law enforcement.

These forms of violence most often occur before the age of 25 for both men and women. Child abuse and related fatalities continue to be significant health concerns. It is well documented that **adverse childhood experiences (ACEs)** such as abuse and neglect can have a major impact on health and well-being throughout one's life. ACE studies have found that as the number of ACE events increases, so do risks for heart disease, asthma, diabetes, cancer, depression, anxiety, post-traumatic stress disorder (PTSD), disability, unemployment, sexually transmitted infections, and other health problems (Centers for Disease Control and Prevention [CDC], 2020a). The impact of trauma on physical, mental, emotional, and spiritual health is one of the primary reasons that nurses need to assess for trauma and provide trauma-informed care.

Child abuse includes physical or sexual abuse, psychological maltreatment, and neglect. Data from the U.S. Department of Health and Human Services (2021) identify that the majority of abused children (61%) are neglected, whereas a smaller percentage are physically abused (10.3%) or sexually abused (7.2%). Nationally, in 2019, an estimated 1,840 children died of abuse or neglect. Human trafficking, which includes sex trafficking is another form of child abuse that is a significant public health concern. Federal law defines human trafficking as

> a commercial sex act [that] is induced by force, fraud, or coercion, or in which the person induced to perform such act has not attained 18 years of age or, the recruitment, harboring, transportation, provision, or obtaining of a person for labor or services, through the use of force, fraud, or coercion for the purpose of subjection to involuntary servitude, peonage, debt bondage, or slavery. (U.S. Department of Education, 2013)

Prevalence statistics are difficult to compile, but sex trafficking of children has been reported in all 50 U.S. states, and traffickers have been known to prey on children as young as 9 years of age.

Elder abuse and neglect are also a significant problem. The CDC (2020b) estimates that 1 in 10 people over the age of 60 and living at home is a victim of physical or sexual abuse, neglect (the most common form of elder abuse), abandonment, and/or financial exploitation. *Institutional abuse* refers to elder adults who live in residential facilities and are victimized by any of the above-mentioned forms of abuse. There is general agreement that statistics underestimate the scope of the problem. Despite mandatory reporting laws in most states and the recent trend toward more reporting of abuse, adult protective services vary markedly from state to state. One study estimated that for every 1 case that came to the attention of these agencies, 24 had not been reported (National Center on Elder Abuse [NCEA], n.d.).

Abuse affects all populations equally. It occurs among all races, religions, economic classes, ages, and educational backgrounds. Many abusers were themselves victims of abuse as children.

Family violence is not a new problem; in fact, it is probably as old as humankind and has been documented as far back as biblical times. Child abuse became a mandatory reportable occurrence in the United States in 1968. Responsibility for the protection of elders from abuse rests primarily with the states. In 1987, Congress passed amendments to the Older Americans Act of 1965 that provide for state Area Agencies on Aging to assess the need for elder abuse prevention services. These events have made it possible for individuals who once felt powerless to stop the abuse against them to come forward and seek advice, support, and protection.

This chapter discusses intimate partner violence, child abuse (including neglect), and sexual assault. Elder abuse is discussed in Chapter 24, "The Aging Individual." Factors that predispose individuals to commit acts of abuse against others, as well as the physical and psychological effects on the survivors, are examined.

Nursing care of individuals who have experienced abusive behavior from others is presented within the context of the nursing process. Various treatment modalities are described.

Predisposing Factors

What predisposes individuals to be abusive? Although no one really knows for sure, several theories have been espoused. As researchers have sought to better understand aggression and violence, two distinct forms of aggression have been identified: *reactive* aggression, which is associated with impulsivity and is more common among people who have a history of being abused, and *proactive* aggression, which is initiated rather than provoked and is more common in psychopathy (Rosell & Siever, 2015). Most research is associated with reactive aggression, and the following is a brief discussion of current evidence associated with biological, psychological, and sociocultural influences.

Biological Theories

Neurophysiological Influences

Research demonstrates consistently that lower volume of the amygdala plays a role in aggression (Rosell & Siever, 2015). The amygdala, which is responsible for impulse control and affective processing, appears to be less well modulated in people with aggression, and responses to fear are reduced. The prefrontal cortex also has a primary role in aggression; smaller volumes of left-sided gray matter and greater right-sided volume have been noted in people with aggressive traits. Evidence has also demonstrated lowered connectivity between the amygdala and the prefrontal cortex as associated with increased aggression. The striatum, an area of the brain that plays a critical role in selection and inhibition of affective, cognitive, and motor responses, has been identified as dysfunctional in aggression (Rosell & Siever, 2015).

Biochemical Influences

Research suggests that serotonin may have both inhibitory and stimulating effects on aggressive behavior, depending on the brain region measured and specific receptors where it acts (Narvaes & Martins de Almeida, 2014). Catecholamines, gamma-aminobutyric acid (GABA), and glutamate are neurotransmitters that modulate the serotonin-influenced increase in aggression (Miczek et al., 2017). The role of testosterone, which has been classically associated with aggression, may be better understood as a complex interaction with other hormones such as serotonin and cortisol (Batrinos, 2012; Dreher et al., 2016). Research is ongoing to explore these mechanisms, their interactions in the brain, and the influence of environmental factors. An explanation of these biochemical influences on violent behavior is presented in Figure 25–1.

Genetic Influences

A recent study by Zhang-James and colleagues (2019) identified that at least 40 genes are associated with aggression, suggesting that the genetics underlying aggression are quite complex. It has also been demonstrated that stressful life events can influence some gene variants in the development of aggressive tendencies. The heritability of aggression is estimated at around 50%. Zhang and associates (2019) add to their findings that aggression in attention deficit-hyperactivity disorder (ADHD) and in adults with major depression share common DNA variants, and the lack of genetic correlations of either dataset with schizophrenia, bipolar disorder, autism, or PTSD suggests that for these disorders, aggression may arise from different causal factors. They conclude that future studies are needed to fully address the genetic bases of the comorbidity between aggression and psychiatric disorders.

Disorders of the Brain

Organic brain syndromes associated with various cerebral disorders have been implicated in the predisposition to aggressive and violent behavior. Brain tumors, particularly in the areas of the limbic system and the temporal lobes; trauma to the brain, resulting in cerebral changes; and diseases such as encephalitis (or medications that may affect this syndrome) and epilepsy, particularly temporal lobe epilepsy, have all been implicated.

Psychological Theories

Psychodynamic Theory

Psychodynamic theorists suggest that unmet needs for satisfaction and security result in an underdeveloped ego and a weak superego. It is thought that when frustration occurs, aggression and violence supply this individual with a dose of power and prestige that boosts the self-image and validates a significance to their life that is lacking. The immature ego cannot prevent dominant id behaviors from occurring, and the weak superego is unable to produce feelings of guilt.

Learning Theory

Children learn to behave by imitating their role models, which are usually their parents. Models are more likely to be imitated when they are perceived

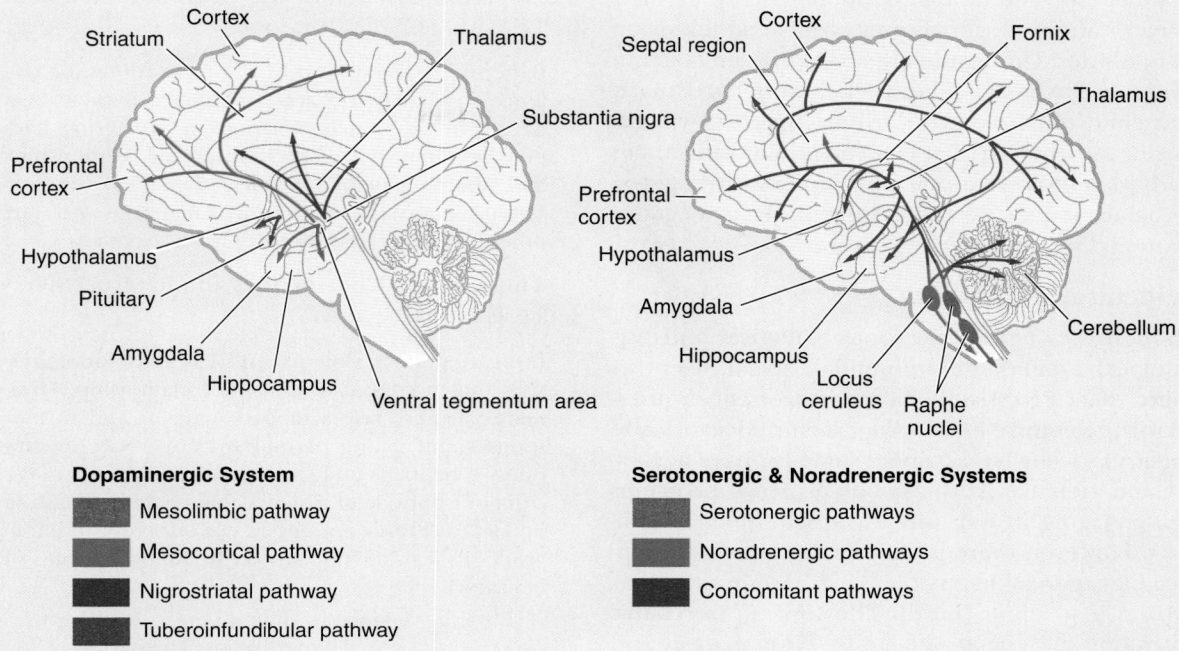

FIGURE 25–1 Neurobiology of violence.

NEUROTRANSMITTERS

Neurotransmitters that have been implicated in the etiology of aggression and violence include serotonin and increases in norepinephrine and dopamine.

ASSOCIATED AREAS OF THE BRAIN

- ***Limbic structures:*** Emotional alterations
- ***Prefrontal and frontal cortices:*** Modulation of social judgment
- ***Amygdala:*** Anxiety, rage, fear
- ***Hypothalamus:*** Stimulates sympathetic nervous system in "fight-or-flight" response
- ***Hippocampus:*** Learning and memory

MEDICATIONS USED TO MODULATE AGGRESSION

1. Studies have suggested that serotonin and selective serotonin reuptake inhibitors (SSRIs) may reduce or increase irritability and aggression depending on the brain region measured and specific receptors where it acts (Narvaes & Martins de Almeida, 2014). In turn, catecholamines, gamma-aminobutyric acid (GABA), and glutamate modulate those effects (Miczek et al., 2017).
2. Mood stabilizers that dampen limbic irritability may be important in reducing the susceptibility to react to provocation or threatening stimuli by overactivation of limbic system structures such as the amygdala (Rosell & Siever, 2015). Carbamazepine (Tegretol), phenytoin (Dilantin), and divalproex sodium (Depakote) have yielded positive results. Lithium has also been used effectively in violent individuals (Schatzberg et al., 2019).
3. Antiadrenergic agents such as beta blockers (e.g., propranolol) have been shown to reduce aggression in some individuals, presumably by dampening excessive noradrenergic activity (Schatzberg et al., 2019).

In their ability to modulate excessive dopaminergic activity, antipsychotics—both typical and atypical—have been helpful in the control of aggression and violence, particularly in individuals with comorbid psychosis.

as prestigious or influential or when the behavior is followed by positive reinforcement. Children may have an idealistic perception of their parents during the very early developmental stages but as they mature may begin to imitate the behavior patterns of their teachers, friends, and others. Individuals who were abused as children or who witnessed domestic violence as children are more likely to manifest reactive aggression as adults (Rosell & Siever, 2015).

Adults and children alike model many of their behaviors after individuals they observe on television and in movies. Unfortunately, modeling can result in maladaptive as well as adaptive behavior, particularly when children view heroes triumphing over villains by using violence. It is also possible that individuals who have a biological predisposition toward aggressive behavior may be more susceptible to negative role modeling.

Sociocultural Theories

Although they agree that some biological and psychological aspects are influential, social scientists believe that aggressive behavior is primarily a product of one's culture and social structure. Historically, American society has accepted some forms of aggression and violence as the means to solve problems (e.g., engaging in war, physical disciplining of children). However, there is widespread general acceptance that aggression or violence in certain situations is wrong (e.g., child abuse). The concept of relative deprivation has been shown to have a profound effect on collective violence within a society. Poverty, prolonged unemployment, family breakdown, emotional distress, lack of access to resources, and exposure to violence in the community and in the family have all been linked to increases in aggression (American Psychological Association, 2021; Espolage et al., 2013).

Application of the Nursing Process

Background Assessment Data

Data related to **intimate partner violence**, child abuse and neglect, and sexual assault are presented in this section. Characteristics of both victim and abuser are addressed. This information may be used as background knowledge in designing plans of care for these patients.

Intimate Partner Violence

CORE CONCEPT

Battering

A pattern of coercive control founded on and supported by physical and/or sexual violence or threat of violence of an intimate partner.

Various terms are used to describe the pattern of violence between intimate partners, including intimate partner violence (IPV), domestic violence, and battering.

Tracy (2019) adds to the definition of battering as follows:

> Battering is also known by the term "domestic violence" and refers to acts of violence between two parties in an intimate relationship. Battering happens in heterosexual and homosexual relationships and either a male or a female can be the batterer or victim. Battering may occur in a marriage or in any other form of relationship.

The CDC (2020c) defines intimate partner violence as follows:

> Intimate partner violence (IPV) is abuse or aggression that occurs in a romantic relationship. "Intimate partner" refers to both current and former spouses and dating partners. IPV can vary in how often it happens and how severe it is. It can range from one episode of violence that could have lasting impact to chronic and severe episodes over multiple years. IPV can include any of the following types of behavior:
>
> **Physical violence** is when a person hurts or tries to hurt a partner by hitting, kicking, or using another type of physical force.
>
> **Sexual violence** is forcing or attempting to force a partner to take part in a sex act, sexual touching, or a non-physical sexual event (e.g., sexting) when the partner does not or cannot consent.
>
> **Stalking** is a pattern of repeated, unwanted attention and contact by a partner that causes fear or concern for one's own safety or the safety of someone close to the victim.
>
> **Psychological aggression** is the use of verbal and non-verbal communication with the intent to harm another person mentally or emotionally and/or to exert control over another person.

The U.S. Department of Justice (2018) defines *intimate partner violence* as such:

> Intimate partner violence (IPV), often called domestic violence, is generally described as abuse within the context of an intimate partner relationship, where one partner asserts power and control over the other. While legal definitions vary by state, IPV can include physical, sexual, and psychological abuse, as well as economic coercion.

Physical abuse between domestic partners may be known as spouse abuse, domestic or family violence, wife or husband battering, or IPV. According to the NISVS (D'Inverno et al., 2019), an estimated 47% of men and women will be victims of psychological aggression in their lifetime; 32% of women will be victims of physical violence; 16% of women and 7% of men will be victims of contact sexual violence;

and 9% of all homicides are committed by an intimate partner. Many victimizations are not reported to the police, and the main reason given for not reporting is that it was "considered a personal matter."

Profile of the Victim

For the purposes of this chapter, women are identified as the victim (and men as the victimizer) because the largest percentage of victims are women and most of the available data speak specifically about female victims. It should be noted, however, that men may also be victims and victimized in similar ways. Likewise, female perpetrators of IPV may share many of the characteristics that are commonly identified as the profile of male victimizers.

Battered women represent all age, racial, religious, cultural, educational, and socioeconomic groups. They may be married or single, non-working, hourly workers, or business executives. Many women who are battered have low self-esteem, commonly adhere to feminine sex-role stereotypes, and often accept the blame for the batterer's actions. Feelings of guilt, anger, fear, and shame are common. They may be isolated from family and support systems.

Some women in violent relationships grew up in abusive homes and may have left those homes and gotten married at a very young age in order to escape the abuse. The battered woman views her relationship as male dominant, and as the battering continues, her ability to see the options available to her and to make decisions concerning her life (and possibly those of her children) decreases. The phenomenon of *learned helplessness* may be applied to the woman's progressing inability to act on her own behalf. Learned helplessness occurs when an individual comes to understand that regardless of their behavior, the outcome is unpredictable and usually undesirable.

Profile of the Victimizer

Batterers are typically characterized as persons with low self-esteem. Pathologically jealous, they present a "dual personality," one to the partner and one to the rest of the world. They are often under a great deal of stress but have limited ability to cope with the stress. The typical abuser is very possessive and perceives his partner as a possession. He becomes threatened when she shows any sign of independence or attempts to share herself and her time with others. Small children are often ignored by the abuser; however, they may also become the targets of abuse as they grow older, particularly if they attempt to protect their mother from abuse. The abuser also may use threats of taking the children away as a tactic of emotional abuse.

The perpetrator of abuse typically wages a continuous campaign of degradation against his partner. He uses insults and humiliations and strives to keep her isolated from others and totally dependent on him. He demands to know where she is at every moment, and when she tells him, he challenges her honesty. He achieves power and control through intimidation.

The Cycle of Battering

In her classic studies of battered women and their relationships, Walker (1979) identified a cycle of predictable behaviors that is repeated over time. These behaviors can be divided into three distinct phases that vary in time and intensity both within the same relationship and among different couples. Figure 25–2 depicts a graphic representation of the **cycle of battering.**

Phase I. The Tension-Building Phase During this phase, the woman senses that the man's tolerance for frustration is declining. He becomes angry with little provocation but, after lashing out at her, may be quick to apologize. The woman may become very nurturing and compliant, anticipating his every whim in an effort to prevent his anger from escalating. She may just try to stay out of his way.

Minor battering incidents may occur during this phase, and in a desperate effort to avoid more serious confrontations, the woman accepts the abuse as legitimately directed toward her. She denies her anger and rationalizes his behavior (e.g., "I need to do better," "He's under so much stress at work," "It's the alcohol—if only he didn't drink"). She

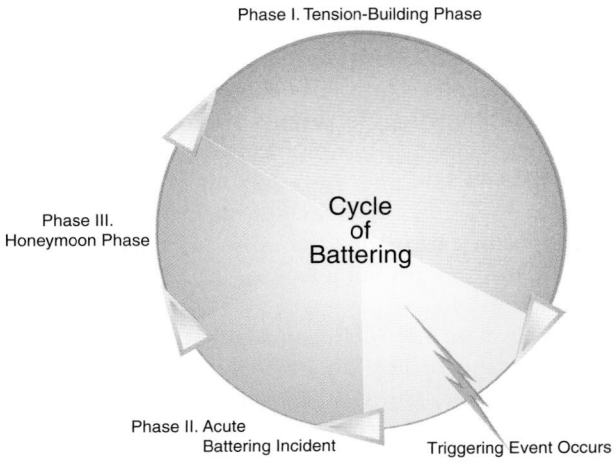

FIGURE 25–2 The cycle of battering.

assumes the guilt for the abuse, even reasoning that perhaps she *did* deserve the abuse, just as her aggressor suggests.

The minor battering incidents continue, and the tension mounts as the woman waits for the impending explosion. The abuser begins to fear that his partner will leave him. His jealousy and possessiveness increase, and he uses threats and brutality to keep her in his captivity. Battering incidents become more intense, after which the woman becomes less and less psychologically capable of restoring equilibrium. She withdraws from him, which he misinterprets as rejection, further escalating his anger toward her. Phase I may last from a few weeks to many months or even years.

Phase II. The Acute Battering Incident This phase is the most violent and the shortest, usually lasting up to 24 hours. It most often begins with the batterer justifying his behavior to himself. By the end of the incident, however, he cannot understand what has happened, only that in his rage he has lost control over his behavior.

This incident may begin with the batterer wanting to "just teach her a lesson." In some instances, the woman may intentionally provoke the behavior. Having come to a point in phase I in which the tension is unbearable, long-term battered women know that once the acute phase is behind them, things will be better.

During phase II, women feel their only option is to find a safe place to hide from the batterer. Many women can describe the violence in great detail, almost as if dissociation from their bodies had occurred. The batterer generally minimizes the severity of the abuse. Help is usually sought only in the event of severe injury or if the woman fears for her life or the lives of her children.

Phase III. Calm, Loving, Respite ("Honeymoon") Phase In this phase, the batterer becomes extremely loving, kind, and contrite. He promises that the abuse will never recur and begs her forgiveness. He is afraid she will leave him and uses every bit of charm he can muster to ensure this does not happen. He believes he now can control his behavior, and because now that he has "taught her a lesson," he believes she will not "act up" again.

He plays on her feelings of guilt, and she desperately wants to believe him. She wants to believe that he *can* change, and that she will no longer have to suffer abuse. During this phase, the woman relives her original dream of ideal love and chooses to believe that *this* is what her partner is *really* like.

This loving phase becomes the focus of the woman's perception of the relationship. She bases her reason for remaining in the relationship on this "magical" ideal phase and hopes against hope that the previous phases will not be repeated. This hope is evident even in those women who have lived through a number of horrendous cycles.

Although phase III usually lasts somewhere between the lengths of time associated with phases I and II, it can be so short as to almost pass undetected. In most instances, the cycle soon begins again with renewed tensions and minor battering incidents. In an effort to "steal" a few precious moments of the phase III kind of loving, the battered woman becomes a collaborator in her own abusive lifestyle. Victim and batterer become locked together in an intense, symbiotic relationship.

Why Do They Stay?

Probably the most common response that battered women give for staying is that they fear for their life and/or the lives of their children. As the battering progresses, the man gains power and control through intimidation and instilling fear with threats such as, "I'll kill you and the kids if you try to leave." Challenged by these threats and dealing with her low self-esteem and sense of powerlessness, the woman sees no way out. In fact, she may try to leave only to return when confronted by her partner and the psychological power he holds over her.

Women have been known to stay in an abusive relationship for many reasons, some of which include the following:

- ***Fear of retaliation:*** A woman may have been threatened with murder of herself and her children. Other perpetrator tactics include sleep deprivation, blackmail, and murdering pets. Each act may be used to increase fear of retaliation. In the lesbian, gay, bisexual, and transgender community, fear of being outed is sometimes used to manipulate the victim.
- ***Fear of losing custody of the children:*** Women are sometimes threatened by the spouse that they will take away the children. There may have been attempts to convince the woman that she is an unfit mother.
- ***Physical or financial dependence:*** Victims may fear that they are unable to care for themselves without the victimizer. Victims with disabilities may also be physically dependent on the victimizer for caregiving and financial support.

- ***Lack of a support network:*** The victim may be under pressure from family members to stay in the marriage and try to work things out. In addition, the victimizer may have isolated the victim from family and friends.
- ***Fears about what others will think:*** Cultural or religious convictions against divorce may dictate trying to save the marriage at all costs. The dual personality exhibited by perpetrators of abuse may lead the victim to think no one will believe them.
- ***Hopefulness:*** The victim remembers good times and love in the relationship and has hope that her partner will change his behavior and they can have good times again.
- ***Lack of attention to the danger:*** Low self-esteem may contribute to victim's belief that they are responsible for being abused and if they just change their behavior the abuse will stop. The honeymoon phase of the battering cycle provides reinforcement for the belief that it won't happen again. The dissociation that accompanies PTSD, may contribute to the victim's numbness or lack of awareness of the reality of the situation. Or, as Leslie Morgan Steiner poignantly states in a TED Talk (cited by Dockterman, 2014):

> Why did I stay? I didn't know he was abusing me. Even though he held those loaded guns to my head, pushed me down stairs, threatened to kill our dog, pulled the key out of the car ignition as I drove down the highway, poured coffee grinds on my head as I dressed for a job interview, I never once thought of myself as a battered wife. Instead I was a very strong woman in love with a deeply troubled man, and I was the only person on earth who could help [him] face his demons.

It is important to recognize that 75% of domestic violence-related homicides occur upon separation and there is a 75% increase of violence for at least two years after the victim leaves an abusive relationship (Center for Relationship Abuse Awareness, 2021). Clients should be empowered to make that decision and provided with resources and referrals to maximize their safety if they choose to leave, but nonetheless, the decision must be theirs to make.

Child Abuse

Erik Erikson (1963) stated, "The worst sin is the mutilation of a child's spirit." Children are vulnerable and relatively powerless, and the effects of maltreatment are deep and long lasting. Child maltreatment typically includes physical or emotional injury, physical or emotional neglect, or sexual acts inflicted upon a child by a caregiver. The federal Child Abuse Prevention and Treatment Act (CAPTA) identifies a minimum set of acts or behaviors that characterize child abuse or neglect. These include "any recent act or failure to act on the part of a parent or caretaker which results in death, serious physical or emotional harm, sexual abuse or exploitation, or an act or failure to act which presents an imminent risk of serious harm." In addition, "a child shall be considered a victim of 'child abuse and neglect' and of 'sexual abuse' if the child is identified, by a State or local agency employee of the State or locality involved, as being a victim of sex trafficking or a victim of severe forms of trafficking in persons" (Child Welfare Information Gateway [CWIG], 2019). States may use these definitions as foundations on which to establish state legislation.

Physical Abuse

Physical abuse of a child includes "any nonaccidental physical injury (ranging from minor bruises to severe fractures or death) as a result of punching, beating, kicking, biting, shaking, throwing, stabbing, choking, hitting (with a hand, stick, strap, or other object), burning, or otherwise harming a child, that is inflicted by a parent, caregiver, or other person who has responsibility for the child" (CWIG, 2019). Maltreatment is considered whether or not the caretaker intended to cause harm or even if the injury resulted from discipline or physical punishment. The most obvious way to detect it is by outward physical signs. However, behavioral indicators also may be evident.

Physical abuse may include any of the following (CWIG, 2019). The child:

- Has unexplained burns, bites, bruises, broken bones, or black eyes.
- Has fading bruises or other marks noticeable after an absence from school.
- Seems frightened of the parents and protests or cries when it is time to go home.
- Shrinks at the approach of adults.
- Reports injury by a parent or another adult caregiver.
- Abuses animals or pets.

Physical abuse may be suspected when the parent or other adult caregiver (CWIG, 2019):

- Offers conflicting, unconvincing, or no explanation for the child's injury.
- Describes the child as "evil" or in some other very negative way.

- Uses harsh, physical discipline with the child.
- Has a history of abuse as a child.
- Has a history of abusing animals or pets.

Emotional Abuse

Emotional abuse involves a pattern of behavior on the part of the parent or caretaker that results in serious impairment of the child's social, emotional, or intellectual functioning. Examples of emotional injury include belittling or rejecting the child, ignoring the child, blaming the child for things over which the child has no control, isolating the child from normal social experiences, and using harsh and inconsistent discipline. Emotional maltreatment may be indicated if the child (CWIG, 2019):

- Shows extremes in behavior, such as overly compliant or demanding behavior, extreme passivity, or aggression.
- Is either inappropriately adult (e.g., parenting other children) or inappropriately infantile (e.g., frequently rocking or head-banging).
- Is delayed in physical or emotional development.
- Has attempted suicide.
- Reports a lack of attachment to the parent.

Emotional abuse may be suspected when the parent or other adult caregiver (CWIG, 2019):

- Constantly blames, belittles, or berates the child.
- Is unconcerned about the child and refuses to consider offers of help for the child's problems.
- Overtly rejects the child.

Physical and Emotional Neglect

CORE CONCEPT

Neglect

Physical neglect of a child includes refusal of or delay in seeking health care, abandonment, expulsion from the home or refusal to allow a runaway to return home, and inadequate supervision.

Emotional neglect refers to a chronic failure by the parent or caretaker to provide the child with the hope, love, and support necessary for the development of a sound, healthy personality.

The possibility of neglect may be considered when the child (CWIG, 2019):

- Is frequently absent from school.
- Begs or steals food or money.
- Lacks needed medical or dental care, immunizations, or glasses.
- Is consistently dirty and has severe body odor.
- Lacks sufficient clothing for the weather.
- Abuses alcohol or other drugs.
- States that there is no one at home to provide care.

The possibility of neglect may be considered when the parent or other adult caregiver (CWIG, 2019):

- Appears to be indifferent to the child.
- Seems apathetic or depressed.
- Behaves irrationally or in a bizarre manner.
- Is abusing alcohol or other drugs.

Sexual Abuse of a Child

Various definitions of **child sexual abuse** are available in the literature. CAPTA defines *sexual abuse* as:

> Employment, use, persuasion, inducement, enticement, or coercion of any child to engage in, or assist any other person to engage in, any sexually explicit conduct or simulation of such conduct for the purpose of producing any visual depiction of such conduct; or the rape, and in cases of caretaker or inter-familial relationships, statutory rape, molestation, prostitution, or other form of sexual exploitation of children, or incest with children. (CWIG, 2019)

Included in the definition is **sexual exploitation of a child,** in which a child is induced or coerced into engaging in sexually explicit conduct for the purpose of promoting any performance, and child sexual abuse, in which a child is being used for the sexual pleasure of an adult (parent or caretaker) or any other person.

Child sexual abuse may be considered a possibility when the child (CWIG, 2019):

- Has difficulty walking or sitting.
- Suddenly refuses to change for gym or to participate in physical activities.
- Reports nightmares or bedwetting.
- Experiences a sudden change in appetite.
- Demonstrates bizarre, sophisticated, or unusual sexual knowledge or behavior.
- Becomes pregnant or contracts a venereal disease, particularly if under age 14.
- Runs away.
- Reports sexual abuse by a parent or another adult caregiver.
- Attaches very quickly to strangers or new adults in their environment.

Sexual abuse may be considered a possibility when the parent or other adult caregiver (CWIG, 2019;

Rape, Abuse & Incest National Network [RAINN], 2021):

- Is unduly protective of the child or severely limits the child's contact with other children, especially of the opposite sex.
- Is secretive and isolated.
- Does not respect boundaries or listen when someone tells them "no."
- Engages in touching that a child or child's parents/guardians have indicated is unwanted.
- Tries to be a child's friend rather than filling an adult role in the child's life.
- Does not seem to have age-appropriate relationships makes up excuses to be alone with the child.
- Expresses unusual interest in child's sexual development, such as commenting on sexual characteristics or sexualizing normal behaviors.
- Gives a child gifts without occasion or reason.

Characteristics of the Abuser

A number of factors have been associated with adults who abuse or neglect their children. Parents who abuse their children were often victims of abuse in their own early lives and have impaired attachment with their child. Substance use disorders also increase the risk for child abuse and neglect. Additional characteristics that may be associated with abusive parents include the following:

- Repetitive shaming, blaming, or teasing in humiliating ways
- Withholding care or demanding that a child earn the ability to have their basic needs met
- Lacking adaptive coping strategies; angers easily; has difficulty trusting others
- Expecting the child to be perfect or showing favoritism to siblings; exclusion or neglect
- Overt or veiled threats of physical injury

Flaherty and Stirling (2010) identify a number of characteristics of children, their parents, and the environment that increase a child's risk for maltreatment. For example, when a child has a chronic illness, disabilities, or behavioral problems and when parents are ill equipped to parent related to their own emotional, behavioral, or substance-use issues, children may become the victim of abuse or neglect. Environmental factors including social isolation, poverty, IPV, and a nonbiologically related male living in the household have also been linked to increased risk. Although individual risk factors don't necessarily predict that a child is in danger, when multiple factors coexist, the risk of child abuse increases.

CORE CONCEPT

Incest

Sexual contact or sexual exploitation of close relatives or participants who are related to each other by a kinship bond that is regarded as a prohibition to sexual relations (e.g., caretakers, stepparents, stepsiblings).

The Incestuous Relationship

A great deal of attention has been given to the study of father-daughter incest but, by definition, incest includes sexual relations between any close relative, including stepparents, adoptive relatives, and siblings. Communication between the parents is typically ineffective and the perpetrator is domineering, impulsive, and physically abusive. The other parent, most often the mother, is passive and submissive even though she may suspect that incest is occurring. At times, this passive response is born from fear of the perpetrator or denial that the child is being harmed. Families in which a single mother invites another man to live in the home or remarries increases the risk for incest by the boyfriend or stepparent (Henderson, 2021).

The child victim may experience a variety of physical ailments connected to this abuse in addition to the conflicting emotions of fear, anger, and helplessness at odds with the desire for a loving relationship with the perpetrator. Often psychological symptoms are the most apparent signs of this child's conflict, including self-harming behaviors, school-related problems, withdrawal or aggression, nightmares, depression, eating disorders, PTSD, and overt sexual behavior with peers.

The incest is typically ongoing and, although the oldest daughter in a family is most vulnerable to becoming a participant in father-daughter incest, some fathers form sequential relationships with several daughters. If incest has been reported with one daughter, it should be suspected with all the daughters.

The Adult Survivor of Incest

Several common characteristics have been identified in adults who have experienced incest as children. Basic to these characteristics is a fundamental lack of trust resulting from an unsatisfactory parent-child relationship, which contributes to low self-esteem and a poor sense of identity. Children of incest often feel trapped, for they have been admonished not to talk about the experience and may be afraid, or even fear for their lives, if they are exposed. If they do muster the courage to report the incest, particularly to the mother, they sometimes are not believed. This is confusing to the child, who is then left with a sense of self-doubt, inability to trust their own feelings, and inability to trust either parent for protection. The child develops feelings of guilt with the realization over the years that the parents are using the child in an attempt to solve their own problems.

Adult survivors of incest who decide to come forward with their stories usually are estranged from nuclear family members. They may be blamed by family members for disclosing the "family secret" and often are accused of overreacting to the incest. Frequently, the estrangement becomes permanent when family members continue to deny the behavior and the individual is accused of lying. In recent years, a number of celebrities have come forward with stories of their childhood sexual abuse. Some have chosen to make the disclosure only after the death of their parents. Revelation of these past activities can be one way of contributing to the healing process for which incest survivors so desperately strive.

Many studies support that there are a multitude of long-term physical and mental consequences in adult survivors of child sexual abuse (Collin-Vézina et al., 2013; Irish et al., 2010) including irritable bowel syndrome, chronic pain, cardiovascular symptoms, obesity, depression, anxiety, eating disorders, and substance use disorders.

The conflicts associated with pain (either physical or emotional) and sexual pleasure experienced by children who are sexually abused are often repeated in adult relationships. Betrayal of trust and violations of personal boundaries in childhood contribute to trust issues and interpersonal difficulties in adulthood that increase risk for re-victimization (Cashmore & Shackel, 2013). Women who were abused as children often enter into relationships with men who abuse them physically, sexually, or emotionally. In addition, studies have shown that childhood sexual abuse victims are at greater risk for instability in adult relationships, more sexual partners and sexual problems, and greater negativity toward partners (Cashmore & Shackel, 2013). The researchers add that, although most childhood abuse victims do not become sex offenders in adulthood, of those who are known to be offenders, as many as 75% report childhood sexual victimization.

Sexual Violence

Sexual violence is often equated with rape, but that is only one type of sexual assault. It is important for nurses and other health-care providers to be aware that sexual violence includes any act of sexual coercion, including penetration, unwanted sexual contact, and noncontact unwanted sexual experiences (CDC, 2020a). All of these experiences can result in trauma, and assessment for history of these events is foundational to providing trauma-informed care. Read about Diana's experiences in this chapter's "Real People, Real Stories" feature.

Sexual assault is any type of sexual act in which an individual is threatened or coerced to submit against their will. Rape, a type of sexual assault, occurs over a broad spectrum of experiences ranging from the surprise attack by a stranger to insistence on sexual intercourse by an acquaintance or spouse. Regardless of the defining source, one common theme always emerges: rape is an act of aggression, not one of passion.

CORE CONCEPT

Rape

The expression of power and dominance by means of sexual violence, most commonly by men over women, although men may also be rape victims.

Acquaintance rape (called **date rape** if the encounter is a social engagement agreed to by the victim) is a term applied to situations in which the rapist is acquainted with the victim. They may be out on a first date, may have been dating for a number of months, or merely may be acquaintances or schoolmates. College campuses are the location for a staggering number of these types of rapes, a great many of which go unreported. An increasing number of colleges and universities are establishing programs for rape prevention and counseling for survivors of rape.

Marital rape, which has been recognized only in recent years as a legal category, is the case in which a spouse may be held liable for sexual abuse directed at a marital partner against that person's will. Historically, with societal acceptance of the concept of women as marital property, the legal definition of rape held an exemption within the marriage relationship. In 1993, marital rape became a crime in all 50 states, under at least one section of the sexual offenses code. In many states, there are no exemptions granted to husbands, but in a significant number of states, there

Real People, Real Stories: Diana's Journey

This individual wished to remain anonymous. Diana is not her real name. Her story is a poignant lesson in the various ways that one can be victimized, the long-term impact of such experiences on one's sense of self-esteem and personal safety, and the importance of nurses' understanding of trauma-informed care.

Karyn: I appreciate your willingness to talk about your experiences. If at any time you become uncomfortable discussing these events we don't need to continue. All right?

Diana: I've had a lot of therapy, and I feel like it's important to tell and keep on telling so that, hopefully, something good will come out of it. When I was 6 years old, I had a crush on my best friend's brother. He was 12 years old, and when he started giving me attention, I thought he liked me; until he took me into a room, took my clothes off, and was touching me. He wanted me to take his clothes off, and I said no. I told my mom, and she intervened with his parents, but when a second incident occurred, my mother stopped me from going to my friend's house. I felt a lot of shame and embarrassment, but I never really talked about my feelings. For a long time, I carried around the belief that it was somehow my fault because I had a crush on him. I found out later that there were several other children who he molested and that his mom had implied they were "making it up."

When I was around 8 years old, I was in a toy store and a man came up from behind me and rubbed my rear end under my dress. I ran to get my father, but the perpetrator ran out of the store, and my parents decided not to call the police. They felt like I'd been scared enough. As an adult, I can understand that. But as a child, I felt like someone did a bad thing to me, and I wished that someone had defended me. As a middle schooler, one of the neighborhood girls wanted to play Truth or Dare. I think she did this with a lot of girls. The dare was to take off my clothes after which she put her hands on me. I said no but felt paralyzed with fear when she touched me anyway. She was a year older, and again, I remember feeling powerless and thinking I didn't know what to do.

In another incident in middle school, one of the boys jumped out in front of me in the school hallway and grabbed my breasts. A teacher saw him do it and was going to send him to the principal's office, but the boy looked scared and I somehow thought it must be my job to protect him . . . or maybe I was trying to act like it was no big deal, so I told the teacher to just let him go. I didn't want to get the boy in trouble, and I was so embarrassed and humiliated, I just wanted it to go away. Part of me wishes the teacher hadn't listened to me, though. I don't think that boy had any idea how much he hurt me and how awful it was.

Karyn: I think that may be a common reaction by girls or women; even though someone has offended against us, we don't want to hurt them in return. And it minimizes the fact that we have been hurt.

Diana: Yes, and my parents were knee deep in the Catholic training that if someone hurts you, you should just walk away or turn the other cheek. That influenced my own thinking, that you don't defend yourself—you should just walk away and avoid conflict. But that's a misunderstanding of the "turn the other cheek" teaching, which is really about showing forgiveness when people demonstrate remorse. It doesn't mean letting people hurt you without consequences. Around this time, I started putting on a lot of weight. I've always felt it was, in part, a reaction meant to keep people at a distance, so they couldn't hurt me.

Karyn: I've heard other people share a similar coping or defense mechanism; doing something simply to keep people away. Was that effective?

Diana: It only added to my self-esteem issues. I struggled with the question of why these things were happening to me. I felt like I must be doing something wrong. As a teenager, I struggled with anxiety and depression, and I was sent to a psychiatrist, but it wasn't helpful. Then when I moved to New York City for college, there were a couple of incidents on the subway. One was a frail-looking elderly man who stuck his hand between my legs, and when I turned around to confront him, he was laughing at me. I felt very powerless. I thought about kicking him, but, again, I didn't want to injure this shriveled-up old man, and I also didn't know if he had a knife, a gun. . . . So there's the fear, the powerlessness, and the anger that someone was touching me and laughing at me, and I could do nothing. I wondered if I was sending out some vibe—i.e., it must be my fault. My friend told me I needed to learn how to put on an angry face and carry an umbrella to better defend myself. I knew I had anxiety and self-esteem issues, and that's when I decided I needed therapy.

Karyn: That took a lot of courage to identify what you needed to do to take some control back. What has been most helpful about that process?

Diana: I explored the underpinnings of my self-esteem issues and identified coping skills, but nonetheless, as an adult many things can trigger the feelings of vulnerability, anxiety, and low self-esteem: news stories about rape or abuse, or times when women or children are demeaned in the media, especially from people manipulating their power or authority. That brings up a lot of "stuff" for me. When my counselor challenged me to identify what was in the way of being able to set all this stuff aside—that's when I had the insight that I just wanted to know something good could come out of all this pain.

Continued

Real People, Real Stories: Diana's Journey—cont'd

Karyn: One of the things you've told me is that you've been able to teach your daughters how to respond in such situations.

Diana: Yes, that was important and felt like a victory. I'm better able to identify potentially harmful situations. I've taught them to listen to that inner voice, where you get that "bad feeling" you can get that warns you when you're in a situation that may require defending or protecting yourself, and I taught my daughters how to be prepared. I've told them that if someone tries to touch them, it's okay to fight back. Its okay to tell me, school officials, tell anyone, and to keep telling until someone believes them and responds. I want them to know that it's safe to talk to me about their feelings and that they are not powerless.

Karyn: I think that's an important message for health-care professionals as well: to listen, to not brush off someone's experiences but rather to explore the events, thoughts, and feelings and identify coping strategies.

Diana: Yes, I think sometimes adults who thought it was less traumatizing for me to walk away or try to forget about it thought they were helping, but that's not the answer. Even now, after all these years, I wasn't sure if you would think my story was important enough to tell, I mean, to some people, it might not seem so bad. I wasn't raped, it wasn't a family member—but it still left me feeling awful.

Karyn: I think your story is very important to tell. You are taking the opportunity to teach others that victimization can occur in a variety of ways, that it can have long-term effects on self-esteem, and that it is important to find ways to regain a sense of control and self-worth. I really appreciate your sharing this. What do you think are the most important things that nurses need to know about your and others' experience with victimization and trauma?

Diana: First of all, that 40 years later, those incidents still affect me. I saw a picture of the boy who molested me on a friend's Facebook page, and I felt sick and afraid all over again. And I beat myself up for still letting it get to me. Nurses need to know that even events that happened years ago can influence one's emotional responses in the present.

Second, the idea of "getting closure," even so many years later, is a misnomer. Certain things can trigger those memories and anxieties, and when they come back, all you can do is drag them out and talk about them again and again and again. It's another version of "you tell and you tell and you don't stop telling" until you remember that you survived it, that it wasn't your fault, and that you don't need to feel ashamed or embarrassed or humiliated (even if part of you still does).

Third, I want nurses to know that they are the front lines, and no matter what clinical area they practice in, a history of sexual trauma or abuse can affect how their patients experience and receive health care. I had a lot of trouble as an adult fertility patient, having to dress and undress so many times and deal with so many invasive procedures. It was important to tell my health-care providers why my heart was pounding, why I seemed so nervous, why I hated mammographies and regular GYN exams a little bit more than the average woman. . . . That, as always, a nurse's ability to care and offer compassion can make the biggest difference, and it all begins with trust and helping your patient to "tell." And I wanted to say thank you for the times those nurses held my hand, and squeezed tight, and told me that I would be okay.

are still some exemptions providing immunity to husbands from being prosecuted for rape. In 13 states (Connecticut, Idaho, Iowa, Maryland, Michigan, Mississippi, Nevada, New Hampshire, Ohio, Oklahoma, Rhode Island, South Carolina, and Washington), spousal rape laws either explicitly require the use of force or provide immunity if one spouse is incapacitated, effectively providing immunity if the spouse was drugged, unconscious, or otherwise unable to give consent (Stanley, 2020). In all states where husbands can be prosecuted, the criteria for proving marital rape are very stringent.

Statutory rape is defined as unlawful intercourse between a person who is over the age of consent with a person who is under the age of consent. In the United States, legal age of consent varies from state to state, ranging from age 16 to 18 (Barnett, 2016). An adult who has intercourse with a person who is under the age of consent can be arrested for statutory rape, even if the interaction occurred between consenting individuals.

Profile of the Victimizer

It is difficult to profile a rapist because rapists comprise a heterogenous group and are not distinguished by looks or intelligence. The majority of rapes are premeditated, and some behavioral characteristics that have been identified as associated with premeditation include the perpetrator seeking out a victim who appears to be vulnerable (capable of being overpowered or in an opportunistic position such as being alone or isolated from others); alcohol and drugs such as Rohypnol (flunitrazepam) may serve the purpose of increasing victim vulnerability. The perpetrator may also violate or ignore others' rights in a way that gives them information about whether a potential victim is passive or tolerant of those behaviors. But again, although these behaviors might be observed more commonly, they do not clearly define the complete profile of these perpetrators.

In 80% of the cases of rape and sexual assault among college-age females, the offender was known to the victim, and 1 in 10 rapes involved the use of a weapon (U.S. Bureau of Justice Statistics, 2014). Although statistics such as these help to describe aspects of the problem, understanding the essence of what defines the perpetrator of aggression and violence is the subject of ongoing research.

The Victim

Rape can occur at any age; however, the most recent statistics suggest that the highest-risk age-group is females younger than age 34 and that most victims tend to have lower incomes and have never married (RAINN, 2021). Rapes are less likely to be reported than other violent crimes. Most sexual assault victims are single women, and the attack frequently occurs in or close to the victim's own neighborhood.

Although women are at highest risk for being victims of rape perpetrated by males, males may also be victimized by women or other men. Rape survivors who present themselves for care shortly after the crime has occurred likely may be experiencing an overwhelming sense of violation and helplessness that began with the powerlessness and intimidation experienced during the rape. Burgess and Holmström (1974), who developed the classical definition of what has been described as **rape-trauma syndrome,** identified two emotional patterns of response that may occur within hours after a rape and with which health-care workers may be confronted in the emergency department or rape crisis center. In the **expressed response pattern,** the survivor expresses feelings of fear, anger, and anxiety through such behaviors as crying, sobbing, restlessness, and tension. In the **controlled response pattern,** the feelings are masked or hidden, and a calm, composed, or subdued affect is seen.

The following manifestations may be evident in the days and weeks after the attack (Burgess, 2010):

- Contusions and abrasions on various parts of the body
- Headaches, fatigue, sleep pattern disturbances
- Stomach pains, nausea, and vomiting
- Vaginal discharge and itching, burning upon urination, rectal bleeding, and pain
- Rage, humiliation, embarrassment, desire for revenge, and self-blame
- Fear of physical violence and death

The long-term effects of sexual assault depend largely on the individual's ego strength, social support system, and the way the person was treated as a victim (Burgess, 2010). Various long-term effects include increased restlessness, dreams and nightmares, and phobias (particularly those having to do with sexual interaction). Some women report that it takes years to get over the experience; they describe a sense of vulnerability and a loss of control over their own lives during this period. They feel defiled and unable to wash themselves clean, and some women are unable to remain living alone in their home or apartment.

Some survivors develop a **compounded rape reaction** in which additional symptoms such as depression and suicide, substance abuse, and even psychotic behaviors may be noted (Burgess, 2010). Another variation has been called the **silent rape reaction** in which the survivor tells no one about the assault. Anxiety is suppressed and the emotional burden may become overwhelming. The unresolved sexual trauma may not be revealed until the woman is forced to face another sexual crisis in her life that reactivates the previously unresolved feelings.

Diagnosis and Outcome Identification

Nursing diagnoses are formulated from the data gathered during the assessment phase and with background knowledge regarding predisposing factors to the situation. Some common nursing diagnoses for survivors of abuse include the following:

- Rape-trauma syndrome related to sexual assault evidenced by verbalizations of the attack; bruises and lacerations over areas of body; severe anxiety
- Powerlessness related to cycle of battering evidenced by verbalizations of abuse; bruises and lacerations over areas of body; fear for her safety and that of her children; verbalizations of no way to get out of the relationship
- Risk for delayed development related to abusive family situation

Outcome Criteria

The following criteria may be used to measure outcomes in the care of abuse survivors. The patient who has been sexually assaulted:

- Is no longer experiencing panic anxiety.
- Demonstrates a degree of trust in the primary nurse.
- Has received immediate attention to physical injuries.
- Has initiated behaviors consistent with the grief response.

The patient who has been physically battered:

- Has received immediate attention to physical injuries.
- Verbalizes assurance of their immediate safety.
- Discusses life situation with primary nurse.
- Can verbalize choices from which they may receive assistance.

The child who has been abused:

- Has received immediate attention to physical injuries.
- Demonstrates trust in primary nurse by discussing abuse through the use of play therapy.
- Is demonstrating a decrease in regressive behaviors.

Planning and Implementation

Table 25–1 provides a plan of care for the patient who is a survivor of abuse. Nursing diagnoses are presented, along with outcome criteria, appropriate nursing interventions, and rationales for each.

Evaluation

Evaluation of nursing actions to assist survivors of abuse must be considered on both a short- and a long-term basis.

Short-term evaluation may be facilitated by gathering information using the following types of questions:

- Has the individual been reassured of their safety?
- Is this evidenced by a decrease in panic anxiety?
- Have wounds been properly cared for and provision made for follow-up care?
- Have emotional needs been attended to?
- Has trust been established with at least one person to whom the patient feels comfortable relating the abusive incident?
- Have available support systems been identified and notified?
- Have options for immediate circumstances been presented?

Long-term evaluation may be conducted by health-care workers who have an ongoing professional relationship with the individual long after the immediate crisis has passed.

- Is the individual able to conduct activities of daily living satisfactorily?
- Have physical wounds healed properly?
- Is the patient appropriately progressing through the behaviors of grieving?
- Is the patient free of sleep disturbances (nightmares, insomnia); psychosomatic symptoms (headaches, stomach pains, nausea/vomiting); regressive behaviors (enuresis, thumb sucking, phobias); and psychosexual disturbances?
- Is the individual free from problems with interpersonal relationships?
- Has the individual considered the alternatives for change in their personal life?
- Has a decision been made relative to the choices available?
- Is the individual satisfied with the decision that has been made?

Forensic Nursing

Forensic nursing is a specialized nursing role in which nurses apply their skills to the care, evaluation, and advocacy for victims of crime in a variety of settings, including primary care facilities, hospitals, and correctional institutions. Catalano (2020) offers the following definition:

> Forensic nursing is an emerging field that forms an alliance between nursing, law enforcement, and the forensic sciences. The term *forensic* means anything belonging to, or pertaining to, the law. . . . Forensic nurses provide a continuum of care to victims and their families beginning in the emergency room or crime scene and leading to participation in the criminal investigation and the courts of law. (p. 700)

The International Association of Forensic Nurses (IAFN) (2021a) states:

> A forensic nurse is a Registered or Advanced Practice nurse who has received specific education and training. Forensic nurses provide specialized care for patients who are experiencing acute and long-term health consequences associated with victimization or violence, and/or have unmet evidentiary needs relative to having been victimized or accused of victimization. In addition, forensic nurses provide consultation and testimony for civil and criminal proceedings relative to nursing practice, care given, and opinions rendered regarding findings.

Table 25–1 | CARE PLAN FOR SURVIVORS OF ABUSE

NURSING DIAGNOSIS: RAPE-TRAUMA SYNDROME

RELATED TO: Sexual assault

EVIDENCED BY: Verbalizations of the attack; bruises and lacerations over areas of body; severe anxiety

OUTCOME CRITERIA	NURSING INTERVENTIONS	RATIONALE
Short-Term Goal ■ Patient's physical wounds will heal without complication. **Long-Term Goal** ■ Patient will begin a healthy grief resolution, initiating the process of physical and psychological healing (time to be individually determined).	1. It is important to communicate the following to the individual who has been sexually assaulted: "You are safe here." "I'm sorry that it happened." "I'm glad you survived." "It's not your fault. No one deserves to be treated this way." "You did the best that you could."	1. The victim of rape or sexual assault is often frightened and must be reassured of their safety. The patient may also be overwhelmed with self-doubt and self-blame, and these statements instill trust and validate self-worth.
	2. Explain every assessment procedure that will be conducted and why it is being conducted. Ensure that data collection is conducted in a caring, collaborative, nonjudgmental manner.	2. This may serve to decrease fear/anxiety and increase trust.
	3. Ensure that the patient has adequate privacy for all immediate post-crisis interventions. Try to have as few people as possible providing the immediate care or collecting immediate evidence.	3. The post-trauma patient typically feels extremely vulnerable. Additional people in the environment increase this feeling of vulnerability and serve to escalate anxiety.
	4. Encourage the patient to give an account of the assault. Listen, but do not probe.	4. Nonjudgmental listening provides an avenue for catharsis to begin healing. A detailed account may be required for legal follow-up, and a caring nurse, as patient advocate, may help to lessen the trauma of evidence collection.
	5. Discuss with the patient whom to call for support or assistance. Provide information about referrals for aftercare.	5. Because of severe anxiety and fear, the patient may need assistance from others during this immediate post-crisis period. Provide referral information in writing for later reference (e.g., psychotherapist, mental health clinic, community advocacy group).

Continued

Table 25–1 | CARE PLAN FOR SURVIVORS OF ABUSE—cont'd

NURSING DIAGNOSIS: POWERLESSNESS

RELATED TO: Cycle of battering

EVIDENCED BY: Verbalizations of abuse; bruises and lacerations over areas of body; fear for own safety and that of children; verbalizations of no way to get out of the relationship

OUTCOME CRITERIA	NURSING INTERVENTIONS	RATIONALE
Short-Term Goal ■ Patient will recognize and verbalize choices available, thereby perceiving some control over life situation.	1. In collaboration with the physician, ensure that all physical wounds, fractures, and burns receive immediate attention. Take photographs if the individual will permit.	1. Patient safety is a nursing priority. Photographs may be called in as evidence if charges are filed.
Long-Term Goal ■ Patient will exhibit control over life situation by making decision about how to maintain personal safety.	2. Take the patient to a private area to do the interview.	2. If the patient is accompanied by the person who did the battering, the patient is not likely to be truthful about the injuries.
	3. If the patient has come alone or with children, reassure them of their safety. Encourage the patient to discuss the battering incident. Ask questions about whether this has happened before, whether the abuser takes drugs, whether the victim has a safe place to go, and whether the victim is interested in pressing charges.	3. Some victims attempt to keep secret how their injuries occurred in an effort to protect the partner or because they are fearful that the partner will kill them if they tell.
	4. Ensure that "rescue" efforts are not attempted by the nurse. Offer support but remember that the final decision must be made by the patient.	4. Making their own decision promotes the patient's sense of control over their life situation. Imposing judgments and giving advice are nontherapeutic.
	5. Stress to the patient the importance of safety. Provide information about available resources. These may include crisis hot lines, community groups for victims of abuse, shelters, counseling services, and information regarding the victim's rights in the civil and criminal justice system. Respect the patient's decision about whether to stay or leave the home or marriage.	5. Knowledge of available choices decreases the individual's sense of powerlessness. Respecting the patient's decision empowers critical thinking and decision making.

Table 25–1 | CARE PLAN FOR SURVIVORS OF ABUSE—cont'd

NURSING DIAGNOSIS: RISK FOR DELAYED DEVELOPMENT
RELATED TO: Child abuse

OUTCOME CRITERIA	NURSING INTERVENTIONS	RATIONALE
Short-Term Goal ■ Patient will develop trusting relationship with nurse and report how evident injuries were sustained. **Long-Term Goal** ■ Patient will demonstrate behaviors consistent with age-appropriate growth and development.	1. Perform complete physical assessment of the child. Take particular note of bruises (in various stages of healing), lacerations, and patient complaints of pain in specific areas. Do not overlook or discount the possibility of sexual abuse. Assess for nonverbal signs of abuse: aggressive conduct, excessive fears, extreme hyperactivity, apathy, withdrawal, age-inappropriate behaviors.	1. An accurate and thorough physical assessment is required to provide appropriate care for the patient.
	2. Conduct an in-depth interview with the parent or adult who accompanies the child. Consider: If the injury is being reported as an accident, is the explanation reasonable? Is the injury consistent with the explanation? Is the injury consistent with the child's developmental capabilities?	2. Fear of imprisonment or loss of child custody may place the abusive parent on the defensive. Discrepancies may be evident in the description of the incident, and lying to cover up involvement is a common defense that may be detectable in an in-depth interview.
	3. Use games or play therapy to gain the child's trust. Use these techniques to assist in describing the child's side of the story.	3. Establishing a trusting relationship with an abused child is extremely difficult. The child may not even want to be touched. These types of play activities can provide a nonthreatening environment that may enhance the child's attempt to discuss these painful issues.

The sexual assault nurse examiner (SANE) is a clinical forensic registered nurse who has received specialized training to care for the sexual assault victim. Responsibilities include interviewing the victim, completing the physical examination, collecting specimens for forensic evidence, and documenting findings. Sexual assault nurse examiners also provide emotional support for victims and family members. The goal is to provide competent evidence collection and compassionate care that reduces psychological trauma. When the case goes to court, the SANE testifies as an expert legal witness regarding how the evidence was collected and the physical and psychological condition of the client. Forensic mental health nurses may also be called upon to assess convicted perpetrators for physical fitness, criminal responsibility, disposition, and early release or to provide treatment for convicted offenders.

Preservation of Evidence

Crime-related evidence is essential to criminal investigation and must be protected in a manner consistent with the investigation. Brown (2013) identifies common types of evidence as clothing, bullets, gunshot powder on the skin, bloodstains, hairs, fibers, grass, and any other debris found on the individual such as fragments of glass, paint, and wood. Often, this type of evidence is destroyed in the clinical setting when health-care personnel are unaware of its potential value in an investigation. This type of evidence must be saved and documented in all medical or accident cases that have legal implications.

Investigation of Wound Characteristics

When clients present in the emergency department with wounds from undiagnosed trauma, the clinical forensic nurse specialist documents the injuries. Failure to do so may interfere with the administration of justice should legal implications later arise. Nurses managing the care of a victim in the emergency department must be able to make assessments about the type of wound, the weapons involved, and an estimated length of time between the injury and presentation for treatment.

One type of wound that may go unnoticed is nonfatal strangulation. The IAFN (2016) notes that 47 to 68% of women who report domestic violence have experienced one or more events of strangulation, and fatalities have occurred in victims who demonstrate no visible external injuries. Serious internal injuries, including fractured trachea, carotid aneurysm, cerebral artery infarct, and death, may occur days or weeks after the event. Child victims of strangulation are at increased risk for spinal cord injuries. The IAFN recommends universal screening for strangulation events using a collaborative, trauma-informed care approach, including protocols for medical/radiological evaluation, danger assessment, and safety plan development. They note that strangulation events are a strong predictor of future violence and risk for homicide. Brown (2019) stresses that direct inquiry about whether an attempt to strangle has occurred (in any assault victim) is essential because physical signs may be absent at the time of presentation, and victims may not be forthcoming with this information unless directly questioned. The IAFN (2021b) publishes a Nonfatal Strangulation Documentation Toolkit that details examples of direct questions and important aspects of documentation.

Treatment Modalities

Trauma-Informed Care

Trauma-informed care is foundational to all treatment modalities when responding to survivors of abuse and neglect. At the outset it requires awareness that trauma can have long-lasting physical, mental, emotional, and spiritual consequences. It will influence the ability to establish a trusting relationship and to collect accurate assessment data.

An individual's response to trauma is rooted in the fight-or-flight mechanism (the autonomic nervous system) that is designed to protect survival. When activated, however, this response disrupts the normal functions of body systems, including the brain. Notably, memories become fragmented and sensory experiences become intensified. When someone has also had previous traumas, the fight-or-flight response is easily reactivated. Thus, when a patient is interviewed immediately following a traumatic event, the patient may have extreme difficulty recalling events in sequence. In this situation, the nurse must recognize that collecting information will take time, and information may be shared in seemingly disconnected parts. Sensory experiences may be so intensified that any loud noise, smell, visual experience, or touch can retrigger intense fear. Assuring the patient of their safety and working to establish trust, empathy, and compassionate care is not only good patient care in general, but for the trauma victim, it reduces the likelihood of retriggering fear, the fight-or-flight response, and its effects on the body and brain; a process called **retraumatization.** Healthcare provider behaviors that may increase the risk for retraumatization include any behavior that violates the patient's trust, care that is imposed rather than collaborative, and punitive or shame-based approaches. Box 25-1 outlines four basic principles of trauma-informed care.

Crisis Intervention

The focus of the initial interview and follow-up with the patient who has been sexually assaulted is on the rape incident alone. Problems not associated with the rape are not dealt with at this time. The goal of crisis intervention is to help survivors return to their previous lifestyle as quickly as possible.

The patient should be involved in the intervention and decision making from the beginning. This involvement promotes a sense of competency, control, and empowerment in decision making. It is the essence of patient-centered care. Because an overwhelming sense of powerlessness accompanies the rape experience, active involvement by the survivor is both a validation of personal worth and the beginning of the recovery process. Crisis intervention is time limited—usually 6 to 8 weeks. If problems resurface beyond this time, the individual is referred for assistance from other agencies (e.g., long-term psychotherapy from a psychiatrist or mental health clinic).

BOX 25–1 Trauma-Informed Care: The Four R's

Four Domains of Trauma-Informed Approaches	Definitions and Activities
REALIZE	**R**ealizes the widespread impact of trauma. Screens for trauma history. Understands potential paths for recovery.
RECOGNIZE	**R**ecognizes the signs and symptoms of trauma in clients, families, staff, and others involved with the system.
RESPOND	**R**esponds by fully integrating knowledge about trauma into policies, procedures, and practices.
RESIST	**R**esists retraumatization. Behaviors include trustworthiness, transparency, assuring client safety, collaboration, and empowerment.

Source: Adapted from Substance Abuse and Mental Health Services Administration. (n.d.). SAMHSA-HRSA integrated health solutions: Trauma. https://www.integration.samhsa.gov/clinical-practice/trauma-informed

During the crisis period, attention is given to coping strategies for dealing with the symptoms common to the post-trauma client. Initially, the individual undergoes a period of disorganization during which there is difficulty making decisions, extreme or irrational fears, and general mistrust. Observable manifestations may range from stark hysteria to expression of anger and rage to silence and withdrawal. Guilt and feelings of responsibility for the rape, as well as numerous physical manifestations, are common. The crisis counselor will attempt to help the individual draw upon previous successful coping strategies to regain control over their life.

If the patient is a victim of domestic violence, the counselor ensures that various resources and options are made known to the individual so that they may make a personal decision regarding next steps. Support groups provide a valuable forum for reducing isolation and learning new strategies for coping with the aftermath of physical or sexual abuse. Particularly for the survivor of rape, the peer support group provides a therapeutic forum for reducing the sense of isolation they may feel in the aftermath of predictable social and interpersonal responses to their experience.

The Safe House or Shelter

Most major cities in the United States now have **safe houses or shelters** where victims can reside temporarily in an environment that assures physical protection for them and their children and resources for emotional healing. Safe houses have historically catered exclusively to the needs of female victims, but recently more safe houses for male victims of domestic violence are surfacing in the United States and in other countries. These shelters provide a variety of services, and the residents receive emotional support from staff and one another. Most shelters provide individual and group counseling; help with bureaucratic institutions such as the police, legal representation, and social services; child care and children's programming; and aid for making future plans, such as employment counseling and linkages with housing authorities. Lengths of stay vary greatly depending on several factors, such as availability of outside support systems, financial resources, and personal resources.

Family-Based Interventions

The focus of therapy with families who experience violence is to help them develop democratic (respectful, interactive) ways of solving problems. The hope is that these interventions will reduce physical violence, but study results are mixed. The variables that influence violence within families are multifaceted, including the presence or absence of substance use disorders, support networks, and consensus about the need for change.

In a systematic review and meta-analysis (Vlahovicova et al., 2017), researchers concluded that there is evidence to support the benefits of social learning theory-based behavioral parenting programs to prevent recurrence of child abuse. The authors caution, though, that the effects were modest (an 11% lower recidivism to child protective services among families who received the training) and very few of the studies included follow-up beyond 6 months.

Karakurt and associates (2016) conducted a systematic review and meta-analysis that supported the view that couples therapy has a positive impact in reducing IPV in certain situations. The authors caution that "further research into what couple and relationship characteristics predict greater effectiveness of couple therapy is necessary before the widespread adoption of conjoint therapy as a standard form of treatment is really feasible."

Summary and Key Points

- Abuse is the maltreatment of one person by another.
- Intimate partner violence, child abuse, and sexual assault are widespread.
- Various factors have been theorized as influential in the predisposition to violent behavior. Physiological and biochemical influences within the brain have been suggested, as has the possibility of genetic links.
- Organic brain syndromes associated with various cerebral disorders and traumatic brain injury have been implicated in the predisposition to aggressive and violent behavior.
- Psychoanalytical theorists relate the predisposition to violent behavior to underdeveloped ego and a poor self-concept.
- Learning theorists suggest that children imitate the abusive behavior of their parents. This theory has been substantiated by studies that show that individuals who were abused as children or whose parents disciplined them with physical punishment are more likely to be abusive as adults.
- Societal influences, such as general acceptance of violence as a means of solving problems, also have been implicated.
- Although domestic violence is more frequently perpetrated by men against women, about 24% of victims are men.
- Victims who are battered often blame themselves for their situation. They may have been reared in abusive families and have come to expect this type of behavior.
- Battered women commonly see no way out of their present situation and may choose to remain in an abusive relationship for a variety of reasons.
- Child abuse includes physical and emotional abuse, physical and emotional neglect, and sexual abuse.
- A child may experience many years of abuse without reporting it because of fear of retaliation by the abuser.
- Some children report incest experiences to their mothers only to be rebuffed and told to remain secretive about the abuse.
- Research has identified a strong link between adverse childhood experiences (ACEs) (including abuse and neglect) and physical, psychosocial, and mental illness in adulthood.
- Sexual assault is identified as an act of aggression, not passion.
- A history of abuse and neglect in childhood increases one's risk of perpetrating abuse and neglect upon others in adulthood.
- Rape is a traumatic experience, and many victims experience flashbacks, nightmares, rage, physical symptoms, depression, and thoughts of suicide for many years after the occurrence.
- Trauma-informed care is foundational to all interventions and treatment modalities for the client who is a survivor of abuse or neglect.
- Nursing behaviors that are untrustworthy, noncollaborative, punitive, or shame-based or that minimize or ignore trauma-associated fears and concerns can be retraumatizing to victims of abuse and neglect.
- Forensic nursing is a specialized field of practice that seeks to provide care with attention to the needs of the victim as well as issues related to criminal proceedings.
- Treatment modalities for survivors of abuse include crisis intervention with the sexual assault victim, safe shelters for battered victims, cognitive behavior therapy or other trauma-specific psychotherapies, and family-based interventions.

Review Questions

Select the answer that is most appropriate for each of the following questions:

1. Trauma-informed care is foundational to all interventions with a victim of violence for which of the following reasons?
   a. It is a legal requirement in all 50 states.
   b. Trauma victims are unaware they have been traumatized until they are so informed.
   c. Victims of violence are at high risk for retraumatization.
   d. The client has a right to know what will happen to the perpetrator.

2. A SANE nurse's primary role when intervening with a victim of violence is to:
   a. Conduct a sexual assault examination and preserve evidence
   b. Conduct a mini mental status examination
   c. Refer the client to a police officer
   d. Determine whether the client is lying about the events
3. A female child, age 5, is sent to the school nurse's office with an upset stomach. She has vomited and soiled her blouse. When the nurse removes her blouse, she notices that the child has numerous bruises on her arms and torso in various stages of healing. She also notices some small scars, and her abdomen protrudes on her small, thin frame. From the objective physical assessment, the nurse should screen further for:
   a. Physical and sexual abuse
   b. Physical abuse and neglect
   c. Emotional neglect
   d. Sexual and emotional abuse
4. A school nurse notices bruises and scars on a 5-year-old child's body, but the child refuses to say how they received them. Which of the following is an evidence-based approach for further assessment by the nurse?
   a. Have the child evaluated by the school psychologist.
   b. Tell the child they may select a "treat" from the treat box (e.g., sucker, balloon, junk jewelry) if they answer the nurse's questions.
   c. Explain to the child that if they answer the questions, they may stay in the nurse's office and not have to go back to class.
   d. Use a "family" of dolls to role-play the child's family with them.
5. The nurse is providing education to a support group for survivors of rape. Which of the following items is evidence-based information to include in this teaching?
   a. Rapists typically drink alcohol and are not in control of their actions.
   b. Rape is usually an event that occurs between two people who are sexually frustrated.
   c. Men who are born into poverty are predisposed to becoming rapists after puberty.
   d. Rape is an expression of power and dominance by means of sexual aggression and violence.

Clinical Judgment Questions

6. A female client arrives at the emergency department and tells the nurse her husband inflicted the cuts to her face that required sutures. She says, "I didn't want to come. I'm really okay. He only does this when he has too much to drink. I just shouldn't have yelled at him." The best response by the nurse is:
   a. "How often does he drink too much?"
   b. "It is not your fault. You did the right thing by coming here."
   c. "How many times has he done this to you?"
   d. "He is not a good husband. You have to leave him before he kills you."
7. A woman who has a long history of being battered by her husband is staying at the woman's shelter. She has received emotional support from staff and peers and has been made aware of the alternatives open to her. Nevertheless, she decides to return to her home and marriage. The best response by the nurse to the woman's decision is:
   a. "I just can't believe you have decided to go back to that horrible man."
   b. "I'm just afraid he will kill you or the children when you go back."
   c. "What makes you think things have changed with him?"
   d. "I hope you have made the right decision. Call this number if you need help."

Continued

8. A school nurse notices suspicious bruises and scars on a child's body. The nurse suspects that the child is being physically abused. Which action by the nurse is a priority at this point?
   a. As a health-care worker, report the suspicion to child protective services.
   b. Check the child again in a week and see if there are any new bruises.
   c. Meet with the child's parents and ask them how the child got the bruises.
   d. Initiate paperwork to have the child placed in foster care.
9. A college-age female client is brought to the emergency department by their roommate after she confided that she was raped by her date who invited her to a frat party. The client says to the nurse, "It's all my fault. I shouldn't have gone to a party where I knew there was going to be alcohol." Which of these is the best response by the nurse?
   a. "Yes, you're right. You put yourself in a very vulnerable position when you allowed him to get you drunk."
   b. "You are not to blame for his behavior. You obviously made some right decisions, because you survived the attack."
   c. "There's no sense looking back now. Just look forward, and make sure you don't put yourself in the same situation again."
   d. "You'll just have to see that he is arrested so he won't do this to anyone else."
10. A young man who has just undergone a sexual assault is brought into the emergency department by a friend. What is the priority nursing intervention?
   a. Help him to bathe and clean himself up.
   b. Provide physical and emotional support during evidence collection.
   c. Provide him with a written list of community resources for survivors of rape.
   d. Discuss the importance of a follow-up visit to evaluate for sexually transmitted diseases.

IMPLICATIONS FOR EVIDENCE-BASED PRACTICE

Daphna-Tekoah, S., Lev-Wiesel, R., Israeli, D., & Balla, U. (2019). A novel screening tool for assessing child abuse: The medical somatic dissociation questionnaire–MSDQ, *Journal of Child Sexual Abuse, 28*(5), 526–543. https//doi.org/10.1080/10538712.2019.1581868

DESCRIPTION OF THE STUDY: Noting that somatic dissociation is associated with a history of childhood abuse, the researchers sought to validate a novel questionnaire that can be used to evaluate somatic dissociation in a health-care setting. The researchers recruited 541 adults from the general population via the Internet and used several measures to validate history of childhood abuse and somatic dissociation. *Somatic dissociation* is defined as somatic manifestations represented in the form of "pseudoneurological" symptoms due to disturbances or alterations of normal integrated functions of consciousness, memory or identity mainly related to trauma and other psychological stressors. The symptoms are otherwise unexplainable.

RESULTS OF THE STUDY: The MSDQ demonstrated "powerful internal consistency, reliability, and convergent validity of the instrument" and correlated highly with the presence of psychological symptoms. In addition, the tool demonstrated validity when differences between adults who experienced child sexual abuse and those who did not were compared.

IMPLICATIONS FOR NURSING PRACTICE: Assessment of the long-term impacts of childhood sexual abuse can be difficult and, as the authors note, the diagnosis of childhood sexual abuse is hampered by the lack of valid tools. For nurses working in primary care settings with adults who have unexplained somatic symptoms, the MSDQ presents an evidence-based option for assisting in the diagnosis of childhood sexual abuse, which then provides a foundation for evaluation of current distress, long-term impacts, and the potential for exploring specialized trauma intervention programs.

TEST YOUR CLINICAL REASONING AND CLINICAL JUDGMENT SKILLS

Sandy is a psychiatric registered nurse who works at a safe house for battered women. Lisa has just been admitted with her two small children after she was treated in the emergency department. She had been beaten severely by her husband while he was intoxicated last night. She escaped with her children after he passed out in their bedroom.

In her initial assessment, Sandy learns from Lisa that she has been battered by her husband for 5 years, beginning shortly after their marriage. She explained that she "knew he drank quite a lot before we were married but thought he would stop after we had kids." Instead, the drinking has increased. Sometimes, he does not even get home from work until 11 o'clock or midnight after stopping to drink at the bar with his buddies.

Lately, he has begun to express jealousy and a lack of trust in Lisa, accusing her of numerous infidelities and indiscretions, none of which is true. Lisa says, "If only he wasn't under so much stress on his job, then maybe he wouldn't drink so much. Maybe if I tried harder to make everything perfect for him at home—I don't know. What do you think I should do to keep him from acting this way?"

Answer the following questions related to Lisa:

1. What is an appropriate response to Lisa's question?
2. Identify the priority psychosocial nursing diagnosis for Lisa.
3. What must the nurse ensure that Lisa learns from this experience?

Communication Exercises

1. Sarah is being treated in the emergency department for wounds inflicted by her husband. Sarah says to the nurse, "He's really not a bad person. He's just under so much stress right now. His company is laying people off, and he thinks he will be next. He drinks a lot when he comes home from work. I just need to make things easier for him at home. I shouldn't have asked him to mow the lawn."
   How would the nurse respond appropriately to this statement by Sarah?
2. Sarah tells the nurse, "I don't know what to do. I'm afraid he will hurt the kids."
   How would the nurse respond appropriately to this statement by Sarah?
3. Sarah also states, "I don't want to press charges. I just want to go home!"
   How would the nurse respond appropriately to this statement by Sarah?

MOVIE CONNECTIONS

The Burning Bed (Domestic violence) ▪ *Life With Billy* (Domestic violence) ▪ *Two Story House* (Child abuse) ▪ *The Prince of Tides* (Domestic violence) ▪ *Radio Flyer* (Child abuse) ▪ *Flowers in the Attic* (Child abuse) ▪ *A Case of Rape* (Sexual assault) ▪ *The Accused* (Sexual assault) ▪ *Spotlight* (Child molestation) ▪ *What's Love Got to Do With It* (Domestic violence)

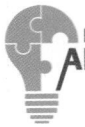

Go to **Davis Advantage** to complete your learning: strengthen understanding, apply your knowledge, and prepare for the Next Gen NCLEX®.

References

American Psychological Association. (2021). *Violence and socioeconomic status.* http://www.apa.org/pi/ses/resources/publications/violence.aspx

Barnett, B. (2016). *What is the age of consent in the United States?* https://www.bhwlawfirm.com/legal-age-consent-united-states-map/

Batrinos M. L. (2012). Testosterone and aggressive behavior in man. *International Journal of Endocrinology and Metabolism, 10*(3), 563–568. https://doi.org/10.5812/ijem.3661

Brown, K. (2013). *Evidence collection and preservation in a healthcare setting.* Gannett Education Course #CE296-60. http://ce.nurse.com/CE296-60/Evidence-Collection-and-Preservation-in-a-Healthcare-Setting

Brown, T. (2019). Strangulation victims: A forensic approach. *Medscape.* https://www.medscape.com/viewarticle/907317

Burgess, A. (2010). Rape violence. *Gannett Education Course #60025.* http://ce.nurse.com/60025/Rape-Violence

Cashmore, J., & Shackel, R. (2013). *The long-term effects of child sexual abuse.* https://aifs.gov.au/cfca/publications/long-term-effects-child-sexual-abuse/introduction

Catalano, J. T. (2020). Developments in current nursing practice. In J. T. Catalano (Ed.), *Nursing now! Today's issues, tomorrow's trends* (8th ed., pp. 700–716). F.A. Davis.

Center for Relationship Abuse Awareness. (2021). *Barriers to leaving an abusive relationship.* http://stoprelationshipabuse.org/educated/barriers-to-leaving-an-abusive-relationship/

Centers for Disease Control and Prevention. (2020a). *Violence prevention: About behavioral risk factor surveillance system ACE data.* https://www.cdc.gov/violenceprevention/acestudy/ace_brfss.html

Centers for Disease Control and Prevention. (2020b). *Preventing elder abuse.* https://www.cdc.gov/violenceprevention/elderabuse/fastfact.html

Centers for Disease Control and Prevention. (2020c). *Preventing intimate partner violence.* https://www.cdc.gov/violenceprevention/intimatepartnerviolence/fastfact.html

Child Welfare Information Gateway. (2019). *What is child abuse and neglect? Recognizing the signs and symptoms.* https://www.childwelfare.gov/pubs/factsheets/whatiscan

Collin-Vézina, D., Daigneault, I., & Hébert, M. (2013). Lessons learned from child sexual abuse research: Prevalence, outcomes, and preventive strategies. *Child and Adolescent Psychiatry and Mental Health, 7*(1), 22. https://doi.org/10.1186/1753-2000-7-22

Daphna-Tekoah, S., Lev-Wiesel, R., Israeli, D., & Balla, U. (2019). A novel screening tool for assessing child abuse: The medical somatic dissociation questionnaire–MSDQ. *Journal of Child Sexual Abuse, 28*(5), 526–543. https://doi.org/10.1080/10538712.2019.1581868

D'Inverno, A. S., Smith, S. G., Zhang, X., & Chen, J. (2019). *The impact of intimate partner violence: A 2015 NISVS research-in brief.* National Center for Injury Prevention and Control, Centers for Disease Control and Prevention. https://www.cdc.gov/violenceprevention/pdf/nisvs/nisvs-impactbrief-508.pdf

Dockterman, E. (2014, September 9). Why women stay: The paradox of abusive relationships. *Time.* https://time.com/3309687/why-women-stay-in-abusive-relationships/

Dreher, J. C., Dunne, S., Pazderska, A., Frodl, T., Nolan, J. J., & O'Doherty, J. P. (2016). Testosterone causes pro- and antisocial behaviors. *Proceedings of the National Academy of Sciences, 113*(41), 11633–11638. https://doi.org 10.1073/pnas.1608085113

Espolage, D. L., Low, S., Mrinalini, A. R., Hong, J. S., & Little, T. D. (2013). Family violence, bullying, fighting, and substance use among adolescents: A longitudinal mediational model. *Journal of Research on Adolescence, 24*(2), 337–349. https://doi.org/10.1111/jora.12060

Flaherty, E. G., Stirling, J.; American Academy of Pediatrics, Committee on Child Abuse and Neglect. (2010). Clinical report—The pediatrician's role in child maltreatment prevention. *Pediatrics, 126*(4), 833–841.

Henderson, R. J. (2021). *Incest.* https://patient.info/doctor/incest

International Association of Forensic Nurses. (2016). *The evaluation and treatment of non-fatal strangulation in the health care setting.* https://cdn.ymaws.com/www.forensicnurses.org/resource/resmgr/education/Strangulation_Position_Paper.pdf

International Association of Forensic Nurses. (2021a). *What is forensic nursing?* https://www.forensicnurses.org/page/WhatisFN

International Association of Forensic Nurses. (2021b). *Non-fatal strangulation documentation toolkit.* https://www.forensicnurses.org/page/STAssessment

Irish, L., Kobayashi, I., & Delahanty, D. L. (2010). Long-term physical health consequences of childhood sexual abuse: A meta-analytic review. *Journal of Pediatric Psychology, 35*(5), 450–461. https://doi.org/10.1093/jpepsy/jsp118

Karakurt, G., Whiting, K., van Esch, C., Bolen, S. D., & Calabrese, J. R. (2016). Couples therapy for intimate partner violence: A systematic review and meta-analysis. *Journal of Marital and Family Therapy, 42*(4), 567–583. https://doi.org/10.1111/jmft.12178

Miczek, K. A., DeBold, J. F., Gobrogge, K., Newman, E. L., & de Almeida, R. M. M. (2017). The role of neurotransmitters in violence and aggression. In P. Sturmey, *The Wiley handbook of violence and aggression.* Wiley-Blackwell. https://doi.org/10.1002/9781119057574.whbva019

Narvaes, R., & Martins de Almeida, R. M. (2014). Aggressive behavior and three neurotransmitters: Dopamine, GABA, and serotonin—A review of the last 10 years. *Psychology & Neuroscience, 7*(4), 601–607. http://doi.org/10.3922/j.psns.2014.4.20

National Center on Elder Abuse. (n.d.). *Elder abuse: Frequently asked questions.* U.S. Administration on Aging. https://ncea.acl.gov/faq/index.html#faq5

Rape, Abuse & Incest National Network. (2021). *Warning signs for young children.* https://www.rainn.org/articles/warning-signs-young-children

Rosell, D. R., & Siever, L. J. (2015). The neurobiology of aggression and violence. *CNS Spectrum, 20*(3), 254–279 http://doi.org/10.1017/S109285291500019X

Schatzberg, A. F., Cole, J. O., & DeBattista, C. (2019). *Manual of clinical psychopharmacology* (9th ed.). American Psychiatric.

Stanley, M. (2020). The bizarre legal loopholes surrounding spousal rape. *Psychology Today.* https://www.psychologytoday.com/us/blog/making-sense-chaos/202005/the-bizarre-legal-loopholes-surrounding-spousal-rape

Substance Abuse and Mental Health Services Administration. (n.d.). SAMHSA-HRSA integrated health solutions: Trauma. https://www.integration.samhsa.gov/clinical-practice/trauma-informe

Tracy, N. (2019). *What is battering?* http://www.healthyplace.com/abuse/domestic-violence/what-is-battering

U.S. Bureau of Justice Statistics. (2014). *Rape and sexual assault among college-age females, 1995–2013.* http://www.bjs.gov/index.cfm?ty=pbdetail&iid=5176

U.S. Department of Education. (2013). *Human trafficking of children in the United States.* http://www2.ed.gov/about/offices/list/oese/oshs/factsheet.html

U.S. Department of Health & Human Services, Administration for Children and Families, Administration on Children, Youth and Families, Children's Bureau. (2021). *Child maltreatment 2019.* https://www.acf.hhs.gov/sites/default/files/documents/cb/cm2019.pdf

U.S. Department of Justice. (2018). *2018 NCVRW resource guide: Intimate partner violence fact sheet.* https://ovc.ncjrs.gov/ncvrw2018/info flyers/fact_sheets/2018NCVRW_IPV_508_QC.pdf

Vlahovicova, K., Melendez-Torres, G. J., Leijten, P., Knerr, W., & Gardner, F. (2017). Parenting programs for the prevention of child physical abuse recurrence: A systematic review and meta-analysis. *Clinical Child and Family Psychology Review, 20*(3), 351–365. https://doi.org/10.1007/s10567-017-0232-7

Zhang-James, Y., Fernàndez-Castillo, N., Hess, J. L., Malki, K., Glatt, S. J., Cormand, B., & Faraone, S. V. (2019). An integrated analysis of genes and functional pathways for aggression in human and rodent models. *Molecular Psychiatry, 24*(11), 1655–1667. https://doi.org/10.1038/s41380-018-0068-7.

Classical References

Burgess, A. W., & Holmström, L. L. (1974). Rape trauma syndrome. *American Journal of Psychiatry, 131*(9), 981–986. https://doi.org/10.1176/appi.ajp.131.9.981. PMID 4415470

Erikson, E. H. (1963). *Childhood and society* (2nd ed.). W. W. Norton.

Walker, L. E. (1979). *The battered woman.* Harper & Row.

Community Mental Health Nursing 26

CHAPTER OUTLINE

Objectives
Introduction
Historical Perspective
The Public Health Model
The Community as Client
Summary and Key Points
Review Questions
Clinical Judgment Questions
Implications of Evidence-Based Practice

KEY TERMS

case management
case manager
deinstitutionalization
diagnosis-related groups (DRGs)
mobile outreach units
prospective payment
serious mental illness (SMI)
shelters
storefront clinics

OBJECTIVES

After reading this chapter, the student will be able to:

1. Discuss the changes in mental health-care delivery.
2. Define the concepts of care associated with the public health model.
3. Discuss primary prevention of mental illness within the community.
4. Identify populations at risk for mental illness within the community.
5. Discuss secondary prevention of mental illness within the community.
6. Describe treatment alternatives related to secondary prevention within the community.
7. Discuss tertiary prevention of mental illness within the community as it relates to the seriously mentally ill and homeless mentally ill.
8. Recognize the history and epidemiology associated with caring for the seriously mentally ill and homeless mentally ill within the community.
9. Identify treatment alternatives for care of the seriously mentally ill and homeless mentally ill within the community.
10. Apply steps of the nursing process to care of the seriously mentally ill and homeless mentally ill within the community.

CORE CONCEPTS

Health Promotion: Primary, secondary, and tertiary prevention
Population Health: Homelessness and mental illness
Health Policy
Professionalism: Nursing process in the care of patients in the community

Introduction

This chapter explores the concepts of primary and secondary prevention of mental illness within communities. Additional focus is placed on tertiary prevention of mental illness: use of community resources to treat individuals with severe and persistent mental illness and homeless persons with mental illness. Emphasis is given to the role of the psychiatric nurse in the various treatment alternatives in the community setting.

Historical Perspective

Before 1840, there was no known treatment for individuals with mental illness. Because mental illness was perceived as incurable, the only "reasonable" intervention was thought to be removing these individuals from the community to a place where they would do no harm to themselves or others.

In 1841, Dorothea Dix, a former schoolteacher, began a personal crusade across the land on behalf of institutionalized individuals with mental illness. Her efforts resulted in more humane treatment of these clients and the establishment of several psychiatric hospitals across the country.

Following the movement initiated by Dix, the number of hospitals for persons with mental illness increased, although unfortunately not as rapidly as did the population with mental illness. The demand soon outgrew the supply, and hospitals became overcrowded and understaffed with conditions that fell far short of Dix's original intentions.

The community mental health movement had its impetus in the 1940s. With establishment of the National Mental Health Act of 1946, the U.S. government awarded grants to the states to develop mental health programs outside of state hospitals. Outpatient clinics and psychiatric units in general hospitals were inaugurated. Then, in 1949, as an outgrowth of the National Mental Health Act, the National Institute of Mental Health (NIMH) was established. The U.S. government has charged this agency with the responsibility for mental health in the United States.

In 1955, the Joint Commission on Mental Health and Illness was established by Congress to identify the nation's mental health needs and to make recommendations for improvement in psychiatric care. In 1961, the Joint Commission published the report *Action for Mental Health* in which recommendations were made for treatment of clients with mental illness, training for caregivers, and improvements in education and research on mental illness. With consideration given to these recommendations, Congress passed the Mental Retardation Facilities and Community Mental Health Centers Construction Act (often called the Community Mental Health Centers Act) of 1963. This act called for the construction of comprehensive community mental health centers, the cost of which would be shared by federal and state governments. The **deinstitutionalization** movement (the closing of state mental hospitals and discharging of individuals with mental illness) had begun.

Unfortunately, many state governments did not have the capability to match the federal funds required for the establishment of these mental health centers. Some communities found it difficult to follow the rigid requirements for services stipulated by the legislation that provided the grant.

In 1980, the Community Mental Health Systems Act, which was to have played a major role in renovation of mental health care, was established. Funding was authorized for community mental health centers, for services to high-risk populations, and for rape research and services. Approval was also granted for the appointment of an associate director for minority concerns at NIMH. However, before this plan could be enacted, the newly inaugurated administration set forth its intention to diminish federal involvement. Budget cuts reduced the number of mandated services, and federal funding for community mental health centers was terminated in 1984.

Meanwhile, costs of care for hospitalized psychiatric clients continued to rise. The problem of the "revolving door" (frequent readmissions) began to intensify. Individuals with severe and persistent mental illness had no place to go when their symptoms exacerbated, except back to the hospital. Individuals without support systems remained in the hospital for extended periods because of lack of appropriate community services. Hospital services were paid for by cost-based, retrospective reimbursement: Medicaid, Medicare, and private health insurance. Retrospective reimbursement encouraged hospital expenditure; the more services that were provided, the more payment was received.

This system of health-care delivery was interrupted in 1983 with the advent of **prospective payment**—the Reagan administration's proposal for cost containment. It was directed at control of Medicare costs by designating pre-established amounts that would be reimbursed for specific diagnoses, or **diagnosis-related groups (DRGs).** Since that time, prospective payment has also been integrated by the states (Medicaid) and by some private insurance companies, drastically affecting the amount of reimbursement for health-care services.

Mental health services have been influenced by prospective payment. General hospital services to psychiatric clients have been severely restricted. Clients who present with acute symptoms, such as acute psychosis, suicidal ideations or attempts, or manic exacerbations, constitute the largest segment of the psychiatric hospital census. Clients with less serious illnesses (e.g., moderate depression or adjustment disorders) often don't meet criteria for hospitalization, and if they do, the length of stay has been shortened considerably by the reimbursement guidelines. Clients are being discharged from the hospital with a greater need for aftercare than in the past when hospital stays were longer.

A positive outgrowth of efforts to reduce costly hospital stays and implement restricted reimbursement has been the development of a broader continuum of outpatient treatment options than what has been available historically. In the past, people who needed psychiatric treatment saw an outpatient therapist or were hospitalized, but today there are partial hospitalization programs, intensive outpatient programs, aftercare programs, and a host of other community-based services available to clients with mental health disorders.

For those with health insurance, inroads have been made to eliminate discrimination against those with mental illness and substance use disorders. The Paul Wellstone and Pete Domenici Mental Health Parity and Addictions Equity Act (2008) required that for health insurance plans that provide mental health and substance use disorder benefits, the plan cannot provide less favorable benefits than those provided for medical/surgical issues. The Affordable Care Act (2010) also required some insurance plans to include mental health and substance use disorder benefits. In reality, however, many people with chronic mental illnesses are uninsured, undertreated, and homeless.

Deinstitutionalization continues to be the focus of mental health care in the United States. Care for the client in the hospital has become cost-prohibitive, whereas care for the client in the community is considered cost-effective. However, as experience with the community mental health movement lengthens, it has also been criticized for being a continuation of an "overly narrow biomedical model" (Vanderplasschen et al., 2013, p. 1). Ironically, the prison populations of homeless persons and those with mental illnesses have risen dramatically during this same time period—one of the problems that Dorothea Dix fought so adamantly against in the first place. The reality of the provision of health-care services today is often more of a political and funding issue than providers would care to admit. Decisions about how to treat are rarely made without consideration of cost and method of payment.

The recovery model (see Chapter 10, "The Recovery Model") promises the hope of integrating the support of community mental health services, peer support, and client empowerment to improve interventions and outcomes as we look to the future. We must serve the consumer by working collaboratively to provide the essential services for health promotion, for early intervention, and to promote improvement in quality of life for this population.

The Public Health Model

The premise of the public health model is based largely on the concepts set forth by Gerald Caplan (1964) during the initial community mental health movement. They include primary prevention, secondary prevention, and tertiary prevention. These concepts have expanded beyond mental health treatment and are now widely accepted as guiding principles in clinical and community settings over a wide range of medical and nursing specialties.

CORE CONCEPT

Primary Prevention

Services aimed at reducing the incidence of mental disorders within the population.

Primary prevention targets both individuals and the environment. Emphasis is twofold:

1. Assisting individuals to increase their ability to cope effectively with stress
2. Targeting and diminishing harmful forces (stressors) within the environment

Nursing in primary prevention is focused on the targeting of groups at risk and the provision of educational programs. Examples include the following:

- Teaching parenting skills and child development to prospective new parents
- Teaching physical and psychosocial effects of alcohol/drugs to elementary school students
- Teaching techniques of stress management to virtually anyone who desires to learn
- Teaching groups of individuals ways to cope with the changes associated with various maturational stages
- Teaching concepts of mental health to various groups within the community
- Providing education and support to unemployed or homeless individuals
- Providing education and support to other individuals in various transitional periods (e.g., widows and widowers, new retirees, and women entering the workforce in middle life)

These are only a few examples of the types of services that nurses provide in primary prevention. Such services can be offered in a variety of settings that are convenient for the public (e.g., churches, schools, colleges, community centers, YMCAs and YWCAs, workplaces of employee organizations, meetings of women's groups, or civic or social organizations such as parent-teacher associations, health fairs, and community shelters).

CORE CONCEPT

Secondary Prevention

Interventions aimed at minimizing early symptoms of psychiatric illness and directed toward reducing the prevalence and duration of the illness.

Secondary prevention is accomplished through early identification of problems and prompt initiation of effective treatment. Nursing in secondary prevention focuses on recognition of symptoms and provision of, or referral for, treatment. Examples include:

- Ongoing assessment of individuals at high risk for illness exacerbation (e.g., during home visits, day care, community health centers, or in any setting where screening of high-risk individuals might occur).
- Provision of care for individuals in whom illness symptoms have been assessed (e.g., individual or group counseling, medication administration, education and support during periods of increased stress [crisis intervention], staffing rape crisis centers, suicide hotlines, homeless shelters, shelters for abused persons, or mobile mental health units).
- Referral for treatment of individuals in whom illness symptoms have been assessed. Referrals may come from support groups, community mental health centers, emergency services, psychiatrists or psychologists, and day or partial hospitalization. Inpatient therapy on a psychiatric unit of a general hospital or in a private psychiatric hospital may be necessary. Psychopharmacology and various adjunct therapies may be initiated as part of the treatment.

Secondary prevention is addressed extensively in Unit 3, "Care of Patients With Psychiatric Disorders." Nursing assessment, diagnosis and outcome identification, planning and implementation, and evaluation are discussed for many of the mental illnesses identified in the *Diagnostic and Statistical Manual of Mental Disorders, Fifth Edition, Text Revision* (*DSM-5-TR*; American Psychiatric Association [APA], 2022). These concepts may be applied in any setting where nursing is practiced.

CORE CONCEPT

Tertiary Prevention

Services aimed at reducing the residual challenges that are associated with severe and persistent mental illness.

Tertiary prevention is accomplished in two ways:

1. Preventing complications of the illness
2. Promoting rehabilitation that is directed toward achievement of each individual's maximum level of functioning

Historically, individuals with severe and persistent mental illness often experienced long hospitalizations that resulted in loss of social skills and increased dependency. With deinstitutionalization, many of these individuals may never have experienced hospitalization, but they still do not possess adequate skills to live productive lives within the community.

Nursing in tertiary prevention focuses on helping patients learn or relearn socially appropriate behaviors so that they may achieve a satisfying role in the community. Examples include:

- Consideration of the rehabilitation process at the time of initial diagnosis and treatment planning.
- Teaching daily living skills and encouraging independence to an individual's maximum ability.
- Referring for various aftercare services (e.g., support groups, day treatment programs, partial hospitalization programs, psychosocial rehabilitation programs, group home or other transitional housing).
- Monitoring effectiveness of aftercare services (e.g., through home health visits or follow-up appointments in community mental health centers).
- Making referrals for support services when required (e.g., some communities have programs linking individuals with serious mental disorders to volunteers who serve to develop friendships with the individuals and who may assist with household chores, shopping, and other activities of daily living with which the individual is having difficulty, in addition to participating in social activities with the individual).
- Providing trauma-informed care and, when health consequences are associated with a history of trauma, making referrals to specialized trauma recovery treatment programs.

Nursing care at the tertiary level of prevention can be administered on an individual or a group basis and in a variety of settings, such as inpatient hospitalization, day or partial hospitalization, group home or halfway house, shelters, home health care, nursing homes, and community mental health centers.

The Community as Client

Primary Prevention

CORE CONCEPT

Community

A group, population, or cluster of people with at least one common characteristic, such as geographic location, occupation, ethnicity, or health concern.

Primary prevention within communities encompasses the twofold emphasis defined earlier in this chapter:

1. Identifying stressful life events that precipitate crises and targeting the relevant populations at high risk
2. Intervening with these high-risk populations to prevent or minimize harmful consequences

Populations at Risk

One way to view populations at risk is to focus on types of crises that individuals typically experience in their lives. Two broad categories are maturational crises and situational crises.

Maturational Crises

Maturational crises are crucial experiences that are associated with various stages of growth and development. Erikson (1963) described eight stages of the life cycle during which individuals struggle with developmental "tasks." Crises can occur during any of these stages, although several developmental periods and life-cycle events have been recognized as having increased crisis potential: adolescence, marriage, parenthood, midlife, and retirement.

Adolescence The task for adolescence, according to Erikson (1963), is *identity versus role confusion.* This is the time in life when individuals ask questions such as "Who am I?" "Where am I going?" and "What is life all about?"

Adolescence is a transition into young adulthood. It is a very volatile time in most families. Commonly, there is conflict over issues of control. Parents sometimes have difficulty relinquishing even a minimal amount of the control they have had throughout their child's infancy, toddler, and school-age years at this time when the adolescent is seeking increased independence. It may seem that the adolescent is 25 years old one day and 5 years old the next. An often-quoted definition of an adolescent, by an anonymous author, is "a toddler with hormones and wheels."

At this time, adolescents are "trying out their wings," although they possess an essential need to know that the parents (or surrogate parents) are available if support is required. In fact, it is believed that the most frequent immediate precipitant to adolescent suicide is loss, threat of loss, or abandonment by parents or closest peer relationship.

Adolescents have many issues to deal with and many choices to make. Some of these include issues that relate to self-esteem and body image (in a body that is undergoing rapid changes), peer relationships, education and career selection, establishing a set of values and ideals, sexuality and sexual experimentation (including issues of birth control and prevention of sexually transmitted infections), drug and alcohol use, and physical appearance.

Nursing interventions with adolescents at the primary level of prevention focus on providing support and accurate information to ease the difficult transition they are undergoing. Educational offerings can be presented in schools, churches, youth centers, or any location in which groups of teenagers gather. Types of programs may include the following:

- Alateen groups for adolescents with alcoholic parent(s)
- Support groups for teenagers who are in need of assistance to cope with specific stressful situations such as pregnancy, abortion, parents' divorce, or death of a loved one.
- Educational programs that inform about and validate body changes and the emotions that may accompany these changes
- Educational programs that inform about positive self-esteem and resilience
- Educational programs that inform about sexuality, pregnancy, contraception, and sexually transmitted infections
- Educational programs that inform about the consequences of alcohol and other drug misuse

Marriage Although there are many culturally accepted choices about the nature of relationships and living arrangements in lieu of marriage in today's society, crises may develop related to conflicting values between generations within a family and related to the many factors influencing those choices, including economic concerns. Ideological changes that stress personal freedom, self-fulfillment, and individual choice have contributed to an increase in people delaying marriage to fulfill career aspirations or leaving marriages that don't fulfill their expectations (Casper & Coritz, 2018).

When young adults do decide to enter into marriage, a crisis may develop associated with unrealistic or uninformed expectations about this institution. It is well understood, too, that children raised in abusive, dysfunctional families are at higher risk for subconsciously choosing partners who perpetuate the negative experiences they were accustomed to while they were growing up. Both of these circumstances can increase the risk for crisis in a marriage.

Nursing interventions at the primary level of prevention with individuals in this stage of development involve education regarding what to expect from marriage and other committed relationships. Educating young adults about assertive communication skills, clarifying each person's expectations for the relationship, healthy boundaries, and, particularly, the risks associated with choosing a partner who perpetuates a cycle of violence are all important aspects of primary prevention.

These interventions can be effective in individual or couple's therapy and in support or educational groups of couples experiencing similar circumstances.

Parenthood There is perhaps no developmental stage that creates an upheaval equal to that of the arrival of a child. Even when the child is desperately wanted and pleasurably anticipated, their arrival usually results in some degree of chaos within the family.

Because the family operates as a system, the addition of a new member influences all parts of the system as a whole. If it is a first child, the relationship between the spouses is likely to be affected by the demands of caring for the infant on a 24-hour basis. If there are older children, they may resent the attention showered on the new arrival and show their resentment in a variety of creative ways.

The concept of having a child (particularly the first one) is often romanticized with little or no consideration given to the realities and responsibilities that accompany this "bundle of joy." Many parents are shocked to realize that such a tiny human can create so many changes in so many lives. It is unfortunate that although parenting is one of the most challenging positions an individual will hold in life, it is one for which new parents are often least prepared.

Nursing intervention at the primary level of prevention with those in the developmental stage of parenthood must begin long before the child is born. How do we prepare individuals for parenthood? *Anticipatory guidance* is a term used to describe interventions designed to help new parents know what they might expect. Volumes have been written on the subject, but it is also important for expectant parents to have a support person or network with whom they can talk and express feelings, excitement, and fears. Nurses can provide the following type of information to help ease the transition into parenthood (Spock & Needlman, 2018; Veltri et al., 2018):

- ***Prepared childbirth classes:*** These classes present what most likely will happen along with information about possible variations from that which is expected.
- ***What to expect after the baby arrives:***
  - *Parent-infant bonding:* Expectant parents should know that it is common for parent-infant bonding not to occur immediately. The strong attachment will occur as parent and infant get to know each other.
  - *Changing communication patterns and relationship styles:* The couple should be encouraged to engage in open, honest communication with each other. Education should be offered about expected changes in communication patterns and the challenges of establishing communication with an infant as well as resources for referral if communication patterns are creating significant role strain. Frustrated attempts to adapt to these challenges can have consequences for the infant as well. In some cases, an infant's need may be neglected if the parents lack skills or resources to navigate communication challenges. "Abusive head trauma, which includes shaken baby syndrome, is an extreme example of an inability to adapt to changed communication patterns with an infant" (Veltri et al., 2018, p. 367). Discuss strategies that family members may consider using to maintain motivation and morale as well as provide for comfort, rest, and self-care for each member.
  - *Clothing and equipment:* Expectant parents need to know what is required to care for a newborn child. Financing childbearing and child rearing, arranging space for a child, and lifestyle should be considered.
  - *Feeding:* Advantages and disadvantages of breastfeeding and formula feeding should be

presented. The couple should be supported in whatever method is chosen. Anticipatory guidance related to technique should be provided for one or both methods, at the expectant parents' request.
  - *Other expectations:* It is important for expectant parents to receive anticipatory guidance about the infant's sleeping and crying patterns, bathing the infant, care of the circumcision and cord, toys that provide stimulation of the newborn's senses, aspects of providing a safe environment, and when to call the physician.
- ***Stages of growth and development:*** It is very important for parents to understand what behaviors should be expected at what stage of development. It is also important to know that their child may not necessarily follow the age guidelines associated with these stages. However, a substantial deviation from these guidelines should be reported to their physician.

Midlife What is middle age? A colleague once remarked that upon turning 50 years of age, "'Now I can say I am officially middle aged' . . . until I began thinking about how few individuals I really knew who were 100!"

Midlife crises are not defined by a specific number. Various sources in the literature identify these conflicts as occurring anytime between ages 35 and 65 years.

What is a midlife crisis? This, too, is very individual, but a number of patterns have been identified within three broad categories:

1. ***An alteration in perception of the self:*** One's perception of self may occur slowly. One may suddenly become aware of being "old" or "middle aged." Other biological changes that occur naturally with the aging process may also affect the crises that occur at this time.
   - In women, a gradual decrease in the production of estrogen initiates the menopause, which results in a variety of physical and emotional symptoms. Some physical symptoms include hot flashes, vaginal dryness, cessation of menstruation, loss of reproductive ability, night sweats, insomnia, headaches, and minor memory disturbances. Emotional symptoms include anxiety, depression, crying for no reason, and temper outbursts.
   - In men, lower testosterone levels may go unnoticed, but some men experience decreased energy, depressed mood, decline in sexual desire and activity, hot flashes, sweating, breast discomfort, and insomnia (Mayo Clinic, 2021). Alteration in sexual functioning is not uncommon.
2. ***An alteration in perception of others:*** A change in relationship with adult children requires a sensitive shift in caring. Shajani and Snell (2019) identify several aspects of this change including:
   - Navigating the new role between parent and adult child in place of the primary parenting role
   - Renegotiating emotional and financial commitments
   - Adjusting to a multitude of exits from and entries into the family system

   These experiences are particularly difficult when parents' values conflict with the relationships and types of lifestyles their children choose. An alteration in perception of one's parents also begins to occur during this time. Having always looked to parents for support and comfort, the middle-aged individual may suddenly find that the roles are beginning to reverse. Aging parents may look to their children for assistance with making decisions regarding their everyday lives and for assistance with chores that they have previously accomplished independently. When parents die, middle-aged individuals must come to terms with their own mortality. The process of recognition and resolution of one's own finitude begins in earnest at this time.
3. ***An alteration in perception of time:*** *Middle age* has been defined as the end of youth and the beginning of old age. Individuals often experience a sense that time is running out: "I haven't done all I want to do or accomplished all I intended to accomplish!" Depression and a sense of loss may occur as individuals realize that some of the goals established in their youth may go unmet.
   - The term *empty nest syndrome* has been used to describe the adjustment period parents experience when the last child leaves home to establish an independent residence. The crisis is often more profound for the mother who has devoted her life to nurturing her family. As the last child leaves, she may perceive her future as uncertain and meaningless.
   - Some women who have devoted their lives to rearing their children decide to develop personal interests and pursue personal goals once the children are grown. This occurs at a time when many husbands have begun to decrease what may have been a compulsive drive for

occupational security during the earlier years of their lives. This disparity in common goals may create conflict and require numerous adaptations on the part of both spouses.

- Finally, an alteration in one's perception of time may be related to the societal striving for eternal youth. The individual may try to delay the external changes that come with aging by the use of cosmetics, hormone creams, or even surgery. This yearning for youth may take the form of sexual promiscuity or extramarital affairs with much younger individuals in an effort to prove that one "still has what it takes." A negative view of oneself as an aging individual may lead to behaviors that are attempts to relive their youth.

Nursing intervention at the primary level of prevention with those in the developmental stage of midlife involves providing accurate information regarding changes that occur during this time of life and support for adapting to these changes effectively. The community is an appropriate place for this education since these experiences are shared by many of its members. These interventions might include the following:

- Nutrition classes to inform individuals in this age-group about the essentials of diet and exercise and the importance of good nutrition. Educational materials on how to avoid obesity or reduce weight can be included.
- Assistance with ways to improve health (e.g., quit smoking, cease or reduce alcohol consumption, reduce fat intake).
- Discussions of the importance of having regular physical examinations, including breast and cervical cancer screening for women and prostate examinations for men.
- Classes and support groups on menopause with information about what to expect.
- Support and information related to physical changes occurring in the body during this time of life and with the grief response that some individuals will experience in relation to loss of youth, "empty nest syndrome," and change in sense of identity.
- Support and information related to care of aging parents. Information and referral to community resources for respite and assistance *before* strain of the caregiver role threatens to disrupt the family system.

Retirement Retirement, which is often anticipated as an achievement in principle, may be met with a great deal of ambivalence when it actually occurs. Our society places a great deal of importance on productivity and on earning as much money as possible at as young an age as possible. These types of values contribute to the ambivalence associated with retirement. Although leisure has been acknowledged as a legitimate reward for workers, leisure during retirement has never been accorded the same social value. Adjustment to this life-cycle event becomes more difficult in the face of societal values that are in direct conflict with the new lifestyle.

Termination of child-rearing activities can result in a loss of self-worth, and individuals who are unable to adapt satisfactorily may become depressed.

It would appear that retirement is becoming, and will continue to become, more accepted by societal standards. With increasing numbers of individuals retiring earlier and living longer, the growing number of aging persons will spend a significantly longer time in retirement. Nursing intervention at the primary level of prevention with the developmental task of retirement involves providing information and support to individuals who have retired or are considering retirement and assessing individual needs with regard to continuing employment in older adulthood. Support can be on a one-to-one basis to assist individuals to sort out their feelings regarding retirement. Well-being in retirement is linked to factors such as stable health status, adequate income, the ability to pursue new goals or activities, extended social network of family and friends, and satisfaction with current living arrangements.

One trend that has been a hallmark of change for many older adults is the increasing numbers of grandparents who are caring for grandchildren and, in many cases, assuming primary responsibility for their care (Casper & Coritz, 2018). Nurses can promote primary prevention of crisis through education about resources for caregiving assistance and sharing what the evidence is teaching us about this new role. In fact, evidence shows that in spite of grief and burdens associated with caregiving, many grandparents identify that this role revealed their inner strength and gave them a sense of accomplishment (White & Cartwright, 2018).

Support can also be provided in a group environment. Support groups of individuals undergoing the same types of experiences can be extremely helpful. Nurses can form and lead these types of groups to assist retiring individuals through this critical period. These groups can also serve to provide information about available resources that offer assistance to individuals in or nearing retirement, such as information concerning Medicare, Social Security, and Medicaid; information related to organizations that specialize in hiring retirees; and information regarding ways to use newly acquired free time constructively.

Situational Crises

Situational crises are acute responses that occur as a result of an external circumstantial stressor. The number and types of situational stressors are limitless and may be real or exist only in the perception of the individual. Some types of situational crises that put individuals at risk for mental illness include the following:

- ***Poverty:*** A number of studies have identified poverty as a direct correlation to emotional illness. This may have to do with the direct consequences of poverty, such as inadequate and crowded living conditions, nutritional deficiencies, medical neglect, unemployment, or being homeless.
- ***High rate of life change events:*** Many studies have found that changes in life patterns due to a large number of significant events occurring in close proximity tend to decrease a person's ability to deal with stress, and physical or emotional illness may be the result (McLeod, 2010). These include life change events such as death of a loved one, divorce, being fired from a job, a change in living conditions, a change in place of employment or residence, physical illness, or a change in body image caused by the loss of a body part or function.
- ***Environmental conditions:*** Environmental conditions can create situational crises. Tornados, floods, hurricanes, and earthquakes have wreaked devastation on thousands of individuals and families in recent years.
- ***Trauma:*** Individuals who have encountered traumatic experiences must be considered at risk for emotional and physical illness. These include traumatic experiences usually considered outside the range of usual human experience, such as rape, war, physical attack, torture, or natural or man-made disaster.

Nursing intervention at the primary level of prevention with individuals experiencing situational crises is aimed at education about how to manage specific situational crises (such as disaster planning) and offering support and assistance with problem-solving during the crisis period. Nursing interventions for patients during a crisis include the following:

- Using a reality-oriented approach. The focus of the problem is on the here and now.
- Remaining with the individual who is experiencing panic anxiety.
- Establishing a rapid working relationship by showing unconditional acceptance, by active listening, and by attending to immediate needs.
- Discouraging lengthy explanations or rationalizations of the situation; promoting an atmosphere for verbalization of true feelings.
- Setting firm limits on aggressive, destructive behaviors. At high levels of anxiety, behavior is likely to be impulsive and regressive. Establish at the outset what is acceptable and what is not and maintain consistency.
- Clarifying the problem that the individual is facing. The nurse does this by describing their perception of the problem and comparing it with the individual's perception of the problem.
- Helping the individual determine what they believe precipitated the crisis.
- Acknowledging feelings of anger, guilt, helplessness, and powerlessness while taking care not to provide positive feedback for these feelings.
- Guiding the individual through a problem-solving process directed toward positive life change:
  - Helping the individual confront the source of the problem that is creating the crisis response.
  - Encouraging the individual to discuss changes they desire to make. Jointly determining whether these desired changes are realistic.
  - Encouraging exploration of feelings about aspects that cannot be changed and explore alternative ways of coping more adaptively in these situations.
  - Discussing alternative strategies for creating change in situations that can realistically be changed.
  - Weighing benefits and consequences of each alternative.
  - Assisting the individual to select alternative coping strategies that will help alleviate future crises.
- Identifying external support systems and new social networks from which the individual may seek assistance in times of stress.

Nursing at the level of primary prevention focuses largely on education of the consumer to prevent initiation or exacerbation of mental illness.

Secondary Prevention

Populations at Risk

Secondary prevention within communities relates to using early detection and prompt intervention with individuals experiencing mental illness symptoms. The same maturational and situational crises that are presented in the previous section on primary prevention are used to discuss intervention at the secondary level of prevention.

Maturational Crises

Adolescence The need for intervention at the secondary level of prevention in adolescence occurs when disruptive and age-inappropriate behaviors become the norm, and the family can no longer cope adaptively with the situation. All levels of dysfunction are considered—from dysfunctional family coping to the need for hospitalization of the adolescent.

Nursing intervention with the adolescent at the secondary level of prevention may occur in the community setting at community mental health centers, physician's offices, schools, public health departments, and crisis intervention centers. Nurses may work with families to problem solve and improve coping and communication skills, or they may work on a one-to-one basis with the adolescent in an attempt to modify behavior patterns.

Adolescents may be hospitalized for a variety of problems, including (but not limited to) conduct disorders, adjustment disorders, eating disorders, substance-related disorders, depression, and anxiety disorders. Inpatient care is determined by severity of symptomatology. Nursing care of adolescents in the hospital setting focuses on problem identification and stabilizing a crisis situation. Once stability has been achieved, patients are commonly discharged to outpatient care. If an adolescent's home situation has been deemed unsatisfactory, the state may take custody, and the child is then discharged to a group or foster home.

Marriage Problems that are not uncommon to the disruption of a marriage relationship include substance abuse on the part of one or both partners and disagreements on issues of sex, money, children, gender roles, and infidelity, among others.

Nursing intervention at the secondary level of prevention with individuals encountering marriage problems may include support groups for newly divorced individuals, referral to couples therapy, or referral to other specific treatment programs as needs are identified.

Divorce typically invokes a spectrum of troubling emotions including anger, mistrust, depression, and grief. Risks for clinical depression and suicide should always be a part of the assessment. Divorce also has an impact on the children involved. Group counseling with children who are manifesting behavioral or emotional problems associated with parental divorce is an important option for secondary prevention.

Parenthood Intervention at the secondary level of prevention with parents can be required for a number of reasons, such as:

- Physical, emotional, or sexual abuse of a child
- Physical or emotional neglect of a child
- Birth of a child with special needs
- Diagnosis of a terminal illness in a child
- Death of a child

Nursing intervention at the secondary level of prevention includes being able to recognize the physical and behavioral signs that indicate possible abuse of a child. The child may be cared for in the emergency department or as an inpatient on the pediatric unit or child psychiatric unit of a general hospital.

Nursing intervention with parents may include teaching effective methods of disciplining children, aside from physical punishment. Methods that emphasize the importance of positive reinforcement for acceptable behavior can be very effective. Family members must be committed to consistent use of this behavior modification technique for it to be successful.

Parents should also be informed about behavioral expectations at the various levels of development. Knowledge of what to expect from children at these various stages may provide needed anticipatory guidance to deal with the crises commonly associated with each stage.

Referral to family therapy may help family members to resolve communication problems. Members are encouraged to express honest feelings in a manner that is nonthreatening to other family members. Active listening, assertiveness techniques, and respect for the rights of others are taught and encouraged. Barriers to effective communication are identified and resolved.

Referrals to agencies that evaluate the family's ability to manage and safely care for each other may be warranted. Alternative agencies that may provide relief from the stress of parenting may also be considered (e.g., "Mom's Day Out" programs, sitter-sharing organizations, and day-care institutions). Support groups for abusive parents may also be helpful, and assistance in locating or initiating such a group may be provided.

The nurse can assist parents who are grieving the loss of a child or the birth of a child with special needs by helping them to express their feelings associated with the loss or by referring them to community support groups. Feelings such as shock, denial, anger, guilt, powerlessness, and hopelessness need to be expressed in order for the parents to progress through the grief response.

Home health care assistance can be provided for the family of a child with special needs. This can be done by making referrals to other professionals, such as speech, physical, and occupational therapists; medical social workers; psychologists; and nutritionists. If the child with special needs is hospitalized, the home health nurse can provide specific information to hospital staff that may be helpful in providing continuity of care for the client and help in the transition for the family.

Midlife Nursing care at the secondary level of prevention during midlife becomes necessary when the individual is unable to integrate all of the changes that are occurring during this period. An inability to accept the physical and biological changes, the changes in relationships between themselves and their adult children and aging parents, and the loss of the perception of youth may result in depression for which the individual may require help to resolve.

Retirement Retirement can also result in depression for individuals who are unable to satisfactorily grieve for the loss of this aspect of their lives. Depression is more likely to occur when individuals have not planned for retirement or when they have derived most of their self-esteem from their employment.

Nursing intervention at the secondary level of prevention with depressed individuals takes place in both inpatient and outpatient settings. Severely depressed patients with suicidal ideations will need close observation in the hospital setting, whereas those with mild to moderate depression may be treated in the community. A plan of care for the patient with depression is found in Chapter 16, "Depressive Disorders." These concepts apply to the secondary level of prevention and may be used in all nursing care settings.

Situational Crises

Nursing care at the secondary level of prevention with patients undergoing situational crises occurs only if crisis intervention at the primary level failed and the individual is unable to function socially or occupationally. Exacerbation of mental illness symptoms requires intervention at the secondary level of prevention. These disorders are addressed in pertinent chapters throughout Unit 3, "Care of Patients With Psychiatric Disorders." Nursing assessment, diagnosis and outcome identification, planning and implementation, and evaluation are discussed for many of the mental illnesses identified in the *DSM-5-TR* (APA, 2022). These skills may be applied in any setting where nursing is practiced.

A case study of nursing care at the secondary level of prevention in a community setting is presented on the next page.

Tertiary Prevention

Individuals With Severe and Persistent Mental Illness

Various terms such as *chronic mental illness, severe and persistent mental illness,* or *serious mental illness* have been used to describe disorders that contribute to significant functional impairment. The term *chronic* has been replaced by the latter two descriptors because "chronic" may have a negative connotation suggesting recovery is not possible (Substance Abuse and Mental Health Services Administration [SAMHSA], 2016). In fact, those with SMI can respond to treatment, services, and recovery-oriented support (SAMHSA, 2016). Furthermore, not all SMIs are severe *and* persistent.

The NIMH (2021) defines **serious mental illness (SMI)** as "a mental, behavioral, or emotional disorder resulting in serious functional impairment, which substantially interferes with or limits one or more major life activities." Those that are identified as "severe and persistent" are characterized by significant, ongoing, functional impairment and major disability. These disorders are identified by criteria listed in the *DSM-5-TR.* Diagnoses may include schizophrenia and related disorders, bipolar disorder, autism spectrum disorders, major depressive disorder, panic disorder, obsessive-compulsive disorder, post-traumatic stress disorder, borderline personality disorder, and attention deficit-hyperactivity disorder. Based on 2019 statistics, SMI affects about 5.2% of the population residing in the United States (NIMH, 2021). The actual number may be significantly higher because this research did not attempt to include the homeless, those in active military duty, or those who were in institutions such correctional facilities, nursing homes, mental institutions, or long-term hospitals for the entire year.

CASE STUDY AT SECONDARY LEVEL OF PREVENTION

PARENTHOOD

The identified patient was a petite, doll-like 4-year-old girl named Tanya. She was the older of two children in a Latino American family. The other child was a boy named Joseph, age 2. The mother was 5 months pregnant with their third child. The family had been referred to the nurse after Tanya was placed in foster care following a report to child protective services by her nursery school teacher that the child had marks on her body suspicious of child abuse.

The parents, Paulo and Annette, were in their mid-20s. Paulo had lost his job at an aircraft plant 3 months ago and had been unable to find work since. Annette brought in a few dollars from cleaning houses for other people, but the family was struggling to survive.

Paulo and Annette were angry at having to see the nurse. After all, "Parents have the right to discipline their children." The nurse did not focus on the *intent* of the behavior but instead looked at factors in the family's life that could be viewed as stressors. This family had multiple stressors: poverty, the father's unemployment, the age and spacing of the children, the mother's chronic fatigue from work at home and in other people's homes, and finally, having a child removed from the home against the parents' wishes.

During therapy with this family, the nurse discussed the behaviors associated with various developmental levels. She also discussed possible deviations from these norms and when they should be reported to the physician. The nurse and the family discussed Tanya's behavior and how it compared with the norms.

The parents also discussed their own childhoods. They were able to relate some of the same types of behaviors that they observed in Tanya. But they both admitted that they came from families whose main method of discipline was physical punishment. Annette had been the oldest child in her large family and had been expected to "keep the younger ones in line." When she had not done so, she was punished with her father's belt. She expressed anger toward her father, although she had never been allowed to express it at the time.

Paulo's father had died when he was a small boy, and Paulo had been expected to be the "man of the family." From the time he was very young, he worked at odd jobs to bring money into the home. Because of this, he had little time for the usual activities of childhood and adolescence. He held much resentment toward the young men who "had everything and never had to work for it."

Paulo and Annette had high expectations for Tanya. In effect, they expected her to behave in a manner well beyond her developmental level. These expectations were based on the reflections of their own childhoods. They were uncomfortable with the spontaneity and playfulness of childhood because they had had little personal experience with these behaviors. When Tanya balked and expressed the verbal assertions common to early childhood, Paulo and Annette interpreted these behaviors as defiance toward them and retaliated with anger in the manner in which they had been parented.

With the parents, the nurse explored feelings and behaviors from their past so that they were able to understand the correlation to their current behaviors. They learned to negotiate ways to deal with Tanya's age-appropriate behaviors. In combined therapy with Tanya, they learned how to relate to her childishness and even how to enjoy playing with both of their children.

The parents ceased blaming each other for the family's problems. Annette had spent a good deal of her time deprecating Paulo for his lack of support of his family, and Paulo blamed Annette for being "unable to control her daughter." Communication patterns were clarified, and life in the family became more peaceful.

Without a need to "prove himself" to his wife, Paulo's efforts to find employment met with success because he no longer felt the need to turn down jobs that he believed his wife would perceive to be beneath his capabilities. Annette no longer works outside the home, and both she and Paulo participate in the parenting chores. Tanya and her siblings continue to demonstrate age-appropriate developmental progression.

History and Epidemiology

The deinstitutionalization that began in the 1960s occurred rapidly and without sufficient planning for the needs of these individuals as they reentered the community. Individuals with support systems that could provide assistance with living arrangements and sheltered employment experiences most often received the outpatient treatment they required. Those without adequate support, however, either managed to survive on a meager income or were forced into homelessness. Some were sent to nursing homes meant to provide care for individuals with physical disabilities.

Certain segments of our population with severe and persistent mental illness have been left untreated: the elderly, the working poor, the homeless, and those individuals previously supported by funds that were cut by various social reforms. These circumstances have promoted a greater number of crisis-oriented emergency department visits and hospital admissions and repeated confrontations with law enforcement officials.

In 2002, President George W. Bush established the New Freedom Commission on Mental Health. This commission was charged with the task of conducting a comprehensive study of the U.S. mental health service delivery system. Members were to identify unmet needs and barriers to services and recommend steps for improvement in services and support for individuals with SMI. In July 2003, the Commission presented its final report (President's New Freedom Commission on Mental Health, 2003). The Commission identified the following five barriers:

1. ***Fragmentation and gaps in care for children:*** About 7% to 9% of children ages 9 to 17 have a serious emotional disturbance (SED). The Commission found that services for children are even more fragmented than those for adults with more uncoordinated funding and differing eligibility requirements. Only a fraction of children with SED appears to have access to school-based or school-linked mental health services. Children with SED who are identified for special education services have higher levels of absenteeism, higher drop-out rates, and lower levels of academic achievement than students with other disabilities.
2. ***Fragmentation and gaps in care for adults with SMI:*** The Commission expressed concern that so many adults with SMI are homeless, dependent on alcohol or drugs, unemployed, and go without treatment. The commission identified public attitudes and the stigma associated with mental illness as major barriers to treatment. Stigma is often internalized by individuals with mental illness, leading to hopelessness, lower self-esteem, and isolation. Stigma deprives these individuals of the support they need to recover.
3. ***High unemployment and disability for people with SMI:*** Undetected, untreated, and poorly treated mental disorders interrupt careers, leading many individuals into lives of disability, poverty, and long-term dependence. The Commission found a 90% unemployment rate among adults with SMI—the worst level of employment of any group of people with disabilities. Some surveys have shown that many individuals with SMI *want* to work—and could with modest assistance. However, the largest "program" of assistance the United States offers for people with mental illness is disability payments. Sadly, societal stigma is also reflected in employment discrimination against people with mental illness.
4. ***Older adults with mental illnesses are not receiving care:*** The Commission reported that about 5% to 10% of older adults have major depression, yet most are not properly recognized and treated. In its Interim Report (2002), the Commission clarified that:

> Older people are reluctant to get care from specialists. They feel more comfortable going to their primary care physician. Still, they are often more sensitive to the stigma of mental illness, and do not readily bring up their sadness and despair. If they acknowledge problems, they are more likely than young people to describe physical symptoms. Primary care doctors may see their suffering as "natural" aging or treat their reported physical distress instead of the underlying mental disorder. What is often missed is the deep impact of depression on older people's capacity to function in ways that are seemingly effortless for others. (p. 13)

5. ***Mental health and suicide prevention are not yet national priorities:*** The United States' failure to prioritize mental health puts many lives at stake. Families struggle to maintain equilibrium, while communities strain (and often fail) to provide needed assistance for adults and children with mental illness. The report noted that over 30,000 lives are lost annually to suicide. (In 2019, those numbers were dramatically higher, rising to 47,511 annual deaths by suicide.) About 90% of those who take their own lives have a mental disorder. Many individuals who die by suicide have not had the care in the months before their death that would have helped them. Both the APA and the National Mental Health Association called on the U.S. Congress to pass parity legislation.

As previously mentioned, in 2008, a federal law known as the Paul Wellstone and Pete Domenici Mental Health Parity and Addiction Equity Act was enacted that generally prevents group health plans and health insurance issuers that provide mental health or substance use disorder benefits from imposing less favorable limitations on those benefits than on medical/surgical benefits. In 2010, the Affordable Care Act amended this provision to include individual insurance plans, and in 2014, a final regulation clarified and expanded the parity law (Centers for Medicare & Medicaid Services [CMS], n.d.).

Many recent national initiatives since the commission's report have attempted to bridge the gaps, particularly with efforts to address the still climbing national suicide rates and the opiate overdose epidemic. Clearly, there is still much work to be done.

The Commission outlined the following goals and recommendations for mental health reform:

- ***Goal 1: Americans will understand that mental health is essential to overall health.***
  - Advance and implement a national campaign to reduce the stigma of seeking care and a national strategy for suicide prevention.
  - Address mental health with the same urgency as physical health.
- ***Goal 2: Mental health care will be consumer and family driven.***
  - Develop an individualized plan of care for every adult with SMI and child with SED.
  - Involve consumers and families fully in orienting the mental health system toward recovery.
  - Align relevant federal programs to improve access and accountability for mental health services.
  - Create a comprehensive state mental health plan.
  - Protect and enhance the rights of people with mental illness.
- ***Goal 3: Disparities in mental health services will be eliminated.***
  - Improve access to quality care that is culturally competent.
  - Improve access to quality care in rural and geographically remote areas.
- ***Goal 4: Early mental health screening, assessment, and referral to services will be common practice.***
  - Promote the mental health of young children.
  - Improve and expand school mental health programs.
  - Screen for co-occurring mental and substance use disorders and link with integrated treatment strategies.
  - Screen for mental disorders in primary health care, across the life span, and connect to treatment and supports.
- ***Goal 5: Excellent mental health care will be delivered and research will be accelerated.***
  - Accelerate research to promote recovery and resilience and ultimately to cure and prevent mental illnesses.
  - Advance evidence-based practices using dissemination and demonstration projects and create a public-private partnership to guide their implementation.
  - Improve and expand the workforce providing evidence-based mental health services and supports.
  - Develop the knowledge base in four understudied areas: mental health disparities, long-term effects of medications, trauma, and acute care.
- ***Goal 6: Technology will be used to access mental health care and information.***
  - Use health technology and telehealth to improve access and coordination of mental health care, especially for Americans in remote areas or in underserved populations.
  - Develop and implement integrated electronic health record and personal health information systems.

SAMHSA, in collaboration with a number of other federal agencies, is actively engaged in initiatives to address mental health issues for specific, underserved populations, for suicide prevention, and for a host of other community and public health concerns. The surgeon general released a landmark report in 2016 identifying substance abuse as a national health priority in response to the rising death toll from opiate overdoses (U.S. Department of Health and Human Services, Office of the Surgeon General, 2016). In 2018, the National Institutes of Health launched the HEAL (Helping End Addictions Long-term) effort that includes 15 initiatives geared toward better treatment of opiate addiction and pain management. There is no doubt much current national attention to mental health and addiction concerns particularly related to epidemic levels of suicide and opiate-related deaths. The solutions to the multitude of SMI and substance use-related issues that affect individuals and communities are complex and will require ongoing individual, local, and nationwide efforts.

Many nurse leaders see this period of health-care reform as an opportunity for nurses to expand their roles and assume key positions in education, prevention, assessment, and referral. Nurses are, and will continue to be, in key positions to assist individuals with severe and persistent mental illness to remain as independent as possible, to manage their illness within the community setting, and to strive to minimize the number of hospitalizations required.

Treatment Alternatives

In the current *Psychiatric-Mental Health Nursing: Scope and Standards of Practice* (American Psychiatric Nurses Association & International Society of Psychiatric-Mental Health Nurses, 2021), community-based care is identified as within the scope of practice for psychiatric mental health registered nurses. They define *community-based care* as potentially including "care delivered in partnership with health-care consumers in their homes, worksites, mental health clinics and programs, health maintenance organizations, shelters and clinics for the homeless, crisis centers, senior centers, group homes, and other community settings" (p. 24). It is clear that psychiatric nurses can and should play an active role in mental health care in the community.

Community Mental Health Centers The goal of community mental health centers in caring for individuals with severe and persistent mental illness is to improve coping ability and prevent exacerbation of acute symptoms. A major obstacle in meeting this goal has been the lack of advocacy or sponsorship for clients who require services from a variety of sources. This has placed responsibility for health care on an individual with mental illness who is often barely able to cope with everyday life. **Case management** (which is discussed in Chapter 6, "The Nursing Process in Psychiatric Mental Health Nursing") has become a recommended method of treatment for individuals with severe and persistent mental illness. Ling and Ruscin (2013) state:

> Nurses may be uniquely qualified to be case managers because of their holistic and broad-based background, understanding of health care, and role in patient education and referrals. Case management is an area of practice that offers nurses an opportunity to build on their clinical knowledge, communication, and nursing process skills to function in an expanded patient care role.

In its standards of practice, the Case Management Society of America (CMSA, 2020) defines case management as "a collaborative practice including patients, caregivers, nurses, social workers, physicians, payers, support staff, other practitioners and the community. The Case Management process facilitates communication and care coordination along a continuum through effective transitional care management" (p. 2). Ling and Ruscin (2013) identify six essential activities and nursing role functions that blend with the steps of the nursing process to form a framework for nursing case management:

1. ***Assessment:*** During the assessment process, the nurse gathers pertinent information about a patient's situation and ability to function. Information may be obtained through physical examination, patient interview, medical records, and reports from significant others. Ling and Ruscin state, "The case manager's goal is to obtain accurate information about the patient's status and identify factors that may significantly affect the patient's recovery and care."
2. ***Planning:*** A service care plan is devised with patient participation. The plan should include mutually agreed-on goals, specific actions directed toward goal achievement, and selection of essential resources and services through collaboration among health-care professionals, the patient, and the family or significant others.
3. ***Implementation:*** In this phase, the patient receives the needed services from the appropriate providers. In some instances, the nursing **case manager** is also a provider of care, whereas in others, they are simply the coordinator of care.
4. ***Coordination:*** The case manager "partners with patients/families/caregivers/community-based organizations and the health care team to jointly communicate, problem solve and share accountability for optimal outcomes" and "respects and incorporates patients' goals of care and treatment preferences while respecting available resources" (CMSA, 2020). This collaborative effort involves the patient, the physician, any other pertinent health-care providers, and family members or significant others concerned with the patient's care. The case manager ensures that all tests and treatments are conducted according to schedule and maintains close communication with all health-care providers to ensure that patient care is proceeding according to the plan.
5. ***Monitoring:*** The case manager monitors the effectiveness of the care plan by gathering pertinent information from various sources at regular intervals to determine the patient's response and ensures revision as needed (CMSA, 2020). If problems are identified, immediate adjustments are made.
6. ***Evaluation:*** The case manager evaluates the patient's responses to interventions and progress toward pre-established goals. Regular contact is maintained with patient, family or significant others, and direct service providers. Ongoing coordination of care continues until outcomes have been achieved. If the expected outcomes are not achieved, the case manager reevaluates the plan to determine the reason and takes steps to intervene and modify the existing plan.

A case study of nursing case management within a community mental health center is presented below.

CASE STUDY IN A COMMUNITY MENTAL HEALTH CENTER

NURSING CASE MANAGEMENT

William is a 63-year-old man with chronic schizophrenia who came into the community mental health center upon the recommendation of a local church where he sometimes attends their meal program. The nurse begins a comprehensive assessment and assures William that she wants to collaborate with him to identify how to best meet his needs. She assesses his basic physical health, management of daily living, family involvement, work history, involvement with any other social agencies, finances, medications, and other concerns identified by William. She determines that William has not been taking antipsychotic medication for at least 3 months. Prior to that, he had been living in a house with several other individuals, most of whom were abusing substances. They were helping him access medications from a community medication program but were often taking or reselling most of his prescription.

When the house was raided by police, William became homeless. He is currently disorganized in his thinking and actively hallucinating. He expresses desire to take medication but feels that finding a place to live is his most important priority. There is no family involvement, and William is unable to identify any support systems.

The nurse contacts the social worker for assistance with housing options and social resources such as food stamps and contacts the physician to schedule an appointment for medication evaluation. The nurse recommends that William attend the partial hospitalization program offered at the community mental health center, and he agrees but says he does not have transportation. The local church has offered to help William in any way they can, so the nurse contacts them and asks about their availability to provide transportation. The church informs her that they can provide transportation on Tuesdays and Thursdays.

During the assessment, William identified that sometimes the "people start fighting" in his mind and when he starts to scream back someone nearby always calls the police because they "don't get that I'm just trying to defend myself." The nurse then engages a peer support specialist who introduces William to Alfonzo, a 65-year-old man with chronic schizophrenia who is willing to provide support to William regarding symptom management. Alfonzo is also willing to provide transportation to the partial hospitalization program on the days when the church resources are not available. The nurse notices that William has some open sores on his feet. She cleans and bandages his feet, orders bloodwork to assess for infection, and accesses socks and footwear from the clothes bank offered through the Salvation Army. She continues to meet regularly with William once a month on a day that he attends a partial hospitalization program and administers the injectable antipsychotic medication (fluphenazine [Prolixin]) ordered by the physician. During her reassessment, William identifies that he has been "hanging out" with Alfonzo and states "he really understands me." He expresses that he still hears people fight sometimes in his head but is not as bothered by them. The social worker has facilitated group home placement, which is not available for another 3 months, but in the meantime the local homeless shelter has arranged for William to stay there. The local church has offered William a small stipend to help with stuffing envelopes, and when the nurse asks him how that job is going, William says, "They are nice people at the church, and they say I really help them, too."

Assertive Community Treatment (ACT) The National Alliance on Mental Illness (NAMI, 2021) defines *ACT* as:

> a team-based treatment model that provides multidisciplinary, flexible treatment and support to people with mental illness 24/7. ACT is based around the idea that people receive better care when their mental health care providers work together. ACT team members help the person address every aspect of their life, whether it be medication, therapy, social support, employment or housing.

This approach includes members from psychiatry, social work, nursing, and substance abuse and vocational rehabilitation. The ACT team provides these services 24 hours a day, 7 days a week, 365 days a year.

The ACT team provides treatment, rehabilitation, and support services to individuals with severe and persistent mental illness who are unable on their own to receive treatment from a traditional model of case management. The team is usually able to provide most services with minimal referrals to other mental health programs or providers. Services are provided within community settings, such as a person's home, local restaurants, parks, nearby stores, and any other place that the individual requires assistance with living skills.

Partial Hospitalization Programs Partial hospitalization programs (also called day or evening treatment programs) are designed to prevent institutionalization or to ease the transition from inpatient hospitalization to community living. Various types of treatment are offered. Many include therapeutic community (milieu) activities; individual, group, and family therapies; psychoeducation; alcohol and drug education; crisis intervention; therapeutic recreational activities; and occupational therapy. Many programs offer medication administration and monitoring as part of their care. Some programs have established medication clinics for individuals on long-term psychopharmacological therapy. These clinics may include educational classes and support groups for individuals with similar conditions and treatments.

Partial hospitalization programs generally offer a comprehensive treatment plan formulated by an interdisciplinary team of psychiatrists, psychologists, nurses, occupational and recreational therapists, and social workers. Nurses take a leading role in the administration of partial hospitalization programs. They lead groups, provide crisis intervention, conduct individual counseling, act as role models, and make necessary referrals for specialized treatment. Use of the nursing process provides continual evaluation of the program, and modifications can be made as necessary.

Partial hospitalization programs are an effective method of preventing hospitalization for many individuals with severe and persistent mental illness. They are a way of transitioning individuals from the acute care setting back into the mainstream of the community. For some individuals who have been deinstitutionalized, they provide structure, support, opportunities for socialization, and an improvement in their overall quality of life.

Community Residential Facilities Community residential facilities for persons with severe and persistent mental illness are known by many names: group homes, halfway houses, foster homes, boarding homes, sheltered care facilities, transitional housing, independent living programs, social rehabilitation residences, and others. These facilities differ by the purpose for which they exist and the activities that they offer.

Some of these facilities provide food, shelter, housekeeping, and minimal supervision and assistance with activities of daily living. Others may also include a variety of therapies and serve as a transition between hospital and independent living. In addition to the basics, services might include individual and group counseling, medical care, job training or employment assistance, and leisure-time activities.

The concept of transitional housing for individuals with SMI is sound and has often been a successful means of therapeutic support and intervention to facilitate residence within the community. However, without guidance and planning, transition to the community can be problematic. These individuals may be ridiculed and rejected by the community or become targets of unscrupulous individuals who take advantage of their inability to care for themselves satisfactorily. A period of structured reorientation to the community in a living situation that is supervised and monitored by professionals is more likely to result in a successful transition for the individual with severe and persistent mental illness.

Psychiatric Home Health Care For the individual with SMI who no longer lives in a structured, supervised setting, home health care may provide the resources needed to live independently. To receive home health care, individuals must validate their homebound status for the prospective payer (Medicare, Medicaid, most insurance companies, and Department of Veterans Affairs [VA] benefits). An acute psychiatric diagnosis is not enough to qualify for the service. The client must be unable to leave the home without considerable difficulty or the assistance of another person. The plan of treatment and subsequent charting must explain why the client's psychiatric disorder keeps them at home and justify the need for home services.

Homebound clients most often have a diagnosis of depressive disorder, neurocognitive disorder, anxiety disorder, bipolar disorder, or schizophrenia. Many older clients are homebound because of medical conditions that impair mobility and necessitate home care.

Nurses who provide psychiatric home care must have an in-depth knowledge of psychopathology, psychopharmacology, and how medical and physical problems can be influenced by psychiatric impairments. These nurses must be highly adept at performing biopsychosocial assessments. They must be sensitive to changes in behavior that signal psychiatric or medical decompensation so that early intervention may be implemented.

Another important job of the psychiatric home health nurse is monitoring the patient's adherence to the regimen of psychotropic medications. Some patients who are receiving injectable medications remain on home health care only until they can be placed on oral medications. Those receiving oral medications require close monitoring for adherence and assistance with the uncomfortable side effects of some of these drugs. Lack of adherence to the medication regimen is responsible for approximately two-thirds of psychiatric hospital readmissions. Home health nurses can assist patients with this problem by helping them to see the relationship between control of their psychiatric symptoms and adherence to their medication regimen.

Patient populations that benefit from psychiatric home health nursing include:

- ***Older adults:*** These individuals may not have a psychiatric diagnosis, but they may be experiencing emotional difficulties that have arisen from medical, sociocultural, or developmental factors. Depressed mood and social isolation are common.
- ***Persons with severe and persistent mental illness:*** These individuals have a history of psychiatric illness and hospitalization. They require long-term medications and continual supportive care. Common diagnoses include recurrent major depressive disorder, schizophrenia, and bipolar disorder.
- ***Individuals in acute crisis situations:*** These individuals are in need of crisis intervention and/or referral for short-term psychotherapy.

Psychiatric home nursing care is typically provided by nurses who have special training and/or experience beyond the standard curriculum require for a registered nurse. Preparation for psychiatric home health nursing, in addition to registered nurse licensure, should include several years of psychiatric inpatient treatment experience. It is also recommended that the nurse have medical-surgical nursing experience because this patient commonly has several medical comorbidities. Additional training and experience in psychotherapy are viewed as helpful but not required. Psychotherapy is not the primary focus of psychiatric home nursing care. In fact, most reimbursement sources do not pay for exclusively insight-oriented therapy. Crisis intervention, patient education, and hands-on care are common interventions in psychiatric home nursing care.

The psychiatric home health nurse provides comprehensive nursing care, incorporating interventions for physical and psychosocial problems into the treatment plan. The interventions are based on the patient's mental and physical health status, cultural influences, and available resources. The nurse is accountable to the patient at all times during the therapeutic relationship. Nursing interventions are carried out with appropriate knowledge and skill, and referrals are made when the need is outside the scope of nursing practice. Continued collaboration with other members of the health-care team (e.g., psychiatrist, social worker, psychologist, occupational therapist, and/or physical therapist) is essential for maintaining continuity of care.

See the following case study on psychiatric home health care and the nursing process. A plan of care for Mrs. C (the client in the case study) is presented in Table 26–1. Nursing diagnoses are presented, along with outcome criteria, appropriate nursing interventions, and rationale for each.

Care for the Caregivers Psychiatric home health care also provides support and assistance to primary caregivers. When family is the provider of care on a 7-day-a-week, 24-hour-a-day schedule for a loved one with a severe and persistent mental disorder, it can be very exhausting and very frustrating. A care plan for primary caregivers is presented in Table 26–2.

The Homeless Population

History and Epidemiology

In 1993, Dr. Richard Lamb, a recognized expert in the field of severe and persistent mental illness, wrote:

> Alec Guinness, in his memorable role as a British Army colonel in *Bridge on the River Kwai*, exclaims at the end of the film when he finally realizes he has been working to help the enemy, "What have I done?" As a vocal advocate and spokesman for deinstitutionalization and community treatment of severely mentally ill patients for well over two decades, I often find myself asking that same question. (p. 1209)

Individuals with SMI are a high-risk population for homelessness. It is difficult to determine the true scope of the problem because even the statisticians who collect the data have difficulty defining *homeless persons.* They have sometimes been identified as "those people who sleep in shelters or public spaces." Since not all those who are homeless are able to access shelters, and public spaces are difficult to define, statistics about the number of homeless individuals with SMI are underestimated.

According to the Stewart B. McKinney Homeless Assistance Act (Govtrack, 1987), a person is considered homeless who

> lacks a fixed, regular, and adequate night-time residence; and . . . has a primary night-time residency that is: (A) a supervised publicly or privately operated shelter designed to provide temporary living accommodations, (B) an institution that provides a temporary residence for individuals intended to be institutionalized, or (C) a public or private place not designed for, or ordinarily used as, a regular sleeping accommodation for human beings.

CASE STUDY FOR PSYCHIATRIC HOME HEALTH CARE

NURSING HISTORY AND ASSESSMENT

Mrs. C, age 76, has been living alone in her small apartment for 6 months since the death of her husband to whom she had been married for 51 years. Mrs. C had been an elementary school teacher for 40 years, retiring at age 65 with an adequate pension. She and her husband had no children. A niece looks in on Mrs. C regularly. It was she who contacted Mrs. C's physician when she observed that Mrs. C was not eating properly, was losing weight, and seemed to be isolating herself more and more. She had not left her apartment in weeks. Her physician referred her to psychiatric home health care.

On her initial visit, Renee, the psychiatric home health nurse, conducted a preliminary assessment, revealing the following information about Mrs. C:

1. Blood pressure 90/60 mm Hg
2. Height 5 ft 5 in.; weight 102 lb
3. Poor skin turgor; dehydration
4. Subjective report of occasional dizziness
5. Subjective report of loss of 20 pounds since the death of her husband
6. Oriented to time, place, person, and situation
7. Memory (remote and recent) intact
8. Flat affect
9. Mood is dysphoric and tearful at times, but client is cooperative
10. Denies thoughts to harm self but states, "I feel so alone; so useless."
11. Subjective report of difficulty sleeping
12. Subjective report of constipation

DIAGNOSIS AND OUTCOME IDENTIFICATION

The following nursing diagnoses were formulated for Mrs. C:

1. Complicated grieving related to death of husband evidenced by symptoms of depression such as withdrawal, anorexia, weight loss, difficulty sleeping, dysphoric/tearful mood
2. Risk for injury related to dizziness and weakness from lack of activity, low blood pressure, and poor nutritional status
3. Social isolation related to depressed mood and feelings of worthlessness, evidenced by staying home alone, refusing to leave her apartment

OUTCOME CRITERIA

The following criteria were selected as measurement of outcomes in the care of Mrs. C:

- Experiences no physical harm/injury
- Is able to discuss feelings about husband's death with nurse
- Sets realistic goals for self
- Is able to participate in problem-solving regarding her future
- Eats a well-balanced diet with snacks to restore nutritional status and gain weight
- Drinks adequate fluids daily
- Sleeps at least 6 hours per night and verbalizes feeling well rested
- Shows interest in personal appearance and hygiene and is able to accomplish self-care independently
- Seeks to renew contact with previous friends and acquaintances
- Verbalizes interest in participating in social activities

PLANNING AND IMPLEMENTATION

A care plan for Mrs. C is presented in Table 26–1.

EVALUATION

Mrs. C started the second week taking trazodone (Desyrel) 150 mg at bedtime. Her sleep was enhanced, and within 2 weeks she showed a noticeable improvement in mood. She began to discuss how angry she felt about being all alone in the world. She admitted that she had felt anger toward her husband but experienced guilt and tried to suppress that anger. As she was assured that these feelings were normal, they became easier for her to express.

The nurse arranged for a local teenager to do some weekly grocery shopping for Mrs. C and contacted the local Meals on Wheels program, which delivered her noon meal to her every day. Mrs. C began to eat more and slowly to gain a few pounds. She still has an occasional problem with constipation but verbalizes improvement with the addition of vegetables, fruit, and a daily stool softener prescribed by her physician.

Mrs. C used her walker until she felt she was able to ambulate without assistance. She reports that she no longer experiences dizziness, and her blood pressure has stabilized at around 100/70 mm Hg.

Mrs. C has joined a senior citizens group and attends activities weekly. She has renewed previous friendships and formed new acquaintances. She sees her physician monthly for medication management and visits a local adult day health center for regular blood pressure and weight checks. Her niece still visits regularly, but her favorite relationship is the one she has formed with her constant canine companion, Molly, whom Mrs. C rescued from the local animal shelter and who continually demonstrates her unconditional love and gratitude.

Table 26–1 | CARE PLAN FOR PSYCHIATRIC HOME HEALTH CARE OF DEPRESSED OLDER ADULT (MRS. C)

NURSING DIAGNOSIS: MALADAPTIVE GRIEVING

RELATED TO: Death of husband

EVIDENCED BY: Symptoms of depression such as withdrawal, anorexia, weight loss, difficulty sleeping, and dysphoric/tearful mood

OUTCOME CRITERIA	NURSING INTERVENTIONS	RATIONALE
Short-Term Goal ■ Mrs. C will discuss any angry feelings she has about the loss of her husband. **Long-Term Goal** ■ Mrs. C demonstrates adaptive grieving behaviors and evidence of progression toward resolution.	1. Assess Mrs. C's position in the grief process.	1. Accurate baseline data are required to plan accurate care for Mrs. C.
	2. Develop a trusting relationship by showing empathy and caring. Be honest and keep all promises. Show genuine positive regard.	2. These interventions provide the basis for a therapeutic relationship.
	3. Explore feelings of anger and help Mrs. C direct them toward the source. Help her understand it is appropriate and acceptable to have feelings of anger and guilt about her husband's death.	3. Knowledge of acceptability of the feelings associated with normal grieving may help to relieve some of the guilt that these responses generate.
	4. Encourage Mrs. C to review honestly the relationship she had with her husband. With support and sensitivity, point out the reality of the situation in areas where misrepresentations may be expressed.	4. Ability to explore positive and negative aspects of the relationship and the loss facilitates grief work.
	5. Determine whether Mrs. C has spiritual needs that are unfulfilled. If so, contact spiritual leader for intervention with Mrs. C.	5. Recovery may be blocked if spiritual distress is present and care is not provided.
	6. Refer Mrs. C to physician for medication evaluation.	6. Antidepressant therapy may be helpful for treating symptoms of major depressive disorder.

NURSING DIAGNOSIS: RISK FOR INJURY

RELATED TO: Dizziness and weakness from lack of activity, low blood pressure, and poor nutritional status

OUTCOME CRITERIA	NURSING INTERVENTIONS	RATIONALE
Short-Term Goals ■ Mrs. C will use walker when ambulating. ■ Mrs. C will not experience physical harm or injury. **Long-Term Goal** ■ Mrs. C will not experience physical harm or injury.	1. Assess vital signs at every visit. Report to physician should they fall below baseline.	1. Patient safety is a nursing priority.
	2. Encourage Mrs. C to use walker until strength has returned.	2. The walker will help prevent Mrs. C from falling.
	3. Visit Mrs. C during mealtimes and sit with her while she eats. Encourage her niece to do the same. Ensure that easy-to-prepare, nutritious foods for meals and snacks are available in the house and that they are items that Mrs. C likes.	3. She is more likely to eat what is convenient and what she enjoys.

Table 26–1 | CARE PLAN FOR PSYCHIATRIC HOME HEALTH CARE OF DEPRESSED OLDER ADULT (MRS. C)—cont'd

OUTCOME CRITERIA	NURSING INTERVENTIONS	RATIONALE
	4. Contact local meal delivery service (e.g., Meals on Wheels) to deliver some of Mrs. C's meals.	4. This would ensure that she receives at least one complete and nutritious meal each day.
	5. Weigh Mrs. C each week.	5. Weight gain is a measurable, objective means of assessing whether Mrs. C is eating.
	6. Ensure that diet contains sufficient fluid and fiber.	6. Adequate dietary fluid and fiber will help to alleviate constipation. She may also benefit from a daily stool softener.

NURSING DIAGNOSIS: SOCIAL ISOLATION
RELATED TO: Depressed mood and feelings of worthlessness
EVIDENCED BY: Staying home alone, refusing to leave apartment

OUTCOME CRITERIA	NURSING INTERVENTIONS	RATIONALE
Short-Term Goal ■ Mrs. C will discuss with nurse feelings about past social relationships and those she may like to renew.	1. As nutritional status improves and strength is gained, encourage Mrs. C to become more active. Take walks with her; help her perform simple tasks around her house.	1. Increased activity enhances both physical and mental status.
Long-Term Goal ■ Mrs. C will renew contact with friends and participate in social activities.	2. Assess lifelong patterns of relationships.	2. Mrs. C will very likely keep the same style of relationship development that she had in the past.
	3. Help her identify present relationships that are satisfying and activities that she considers interesting.	3. She is the person who truly knows what she likes, and these personal preferences will facilitate success in reversing social isolation.
	4. Assess mental status for mood changes and risk for suicide.	4. Mrs. C. has expressed feelings of depression and worthlessness, so her mental status should be assessed regularly to identify any worsening of symptoms and risk for suicide.
	5. Consider the feasibility of a pet.	5. There are many documented studies of the benefits to elderly individuals of companion pets.
	6. Suggest possible alternatives that Mrs. C may consider as she seeks to participate in social activities. These may include foster grandparent programs, senior citizens centers, church activities, craft groups, and volunteer activities. Help her to locate individuals with whom she may attend some of these activities.	6. These interventions facilitate goal-directed task completion.

Table 26–2 | CARE PLAN FOR PRIMARY CAREGIVER OF INDIVIDUAL WITH SEVERE AND PERSISTENT MENTAL ILLNESS

NURSING DIAGNOSIS: CAREGIVER ROLE STRAIN

RELATED TO: Severity and duration of the care receiver's illness and lack of respite and recreation for the caregiver

EVIDENCED BY: Feelings of stress in relationship with care receiver, feelings of depression and anger, family conflict around issues of providing care

OUTCOME CRITERIA	NURSING INTERVENTIONS	RATIONALE
Short-Term Goal ■ Caregivers will verbalize understanding of ways to facilitate the caregiver role. **Long-Term Goal** ■ Caregivers will demonstrate effective problem-solving skills and develop adaptive coping mechanisms to regain equilibrium.	1. Assess caregivers' abilities to anticipate and fulfill the individual's unmet needs. Provide information to assist caregivers with this responsibility. Ensure that caregivers encourage individual to be as independent as possible.	1. Caregivers may be unaware of what their loved one can realistically accomplish. They may be unaware of the nature of the illness.
	2. Ensure that caregivers are aware of available community support systems from which they may seek assistance when required. Examples include respite care services, day treatment centers, and adult day-care centers.	2. Referral to community support resources facilitates stress reduction in the caregiver. Studies have shown that abuse risk increases in situations where the caregiver is highly stressed and overwhelmed (Patel et al., 2021).
	3. Encourage caregivers to express feelings, particularly anger.	3. Accepting the caregiver's discussion of feelings promotes exploring adaptive coping behaviors.
	4. Encourage participation in support groups composed of members with similar life situations. Provide information about support groups that may be helpful: a. National Alliance on Mental Illness (NAMI) b. American Association on Intellectual and Developmental Disabilities (AAIDD) c. Alzheimer's Association	4. Hearing others who are experiencing the same problems discuss ways in which they have coped may help caregiver adopt more adaptive strategies. Individuals who are experiencing similar life situations provide empathy and support for each other.

The National Alliance to End Homelessness (2020) reports that overall homelessness declined by 12% since 2007, but this trend may be changing since 2019 marked annual increases for the third year in a row. The largest reductions have occurred among veterans in which homelessness has decreased by 50%. However, about 33% of the current homeless population have some form of SMI (National Coalition for the Homeless [NCH], 2017) and one of the cited contributing factors is limited access to inpatient psychiatric treatment. Homelessness among the mentally ill continues to be a significant concern for this vulnerable population.

Many homeless individuals are children and young adults. Some are homeless because of their dependence on a parent who is homeless, but many are trauma victims who have left their homes to avoid physical or sexual abuse and neglect. Some are LGBTQ (lesbian, gay, bisexual, transgender, or questioning) youth who have become homeless secondary to family intolerance about their sexual orientation and identity (Safe horizon, 2018).

On a single night in 2020, there were reported 34,210 unaccompanied homeless youths, representing just over 6% of the total homeless population, and just over 50% of those youths were unsheltered (U.S. Department of Housing and Urban Development [HUD], 2021). Many initiatives have sought to reduce these numbers and to provide resources to minimize disruptions posed by homelessness. In October 2016, amendments to the McKinney-Vento Act went into effect that include provisions for homeless children and young adults to receive adequate and accessible education. However, these provisions do not address the child who is "on the run." These children remain a high-risk, vulnerable population who often have a history of trauma as well as additional trauma posed by homelessness and sex trafficking.

Mental Illness and Homelessness

Demographics The prevalence of SMI among the homeless population is difficult to clarify. SAMHSA (2020) provides the following demographics through statistics gathered from Projects for Assistance in Transition from Homelessness (PATH), which was specifically established for funding services to people with SMI. Thus, these statistics are based on the makeup of PATH clients:

- ***Age:*** Approximately 19.9% of PATH clients with SMI are younger than age 30; individuals between the ages of 31 and 61 make up the bulk of this population at 72.4%; about 7.7% are 62 years or older.
- ***Gender:*** Male individuals comprise approximately 59.1% of the homeless population with SMI; 39.9% are female; 0.5% are transgender or gender nonconforming.
- ***Ethnicity and race:*** The homeless SMI population is estimated to be 55.4% white, 34.4% African American, 14.4% Hispanic/Latino, 3.8% American Indian or Alaska Native, and 0.9% Asian. The ethnic makeup of homeless populations varies according to geographic location.

A reported 33% of the homeless population are individuals with untreated SMI (Treatment Advocacy Center, 2018). Who are these individuals, and why are they homeless? Some blame the deinstitutionalization movement. Persons with mental illness who were released from state and county mental hospitals and who did not have families with whom they could reside sought residence in board and care homes of varying quality. Halfway houses and supportive group living arrangements were helpful but scarce. Many of those with families returned to their homes, but because families received little, if any, instruction or support, the consequences of their mentally ill loved one returning to live at home were often turbulent, resulting in the individual frequently leaving home.

Types of Mental Illness Among the Homeless Several studies have been conducted (primarily in large, urban areas) that have addressed the most common types of mental illness identified among homeless individuals. Schizophrenia is frequently described as the most common diagnosis. Other prevalent disorders include bipolar disorder, substance addiction, depression, personality disorders, and neurocognitive disorders. Many exhibit psychotic symptoms, are former residents of long-term care institutions for the mentally ill, and have isolated themselves in an effort to avoid being identified as a part of the mental health system. Many are a danger to themselves or others, yet they often do not even see themselves as ill. Substance use disorders are a common comorbidity.

Contributing Factors to Homelessness Among Individuals With Mental Illness

Deinstitutionalization As previously stated, deinstitutionalization is frequently implicated as a contributing factor to homelessness among individuals with mental illness. Deinstitutionalization began out of expressed concern by mental health professionals and others who described the "deplorable conditions" under which mentally ill individuals were housed.

Certainly another motivating factor for deinstitutionalization was the financial burden these clients placed on state governments.

Although the deinstitutionalization movement has prompted an expansion of community mental health resources, the number of people with mental illness being incarcerated in correctional facilities has skyrocketed and is now estimated to be two to four times that of the general population (National Institute of Corrections, n.d.). Supporters of the community mental health movement have argued that ongoing problems for those with severe mental illness are related to lack of compliance with medications, but critics have argued that the community mental health model has been too narrowly focused on a biomedical approach and must revise and expand its model of services to meet the complex needs of this population going forward.

Deinstitutionalization has been criticized for contributing to both homelessness rates and criminalization of people with mental illnesses, but several other factors have been implicated as well.

Poverty Cuts in various government entitlement programs have depleted the allotments available for individuals with severe and persistent mental illness living in the community. The job market is prohibitive for individuals whose behavior is incomprehensible or even frightening to many. The stigma and discrimination associated with mental illness may be diminishing slowly, but it is highly visible to those who suffer from its effects.

Scarcity of Affordable Housing Not only is there a scarcity of affordable housing, but the number of single-room-occupancy (SRO) hotels has diminished drastically. These SRO hotels provided a means of relatively inexpensive housing, and although some people believe that these facilities nurtured isolation, they provided adequate shelter from the elements for their occupants. Because so many mentally ill individuals rely on homeless shelters, there is concern that shelters are becoming mini-institutions for individuals with SMI.

Other Factors Several other factors that may contribute to homelessness have been identified:

- ***Lack of affordable health care:*** For families barely able to pay for their day-to-day living expenses, a catastrophic illness can start the downward spiral to homelessness.
- ***Domestic violence:*** According to a Family and Youth Services Report (2016) up to 57% of homeless women identify domestic violence as the primary reason for homelessness. Other research has found that 93% of homeless mothers had a history of trauma, 79% experienced trauma as children, and 81% experienced multiple traumatic events (NCH, 2015). The need for trauma-informed care in this population cannot be overstated.
- ***Substance use disorders:*** For individuals with alcohol or drug addictions, in the absence of appropriate treatment, the chances increase for being forced into life on the street. The following have been cited as obstacles to addiction treatment for homeless persons: lack of health insurance, lack of documentation, waiting lists, scheduling difficulties, daily contact requirements, lack of transportation, ineffective treatment methods, lack of supportive services, and cultural insensitivity.

Challenges in Caring for Homeless Individuals With SMI

Interfering Factors Among the many issues that complicate service planning for homeless individuals with mental illness is this population's mobility. Frequent relocation confounds service delivery and interferes with providers' efforts to ensure appropriate care. Some individuals with SMI may be affected by homelessness only temporarily or intermittently. These individuals are sometimes called the "episodically homeless." Others move around within neighborhoods or cities as needs change and based on whether or not they can obtain needed services. Many homeless individuals with SMI exhibit continuous unbounded movement over wide geographical areas.

Not all homeless individuals with mental illness are mobile. Health-care workers must identify movement patterns of homeless people in their area to at least try to bring the best care possible to this unique population. This effort may mean delivering services to those individuals who do not seek out services on their own.

Health Issues Life as a homeless person can have severe consequences in terms of health. Exposure to the elements, poor diet, sleep deprivation, risk of violence, injuries, and little or no health care can all lead to a precarious state of health and exacerbate any pre-existing illnesses. Compared with other homeless individuals, those who abuse alcohol are at greater risk for neurological impairment, heart disease and hypertension, chronic lung disease, gastrointestinal disorders, hepatic dysfunction, and trauma.

Thermoregulation is a health problem for all homeless individuals because of their exposure to all kinds of weather and a compounded problem for the homeless alcoholic who is at higher risk for hypothermia.

It is difficult to determine whether mental illness is a cause or an effect of homelessness. Some behaviors that may seem deviant may be adaptations to life on the street. It has been suggested that some homeless individuals may even seek hospitalization in psychiatric institutions in an attempt to get off the streets for a short time.

Whereas tuberculosis (TB) rates in the United States have been on the decline for several years, the homeless remain an at-risk population; 5% of those with TB reported homelessness within the prior year (Centers for Disease Control and Prevention, 2020).

Crowded shelters provide ideal conditions for spread of respiratory infections among their inhabitants. These concerns have been amplified during the global COVID pandemic prompting the CDC to reinforce the critical need to maintain shelter services for the homeless population and to identify guidelines for minimizing spread of infections, including the recommendation that communities identify the need for overflow sites to maintain safe distancing in shelters (CDC, 2022). The risk of acquiring TB is also increased by the prevalence of alcoholism, drug addiction, HIV infection, poor nutrition, and lack of access to medical care among homeless individuals.

Dietary deficiencies are a continuing problem for homeless individuals. Not only is the homeless person commonly in a poor nutritional state, but the condition itself exacerbates a number of other health problems. Homeless people have higher mortality rates and a greater number of serious disorders than their counterparts in the general population.

Sexually transmitted infections (STIs), such as gonorrhea and syphilis, are a serious problem for the homeless. One of the most serious STIs prevalent among homeless individuals is HIV infection. Street life is precarious for individuals who are immunosuppressed by HIV. Rummaged food scraps are often spoiled, and exposure to the elements is a continuous threat. Individuals with HIV disease who stay in shelters often are exposed to the infectious diseases of others, which can be life threatening in their vulnerable condition.

Homeless children have special health needs. Children without a home are more vulnerable to asthma, ear infections, stomach problems, and speech problems than their counterparts who are not homeless. They also experience more mental health problems, such as anxiety, depression, and withdrawal. They are twice as likely to experience hunger and four times as likely to have delayed development.

A growing problem, which has captured national attention, is the increasing number of hate crimes perpetrated against the homeless. These attacks do not appear to be specifically directed toward the mentally ill but rather reflect a primary bias against homeless people. Based on the most recent report by NCH (2018), most of the victims (83%) are male, 69% are 40 years of age or older, and almost 43% of the attacks are fatal. Most of the perpetrators were male and 67% were younger than age 30. The NCH adds that there is a documented correlation between laws that criminalize homelessness and increases in attacks on the homeless, possibly because it sends a message to the public that "'homeless people do not matter and are not worthy of living in our city.' This message is blatant in the attitudes many cities have toward homeless people and can be used as an internal justification for attacking someone" (2018, p. 17). Many attacks are not even reported, and those who survive the attacks are vulnerable to post-traumatic stress disorder. Community mental health nurses have an opportunity and a responsibility to assess and intervene for homeless people, who are a vulnerable population on so many levels.

Community Resources for the Homeless

Homeless Shelters The system of **shelters** for the homeless in the United States varies widely from converted warehouses that provide cots or floor space on which to sleep overnight to significant operations that provide a multitude of social and health-care services. They are run by volunteers and paid professionals and are sponsored by churches, local governments, and a variety of social agencies.

It is impossible, then, to describe a "typical" shelter. One profile may be described as the provision of lodging, food, and clothing to individuals who are in need of these services. Some shelters also provide medical and psychiatric evaluations, first aid and other health-care services, and referral for case management services by nurses or social workers.

Individuals who seek services from the shelter are generally assigned a bed or cot, issued a set of clean linen, provided a place to shower, given access to laundry facilities, and offered a meal in the shelter kitchen or dining hall. Most shelters attempt to separate dormitory areas for men and women with various consequences for those who violate the rules.

Shelters cover expenses through private and corporate donations, church sponsorships, and government grants. From the outset, shelters were conceptualized as "temporary" accommodations for individuals who needed a place to spend the night. Realistically, they have become permanent lodging for some homeless individuals with little hope for improving their situation. Some individuals use shelters for their mailing address.

Shelters provide a safe and supportive environment for homeless individuals who have no other place to go. Some homeless people who inhabit shelters use the resources offered to improve their lot in life, whereas others become dependent on the shelter's provisions.

Health-Care Centers and Storefront Clinics Some communities have established "street clinics" to serve the homeless population. Many of these clinics are operated by nurse practitioners who work in consultation with physicians in the area. In recent years, some of these health-care clinics have provided clinical sites for nursing students in their community health rotation. Some have been staffed by faculties of nursing schools that have established group practices in the community setting.

A wide variety of services are offered at these clinics, including administering medications, assessing vital signs, screening for TB and other communicable diseases, giving immunizations and flu shots, changing dressings, and administering first aid. Physical and psychosocial assessments, health education, and supportive counseling are also frequent interventions.

Nursing in **storefront clinics** for the homeless provides many special challenges, not the least of which is poor working conditions. These clinics often operate under severe budgetary constraints with inadequate staffing, supplies, and equipment in rundown facilities located in high-crime neighborhoods. Frustration is often high among nurses who work in these clinics because they are seldom able to see measurable progress in their homeless patients. Maintenance of health management is virtually impossible for many individuals who have no resources outside the health-care setting. When return appointments for preventive care are made, the lack of follow-through is high.

Mobile Outreach Units **Mobile outreach units** literally reach out to the homeless in their own environment in an effort to provide health care. Volunteers and paid professionals form teams to drive or walk around and seek out homeless individuals who are in need of assistance. They offer coffee, sandwiches, and blankets in an effort to show concern and establish trust. If assistance can be provided at the site, it is done so. If not, every effort is made to ensure that the individual is linked with a source that can provide the necessary services.

Mobile outreach units provide assistance to homeless individuals who are in need of physical or psychological care. The emphasis of outreach programs is to accommodate the homeless who refuse to seek treatment elsewhere. Most target those with SMI. When trust has been established and the individual agrees to come to the team's office, medical and psychiatric treatment is initiated. Involuntary hospitalization is initiated when an individual is deemed harmful to self or others or otherwise meets the criteria for being considered "gravely disabled."

The Homeless Client and the Nursing Process

Following is a case study demonstrating nursing process with a client experiencing homelessness.

Summary and Key Points

- Psychiatric care has shifted from primarily inpatient hospitalization to a continuum of services within the community. This trend is largely due to the need for greater cost-effectiveness in the provision of care to individuals with mental illness.
- The community mental health movement began in the 1960s with the closing of state hospitals and the deinstitutionalization of many individuals with severe and persistent mental illness.
- Mental health care within the community targets primary prevention (reducing the incidence of mental disorders within the population), secondary prevention (reducing the prevalence of psychiatric illness by shortening the course of the illness), and tertiary prevention (reducing the residual defects that are associated with severe and persistent mental illness).
- Primary prevention focuses on identification of populations at risk for mental illness, increasing their ability to cope with stress, and targeting and diminishing harmful forces within the environment.
- Secondary prevention is accomplished through early identification of problems and prompt initiation of effective treatment.
- Tertiary prevention focuses on preventing complications of the illness and promoting rehabilitation that is directed toward achievement of the individual's maximum level of functioning.
- Registered nurses serve as providers of psychiatric mental health care in the community setting.
- Nurses provide outpatient care for individuals with severe and persistent mental illness in community mental health centers, partial hospitalization programs, community residential facilities, clinics, and through psychiatric home health care.
- Homeless persons with mental illness provide a special challenge for the community mental health nurse. Care is provided within homeless shelters, at health-care centers or storefront clinics, and through mobile outreach programs.

CASE STUDY: NURSING PROCESS WITH A HOMELESS PATIENT

NURSING HISTORY AND ASSESSMENT

Joe, age 68, is brought to the community health clinic by two of his peers, who report: "He just had a fit. He needs a drink bad!" Joe is dirty and unkempt, has visible tremors of the upper extremities, and is weak enough to require assistance when ambulating. He is cooperative as the nurse completes the intake assessment. He is coherent, although thought processes are slow. He is disoriented to time and place. He appears somewhat frightened as he scans the unfamiliar surroundings. He is unable to tell the nurse when he had his last drink. He reports no physical injury, and none is observable.

Joe carries a small bag with a few personal items inside, including a Department of Veterans Affairs (VA) benefit card, identifying him as a veteran of the Vietnam War. The nurse finds a cot for Joe to lie down, ensures that his vital signs are stable, and telephones the number on the VA card. The clinic nurse discovers that Joe is well known to the admissions personnel at the VA. He has a 35-year history of schizophrenia with numerous hospitalizations. At the time of his last discharge, he was taking fluphenazine (Prolixin) 10 mg twice a day. He told the clinic nurse that he took the medication for a few months after he got out of the hospital but then did not have the prescription refilled. He could not remember when he had last taken fluphenazine.

Joe also has a long history of alcohol-related disorders and has participated in the VA substance rehabilitation program three times. He has no home address and receives his VA disability benefit checks at a shelter address. He reports that he has no family. The nurse makes arrangements for VA personnel to drive Joe from the clinic to the VA hospital, where he is admitted for detoxification. She sets up a case management file for Joe and arranges with the hospital to have Joe return to the clinic after discharge.

DIAGNOSIS AND OUTCOME IDENTIFICATION

The following nursing diagnosis was formulated for Joe:

Ineffective health maintenance related to ineffective coping skills evidenced by abuse of alcohol, lack of follow-through with antipsychotic medication, and lack of personal hygiene

Ongoing criteria were selected as outcomes for Joe:

- Follows the rules of the group home and maintains his residency status
- Attends weekly sessions of group therapy at the VA day treatment program
- Attends weekly sessions of Alcoholics Anonymous and maintains sobriety
- Reports regularly to the health clinic for injections of fluphenazine
- Volunteers at the VA hospital 3 days a week
- Secures and retains permanent employment

PLANNING AND IMPLEMENTATION

During Joe's hospitalization, the clinic nurse remained in contact with his case. Joe received complete physical and dental examinations and treatment during his hospital stay. The clinic nurse attended the treatment team meeting for Joe as his outpatient case manager. It was decided at the meeting to try giving Joe injections of fluphenazine decanoate because of his history of lack of adherence to his daily oral medication regimen. The clinic nurse would administer the injection every 4 weeks.

At Joe's follow-up clinic visit, the nurse explains to Joe that she has found a group home where he may live with others who have personal circumstances similar to his. At the group home, meals will be provided and the group home manager will ensure that Joe's basic needs are fulfilled. A criterion for remaining at the residence is for Joe to remain alcohol free. Joe is agreeable to these living arrangements.

With Joe's concurrence, the clinic nurse also performs the following interventions:

- Goes shopping with Joe to purchase some new clothing, allowing Joe to make decisions as independently as possible
- Helps Joe move into the group home and introduces him to the manager and residents
- Helps Joe change his address from the shelter to the group home so that he may continue to receive his VA benefits
- Enrolls Joe in the weekly group therapy sessions of the day treatment facility connected with the VA hospital
- Helps Joe locate the nearest Alcoholics Anonymous group and identifies a sponsor who will ensure that Joe gets to the meetings
- Sets up a clinic appointment for Joe to return in 4 weeks for his fluphenazine injection; telephones Joe 1 day in advance to remind him of his appointment
- Instructs Joe to return to or call the clinic if any of the following symptoms occur: sore throat, fever, nausea and vomiting, severe headache, difficulty urinating, tremors, skin rash, or yellow skin or eyes
- Assists Joe in securing transportation to and from appointments
- Encourages Joe to set realistic goals for his life and offers recognition for follow-through
- When Joe is ready, discusses employment alternatives with him; suggests the possibility of starting with a volunteer job (perhaps as a VA hospital volunteer)

EVALUATION

Evaluation of the nursing process with homeless individuals who have mental illness must be highly individualized. Statistics show that chances for relapse with this population are high. Therefore, it is extremely important that outcome criteria be realistic so as not to set the patient up for failure.

Review Questions

Select the answer that is most appropriate for each of the following questions:

1. Which represents a nursing intervention at the primary level of prevention?
   a. Teaching a class in parent effectiveness training
   b. Leading a group of adolescents in drug rehabilitation
   c. Referring a married couple for sex therapy
   d. Leading a support group for battered women
2. Which represents a nursing intervention at the secondary level of prevention?
   a. Teaching a class about menopause to middle-aged women
   b. Providing support in the emergency department to a rape victim
   c. Leading a grief support group for widows and widowers
   d. Making monthly visits to the home of a client with schizophrenia to ensure medication compliance
3. Which represents a nursing intervention at the tertiary level of prevention?
   a. Serving as case manager for a mentally ill homeless client
   b. Leading a support group for newly retired men
   c. Teaching prepared childbirth classes
   d. Caring for a depressed widow in the hospital
4. A 78-year-old widow who lives alone has been diagnosed with depression. Which criterion would qualify this client for home health visits?
   a. The client doesn't like to drive on busy roads.
   b. The client is physically too weak to travel without risk of injury.
   c. The client refuses to seek assistance as suggested by their physician, "because I don't have a psychiatric problem."
   d. The client says they would rather have home visits than go to the physician's office.
5. Which issue has been identified as contributing to the increase in the population of those who are homeless? (Select all that apply.)
   a. Poverty
   b. Lack of affordable health care
   c. Substance abuse
   d. Severe and persistent mental illness
   e. Growth in the number of family members living together

Clinical Judgment Questions

6. A homeless person has just come to live in a shelter. The shelter nurse is assigned to their care. Which is a priority intervention on the part of the nurse?
   a. Referring them to a social worker
   b. Developing a plan of care
   c. Conducting a behavioral and needs assessment
   d. Helping them apply for Social Security benefits
7. A psychiatric home health nurse has received an order to begin regular visits to a client diagnosed with depression. Which potential problems is a priority to evaluate during the first home visit?
   a. Maladaptive grieving
   b. Social isolation
   c. Risk for injury
   d. Sleep pattern disturbance

8. The home health nurse is assessing an 87-year-old man who states, "I've lived long enough and there's just nothing left for me." Which is the best response on the part of the nurse?
   a. "Of course there is; why would you say such a thing?"
   b. "You seem so sad. I'm going to do my best to cheer you up."
   c. "Let's talk about why you are feeling this way."
   d. "Are you having any thoughts of suicide?"
9. The physician has ordered trazodone 150 mg to be taken at bedtime for a 75-year-old widow with co-occurring insomnia and a history of depression. Which statement about this medication is a priority for the home health nurse to make in teaching the client about trazodone?
   a. "You may feel dizzy when you stand up, so go slowly when you get up from sitting or lying down."
   b. "Make sure you let me know if you're getting adequate sleep. Trazodone sometimes interferes with sleep."
   c. "Don't get out of bed unless someone is available to assist you."
   d. "This medication takes around four to six weeks before you will notice any therapeutic effect."
10. The community mental health nurse is assessing a homeless woman who left her husband and "had nowhere else to go." She was referred to the clinic from the homeless shelter for an evaluation to rule out depression. Which priority action should the nurse include in the initial assessment? (Select all that apply.)
    a. Ask about trauma history.
    b. Assess risk for suicide.
    c. Assess her comfort level with the accommodations at the homeless shelter.
    d. Explore her financial resources.

IMPLICATIONS OF EVIDENCE-BASED PRACTICE

Moreno, C., Wykes, T., Galderisi, S., Nordentoft, M., Crossley, N., Jones, N., Cannon, M., Correll, U. C., Byrne, L., Carr, S., Chen, E. Y. H., Gorwood, P., Johnson, S., Kärkkäinen, H., Krystal, J. H., Lee, J., Lieberman, J., López-Jaramillo, C., Männikkö, M., . . . Arango, C. (2020). How mental health care should change as a consequence of the COVID-19 pandemic. *Lancet Psychiatry*, *7*(9), 813–824. https://doi.org/10.1016/S2215-0366(20)30307-2

DESCRIPTION OF THE STUDY: This study was conducted by a panel of experts worldwide and involved a review of available literature on mental health consequences associated with the COVID-19 pandemic with the intent to develop a position paper on emerging mental health priorities going forward. The authors note that most research is preliminary and that longitudinal studies will be needed to confirm the ongoing relevance of current priorities.

RESULTS OF THE STUDY: Several findings relevant to mental health priorities in the COVID-19 pandemic were identified. Selected findings include:

- Most surveys identified increases in depression, anxiety, and stress related to fear of illness, fear of life disruptions, and fear of economic distress.
- Social media exposure has been associated with increased anxiety, and comorbid anxiety and depression.
- Emerging reports have identified a 33% incidence of dysexecutive syndrome (a syndrome of emotional, behavioral, and cognitive deficits) after discharge among patients hospitalized in the ICU with COVID-19.
- Risk factors for infection and a severe course of illness include those with SMI, substance use disorders, and homelessness.
- People with pre-existing mental health disorders have reported increased symptoms and poorer access to

Continued

IMPLICATIONS OF EVIDENCE-BASED PRACTICE—cont'd

services and supports since the onset of the COVID-19 pandemic.

The authors conclusions include:

- Retaining existing services and promoting new practices that expand access and provide cost-effective delivery of effective mental health services to individuals who already have mental disorders or who have developed them during the pandemic should be a priority.
- Ongoing community assessment to identify post-COVID mental health and neurological issues needs to be systematically conducted.
- Service provision that targets health needs and reduces disparities, both globally and within individual countries needs to be put in place.

IMPLICATIONS FOR NURSING PRACTICE: Nurses who work in community mental health can be instrumental in identifying and responding to immediate and long-term mental health needs associated with this pandemic. The findings and position paper that resulted from this study clarified some associated mental health needs and disparities for those with pre-existing SMI and for those in the general population.

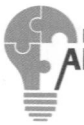

Go to **Davis Advantage** to complete your learning: strengthen understanding, apply your knowledge, and prepare for the Next Gen NCLEX®.

References

American Psychiatric Association. (2022). *Diagnostic and statistical manual of mental disorders* (5th ed., text rev.) American Psychiatric Association.

American Psychiatric Nurses Association & International Society of Psychiatric-Mental Health Nurses. (2021). *Psychiatric-mental health nursing: Scope and standards of practice* (3rd ed.). American Nurses Association.

Case Management Society of America. (2020). *Case management standards of practice & scope of services.*

Casper, L. M., & Coritz, A. (2018). Family demography: Continuity and change in north American families. In J. R. Kaakinen, D. P. Coehlo, R. Steele, & M. Robinson (Eds.), *Family health care nursing* (6th ed., pp. 53–81). F.A. Davis.

Centers for Disease Control and Prevention. (2020). *TB in the homeless population.* https://www.cdc.gov/tb/topic/populations/Homelessness/default.htm

Centers for Disease Control and Prevention. (2022). *Interim guidance for homeless service providers to plan and respond to coronavirus disease 2019 (COVID-19).* https://www.cdc.gov/coronavirus/2019-ncov/community/homeless-shelters/plan-prepare-respond.html

Centers for Medicare & Medicaid Services. (n.d.). *The mental health parity and addiction equity act.* https://www.cms.gov/CCIIO/Programs-and-Initiatives/Other-Insurance-Protections/mhpaea_factsheet.html

Family and Youth Services Bureau. (2016). *Domestic violence and homelessness: Statistics (2016).* https://www.acf.hhs.gov/fysb/resource/dv-homelessness-stats-2016

Ling, C., & Ruscin, C. (2013). *Case management basics.* Gannett Education Course #60102. http://ce.nurse.com/60102/Case-Management-Basics

Mayo Clinic. (2021). *Male menopause: Myth or reality?* https://www.mayoclinic.org/healthy-lifestyle/mens-health/in-depth/male-menopause/art-20048056

McLeod, S. A. (2010). *SRRS—Stress of life events.* http://www.simplypsychology.org/SRRS.html

Moreno, C., Wykes, T., Galderisi, S., Nordentoft, M., Crossley, N., Jones, N., Cannon, M., Correll, U. C., Byrne, L., Carr, S., Chen, E. Y. H., Gorwood, P., Johnson, S., Kärkkäinen, H., Krystal, J. H., Lee, J., Lieberman, J., López-Jaramillo, C., Männikkö, M., . . . Arango, C. (2020). How mental health care should change as a consequence of the COVID-19 pandemic. *Lancet Psychiatry, 7*(9), 813–824. https://doi.org/10.1016/S2215-0366(20)30307-2

National Alliance on Mental Illness. (2021). *Psychosocial treatments: Assertive community treatment.* https://www.nami.org/Learn-More/Treatment/Psychosocial-Treatments

National Alliance to End Homelessness. (2020). *The state of homelessness in America: 2020 edition.* https://endhomelessness.org/homelessness-in-america/homelessness-statistics/state-of-homelessness-2020/

National Coalition for the Homeless. (2015). *How trauma-informed care is helping homeless families.* http://nationalhomeless.org/category/domestic-violence/

National Coalition for the Homeless. (2017). *Mental illness and homelessness.* http://nationalhomeless.org/wp-content/uploads/2017/06/Mental-Illness-and-Homelessness.pdf

National Coalition for the Homeless. (2018). *Vulnerable to hate: A survey of bias-motivated violence against people experiencing homelessness in 2016–2017.* https://nationalhomeless.org/wp-content/uploads/2018/12/hate-crimes-2016-17-final_for-web.pdf

National Institute of Corrections. (n.d.). *Mentally ill persons in corrections.* http://nicic.gov/mentalillness

National Institute of Mental Health. (2021). *Mental illness.* https://www.nimh.nih.gov/health/statistics/mental-illness

National Institutes of Health. (2018). *The helping to end addiction long-term® initiative.* https://heal.nih.gov/

Patel, K., Bunachita, S., Chiu, H., Suresh, P., & Patel, U. K. (2021). Elder abuse: A comprehensive overview and physician-associated challenges. *Cureus, 13*(4), e14375. https://doi.org/10.7759/cureus.14375

President's New Freedom Commission on Mental Health. (2002). *Interim report: Older adults with mental illnesses are not receiving care.* http://govinfo.library.unt.edu

President's New Freedom Commission on Mental Health. (2003). *Achieving the promise: Transforming mental health care in America.* http://govinfo.library.unt.edu/mentalhealthcommission/reports/reports.htm

Safe Horizon. (2018). *Youth homelessness statistics and facts.* https://www.safehorizon.org/get-informed/homeless-youth-statistics-facts/#definition/

Shajani, Z., & Snell, D. (2019). *Nurses and families: A guide to family assessment and intervention* (7th ed.). F.A. Davis.

Spock, B., & Needlman, R. (2018). *Dr. Spock's baby and child care* (10th ed.). Gallery Books.

Substance Abuse and Mental Health Services Administration. (2016). *Behind the term serious mental illness.* https://www.hsdl.org/?abstract&did=801613

Substance Abuse and Mental Health Services Administration. (2020). *PATH annual report data: 2019.* https://pathpdx.samhsa.gov/Content/preGen/national/24/PATH_Annual_Report_For_FY_2019.pdf

Treatment Advocacy Center. (2018). *Eliminating barriers to the treatment of mental illness.* https://www.treatmentadvocacycenter.org/fixing-the-system/features-and-news/2596-how-many-people-with-serious-mental-illness-are-homeless

U.S. Department of Health and Human Services, Office of the Surgeon General. (2016). *Facing addiction in America: Report on alcohol, drugs, and health.* https://addiction.surgeongeneral.gov/sites/default/files/surgeon-generals-report.pdf

U.S. Department of Housing and Urban Development. (2021). *The 2020 Annual Homeless Assessment Report (AHAR) to Congress.* https://www.huduser.gov/portal/sites/default/files/pdf/2020-AHAR-Part-1.pdf

Vanderplasschen, W., Rapp, R. C., Pearce, S., Vandevelde, S., & Broekaert, E. (2013). Mental health, recovery, and the community. *Scientific World Journal, 2013*(4), 1–3. https://doi.org/10.1155/2013/926174

Veltri, L., Wilson-Mitchell, K., & O'Mahony, J. M. (2018). Family nursing with childbearing families. In J. R. Kaakinen, D. P. Coehlo, R. Steele, & M. Robinson (Eds.), *Family health care nursing* (6th ed., pp. 357–387). F.A. Davis.

White, D. L., & Cartwright, J. C. (2018). Family health in mid- and later life. In J. R. Kaakinen, D. P. Coehlo, R. Steele, & M. Robinson (Eds.), *Family health care nursing* (6th ed., pp. 457–496). F.A. Davis.

Classical References

Caplan, G. (1964). *Principles of preventive psychiatry.* Basic Books.

Erikson, E. (1963). *Childhood and society* (2nd ed.). W. W. Norton.

Govtrack. (1987). *H.R. 558 (100th): Stewart B. McKinney Homeless Assistance Act.* https://www.govtrack.us/congress/bills/100/hr558/text

Lamb, H. R. (1993). Perspectives on effective advocacy for homeless mentally ill persons. *Hospital and Community Psychiatry, 43*(12), 1209–1212.

27 The Bereaved Individual

CORE CONCEPTS
Grief and Loss
Self
Stress and Coping

CHAPTER OUTLINE

Objectives
Introduction
Theoretical Perspectives on Loss and Bereavement
Length of the Grief Process
Anticipatory Grief
Maladaptive Responses to Loss
Application of the Nursing Process
End-of-Life Resources
Summary and Key Points
Review Questions
Clinical Judgment Questions
Implications of Evidence-Based Practice
Communication Exercises
Movie Connections

KEY TERMS

advance directive
anticipatory grieving
bereavement
bereavement overload
grief
hospice
maladaptive grief
mourning

OBJECTIVES

After reading this chapter, the student will be able to:

1. Describe various types of loss that trigger the grief response in individuals.
2. Discuss theoretical perspectives of grieving as proposed by Elisabeth Kübler-Ross, John Bowlby, George Engel, and J. William Worden.
3. Differentiate between normal and maladaptive responses to loss.
4. Discuss grieving behaviors common to individuals at various stages across the life span.
5. Formulate nursing diagnoses and goals of care for individuals experiencing the grief response.
6. Describe appropriate nursing interventions for individuals experiencing the grief response.
7. Identify relevant criteria for evaluating nursing care of individuals experiencing the grief response.
8. Describe the concept of hospice care for people who are dying and their families.
9. Discuss the use of advance directives for individuals to provide directions about their future medical care.

Introduction

CORE CONCEPT

Loss

The experience of separation from something of personal importance.

Loss is anything that is perceived as such by the individual. The separation from loved ones or the giving up of treasured possessions for whatever reason; the experience of failure, either real or perceived; or life events that create change in a familiar pattern of existence—all can be experienced as loss, and all can trigger behaviors associated with the grieving process. Loss and bereavement are universal events encountered by all beings that experience emotions. Following are examples of some notable forms of loss:

- A significant other (person or pet), through death, divorce, or separation for any reason.
- Illness or debilitating conditions. Examples include (but are not limited to) diabetes, stroke, cancer, rheumatoid arthritis, multiple sclerosis, Alzheimer's disease, hearing or vision loss, and spinal cord or head injuries. Some of these conditions not only incur a loss of physical and/or emotional wellness but may also result in the loss of personal independence.
- Developmental/maturational changes or situations, such as menopause, andropause, infertility, "empty nest syndrome," aging, impotence, or hysterectomy.
- A decrease in self-esteem due to inability to meet self-expectations or the expectations of others (even if these expectations are only perceived by the individual as unfulfilled). This includes a real or perceived loss of potential hopes and dreams.
- Personal possessions that symbolize familiarity and security in a person's life. Separation from these familiar and personally valued external objects represents a loss of material extensions of the self.

CORE CONCEPT

Grief

Deep mental and emotional anguish that is a response to the subjective experience of loss of something significant.

Some texts differentiate the terms **mourning** and **grief** by describing mourning as the psychological process (or stages) through which the individual passes on the way to successful adaptation to the loss of a valued object. Grief may be viewed as the subjective states that accompany mourning or the emotional work involved in the mourning process. Similarly, **bereavement** is described as the period of grief and sadness that is the normal process of reacting to a loss and may include mental, physical, social, and emotional reactions (MedlinePlus, 2020). For purposes of this text, grief work, bereavement, and the process of mourning are collectively referred to as the *grief response.*

This chapter examines human responses to the experience of loss. Care of bereaved individuals is presented in the context of the nursing process.

Theoretical Perspectives on Loss and Bereavement

Stages of Grief

Behavior patterns associated with the grief response include many individual variations. However, sufficient similarities have been observed to warrant characterization of the grief response as a syndrome that has a predictable course with an expected resolution. Early theorists, including Kübler-Ross (1969), Bowlby (1961), and Engel (1964), described behavioral stages through which individuals advance in their progression toward resolution. A number of variables influence one's progression through the grief process, and it should not be understood as a linear process. Some individuals may reach acceptance only to revert to an earlier stage, some may never complete the sequence, and some may never progress beyond the initial stage.

A more contemporary grief specialist, J. William Worden (2009), offers a set of tasks that must be processed in order to complete the grief response. He suggests that it is possible for a person to accomplish some of these tasks and not others, resulting in an incomplete bereavement and thus impairing further growth and development. A comparison of the similarities among these four models is presented in Table 27–1.

Elisabeth Kübler-Ross

These well-known stages of the grief process were identified by Kübler-Ross in her extensive work with

TABLE 27–1 Stages and Tasks of the Normal Grief Response

A COMPARISON OF MODELS BY ELISABETH KÜBLER-ROSS, JOHN BOWLBY, GEORGE ENGEL, AND WILLIAM WORDEN

STAGES/TASKS					
KÜBLER-ROSS	BOWLBY	ENGEL	WORDEN	POSSIBLE TIME DIMENSION	BEHAVIORS
I. Denial	I. Numbness/protest	I. Shock/ disbelief	I. Accepting the reality of the loss	Occurs immediately on experiencing the loss. Usually lasts no more than a few weeks.	Individual has difficulty believing that the loss has occurred.
II. Anger	II. Disequilibrium	II. Developing awareness		In most cases begins within hours of the loss. Peaks within a few weeks.	Anger is directed toward self or others. Ambivalence and guilt may be felt toward the lost entity.
III. Bargaining					The individual fervently seeks alternatives to improve current situation.
		III. Restitution			Attends to various rituals associated with the culture in which the loss has occurred.
IV. Depression	III. Disorganization and despair	IV. Resolution of the loss	II. Processing the pain of grief	Very individual. Commonly 6 to 12 months. Longer for some.	The actual work of grieving. Preoccupation with the lost entity. Feelings of helplessness and loneliness occur in response to realization of the loss. Feelings associated with the loss are confronted.
			III. Adjusting to a world without the lost entity	Ongoing.	How the environment changes depends on the roles the lost entity played in the life of the bereaved person. Adaptations will have to be made as the changes are presented in daily life. New coping skills will have to be developed.
IV. Acceptance	IV. Reorganization	V. Recovery	IV. Finding an enduring connection with the lost entity in the midst of embarking on a new life		Resolution is complete. The bereaved person experiences a reinvestment in new relationships and new goals. The lost entity is not purged or replaced but relocated in the life of the bereaved. At this stage, terminally ill persons express a readiness to die.

dying patients. Behaviors associated with each of these stages can be observed in individuals experiencing the loss of any concept of personal value.

- ***Stage I: Denial:*** In this stage, individuals have difficulty believing that the loss has occurred. They may say, "No, it can't be true!" or "It's just not possible." This stage may protect individuals from the psychological pain of reality.
- ***Stage II: Anger:*** This is the stage when reality sets in. Feelings associated with this stage include sadness, guilt, shame, helplessness, and hopelessness. Self-blame or blaming of others may lead to feelings of anger toward the self and others. Anxiety levels may be elevated, and individuals may experience confusion and a decreased ability to function independently. They may be preoccupied with an idealized image of what has been lost. Numerous somatic complaints are common.
- ***Stage III: Bargaining:*** At this stage in the grief response, individuals attempt to strike a bargain with God for a second chance or for more time. They acknowledge the loss, or impending loss, but hold out hope for additional alternatives, as evidenced by statements such as, "If only I could . . ." or "If only I had . . ."
- ***Stage IV: Depression:*** In this stage, individuals mourn for that which has been or will be lost. This is a very painful stage during which individuals must confront feelings associated with having lost someone or something of value (called *reactive depression*). An example might be the individual who is mourning a change in body image. Feelings associated with an impending loss (called *preparatory depression*) are also confronted. Examples include permanent lifestyle changes related to the altered body image or even an impending loss of life itself. Regression, withdrawal, and social isolation may be observed behaviors with this stage. Therapeutic intervention should be available, but not imposed, and with guidelines for implementation based on individual readiness.
- ***Stage V: Acceptance:*** At this time, individuals have worked through the behaviors associated with the other stages and accept or are resigned to the loss. Anxiety decreases, and methods for coping with the loss have been established. Individuals at this stage are less preoccupied with what has been lost and increasingly interested in other aspects of the environment. If this is an impending death of self, the individual is ready to die. The person may become very quiet and withdrawn, seemingly devoid of feelings. These behaviors are an attempt to facilitate the passage by slowly disengaging from the environment.

David Kessler, who collaborated with Kübler-Ross, recently advanced the concept of a sixth stage of grief that he labels *finding meaning* (Kessler, 2019). He advances the idea that grief is transformed into peace and a renewed sense of hopefulness when meaning, rather than closure, is sought.

John Bowlby

John Bowlby hypothesized four stages in the grief process. He implies that these behaviors can be observed in all individuals who have experienced the loss of something or someone of value, even in babies as young as 6 months of age.

- ***Stage I: Numbness or protest:*** This stage is characterized by a feeling of shock and disbelief that the loss has occurred. Reality of the loss is not acknowledged.
- ***Stage II: Disequilibrium:*** During this stage, the individual has a profound urge to recover what has been lost. Behaviors associated with this stage include a preoccupation with the loss, intense weeping and expressions of anger toward the self and others, and feelings of ambivalence and guilt associated with the loss.
- ***Stage III: Disorganization and despair:*** Feelings of despair occur in response to realization that the loss has occurred. Activities of daily living become increasingly disorganized, and behavior is characterized by restlessness and aimlessness. Efforts to regain productive patterns of behavior are ineffective, and the individual experiences fear, helplessness, and hopelessness. Somatic complaints are common. Perceptions of visualizing or being in the presence of that which has been lost may occur. Social isolation is common, and the individual may feel a great deal of loneliness.
- ***Stage IV: Reorganization:*** The individual accepts or becomes resigned to the loss. New goals and patterns of organization are established. The individual begins a reinvestment in new relationships and indicates a readiness to move forward within the environment. Grief subsides and recedes into valued remembrances.

George Engel

Engel describes the grief process in five stages that include emotions, behaviors, and tasks associated with each stage.

- ***Stage I: Shock and disbelief:*** The initial reaction to a loss is a stunned, numb feeling and refusal by the individual to acknowledge the reality of the loss. Engel states that this stage is an attempt by the individual to protect the self "against the effects of the overwhelming stress by raising the threshold against its recognition or against the painful feelings evoked thereby."

- ***Stage II: Developing awareness:*** This stage begins within minutes to hours of the loss. Behaviors associated with this stage include excessive crying and regression to a state of helplessness and a child-like manner. Awareness of the loss creates feelings of emptiness, frustration, anguish, and despair. Anger may be directed toward the self or toward others in the environment who are held accountable for the loss.
- ***Stage III: Restitution:*** In this stage, the various rituals associated with loss within a culture are performed. Examples include funerals, wakes, special attire, a gathering of friends and family, and religious practices customary to the spiritual beliefs of the bereaved. Participation in these rituals is thought to assist the individual to accept the reality of the loss and to facilitate the recovery process.
- ***Stage IV: Resolution of the loss:*** This stage is characterized by a preoccupation with the loss. The concept of the loss is idealized, and the individual may even imitate admired qualities of the lost entity. Preoccupation with the loss gradually decreases over a year or more, and the individual eventually begins to reinvest feelings in others.
- ***Stage V: Recovery:*** Obsession with the loss has ended, and the individual is able to go on with life.

J. William Worden

Worden views the bereaved person as active and self-determining rather than as a passive participant in the grief process. He proposes that bereavement includes a set of tasks that must be reconciled in order to complete the grief process. Worden's four tasks of mourning include the following:

- ***Task I: Accepting the reality of the loss:*** When something of value is lost, it is common for individuals to refuse to believe that the loss has occurred. Behaviors include misidentifying individuals in the environment as their lost loved one, retaining possessions of the lost loved one as though they have not died, and removing all reminders of the lost loved one so as not to have to face the reality of the loss. Worden (2009) stated:

> Coming to an acceptance of the reality of the loss takes time since it involves not only an intellectual acceptance but also an emotional one. The bereaved person may be intellectually aware of the finality of the loss long before the emotions allow full acceptance of the information as true. (p. 42)

Belief and denial are intermittent while grappling with this task. It is thought that traditional rituals such as the funeral help some individuals move toward acceptance of the loss.

- ***Task II: Processing the pain of grief:*** Pain associated with a loss includes both physical and emotional pain. This pain must be acknowledged and worked through. To avoid or suppress it serves only to delay or prolong the grieving process. People do this by refusing to allow themselves to think painful thoughts, by idealizing or avoiding reminders of the lost entity, and by using alcohol or drugs. The intensity of the pain and the manner in which it is experienced are different for all individuals. However, the commonality is that it *must* be experienced. Failure to do so generally results in some form of depression that commonly requires therapy, which then focuses on working through the pain of grief that the individual failed to work through at the time of the loss. In this very difficult task II, individuals must "allow themselves to process the pain—to feel it and to know that one day it will pass" (Worden, 2009, p. 45).
- ***Task III: Adjusting to a world without the lost entity:*** It usually takes months for bereaved persons to realize what their world will be like without the lost entity. In the case of a lost loved one, how the environment changes will depend on the types of roles that person fulfilled in life. In the case of a changed lifestyle, individuals will be required to make adaptations to their environment in terms of the changes as they are presented in daily life. In addition, those individuals who had defined their identity through the lost entity will require an adjustment to their own sense of self. Worden identifies that successful completion of task III entails redefining the loss in a way that is beneficial to the survivor.

If the bereaved person experiences failures in their attempt to adjust in an environment without the lost entity, feelings of low self-esteem may result. Regressed behaviors and feelings of helplessness and inadequacy are not uncommon. Worden states:

> [Another] area of adjustment is to one's sense of the world. Loss through death can challenge one's fundamental life values and philosophical beliefs—beliefs that are influenced by our

> families, peers, education, and religion as well as life experiences. The bereaved person searches for meaning in the loss and its attendant life changes to make sense of it and to regain some control of their life. (pp. 48–49)

To be successful in task III, bereaved individuals must develop new skills to cope and adapt to their new environment without the lost entity. Achievement of this task determines the outcome of the mourning process—that of continued growth or a state of arrested development.

- ***Task IV: Finding an enduring connection with the lost entity in the midst of embarking on a new life:*** This task allows the bereaved person to identify a special place for the lost entity. Individuals need not purge from their history or find a replacement for that which has been lost. Instead, there is a kind of continued presence of the lost entity that only becomes *relocated* in the life of the bereaved. Successful completion of task IV involves letting go of past attachments and forming new ones. However, there is also the recognition that although the relationship between the bereaved and what has been lost is changed, it is nonetheless still a relationship. Worden suggested that one never loses memories of a significant relationship. He states:

> For many people, Task IV is the most difficult one to accomplish. They get stuck at this point in their grieving and later realize that their life in some way stopped at the point the loss occurred. (p. 52)

Worden related the story of a teenage girl who had a difficult time adjusting to the death of her father. After 2 years, when she began to finally fulfill some of the tasks associated with successful grieving, she wrote these words that express rather clearly what bereaved people in task IV are struggling with: "There are other people to be loved, and it doesn't mean that I love Dad any less". (p. 52)

Length of the Grief Process

Stages of grief describe an orderly approach to the resolution of mourning. Each stage presents tasks that must be overcome through a painful experiential process. Engel (1964) stated that successful resolution of the grief response is thought to have occurred when a bereaved individual is able "to remember comfortably and realistically both the pleasures and disappointments of the lost relationship" (p. 96). The length of the grief process depends on the individual and can last for years without being maladaptive. The acute phase of normal grieving usually lasts about 6 to 8 weeks—longer in older adults—but complete resolution of the grief response may take much longer. Boland and Verduin (2022) state:

> Ample evidence suggests that the bereavement process does not end within a prescribed interval; certain aspects persist indefinitely for many otherwise high-functioning, normal individuals. Common manifestations of protracted grief occur intermittently. . . . [M]ost grief does not fully resolve or permanently disappear; rather grief becomes circumscribed and submerged only to reemerge in response to certain triggers. (p. 850)

A number of factors influence the eventual outcome of the grief response. The grief response can be more difficult if:

- The bereaved person was strongly dependent on or perceived the lost entity as an important means of physical and/or emotional support.
- The relationship with the lost entity was highly ambivalent. A love-hate relationship may instill feelings of guilt that can interfere with the grief work.
- The individual has experienced a number of recent losses. Grief tends to be cumulative, and if previous losses have not been resolved, each succeeding grief response becomes more difficult for that individual to handle.
- The loss is that of a young person. Grief over loss of a child is often more intense than it is over the loss of an elderly person. Traumatic death, in general, increases the likelihood of maladaptive grief, but when a child dies a violent death, studies have found an increased incidence of post-traumatic stress disorder (PTSD) in parents and particularly among mothers. One study found PTSD symptoms in over 25% of mothers up to 5 years after the violent death of a child (Murphy et al., 2003).
- The state of the person's physical or psychological health is unstable at the time of the loss.
- The bereaved person perceives (whether real or imagined) some responsibility for the loss.
- The loss is secondary to suicide.
- The loss is a traumatic death such as murder.

The grief response may be facilitated if:

- The individual has the support of significant others to assist them through the mourning process.
- The individual has the opportunity to prepare for the loss. Grief work is more intense when the loss is sudden and unexpected. The experience of *anticipatory grieving* is thought to facilitate the grief response that occurs at the time of the actual loss.

Worden (2009) states:

> There is a sense in which mourning can be finished, when people regain an interest in life, feel more hopeful, experience gratification again, and adapt to new roles. There is also a sense in which mourning is never finished. [People must understand] that mourning is a long-term process and that the culmination will not be a pre-grief state. (p. 77)

Anticipatory Grief

Anticipatory grieving is the experiencing of the feelings and emotions associated with the normal grief response before the loss actually occurs. It is different in several ways from conventional grief. For example, conventional grief tends to diminish in intensity with time. Anticipatory grief can become more intense as the expected loss becomes imminent.

Although anticipatory grief is thought to facilitate the actual mourning process following the loss, it may be problematic. In the case of a dying person, difficulties can arise when the family members complete the process of anticipatory grief, and detachment from the dying person occurs prematurely. The person who is dying may experience feelings of loneliness and isolation as the psychological pain of imminent death is faced without family support. Another example of difficulty associated with premature completion of the grief response is one that can occur on the return of persons long absent and presumed dead (e.g., soldiers missing in action or prisoners of war). In this instance, resumption of the previous relationship may be difficult for the bereaved person.

Anticipatory grieving may serve as a defense for some individuals to ease the burden of loss when it actually occurs. It may prove to be less functional for others who, because of interpersonal, psychological, or sociocultural variables, are unable in advance of the actual loss to express the intense feelings that accompany the grief response.

One qualitative study examined the unique process of grief for family caregivers of a relative who has dementia. A common theme was that in addition to anticipatory grief related to the final loss, these family members were, at the same time, grieving *actual* losses throughout the journey of their family member's illness (Peacock et al., 2014). These included grieving the loss of the ill person's personality, companionship, social self, and cognition as the disease progressed. The grief reactions of these active caregivers were similar to those of bereaved caregivers, although their family member was still alive. This study highlights the multiplicity of factors that can influence the grieving process.

Maladaptive Responses to Loss

When, then, is the grieving response considered to be maladaptive? Three types of pathological grief reactions have been described. **Maladaptive grief** includes delayed or inhibited grief, an exaggerated or distorted grief response, and chronic or prolonged grief.

Delayed or Inhibited Grief

Delayed or inhibited grief refers to the absence of evidence of grief when it ordinarily would be expected. Many times, cultural influences, such as the expectation to keep a "stiff upper lip," contribute to the delayed response.

Delayed or inhibited grief is potentially pathological because clients are simply not dealing with the reality of the loss. They remain fixed in the denial stage of the grief process, sometimes for many years. When this occurs, the grief response may be triggered, sometimes many years later, when individuals experience a subsequent loss. Sometimes the grief process is triggered spontaneously or in response to a seemingly insignificant event. Overreaction to another person's grief process may be one manifestation of delayed grief.

The recognition of delayed grief is critical because, depending on the profundity of the loss, the lack of mourning may prevent assimilation of the loss and thereby delay a return to satisfying living. Without the understanding and assimilation that the grief process can provide, subsequent losses may be compounded by previously unresolved grief work. Delayed grieving most commonly occurs because of ambivalent feelings toward the lost entity, outside pressure to resume normal function, or perceived lack of internal and external resources to cope with a profound loss.

Distorted (Exaggerated) Grief Response

In the distorted grief reaction, all of the symptoms associated with normal grieving are exaggerated. Feelings of sadness, helplessness, hopelessness, powerlessness, anger, and guilt, as well as numerous somatic complaints, render the individual dysfunctional in terms of management of daily living. Morrow (2022) describes this as complicated grief in which "the usual responses to the death of a loved one do not fade over time and can impair or prevent them from leading their normal lives."

When the exaggerated grief reaction occurs, the individual remains fixed in the anger stage of the grief response. This anger may be directed toward others in the environment to whom the individual may be attributing the loss. However, many times the anger is turned inward to the self. When this occurs, depression is the result. Depressive mood disorder is a type of exaggerated grief reaction. This should be distinguished from the depression that is considered part of the normal grieving process (see Table 27–2).

Chronic or Prolonged Grieving

Some authors have discussed a chronic or prolonged grief response as a type of maladaptive grief response. Caution must be taken in making this determination because, as stated previously, length of the grief response depends on the individual. An adaptive response may take years for some people. A prolonged process may be considered maladaptive when enduring thoughts, emotions, and behaviors prevent the bereaved person from adaptively performing activities of daily living. An example is a widow who refused to participate in family gatherings following the death of her husband, but instead, for many years until her own death, took a sandwich to the cemetery on holidays, sat on the tombstone, and ate her "holiday meal." Whether one's behaviors constitute prolonged or chronic grieving must be considered in a cultural context. In some cultures, establishing a memorial ritual to the deceased is the norm, whereas in other cultures, it might be perceived as prolonged grieving.

Normal Versus Maladaptive Grieving

Although Morrow (2022) identifies that it is difficult to establish a time frame signaling the difference between normal and maladaptive (or complicated) grieving, several symptoms are red flags of complicated grief. These include the following:

- Episodes of rage, or prolonged, unresolved anger
- Inability to focus on anything but the loss
- Intense focus on or avoidance of any reminders of the lost entity
- Prolonged difficulty accepting the reality of the loss
- Self-destructive behavior, including alcohol and drug abuse
- Suicidal thoughts and actions

A crucial difference between normal and maladaptive grieving is the loss of self-esteem. Marked feelings of worthlessness are indicative of depression rather than uncomplicated, normal bereavement.

Hensley and Clayton (2013) add that when depressed inpatients were compared with individuals who were experiencing depression associated with bereavement, four symptoms were absent in the bereavement population: suicidal thoughts, feeling they were a burden to others, feeling they would rather be dead, and psychomotor retardation. These may be considered associated symptoms of low self-esteem and feelings of worthlessness. The presence of suicide ideation is clear evidence of an abnormal

TABLE 27–2 Normal Grief Reactions Versus Symptoms of Clinical Depression

NORMAL GRIEF	CLINICAL DEPRESSION
Self-esteem intact	Self-esteem is disturbed
May openly express anger	Usually does not directly express anger
Experiences a mixture of "good and bad days"	Persistent state of dysphoria
Able to experience moments of pleasure	Anhedonia is prevalent
Accepts comfort and support from others	Does not respond to social interaction and support from others
Maintains feeling of hope	Feelings of hopelessness prevail
May express guilt feelings over some aspect of the loss	Has generalized feelings of guilt
Relates feelings of depression to specific loss experienced	Does not relate feelings to a particular experience
May experience transient physical symptoms	Expresses chronic physical complaints

Sources: Compiled from Boland & Verduin (2022); Corr & Corr (2013); Pies (2013).

grief reaction and requires careful assessment and intervention to prevent suicide.

Studies have identified the incidence of major depressive disorder among the bereaved to be at around 35% at 1 month following a loss, and although the incidence tends to decrease over time, 8% to 11% develop chronic depression (Hensley & Clayton, 2013). The authors add that factors such as poor physical health, poor mental health, and substance use disorders prior to a loss increase the risk for chronic depression following loss. A summary of differences between normal grieving and clinical depression is presented in Table 27–2.

Application of the Nursing Process

Background Assessment Data

Concepts of Death—Developmental Issues

All individuals have their own unique concept of death, which is influenced by past experiences with death as well as age and level of emotional development. This section addresses the various perceptions of death according to developmental age.

Children

- ***Birth to Age 2:*** Infants are unable to recognize and understand death, but they can experience the feelings of loss and separation. Infants who are separated from their mother may become quiet, lose weight, and sleep less. Children at this age will likely sense changes in the atmosphere of the home where a death has occurred. They often react to the emotions of adults by becoming irritable and crying more than usual.
- ***Ages 3 to 5:*** Preschoolers and kindergartners have some understanding about death but often have difficulty distinguishing between fantasy and reality. They believe death is reversible, and their thoughts about death may include magical thinking. For example, they may believe that their thoughts or behaviors caused a person to become sick or to die. Children of this age are capable of understanding at least some of what they see and hear from adult conversations or media reports. They become frightened if they feel a threat to themselves or their loved ones. They are concerned with safety issues and require a great deal of personal reassurance that they will be protected. Regressive behaviors such as loss of bladder or bowel control, thumb sucking, and temper tantrums are common. Changes in eating and sleeping patterns may also occur.
- ***Ages 6 to 9:*** Children at this age are beginning to understand the finality of death. They are able to understand a more detailed explanation of why or how a person died, although the concept of death is often associated with old age or with accidents. They may believe that death is contagious and avoid association with individuals who have experienced a loss by death. Death is often personified in the form of a "bogey man" or a monster—someone who takes people away or someone whom they can avoid if they try hard enough. It is difficult for them to perceive their own death. Normal grief reactions at this age include regressive and aggressive behaviors, withdrawal, school phobias, somatic symptoms, and clinging behaviors.
- ***Ages 10 to 12:*** Preadolescent children are able to understand that death is final and eventually affects everyone, including themselves. They are interested in the physical aspects of dying and the final disposition of the body. They may ask questions about how the death will affect them personally. Feelings of anger, guilt, and depression are common. Peer relationships and school performance may be disrupted. There may be a preoccupation with the loss and a withdrawal into the self. Adams (2014) states that evidence supports that young people who are bereaved are more likely to be poor school attenders, change schools, and be excluded and are less likely to be involved in activities both in and out of school, which puts them at higher risk for underperformance, health problems, and feelings of hopelessness. They will require support, flexibility in management of anger responses, and reassurance of their own safety and self-worth.

Adolescents

Adolescents are usually able to view death on an adult level. They understand death to be universal and inevitable; however, they have difficulty tolerating the intense feelings associated with the death of a loved one. They may or may not cry. They may withdraw into themselves or attempt to go about usual activities to avoid dealing with the pain of the loss. Some teens exhibit acting-out behaviors, such as aggression and defiance. It is often easier for adolescents to discuss their feelings with peers than with their parents or other adults. Some adolescents may show regressive behaviors, whereas others react by trying to take care of their loved ones who are also grieving. In general, individuals of this age-group have an attitude of immortality. Although they understand that their own death is inevitable, the concept is so far reaching as to be imperceptible.

Adults

The adult's concept of death is influenced by experiential, cultural, and religious backgrounds. Behaviors associated with grieving in the adult are discussed in the section "Theoretical Perspectives on Loss and Bereavement."

Older Adults

Philosophers and poets have described late adulthood as the "season of loss." By the time individuals reach their 60s and 70s, they have experienced numerous losses, and mourning has become a lifelong process. Those who are most successful at adapting earlier in life will similarly cope better with the losses and grief inherent in aging. Unfortunately, with the aging process comes a convergence of losses, the timing of which makes it impossible for the aging individual to complete the grief process in response to one loss before another occurs. Because grief is cumulative, multiple losses can result in **bereavement overload.** The person is less able to adapt and reintegrate, complicated grief responses ensue, and mental and physical health may be jeopardized (Tousley, 2020). Bereavement overload has been implicated as a predisposing factor in the development of depressive disorder in older adults.

Some believe that bereavement among elderly couples is also associated with increased risk for mortality. Although many variables influence mortality in this population, evidence suggests that, in cases where the loss is anticipated, there is not an increased risk for mortality; conversely, when the loss is unexpected, including significant financial losses, there is an increased risk (King et al., 2013; Pool et al., 2018; Shah et al., 2013). This research highlights the need for additional assessment and support during the bereavement period when loss is unexpected.

Bereavement Risk Assessment

Several tools have been developed to assess the risk for maladaptive grief responses. They incorporate many of the issues previously discussed and are framed to identify multiple risk factors commonly associated with maladaptive grief reactions that may require additional resources and intervention. Some potential indicators of increased risk for maladaptive grief follow:

- Additional financial problems posed by the loss
- Lack of coping skills or lack of experience in responding to loss
- Emotional or physical dependence on the lost person or item
- History of mental illness or substance abuse
- History of trauma, including abuse
- Multiple losses within a short time frame

Although formalized tools are more often used in palliative care settings, they constitute an important aspect of assessment for all nurses responding to the needs of the bereaved patient.

Concepts of Death—Cultural Issues

As previously stated, bereavement practices are greatly influenced by cultural and religious backgrounds. It is important for health-care professionals to have an understanding of these individual differences in order to provide culturally sensitive care to their patients. Clinicians must be able to identify and appreciate what is culturally expected or required, because failure to carry out expected rituals may hinder the grief process and result in unresolved grief for some bereaved individuals. Box 27–1 provides a set of guidelines for assessing individual preferences and practices with regard to death rituals.

Nursing Diagnosis and Outcome Identification

From the analysis of the assessment data, appropriate nursing diagnoses are formulated for the patient and family experiencing grief and loss. From these identified diagnoses, accurate planning of nursing care is executed. Possible nursing diagnoses for grieving persons include the following:

- Risk for maladaptive grieving related to loss of a valued entity/concept; loss of a loved one
- Risk for spiritual distress related to maladaptive grief responses

BOX 27–1 Guidelines for Assessing Preferences Related to Death Rituals

DEATH RITUALS AND EXPECTATIONS

1. Identify specific death rituals and expectations.
2. Encourage individual to describe death rituals and mourning practices.
3. What are preferences regarding burial practices, such as cremation?

RESPONSES TO DEATH AND GRIEF

1. Identify values and beliefs about death and grief.
2. Explore the individual's perceptions about death, dying, and the afterlife.

The following criteria may be used for measurement of outcomes in the care of the grieving patient. The patient:

- Acknowledges awareness of the loss.
- Is able to express feelings about the loss.
- Verbalizes stages of the grief process and behaviors associated with each.
- Expresses personal satisfaction and support from spiritual practices.

Planning and Implementation

Table 27–3 provides a plan of care for the grieving person. Selected nursing diagnoses are presented, along with outcome criteria, appropriate nursing interventions, and rationales for each.

Evaluation

In the final step of the nursing process, a reassessment is conducted to determine whether the nursing actions have been successful in achieving the objectives of care. Evaluation of the nursing actions for the grieving patient may be facilitated by gathering information using the following types of questions:

- Has the patient discussed the recent loss with staff and family members?
- Is the patient able to verbalize feelings and behaviors associated with each stage of the grieving process and recognize their own position in the process?
- Has obsession with and idealization of the lost entity subsided?
- Is anger toward the loss expressed appropriately?
- Is the patient able to participate in usual religious practices and feel satisfaction and support from them?
- Is the patient seeking out interaction with others in an appropriate manner?
- Is the patient able to verbalize positive aspects about their life, past relationships, and prospects for the future?

End-of-Life Resources

Hospice

Hospice is a program that provides palliative and supportive care to meet the special needs of people who are dying and their families. Hospice care provides physical, psychological, spiritual, and social care for the person for whom aggressive treatment is no longer appropriate. Various models of hospice exist, including freestanding institutions that provide both inpatient and home care, those affiliated with hospitals and nursing homes in which hospice services are provided in the institutional setting, and hospice organizations that provide home care only. Historically, the hospice movement in the United States has evolved mainly as a system of home-based care.

Hospice helps patients achieve physical and emotional comfort so that they can concentrate on living life as fully as possible. Patients are urged to stay active for as long as they are able—to take part in activities they enjoy and to focus on the quality of life.

Hospice follows an interdisciplinary team approach to provide care for the terminally ill individual in the familiar surroundings of the home environment. The interdisciplinary team consists of nurses, attendants (homemakers, home health aides), physicians, social workers, volunteers, and other health-care workers from other disciplines as required for individual patients.

The hospice approach is based on seven components:

1. The interdisciplinary team
2. Pain and symptom management
3. Emotional support to patient and family
4. Pastoral and spiritual care
5. Bereavement counseling
6. 24-hour on-call nurse/counselor
7. Staff support

These are the ideal, and some hospice programs may not include all of these services. The National Hospice and Palliative Care Organization (NHPCO) publishes standards of care based on principles that are directed at the hospice program concept.

Interdisciplinary Team

- ***Nurses:*** A registered nurse usually acts as case manager for care of hospice patients. The nurse assesses the patient's and family's needs, establishes the goals of care, supervises and assists caregivers, evaluates care, serves as patient advocate, provides educational information as needed to patient, family, and caregivers, and provides physical care when needed, including IV therapy.
- ***Attendants:*** These individuals are usually the members of the team who spend the most time with the patient. They assist with personal care and all activities of daily living. Without these daily attendants, many individuals would be unable to spend their remaining days in their home. Attendants may be noncertified and provide basic housekeeping services; they may be certified nursing assistants who assist with personal care; or they may be licensed

Table 27–3 | CARE PLAN FOR THE GRIEVING PERSON

NURSING DIAGNOSIS: RISK FOR MALADAPTIVE GRIEVING

RELATED TO: Loss of a valued entity/concept; loss of a loved one

OUTCOME CRITERIA	NURSING INTERVENTIONS	RATIONALE
Short-Term Goals ■ Patient will acknowledge awareness of the loss. ■ Patient will express feelings about the loss. ■ Patient will verbalize own position in the grief process. **Long-Term Goal** ■ Patient will progress through the grief process in a healthful manner toward resolution.	1. Assess the patient's current grief process.	1. Accurate baseline data are required to provide appropriate assistance.
	2. Develop trust. Show empathy, concern, and unconditional positive regard.	2. Developing trust provides the basis for a therapeutic relationship.
	3. Help the patient actualize the loss by talking about it. "When did it happen?" "How did it happen?" and so forth.	3. Reviewing the events of the loss can help the patient come to full awareness of the loss.
	4. Help the patient identify and express feelings. Some potentially problematic feelings include:	4. Until the patient can recognize and accept personal feelings regarding the loss, grief work cannot progress.
	a. Anger. The anger may be directed at the deceased, at God, displaced onto others, or retroflected inward on the self. Encourage client to examine this anger and validate the appropriateness of this feeling.	a. Many people will not admit to angry feelings, believing it is inappropriate and unjustified. Expression of this emotion is necessary to prevent fixation in this stage of grief.
	b. Guilt. The patient may feel that they did not do enough to prevent the loss. Help patient by reviewing the circumstances of the loss and the reality that it could not be prevented.	b. Feelings of guilt prolong resolution of the grief process.
	c. Anxiety and helplessness. Help the patient to recognize the way that life was managed before the loss. Help the patient to put the feelings of helplessness into perspective by pointing out ways that they managed situations effectively without help from others. Role-play life events and assist with decision-making situations.	c. The patient may have fears that they may not be able to carry on alone.
	5. Interpret normal behaviors associated with grieving and provide the patient with adequate time to grieve.	5. Understanding of the grief process will help prevent feelings of guilt generated by these responses. Individuals need adequate time to adjust to the loss and all its ramifications. This involves getting past birthdays and anniversaries of which the deceased was a part.

Continued

Table 27–3 | CARE PLAN FOR THE GRIEVING PERSON—cont'd

OUTCOME CRITERIA	NURSING INTERVENTIONS	RATIONALE
	6. Provide continuing support. If this is not possible by the nurse, then offer referrals to support groups. Support groups of individuals going through the same experiences can be very helpful for the grieving individual.	6. The availability of emotional support systems facilitates the grief process.
	7. Identify pathological defenses that the patient may be using (e.g., drug/alcohol use, somatic complaints, social isolation). Educate the patient as to how these unhealthy defense mechanisms delay the process of grieving.	7. The bereavement process is impaired by behaviors that mask the pain of the loss.
	8. Encourage the patient to make an honest review of the relationship with the lost entity. Journal keeping is a facilitative tool with this intervention.	8. Only when the patient is able to see both positive and negative aspects related to the loss will the grieving process be complete.

NURSING DIAGNOSIS: RISK FOR SPIRITUAL DISTRESS

RELATED TO: Maladaptive grief process

OUTCOME CRITERIA	NURSING INTERVENTIONS	RATIONALE
Short-Term Goal ■ Patient will identify meaning and purpose in life, moving forward with hope for the future.	1. Be accepting and nonjudgmental when the patient expresses anger and bitterness toward God. Stay with the patient.	1. The nurse's presence and nonjudgmental attitude promote patient's feelings of self-worth and promote trust in the relationship.
Long-Term Goal ■ Patient will express achievement of support and personal satisfaction from spiritual practices.	2. Encourage the patient to vent feelings related to meaning of own existence in the face of current loss.	2. The patient may believe they cannot go on living without lost object. Catharsis can provide relief and put life back into realistic perspective.
	3. Encourage the patient as part of grief work to reach out to previously used religious practices for support. Encourage the patient to discuss these practices and how they provided support in the past.	3. The patient may find comfort in religious rituals with which they are familiar.
	4. Assure the patient that they are not alone when feeling inadequate in the search for life's answers.	4. Validation of the patient's feelings and assurance that they are shared by others. Offer encouragement and an affirmation of acceptability.
	5. Contact spiritual leader of the patient's choice if requested.	5. These individuals serve to provide relief from spiritual distress and often can do so when other support persons cannot.

vocational or practical nurses who provide more specialized care, such as dressing changes or tube feedings.

- ***Physicians:*** The patient's primary physician and the hospice medical consultant have input into the care of the hospice patient. Orders may continue to come from the primary physician, whereas pain and symptom management may come from the hospice consultant. Ideally, these physicians attend weekly patient care conferences and provide in-service education for hospice staff as well as others in the medical community.
- ***Social workers:*** The social worker assists the patient and family members with psychosocial issues, including those associated with the patient's condition, financial issues, legal needs, and bereavement concerns. The social worker provides information on community resources from which the patient and family may receive support and assistance. Some of the functions of the nurse and social worker may overlap at times.
- ***Trained volunteers:*** Volunteers are vital to the hospice concept. They provide services that may otherwise be financially impossible. They are specially selected and extensively trained, and they provide services such as transportation, companionship, respite care, recreational activities, and light housekeeping, and in general, they are sensitive to the needs of families in stressful situations.
- ***Rehabilitation therapists:*** Physical therapists may assist hospice patients in an effort to minimize physical disability. They may assist with strengthening exercises and provide assistance with special equipment needs. Occupational therapists may help the debilitated patient learn to accomplish activities of daily living as independently as possible. Other consultants, such as speech therapists, may be called upon for the patient with special needs.
- ***Dietitian:*** A nutritional consultant may be helpful to the hospice patient who is experiencing nausea and vomiting, diarrhea, anorexia, and weight loss. A nutritionist can ensure that the patient is receiving the proper balance of calories and nutrients.
- ***Counseling services:*** The hospice patient may require the services of a psychiatrist or psychologist if there is a history of mental illness or if neurocognitive disorder or depression has become a problem. Other types of counseling services are available to provide assistance in dealing with the special needs of each patient.

Pain and Symptom Management

Improved quality of life is a primary goal of hospice care. Thus, a major intervention for all caregivers is to ensure that the patient is as comfortable as possible, whether experiencing pain or other types of symptoms common in the terminal stages of an illness.

Emotional Support

Members of the hospice team encourage patients and families to discuss the eventual outcome of the disease process. Some individuals find discussing issues associated with death and dying uncomfortable, and if so, their decision is respected. However, honest discussion of these issues provides a sense of relief for some people, and they are more realistically prepared for the future. It may even draw some families closer together during this stressful time.

Pastoral and Spiritual Care

Hospice philosophy supports the individual's right to seek guidance or comfort in the spiritual practices most suited to that person. The hospice team members help patients obtain the spiritual support and guidance for which they express a preference.

Bereavement Counseling

Hospice provides a service to surviving family members or significant others after the death of their loved one. This service is usually provided by a bereavement counselor, but when one is not available, volunteers with special training in bereavement care may be of service. A grief support group may be helpful for the bereaved and provide a safe place for them to discuss their own fears and concerns about the death of a loved one.

24-Hour On-Call

The standards of care set forth by NHPCO state that care shall be available 24 hours a day, 7 days a week. A nurse or counselor is usually available by phone or for home visits around the clock. The knowledge that emotional or physical support is available at any time, should it be required, provides considerable support and comfort to significant others or family caregivers.

Staff Support

Team members (all of those who work closely and frequently with the patient) often experience emotions similar to those of the patient or their family and/or significant others. They may experience anger, frustration, or fears of death and dying—all of which must be addressed through staff support groups, team conferences, time off, and adequate and effective supervision. Burnout is a common concern among hospice staff. Stress can be reduced, trust enhanced, and team functioning made more effective if lines of communication are kept open among all members (medical director through volunteer), if information is readily accessible through staff conferences and in-service education, and if staff know they are appreciated and feel good about what they are doing. Each of these roles and services is designed to promote adaptive coping in loss and bereavement.

Advance Directives

The term **advance directive** refers to a living will (which specifies what types of medical treatment are desired should the individual become incapacitated), a durable power of attorney (which designates who can make and handle financial affairs if the individual is incapacitated), and a health-care proxy (which designates who can make health-care decisions for the person if they are unable to make their wishes known). These legal documents allow individuals to provide directions about their future medical care. Advance directives are legally binding in all 50 states (Boland & Verduin, 2022).

Doctors usually follow clearly stated directives. It is important that the physician be informed that an advance directive exists and what the specific wishes of the patient are. In 1991, the U.S. Congress passed the Patient Self-Determination Act, which mandates that all health-care facilities must advise patients of their rights to refuse treatment, must make advance directives available to patients on admission, and must keep records of whether a patient has an advance directive or a designated health-care proxy. State laws also define how and under what circumstances individuals can refuse life-sustaining medical interventions. These are generally referred to as *natural death acts.* Nurses need to be aware of both federal law and the applicable state laws in the state where they practice nursing.

Despite the existence of laws allowing for an advance directive document, many people have not established this document for themselves, and even when advance directives exist, they may not be honored when the circumstances are confusing or unclear. Catalano and Catalano (2020) identify additional reasons why advance directives are sometimes not honored:

- Advance directives that were formulated long before their implementation may call into question whether clients understood the ramifications of their decisions for future medical problems and interventions at that time.
- In general, the language used in standard living will documents is not specific enough to cover all health-care circumstances. Consequently, health-care providers may lack clarity about how to proceed because the advance directive itself lacks clarity.
- Because state laws vary, when patients are in a state other than the one where the advance directive was established, it may raise questions about the document's legality.

Advance directives are designed to allow patients to be in control of decisions about their right to live or die. It is also a way to spare family and loved ones the burden of making choices without knowing the wishes of the person who is dying. Nurses can play an active role in discussing advance directives within a culturally sensitive framework and encouraging patients who have advance directives to review and update them periodically to ensure that their wishes remain clear.

Summary and Key Points

- Loss is the experience of separation from something of personal importance.
- Loss is anything that is perceived as such by the individual.
- Loss of any concept of value to an individual can trigger the grief response.
- Elisabeth Kübler-Ross identified five stages that individuals pass through on their way to resolution of a loss: denial, anger, bargaining, depression, and acceptance.
- John Bowlby described similar stages that he identified in the following manner: stage I, numbness or protest; stage II, disequilibrium; stage III, disorganization and despair; and stage IV, reorganization.
- George Engel's stages include shock and disbelief, developing awareness, restitution, resolution of the loss, and recovery.
- J. William Worden, a more contemporary clinician, has proposed that bereaved individuals must accomplish a set of tasks to complete the grief process. These four tasks include accepting the reality of the loss, processing the pain of grief, adjusting to a world without the lost entity, and finding an enduring connection with the lost entity in the midst of embarking on a new life.

- The length of the grief process is highly individual, and it can last for years without being maladaptive.
- The acute stage of the grief process typically lasts a couple of months, but resolution usually takes much longer.
- Anticipatory grieving is the experiencing of the feelings and emotions associated with the normal grief process in response to anticipation of the loss.
- Anticipatory grieving is thought to facilitate the grief process when the actual loss occurs.
- Three types of maladaptive grief reactions have been described:
  1. Delayed or inhibited grief in which there is absence of evidence of grief when it ordinarily would be expected
  2. Distorted or exaggerated grief response in which the individual remains fixed in the anger stage of the grief process and all of the symptoms associated with normal grieving are exaggerated
  3. Chronic or prolonged grieving in which the individual is unable to let go of grieving behaviors after an extended period and in which behaviors are evident that indicate the bereaved individual is not accepting that the loss has occurred
- One crucial difference between normal and maladaptive grieving is the loss of self-esteem. Loss of self-esteem is more symptomatic of clinical depression.
- Feelings of worthlessness, feeling that one is a burden to others, suicidal ideas, and psychomotor retardation are indicative of clinical depression rather than uncomplicated bereavement.
- Very young children do not understand death but often react to the emotions of adults by becoming irritable and crying more than usual. They often believe death is reversible.
- School-age children understand the finality of death. Grief behaviors may reflect regression or aggression, school phobias, or sometimes a withdrawal into the self.
- Adolescents are usually able to view death on an adult level. Grieving behaviors may include withdrawal or acting out. Although they understand that their own death is inevitable, the concept is so far-reaching as to be imperceptible.
- By the time people have reached their 60s or 70s, they have experienced numerous losses. Because grief is cumulative, multiple losses can result in bereavement overload. Depression is a common response.
- Nurses should assess a patient's bereavement needs within a culturally sensitive context.
- Hospice is a program that provides palliative and supportive care to meet the special needs of people who are dying and their families.
- The term *advance directive* refers to a living will, a durable power of attorney for health care, or a health-care proxy. Advance directives allow patients to be in control of decisions at the end of life and spare family and loved ones the burden of making choices without knowing what is most important to the person who is dying.

Review Questions

Select the answer that is most appropriate for each of the following questions:

1. Which of the following is most likely to initiate a grief response in an individual? (Select all that apply.)
   a. Death of a pet dog
   b. Onset of menopause
   c. Failing an examination
   d. Divorce
2. A client, who is dying of cancer, says to the nurse, "I just want to see my new grandbaby. If only God will let me live until she is born. Then I'll be ready to go." This is an example of which of Kübler-Ross's stages of grief?
   a. Denial
   b. Anger
   c. Bargaining
   d. Acceptance

Continued

3. A recent widow, states, "I'm going to have to learn to pay all the bills. Hank always did that. I don't know if I can handle all of that." This is an example of which of the tasks described by Worden?
   a. Task I. Accepting the reality of the loss
   b. Task II. Processing the pain of grief
   c. Task III. Adjusting to a world without the lost entity
   d. Task IV. Finding an enduring connection with the lost entity in the midst of embarking on a new life
4. Engel identifies which of the following as successful resolution of the grief process?
   a. When the bereaved person can talk about the loss without crying
   b. When the bereaved person no longer talks about the lost entity
   c. When the bereaved person puts all remembrances of the loss out of sight
   d. When the bereaved person can discuss both positive and negative aspects about the lost entity
5. Which of the following is thought to facilitate the grief process?
   a. The ability to grieve in anticipation of the loss
   b. The ability to grieve alone without interference from others
   c. Having recently grieved for another loss
   d. Taking personal responsibility for the loss

Clinical Judgment Questions

6. A client who lost his wife after 35 years of marriage presents at his primary care physician's office 10 months later. He has lost 20 pounds and tells the nurse, "I just don't want to eat or do anything else for that matter." Which action by the nurse is a priority?
   a. Assess the client for depression and suicide risk.
   b. Ask the physician to order gastrointestinal studies.
   c. Encourage the client to talk about his relationship with his deceased wife.
   d. Instruct the client that the doctor will be in shortly, but right now the physical assessment must be completed.
7. An 80-year-old client arrives at the emergency department accompanied by her daughter. The daughter tells the nurse that her mom lost her husband 2 months ago and since then her mom has complained of feeling depressed and anxious. Earlier today, she began complaining of chest pain. Which action by the nurse is a priority?
   a. Instruct the daughter not to worry; these are common grief responses in the elderly.
   b. Assess vital signs and obtain an ECG.
   c. Refer the client to grief support groups in the area.
   d. Educate the client in relaxation and deep breathing exercises and evaluate whether this helps resolve the chest pain.
8. A 10-year-old child returns to school after the death of his mother. The school nurse becomes aware that this child is frequently talking in the classroom about fears that he will die, too. The classroom teacher is asking for recommendations about how to handle this situation. Which action by the nurse is most appropriate?
   a. Instruct the teacher to refer the child for psychological evaluation because this is a warning sign of depression and possible suicide.
   b. Encourage the teacher to redirect the child to activities that are focused on school performance.
   c. Educate the teacher that this a common reaction in children of this age and it is best for the teacher to offer reassurance that he is safe.
   d. Instruct the teacher to prohibit discussion of this topic in class because children in this age-group cannot understand the finality of death.

9. A client whose husband died from cancer 1 month ago attends a grief support group being conducted by the hospice nurse. During the group this client states, "Sometimes I wish I could go be with my husband. I just want to die." Which action by the nurse is a priority?
   a. Ask the client if she is having thoughts of harming or killing herself.
   b. Instruct the client and the other group members that this is a normal part of the grieving process.
   c. Make arrangements for the client to be evaluated by a psychiatrist.
   d. Elicit support from other group members by asking them if any of them have had similar feelings.
10. An adolescent who recently lost his brother in a fatal accident is referred to the school nurse following a physical fight with a peer. After attending to the client's bleeding lip, the parents ask the nurse for recommendations because their son has had several physical confrontations after the death of his brother. Which action by the nurse is most beneficial?
   a. Encourage the parents to set more limits because adolescents need more structure as they work through their grief.
   b. Encourage the parents to schedule an appointment with a psychiatrist because his behavior is a sign of a developing conduct disorder.
   c. Provide information about available support groups for adolescents who have also experienced the loss of a loved one.
   d. Instruct the parents that making their son accept legal consequences for his behavior will likely resolve the problem behavior.

IMPLICATIONS OF EVIDENCE-BASED PRACTICE

Verdery, A. M., Smith-Greenaway, E., Margolis, R., & Daw, R. (2020). Tracking the reach of COVID-19 kin loss with a bereavement multiplier applied to the United States. *Proceedings of the National Academy of Sciences, 117*(30), 17695–17701. https//:doi.org/10.1073/pnas.2007476117

DESCRIPTION OF THE STUDY: Noting that COVID-19 has created a mortality shock throughout the world and may yield a second wave of population health concerns tied to bereavement and social support reductions, the researchers sought to project the magnitude of potential bereavement-related concerns in the United States associated with COVID-19-related losses. An indicator, which the researchers identified as a "bereavement multiplier," was used to estimate the average number of people who will experience the loss of a close relative.

RESULTS OF THE STUDY: Analysis demonstrated that for every COVID-19 death, approximately nine surviving Americans will lose a grandparent, parent, sibling, spouse, or child. The researchers report that estimates of the bereavement multiplier are stable across epidemiological realities, including infection scenarios, total number of deaths, and the distribution of deaths, which means this indicator can estimate the bereavement burden over the course of the epidemic in lockstep with rising death tolls. The researchers conclude that the bereavement multiplier is a useful indicator for tracking COVID-19's multiplicative impact as it reverberates across American families and can be tailored to other causes of death.

IMPLICATIONS FOR NURSING PRACTICE: Understanding and projecting the magnitude of bereavement in circumstances like the COVID-19 pandemic can inform nurses and other health-care professionals about the potential needs for additional resources in caring for bereaved individuals. Recognizing that other research (as discussed earlier in this chapter) supports that particularly sudden, unanticipated loss is associated with both physical and mental consequences, these findings suggest that nurses will need to be prepared to address a variety of grief reactions in a variety of health-care settings following the acute period of mortality associated with this pandemic.

Communication Exercises

1. Jane's husband has been hospitalized for several days in end-stage congestive heart failure and she has just been told that he has died. She begins sobbing and screams at the nurse, "You killed my husband! I should have never brought him to the hospital!"
   What would be an appropriate, empathic response by the nurse?
2. The doctor has shared test results with David revealing that his terminal cancer is not responding to treatment. David looks to the nurse and asks, "Am I dying?"
   What would be an appropriate response by the nurse?
3. Paula has been told that she has a terminal illness. She says to the nurse, "Why would God do this to me?"
   What response by the nurse would demonstrate sensitivity to Paula's spiritual distress?

MOVIE CONNECTIONS

Steel Magnolias ▪ *My Girl* ▪ *Up* ▪ *Rabbit Hole* ▪ *Stepmom* ▪ *The Bucket List* ▪ *Tig*

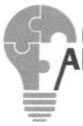

Go to **Davis Advantage** to complete your learning: strengthen understanding, apply your knowledge, and prepare for the Next Gen NCLEX®.

References

Adams, J. (2014). Death and bereavement: A whole-school approach. *Community Practitioner, 87*(8), 35–36.

Boland, R., & Verduin, M. L. (2022). *Kaplan & Sadock's synopsis of psychiatry* (P. Ruiz, Ed.). (12th ed.). Wolters Kluwer.

Catalano, J. T., & Catalano, S. (2020). Bioethical issues. In J. T. Catalano (Ed.), *Nursing now! Today's issues, tomorrow's trends* (8th ed., pp. 148–182). F.A. Davis.

Corr, C. A., & Corr, D. M. (2013). *Death and dying: Life & living* (7th ed.). Wadsworth.

Hensley, P. L., & Clayton, P. J. (2013). Why the bereavement exclusion was introduced in DSM-III. *Psychiatric Annals, 43*(6), 256–260.

Kessler, D. (2019). *Finding meaning: The sixth stage of grief.* Scribner.

King, M., Vasanthan, M., Petersen, I., Jones, L., Marston, L., & Nazareth, I. (2013). Mortality and medical care after bereavement: A practical cohort study. *PLoS ONE, 8*(1), 1–7. https://doi.org/10.1371/journal.pone.0052561

MedlinePlus. (2020). *Bereavement.* https://medlineplus.gov/bereavement.html

Morrow, A. (2022). Differences between normal and complicated grief. https://www.verywell.com/grief-and-mourning-process-1132545

Murphy, S. A., Johnson, L. C., Chung, I. J., & Beaton, R. D. (2003). The prevalence of PTSD following the violent death of a child and predictors of change 5 years later. *Journal of Traumatic Stress, 16*(1), 17–25. https://doi.org/10.1023/A:1022003126168

Peacock, S. C., Hammond-Collins, K., & Ford, D. A. (2014). The journey with dementia from the perspective of bereaved caregivers: A qualitative descriptive study. *BioMed Central Nursing, 13*(42), 1–10.

Pies, R. W. (2013). Grief and depression: The sages knew the difference. *Psychiatric Times, 30*(6). http://www.psychiatrictimes.com/display/article/10168/2140230

Pool, L. R., Burgard, S. A., Needham, B. L., Elliott, M. R., Langa, K. M., & Mendes de Leon, C. F. (2018). Association of a negative wealth shock with all-cause mortality in middle-aged and older adults in the United States. *JAMA, 319*(13), 1341–1350. https://doi.org/10.1001/jama.2018.2055

Shah, S. M., Carey, I. M., Harris, T., DeWilde, S., Victor, C. R., & Cook, D. G. (2013). The effect of unexpected bereavement on mortality in older couples. *American Journal of Public Health, 103*(6), 1140–1145.

Tousley, M. (2020). Coping with cumulative losses. *Grief Healing.* http://www.griefhealingblog.com/2013/02/coping-with-cumulative-losses.html

Worden, J. W. (2009). *Grief counseling and grief therapy: A handbook for the mental health practitioner* (4th ed.). Springer.

Verdery, A. M., Smith-Greenaway, E., Margolis, R., & Daw, R. (2020). Tracking the reach of COVID-19 kin loss with a bereavement multiplier applied to the United States. *Proceedings of the National Academy of Sciences, 117*(30), 17695–17701. https://doi.org/10.1073/pnas.2007476117

Classical References

Bowlby, J. (1961). Processes of mourning. *International Journal of Psychoanalysis, 42,* 22.

Engel, G. (1964). Grief and grieving. *American Journal of Nursing, 64,* 93.

Kübler-Ross, E. (1969). *On death and dying.* Macmillan.

28 Military Families

CHAPTER OUTLINE

Objectives
Introduction
Historical Perspective
Epidemiology
Application of the Nursing Process
Treatment Modalities
Summary and Key Points
Review Questions
Clinical Judgment Questions
Movie Connections

CORE CONCEPTS

Stress and Coping
Behaviors: Maladaptive behaviors
Professionalism: Nursing process in the care of military families

KEY TERMS

military deployment
post-traumatic stress disorder
traumatic brain injury
veterans

OBJECTIVES

After reading this chapter, the student will be able to:

1. Discuss the history and epidemiology associated with mental health in members and veterans of the U.S. military.
2. Describe the lifestyle of career military families.
3. Discuss the impact of deployment on families of service members.
4. Discuss concerns of women in the military.
5. Describe combat-related illnesses common in members and veterans of the U.S. military.
6. Apply steps of the nursing process in care of veterans with traumatic brain injury and post-traumatic stress disorder.
7. Discuss various modalities relevant to treatment of traumatic brain injury and post-traumatic stress disorder.

Introduction

Because of U.S. involvement in Iraq and Afghanistan, perhaps at no time in modern history has so much attention been given to what individuals and families experience as a result of their lives in the military. Services to meet the needs of active-duty military personnel and **veterans** (individuals who have served but are no longer serving) are in great demand, and resources for these services will be required for many years to come. More mental health-care practitioners will be needed as the increasing numbers of veterans and their family members struggle to cope with the effects of **military deployment** (movement into active tours of duty).

This chapter addresses issues associated with the lives of military families and veterans of military combat. A discussion of nursing care for these individuals is presented and selected medical treatment modalities are described.

Historical Perspective

To care for him who shall have borne the battle
and for his widow and his orphan.
—Abraham Lincoln, 1865

There is little doubt that individuals who survive military combat return from battle with scars—physical or psychological, or both. Reports of war-related psychological symptoms have existed in writing throughout the centuries and have been identified by terms such as *shell shock* and *battle fatigue*. Many veterans of World War I and World War II were expected to be stoic, to lock up their feelings, and to never speak of the scenes of carnage and combat that they witnessed. Misuse of alcohol became a common way to deal with the emotions and experiences that were uncomfortable to discuss. **Post-traumatic stress disorder** (PTSD) (a psychiatric disorder associated with exposure to one or more traumatic events) has been associated with high rates of alcoholism among veterans, particularly those who have experienced active-duty combat. Only in recent history have the invisible wounds of combat veterans received the attention they desperately require.

Very little was written about PTSD during the years between 1950 and 1970. This absence was followed in the 1970s and 1980s by a significant increase in the amount of research and writing on the subject. Many of the papers written during this time were about Vietnam veterans. Clearly, the renewed interest in PTSD was linked to the psychological casualties of the Vietnam War. The diagnostic category of PTSD did not appear until the third edition of the *Diagnostic and Statistical Manual of Mental Disorders* (3rd ed.; *DSM-III*; American Psychiatric Association [APA]) in 1980, after a need was indicated by increasing numbers of problems experienced by Vietnam veterans and victims of multiple disasters.

Epidemiology

Currently, the military comprises more than 1.3 million individuals on active duty in the U.S. armed forces in more than 150 countries around the world. Reserve forces number over 1.2 million and the overall total number of military personnel (including civilian personnel) is over 3.5 million (Department of Defense [DoD], 2019). Approximately 16.9% of those in active duty are women and they comprise roughly 18.4% of active-duty officers. Veterans currently number more than 18 million (U.S. Census Bureau, 2019).

Since the beginning of the wars in Afghanistan and Iraq in 2001, more than 2.2 million U.S. military personnel have been deployed in 3 million tours of duty lasting more than 30 days as part of Operation Enduring Freedom (OEF) and Operation Iraqi Freedom (OIF) (Institute of Medicine [IOM], 2013). According to the IOM report *Returning Home from Iraq and Afghanistan*, 44% of these military personnel identified difficulty readjusting to daily living upon return from deployment, and 30% reported unemployment, which is twice the percentage of their nonveteran counterparts. The cost in deaths and physical and psychological injuries cannot be measured.

Application of the Nursing Process

Background Assessment Data

The Military Family

The military lifestyle offers both positive and negative aspects to those who choose this way of life. Hall (2011) summarizes several pros and cons about what has come to be known as the Warrior Society. Advantages include:

- Early retirement compared to civilian counterparts
- A vast resource system to meet family needs
- Job security with a guaranteed paycheck
- Health-care benefits
- Opportunities to see different areas of the world
- Educational opportunities

Disadvantages include:

- Frequent separations and reunions
- Regular household relocations
- Living life under the maxim of "the mission must always come first"
- A pattern of rigidity, regimentation, and conformity in family life
- Feelings of detachment from the nonmilitary community
- The social effects of "rank"
- The lack of control over pay, promotion, and other benefits

Mary Wertsch (1996), who conducted a vast amount of research on the culture of the military family, stated, "The great paradox of the military is that its members, the self-appointed front-line guardians of our cherished American democratic values, do not live in democracy themselves" (p. 15). The military is maintained by a rigid authoritarian structure, and these characteristics often extend into the structure of the home.

A class system is strikingly evident in the military with two distinct subcultures: that of the officer and that of the enlisted ranks. Hall (2011) states:

> The United States has made great strides in the past five decades to affirm and equalize the differences in

> society, but the assumption of all military systems in the world is that it is essential for the functioning of the organization to maintain a rigid hierarchical system based on dominance and subordination. (p. 38)

Isolation and alienation are common facets of military life. To compensate for the extreme mobility, the focus of this lifestyle turns inward to the military world rather than outward to the local community. Children of military families almost always report that no matter what school they attend, they feel "different" from the other students (Wertsch, 1996).

These descriptions apply principally to "career" military families. Another type of military family, those in the all-volunteer military, have become a familiar part of the American culture in recent years. The military campaigns of OEF and OIF together make up the longest sustained U.S. military operation since the Vietnam War, and they are the first extended conflicts to depend on an all-volunteer military (IOM, 2013). There has been heavy dependence on the National Guard and Reserves and an escalation in the pace, duration, and number of deployments and redeployments experienced by these individuals. Many had joined the National Guard or Reserves as a second job for financial reasons or for the educational opportunities available to them. Little thought had been given to the possibility of actually fighting in a war. As one anonymous reservist posted on his blog:

> The active forces have the harder role. They're required to be fully ready 24/7/365, and to deploy and fight on much shorter notice than the Reserve [forces] . . . it's their livelihood and (for many) their career. They're serving full-time; reservists aren't. But is that really quite true anymore? . . . Many reservists have already served multiple years on active duty since 9/11, away from home/job/family. And this situation doesn't look to change anytime soon. (Kelly Temps in Uniform, 2012)

In recent years, enlistees in the National Guard and Reserves are being told that they should expect to serve an interval of active duty. The Iraq and Afghanistan conflicts have engaged more National Guard and Reserve forces members than previous conflicts, and perhaps associated with this is the finding that more women and parents of young children are being deployed as well (IOM, 2013). Most individuals in the National Guard and Reserves are willing to serve when and where they are needed. However, they consider themselves "part-timers." The extended campaigns of OEF and OIF have changed this part-time concept for many who have served multiple tours of duty, creating a hardship on their families and their civilian careers. The IOM reports that recent military tours of duty, in general, are marked by longer deployments and shorter intervals at home. Many of these "temporary citizen soldiers," as well as their full-time military counterparts, now carry the physical and psychological scars of battle.

Military Spouses and Children

A military spouse inherently knows and lives with the concept of "mission first." Devries and colleagues (2012) state, "While the military works hard to value the family lives of service members and their welfare, the nature of the job is that the mission trumps all other concerns" (p. 11). However, times have changed from the days when life in the military was viewed as a two-person career, in which a woman was expected to "create the right family setting so that her husband's work reflected his life at home, by staying positive, being interested in his duty, and being flexible and adaptable" (Hall, 2012, p. 148). Many of today's military spouses have their own careers or are pursuing higher levels of education. They do not view the military as a joint career with their service member spouse.

The lives of military spouses and children are clearly affected when the service member's active-duty assignments require frequent family moves. In most instances, when the service member receives orders for a new geographical assignment, the spouse's education or career, or both, is put on hold and the entire family is relocated. Other occasions may arise when the family is unable to immediately follow the service member to the new location. In certain instances, such as when a student may be about to complete a semester or is about to graduate, the service member may proceed to the new assignment without the family. This is difficult for the military spouse who is left alone to care for children as well as to deal with all aspects of the move. Among active-duty members, almost 37% have children (DoD, 2019).

Military children and their parents face unique challenges. There are over 977,000 children and youth in military families, and approximately 42.1% of the children of active-duty members are 5 years of age or younger (DoD, 2019). School-age children primarily attend civilian public schools where they form a unique subculture among staff and peers who often do not understand their life experiences. Children who grow up in a career military family learn to adapt to changing situations very quickly and to hide a certain level of fear associated with the nomadic lifestyle. Hall (2008) states:

> It is not just a fear of what might happen to their family or their military parents but a fear of the unknown, of not being accepted, of being behind, of not finding friends, or of not being cool. One of the most common concerns expressed by students when they arrive in a new school is who they will eat lunch with. Another reality for student athletes is that a student could be the star of the basketball team in one school and be sitting on the bench at the next. (p. 103)

The Impact of Deployment

Not since the Vietnam War have so many U.S. military families been affected by deployment-related family separation, combat injury, and death. Many service members have been deployed multiple times. Those who are deployed most frequently describe their greatest fear as that of having to leave their spouse and children. Lengthy separations pose many challenges to all members of the family. Spouses undertake all the challenges of managing the household in addition to assuming the role of the singular parent. The pressure and stress are intense as the spouse attempts to maintain an atmosphere of strength for the children while experiencing the fears and anxiety associated with the life-threatening conditions facing their service member partner.

Millions of American children have experienced the deployment of a parent to Iraq or Afghanistan and thousands have either lost a parent or have a parent who was wounded in these conflicts. Smith (2012) states:

> The stress that comes when a family member is deployed is significant, and that stress is multiplied when a loved one is wounded or killed. When parents return from deployment, they are not always the same as they were before. Major injuries, such as loss of a limb, traumatic brain injury, or posttraumatic stress disorder are life-altering, and children often have a hard time understanding the reason for a significant change in the appearance, personality, or behavior of a parent.

The following behaviors have been reported in children in response to the deployment of a parent (American Academy of Child & Adolescent Psychiatry, n.d.):

- ***Infants (birth to 12 months)*** may respond to disruptions in their schedule with decreased appetite, weight loss, irritability, and/or apathy.
- ***Toddlers (1 to 3 years)*** may become sullen, tearful, throw temper tantrums, or develop sleep problems.
- ***Preschoolers (3 to 6 years)*** may regress in areas such as toilet training, sleep, separation fears, physical complaints, or thumb sucking. They may assume blame for parent's departure.
- ***School-age children (6 to 12 years)*** are more aware of potential dangers to parent. They may exhibit irritable behavior, aggression, or whininess and may become more regressed and fearful about parent's safety.
- ***Adolescents (13 to 18 years)*** may be rebellious, irritable, or more challenging of authority. Parents need to be alert to high-risk behaviors, such as problems with the law, sexual acting out, and drug or alcohol abuse.

A recent meta-analysis (Cunitz et al., 2019) of studies on the impact of deployment as a risk factor for children's mental health reports that the reduced contact with the deployed parent, concerns about that parent's safety, and the role confusion brought on by taking on too-early and possibly age-inappropriate family responsibilities can lead to physical and mental overload and result in less family involvement, reduced emotional warmth and responsiveness, controlling or rejecting behaviors, and even hostility.

Pincus and associates (2007) describe the cycle of deployment in five distinct stages: predeployment, deployment, sustainment, redeployment, and postdeployment.

1. ***Predeployment:*** The time frame for this stage is variable, beginning with the receipt of the orders and ending when the service member departs. Family members alternate with feelings of denial and anticipation of loss. The soldier and family get their affairs in order, extended training periods result in long hours apart, and the anxiety of the anticipated departure promotes stress and irritability among family members.
2. ***Deployment:*** This stage includes the time from actual deployment through the first month of separation. Military spouses report feeling disoriented and overwhelmed, and they experience a range of emotions, including numbness, sadness, loneliness, and abandonment. It is a time of disorganization as the spouse struggles to take charge of the details of living without his or her partner.
3. ***Sustainment:*** Sustainment begins about 1 month into the deployment until about a month before the service member's expected return. During this stage, the spouse and children establish new support systems and institute new family routines.

Technology makes it possible for the family and service member to keep in touch with each other by phone, video, and e-mail. Despite the difficulties and obstacles encountered, most military families successfully negotiate this stage and anxiously anticipate their loved one's return.

4. ***Redeployment:*** This stage is defined as the month before the service member is scheduled to return home. There is excitement and apprehension associated with the homecoming. Pincus and associates (2007) identify concerns such as, "Will he (she) agree with the changes I have made?" "Will I have to give up my independence?" "Will we get along?"
5. ***Postdeployment:*** This stage typically lasts 3 to 6 months and begins with the return of the service member to the home station. There is a period of adjustment beginning with the "honeymoon" period when the spouses reconnect physically but not necessarily emotionally. The returning service member may desire to "pick up where they left off," only to encounter resistance from the spouse, who expresses a reluctance to relinquish the degree of independence and autonomy to which they have become accustomed during the separation. Pincus and associates (2007) state:

> Postdeployment is probably the most important stage for both soldier and spouse. Patient communication, going slow, lowering expectations, and taking time to get to know each other again is critical to the task of successful reintegration of the soldier back into the family.

Counseling may be required if the service member has been injured or experiences a traumatic stress reaction. In addition, the fact that many service members are redeployed back into active duty creates unique challenges in a family's attempts to re-establish roles and relationships postdeployment. Children may express a variety of emotions and behaviors including numbness rejection, or hostility.

Women in the Military

Women make up approximately 16.9% of the U.S. military and 20.6% of National Guard and Reserve members (DoD, 2019). Women have been serving in the military since the time of the Civil War, mostly in the roles of nurses, spies, and support persons. More recently the Pentagon relaxed its ban on women serving in combat roles, and "women began to fly combat aircraft, staff missile placements, drive convoys in the desert, and participate in other roles that involved potential combat exposure" (Mathewson, 2011, p. 217). Early in 2013, the secretary of defense lifted the ban on combat jobs to women, gradually opening direct combat units to female troops. At the present time, certain specialty positions continue to remain off limits, although the plan is to integrate women into these positions. Flexibility in the new law exists for exemptions to occur if further assessment reveals that some jobs are inappropriate for women.

A number of issues are of special concern to women in the military, including sexual harassment, sexual assault, differential treatment and conditions, and being a parent.

- ***Sexual harassment:*** Sexual harassment includes "unwelcome sexual advances, requests for sexual favors, and other verbal or physical harassment of a sexual nature (U.S. Equal Employment Opportunity Commission [EEOC], n.d.). In addition to overt sexual behavior, sexual harassment includes making offensive comments about a person's sex/gender. From statements such as "You look nice this morning" or "Hey, you smell good" to blatant suggestions or requests for sexual interactions, Wolfe and associates (1998), in a study of women on active duty during the Persian Gulf War, found that rates of both physical and sexual harassment were higher than are typically found in peacetime military samples. Reports by military therapists conveyed that women who were sexually harassed while in the military suffer high rates of a range of problems following discharge, including poor self-image, relationship problems, drug use, depression, and PTSD.
- ***Sexual assault:*** The DoD (Department of Defense [2021a]) received reports of 7,816 cases of sexual assault in 2020 with 6,290 involving allegations from service members for incidents that occurred during military service (a 1% increase from the previous year); 81% of the victims were females. The DoD defines *sexual assault* as "unwanted sexual contact," and Congress now requires annual tracking of reported events. In each subsequent year for the past several reporting periods, there has been an increase in reporting. The DoD, in addition to collecting data on reports of sexual assaults, now collects data on reports of retaliation associated with reporting. In its latest report, the DoD (2021a) notes that, in most cases, the reports of retaliation were from women and the retaliation was most often from a superior in the chain of command rather than the perpetrator of the sexual assault. Clearly, the culture within the military continues to reinforce

that there are consequences when events such as these are reported.

In 2000, following incidents of military sexual assault that were made public, the Veterans Health Administration mandated universal health screening for sexual trauma among military personnel. But despite the efforts within the DoD to identify and correct this problem, incidents continue, suggesting that sexual assault remains a part of military culture and is likely underreported.

Some women who report their sexual assaults are discharged from the service with psychiatric diagnoses of personality disorder or adjustment disorder. Vlahos (2012) reports:

> For the veteran, getting a personality disorder or adjustment disorder discharge can be catastrophic. Not only does it carry a stigma for future employers, it cuts the veteran off from a series of benefits, including health care and service-related disability compensation.

- Survivors of sexual assault in the military report long-lasting effects, including PTSD, depression, suicidal ideation and attempts, eating disorders, anxiety disorders, relationship difficulties, and substance abuse. Wolf (2012) notes that, among military veterans, the leading cause of PTSD for men is combat trauma, whereas for women it is sexual trauma. She states, "Our women veterans are more likely to be traumatized by a sexual assault by a fellow soldier, or a commander, than by their own battlefield or war experiences."
- ***Differential treatment and conditions:*** Although their numbers have increased, women still constitute a minority in the military. One female officer stated that because of the small number of women in any given unit, officers and enlisted personnel are often housed together. She indicated that she missed being with other officers to discuss work and being able to spend time with her peers. She also reported that the enlisted women were uncomfortable with an officer in their presence. Burgess and colleagues (2013) add that when sexual trauma occurs among military personnel, it is occurring in the workplace and, consequently, the victim is often in a position of having ongoing contact with the perpetrator and may also be in a dependent position if the perpetrator is in a supervisory role.

  Women's military careers are often limited by their exclusions from occupational specialties. These sanctions often preclude female officers and enlisted personnel from the most prestigious units and occupations in the military, their participation in which is essential to ascending in the ranks should they choose to make the military a career. Fears of additional occupational discrimination may prevent women from reporting incidents of sexual harassment and assault. Many bans have been lifted, and occupations that historically have been off limits are now open to women. However, the manner in which the culture within the military responds to those changes remains to be seen.
- ***Parenting issues:*** Women's feelings associated with leaving their children often differ from those of men. Women seem to struggle more with guilt feelings for "abandoning" their children, whereas men have stronger emotions tied to a sense of doing their duty. Although men also experience regret at leaving their children, they often rely on the assurance that the children have their mothers to care for them.

Veterans

Most veterans returning from a combat zone undergo a period of adjustment. A study of young veterans (Pedersen et al., 2016) identified that 70% screened as positive for behavioral health problems, less than a third of whom received adequate psychotherapy or psychotropic treatment. Many veterans have migraine headaches and experience cognitive difficulties, such as memory loss. Hypervigilance, insomnia, and jitteriness are common. The Substance Abuse and Mental Health Services Administration (SAMHSA) (Pemberton et al., 2016) reported that, particularly in the 18 to 25 age-group of veterans, there was a higher incidence of nonmedical use of pain relievers, amphetamine use, and alcohol abuse or dependence than for nonveterans and higher incidence of mental illness including major depressive episodes and severe mental illnesses. Plach and Sells (2013) identified in a study of veterans, that over 50% screened positive for problem drinking, and over 90% had engaged in hazardous drinking.

Traumatic Brain Injury

The incidence of **traumatic brain injury** (TBI) is a significant sequela of the Iraq and Afghanistan conflicts. Mild TBI is so frequent that it has been referred to as the "signature injury" of the wars in these countries (Cogan, 2014). The DoD (2021b) reports a total of 434,618 TBIs since 2000, and over 16,000 in 2020 alone.

The Department of Veterans Affairs and Department of Defense (VA/DoD, 2016) offer the following definition of TBI:

> A traumatically induced structural injury and/or physiological disruption of brain function as a result of an external force that is indicated by new onset or worsening of at least one of the following clinical signs, immediately following the event:
> - Any period of loss of or a decreased level of consciousness
> - Any loss of memory for events immediately before or after the injury (post-traumatic amnesia)
> - Any alteration in mental state at the time of the injury (confusion, disorientation, slowed thinking, etc.) (Alteration of consciousness/mental state)
> - Neurological deficits (weakness, loss of balance, change in vision, praxis, paresis/plegia, sensory loss, aphasia, etc.) that may or may not be transient
> - Intracranial lesion

Symptoms may be classified as mild, moderate, or severe, according to their severity. In the civilian population, the most common causes of TBI include child abuse in infants and toddlers, motor vehicle accidents in adolescents and young adults, and falls and associated subdural hematomas in older adults (Strong & Donders, 2012). Blasts from explosive devices are the leading cause of TBI for active-duty military personnel in combat (Birk, 2010; Cogan, 2014). Although the mechanism of damage from explosive blasts is not completely understood, researchers believe that it is "the pressure wave passing through the brain that significantly disrupts brain function" (Mayo Clinic, 2021). TBI also results from penetrating wounds, severe blows to the head with shrapnel or debris, and falls or bodily collisions with objects following a blast. Symptoms of TBI according to level of severity are presented in Table 28–1.

Most soldiers who have sustained a mild TBI improve with no lasting clinical sequelae (VA/DoD, 2016). Many recover within hours to days, or, at most, weeks. In a small minority, symptoms persist from 6 months to a year. The location and severity of the injury are factors that determine the long-term outcome for individuals with TBI. Severity is determined by the nature, speed, and location of the impact and by complications such as hypoxemia, hypotension, intracranial hemorrhage, and increased intracranial pressure.

The most common long-term consequences of TBI include problems with cognition (e.g., thinking, memory, and reasoning) and behavior or mental health (e.g., depression, anxiety, personality changes, aggression, acting out, and social inappropriateness). Seizures occur in about 15% to 20% of individuals with TBI and commonly develop within the first 24 hours following the injury. With mild TBI, seizures usually subside within a week after the initial trauma. The potential for chronic epilepsy increases with severity of the injury.

Language and communication problems, such as aphasia, dysarthria, and dysphasia, can result from TBI (Byers & Jorge, 2017). Difficulties may also exist in the subtler aspects of communication, such as body language and nonverbal expression.

Studies show that TBI can have long-term adverse effects on social functioning and productivity. Temkin and colleagues (2009) stated:

> Penetrating head injury sustained in wartime is clearly associated with increased unemployment. TBI also adversely affects leisure and recreation, social relationships, functional status, quality of life, and independent living. Although there is a dose-response relationship between severity of injury and social outcomes, there is insufficient evidence to determine at what level of severity the adverse effects are demonstrated. (p. 460)

Risk for degenerative brain diseases such as Alzheimer's disease (AD), Parkinson's disease, and dementia pugilista (dementia associated with repetitive blows to the head) are increased with severe or repeated TBI (Mayo Clinic, 2021). The risk for AD in individuals with moderate TBI is 2.3 times greater than it is in the general population. More research is needed to identify why and how TBI increases these risks.

Several factors have also been identified that may worsen the condition of military personnel who sustain a TBI. Being in a high-stress environment, being in extreme temperatures such as the 120°F temperatures common in Iraq, and having a TBI that is not recognized until the postdeployment period may all interfere with healing (Cogan, 2014). The prevalence as well as short- and long-term consequences suggest that screening for TBI should be conducted for all military personnel returning from active duty who present with physical, cognitive, or emotional symptoms. Emotional symptoms of TBI may be misdiagnosed (particularly in women) as a psychiatric disorder and since there are many service-related injuries beyond exposure to explosive blasts that can result in TBIs, assessment should always attempt to rule out TBI before finalizing a diagnosis (Bolster, 2019).

TABLE 28–1 Criteria and Symptomatology of Traumatic Brain Injury (TBI) According to Level of Severity

MILD	MODERATE	SEVERE
CRITERIA		
Structural imaging = normal	Structural imaging = normal or abnormal	Structural imaging = normal or abnormal
Loss of consciousness 0–30 min	Loss of consciousness >30 min and <24 hr	Loss of consciousness >24 hr
Alteration of consciousness/mental state = a moment up to 24 hr	Alteration of consciousness/mental state >24 hr; severity based on other criteria	Alteration of consciousness/mental state >24 hr; severity based on other criteria
Post-traumatic amnesia = 0–1 day	Post-traumatic amnesia = >1 and <7 days	Post-traumatic amnesia >7 days
Glasgow Coma Scale = 13–15 (best available score within first 24 hr)*	Glasgow Coma Scale = 9–12	Glasgow Coma Scale <9
SYMPTOMS		
Headache	Any of the symptoms of mild TBI	Any of the symptoms of mild TBI
Dizziness, ringing in the ears	Headache that gets worse or does not go away	Headache that gets worse or does not go away
Nausea	Repeated nausea and vomiting	Repeated nausea and vomiting
Trouble concentrating, confusion	Seizures	Seizures
Blurred vision	Difficulty awakening from sleep	Inability to awaken from sleep
Changes in sleep patterns	Dilation of one or both pupils of the eyes	Dilation of one or both pupils of the eyes
Mood changes	Slurred speech	Slurred speech
Sensitivity to light or sound	Weakness or numbness in the extremities Loss of coordination Increased confusion Restlessness Agitation	Weakness or numbness in the extremities Loss of coordination Profound confusion Restlessness Agitation

Source: Compiled from Department of Veterans Affairs & Department of Defense (2016); Mayo Clinic (2021); National Institute of Neurological Disorders and Stroke (2020).
*In 2015, the DoD recommended against using the Glasgow Coma Scale to diagnose TBI.

Post-traumatic Stress Disorder

PTSD is the most common mental disorder among veterans returning from military combat. The lifetime prevalence for PTSD in the general population is 6.8%; among military veterans, estimates range from 13.8% to 30% (Gradus, 2020).

The diagnostic criteria for PTSD from the *Diagnostic and Statistical Manual of Mental Disorders, Fifth Edition, Text Revision* (*DSM-5-TR*; American Psychiatric Association [APA], 2022) are presented in Chapter 19, "Trauma- and Stressor-Related Disorders." The disorder can occur when an individual is exposed to an accident or violence in which there is actual or threatened death or serious injury to the self or others. Symptoms of PTSD include the following:

- Reexperiencing the trauma through flashbacks, nightmares, and intrusive thoughts
- Intensive efforts to avoid activities, people, places, situations, or objects that arouse recollections of the trauma
- Chronic negative emotional state and diminished interest or participation in significant activities
- Aggressive, reckless, or self-destructive behavior

- Hypervigilance and exaggerated startle response
- Angry outbursts, problems with concentration, and sleep disturbances

Symptoms of PTSD may be delayed, in some instances for years. When emotions regarding the trauma are constricted, they may suddenly appear at some time in the future following a major life event, stressor, or an accumulation of stressors with time that challenge the person's defenses. Symptoms also may be masked by other physical or mental health problems that the veteran may be experiencing. In some instances, the symptoms do not appear to be problematic until the individual begins a readjustment to routine occupational or social functioning.

Reports indicate that many veterans decades after returning from combat have been diagnosed with PTSD (U.S. Department of Veteran Affairs, 2020). At the time of their return, rarely did these veterans speak of their war experiences. But in many, the visions of horror have seeped to the surface in nightmares, flashbacks, anxiety, and emotional numbness. Langer (2011) reported that the PTSD symptoms for these veterans seemed to become more prominent in midlife and that the most significant precipitant was retirement. For many, their work gave meaning to their lives, and without it the symptoms of depression, anxiety, substance abuse, and PTSD began to emerge. Langer stated:

> Besides retirement, other precipitants [to PTSD in midlife] include the deaths of friends, one's own deteriorating health, children becoming autonomous, divorce, and other losses associated with aging. Other precipitants include current events that trigger memories of one's own combat experience, e.g., 9/11 and other wars.

Soldiers with PTSD, TBI, or depression have all been identified as high risk for partner abuse (Slosson, 2012), and research has identified "severe and pervasive negative effects on marital adjustment, general family functioning, and mental health of partners" (Price & Stevens, 2019) contributing to parenting problems, caregiver burden, and divorce. In its report on the readjustment needs of veterans, the IOM (2013) identified a significant rise in domestic violence among veterans of the Iraq and Afghanistan wars, and recommended this issue be a high priority for assessment and intervention. The burden of caregiving to a partner with PTSD has been noted as a contributing factor in relationship difficulties. Some caregivers may experience what has been termed as *secondary trauma* or *vicarious traumatization*, a condition in which somatic symptoms and emotional distress occur as a response to caring for an individual who exhibits the symptoms of PTSD. Secondary symptoms are also common in children with a parent suffering from PTSD. Family members sometimes report having nightmares that mimic feelings and experiences of the veteran, difficulty sleeping, depression, and even visual hallucinations that are similar to the veteran's flashbacks.

Co-occurring disorders are common in individuals with PTSD, including major depressive disorder, substance use disorders, and anxiety disorders. Individuals with TBI may develop PTSD, depending on the degree of amnesia experienced immediately following the cerebral trauma. In addition, evidence supports that PTSD increases the risk for dementia (Desmarais et al., 2020).

Depression and Suicide

Depressive disorder has been identified as one of the most common mental health disorders among veterans and among those who were diagnosed with depression, 33.2% of them also had a PTSD diagnosis (Close, 2020). Both disorders are associated with impairment in interpersonal relationships, occupational and social functioning, increased risk for substance use disorders, and increased risk for suicide.

Reports by the DoD and VA indicate that the number of suicides among veterans and active-duty military has risen dramatically since 2001, the year that detailed record-keeping began. This number reached an all-time high in 2012 with a rate of 22.7 suicides per 100,000 population (319) of active-duty military personnel, and although that number declined somewhat in 2013 to 18.7 per 100,000 (259), the number of suicides among Reservists and National Guard members remained alarmingly high at 23.4 to 28.9 per 100,000, respectively (Kime, 2015). Currently suicide rates among active-duty members continue to rise, and when suicides among veterans are added to the numbers, the incidence is even higher. In 2019, the year for which the most recent data are available, suicide rates climbed to 25.9 per 100,000 among active-duty members, an increase from 20.4 per 100,000 in 2014 (DoD, 2020). The DoD reports that when statistics are adjusted for age and sex, these numbers approximate suicide rates in the general population, but in any scenario, the numbers are climbing and underscore the need for intensive and ongoing suicide prevention initiatives.

In 2017 the U.S. Department of Veterans Affairs released a report that examined suicide rates among veterans from 1979 to 2014. One significant finding was that the incidence of suicide among veterans was 22% higher than the general population and 65% of all military personnel who died by suicide were veterans age 50 or older. For female veterans, the highest suicide rate was among those ages 18 to 29.

Access to firearms has been identified as increasing the risk for suicide among vulnerable military personnel. Whereas the use of firearms as a method for suicide has declined in the civilian population, it remains high among veterans and has increased among female veterans. The U.S. Department of Veterans Affairs (2017) concludes that "these results strongly suggest that firearms safety initiatives are likely an important component of an effective suicide prevention strategy for male and female veterans" (p. 47). The latest annual report on suicide (DoD, 2020) clarifies further that 83% of firearm deaths among active service members are related to suicide, compared to 3.5% that are related to combat.

The IOM report (2013) identified that compounding the risks for suicide is the fact that the VA has had a policy against restricting access to privately owned weapons. In 2014, VA policies were expanded to allow commanders to discuss access to firearms with at-risk populations and to provide for voluntary surrender of their firearms if they request it (Kime, 2015). The latest DoD annual report (2020) identifies several initiatives focused on suicide prevention, one of which is a pilot program called CALM (Counseling on Access to Lethal Means) that trains nonmedical military providers on strategies to reduce access to and safely store lethal weapons.

Suicide among military personnel is closely associated with the diagnoses of substance use disorder, major depressive disorder, anxiety disorders, PTSD, and TBI. A common theme among investigations of suicide attempts and completed suicides by military service members includes marital/relationship distress. Devries and associates (2012) found that relationship problems were a factor in over 50% of suicides in the Army.

A study by Ravindran and associates (2020) found that veterans who were never married or who were divorced, separated, or widowed at the time of transition from active duty were at higher risk for suicide. Conversely, a study of National Guard members (Blow et al., 2018) found that, in the postdeployment period, a strong intimate relationship decreased suicide rates in members who had PTSD, depression, and anxiety (a group that has been identified at particularly high risk for suicide).

The multiplicity of factors influencing these dramatic suicide rates makes it hard to pinpoint a specific cause, but it has captured the attention of the government and the general public. President Obama signed into law the Clay Hunt Suicide Prevention for American Veterans (SAV) Act (2015), which, among other things, intends to expand peer support for troubled veterans, streamline transitions for exiting service people, and mandate annual surveying of VA mental health and suicide prevention programs. Clayton Hunt was a decorated Marine who struggled with PTSD and depression after returning home from active duty and took his own life in 2011.

Substance Use Disorder

In addition to rising suicide rates, alcohol and drug misuse is a significant problem in the military with more than 1 in 10 veterans being diagnosed with a substance use disorder (National Institute on Drug Abuse [NIDA], 2019). About 30% of Army suicides and over 45% of suicide attempts since 2003 involved alcohol or drug use and an estimated 20% of high-risk behavior deaths were attributed to alcohol or drug overdose (NIDA, 2019).

Substance use disorder (SUD) is a common co-occurring condition with PTSD. Among OEF/OIF veterans, 63% diagnosed with an SUD also met criteria for PTSD, and veterans dually diagnosed with PTSD and SUDs are more likely to have additional co-occurring psychiatric and medical conditions, such as seizures, liver disease, HIV, schizophrenia, anxiety disorders, and bipolar disorder (Teeters et al., 2017). One study found that around 22% of all service members report heavy alcohol use (Herberman Mash et al., 2016). The combination of substance use, PTSD, depression, and TBI contributes to a significant risk for mental illness, relationship problems, difficult readjustment to home life, and, in many cases, suicide.

Among veterans who sought treatment for substance use disorder, 65% (almost double that of the nonveteran population) identified alcohol as their primary substance of misuse (SAMHSA, 2015).

As with U.S. civilians, opioid pain medication use and abuse among military personnel has increased. NIDA (2019) reported that from 2005 to 2009, prescriptions for pain medications prescribed by military physicians quadrupled. Since 2011, opioid prescriptions have declined in military and civilian populations yet one study found that 46.2% of combat-wounded veterans were misusing opioids and 21.7% were misusing sedatives (Kelley et al., 2019).

According to a 2018 analysis, 30% of veterans and 14% of active-duty members report using tobacco, and e-cigarette use is increasing (U.S. Food and Drug Administration, 2020). The IOM report (2013) on readjustment needs of veterans identified that as many as 39% of veterans are struggling with substance use issues, and their recommendations included supporting research to identify evidence-based treatments for substance use disorders as well as reevaluating policies about access to substances of abuse within the military. A firsthand account of what it was like for Sean, a soldier who served in Iraq, and his experience afterward, is presented in "Real People Real Stories: The Military Experience."

Diagnosis and Outcome Identification

Nursing diagnoses are formulated from the data gathered during the assessment phase and with background knowledge regarding predisposing factors to the disorder. Table 28–2 presents a list of selected patient behaviors and the NANDA-International nursing diagnoses (Herdman et al., 2021) that correspond to those behaviors, which may be used in planning assistance for families as they confront the unique challenges associated with military life. Outcome criteria are presented for each.

Planning, Implementation, and Evaluation

Nurses provide care for service members, veterans, and their families in a variety of settings, including general hospitals, VA hospitals, community health centers, doctors' offices, long-term care centers, and community-based clinics. The care required by the veterans returning from combat in the war on terrorism is complex and multifaceted. War-related physical injuries are often striking and conspicuous in their visibility. However, it is the veteran's *invisible* injuries with which psychiatric mental health nurses are most often called upon for treatment. The need for nurses to provide care for the increasing number of veterans with these invisible injuries is intensifying, and the VA continues to search for more effective ways to ensure that military veterans and families receive the care that they desperately need and deserve. Clever and Segal (2013) caution that even though military families have some unique challenges, including compounding issues when both spouses are in the military, they are a diverse group and their needs are dynamic as they move through the transitions in their military career and family life.

Interventions for a selected number of nursing diagnoses relevant to veterans and military families are presented in Table 28–3. Evaluation is conducted by reassessing to determine whether the nursing actions have been successful in meeting the outcome criteria.

Treatment Modalities

Treatment for PTSD and TBI includes psychosocial, rehabilitative, and medical approaches, which often can be combined for optimal response. Selection of appropriate therapy depends on accurate diagnosis and symptom assessment.

Post-traumatic Stress Disorder

Psychosocial Therapies

Cognitive therapy, prolonged exposure therapy, group and family therapy, and eye movement desensitization and reprocessing have all been used successfully in the treatment of PTSD.

Psychopharmacology

Selective serotonin reuptake inhibitors (SSRIs) are now considered first-line treatment of choice for PTSD because of their efficacy, tolerability, and safety ratings. Other antidepressants that have also been effective include trazadone, the tricyclics amitriptyline and imipramine, and the monoamine oxidase inhibitor (MAOI) phenelzine. Benzodiazepines are sometimes prescribed for their antipanic effects, although their addictive properties make them less desirable. Antihypertensives, such as propranolol and clonidine, have been successful in alleviating symptoms such as nightmares, intrusive recollections, hypervigilance, insomnia, startle responses, and angry outbursts. More recently, intravenous ketamine, an *N*-methyl-D-aspartate receptor antagonist, has demonstrated efficacy (along with psychotherapy) in treating PTSD (Greenway et al., 2020). Das and associates (2019) in their research on ketamine as a pharmacological treatment for problem drinking, found that ketamine was able to disrupt maladaptive memories when administered immediately after those memories were retrieved. Such findings offer hope for the same benefits in the treatment of PTSD. Although the mechanisms of action are not yet clearly understood, research supports that it may be a very beneficial treatment option for PTSD (Feder et al., 2021).

Real People, Real Stories: The Military Experience

(The individual requested that his real name not be used.)

Karyn: What was it like for you when you returned from your tour of duty?

Sean: I was in Iraq for 360 days, and when we landed in the U.S., there was a little welcome home ceremony, and then we went to hang out at the NCO club. The next day, there was a lot of paper to process for benefits and release forms. There was an assessment by a doctor that was about 5 minutes. Basically, they ask if you're okay and they take your word for it. If you say you're not okay, then you can't leave with everyone else. The third day, they encouraged us to join the American Legion and VFW clubs and then bussed us home.

Karyn: You've mentioned before that you had postconcussion headaches and some nightmares. Were you still having these symptoms when you got home?

Sean: Yeah, I had been in an area, during my tour of duty, where a roadside bomb detonated. At the time, I was having extreme headaches, and I got pain medications, but no one talked about what had happened or how I was handling that. The role of the military was to make the soldier mission-capable, so that meant just treating the symptoms. When I got home, I was still having some nightmares and headaches, but I couldn't talk about it. My wife was in the military too, so we had both learned not to talk about emotions. Within a year, I was drinking heavily and separated from my wife. I sought out treatment at the VA, but I only went three times. I felt like they were primarily trying to validate my story as if they wanted to defend themselves against a potential claim. They never asked about alcohol use. I felt angry, and I had some aggression. I felt abandoned. Then I found out my mom had stolen my military checks and had spent them. At that point, I lost faith in everything. All of my core beliefs were gone. The only thing I had faith in was my fellow soldiers, and now that we were back home, they weren't there.

Karyn: Do you get together with any fellow vets?

Sean: Mostly people connect over Facebook, so they don't really get together. The military clubs are all about drinking, so there aren't any healthy options. I do know, though, that sometimes when vets have gotten wind through Facebook that one of us is suicidal, they've travelled across the country to track them down and try to get them help.

Karyn: The suicide rates have been tragically high among vets. Have you ever had thoughts yourself about suicide?

Sean: I have. I was in a very dark place. I thought I was such an awful person that the best option was to kill myself. I was drinking, I was making bad moral decisions, and I was nasty to friends. I didn't care about anything or any consequences. I just wanted momentary relief so I drank more, but, of course, that increased the depression. And it seems like every time we go to military exercises, we hear of another loss of someone to suicide. Last week, it was a fellow soldier who was a decorated hero for saving the lives of many of our guys. [Tearful.] So how do you rectify that someone saved all those lives and then comes home and takes their own life?

Karyn: It does seem like senseless, tragic loss. What has helped you get out of that dark place?

Sean: I have a brother who, even though he couldn't understand what I was going through, he kept checking in on me and repeatedly told me he was praying for me. He just kept showing up and telling me I had to get God back in my life. I knew he cared. I had a DUI and an accident, but I kept thinking "I just have to suck it up and be stronger than this." Instead, the drinking just increases exponentially faster than you can respond or try to control it. One night, I went home and trashed my house. I was ripping sinks out of walls. I remember a neighbor came over and told me I just needed to sober up, but I called the police and told them to take me in. I knew I was out of control.

When I got to the psych unit, I knew I wanted to be "fixed," but that mainly meant I wanted to be under control. I don't remember being asked if I wanted pills, but they gave me pills, and I didn't want to take them because it just made me feel less in control. There was an LPN there who told me that her husband was a vet and that she knew he was a good person. She said she never let his behavior define who he was. That gave me a lot of hope, like maybe I wasn't such an awful person. I reached out to God, and things started to change. I acknowledged that drinking was a primary issue, I cut ties with several unhealthy relationships, and there were supportive friends who came to visit me in the hospital, so I started to see that there were people who genuinely cared about me.

Karyn: What do you want health-care providers and fellow soldiers to learn from your experience?

Sean: First, a soldier is not who you are; it's a job you do. I wish I had spent more time before my deployment literally writing down all those things that define who I am, like, I'm a loving father and a good friend and what is most important to me; what am I willing to die for. I think it would have helped me, when I came back home, to concretely remind myself of who I am. It's easy to lose all sense of that in the military.

Second, no mood-altering chemicals. There are a lot of things within the military that promote the use of chemicals such as alcohol and pain medication, and while it may keep people mission-ready or temporarily numb you, it becomes disastrous.

Third, reach out for support or, if you are a health-care provider, help someone identify those people who will provide ongoing support. Supportive people and reaching out to God have been my lifelines.

TABLE 28–2 Nursing Diagnoses: Planning Care for Military Families

RISK FACTORS/DEFINING CHARACTERISTICS	NURSING DIAGNOSES	OUTCOME CRITERIA
POST-TRAUMATIC STRESS DISORDER		
Rage reactions, aggression, irritability, substance use, flashbacks, startle reaction	Risk for other-directed violence	Patient will demonstrate appropriate coping behaviors. Patient will not harm others.
Depression, perception of lack of social support, physical disabilities from combat injuries, feelings of hopelessness	Risk for suicidal behavior	Patient will not harm self.
Anger, aggression, depression, difficulty concentrating, flashbacks, guilt, headaches, hypervigilance, intrusive thoughts and dreams, nightmares, emotional numbness, panic attacks, substance abuse	Post-trauma syndrome related to having experienced the trauma of military combat	Patient will begin a healthy grief resolution, initiating the process of psychological healing. Patient will demonstrate ability to deal with emotional reactions in an individually appropriate manner.
Substance abuse	Ineffective coping; denial	Patient will verbalize understanding of the destructiveness of substance abuse and demonstrate a more adaptive method of coping.
Confusion, fear, and anxiety among family members and their inability to deal with the affected member's unpredictable behavior; ineffective family decision-making process	Interrupted family processes related to crisis associated with veteran member's illness	Family will verbalize understanding of trauma-related illness, demonstrate ability to maintain anxiety at manageable level, and make appropriate decisions to stabilize family functioning.
TRAUMATIC BRAIN INJURY		
Impaired physical mobility, limited range of motion, decreased muscle strength and control, perceptual or cognitive impairment, seizures	Risk for injury	Patient will remain free of physical injury.
Memory deficits; distractibility; altered attention span or concentration; impaired ability to make decisions, problem solve, reason, or conceptualize; personality changes	Disturbed thought processes	Patient will regain cognitive ability to execute mental functions realistic with the extent of the injury.
Inability to perform desired or appropriate activities of daily living	Self-care deficit (specify)	Patient performs self-care activities within level of own ability.
Confusion, fear, and anxiety among family members and the inability to adapt to changes associated with veteran member's injury; difficulty accepting/receiving help; inability to express or to accept each other's feelings	Interrupted family processes related to situational transition and crisis; uncertainty about expectations and ultimate outcome	Family will verbalize understanding of trauma-related illness, demonstrate ability to maintain anxiety at manageable level, and make appropriate decisions to stabilize family functioning.
FAMILY MEMBERS' ISSUES		
Regressive behaviors, loss of appetite, temper tantrums, clinging behaviors, guilt and self-blame, sleep problems, irritability, aggression (children)	Risk for delayed child development related to feelings of abandonment associated with parent's deployment	Parent/caregiver will identify behaviors at risk and initiate interventions to promote appropriate development. Child will develop healthy coping strategies and resume normal developmental progression.

Continued

TABLE 28–2 Nursing Diagnoses: Planning Care for Military Families—cont'd

RISK FACTORS/DEFINING CHARACTERISTICS	NURSING DIAGNOSES	OUTCOME CRITERIA
Rebelliousness, irritability, acting-out behaviors, promiscuity, substance use (adolescents)	Ineffective coping related to feelings of abandonment associated with parent's deployment	Patient will work through stages of grief associated with the perceived loss and demonstrate healthy, age-appropriate coping strategies.
Depression, anxiety, loneliness, fear, feeling overwhelmed and powerless, anger (spouse/partner)	Risk for maladaptive grieving related to military deployment of spouse/partner	Patient will work through stages of grief, achieve a healthy acceptance, and express a sense of control over the present situation and future outcome.
Anger, anxiety, frustration, ineffective coping, sleep deprivation, somatic symptoms, fatigue (spouse/partner/caregiver)	Caregiver role strain related to complexity of caregiving responsibilities; lack of respite	Caregiver will demonstrate effective problem-solving skills and develop adaptive coping mechanisms to regain equilibrium.

TABLE 28–3 Nursing Interventions for Veteran Patients and Military Families

Post-traumatic stress syndrome (PTSD)	Stay with patients during periods of flashbacks and nightmares and offer reassurance of personal safety. Encourage patients to talk about the traumatic experience at their own pace. Discuss maladaptive coping mechanisms being employed. Assist patients in their effort to use more adaptive strategies. Include available support systems and make referrals for additional assistance where required. Help patients understand that use of substances merely numbs feelings and delays healing. Refer for treatment of substance use disorder. Discuss use of stress-management techniques, such as deep breathing, meditation, relaxation, and exercise. Administer medications as prescribed and provide medication education.
Risk for suicide (post-traumatic stress disorder [PTSD], traumatic brain injury [TBI])	Assess degree of risk according to seriousness of threat, existence of a plan, and availability and lethality of the means. Ask directly if patients are thinking of acting on thoughts or feelings. Ascertain presence of significant others for support. Determine whether substance use is a factor. Encourage expression of feelings, including appropriate expression of anger. Ensure that environment is safe. Help patients identify more appropriate solutions and offer hope for the future. Collaborate with patients to develop an ongoing plan for safety.
Disturbed thought processes (TBI)	Evaluate mental status, including extent of impairment in thinking ability; remote and recent memory; orientation to person, place, and time; insight and judgment; changes in personality; attention span, distractibility, and ability to make decisions or problem solve; ability to communicate appropriately; anxiety level; evidence of psychotic behavior. Report to physician any cognitive changes that become obvious. Note behaviors indicative of potential for violence and take appropriate action to prevent harm to clients and others. Provide safety measures as required. Institute seizure precautions if indicated. Assist with limited mobility issues. Monitor medication regimen. Refer to appropriate rehabilitation providers.

TABLE 28–3 Nursing Interventions for Veteran Patients and Military Families—cont'd

Interrupted family processes (PTSD, TBI)	Emphasize the importance of and encourage continuous, open communication between family members to facilitate ongoing problem-solving. Assist families to identify and use previously successful coping strategies. Encourage family participation in multidisciplinary team conference or group therapy. Involve families in social support and community activities of their interest and choice. Encourage use of stress-management techniques. Make necessary referrals (e.g., parent effectiveness, specific disease or disability support groups, self-help groups, clergy, psychological counseling, family therapy). Assist families to identify situations that may lead to fear or anxiety. Involve families in mutual goal setting to plan for the future. Identify community agencies from which families may seek assistance (e.g., Meals on Wheels, visiting nurse, trauma support group, American Cancer Society, Veterans Administration).
Risk for maladaptive grieving (family of deployed service member)	Help family members to realize that all the feelings they are having are a normal part of the grieving process. Validate their feelings of anger, loneliness, fear, powerlessness, dysphoria, and distress at separation from their loved one.
	Help parents to understand that children's and adolescents' problematic behaviors are symptoms of grieving and that they should not be deemed unacceptable and result in punishment but rather be recognized as having their basis in grief. Children should be allowed an appropriate amount of time to grieve. Some experts believe that children need at least 4 weeks to adjust to a parent's deployment (Gabany & Shellenbarger, 2010). Refer for professional help if improvement is not observed in a reasonable period. Assess if maladaptive coping strategies, such as substance abuse, are being used. Identify and encourage patients to employ previously used successful coping strategies. Encourage resuming involvement in usual activities. Caution against spending too much time alone. Suggest keeping a journal of experiences and feelings. Refer to other resources, as needed, such as psychotherapy, family counseling, religious references or pastor, or grief support group.
Caregiver role strain (spouse/caregiver of injured service member)	Assess spouse/caregivers ability to anticipate and fulfill the injured service member's unmet needs. Provide information to assist caregivers with this responsibility. Ensure that caregivers encourage injured service members to be as independent as possible. Encourage caregivers to express feelings and to participate in a support group. Provide information or demonstrate techniques for dealing with acting-out, violent, or disoriented behavior by injured service members. Identify additional needs, and ensure that resources are provided (e.g., physical therapy, occupational therapy, nutritionist, financial and legal help, and respite care). Assess for abuse of substances as a coping strategy. Refer to counseling or psychotherapy as needed.

Complementary Therapies

Several complementary and alternative medicine therapies have demonstrated some efficacy in treating symptoms of PTSD including acupuncture, moxibustion (a type of traditional Chinese medicine that involves burning moxa, a cone or stick made of ground mugwort leaves, on or near acupuncture points), Chinese herbal medicines, meditation, yoga, deep-breathing exercises, progressive relaxation, and tai chi (Song et al., 2020). The authors note, though, that more research is needed.

Traumatic Brain Injury

Type of care for the client with TBI depends on severity of the injury and area of the brain involved. Those with mild TBI most often achieve full recovery without ongoing treatment. Symptom treatment and rest may be adequate for a full recovery. For those with moderate or severe TBI, several treatment options are listed below.

Psychosocial Therapies

Cognitive behavioral therapy (CBT) has been shown to be helpful to individuals with TBI. Scorer (2013) states, "An advantage of [CBT] interventions is that, given their highly structured content, they are amenable to specialized adaptation for memory, attention, and problem-solving impairments, reflecting the difficulties people with TBI often experience."

Rehabilitation Therapies

Rehabilitation therapy is multifaceted and determined by severity and location of the brain damage. Cognitive rehabilitation therapy (CRT) is one strategy designed to help individuals regain their normal brain function through an individualized training program that incorporates learning compensatory strategies for coping with persistent deficiencies involving memory, problem-solving, and the thinking skills to get things done (National Institute of Neurological Disorders and Stroke [NINDS], 2020).

Specialists in the care of the individual with TBI may include any or all of the following (Mayo Clinic, 2021):

- ***Physiatrist:*** A physician trained in the medical specialty of physical medicine and rehabilitation. This physician oversees other professionals involved in the rehabilitation process.
- ***Occupational therapist:*** Helps the individual learn, relearn, or improve skills for everyday living.
- ***Physical therapist:*** Assists the veteran with mobility and relearning movement patterns, balance, and walking.
- ***Recreational therapist:*** Assists with leisure activities.
- ***Speech and language pathologist:*** Helps the person improve communication skills and use assistive communication devices, if necessary.
- ***Neuropsychologist or psychiatrist:*** Helps the veteran manage behaviors or learn coping strategies, provides talk therapy as needed for emotional and psychological well-being, and prescribes medication as needed.
- ***Social worker or case manager:*** Coordinates access to services, assists with care decisions and planning, and facilitates communication among various professionals, care providers, and family members.

Psychopharmacology

Medications for the individual with TBI are given to ameliorate specific symptoms. Antidepressants are prescribed for depression, which is very prevalent in individuals with TBI. SSRIs are commonly the antidepressants of choice, although tricyclics and others, such as venlafaxine, trazodone, bupropion, and duloxetine, are also used. Benzodiazepines or SSRIs may be administered for treatment of anxiety symptoms, and antipsychotics are prescribed if aggression, agitation, or psychotic behaviors occur. Anticonvulsants are given if seizures are a problem, and the physician may prescribe skeletal muscle relaxants for muscle spasms or spasticity. Methylphenidate or modafinil has been used to treat attention deficits and hyperactivity (Huang et al., 2016), and donepezil has been shown to be effective in enhancing cognitive performance of individuals with TBI (Foster & Spiegel, 2008).

Summary and Key Points

- Military personnel (including civilian personnel) number over 3.5 million. More than 1.3 million are active-duty members.
- Veterans currently number more than 18 million.
- The military lifestyle offers both positive and negative aspects to those who choose this way of life.
- To compensate for the extreme mobility, the focus of the military lifestyle turns inward to the military world rather than outward to the local community.
- In the Operation Enduring Freedom (OEF) and Operation Iraqi Freedom (OIF) campaigns, there has been heavy dependence on the National Guard and Reserves and an escalation in the pace, duration, and number of deployments and redeployments experienced by these individuals.
- Military families face unique challenges, including frequent moves and many separations.
- Children and adolescents exhibit a number of problematic behaviors in response to the separation from a deployed parent.
- The cycle of deployment is described in five distinct stages: predeployment, deployment, sustainment, redeployment, and postdeployment.
- Special concerns of women in the military include sexual harassment, sexual assault, differential treatment and conditions, and issues related to being a parent.

- Evidence supports that a majority of young veterans screen positive for behavioral health problems and a third or less of those have had adequate treatment. Returning from a combat zone causes feelings and reactions that may contribute to difficulties with reintegration into civilian life.
- Traumatic brain injury (TBI) is a traumatically induced structural injury and/or physiological disruption of brain function as a result of an external force to the head that has been associated with risk for mental illness, relationship problems, difficult readjustment to home life, and, in many cases, suicide.
- Symptoms of TBI are related to the severity of the injury and the area of the brain that has been injured.
- The most common long-term consequences of TBI include problems with cognition and behavior or mental health.
- Post-traumatic stress disorder (PTSD) is the most common mental disorder among veterans returning from military combat.
- Symptoms of PTSD may occur shortly after the trauma, or they may be delayed, in some instances for years.
- Depression among military veterans is common, and suicide rates among veterans and service members have continued to be higher than in the general population.
- Substance use disorder and depression are common co-occurring conditions with PTSD.
- Nursing care of military families and veterans is presented in the context of the six steps of the nursing process.
- Treatment modalities for PTSD and TBI include psychosocial therapies, psychopharmacology, complementary therapies, and rehabilitation therapies.

Review Questions

Select the answer that is most appropriate for each of the following questions:

1. A soldier who was deployed to Afghanistan a year ago is returning home this week. Which of the following postdeployment situations may be likely to occur during the first few months after returning home to his spouse and family? (Select all that apply.)
   a. A honeymoon period of physical reconnection
   b. Resistance from the spouse regarding possible loss of autonomy
   c. Rejection by the children for perceived abandonment
   d. A period of adjustment to reconnect emotionally
2. Which of the following is the leading cause of traumatic brain injury (TBI) in active-duty military personnel in combat?
   a. Military vehicle accidents
   b. Blasts from explosive devices
   c. Falls
   d. Blows to the head from falling debris
3. A veteran of the war in Iraq has been diagnosed with post-traumatic stress disorder (PTSD). He is a client of a VA outpatient clinic. He tells the nurse during his outpatient clinic visit that he experiences panic attacks. Which of the following medications may be prescribed to treat his panic attacks?
   a. Alprazolam
   b. Lithium
   c. Carbamazepine
   d. Haldol
4. Which of the following psychosocial therapies has been shown to be helpful for clients with TBI?
   a. Eye movement desensitization
   b. Psychoanalysis
   c. Reality therapy
   d. Cognitive behavior therapy

Continued

5. A client who was injured during combat in Afghanistan has a diagnosis of TBI. Which of the following medications might the physician prescribe to improve his memory and thinking capability?
   a. Carbamazepine
   b. Duloxetine
   c. Donepezil
   d. Bupropion

Clinical Judgment Questions

6. A veteran of the war in Iraq has been diagnosed with PTSD. He has been hospitalized after swallowing a handful of his antianxiety medication. His physical condition was stabilized in the emergency department, and he has been admitted to the psychiatric unit. In developing his initial plan of care, which is the priority nursing diagnosis?
   a. Post-trauma syndrome
   b. Risk for suicide
   c. Complicated grieving
   d. Disturbed thought processes
7. A veteran of the war in Iraq has been diagnosed with PTSD. He has been hospitalized on the psychiatric unit following an attempted suicide. In the middle of the night, he wakes up yelling and tells the nurse he was having a flashback to when his unit transport drove over an improvised explosive device and most of his fellow soldiers were killed. He is breathing heavily and perspiring, and his heart is pounding. Which is the nurse's most appropriate initial intervention?
   a. Contact the doctor on call to report the incident.
   b. Administer the prn order for chlorpromazine.
   c. Stay with the client and reassure him of his safety.
   d. Instruct him to sit outside the nurses' station until he is calm.
8. Mike, a veteran of combat in Afghanistan, has a diagnosis of mild TBI. The psychiatric home health nurse from the VA medical center is assigned to make home visits to Mike and his wife, Marissa, who is his caregiver. Which of the following would be an appropriate nursing intervention by the home health nurse? (Select all that apply.)
   a. Assess for the use of substances by Mike or Marissa.
   b. Encourage Marissa to do everything for Mike to prevent further deterioration in his condition.
   c. Assess Marissa's level of stress and potential for burnout.
   d. Encourage Marissa to allow Mike to be as independent as possible.
   e. Suggest that Marissa ask the physician for a nursing home placement for Mike.
9. A veteran who has returned 6 months ago reports to the mental health clinic, stating, "I'm falling apart. I think I'm losing it." Based on an understanding of common problems among military personnel and veterans, which item should the nurse prioritize in conducting an assessment? (Select all that apply.)
   a. Screen for alcohol and other drug abuse.
   b. Assess for suicide risk.
   c. Evaluate for evidence of TBI.
   d. Assess for signs and symptoms of PTSD.
   e. Assess whether the client had evidence of any mental illness symptoms before entry in the military.

MOVIE CONNECTIONS

The Best Years of Our Lives (1946) ▪ *The Deer Hunter* (1978) ▪ *Jarhead* (2005) ▪ *In the Valley of Elah* (2007) ▪ *The Lucky Ones* (2008) ▪ *A Walk in My Shoes* (2010) ▪ *Thank-You for Your Service* (2017) ▪ *SGT. Will Gardner* (2019)

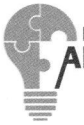

Go to **Davis Advantage** to complete your learning: strengthen understanding, apply your knowledge, and prepare for the Next Gen NCLEX®.

References

American Academy of Child & Adolescent Psychiatry. (n.d.). *Military families.* https://www.aacap.org/AACAP/Families_and_Youth/Facts_for_Families/FFF-Guide/Families-In-The-Military-088.aspx

American Psychiatric Association. (1980). *Diagnostic and statistical manual of mental disorders* (3rd ed.).

American Psychiatric Association. (2022). *Diagnostic and statistical manual of mental disorders* (5th ed., text rev.).

Birk, M. (2010). Traumatic brain injury. *Army Medicine.* http://www.armymedicine.army.mil/hc/healthtips/08/201003mtbi.cfm

Blow, A. J., Farero, A., Ganoczy, D., Walters, H., & Valenstein, M. (2018). Intimate relationships buffer suicidality in National Guard service members: A longitudinal study. *Suicide and Life-Threatening Behavior, 49*(6), 1523–1540. https://doi.org/10.1111/sltb.12537

Bolster, M. (2019, October/November). Moving ahead. *Brain & Life,* 38.

Burgess, A. W., Slattery, D. M., & Herlihy, P. A. (2013). Military sexual trauma: A silent syndrome. *Journal of Psychosocial Nursing, 51*(2), 20–26.

Byers, J. A., & Jorge, R. E. (2017). Neuropsychiatric consequences of traumatic brain injury. In B. J. Sadock, V. A. Sadock, & P. Ruiz (Eds.), *Comprehensive textbook of psychiatry* (pp. 522–540). Wolters Kluwer.

Clay Hunt Suicide Prevention for American Veterans Act of 2015, 38 U.S.C. § 1709B *et seq.* (2015). https://www.congress.gov/bill/114th-congress/house-bill/203

Close, L. (2020). *Veterans' mental health issues.* https://veteranaddiction.org/veterans-mental-health-issues/#:~:text=PTSD

Clever, M., & Segal, D. R. (2013). The demographics of military children and families. *The Future of Children, 23*(2), 13–39. https://doi.org/10.1353/foc.2013.0018

Cogan, A. M. (2014). Occupational needs and intervention strategies for military personnel with mild traumatic brain injury and persistent post-concussion symptoms: A review. *OTJR: Occupation, Participation, and Health, 34*(3), 150–159.

Cunitz, K., Dölitzsch, C., Kösters, M., Willmund, G. D., Zimmermann, P., Bühler, A. H., Fegert, J. M., Ziegenhain, U., & Kölch, M. (2019). Parental military deployment as risk factor for children's mental health: A meta-analytical review. *Child and Adolescent Psychiatry and Mental Health, 13*(26). https://doi.org/10.1186/s13034-019-0287-y

Das, R. K., Gale, G., Walsh, K., Hennessy, V. E., Iskandar, G., Mordecai, L. A., Brandner, B., Kindt, M., Curran, H. V., & Kamboj, S. K. (2019). Ketamine can reduce harmful drinking by pharmacologically rewriting drinking memories. *Nature Communications, 10*(1), 5187. https://doi.org/10.1038/s41467-019-13162

Department of Defense. (2019). *2019 demographics: Profile of the military community.* https://download.militaryonesource.mil/12038/MOS/Reports/2019-demographics-report.pdf

Department of Defense. (2020). *Annual suicide report: 2019.* https://www.dspo.mil/Portals/113/Documents/CY2019%20Suicide%20Report/DoD%20Calendar%20Year%20CY%202019%20Annual%20Suicide%20Report.pdf?ver=YOA4IZVcVA9mzwtsfdO5Ew%3d%3d

Department of Defense. (2021a). *Department of Defense annual report on sexual assault in the military, Fiscal year 2020.*

Department of Defense. (2021b). *DoD worldwide numbers for TBI.* https://health.mil/About-MHS/OASDHA/Defense-Health-Agency/Research-and-Development/Traumatic-Brain-Injury-Center-of-Excellence/DOD-TBI-Worldwide-Numbers

Department of Veterans Affairs & Department of Defense. (2016). *Clinical practice guideline for management of concussion/mild traumatic brain injury.* https://www.healthquality.va.gov/guidelines/Rehab/mtbi/mTBICPGClinicianSummary50821816.pdf

Desmarais, P., Weidman, D., Wassef, A., Bruneau, M. A., Friedland, J., Bajsarowicz, P., Thibodeau, M. P., Herrmann, N., & Nguyen, Q. D. (2020). The interplay between post-traumatic stress disorder and dementia: A systematic review. *The American Journal of Geriatric Psychiatry, 28*(1), 48–60. https://doi.org/10.1016/j.jagp.2019.08.006

Devries, M. R., Hughes, H. K., Watson, H., & Moore, B. A. (2012). Understanding the military culture. In B. A. Moore (Ed.), *Handbook of counseling military couples* (pp. 7–18). Routledge.

Feder, A., Costi, S., Rutter, S. B., Collins, A. B., Govindarajulu, U., Jha, M. K., Horn, S. R., Kautz, M., Corniquel, M., Collins, K. A., Bevilacqua, L., Glasgow, A. M., Brallier, J., Pietrzak, R. H., Murrough, J. W., & Charney, D. S. (2021). A randomized controlled trial of repeated ketamine administration for chronic posttraumatic stress disorder. *American Journal of Psychiatry, 178*(2), 193–202. https://doi.org/10.1176/appi.ajp.2020.20050596

Foster, M., & Spiegel, D. R. (2008). Use of donepezil in the treatment of cognitive impairments of moderate traumatic brain injury. *Journal of Neuropsychiatry and Clinical Neurosciences, 20*(1), 106.

Gabany, E., & Shellenbarger, T. (2010). Caring for families with deployment stress: How nurses can make a difference in the lives of military families. *American Journal of Nursing, 110*(11), 36–41.

Gradus, J. L. (2020). Epidemiology of PTSD. *National Center for PTSD.* https://www.ptsd.va.gov/professional/treat/essentials/epidemiology.asp#three

Greenway, K. T., Garel, N., Jerome, L., & Feduccia, A. A. (2020). Integrating psychotherapy and psychopharmacology: Psychedelic-assisted psychotherapy and other combined treatments. *Expert Review of Clinical Pharmacology, 13*(6), 655–670. https://doi.org/10.1080/17512433.2020.1772054.

Hall, L. K. (2008). *Counseling military families.* Taylor & Francis.

Hall, L. K. (2011). The military culture, language, and lifestyle. In R. B. Everson & C. R. Figley (Eds.), *Families under fire* (pp. 31–52). Routledge.

Hall, L. K. (2012). The military lifestyle and the relationship. In B. A. Moore (Ed.), *Handbook of counseling military couples* (pp. 137–156). Routledge.

Herberman Mash, H. B., Fullerton, C. S., Ng, T. H. H., Nock, M. K., Wynn, G. H., & Ursano, R. J. (2016). Alcohol use and reasons for drinking as risk factors for suicidal behavior in the U.S. army. *Military Medicine, 181*(8), 811.

Herdman, T. H., Kamitsuru, S., & Lopes, C. T. (2021). *NANDA International, Inc. nursing diagnoses: Definitions and classifications 2020–2023* (12th ed.). Thieme.

Huang, C. H., Huang, C. C., Sun, C. K., Lin, G. H., & Hou, W. H. (2016). Methylphenidate on cognitive improvement in patients with traumatic brain injury: A meta-analysis. *Current Neuropharmacology, 14*(3), 272–281. https://doi.org/10.2174/1570159X13666150514233033

Institute of Medicine. (2013). *Returning home from Iraq and Afghanistan: Readjustment needs of veterans, service members, and their families.* National Academies Press.

Kelley, M. L., Bravo, A. J., Votaw, V. R., Stein, E., Redman, J. C., & Witkiewitz, K. (2019). Opioid and sedative misuse among veterans wounded in combat. *Addictive Behaviors, 92*, 168–172. https://doi.org/10.1016/j.addbeh.2018.12.007

Kelly Temps in Uniform. (2012). *This ain't Hell, but you can see it from here.* http://thisainthell.us/blog/?p=30410

Kime, P. (2015, January 16). DoD military suicide rate declining. *Military Times.* http://www.militarytimes.com/story/military/pentagon/2015/01/16/defense-department-suicides-2013-report/21865977

Langer, R. (2011). Combat trauma, memory, and the World War II veteran. *War, Literature & the Arts, 23*(1). http://wlajournal.com/23_1/images/langer.pdf

Mathewson, J. (2011). In support of military women and families. In R. B. Everson & C. R. Figley (Eds.), *Families under fire* (pp. 215–235). Routledge.

Mayo Clinic. (2021). *Traumatic brain injury.* http://www.mayoclinic.com/health/traumatic-brain-injury/DS00552

National Institute on Drug Abuse. (2019). Substance use and military life: Drug facts. https://www.drugabuse.gov/publications/drugfacts/substance-use-military-life

National Institute of Neurological Disorders and Stroke. (2020). *Traumatic brain injury: Hope through research.* https://www.ninds.nih.gov/Disorders/Patient-Caregiver-Education/Hope-Through-Research/Traumatic-Brain-Injury-Hope-Through

Pedersen, E. R., Marshall, G. N., & Kurz, J. (2016). Behavioral health treatment receipt among a community sample of young adult veterans. *Journal of Behavioral Health Services & Research.* https://doi.org/10.1007/s11414-016-9534-7

Pemberton, M. R., Forman-Hoffman, V. L., Lipari, R. N., Ashley, O. S., Heller, D. C., & Williams, M. R. (2016). *Prevalence of past year substance use and mental illness by veteran status in a nationally representative sample.* https://www.samhsa.gov/data/sites/default/files/NSDUH-DR-VeteranTrends-2016/NSDUH-DR-VeteranTrends-2016.htm

Pincus, S. H., House, R., Christenson, J., & Alder, L. E. (2007). *The emotional cycle of deployment: A military family perspective.* https://www.west-point.org/parent/wppc-st_louis/Deployment/TheEmotionalCycleofDeployment.pdf

Plach, H. L., & Sells, C. H. (2013). Occupational performance needs of young veterans. *American Journal of Occupational Therapy, 67*, 73–81. https://doi.org/10.5014/ajot.2013.003871

Price, J. L., & Stevens, S. P. (2019). *Partners of veterans with PTSD: Research findings.* https://www.ptsd.va.gov/professional/treat/specific/vet_partners_research.asp

Ravindran, C., Morley, S. W., Stephens, B. M., Stanley, I. H., & Reger, M. A. (2020). Association of suicide risk with transition to civilian life among us military service members. *JAMA Network Open, 3*(9), e2016261. https://doi.org/10.1001/jamanetworkopen.2020.16261

Scorer, R. (2013). *Psychological therapies for victims of traumatic brain injury.* http://www.pannone.com/media/articles/clinical-negligence/medical-negligence/psychological-therapies-for-victims-of-traumatic-brain-injury-and-how-medical-evidence-plays-a-crucial-role

Slosson, M. (2012). Violent sex crimes by U.S. Army soldiers rise: Report. *Reuters.* https://www.reuters.com/article/us-army-health-report/violent-sex-crimes-by-u-s-army-soldiersrise-report-idUSTRE80J01C20120120

Smith, R. (2012). Military children and families. *Helping Hands for Freedom.* http://helpinghandsforfreedom.org/remaining-programs-2012-arizona-military-children-families/#more-567

Song, K., Xiong, F. M., Ding, N., Huang, A., & Zhang, H. (2020). Complementary and alternative therapies for post-traumatic stress disorder: A protocol for systematic review and network meta-analysis. *Medicine, 99*(28), e21142. https://doi.org/10.1097/MD.0000000000021142

Strong, C. H., & Donders, J. (2012). Traumatic brain injury. In B. A. Moore (Ed.), *Handbook of counseling military couples* (p. 279–294). Routledge.

Substance Abuse and Mental Health Services Administration. (2015). Veterans' primary substance of abuse is alcohol in treatment admissions. *The CBHSQ Report.* http://www.samhsa.gov/data/sites/default/files/report_2111/Spotlight-2111.pdf

Teeters, J. B., Lancaster, C. L., Brown, D. G., & Back, S. E. (2017). Substance use disorders in military veterans: Prevalence and treatment challenges. *Substance Abuse and Rehabilitation, 8*, 69–77. https://doi.org/10.2147/SAR.S116720

Temkin, N. R., Corrigan, J. D., Dikmen, S. S., & Machamer, J. (2009). Social functioning after traumatic brain injury. *Journal of Head Trauma Rehabilitation, 24*(6), 460–467.

U.S. Census Bureau. (2019). *Quick facts United States.* http://www.census.gov/quickfacts/table/PST045219

U.S. Department of Veteran Affairs. (2017). *VA releases veteran suicide statistics by state.* https://www.va.gov/opa/pressrel/pressrelease.cfm?id=2951

U.S. Department of Veteran Affairs. (2020). *Aging veterans and post-traumatic stress symptoms.* https://www.ptsd.va.gov/understand/what/aging_veterans.asp

U.S. Food and Drug Administration. (2020). *Tobacco use in the military: A danger for those who keep us safe.* https://www.fda.gov/tobacco-products/health-information/tobacco-use-military-danger-those-who-keep-us-safe

U.S. Equal Employment Opportunity Commission. (n.d.). *Sexual harassment.* https://www.eeoc.gov/laws/types/sexual_harassment.cfm

Vlahos, K. B. (2012). The rape of our military women. *Anti-War.Com.* http://original.antiwar.com/vlahos/2012/05/14/the-rape-of-our-military-women

Wolf, N. (2012, June 14). A culture of cover-up: Rape in the ranks of the U.S. military. *The Guardian.* http://www.guardian.co.uk/commentisfree/2012/jun/14/culture-coverup-rape-ranks-us-military

Classical References

Wertsch, M. E. (1996). *Military brats: Legacies of childhood inside the fortress.* Brightwell.

Wolfe, J., Sharkansky, E. J., Read, J. P., Dawson, R., Martin, J. A., & Oimette, P. C. (1998). Sexual harassment and assault as predictors of PTSD symptomatology among U.S. female Persian Gulf military personnel. *Journal of Interpersonal Violence, 13*(1), 40–57.

Appendix A

Mental Status Assessment

Gathering the correct information about the patient's mental status is essential to the development of an appropriate plan of care. The mental status examination is a description of all the areas of the patient's mental functioning. The following are the components that are considered critical in the assessment of a patient's mental status. Examples of interview questions and criteria for assessment are included.

Identifying Data

1. Name
2. Gender
3. Age
   a. How old are you?
   b. When were you born?
4. Race/culture
   a. What country did you (your ancestors) come from?
5. Occupational/financial status
   a. How do you make your living?
   b. How do you obtain money for your needs?
6. Educational level
   a. What was the highest grade level you completed in school?
7. Significant other
   a. Are you married?
   b. Do you have a significant relationship with another person?
8. Living arrangements
   a. Do you live alone?
   b. With whom do you share your home?
9. Religious preference
   a. Do you have a religious preference?
10. Allergies
    a. Are you allergic to anything?
    b. Foods? Medications?
11. Special diet considerations
    a. Do you have any special diet requirements?
    b. Diabetic? Low sodium?
12. Chief complaint
    a. For what reason did you come for help today?
    b. What seems to be the problem?
13. Medical diagnosis

General Description

Appearance

1. Grooming and dress
   a. Note unusual modes of dress.
   b. Evidence of soiled clothing?
   c. Use of makeup?
   d. Neat; unkempt?
2. Hygiene
   a. Note evidence of body or breath odor.
   b. Note condition of skin, fingernails.
3. Posture
   a. Note if standing upright, rigid, slumped over.
4. Height and weight
   a. Perform accurate measurements.
5. Level of eye contact
   a. Intermittent?
   b. Occasional and fleeting?
   c. Sustained and intense?
   d. No eye contact?
6. Hair color and texture
   a. Is hair clean and healthy looking?
   b. Greasy, matted, tangled?
7. Evidence of scars, tattoos, or other distinguishing skin marks
   a. Note any evidence of swelling or bruises.
   b. Birthmarks?
   c. Rashes?
8. Evaluation of patient's appearance compared with chronological age

Motor Activity

1. Tremors
   a. Do hands or legs tremble?
   b. Continuously?
   c. At specific times?
2. Tics or other stereotypical movements
   a. Any evidence of facial tics?
   b. Jerking or spastic movements?
3. Mannerisms and gestures
   a. Specific facial or body movements during conversation?
   b. Nail biting?

   c. Covering face with hands?
   d. Grimacing?
4. Hyperactivity
   a. Gets up and down out of chair.
   b. Paces.
   c. Unable to sit still.
5. Restlessness or agitation
   a. Lots of fidgeting.
   b. Clenching hands.
6. Aggressiveness
   a. Overtly angry and hostile.
   b. Threatening.
   c. Uses sarcasm.
7. Rigidity
   a. Sits or stands in a rigid position.
   b. Arms and legs appear stiff and unyielding.
8. Gait patterns
   a. Any evidence of limping?
   b. Limitation of range of motion?
   c. Ataxia?
   d. Shuffling?
9. Echopraxia
   a. Evidence of mimicking the actions of others?
10. Psychomotor retardation
   a. Movements are very slow.
   b. Thinking and speech are very slow.
   c. Posture is slumped.
11. Freedom of movement (range of motion)
   a. Note any limitation in ability to move.

Speech Patterns

1. Slowness or rapidity of speech
   a. Note whether speech seems very rapid or slower than normal.
2. Pressure of speech
   a. Note whether speech seems frenzied.
   b. Unable to be interrupted?
3. Intonation
   a. Are words spoken with appropriate emphasis?
   b. Are words spoken in monotone, without emphasis?
4. Volume
   a. Is speech very loud? Soft?
   b. Is speech low-pitched? High-pitched?
5. Stuttering or other speech impairments
   a. Hoarseness?
   b. Slurred speech?
6. Aphasia
   a. Difficulty forming words.
   b. Use of incorrect words.
   c. Difficulty thinking of specific words.
   d. Making up words (neologisms).

General Attitude

1. Cooperative/uncooperative
   a. Answers questions willingly.
   b. Refuses to answer questions.
2. Friendly/hostile/defensive
   a. Is sociable and responsive.
   b. Is sarcastic and irritable.
3. Uninterested/apathetic
   a. Refuses to participate in interview process.
4. Attentive/interested
   a. Actively participates in interview process.
5. Guarded/suspicious
   a. Continuously scans the environment.
   b. Questions motives of interviewer.
   c. Refuses to answer questions.

Emotions

Mood

1. Depressed; despairing
   a. Reports overwhelming feeling of sadness.
   b. Reports loss of interest in regular activities.
2. Irritable
   a. Easily annoyed and provoked to anger.
3. Anxious
   a. Demonstrates or verbalizes feeling of apprehension.
4. Elated
   a. Expresses feelings of joy and intense pleasure.
   b. Is intensely optimistic.
5. Euphoric
   a. Demonstrates a heightened sense of elation.
   b. Expresses feelings of grandeur ("Everything is wonderful!").
6. Fearful
   a. Demonstrates or verbalizes feeling of apprehension associated with real or perceived danger.
7. Guilty
   a. Expresses a feeling of discomfort associated with real or perceived wrongdoing.
   b. Expresses associated feelings of sadness and despair.
8. Labile
   a. Exhibits mood swings that range from euphoria to depression or anxiety.

Affect

1. Congruence with mood
   a. Outward emotional expression is consistent with mood (e.g., if depressed, emotional expression is sadness, eyes downcast, may be crying).

2. Constricted or blunted
   a. Minimal outward emotional expression is observed.
3. Flat
   a. There is an absence of outward emotional expression.
4. Appropriate
   a. The outward emotional expression is what would be expected in a certain situation (e.g., crying upon hearing of a death).
5. Inappropriate
   a. The outward emotional expression is incompatible with the situation (e.g., laughing upon hearing of a death).

Thought Processes

Form of Thought

1. Flight of ideas
   a. Verbalizations are continuous and rapid and flow from one to another.
2. Loose association
   a. Verbalizations shift from one unrelated topic to another.
3. Circumstantiality
   a. Verbalizations are lengthy and tedious and, because of numerous details, are delayed in reaching the intended point.
4. Tangentiality
   a. Verbalizations that are lengthy and tedious and never reach an intended point.
5. Neologisms
   a. The individual is making up nonsensical-sounding words, which have meaning only to him or her.
6. Concrete thinking
   a. Thinking is literal; elemental.
   b. Absence of ability to think abstractly.
   c. Unable to translate simple proverbs.
7. Clang associations
   a. Speaking in puns or rhymes; using words that sound alike but have different meanings.
8. Word salad
   a. Using a mixture of words that have no meaning together; sounding incoherent.
9. Perseveration
10. Repetition of words or phrases in the absence or cessation of socially appropriate context. Echolalia
    a. Persistently repeating what another person says.
11. Mutism
    a. Does not speak (either cannot or will not).
12. Poverty of speech
    a. Speaks very little; may respond in monosyllables.
13. Ability to concentrate and disturbance of attention
    a. Does the person hold attention to the topic at hand?
    b. Is the person easily distractible?
    c. Is there selective attention (e.g., blocks out topics that create anxiety)?

Content of Thought

1. Delusions (Does the person have unrealistic ideas or beliefs?)
   a. Persecutory: A belief that someone is out to get him or her is some way (e.g., "The FBI will be here at any time to take me away").
   b. Grandiose: An idea that he or she is all-powerful or of great importance (e.g., "I am the king, and this is my kingdom! I can do anything!").
   c. Reference: An idea that whatever is happening in the environment is about him or her (e.g., "Just watch the movie on TV tonight. It is about my life").
   d. Control or influence: A belief that their behavior and thoughts are being controlled by external forces (e.g., "I get my orders from Channel 27. I do only what the forces dictate").
   e. Somatic: A belief that he or she has a dysfunctional body part (e.g., "My heart is at a standstill. It is no longer beating").
   f. Nihilistic: A belief that he or she, a part of the body, or even the world does not exist or has been destroyed (e.g., "I am no longer alive").
2. Suicidal or homicidal ideas
   a. Is the individual expressing ideas of harming self or others?
   b. Does the individual express plans and intentions to die? Or plans and intentions to harm another? How strong are these intentions?
   c. Does the individual have access to their chosen means of suicide?
3. Obsessions
   a. Is the person verbalizing about a persistent thought or feeling that the person is unable to eliminate from their consciousness?
4. Paranoia/suspiciousness
   a. Continuously scans the environment.
   b. Questions motives of interviewer.
   c. Refuses to answer questions.

5. Magical thinking
   a. Is the person speaking in a way that indicates belief that their words or actions have the ability to cause and effect that is, in fact, irrational? (e.g., "If you step on a crack, you break your mother's back!" or "If I raise my hand the rain pours down.")
6. Impaired religiosity
   a. Is the individual demonstrating obsession with religious ideas and behavior that is causing marked distress and impairing ability to function?
7. Phobias
   a. Is there evidence of irrational fears (of a specific object or a social situation)?
8. Poverty of thought
   a. Is the individual vague, stereotypical, or limited in ability to share information? Does the patient express feeling of emptiness or being devoid of thought?

Perceptual Disturbances

1. Hallucinations (Is the person experiencing unrealistic sensory perceptions?)
   a. Auditory (Is the individual hearing voices or other sounds that do not exist?)
   b. Visual (Is the individual seeing images that do not exist?)
   c. Tactile (Does the individual feel unrealistic sensations on the skin?)
   d. Olfactory (Does the individual smell odors that do not exist?)
   e. Gustatory (Does the individual have a false perception of an unpleasant taste?)
2. Illusions
   a. Does the individual misperceive or misinterpret real stimuli within the environment (e.g., sees something and thinks it is something else)?
3. Depersonalization (altered perception of the self)
   a. The individual verbalizes feeling "outside the body"; visualizing himself or herself from afar.
4. Derealization (altered perception of the environment)
   a. The individual verbalizes that the environment feels "strange or unreal." A feeling that the surroundings have changed.

Sensorium and Cognitive Ability

1. Level of alertness/consciousness
   a. Is the individual clear-minded and attentive to the environment?
   b. Or is there disturbance in perception and awareness of the surroundings?
2. Orientation. Is the person oriented to the following?
   a. Time
   b. Place
   c. Person
   d. Circumstances
3. Memory
   a. Recent (Is the individual able to remember occurrences of the past few days?)
   b. Remote (Is the individual able to remember occurrences of the distant past?)
   c. Confabulation (Does the individual fill in memory gaps with experiences that have no basis in fact?)
4. Capacity for abstract thought
   a. Can the individual interpret proverbs correctly? For example, "What does 'no use crying over spilled milk' mean?"

Impulse Control

1. Ability to control impulses (Does psychosocial history reveal problems with any of the following?)
   a. Aggression
   b. Hostility
   c. Fear
   d. Guilt
   e. Affection
   f. Sexual feelings

Judgment

1. Ability to solve problems and make decisions
   a. What are your plans for the future?
   b. What do you plan to do to reach your goals?
2. Adaptive versus maladaptive use of coping strategies.

Insight

1. Knowledge about self
   a. Awareness of limitations.
   b. Awareness of consequences of actions.
   c. Awareness of illness.
      i. "Do you think you have a problem?"
      ii. "Do you think you need treatment?"
   d. Awareness of use of ego defense mechanisms (e.g., rationalization, projection, displacement, denial).

Appendix B

Glossary

A

abandonment. A unilateral severance of the professional relationship between a health-care provider and a client without reasonable notice at a time when there is still a need for continuing health care.

abreaction. "Remembering with feeling"; bringing into conscious awareness painful events that have been repressed and reexperiencing the emotions that were associated with the events.

abuse. To use wrongfully or in a harmful way. The maltreatment of one person by another. Improper treatment or conduct that may result in injury.

acculturation. To change one's cultural beliefs, behaviors, and/or values as a result of engagement with people of a different culture.

acquaintance rape. Rape perpetrated by someone with whom the victim has met or priorly been acquainted.

acupoints. In Chinese medicine, areas along the body that link pathways of healing energy.

acupressure. A technique in which the fingers, thumbs, palms, or elbows are used to apply pressure to certain points along the body. This pressure is thought to dissolve any obstructions in the flow of healing energy and to restore the body to a healthier functioning.

acupuncture. A technique in which hair-thin, sterile, disposable, stainless-steel needles are inserted into points along the body to dissolve obstructions in the flow of healing energy and restore the body to a healthier functioning.

acute mania. A primary symptom of bipolar disorder characterized by euphoria and elation. The person may appear to be on a continuous "high." However, the mood is always subject to frequent variation, easily changing to irritability and anger or even to sadness and crying.

acute stress disorder. The *DSM-5* diagnostic category describing a trauma- and stressor-related disorder that is short term (from 3 days to 1 months duration) and results in significant distress or impairment in function. (For a complete list of diagnostic criteria, refer to Chapter 19, "Trauma- and Stressor-Related Disorders.")

adaptation. Restoration of the body to homeostasis following a physiological and/or psychological response to stress.

addiction. A compulsive or chronic requirement. The need is so strong as to generate distress (either physical or psychological) if left unfulfilled.

adjustment. The process of modifying one's behavior in changed circumstances or an altered environment in order to fulfill psychological, physiological, and social needs.

adjustment disorder. A maladaptive reaction to an identifiable psychosocial stressor that occurs within 3 months after onset of the stressor. The individual shows impairment in social and occupational functioning or exhibits symptoms that are in excess of a normal and expectable reaction to the stressor.

advance directive. A legal document that competent individuals may sign to convey wishes regarding future health-care decisions intended for a time when they are no longer capable of informed consent. It may include one or both of the following: (1) a living will, in which individuals identify the type of care that they do or do not wish to have performed and (2) a durable power of attorney for health care, in which individuals name another person who is given the right to make health-care decisions for the individual who is incapable of doing so.

adverse childhood experiences (ACEs). Potentially traumatic events that occur in childhood (0–17 years) including witnessing or experiencing violence, abuse, neglect, or death of a family member by suicide.

advocacy. The act of pleading for, supporting, or representing a cause or individual. Advocacy in nursing applies to any act in which the nurse is serving in the best interests of the patient, from simple procedures such as hand washing to protect the patient from infection to complex ethically and morally charged issues in which certain clients are unable to advocate for themselves.

affect. The behavioral expression of emotion; may be appropriate (congruent with the situation), inappropriate (incongruent with the situation), constricted or blunted (diminished range and intensity), or flat (absence of emotional expression).

affective domain. A category of learning that includes attitudes, feelings, and values.

aggression. Harsh physical or verbal actions intended (either consciously or unconsciously) to harm or injure another.

aggressive. Behavior that defends an individual's own basic rights by violating the basic rights of others (as contrasted with **assertive**).

agonist. A drug that activates specific receptors in the brain thereby increasing a biological reaction.

agoraphobia. The fear of being in places or situations from which escape might be difficult (or embarrassing) or in which help might not be available in the event of a panic attack.

agranulocytosis. Extremely low levels of white blood cells. Symptoms include sore throat, fever, and malaise. This may be a side effect of long-term therapy with some antipsychotic medications.

akathisia. Restlessness; an urgent need for movement; a type of extrapyramidal side effect associated with some antipsychotic medications.

akinesia. Muscular weakness or a loss or partial loss of muscle movement; a type of extrapyramidal side effect associated with some antipsychotic medications.

Alcoholics Anonymous (AA). A major self-help organization for the treatment of alcoholism. It is based on a 12-step program to help members attain and maintain sobriety. Once individuals have achieved sobriety, they in turn are expected to help other persons attending AA.

allopathic medicine. Traditional medicine; the type of medicine traditionally and currently practiced in the United States and taught in U.S. medical schools.

alternative medicine. Practices that differ from usual traditional (allopathic) medicine.

altruism. One therapeutic factor of group therapy (identified by Irvin Yalom) in which individuals gain self-esteem through mutual sharing and concern. Providing assistance and support to others creates a positive self-image and promotes self-growth.

amenorrhea. Cessation of the menses; may be a side effect of some antipsychotic medications and may be a symptom in anorexia nervosa.

amnesia. An inability to recall important personal information that is too extensive to be explained by ordinary forgetfulness.

amnesia, generalized. The inability to recall anything that has happened during the individual's entire lifetime.

amnesia, localized. The inability to recall all incidents associated with a traumatic event for a specific time period following the event.

amnesia, selective. The inability to recall only certain incidents associated with a traumatic event for a specific time period following the event.

amphetamine. A racemic sympathomimetic amine that acts as a central nervous system stimulant. It (and its derivatives such as methamphetamine and dextroamphetamine) is a commonly abused substance but has therapeutic use in the treatment of narcolepsy and attention deficit-hyperactivity disorder.

andropause. Also called *male menopause.* A syndrome of symptoms related to the decline of testosterone levels in men. Some symptoms include depression, weight gain, insomnia, hot flashes, decreased libido, mood swings, decreased strength, and erectile dysfunction.

anger. An emotional response to one's perception of a situation. Anger has both positive and negative functions.

anger management. The use of various techniques and strategies to control responses to anger-provoking situations. The goal of anger management is to reduce both the emotional feelings and the physiological arousal that anger engenders.

anhedonia. The inability to experience or even imagine any pleasant emotion.

anorexia nervosa. An illness characterized by morbid fear of obesity, distorted body image, preoccupation with food, and refusal to eat.

anorexiants. Drugs that suppress appetite.

anorgasmia. Inability to achieve orgasm.

anosmia. Inability to smell.

anosognosia. A symptom of some mental illnesses, such as schizophrenia, in which the individual is manifesting overt symptoms of illness but is unaware of the presence of symptoms/unaware that there is anything wrong.

antagonist. A drug that blocks a receptor thereby dampening a biological reaction.

anticipatory grief. A subjective state of emotional, physical, and social responses to an anticipated loss of a valued entity. The grief response is repeated once the loss actually occurs, but it may not be as intense as it might have been if anticipatory grieving has not occurred.

antisocial personality disorder. A pattern of socially irresponsible, exploitative, and guiltless behavior, evident in the tendency to fail to conform to the law, develop stable relationships, or sustain consistent employment; exploitation and manipulation of others for personal gain is common.

anxiety. Vague, diffuse apprehension that is associated with feelings of uncertainty and helplessness.

aphasia. Inability to communicate through speech, writing, or signs, caused by dysfunction of brain centers.

aphonia. Inability to speak.

apraxia. Inability to carry out motor activities despite intact motor function or inability to use objects properly.

arbitrary inference. In cognitive behavior therapy, this is a type of thinking error in which the individual automatically comes to a conclusion about an incident without the facts to support it or even sometimes despite contradictory evidence to support it.

ascites. Excessive accumulation of serous fluid in the abdominal cavity, occurring in response to portal hypertension caused by cirrhosis of the liver.

assault. An act that results in genuine fear and apprehension that an individual will be touched without consent. Nurses may be guilty of assault for threatening to place an individual in restraints against their will.

assertive. Behavior that enables individuals to act in their own best interests, to stand up for themselves without undue anxiety, to express their honest feelings comfortably, or to exercise their own rights without denying those of others.

assessment. A systematic, dynamic process by which the registered nurse, through interaction with the patient, family, groups, communities, populations, and health-care providers, collects and analyzes data. Assessment may include the following dimensions: physical, functional, psychosocial, emotional, cognitive, sexual, cultural, age-related, environmental, spiritual/transpersonal, and economic.

assimilation. Adopting the behaviors, beliefs, and values of the majority culture.

associative looseness. Sometimes called *loose associations*, a thinking process characterized by speech in which ideas shift from one unrelated subject to another. The individual is unaware that the topics are unconnected.

ataxia. Muscular incoordination.

attachment. Connectedness with others in interpersonal relationship.

attachment theory. The hypothesis that individuals who maintain close relationships with others into old age are more likely to remain independent and less likely to be institutionalized than those who do not.

attention deficit-hyperactivity disorder (ADHD). A disorder characterized by inattention and/or hyperactivity and impulsivity. Frequently the disorder is not recognized until a child begins attending school.

attitude. A frame of reference around which individuals organize knowledge about their world. It includes an emotional element and can have a positive or negative connotation.

autism spectrum disorder. An array of disorders that are characterized by impairment in social interaction skills and interpersonal communication and a restricted repertoire of activities and interests.

autocratic. A leadership style in which the leader makes all decisions for the group. Productivity is very high with this type of leadership, but morale is often low because of the lack of member input and creativity.

autoimmunity. A condition in which the body produces a disordered immunological response against itself. In this situation, the body fails to differentiate between what is normal and what is a foreign substance. When this occurs, the body produces antibodies against normal parts of the body to such an extent as to cause tissue injury.

automatic thoughts. Thoughts that occur rapidly in response to a situation and without rational analysis. They are often negative and based on erroneous logic.

autonomy. Independence; self-governance. An ethical principle that emphasizes the status of persons as autonomous moral agents whose right to determine their destinies should always be respected.

aversive stimulus. A stimulus that follows a behavioral response and decreases the probability that the behavior will recur. (Also called *punishment.*)

avoidant personality disorder. A personality disorder characterized by social withdrawal rooted in extreme fear of rejection and feelings of inadequacy.

axon. The cellular process of a neuron that carries impulses away from the cell body.

B

battering. A pattern of repeated physical assault, usually of a woman by her spouse or intimate partner. Men are also battered, although this occurs much less frequently.

battery. The unconsented touching of another person. Nurses may be charged with battery should they participate in the treatment of a client without their consent and outside of an emergency situation.

behavior modification. A treatment modality aimed at changing undesirable behaviors using a system of reinforcement to bring about the modifications desired.

behavior therapy. A form of psychotherapy, the goal of which is to modify maladaptive behavior patterns by reinforcing more adaptive behaviors.

behavioral objectives. Statements that indicate to individuals what is expected of them. Behavioral objectives are a way of measuring learning outcomes and are based on the affective, cognitive, and psychomotor domains of learning.

belief. A belief is an idea that one holds to be true. It can be rational, irrational, taken on faith, or a stereotypical idea.

beneficence. An ethical principle that refers to one's duty to benefit or promote the good of others.

bereavement. The period of grief and sadness that is the normal process of reacting to a loss and may include mental, physical, social, and emotional reactions.

bereavement overload. An accumulation of grief that occurs when an individual experiences many losses over a short period and is unable to resolve one before another is experienced. This phenomenon is common among the older adults.

binging. A symptom of some eating disorders, notably binge eating disorder and bulimia nervosa in which an individual consumes thousands of calories at one sitting.

binge eating disorder. An illness characterized by recurrent episodes of binging on food.

bioethics. The term used with ethical principles that refer to concepts within the scope of medicine, nursing, and allied health.

biofeedback. The use of instrumentation to become aware of processes in the body that usually go unnoticed and to bring them under voluntary control (e.g., the blood pressure or pulse); used as a method of stress reduction.

bipolar disorder. Characterized by mood swings from profound depression to extreme euphoria (mania) with intervening periods of normalcy. Psychotic symptoms may or may not be present.

black box warning. Formally called a *boxed warning* by the U.S. Food and Drug Administration (FDA), this is a designation which appears on a prescription drug label to call attention to serious or life-threatening risks.

body dysmorphic disorder. An exaggerated belief that the body is deformed or defective in some specific way.

body image. One's perception of their own body. It may also be how one believes others perceive their body. (See also **physical self**.)

borderline personality disorder. A disorder characterized by a pattern of intense and chaotic relationships with affective instability; fluctuating and extreme attitudes regarding other people; impulsivity; direct and indirect self-destructive behavior; and lack of a clear or certain sense of identity, life plan, or values.

boundaries. The level of participation and interaction between individuals and between subsystems. Boundaries denote physical and psychological space that individuals identify as their own. They are sometimes referred to as *limits*. Boundaries are appropriate when they permit appropriate contact with others while preventing excessive interference. Boundaries may be clearly defined (healthy) or rigid or diffuse (unhealthy).

bulimia nervosa. An illness characterized by recurrent binge eating followed by compensatory purging behaviors, such as vomiting, laxative use, excessive exercise, medication use, and others, to prevent weight gain.

C

cachexia. A state of ill health, malnutrition, and wasting; extreme emaciation.

cannabis. The dried flowering tops of the hemp plant. It produces euphoric effects when ingested or smoked and is commonly used in the form of marijuana or hashish.

case management. A health-care delivery process, the goals of which are to provide quality health care, decrease fragmentation, enhance the client's quality of life, and contain costs. A case manager coordinates the client's care from admission to discharge and sometimes following discharge. Critical pathways of care are the tools used for the provision of care in a case management system.

case manager. The individual responsible for negotiating with multiple health-care providers to obtain a variety of services for a client.

catastrophic thinking. Always thinking that the worst will occur without considering the possibility of more likely, positive outcomes.

catatonia. A type of psychological disturbance that is typified by stupor or excitement. Stupor is characterized by extreme psychomotor retardation, mutism, negativism, and posturing; excitement, by psychomotor agitation, in which the movements are frenzied and purposeless. Catatonic symptoms may be associated with other mental or physical disorders.

catharsis. One curative factor of group therapy (identified by Irvin Yalom), in which members in a group can express both positive and negative feelings in a nonthreatening atmosphere.

cell body. The part of the neuron that contains the nucleus and is essential for the continued life of the neuron.

child abuse. Physical or sexual abuse, psychological maltreatment, or neglect of a child.

child sexual abuse. Any sexual act, such as indecent exposure or improper touching to penetration (sexual intercourse), that is carried out with a child.

chiropractic medicine. A system of alternative medicine based on the premise that the relationship between structure and function in the human body is a significant health factor and that such relationships between the spinal column and the nervous system are important because the normal transmission and expression of nerve energy are essential to the restoration and maintenance of health.

Christian ethics. The ethical philosophy, based on Christian doctrine stating that we should treat others as moral equals and treat others as we would want to be treated were we in similar situations; sometimes referred to as the *ethic of the golden rule.*

circadian rhythm. A 24-hour biological rhythm controlled by a "pacemaker" in the brain that sends messages to other systems in the body. Circadian rhythm influences various regulatory functions, including the sleep–wake cycle, body temperature regulation, patterns of activity such as eating and drinking, and hormonal and neurotransmitter secretion.

circumstantiality. In speaking, the delay of an individual to reach the point of a communication, owing to unnecessary and tedious details.

civil law. Law that protects the private and property rights of individuals and businesses.

clang association. A pattern of speech in which the choice of words is governed by sounds. Clang associations often take the form of rhyming.

classical conditioning. A type of learning that occurs when an unconditioned stimulus (UCS) that produces an unconditioned response (UCR) is paired with a conditioned stimulus (CS), until the CS alone produces the same response, which is then called a conditioned response (CR). Pavlov's example: food (i.e., UCS) causes salivation (i.e., UCR); ringing bell (i.e., CS) with food (i.e., UCS) causes salivation (i.e., UCR), ringing bell alone (i.e., CS) causes salivation (i.e., CR).

clinging. A common symptom of separation anxiety disorders in which a child excessively clings to the mother or other individual from whom the child fears being separated.

codependency. An exaggerated dependent pattern of learned behaviors, beliefs, and feelings that make life painful. It is a dependence on people and things outside the self, along with neglect of the self to the point of having little self-identity.

cognition. Mental operations that relate to logic, awareness, intellect, memory, language, and reasoning powers.

cognitive. Relating to the mental processes of thinking and reasoning.

cognitive behavior therapy. A type of therapy in which the individual is taught to control thought distortions that are considered to be a factor in the development and maintenance of emotional disorders.

cognitive development. A series of stages described by Piaget through which individuals progress, demonstrating at each successive stage a higher level of logical organization than at each previous stage.

cognitive domain. A category of learning that involves knowledge and thought processes within the individual's intellectual ability. The individual must be able to synthesize information at an intellectual level before the actual behaviors are performed.

cognitive maturity. The capability to perform all mental operations needed for adulthood.

collaborative safety plan. A plan that is developed in collaboration with a patient who is at risk for suicide to identify strategies for maintaining ongoing safety and prevention of suicide.

collectivist culture. A type of culture that highly values interdependence among its members.

colposcope. An instrument that contains a magnifying lens and to which a 35-mm camera can be attached. A colposcope is used to examine for tears and abrasions inside the vaginal area of a sexual assault victim.

common law. Laws that are derived from decisions made in previous cases.

communication. An interactive process of transmitting information between two or more entities.

community. A group of people living close to and depending to some extent on each other.

compensation. An ego defense mechanism in which an individual covers up a real or perceived weakness by emphasizing a trait that one considers more desirable.

complementary medicine. Practices that differ from usual traditional (allopathic) medicine but may in fact supplement it in a positive way.

compounded rape reaction. Symptoms that are in addition to the typical rape response of physical complaints, rage, humiliation, fear, and sleep disturbances. They include depression and suicide, substance abuse, and even psychotic behaviors.

compulsions. Unwanted repetitive behavior patterns or mental acts (e.g., praying, counting, repeating words silently) that are intended to reduce anxiety, not to provide pleasure or gratification. They may be performed in response to an obsession or in a stereotyped fashion.

concept mapping. A diagrammatic teaching and learning strategy that allows students and faculty to visualize interrelationships between medical diagnoses, nursing diagnoses, assessment data, and treatments. A diagram of client problems and interventions.

concrete thinking. Thought processes that are focused on specifics rather than on generalities and immediate issues rather than eventual outcomes. Individuals who are experiencing concrete thinking are unable to comprehend abstract terminology.

conditioned response. In classical conditioning, a response that is a *learned* response (not reflexive) following repeated exposure to a target stimulus.

conditioned stimulus. In classical conditioning, an unrelated stimulus that is presented to a subject with a target stimulus and that, with repeated exposure, comes to elicit the same response as the original target stimulus.

conduct disorder. A disorder characterized by repetitive and persistent patterns of behavior in which the basic rights of others or major age-appropriate societal norms or rules are violated. It is identified as a disorder of childhood and adolescence and is associated with increased risk for antisocial personality disorder in adulthood.

confabulation. Creating imaginary events to fill in memory gaps.

confidentiality. The rights of individuals to the assurance that their case will not be discussed outside the boundaries of the health-care team.

contextual stimuli. Conditions present in the environment that support a focal stimulus and influence a threat to self-esteem.

contingency contracting. A written contract between individuals used to modify behavior. Benefits and consequences for fulfilling the terms of the contract are delineated.

controlled response pattern. The response to rape in which feelings are masked or hidden, and a calm, composed, or subdued affect is seen.

counselor. Nurses who listen as clients review feelings related to difficulties they are experiencing in any aspect of life; one of the nursing roles identified by H. Peplau.

countertransference. In psychoanalytic theory, countertransference refers to the counselor's behavioral and emotional response to the client. These responses may be related to unresolved feelings toward significant others from the counselor's past or they may be generated in response to the client's behavior toward the counselor.

covert sensitization. An aversion technique used to modify behavior that relies on individuals' imagination to produce unpleasant symptoms. When individuals are about to succumb to undesirable behavior, they visualize something that is offensive or even nauseating in an effort to block the behavior.

criminal law. Law that provides protection from conduct deemed injurious to the public welfare. It provides for punishment of those found to have engaged in such conduct.

crisis. Psychological disequilibrium in individuals who confront a hazardous circumstance that constitutes an important problem that they can neither escape nor solve with their usual problem-solving resources.

crisis intervention. An emergency type of assistance in which the intervener becomes a part of the individual's life situation. The focus is to provide guidance and support to help mobilize the resources needed to resolve the crisis and restore or generate an improvement in previous level of functioning. Usually lasts no longer than 6 to 8 weeks.

critical pathways of care (CPCs). An abbreviated plan of care that provides outcome-based guidelines for goal achievement within a designated length of time.

cultural syndromes. Syndromes that are specific to a cultural group.

culture. A particular society's entire way of living, encompassing shared patterns of belief, feeling, and knowledge that guide people's conduct and are passed down from generation to generation.

cycle of battering. Three phases of predictable behaviors that are repeated over time in a relationship between a batterer and a victim: tension-building phase; the acute battering incident; and the calm, loving, respite (honeymoon) phase.

cyclothymic disorder. A chronic mood disturbance involving numerous episodes of hypomania and depressed mood of insufficient severity or duration to meet the criteria for bipolar disorder.

D

date rape. A situation in which the rapist is known to the victim. This may occur during dating or with acquaintances or schoolmates. (Also called *acquaintance rape.*)

decatastrophizing. In cognitive behavior therapy, with this technique the therapist assists the client to examine the validity of a negative automatic thought. Even if some validity exists, the client is then encouraged to review ways to cope adaptively, moving beyond the current crisis situation.

defamation of character. An individual may be liable for defamation of character by sharing with others information about a person that is detrimental to that person's reputation.

deinstitutionalization. The removal of mentally ill individuals from institutions and the subsequent plan to provide care for these individuals in the community setting.

delayed grief. The absence of evidence of grief when it ordinarily would be expected.

delayed ejaculation. Delayed or absent ejaculation, even though the man has a firm erection and has had more than adequate stimulation.

delirious mania. A grave form of mania characterized by severe clouding of consciousness and representing an intensification of the symptoms associated with mania. The symptoms of delirious mania have become relatively rare since the availability of antipsychotic medications.

delirium. A state of mental confusion and excitement characterized by disorientation for time and place, often with hallucinations, incoherent speech, and a continual state of aimless physical activity.

delusions. False personal beliefs not consistent with a person's intelligence or cultural background. The individual continues to have the belief in spite of obvious proof that it is false and/or irrational.

dementia. See **neurocognitive disorder (NCD).**

democratic leadership. A leadership style employed in group interventions that focuses on full participation of the members in decision making and problem-solving.

dendrites. The cellular processes of a neuron that carry impulses toward the cell body.

denial. Refusal to acknowledge the existence of a real situation and/or the feelings associated with it.

density. The number of people in a given environmental space, influencing interpersonal interaction.

dependent personality disorder. A personality disorder characterized by pervasive, excessive dependency needs, submissiveness, and exaggerated fears of inability to care for oneself.

depersonalization. An alteration in the perception or experience of the self so that the feeling of one's own reality is temporarily lost.

deployment. A term used in the military to describe movement of troops into an active-duty environment.

depression. An alteration in mood that is expressed by feelings of sadness, despair, and pessimism. There is a loss of interest in usual activities, and somatic symptoms may be evident. Changes in appetite and sleep patterns are common.

derealization. An alteration in the perception or experience of the external world so that it seems strange or unreal.

detoxification. The process of managed withdrawal from a substance to which one has become addicted.

diagnosis related groups (DRGs). A system used to determine prospective payment rates for reimbursement of hospital care based on the client's diagnosis.

***Diagnostic and Statistical Manual of Mental Disorders* (5th ed.; *DSM-5*).** Standard nomenclature of emotional illness published by the American Psychiatric Association (APA) and used by all health-care practitioners. It classifies mental illness and presents guidelines and diagnostic criteria for various mental disorders.

diagnostic overshadowing. A phenomenon in which individuals' physical symptoms are assumed to be attributed to their mental illness.

dichotomous thinking. In this type of thinking, situations are viewed in all-or-nothing, black-or-white, good-or-bad terms.

directed association. A technique used to help clients bring into consciousness events that have been repressed. Specific thoughts are guided and directed by the psychoanalyst.

disaster. A natural or man-made occurrence that overwhelms the resources of an individual or community and increases the need for emergency evacuation and medical services.

discriminative stimulus. A stimulus that precedes a behavioral response and predicts that a particular reinforcement will occur. Individuals learn to discriminate between various stimuli that will produce the responses they desire.

disengagement. In family theory, disengagement refers to extreme separateness among family members. It is promoted by rigid boundaries or lack of communication among family members.

disengagement theory. This theory suggests there is a process of mutual withdrawal of aging persons and society from each other that is correlated with successful aging. This theory has been challenged by many investigators.

displacement. Feelings that are transferred from one target to another that is considered less threatening or neutral.

dissociation. The splitting off of clusters of mental contents from conscious awareness, a mechanism central to hysterical conversion and dissociative disorder.

distance. A cultural characteristic that defines the means by which various cultures use interpersonal space to communicate.

distraction. In cognitive behavior therapy, when dysfunctional cognitions have been recognized, activities are identified that can be used to distract clients and divert them from the intrusive thoughts or depressive ruminations that are contributing to their maladaptive responses.

disulfiram. A drug that is administered to individuals who abuse alcohol as a deterrent to drinking. Ingestion of alcohol while disulfiram is in the body results in a syndrome of symptoms that can produce a great deal of discomfort and can even result in death if the blood alcohol level is high.

double-bind communication. An emotionally distressing situation in which an individual receives conflicting messages in the communication process, whereby one message is negated by another. This creates a condition in which a successful response to one message results in a failed response to the other.

dual diagnosis. Clients have a dual diagnosis when it is determined that they have a co-existing substance disorder and mental illness. Treatment is designed to target both problems.

dysthymia. A depressive neurosis. The symptoms are similar to, if somewhat milder than, those ascribed to major depressive disorder. There is no loss of contact with reality.

dystonia. Involuntary muscular movements (spasms) of the face, arms, legs, and neck; may occur as an extrapyramidal side effect of some antipsychotic medications.

E

echolalia. Repetition of words or phrases, spoken by another. This is a common occurrence in toddlers as children begin to develop language skills. In children over 3 years old and in adults, echolalia may be a symptom associated with autism, schizophrenia, amnesia, head trauma, or other neurological disorders.

echopraxia. Involuntary imitation of movements made by another person. Echopraxia is a symptom associated with schizophrenia, Tourette's syndrome, and some other neurological disorders.

ego. One of the three elements of the personality identified by Freud as the rational self or "reality principle." The ego seeks to maintain harmony between the external world, the id, and the superego.

ego defense mechanisms. Strategies employed by the ego for protection in the face of threat to biological or psychological integrity. (See **compensation, denial, displacement, identification, intellectualization, introjection, isolation, projection, rationalization, reaction formation, regression, repression, sublimation, suppression**, and **undoing.**)

elder abuse. Psychological, physical, or financial abuse, or intentional or unintentional neglect, of an older adult.

electroconvulsive therapy (ECT). A type of somatic treatment in which electric current is applied to the brain through electrodes placed on the temples. A grand mal seizure produces the desired effect. This is used with severely depressed patients' refractory to antidepressant medications.

emaciated. The state of being excessively thin or physically wasted.

emotional abuse. A pattern of behavior on the part of the parent or caretaker that results in serious impairment of the child's social, emotional, or intellectual functioning.

emotional neglect. A chronic failure by the parent or caretaker to provide the child with the hope, love, and support necessary for the development of a sound, healthy personality.

empathy. The ability to see beyond outward behavior and sense accurately another's inner experiencing. With empathy, one can accurately perceive and understand the meaning and relevance in the thoughts and feelings of another.

enculturation. The process of learning the norms within a culture.

enmeshment. Exaggerated connectedness among family members. It occurs in response to diffuse boundaries in which there is overinvestment, overinvolvement, and lack of differentiation between individuals or subsystems.

esophageal varices. Veins in the esophagus that become distended because of excessive pressure from defective blood flow through a cirrhotic liver.

ethical dilemma. A situation that arises when, based on moral considerations, an appeal can be made for taking each of two opposing courses of action.

ethical egoism. An ethical theory espousing that what is "right" and "good" is what is best for the individual making the decision.

ethics. A branch of philosophy dealing with values related to human conduct, to the rightness and wrongness of certain actions, and to the goodness and badness of the motives and ends of such actions.

ethnicity. The concept of people identifying with each other because of a shared heritage.

exhibitionistic disorder. A paraphilic disorder characterized by a recurrent urge to expose one's genitals to a stranger.

expressed response pattern. Pattern of behavior in which the victim of rape expresses feelings of fear, anger, and anxiety through such behavior as crying, sobbing, restlessness, and tenseness; in contrast to the rape victim who withholds feelings in the controlled response pattern.

extinction. In behavior therapy, the gradual decrease in frequency or disappearance of a response when the positive reinforcement is withheld.

extrapyramidal symptoms (EPS). A variety of responses that originate outside the pyramidal tracts and in the basal ganglion of the brain. Symptoms may include tremors, chorea, dystonia, akinesia, akathisia, and others. May occur as a side effect of some antipsychotic medications.

F

factitious disorder. Disorders that involve conscious, intentional feigning of physical or psychological symptoms. Individuals with factitious disorder pretend to be ill in order to receive emotional care and support commonly associated with the role of "patient."

false imprisonment. The deliberate and unauthorized confinement of a person within fixed limits by the use of threat or force. A nurse may be charged with false imprisonment by placing a patient in restraints against their will in a nonemergency situation.

family. Two or more individuals who depend on one another for emotional, physical, and economical support. The members of the family are self-defined.

family structure. A set of invisible principles that influence the interaction among family members. These principles are established over time and become the "laws" that govern the conduct of various family members.

family system. A system in which the parts of the whole may be the marital dyad, parent-child dyad, or sibling groups. Each of these subsystems is further divided into subsystems of individuals.

family therapy. A type of therapy in which the focus is on relationships within the family. The family is viewed as a system in which the members are interdependent, and a change in one creates change in all.

fear. An emotion that is based on a cognitive appraisal of a stimulus perceived to be threatening. Fear is differentiated from anxiety in that anxiety is a more diffuse sense of tension and worry that is more internal than tied to an external cause.

fetishistic disorder. A paraphilic disorder characterized by recurrent sexual urges and sexually arousing fantasies involving the use of nonliving objects.

fight-or-flight syndrome. A syndrome of physical symptoms that results from an individual's real or perceived notion that harm or danger is imminent.

flexible boundary. A personal boundary is flexible when, because of unusual circumstances, individuals can alter limits that they have set for themselves. Flexible boundaries are healthy boundaries.

flight of ideas. A symptom common in bipolar manic episodes in which the individual's thoughts are racing and they rapidly switch topics when communicating.

flooding. Sometimes called *implosion therapy*, this technique is used to desensitize individuals to phobic stimuli. The individual is "flooded" with a continuous presentation (usually through mental imagery) of the phobic stimulus until it no longer elicits anxiety.

focal stimulus. A situation of immediate concern that results in a threat to self-esteem.

Focus Charting®. A type of documentation that follows a data, action, and response (DAR) format. The main perspective is a client "focus," which can be a nursing diagnosis, a client's concern, a change in status, or a significant event in the client's therapy. The focus cannot be a medical diagnosis.

forensic. Pertaining to the law; legal.

forensic nursing. The application of forensic science combined with the biopsychological education of the registered nurse in the scientific investigation, evidence collection and preservation, analysis, prevention, and treatment of trauma- and/or death-related medical-legal issues.

free association. A technique used to help individuals bring to consciousness material that has been repressed. The individual is encouraged to verbalize whatever comes into their mind, drifting naturally from one thought to another.

frotteuristic disorder. A paraphilic disorder characterized by the recurrent preoccupation with intense sexual urges or fantasies involving touching or rubbing against a nonconsenting person.

fugue. A sudden, unexpected travel away from home or customary work locale with the assumption of a new identity and an inability to recall one's previous identity; usually occurring in response to severe psychosocial stress.

G

gains. The reinforcements an individual receives for somaticizing.

Gamblers Anonymous (GA). An organization of inspirational group therapy, modeled after Alcoholics Anonymous (AA), for individuals who desire to, but cannot, stop gambling.

gender. The condition of being either male or female.

gender dysphoria. A sense of marked distress and mood disturbances associated with an incongruence between biologically assigned gender and subjectively experienced gender.

general adaptation syndrome. The general biological reaction of the body to a stressful situation, as described by Hans Selye. It occurs in three stages: the alarm reaction stage, the stage of resistance, and the stage of exhaustion.

generalized anxiety disorder. A disorder characterized by chronic (at least 6 months), unrealistic, and excessive anxiety and worry.

genetics. Study of the biological transmission of certain characteristics (physical and/or behavioral) from parent to offspring.

genogram. A graphic representation of a family system. It may cover several generations. Emphasis is on family roles and emotional relatedness among members. Genograms facilitate recognition of areas requiring change.

genotype. The total set of genes present in an individual at the time of conception and coded in the DNA.

genuineness. The ability to be open, honest, and "real" in interactions with others; the awareness of what one is experiencing internally and the ability to project the quality of this inner experiencing in a relationship.

geriatrics. The branch of clinical medicine specializing in the care of older adults and concerned with the problems of aging.

gerontology. The study of normal aging.

geropsychiatry. The branch of clinical medicine specializing in psychopathology of older adults.

grief. A subjective state of emotional, physical, and social responses to the real or perceived loss of a valued entity. Change and failure can also be perceived as losses. The grief response consists of a set of relatively predictable behaviors that describe the subjective state that accompanies mourning.

grief, distorted. A reaction in which all of the symptoms associated with normal grieving are exaggerated out of proportion. Pathological depression is a type of distorted grief. (Also called *exaggerated grief.*)

grief, inhibited. The absence of evidence of grief when it ordinarily would be expected. (Also called *delayed grief.*)

grief, maladaptive. A grief process that it delayed, exaggerated, or chronic and interferes with an individual's ability to function socially, emotionally, and in activities of daily living.

group. A collection of individuals whose association is founded on shared commonalities of interest, values, norms, or purpose. Membership in a group is generally by chance (born into the group), by choice (voluntary affiliation), or by circumstance (the result of life-cycle events over which an individual may or may not have control).

group therapy. A therapy group, founded in a specific theoretical framework, led by a person with an advanced degree in psychology, social work, nursing, or medicine. The goal is to encourage improvement in interpersonal functioning.

gynecomastia. Enlargement of the breasts in men; may be a side effect of some antipsychotic medications.

H

habit-reversal therapy. A type of behavior therapy in which the individual develops awareness of unhealthy habits and learns to substitute more adaptive coping strategies in an effort to extinguish unwanted behaviors.

hallucinations. False sensory perceptions not associated with real external stimuli. Hallucinations may involve any of the five senses.

hepatic encephalopathy. A brain disorder resulting from the inability of the cirrhotic liver to convert ammonia to urea for excretion. The continued rise in serum ammonia results in progressively impaired mental functioning, apathy, euphoria or depression, sleep disturbances, increasing confusion, and progression to coma and eventual death.

histrionic personality disorder. A type of personality disorder characterized by excessively emotional and attention-seeking behavior, often presented in a very colorful and dramatic fashion.

HIV-associated neurocognitive disorder. A neuropathological syndrome, possibly caused by chronic HIV encephalitis and myelitis and manifested by cognitive, behavioral, and motor symptoms that become more severe with progression of the disease.

hoarding disorder. A disorder in which the individual has extreme difficulty parting with possessions, regardless of their value, and may also be accompanied by excessive acquisition of material possessions.

home care. A wide range of health and social services that are delivered at home to recovering, disabled, and chronically or terminally ill persons in need of medical, nursing, social, or therapeutic treatment and/or assistance with essential activities of daily living.

homocysteine. An amino acid produced by the catabolism of methionine. Elevated levels may be linked to increased risk of cardiovascular disease.

hope. A guiding principle of the Recovery Model that stresses potential for improved quality of life and recovery from illness.

hospice. A program that provides palliative and supportive care to meet the special needs arising out of the physical, psychosocial, spiritual, social, and economic stresses that are experienced during the final stages of illness and during bereavement.

hyperactivity. Excessive psychomotor activity that may be purposeful or aimless, accompanied by physical movements and verbal utterances that are usually more rapid than normal. Inattention and distractibility are common with hyperactive behavior.

hypersomnia. Excessive sleepiness or seeking excessive amounts of sleep.

hypertensive crisis. A potentially life-threatening syndrome that results when an individual taking monoamine oxidase inhibitors (MAOIs) eats a product high in tyramine. Symptoms include severe occipital headache, palpitations, nausea and vomiting, nuchal rigidity, fever, sweating, marked increase in blood pressure, chest pain, and coma. (See also **tyramine.**)

hypnosis. A treatment for disorders brought on by repressed anxiety. The client is directed into a state of subconsciousness and assisted, through suggestions, to recall certain events that they cannot recall while conscious.

hypomania. A mild form of mania. Symptoms are excessive hyperactivity but not severe enough to cause marked impairment in social or occupational functioning or to require hospitalization.

I

id. One of the three components of the personality identified by Freud as the "pleasure principle." The id is the locus of instinctual drives; is present at birth; and compels the infant to satisfy needs and seek immediate gratification.

identification. An attempt to increase self-worth by acquiring certain attributes and characteristics of an individual one admires.

illusion. A misperception of a real external stimulus.

implosion therapy. See **flooding.**

impulsivity. The urge or inclination to act without consideration of the possible consequences of one's behavior.

incest. Sexual exploitation of a child under 18 years of age by a relative or nonrelative who holds a position of trust in the family.

informed consent. Permission granted to a healthcare provider (typically the physician) by a client to perform a therapeutic procedure, prior to which information about the procedure has been presented to the client with adequate time given for consideration about the pros and cons.

insomnia. Difficulty initiating. or maintaining sleep.

integration. The process used with individuals with dissociative identity disorder in an effort to bring all the subpersonalities together into one; usually achieved through hypnosis.

integrative health. A holistic approach that incorporates complementary and conventional practices in a coordinated, comprehensive treatment plan.

intellectual disability. A disorder of intellectual and adaptive functioning with onset during the developmental period.

intellectualization. An attempt to avoid expressing actual emotions associated with a stressful situation by using the intellectual processes of logic, reasoning, and analysis.

interdisciplinary care. A concept of providing care for a client in which members of various disciplines work together with common goals and shared responsibilities for meeting those goals.

intimate distance. The closest distance that individuals will allow between themselves and others. In the United States, this distance is 0 to 18 inches.

intimate partner violence. A pattern of abusive behavior that is used by an intimate partner to gain or maintain power and control over the other intimate partner.

intoxication. A physical and mental state of exhilaration and emotional frenzy or lethargy and stupor.

introjection. The beliefs and values of another individual are internalized and symbolically become a part of the self to the extent that the feeling of separateness or distinctness is lost.

isolation. The separation of a thought or a memory from the feeling tone or emotions associated with it (sometimes called *emotional isolation*).

J

justice. An ethical principle reflecting that all individuals should be treated equally and fairly.

K

Kantianism. The ethical principle espousing that decisions should be made and actions taken out of a sense of duty.

kleptomania. A recurrent failure to resist impulses to steal objects not needed for personal use or monetary value.

Korsakoff's psychosis. A syndrome of confusion, loss of recent memory, and confabulation in alcoholics caused by a deficiency of thiamine. It often occurs together with Wernicke's encephalopathy and may be termed *Wernicke-Korsakoff syndrome.*

L

laissez-faire leadership. A leadership type in which the leader lets group members do as they please. There is no direction from the leader. Member productivity and morale may be low owing to frustration from lack of direction.

lanugo. Fine, neonatal-like hair growth on the body and a symptom sometimes seen in individuals with anorexia nervosa.

libel. An action with which an individual may be charged for sharing with another individual, in writing, information that is detrimental to someone's reputation.

libido. Freud's term for the psychic energy used to fulfill basic physiological needs or instinctual drives, such as hunger, thirst, and sexuality.

limbic system. Parts of the brain that collectively make up what is often called the *emotional brain.* The limbic system is associated with feelings such as fear, anger, love, joy, hope, and with sexuality, and social behavior. As research has progressed it has become more difficult to define the boundaries of the limbic system.

long-term memory. Memory for remote events or those that occurred many years ago. The type of memory that is preserved in older individuals.

loose association. A thinking process characterized by speech in which ideas shift from one unrelated topic to another. The individual is unaware that topics are unconnected. (See also **associative looseness.**)

loss. The experience of separation from something of personal importance.

M

magical thinking. A primitive form of thinking in which an individual believes that thinking about a possible occurrence can make it happen.

magnification. A type of thinking in which the negative significance of an event is exaggerated.

maladaptation. A failure of the body to return to homeostasis following a physiological and/or psychological response to stress, disrupting the individual's integrity.

maladaptive grief. A grief process that it delayed, exaggerated, or chronic and interferes with an individual's ability to function socially, emotionally, and in activities of daily living.

malpractice. The failure of one rendering professional services to exercise that degree of skill and learning commonly applied under all the circumstances in the community by the average prudent reputable member of the profession, with the result of injury, loss, or damage to the recipient of those services or to those entitled to rely upon them.

managed care. A concept purposefully designed to control the balance between cost and quality of care. Examples of managed care are health maintenance organizations (HMOs) and preferred provider organizations (PPOs). The amount and type of health care that the individual receives is determined by the organization providing the managed care.

mania. An alteration in mood that may be expressed by feelings of elation, inflated self-esteem, grandiosity, hyperactivity, agitation, racing thoughts, and accelerated speech. Mania can occur as part of bipolar disorder, as part of other medical conditions, or in response to some substances.

marital rape. Sexual violence directed at a marital partner against that person's will.

marital schism. A state of severe chronic disequilibrium and discord within the marital dyad with recurrent threats of separation.

marital skew. A marital relationship in which there is lack of equal partnership. One partner dominates the relationship and the other partner.

Medicaid. A system established by the federal government to provide medical care benefits for indigent Americans. The Medicaid program is jointly funded by state and federal governments, and coverage varies significantly from state to state.

Medicare. A system established by the federal government to provide medical care benefits for older Americans.

medication-assisted treatment. The use of medications to decrease the intensity of symptoms in an individual who is withdrawing from or who is experiencing the effects of excessive use of alcohol and other drugs. Cravings are decreased by administering a controlled dose of another medication.

meditation. A method of relaxation in which an individual sits in a quiet place and focuses total concentration on an object, a word, or a thought.

melancholia. A severe form of major depressive episode. Symptoms are exaggerated, and interest or pleasure in virtually all activities is lost.

mental health. The successful adaptation to stressors from the internal or external environment, evidenced by thoughts, feelings, and behaviors that are age-appropriate and congruent with local and cultural norms.

mental illness. Maladaptive responses to stressors from the internal or external environment, evidenced by thoughts, feelings, and behaviors that are incongruent with the local and cultural norms and interfere with the individual's social, occupational, and/or physical functioning.

mental imagery. A method of stress reduction that employs the imagination. Individuals focus imagination on a scenario that is particularly relaxing to them (e.g., a scene on a quiet seashore, a mountain atmosphere, or floating through the air on a fluffy white cloud).

meridians. In Chinese medicine, pathways along the body in which the healing energy (qi) flows and that are links between acupoints.

milieu. French for "middle"; the English translation connotes "surroundings or environment."

milieu therapy. Also called *therapeutic community* or *therapeutic environment*, this type of therapy consists of a scientific structuring of the environment to effect behavioral changes and to improve the individual's psychological health and functioning.

minimization. A type of thinking in which the positive significance of an event is minimized or undervalued.

misuse *(of substances)*. Overuse of substances with potential for harmful consequences. Equivalent to the term *abuse* but preferred in some contexts to reduce the shaming and stigma associated with referring to individuals as "abusers."

mobile outreach units. Programs in which volunteers and paid professionals drive or walk around and seek out homeless individuals who need assistance with physical or psychological care.

modeling. Learning new behaviors by imitating the behaviors of others.

mood. An individual's sustained emotional tone, which significantly influences behavior, personality, and perception.

moral behavior. Conduct that results from serious critical thinking about how individuals ought to treat others; reflects respect for human life, freedom, justice, or confidentiality.

moral-ethical self. The aspect of personal identity that functions as observer, standard setter, dreamer, comparer, and most of all, evaluator of who individuals say they are. This component of personal identity makes judgments that influence an individual's self-evaluation.

mourning. The psychological process (or stages) through which the individual passes on the way to successful adaptation to the loss of a valued entity.

multidisciplinary care. A concept of providing care for a client in which individual disciplines provide specific services for the client without formal arrangement for interaction between the disciplines.

Munchausen syndrome. See **factitious disorder.**

N

narcissism. Self-love or self-admiration.

narcissistic personality disorder. A disorder characterized by an exaggerated sense of self-worth. These individuals lack empathy and are hypersensitive to the evaluation of others.

narcolepsy. A disorder in which the characteristic manifestation is sleep attacks. The individual cannot prevent falling asleep even in the middle of a sentence or performing a task.

National Standards for Culturally and Linguistically Appropriate Services. A set of standards established by the U.S. Department of Health and Human Services Office of Minority Health for health-care organizations and providers focusing on culturally competent care.

natural law theory. The ethical theory that has as its moral precept to "do good and avoid evil" at all costs. Natural law ethics are grounded in a concern for the human good that is based on people's ability to live according to the dictates of reason.

negative reinforcement. Increasing the probability that a behavior will recur by removal of an undesirable reinforcing stimulus.

negative symptoms. A group of symptoms in schizophrenia that are deficits posed by the disorder. Examples include lack of motivation to complete goal directed activities (avolition), lack of energy (anergia), lack of interest in social relationships (asociality), and others.

negativism. Strong resistance to suggestions or directions; exhibiting behaviors contrary to what is expected.

neglect of a child. *Physical neglect* of a child includes refusal of or delay in seeking health care, abandonment, expulsion from the home or refusal to allow a runaway to return home, and inadequate supervision. *Emotional neglect* refers to a chronic failure by the parent or caretaker to provide the child with the hope, love, and support necessary for the development of a sound, healthy personality.

negligence. The failure to do something that a reasonable person, guided by those considerations that ordinarily regulate human affairs, would do or doing something that a prudent and reasonable person would not do.

neologism. New words that an individual invents that are meaningless to others but have symbolic meaning to the person with psychosis.

neurocognitive disorder (NCD). The *DSM-5* diagnostic label for disorders of global impairment of cognitive functioning that is progressive and interferes with social and occupational abilities. These disorders include Alzheimer's disease and Lewy body dementia among others.

neuroendocrinology. The study of hormones functioning within the neurological system.

neuroleptic. Antipsychotic medication used to prevent or control psychotic symptoms.

neuroleptic malignant syndrome (NMS). A rare but potentially fatal complication of treatment with neuroleptic drugs. Symptoms include severe muscle rigidity, high fever, tachycardia, fluctuations in blood pressure, diaphoresis, and rapid deterioration of mental status to stupor and coma.

neuron. A nerve cell; consists of a cell body, an axon, and dendrites.

neurosis. An unconscious conflict that produces anxiety and other symptoms and leads to maladaptive use of defense mechanisms.

neurotransmitter. A chemical that is stored in the axon terminals of the presynaptic neuron. An electrical impulse through the neuron stimulates the release of the neurotransmitter into the synaptic cleft, which in turn determines whether or not another electrical impulse is generated.

nonassertive. Individuals who are nonassertive (sometimes called *passive*) seek to please others at the expense of denying their own basic human rights.

nonmaleficence. The ethical principle that espouses abstaining from negative acts toward another, including acting carefully to avoid harm.

nonsuicidal self-injuring behavior (NSSIB). Repetitive, nonlethal forms of self-injury that are not intended to end one's life but instead are intended to reduce emotional distress. Examples of NSSIB include "cutting" (cutting oneself with a sharp object), burning, self-hitting, or head banging.

nursing diagnosis. A clinical judgment about individual, family, or community responses to actual and potential health problems/life processes. Nursing diagnoses provide the basis for selection of nursing interventions to achieve outcomes for which the nurse is accountable.

Nursing Interventions Classification (NIC). A comprehensive, research-based, standardized classification of interventions that nurses perform.

Nursing Outcomes Classification (NOC). A comprehensive, standardized classification of patient outcomes developed to evaluate the effects of nursing interventions.

Nursing process. A dynamic, systematic process by which nurses assess, diagnose, identify outcomes, plan, implement, and evaluate nursing care. It has been called *nursing's scientific methodology*. Nursing process gives order and consistency to nursing intervention.

O

obesity. The state of having a body mass index of 30 or above.

object constancy. The phase in the separation/individuation process when the child learns to relate to objects in an effective, constant manner. A sense of separateness is established, and the child is able to internalize a sustained image of the loved object or person when out of sight.

obsessions. Unwanted, intrusive, persistent ideas, thoughts, impulses, or images that cause marked anxiety or distress. Common ones include repeated thoughts about contamination, repeated doubts, a need to have things in a particular order, aggressive or sexual impulses, and fears of harm to oneself or others.

obsessive-compulsive disorder. A disorder in which individuals have recurrent thoughts or ideas (obsessions) that they are unable to put out of their mind and actions that they are unable to refrain from performing (compulsions). The obsessions and compulsions are severe enough to interfere with social and occupational functioning.

obsessive-compulsive personality disorder. A type of personality disorder in which the individual has an intense fear of making mistakes, which manifests in inflexible and perfectionistic behavior. It is differentiated from obsessive-compulsive disorder in that there is no evidence of the obsessive-compulsive rituals in the individual with this personality disorder.

oculogyric crisis. An attack of involuntary deviation and fixation of the eyeballs, usually in the upward position. It may last for several minutes or hours and may occur as an extrapyramidal side effect of some antipsychotic medications.

operant conditioning. The learning of a particular action or type of behavior that is followed by a reinforcement.

opioids. A synthetic or naturally occurring substance that acts on opiate receptors to produce opiate-like effects.

oppositional defiant disorder (ODD). A disorder characterized by a persistent pattern of angry mood and defiant behavior that interferes with social, educational, occupational, or other important areas of functioning. The age of onset is typically around 8 years of age.

orgasm. A peaking of sexual pleasure with release of sexual tension and rhythmic contraction of the perineal muscles and pelvic reproductive organs.

osteoporosis. A reduction in the mass of bone per unit of volume that interferes with the mechanical support function of bone. This process occurs because of demineralization of the bones and is escalated in women about the time of menopause.

outcomes. End results that are measurable, desirable, and observable and translate into observable behaviors.

overgeneralization. Also called *absolutistic thinking*. In cognitive behavior therapy, this refers to a distorted thinking pattern in which sweeping conclusions are made based on one incident—an "all-or-nothing" type of thinking.

overt sensitization. A type of aversion therapy that produces unpleasant consequences for undesirable behavior. An example is the use of disulfiram therapy with alcoholics, which induces an undesirable physical response if the individual has consumed any alcohol.

P

palilalia. Repeating one's own sounds or words (a type of vocal tic associated with Tourette's disorder).

panic. A sudden overwhelming feeling of terror or impending doom. This most severe form of emotional anxiety is usually accompanied by behavioral, cognitive, and physiological signs and symptoms considered to be outside the expected range of normalcy.

panic disorder. A disorder characterized by recurrent panic attacks, the onset of which are unpredictable and manifested by intense apprehension, fear, or terror, often associated with feelings of impending doom and accompanied by intense physical discomfort.

paradoxical intervention. In family therapy, "prescribing the symptom." The therapist requests that the family continue to engage in the behavior that they are trying to change. Tension is relieved, and the family is able to view more clearly the possible solutions to their problem.

paralanguage. The gestural component of the spoken word. It consists of pitch, tone, loudness of spoken messages, the rate of speaking, expressively placed pauses, and emphasis assigned to certain words.

paranoia. A term that implies extreme suspiciousness. In schizophrenia, paranoia is characterized by persecutory delusions and hallucinations of a threatening nature.

paranoid personality disorder. A type of personality disorder in which the individual intensely mistrusts others and assumes that they have malevolent intentions toward them.

paraphilic disorder. Repetitive behaviors or fantasies that involve nonhuman objects, real or simulated suffering or humiliation, or nonconsenting partners.

parasomnia. Unusual or undesirable behaviors that occur during sleep (e.g., nightmares, sleep terrors, and sleepwalking).

passive-aggressive. Behavior that defends an individual's own basic rights by expressing resistance to social and occupational demands. Sometimes called *indirect aggression*, this behavior takes the form of sly, devious, and undermining actions that express the opposite of what the person is really feeling.

pathological gambling. A failure to resist impulses to gamble and gambling behavior that compromises; disrupts; or damages personal, family, or vocational pursuits.

patient-centered care. An approach to patient care that focuses on listening to patients, empowering them as central to decision making about their care, developing a collaborative partnership, and making decisions for patients (such as involuntary hospitalization) only when they are clearly unable to and when it is necessary to protect their safety.

pedophilic disorder. Recurrent urges and sexually arousing fantasies involving sexual activity with a prepubescent child.

peer assistance programs. Programs established by the American Nurses Association to assist impaired nurses. The individuals who administer these efforts are nurse members of the state associations as well as nurses who are in recovery themselves.

perseveration. Persistent repetition of the same word or idea in response to different questions.

personal distance. The distance between individuals who are having interactions of a personal nature, such as a close conversation. In the U.S. culture, personal distance is approximately 18 to 40 inches.

personal identity. The self-perception of individuals that define their functions as observer, standard setter, and self-evaluator. Personal identity helps to maintain a stable self-image and relates to what individuals strive to become.

personal self. See **personal identity.**

personality. Deeply ingrained patterns of behavior, which include the way one relates to, perceives, and thinks about the environment and oneself.

personalization. Taking complete responsibility for situations without considering that other circumstances may have contributed to the outcome.

phencyclidine. An anesthetic used in veterinary medicine; used illegally as a hallucinogen, referred to as *PCP* or *angel dust.*

phenotype. Characteristics of physical manifestations that identify a particular genotype. Examples of phenotypes include eye color, height, blood type, language, and hairstyle. Phenotypes may be genetic or acquired.

phobia. An irrational fear.

physical neglect of a child. The failure on the part of the parent or caregiver to provide for a child's basic needs, such as food, clothing, shelter, medical and dental care, and supervision.

physical self. A personal appraisal by individuals of their physical being; includes physical attributes, functioning, sexuality, wellness-illness state, and appearance.

PIE charting. More specifically called *APIE*, this method of documentation has an **A**ssessment, **P**roblem, **I**ntervention, and **E**valuation (APIE) format and is a problem-oriented system used to document nursing process.

positive reinforcement. A reinforcement stimulus that increases the probability that the behavior will recur.

positive symptoms. A group of symptoms in schizophrenia that are present because of the disorder. Examples include delusions, hallucinations, and disorganized thinking, speech, and behavior.

postpartum depression. Depression that occurs during the postpartum period. It may be related to hormonal changes, tryptophan metabolism, or alterations in membrane transport during the early postpartum period. Other predisposing factors may also be influential.

post-traumatic stress disorder (PTSD). A syndrome of symptoms that can develop following a psychologically distressing event that is outside the range of usual human experience (e.g., rape, war). The individual is unable to cope with the associated anxiety and has nightmares, flashbacks, and panic attacks.

posturing. The voluntary assumption of inappropriate or bizarre postures.

preassaultive tension state. Behaviors predictive of potential violence. They include excessive motor activity; tense posture; defiant affect; clenched teeth and fists; and other arguing, demanding, and threatening behaviors.

precipitating event. A stimulus arising from the internal or external environment that is perceived by individuals as taxing or exceeding their resources and endangering their well-being.

predisposing factors. A variety of elements that influence how an individual perceives and responds to a stressful event. Types of predisposing factors include genetic influences, past experiences, and existing conditions.

Premack principle. This principle states that a frequently occurring response (R1) can serve as a positive reinforcement for a response (R2) that occurs less frequently. For example, a girl may talk to friends on the phone (R2) only if she does her homework (R1).

premature ejaculation. Ejaculation that occurs with minimal sexual stimulation or before, upon, or shortly after penetration and before the person wishes it.

premenstrual dysphoric disorder. A disorder that is characterized by depressed mood, anxiety, mood swings, and decreased interest in activities during the week prior to menses and subsiding shortly after the onset of menstruation.

pressured speech. Rapid, frenetic speech that often occurs as a symptom of bipolar disorder.

priapism. Prolonged painful penile erection, may occur as an adverse effect of some antidepressant medications, particularly trazodone.

primary gain. The receipt of positive reinforcement for somaticizing by being able to avoid difficult situations because of physical complaint.

primary neurocognitive disorder. A neurocognitive disorder (NCD), such as Alzheimer's disease, in which the NCD itself is the major sign of some organic brain disease not directly related to any other organic illness.

primary prevention. Reduction of the incidence of mental disorders within the population by helping individuals to cope more effectively with stress and by trying to diminish stressors within the environment.

privileged communication. A doctrine common to most states that grants certain privileges under which health-care professionals may refuse to reveal information about and communications with clients.

problem-oriented recording (POR). A system of documentation that follows a subjective data, objective data, assessment, plan, implementation, and evaluation (SOAPIE) format. It is based on a list of identified patient problems to which each entry is directed.

prodromal syndrome. A syndrome of symptoms that often precede the onset of aggressive or violent behavior. These symptoms include anxiety and tension, verbal abuse and profanity, and increasing hyperactivity.

progressive relaxation. A method of deep muscle relaxation in which each muscle group is alternately tensed and relaxed in a systematic order with the person concentrating on the contrast of sensations experienced from tensing and relaxing.

projection. Attributing to another person feelings or impulses unacceptable to oneself.

prospective payment. The program of cost containment within the health-care profession directed at setting forth pre-established amounts that would be reimbursed for specific diagnoses.

pseudocyesis. A condition in which an individual has nearly all the signs and symptoms of pregnancy but is not pregnant; a conversion reaction.

pseudodementia. Symptoms of depression that mimic those of neurocognitive disorder.

pseudohostility. A family interaction pattern characterized by a state of chronic conflict and alienation among family members. This relationship pattern allows family members to deny underlying fears of tenderness and intimacy.

pseudomutuality. A family interaction pattern characterized by a façade of mutual regard with the purpose of denying underlying fears of separation and hostility.

pseudoparkinsonism. A side effect of some antipsychotic medications. Symptoms mimic those of Parkinson's disease, such as tremor, shuffling gait, drooling, and rigidity.

psychiatric home care. Care provided by psychiatric nurses in the client's home. Psychiatric home-care nurses must have physical and psychosocial nursing skills to meet the demands of the client population they serve.

psychoanalysis. An approach to treatment of mental and emotional distress, originated by Freud, that focuses on bringing unconscious thoughts and drives into conscious awareness.

psychobiology. The study of the biological foundations of cognitive, emotional, and behavioral processes.

psychodrama. A specialized type of group therapy that employs a dramatic approach in which patients become "actors" in life situation scenarios. The goal is to resolve interpersonal conflicts in a less-threatening atmosphere than the real-life situation would present.

psychodynamic nursing. Being able to understand one's own behavior, to help others identify felt difficulties, and to apply principles of human relations to the problems that arise at all levels of experience.

psychoimmunology. The study of the implications of the immune system in psychiatry.

Psychological Recovery Model. A model of treatment that focuses on the importance of hopefulness, self-determination, and positive self-concept in recovery from mental illnesses or emotional stress.

psychomotor domain. A category of learning in which the behaviors are processed and demonstrated. The information has been intellectually processed, and the individual is displaying motor behaviors.

psychomotor retardation. Extreme slowdown of physical movements that is common in severe depression. Posture slumps, speech is slowed, and digestion becomes sluggish.

psychophysiological. Referring to psychological factors contributing to the initiation or exacerbation of a physical condition. Either a demonstrable organic pathology or a known pathophysiological process is involved.

psychosis. A mental state in which there is a severe loss of contact with reality. Symptoms may include delusions, hallucinations, disorganized speech patterns, and bizarre or catatonic behaviors.

psychosomatic. See **psychophysiological.**

psychotic disorder. A serious psychiatric disorder in which there is a gross disorganization of the personality, a marked disturbance in reality testing, and the impairment of interpersonal functioning and relationship to the external world.

psychotropic medication. Medication that affects psychic function, behavior, or experience.

public distance. Appropriate interactional distance for speaking in public or yelling to someone some distance away. U.S. culture defines this distance as 12 feet or more.

purging. The act of attempting to rid the body of calories by self-induced vomiting or excessive use of laxatives or diuretics.

purpose. A guiding principle in the Psychological Recovery Model that stresses the importance of finding purpose in life for the process of recovery from mental illness.

pyromania. An inability to resist the impulse to set fires.

Q

qi. In Chinese medicine, the healing energy that flows through pathways in the body called *meridians.* (Also called *chi.*)

R

rape. The expression of power and dominance by means of sexual violence, most commonly by men over women, although men may also be raped. Rape is considered an act of aggression, not of passion.

rape-trauma syndrome. A variable group of symptoms that are indicative of the trauma associated with rape. Symptoms may include expressed response patterns, controlled responses, or silent reactions.

rapport. The development between two people in a relationship of special feelings based on mutual acceptance, warmth, friendliness, common interest, a sense of trust, and a nonjudgmental attitude.

rationalization. Attempting to make excuses or formulate logical reasons to justify unacceptable feelings or behaviors.

reaction formation. Preventing unacceptable or undesirable thoughts or behaviors from being expressed by exaggerating opposite thoughts or types of behaviors.

reality therapy. A type of therapy developed by William Glasser, rooted in control theory, which stresses individual responsibility for choosing how to respond to present situations.

receptor sites. Molecules that are situated on the cell membrane of the postsynaptic neuron that will accept only molecules with a complementary shape. These complementary molecules are specific to certain neurotransmitters that determine whether an electrical impulse will be excited or inhibited.

reciprocal inhibition. Also called *counterconditioning,* this technique serves to decrease or eliminate a behavior by introducing a more adaptive behavior but one that is incompatible with the unacceptable behavior (e.g., introducing relaxation techniques to an anxious person; relaxation and anxiety are incompatible behaviors).

recovery. An ongoing process of movement toward improvement in health and quality of life. Originally used to describe the lifelong process of recovering from an addiction, recovery has evolved into a similar ongoing process for those with serious mental illness.

Recovery Model. Refers to several approaches to treatment that share in common a focus on connectedness, hope, optimism about the future, identity, meaning in life, and empowerment in recovery from mental illnesses or emotional stress.

referral. The process of connecting patients with appropriate and specialized health services when screening indicates the need.

reframing. Changing the conceptual or emotional setting or viewpoint in relation to which a situation is experienced and placing it in another frame that fits the "facts" of the same concrete situation equally well or even better and thereby changing its entire meaning. The behavior may not actually change, but the consequences of the behavior may change because of a change in the meaning attached to the behavior.

regression. A retreat to an earlier level of development and the comfort measures associated with that level of functioning.

relaxation. A decrease in tension or intensity, resulting in refreshment of body and mind. A state of refreshing tranquility.

religion. A set of beliefs, values, rites, and rituals adopted by a group of people. The practices are usually grounded in the teachings of a spiritual leader.

religiosity. When identified as a symptom of illness, refers to excessive demonstration of or obsession with religious ideas and behavior that causes marked distress and impairs ability to function; common in schizophrenia.

reminiscence therapy. A process of life review by older individuals that promotes self-esteem and provides assistance in working through unresolved conflicts from the past.

repression. The involuntary blocking of unpleasant feelings and experiences from one's awareness.

residual stimuli. Certain beliefs, attitudes, experiences, or traits that may contribute to an individual's low self-esteem.

retraumatization. Any situation that consciously or unconsciously triggers a reminder of previous trauma and associated symptoms such as anxiety, fear, and feeling unsafe. Retraumatization can exacerbate physical, mental, and emotional consequences of previous trauma.

retrograde ejaculation. Ejaculation of the seminal fluid backward into the bladder; may occur as a side effect of antipsychotic medications.

reuptake. The process of neurotransmitter inactivation by which the neurotransmitter is reabsorbed into the presynaptic neuron from which it had been released.

right. That which an individual is entitled (by ethical, legal, or moral standards) to have, or to do, or to receive from others within the limits of the law.

rigid boundaries. A person with rigid boundaries is "closed" and difficult to bond with. Such individuals have a narrow perspective on life, see things one way, and cannot discuss matters that lie outside their perspective.

ritualistic behavior. Purposeless activities that an individual performs repeatedly in an effort to decrease anxiety (e.g., hand washing); common in obsessive-compulsive disorder.

S

safe house or shelter. An establishment set up by local governments or nonprofit agencies to provide protection for battered women and their children.

SBIRT. An acronym for Screening, Brief Intervention, and Referral for Treatment, SBIRT is an evidence-based approach that can be used in emergency departments, trauma centers, primary care, and other community settings to quickly identify the severity of substance use disorders and refer for treatment as necessary.

scapegoating. Occurs when hostility exists in a marriage dyad and an innocent third person (usually a child) becomes the target of blame for the problem.

schemas. Also called *core beliefs*, cognitive structures that consist of the individual's fundamental beliefs and assumptions, which develop early in life from personal experiences and identification with significant others. These concepts are reinforced by further learning experiences and, in turn, influence the formation of other beliefs, values, and attitudes.

schizoid personality disorder. A type of personality disorder characterized by extreme detachment from personal relationships and restricted expression of emotions.

schizophrenia. One of the schizophrenia spectrum disorders characterized by disturbance in thinking, cognition, emotions, and behavior. Considered a serious mental illness, the course is chronic with episodes of exacerbation and remission. Its causes are likely a combination of genetic, neurodevelopmental, and environmental factors.

schizotypal personality disorder. A disorder characterized by odd and eccentric behavior, not decompensating to the level of schizophrenia.

screening. An aspect of the assessment process in which broad questions are used to identify issues requiring further evaluation.

secondary gain. The receipt of positive reinforcement for somaticizing through added attention, sympathy, and nurturing.

secondary neurocognitive disorder. Neurocognitive disorder that is caused by or related to another disease or condition, such as HIV disease or a cerebral trauma.

secondary prevention. Health care that is directed at reduction of the prevalence of psychiatric illness by shortening the course (duration) of the illness. This is accomplished through early identification of problems and prompt initiation of treatment.

selective abstraction. Sometimes called *mental filter*, a type of thinking in which a conclusion is drawn based on only a selected portion of the evidence.

self-concept. The composite of beliefs and feelings that one holds about oneself at a given time, formed from perceptions of others' reactions. The self-concept consists of the physical self or body image, the personal self or identity, and the self-esteem.

self-consistency. The component of the personal identity that strives to maintain a stable self-image.

self-esteem. The degree of regard or respect that individuals have for themselves. It is a measure of worth that they place on their abilities and judgments.

self-expectancy. A component of personal identity that is the individual's perception of what they want to be, to do, or to become.

self-ideal. See **self-expectancy.**

sensate focus. A therapeutic technique used to treat individuals and couples with sexual dysfunction. The technique involves touching and being touched by another and focusing attention on the physical sensations encountered thereby. Clients gradually move through various levels of sensate focus that progress from nongenital touching to touching that includes the breasts and genitals; touching done in a simultaneous, mutual format rather than by one person at a time; and touching that extends to and allows eventually for the possibility of intercourse.

separation anxiety disorder. A disorder characterized by excessive fear or anxiety concerning separation from those to whom the individual is attached. Its onset may occur at any age but is most commonly diagnosed around the age of 5 or 6 when a child begins attending school.

serious mental illness (SMI). a mental, behavioral, or emotional disorder resulting in serious functional impairment that substantially interferes with or limits one or more major life activities.

serotonin syndrome. A syndrome that is an adverse reaction to serotonergic medications. It may range from mild to severe and is potentially fatal. Symptoms may include significantly elevated temperature, agitation, muscle rigidity or twitching, sweating, irregular heartbeat, and seizures.

sexual assault. Any type of contact or behavior in which a person is forced, coerced, or manipulated into unwanted sexual activity.

sexual assault nurse examiner (SANE). A clinical forensic registered nurse who has received specialized training to provide care to patients who have experienced sexual assault.

sexual exploitation of a child. The inducement or coercion of a child into engaging in sexually explicit conduct for the purpose of promoting any performance (e.g., child pornography).

sexual masochism disorder. Sexual stimulation derived from being humiliated, beaten, bound, or otherwise made to suffer.

sexual sadism disorder. Recurrent urges and sexually arousing fantasies involving acts (real, not simulated) in which the psychological or physical suffering (including humiliation) of the victim is sexually exciting.

sexuality. Sexuality is the constitution and life of an individual relative to characteristics regarding intimacy. It reflects the totality of the person and does not relate exclusively to the sex organs or sexual behavior.

shaping. In learning, one shapes the behavior of another by giving reinforcements for increasingly closer approximations to the desired behavior.

shelters. A variety of places designed to help people experiencing homelessness, ranging from converted warehouses that provide cots or floor space on which to sleep overnight to significant operations that provide a multitude of social and health-care services.

short-term memory. The ability to remember events that occurred very recently. This ability deteriorates with age.

silent rape reaction. The response of a rape victim in which they tell no one about the assault.

slander. An action with which an individual may be charged for orally sharing information that is detrimental to a person's reputation.

social anxiety disorder. A disorder in which the individual experiences extreme fear of doing something embarrassing or being negatively evaluated by others in a social situation.

social distance. The distance considered acceptable in interactions with strangers or acquaintances, such as at a cocktail party or in a public building. U.S. culture defines this distance as 4 to 12 feet.

social distancing. An aspect of stigma that refers to the tendency of health-care workers and others to avoid people with mental illness or addiction.

social phobia. The fear of being humiliated in social situations.

social skills training. Educational opportunities through role play for the person with schizophrenia to learn appropriate social interaction skills and functional skills that are relevant to daily living.

somatization. A method of coping with psychosocial stress by developing physical symptoms.

specific phobia. A persistent fear of a specific object or situation, other than the fear of being unable to escape from a situation (agoraphobia) or the fear of being humiliated in social situations (social phobia).

spirituality. The human quality that gives meaning and sense of purpose to an individual's existence. Spirituality exists within each individual regardless of belief system and serves as a force for interconnectedness between the self and others, the environment, and a higher power.

splitting. A primitive ego defense mechanism in which the person is unable to integrate and accept both positive and negative feelings. In the view of these individuals, people—including themselves—and life situations are either all good or all bad. This trait is common in borderline personality disorder.

statutory law. A law that has been enacted by legislative bodies, such as a county or city council, state legislature, or the U.S. Congress.

statutory rape. Unlawful intercourse between a person who is over the age of consent and a person who is under the age of consent. Legal age of consent varies from state to state. An individual can be arrested for statutory rape even when the interaction has occurred between consenting individuals.

stereotyping. The process of classifying all individuals from the same culture or ethnic group as identical.

stigmatization. The devaluing, marginalizing, and disenfranchising of certain patients because of symptoms or conditions.

stimulus. In classical conditioning, that which elicits a response.

stimulus generalization. The process by which a conditioned response is elicited from all stimuli *similar* to the one from which the response was learned.

storefront clinics. Establishments that have been converted into clinics that serve people experiencing homelessness.

stress. A state of disequilibrium or tension that occurs when there is disharmony between demands occurring within an individual's internal or external environment and their ability to cope with those demands.

stress management. Various methods used by individuals to reduce tension and other maladaptive responses to stress in their lives; includes relaxation exercises, physical exercise, music, mental imagery, or any other technique that is successful for a person.

stressor. A demand from within an individual's internal or external environment that elicits a physiological and/or psychological response.

sublimation. The rechanneling of personally and/or socially unacceptable drives or impulses into activities that are more tolerable and constructive.

subluxation. The term used in chiropractic medicine to describe vertebrae in the spinal column that have become displaced, possibly pressing on nerves and interfering with normal nerve transmission.

substance abuse. Use of psychoactive drugs that poses significant hazards to health and interferes with social, occupational, psychological, or physical functioning.

substance addiction. Physical addiction is identified by the inability to stop using a substance despite attempts to do so; a continual use of the substance despite adverse consequences; a developing tolerance; and the development of withdrawal symptoms upon cessation or decreased intake. Psychological addiction is said to exist when a substance is perceived by the user to be necessary to maintain an optimal state of personal well-being, interpersonal relations, or skill performance.

substitution therapy. The use of various medications to decrease the intensity of symptoms in an individual who is withdrawing from, or experiencing the effects of excessive use of, substances.

subsystems. The smaller units of which a system is composed. In family systems theory, the subsystems are composed of husband–wife, parent–child(ren), or sibling–sibling.

suicide. The act of taking one's own life. Suicide is most often associated with severe depression but there is increased risk of suicide in many mental illnesses including substance use disorders, bipolar disorders, schizophrenia, anxiety disorders, and eating disorders.

suicide prevention. The collective efforts including screening, assessment, referral for treatment, and collaborative partnership with the patient to prevent suicide as an outcome.

suicide risk factors. Situations, stressors, or demographics that have been statistically related to increased vulnerability toward suicide.

suicide warning signs. Behaviors and communication that are associated with more imminent risk for suicide and requiring immediate intervention. These include threats of suicide, a plan with access to means, hopelessness, and others.

sundowning. A phenomenon in patients with neurocognitive disorder in which the symptoms seem to worsen in the late afternoon and evening.

superego. One of the three elements of the personality identified by Freud that represents the conscience and the culturally determined restrictions that are placed on an individual.

suppression. The voluntary blocking from one's awareness of unpleasant feelings and experiences.

surrogate. One who serves as a substitute figure for another.

symbiosis. One of the stages of development in Object Relations Theory in which children view themselves as extensions of their mother rather than a separate entity.

symbiotic relationship. A type of "psychic fusion" that occurs between two people; it is unhealthy in that severe anxiety is generated in either or both if separation is indicated. A symbiotic relationship is normal between infant and mother.

sympathy. The actual sharing of another's thoughts and behaviors. Differs from ***empathy*** in that with empathy one experiences an objective understanding of what another is feeling rather than actually sharing those feelings.

synapse. The junction between two neurons. The small space between the axon terminals of one neuron and the cell body or dendrites of another is called the *synaptic cleft.*

systematic desensitization. A treatment for phobias in which the individual is taught to relax and then asked to imagine various components of the phobic stimulus on a graded hierarchy, moving from that which produces the least fear to that which produces the most.

T

tangentiality. The inability to get to the point of a story. The speaker introduces many unrelated topics until the original topic of discussion is lost. Tangentiality can be symptomatic of cognitive disruptions common in schizophrenia.

tardive dyskinesia. Syndrome of symptoms characterized by bizarre facial and tongue movements, a stiff neck, and difficulty swallowing. It may occur as an adverse effect of long-term therapy with some antipsychotic medications.

technical expert. Peplau's term for one who understands various professional devices and possesses the clinical skills necessary to perform the interventions that are in the best interest of the client.

temperament. A set of inborn personality characteristics that influence an individual's manner of reacting to the environment and ultimately influences their developmental progression.

territoriality. The innate tendency of individuals to own space. Individuals lay claim to areas around them as their own. This phenomenon can have an influence on interpersonal communication.

tertiary gain. The receipt of positive reinforcement for somaticizing by causing the focus of the family to switch to the individual and away from conflict that may be occurring within the family.

tertiary prevention. Health care that is directed toward reduction of the residual effects associated with severe or chronic physical or mental illness.

therapeutic communication. Caregiver verbal and nonverbal techniques that focus on the care receiver's needs and advance the promotion of healing and change. Therapeutic communication encourages exploration of feelings and fosters understanding of behavioral motivation. It is nonjudgmental, discourages defensiveness, and promotes trust.

therapeutic community. Also called *milieu therapy,* this approach strives to manipulate the environment so that all aspects of the client's hospital experience are considered therapeutic.

therapeutic group. Differs from group therapy in that there is a lesser degree of theoretical foundation. Focus is on group relations, interactions between group members, and the consideration of a selected issue. Leaders of therapeutic groups do not require the degree of educational preparation required of group therapy leaders.

therapeutic relationship. An interaction between two people (usually a caregiver and a care receiver) in which input from both participants contributes to a climate of healing, growth promotion, and/or illness prevention.

Tidal Model. A nursing-developed, person-centered approach to the Recovery Model, which stresses the individual's personal story as significant to working on recovery.

time out. An aversive stimulus or punishment during which the individual is removed from the environment where the unacceptable behavior is being exhibited.

token economy. In behavior modification, a type of contracting in which the reinforcers for desired behaviors are presented in the form of tokens, which may then be exchanged for designated privileges.

tolerance. The need for increasingly larger or more frequent doses of a substance in order to obtain the desired effects originally produced by a lower dose.

tort. The violation of a civil law in which an individual has been wronged. In a tort action, one party asserts that wrongful conduct on the part of the other has caused harm, and compensation for harm suffered is sought.

Tourette's disorder. A disorder characterized by the presence of multiple motor tics and one or more vocal tics, which may appear simultaneously or at different periods during the illness. The most common age of onset is around 6 to 7 years of age,

transcendence. A developmental task more recently identified by Eric Erikson and associate in which the older adult must learn to move from materialistic, rational thinking to a broader worldview that includes increased sense of meaning in life, well-being, and a sense of satisfaction.

transference. Transference occurs when a client unconsciously displaces (or "transfers") to the nurse or therapist feelings formed toward a person from their past.

transgender. Describes individuals whose gender identity does not match their assigned sex at birth. Transgender individuals have the self-perception of being of the opposite gender and may seek gender-affirming treatments.

transvestic disorder. A *DSM-5* diagnostic category identified as one of a group of paraphilic disorders in which recurrent sexual urges, sexually arousing fantasies or behaviors arise from dressing in the clothes of the opposite gender *and* the outcome is clinically significant distress or impairment in social, occupational, or other important areas of functioning.

trauma-informed care. An approach to care that assesses for history of physical, sexual, or psychosocial trauma and provides care with consideration for how trauma history may influence an individual's response to interventions and treatments.

traumatic brain injury (TBI). Injury to the brain that is the result of head trauma.

triangles. A three-person emotional configuration that is considered the basic building block of the family system. When anxiety becomes too great between two family members, a third person is brought in to form a triangle. Triangles are dysfunctional in that they offer relief from anxiety through diversion rather than through resolution of the issue.

trichotillomania (hair-pulling disorder). The recurrent failure to resist impulses to pull out one's own hair.

tyramine. An amino acid found in aged cheeses or other aged, overripe, and fermented foods; broad beans; pickled herring; beef or chicken liver; preserved meats; beer and wine; yeast products; chocolate; caffeinated drinks; canned figs; sour cream; yogurt; soy sauce; and some over-the-counter cold medications and diet pills. If foods high in tyramine content are consumed while an individual is taking monoamine oxidase inhibitors, a potentially life-threatening syndrome called *hypertensive crisis* can result.

U

unconditional positive regard. Carl Rogers's term for the respect and dignity of individuals regardless of their unacceptable behavior.

unconditioned response. In classical conditioning, an unconditioned response refers to a reflexive response to a specific target stimulus.

unconditioned stimulus. In classical conditioning, a specific stimulus that elicits an unconditioned, reflexive response.

undoing. A mechanism used to symbolically negate or cancel out a previous action or experience that one finds intolerable.

universality. One curative factor of groups (identified by Irvin Yalom) in which individuals realize that they are not alone in a problem and in the thoughts and feelings they are experiencing. Anxiety is relieved by the support and understanding of others in the group who share similar experiences.

utilitarianism. The ethical theory that espouses the greatest happiness for the greatest number. Under this theory, action would be taken based on the end results that will produce the most good (happiness) for the most people.

V

values. Personal beliefs about the truth; beauty; or worth of a thought, object, or behavior that influences an individual's actions.

values clarification. A process of self-discovery by which people identify their personal values and their value rankings. This process increases awareness about why individuals behave in certain ways.

veracity. An ethical principle that refers to one's duty to always be truthful.

veterans. Individuals who have served in the military.

voyeuristic disorder. Recurrent urges and sexually arousing fantasies involving the act of observing unsuspecting people, usually strangers, who are either naked, in the process of disrobing, or engaging in sexual activity.

W

waxy flexibility. A condition by which the individual with schizophrenia passively yields all movable parts of the body to any efforts made at placing them in certain positions.

Wernicke's encephalopathy. A brain disorder caused by thiamine deficiency and characterized by visual disturbances, ataxia, somnolence, stupor, and, without thiamine replacement, death.

withdrawal. The physiological and mental readjustment that accompanies the discontinuation of an addictive substance.

word salad. A group of words that are put together in a random fashion without any logical connection.

WRAP Model. An approach to the Recovery Model (Wellness Recovery Action Plan) that stresses learning a distinct set of skills necessary for managing symptoms of mental illness or emotional distress in everyday life.

Y

yoga. A system of beliefs and practices, the ultimate goal of which is to unite the human soul with the universal spirit. In Western countries, yoga uses body postures, along with meditation and breathing exercises, to achieve a balanced, disciplined workout that releases muscle tension, tones the internal organs, and energizes the mind, body, and spirit so that natural healing can occur.

Appendix C

Answers to Review Questions

CHAPTER 1. **Mental Health and Mental Illness**
1. a **2.** c **3.** a, b, c **4.** b **5.** d
6. c **7.** b **8.** c **9.** a **10.** b

CHAPTER 2. **Biological Implications**
1. d **2.** d **3.** a **4.** b **5.** c **6.** a
7. d **8.** c **9.** b **10.** a **11.** a, b, c
12. b, c, d

CHAPTER 3. **Ethical and Legal Issues**
1. b **2.** a **3.** c **4.** b **5.** c **6.** d
7. d **8.** b **9.** a **10.** a

CHAPTER 4. **Psychopharmacology**
1. a **2.** b **3.** c **4.** b **5.** a **6.** b
7. a **8.** b **9.** d **10.** b

CHAPTER 5. **Relationship Development and Therapeutic Communication**
1. a, b, c **2.** b **3.** c **4.** a **5.** d **6.** b
7. a **8.** c **9.** d **10.** c **11.** a **12.** b

CHAPTER 6. **The Nursing Process in Psychiatric Mental Health Nursing**
1. b **2.** a **3.** d **4.** a **5.** c **6.** b
7. a, b, c, d **8.** d **9.** c **10.** a

CHAPTER 7. **Psychosocial Interventions and Spiritual Care**
1. c **2.** a, b, c **3.** a, b, d, e **4.** b **5.** b
6. a **7.** b **8.** d **9.** c **10.** d **11.** a
12. d

CHAPTER 8. **Intervention in Groups**
1. b **2.** d **3.** a **4.** c **5.** c **6.** d
7. b **8.** c. **9.** a **10.** c

CHAPTER 9. **Crisis Intervention**
1. c **2.** d **3.** c **4.** c **5.** b, c, d, e
6. d **7.** b **8.** a **9.** c **10.** b **11.** c
12. b

CHAPTER 10. **The Recovery Model**
1. b, d **2.** c **3.** d **4.** a **5.** c **6.** d
7. b

CHAPTER 11. **Suicide Prevention**
1. a **2.** a, c, d, e **3.** d **4.** a, b, c **5.** b
6. c **7.** a **8.** c **9.** b **10.** b, e

CHAPTER 12. **Caring for Patients With Mental Illness and Substance Use Disorders in General Practice Settings**
1. c **2.** d **3.** a **4.** d **5.** a, b, c
6. a, d **7.** b **8.** d

CHAPTER 13. **Neurocognitive Disorders**
1. c, e **2.** d **3.** a, b, e **4.** a **5.** a, c, e
6. b **7.** d **8.** c **9.** b **10.** c

CHAPTER 14. **Substance Use and Addiction Disorders**
1. a **2.** c **3.** b **4.** a **5.** a **6.** c
7. d **8.** c **9.** a **10.** a, b, c, d, e

CHAPTER 15. **Schizophrenia Spectrum and Other Psychotic Disorders**
1. a, b, e **2.** b **3.** a **4.** a **5.** d
6. c **7.** d **8.** d **9.** c **10.** b **11.** c
12. b

CHAPTER 16. **Depressive Disorders**
1. c **2.** a **3.** a, b, d **4.** a, c, e **5.** a
6. b **7.** b **8.** d **9.** c **10.** a, b, d
11. d

CHAPTER 17. **Bipolar and Related Disorders**
1. c **2.** a **3.** a, c, d **4.** a **5.** d **6.** b
7. b **8.** c **9.** a, c, d **10.** b

CHAPTER 18. **Anxiety, Obsessive-Compulsive, and Related Disorders**
1. d **2.** c **3.** d **4.** a **5.** a, b, c **6.** b
7. c **8.** c **9.** a **10.** b

CHAPTER 19. **Trauma- and Stressor-Related Disorders**
1. b **2.** a **3.** d **4.** c **5.** a **6.** a, c
7. c **8.** d **9.** b **10.** d

CHAPTER 20. **Somatic Symptom and Dissociative Disorders**

1. a **2.** b **3.** d **4.** b **5.** a **6.** b
7. d **8.** c **9.** d **10.** b

CHAPTER 21. **Eating Disorders**

1. c **2.** a **3.** b **4.** c **5.** c **6.** b
7. b **8.** b **9.** c **10.** a, b, c, d

CHAPTER 22. **Personality Disorders**

1. a **2.** a **3.** b **4.** d **5.** a **6.** b
7. d **8.** d **9.** c **10.** b

CHAPTER 23. **Children and Adolescents**

1. b **2.** c **3.** d **4.** a **5.** b **6.** b, c, d
7. b **8.** c **9.** a **10.** b

CHAPTER 24. **The Aging Individual**

1. c **2.** d **3.** b **4.** a **5.** d **6.** a
7. d **8.** b **9.** a **10.** c

CHAPTER 25. **Survivors of Abuse or Neglect**

1. c **2.** a **3.** b **4.** d **5.** d **6.** b
7. d **8.** a **9.** b **10.** b

CHAPTER 26. **Community Mental Health Nursing**

1. a **2.** b **3.** a **4.** b **5.** a, b, c, d
6. c **7.** c **8.** d **9.** a **10.** a, b

CHAPTER 27. **The Bereaved Individual**

1. a, b, c, d **2.** c **3.** c **4.** d **5.** a
6. a **7.** b **8.** c **9.** a **10.** c

CHAPTER 28. **Military Families**

1. a, b, c, d **2.** b **3.** a **4.** d **5.** c
6. b **7.** c **8.** a, c, d **9.** a, b, c, d

CHAPTER 29. **Concepts of Personality Development**

1. b **2.** c **3.** d **4.** b **5.** b **6.** b
7. a **8.** c **9.** a **10.** b

CHAPTER 30. **Complementary and Integrative Therapies**

1. a, c, e, f **2.** a, b, d **3.** c, d **4.** a, d, e
5. c **6.** d **7.** c **8.** b **9.** a **10.** c

CHAPTER 31. **Cultural Concepts Relevant to Psychiatric Mental Health Nursing**

1. c **2.** d **3.** a **4.** d **5.** b **6.** c
7. b **8.** b **9.** d **10.** c

CHAPTER 32. **Issues Related to Human Sexuality and Gender Dysphoria**

1. d **2.** b **3.** a, b, d, e **4.** a **5.** c
6. a, b, c, d **7.** b **8.** b **9.** c

Appendix D

Examples of Answers to Communication Exercises

CHAPTER 9 Crisis Intervention

1. "I'll try to help you to the best of my ability. Please tell me what is upsetting you." Establish rapport, convey respect, and assess precipitating events.
2. "Hi Shelley, my name is Mrs. Smith, and I am a registered nurse here to help you. I'm so glad you came in to seek help. I'd like to ask you some questions about the events you've experienced. All right?" Convey respect, reassurance of help, and empower the client to be involved in decision making.
3. "Thomas, last evening you became very upset, stating you thought the FBI was trying to kill you, and you struck another patient." (Giving information) "Do you remember any of those events?" (Assessing the patient's perception and memory) "Restraint is an intervention that we only use when other efforts have failed to protect your safety and the safety of others." (Giving information) "Let's talk about what you think would be helpful in preventing that from happening again." (Formulating a plan, empowering the client to be involved in problem-solving)

CHAPTER 10 The Recovery Model

1. Because inability to sit still may be a side effect of many antipsychotic medications, one response is to assess the client's medications, assess the client's symptoms, and educate him about akathisia as appropriate. This response supports the principle that recovery should empower the client to make informed decisions through providing information and resources. Asking the client how he wishes to proceed supports the principle that recovery is person driven.
   For example:

   > "Joshua, I see that you are taking Thorazine, and the inability to sit still may be a side effect of this medication. There are other medications that will treat your symptoms and that don't have the same risk for this side effect. Would you like to explore these options further?"

2. Using the recovery model principles of respect and the importance of support through peers and allies, one possible response may be, "Kelly, I haven't been in an active combat situation, but I hope to earn your trust as a mental health professional and try to understand, to the best of my ability, the issues you've been struggling with. Many veterans identify, as you have, that fellow veterans are better able to provide ongoing support with an appreciation for the shared experiences you've endured. Are you interested in exploring some of those options, too?"

CHAPTER 11 Suicide Prevention

1. "Mr. J, it sounds like you have been feeling hopeless; this is a common symptom of depression." (Giving information) "Have you been having any thoughts of taking your own life?" (Closed-ended, directive questioning to assess for the presence of suicide ideation)
2. Communication at this point should be focused on thorough assessment of Mr. J's expressed suicide ideas. Assessment questions include (but are not comprehensive):

   "When you have these ideas, do you have a plan in mind?"

   "How strong is your intention to die?"

   "Do you have access to the means for implementing this plan?"
3. "It sounds like you are grieving; that must be very painful. Tell me more about your experience and feelings related to losing your wife." (Empathy, exploring/encouraging description)

CHAPTER 13 Neurocognitive Disorders

1. "Mrs. B, you are not in a restaurant. This is the General Hospital. I am your nurse, Mary. How may I help you?" (Reality orientation)
2. "Mrs. B, you have already eaten your breakfast. Would you like a snack?"

   "Please tell me what it was like when you lived on the farm." (Reminiscing)

CHAPTER 14 Substance Use and Addiction Disorders

1. "Tom, you are here because it has been determined that drinking alcohol is causing problems for you at home and at your work." (Confronting reality)
2. "Tom, you are experiencing symptoms related to your body's withdrawal from alcohol. When did you have your last drink? I will bring you a cup of coffee." (Confrontation with caring)
3. "You are feeling angry toward your boss and your wife, but your drinking is apparently interfering with your job and your marriage. Unless you abstain from alcohol, you are at risk of losing both." (Confronting reality)

CHAPTER 15 Schizophrenia Spectrum and Other Psychotic Disorders

1. "I know that you believe what you are saying is true, but I find it very hard to accept." (Voicing doubt)

   "Please understand that you are safe here." (Reassurance of safety)

2. The nurse should slowly and carefully approach Hal so that he is not startled by his or her presence.

   "Hal, are you hearing the voices again? What do you hear the voices saying to you?" (Encouraging description of perceptions. This type of information may help to protect the client and others from potential violence associated with command hallucinations.)

   "I know the voices seem real to you, but I do not hear any voices speaking." (Presenting reality)

3. "I don't understand what you are saying, Hal. What message do you want to give me? Might you be telling me that you are lonely?" (Seeking clarification; attempting to translate words into feelings)

CHAPTER 16 Depressive Disorders

1. "You have had a lot of losses. You are feeling very much alone right now." (Verbalizing the implied)
2. "You feel sad because you can no longer do the things that you used to do . . . the things that made you feel good about yourself." (Statement that focuses on feelings)
3. Direct questions assessing suicide potential: "Are you or have you been thinking about harming yourself? Do you have a plan for doing so? Have you ever acted on that plan?"

   Demonstrations of genuine concern and caring: "I care about you. I will stay here with you."

   Expressions of empathy: "It must be frightening to feel so all alone. But you are not alone. There are many people who care about you, and I am one of those people."

CHAPTER 17 Bipolar and Related Disorders

1. "Bob, I'm not sure I understand what you are saying. Are your thoughts racing?" (Clarifying, assessing)
2. "John, I have an activity in the next room that I could use your help with. Would you please come with me?" (Offering an alternative activity, redirecting, reducing stimulation)

CHAPTER 18 Anxiety, Obsessive-Compulsive, and Related Disorders

1. "John, I'd like to check your vital signs and then discuss how I can best help you feel more comfortable."
2. "Often, when people become very anxious they develop irrational thinking patterns that contribute to worsening their mood and impacting their behavior in negative ways. By becoming aware of thought patterns that increase your anxiety, you can learn how to replace those automatic thoughts with more rational patterns in a way that improves your mood, symptoms, and behavior."

CHAPTER 21 Eating Disorders

1. "Helena, we've established a treatment plan that limits going to the restroom immediately after a meal because we are trying to help you avoid the urge to purge the food you just ate. Let's talk about how you are feeling right now and see if we can identify some other options for your behaviors before and after meals."
2. "John, many people with this kind of eating disorder report feeling a loss of control, and I understand how that can alter your self-esteem. These are symptoms of an illness with many contributing factors. I want to support you in your efforts to manage this illness, and there is good evidence that recovery is achievable."

CHAPTER 22 Personality Disorders

1. "My name is Nancy. I am your nurse on this shift, and you will be in my care until 11 p.m. You may ask for me by my name if you have any requests." (Giving information)
2. "You were arrested because you broke the law." (Confronting reality)

3. "I do not give out personal information to patients, and I do not go out with patients. I hope that you will be able to get your life straightened out in a positive way." (Confrontation with caring)

CHAPTER 25 Survivors of Abuse or Neglect

1. "You are not to blame, Sarah. You do not deserve to be abused in this way. He is responsible for his behavior."
2. "There are places you can go where you and your children will be safe. I will give you that information."

   "You need to consider whether you want to press charges against him."
3. "You must consider the safety of yourself and your children. You have the phone number of the safe house. It is your decision what to do now."

CHAPTER 27 The Bereaved Individual

1. "I believe we did everything we could to provide care for your husband, and it's so hard to lose someone you love even when they are terminally ill. I'll stay with you and try to answer any questions you have."
2. "Yes, John, it's probable that you are in the end stage of life. Let's talk about how to prepare for this."
3. "Nancy, these are difficult spiritual questions. Would you like to talk more with the chaplain?"

CHAPTER 32 Issues Related to Human Sexuality and Gender Dysphoria

1. "Are you having thoughts of taking your own life?" (Assessment for suicide ideation and intentions are the priority because Jamie has expressed feeling that he wants to die)
2. "I'd be glad to discuss with you the benefits and disadvantages of this option. What do you already know about hormone treatments?" (Conveys respect, collaboration, assessment)

Index

Page numbers followed by "f" denote figures, "t" denotes tables, and "b" denotes boxes.

A

ABA behavior therapy, 660, 662
Abilify. *See* Aripiprazole
Abnormal Involuntary Movement Scale (AIMS), 84, 85–86b
Abreaction, 554
Abstract thinking, 134, 376
Abuse and neglect, 700–724. *See also* Child abuse; Elder abuse; Intimate partner violence (IPV); Sexual assault
  assessment of, 704–713, 705f
  crisis intervention for, 718–719
  definitions in, 701
  diagnosis and outcome identification for, 713–714
  elder, 683–685, 684b, 701
  evaluation of care for, 714
  family-based interventions for, 719–720
  forensic nursing and, 714
  incest, 709–710
  planning and implementation for, 714, 715–717t
  predisposing factors for, 702–704, 703f
  real story on, 711–712
  safe houses/shelters for victims of, 719
  trauma-informed care for, 718, 719b
  treatment modalities for, 718–720, 719b
Acamprosate, 350
Acceptance, in grief process, 759
Acculturation, 836
Acetylcholine, 19, 21t
  aging and, 676
  Alzheimer's disease (AD) and, 269, 270
  basal ganglia and, 19, 21t
  bipolar disorder and, 450
  in REM sleep, 29
  schizophrenia and, 367
  somatostatin and, 24
Acquaintance rape, 710, 880
ACTH. *See* Adrenocorticotropic hormone
Action for Mental Health, 726
Active listening, 111
Activities of daily living (ADLs), 170
Activity theory of aging, 674
Acupressure, 816t, 819, 822
Acupuncture, 819, 822
Acute mania, 452–453
Acute stress disorder, 511, 513b
AD. *See* Alzheimer's disease
Addiction, 300–301. *See also* Substance use disorders
  gambling, 352–353
  medication-assisted treatment of, 348–351
  self-help groups for, 349t
Addison's disease, 28, 412
Adenohypophysis, 26–28
ADH. *See* Antidiuretic hormone
ADHD. *See* Attention deficit-hyperactivity disorder
Adjustment disorders
  assessment of, 518–519
  diagnosis and outcome identification, 519–520
  evaluation of care for, 520
  planning and implementation for, 520, 520–522t
  predisposing factors to, 519
  treatment for, 526–527
ADLs. *See* Activities of daily living
Adolescents, 624–668. *See also* Children
  alcohol use by, 304
  anxiety disorders in, 656–660, 657–658t, 660b
  attention deficit-hyperactivity disorder (ADHD) in, 29, 30, 89–92, 451–452, 635–643, 638f, 640b, 642–643t, 644f
  bipolar disorder in, 451
  depression in, 415–416
  disruptive behavior disorders in, 646b, 649–655, 651b, 652–653t
  gambling behavior in, 352
  gender dysphoria in, 850, 852
  grief in, 764–765
  inhalant use disorder in, 319
  intellectual developmental disorder in, 625–627, 626t
  maturational crisis in, 729, 734
  persistent depressive disorder in, 405, 408b
  personality development in, 588, 589t
  statutory rape and, 712
  suicide by, 222
  vaping by, 317
Adoption studies, 30, 31t
  on depression, 409
Adrenocorticotropic hormone (ACTH), 4–5, 26t, 28
  oxytocin and, 25–26
Adults
  gender dysphoria in, 850, 852
  grief in, 765
Advance directives, 770
Adverse childhood experiences (ACEs), 701
Advocacy, 41
Affect, 403, 446
  disturbances in, 376
Afferent neurons, 17
Affordable Care Act of 2010, 727
Age. *See also* Adolescents; Adults; Children; Elderly
  classification of, 670
  communication and, 109
  depression and, 403–404
  economic status and, 671
  homelessness and, 746
  suicide and, 222–223
Aggression (violence). *See also* Abuse and neglect; Intimate partner violence (IPV)
  amygdala and, 702
  antipsychotics for, 290–291
  crisis, 186–192, 188b, 189–191t
  risk for other-directed, 190–191t, 455–456t, 609–610t, 647t, 657t
  risk for self-directed, 190–191t, 455–456t, 647t, 657t
  suicide and, 225
  symptoms of, 187
  toxoplasmosis and, 32
Aging, 669–699. *See also* Elderly
  adaptation to tasks of, 677–678
  biological aspects of, 674–677
  classification of, 670
  elder abuse and, 683–685, 684b
  employment and, 671, 682
  epidemiology of, 670–672, 671f
  health status and, 672
  life expectancy and, 670
  living arrangements and, 671, 671f
  long-term care and, 683
  marital status and, 671
  normal process of, 674–682, 681t
  nursing process and, 686–688
  psychiatric disorders with, 678–679
  psychological aspects of, 677–679
  sexual aspects of, 680–682, 681t
  sociocultural aspects of, 680
  suicide and, 685–686
  theories of, 672–674
Agitation, antipsychotics for, 290–291
Agonist drugs, 64
Agoraphobia, 480, 481, 481b, 483t, 490t
Agranulocytosis, 80
  Clozaril and risk for, 83–84
AIDS. *See* HIV/AIDS
Akathisia, 84
Akinesia, 84
  conversion disorder and, 538
Alarm reaction stage, 4
Alcohol, 301
  antianxiety agents and, 67–68
  barbiturates and, 88
  benzodiazepines and, 71t
  carbamazepine and, 71t

Alcohol (*continued*)
delirium from, 265
effects on the body, 305–307
historical perspectives on, 304
intoxication from, 308, 332t
medication-assisted treatment of, 349–350
patterns of use of, 304–305
profile of, 303–304, 330t
use during pregnancy, 307–308, 308f
withdrawal from, 309, 332t, 349
Alcoholic cardiomyopathy, 306
Alcoholic hepatitis, 307
Alcoholic myopathy, 306
Alcoholics Anonymous (AA), 346–347, 348b
Alcohol-related birth defects (ARBD), 307–308
Alcohol-related neurodevelopmental disorder (ARND), 307–308
Alcohol use disorder/alcoholism
aging and, 679
Alcoholics Anonymous (AA) for, 346–347, 348b
case study and sample care plan for, 353–354
development of, 305
disulfiram (Antabuse) for deterrence of, 347–348
genetics and, 29, 30
immunological abnormalities and, 32
medication-assisted treatment of, 349
naltrexone for treatment of, 350
vitamin replacement in, 348
Alexithymia, 302, 536
Allopathic medicine, 813
Alpha agonists, 90
for attention deficit-hyperactivity disorder (ADHD), 645t
for Tourette's disorder, 649
Alpha-PVP, 313
Alprazolam (Xanax), 309t, 500t, 525
Alternative medicine, 813, 814t
Altruism, 173
Altruistic suicide, 225
Alzheimer's disease (AD)
adrenocorticotropic hormone (ACTH) and, 28
biological implications in, 31t
clinical findings, epidemiology, and course, 265–268
depression and, 291, 412
genetics and, 29
neurocognitive disorder due to, 268–271, 269f, 270f
stages of, 267–268
traumatic brain injury (TBI) and, 781
treatment for, 287
Ambien. *See* Zolpidem
Amenorrhea
as side effect of antipsychotic agents, 86
American Hospital Association (AHA)
patient Bill of Rights, 42
American Nurses Association (ANA)
on chemically impaired nurses, 345
Code of Ethics for Nurses, 39, 107
definition of nursing, 136–137
Psychiatric-Mental Health Nursing Scope and Standards of Practice, 177
Scope and Standards of Practice, 107, 126
American Nurses Credentialing Center (ANCC), 138
American Psychiatric Association (APA), 4
American Psychiatric Nurses Association (APNA), 39, 126
Amino acids, 21–22t, 23
Amitryptyline, 435t
Amnesia, 540, 540b, 554
Amobarbital, 88t, 309t
Amok, 841t
Amotivational syndrome, 329
Amoxapine, 435t
Amphetamines, 89–92, 313t, 330t
for attention deficit-hyperactivity disorder (ADHD), 645t
delirium from, 265
effects on the body, 318
historical perspectives on, 314
intoxication from, 318, 332t
patterns of use of, 314–315
Amygdala, 16, 17f
aggression and, 702
Alzheimer's disease (AD) and, 270
anxiety disorders and, 477, 483
attention deficit-hyperactivity disorder (ADHD) and, 638
autism spectrum disorder (ASD) and, 629
bipolar disorder and, 450
borderline personality disorder (BPD) and, 598
conduct disorder (CD) and, 654
depression and, 410
schizophrenia and, 368
somatoform disorders and, 539, 542
trauma and, 514
AN. *See* Anorexia nervosa
ANA. *See* American Nurses Association
Anaclitic depression, 413
Analgesics, 90
black box warnings on, 310
delirium induced by, 265
depression induced by, 408
mood symptoms induced by, 449
Anal stage in psychosexual development, 798, 798t
ANCC. *See* American Nurses Credentialing Center
Anergia, 376
Anger
crisis, 186–192, 188b, 189–191t
in grief process, 759
symptoms of, 187
turned inward, 224
Anhedonia, 376
Animal-assisted therapy, 829–830, 830f
Anomic suicide, 225
Anorexia nervosa (AN), 562
assessment of, 564–565, 565b
biological implications in, 31t
care plan for, 542–574t
concept care mapping for, 576, 577f
evaluation of care for, 576, 579
familial tendencies and, 29
luteinizing hormone and follicle-stimulating hormone and, 28
predisposing factors for, 566–568
treatment for, 579–581
Anorgasmia, 860
Anosmia, 538
Anosognosia, 8, 249, 376
ANS. *See* Autonomic nervous system
Antagonists drugs, 64
Anterior pituitary, 26–28, 27f
Antianxiety agents. *See* Anxiolytics
Anticathexis, 797–798
Anticipated life transitions, crises of, 185
Anticipatory grieving, 761, 762
Anticipatory guidance, 730
Antidepressants, 68–73, 71–72t, 74t, 434–437, 435t
for anxiety, 499
for body dysmorphic disorder, 501
for eating disorders, 581
for neurocognitive disorders (NCD), 291
for obsessive-compulsive disorder, 501
for phobic disorders, 501
for post-traumatic stress disorder (PTSD), 525, 785
Antidiuretic hormone (ADH), 24–25, 26t
Antihypertensive agents, 501
for phobic disorders, 501
for post-traumatic stress disorder (PTSD), 525, 785
Antiparkinsonian agents
for antipsychotic side effects, 84, 93
depression induced by, 408
mood symptoms induced by, 449
Antipsychotic agents, 64, 65–66t, 66, 79–87
for agitation, aggression, hallucinations, thought disturbances, and wandering, 290–291
for delirium, 287
mood-stabilizers and, 77t
patient and family education on, 393–394, 468
QT intervals and, 80, 81t, 82t
for schizophrenia, 391–394, 392t, 393t
schizophrenia and, 86–87
for Tourette's disorder, 648–649
Antisocial personality disorder, 29, 30, 592
assessment of, 604–608, 606b
concept care mapping for, 608, 612–613, 612f
conduct disorder (CD) and, 654
diagnosis and outcome identification for, 608
evaluation of care for, 608
familial tendencies and, 29
genetics and, 30
planning and implementation for, 608, 609–611t
treatment for, 615
Anxiety, 5–6, 5f, 476–507. *See also* Generalized anxiety disorder; Obsessive-compulsive disorder; Panic disorder
adjustment disorder with, 518
aging and, 679
assessment of, 479–480, 488, 489b
attention deficit-hyperactivity disorder (ADHD) and, 639
brain and, 476–478, 477f
case study and sample care plan for, 502–503

concept care mapping for, 489, 496f
death, 678
defined, 476
diagnosis and outcomes identification, 488, 490t
due to another medical condition, 484
epidemiology of, 478
evaluation of care for, 495
from hallucinogens, 326
historical perspectives on, 476
in interpersonal theory of personality, 799
medications for, 499–501, 500t
mild, 5f, 6
mild to moderate, 5f, 6
moderate to severe, 5f, 6
in neurocognitive disorders, 291
normal versus abnormal, 478
panic, 8, 490–492t
patient and family education on, 489, 497b
planning and implementation for, 489, 490–495t
prolactin and, 28
sedative-hypnotics and, 87
severe, 5f, 6, 8, 661t
substance/medication-induced, 484
treatment for, 495, 497–501, 500t
Anxiety disorders, 8
in children and adolescents, 656–660, 657–658t, 660b
separation anxiety disorder, 656, 660b
Anxiolytics, 66t, 67–68, 69t, 309t
for anxiety, 499–501, 500t
delirium from, 265
intoxication from, 312, 333t
for phobic disorders, 501
for post-traumatic stress disorder (PTSD), 525
withdrawal from, 312, 333t
Apathy, 376
Aphonia, 537
APIE. *See* Assessment, problem, intervention, and evaluation
APNA. *See* American Psychiatric Nurses Association
Appetite regulation, 16
Apple Watch, 525
Apraxia, 267
Aricept. *See* Donepezil
Aripiprazole (Abilify), 66t, 69, 466t
for autism spectrum disorder (ASD), 632
mood-stabilizers and, 77t
for schizophrenia, 392t
for Tourette's disorder, 648
Ascites, 307
ASD. *See* Autism spectrum disorder
Asenapine (Saphris), 66t, 467t
mood-stabilizers and, 77t
for schizophrenia, 392t
Aspartate, 21t, 23
Assault, 54. *See also* Sexual assault
against homeless persons, 749
risk factors for, 187–188, 188b
of women in the military, 779–780
Assertive community treatment (ACT), 389–390, 740
Assessment. *See also* Diagnosis
of abuse and neglect, 704–713, 705f
anxiety disorders in children, 659
attention deficit-hyperactivity disorder (ADHD), 637–639, 638f
autism spectrum disorder (ASD), 630–631
brief mental status examination, 127, 134t
conduct disorder (CD), 655, 656b
in crisis intervention, 193
cultural, 840, 842, 843–844b
defined, 127
in disaster nursing, 194–195
of elderly, 686
gender dysphoria, 549
of grief, 764–765
ineffective coping, 189t
of intellectual developmental disorder, 626, 626t
of military families, 776–785, 782t
nursing, 136–137
nursing history and assessment tool, 127–133b
oppositional defiant disorder (ODD), 650
psychopharmacology, 61, 61–62b, 63, 63t
sexual dysfunction, 862, 863b
standard of practice, 126–133
Tourette's disorder, 646
Assessment, problem, intervention, and evaluation, 141, 144–145, 145t
Assimilation, 836
Ataque de nervios, 840
Ativan. *See* Lorazepam
Atomoxetine, 90
for attention deficit-hyperactivity disorder (ADHD), 645t
Attachment
aging and, 677
anxiety disorders in children and, 659
autism spectrum disorder (ASD) and, 630
borderline personality disorder and, 599
conduct disorder (CD) and, 654
dependent personality disorder and, 595
emotional abuse and, 708
grief and, 761
love-intimacy, 110
object loss theory and, 413
paraphilic disorders and, 853
phobias and, 484
somatic symptom disorder and, 536
Attention deficit-hyperactivity disorder (ADHD)
agents for, 89–92
assessment of, 637–639, 638f
bipolar disorder and, 451–452
clinical finding, epidemiology, and course of, 635–636
concept care mapping for, 641, 644f
conduct disorder (CD) and, 654
diagnosis of, 639, 640b
evaluation of care for, 641
genetics and, 29, 30
oppositional defiant disorder (ODD) and, 649
outcome identification for, 641
planning and implementation for, 641, 642–643t
predisposing factors for, 636–637
real story on, 635–636
Attitudes, communication and, 108
Atypical antidepressants, 435t
Auditory hallucinations, 375
Autism spectrum disorder (ASD)
assessment of, 630–631
diagnosis of, 631, 631b, 632
epidemiology and course of, 629
evaluation of care for, 632
genetics and, 29
immunological abnormalities and, 32
nonpharmacological treatments for, 632–634
outcome identification for, 632
oxytocin and, 25, 26–27
planning and implementation for, 632, 633–634t
predisposing factors for, 629–630
psychopharmacological intervention for, 632
Autistic phase of infant development, 804, 804t
Autocratic leaders, 175, 175t
Autoimmune theory of aging, 672–673
Autonomic nervous system (ANS), 16, 19, 20f
Autonomy, 41
Autonomy versus shame and doubt stage, 801t, 802
Avanafil (Stendra), 868
Avoidant personality disorder, 594
Avolition, 376
Awareness development, in grief process, 760
Ayahuasca, 70

B

Bagging, 319
Balancing factors, 184, 184f
Barbiturates, 88, 88t, 309t, 330t
effects on the body, 311
medication-assisted treatment of addiction to, 351
withdrawal from, 351
Bargaining, in grief process, 759
Basal ganglia, 13
acetylcholine and, 19, 21t
Alzheimer's disease (AD) and, 270
antipsychotics and, 80, 391
anxiety disorders and, 477
attention deficit-hyperactivity disorder (ADHD) and, 638
bipolar disorder and, 450
dopamine and, 22
gamma-aminobutyric acid and, 23
Huntington's disease and, 273
schizophrenia and, 368
somatostatin and, 24
stimulants and, 89
substance P and, 24
Tourette's disorder and, 646
Bath salts, 313
Battering, 704
cycle of, 705–706, 705f, 716t

Battery, 54
Battle fatigue, 776
Beck Anxiety Inventory, 488
Beck Depression Inventory, 418
Behavior therapy. *See also* Cognitive behavior therapy (CBT)
  for adjustment disorders, 526
  for anxiety, obsessive-compulsive, and related disorders, 498–499
  for children, 660
  for eating disorders, 580
  for schizophrenia, 388
  for Tourette's disorder, 649
Beliefs, communication and, 108
Beneficence, 41
Benzodiazepines, 66t, 67–68, 88, 88t
  for alcohol withdrawal, 349
  for anxiety, 499, 500t
  for delirium, 287
  for phobic disorders, 501
  for post-traumatic stress disorder (PTSD), 525, 785
Bereavement, 756. *See also* Grief
Bereavement counseling, 769
Bereavement overload, 765
Beta blockers, 67, 88, 90
  anxiety and, 501
  depression and, 412
  post-traumatic stress disorder (PTSD) and, 525
Binge eating disorder (BED), 562
  assessment of, 566, 567b
  care plan for, 574–576t
  predisposing factors for, 566–568
  treatment for, 579–581
Biochemical factors
  in abuse and neglect, 702
  in attention deficit-hyperactivity disorder (ADHD), 637
  in bipolar disorder, 450
  in borderline personality disorder (BPD), 598
  in depression, 409–411, 410f
  in obsessive-compulsive and related disorders and, 488
  in panic and generalized anxiety disorders and, 480
  in schizophrenia, 367–369
  in somatic symptom disorders, 539
  in substance-related disorders, 302
  in Tourette's disorder, 645–646
Bioethics, 39
Biological factors and theories
  in abuse and neglect, 702, 703f
  in adjustment disorders, 519
  in aging, 672–673, 674–677
  in antisocial personality disorder, 607
  anxiety disorders in children, 658–659
  in attention deficit-hyperactivity disorder (ADHD), 636–637
  in bipolar disorder, 449–451
  in borderline personality disorder (BPD), 598
  in conduct disorder (CD), 654
  in depression, 409–413, 410f
  in gambling disorder, 353
  in oppositional defiant disorder (ODD), 649–650
  in paraphilias, 857
  in post-traumatic stress disorder (PTSD), 514
  in schizophrenia, 365–370, 368–369f, 370b
  sexual dysfunction, 861–862
  in substance-related disorders, 301–302
  in suicide, 226
  in Tourette's disorder and, 645–646
  in transgender identity, 849
Biologically based therapies, 814–816t
Biological variations and culture, 839
Bipolar disorder, 445–474
  assessment of, 452–453
  attention deficit-hyperactivity disorder (ADHD) and, 639
  biological implications in, 31t
  borderline personality disorder (BPD) and, 596–597
  case study and sample care plan for, 469
  circadian rhythms and, 28
  concept care mapping for, 457, 459f
  developmental implications of, 451–452
  diagnosis and outcome identification in, 453, 454t
  due to another medical condition, 449
  epidemiology of, 446–447
  evaluation of care for, 457, 459
  genetics and, 29, 30
  historical perspective on, 446
  as medication side effect, 450–451
  mood-stabilizing agents for, 73, 75
  patient and family education on, 457, 459b
  planning and implementation for, 453, 454–457t
  predisposing factors for, 449–451
  real story on, 461–462
  recovery models for, 390, 460, 462
  substance/medication-induced, 448–449
  toxoplasmosis and, 32
  treatment for, 451–452, 459–468, 464–467t
  types of, 447–449, 447b, 448b, 449b
Bipolar I disorder, 447–448
Bipolar II disorder, 448
Black box warnings, 68
Black cohosh, 820t
Blood pressure regulation, 16
Body dysmorphic disorder, 485–486, 493–494t
  medications for, 501
Body image, 564
Body mass index (BMI), 568, 569t
Body movement and posture, 110
Body temperature
  eating disorders and, 568
  sedative-hypnotics and, 311
Borderline personality disorder (BPD), 592
  assessment of, 596–599, 597b
  concept care mapping for, 600, 605f
  diagnosis and outcome identification for, 599, 600t
  evaluation of care for, 604
  predisposing factors for, 598–599
  treatment for, 613–615
Boundaries in therapeutic relationship, 106–107
Bowlby, John, 759
Bradycardia, 90, 91
  ADHD medications and, 639
  anorexia nervosa and, 564, 570t
  electroconvulsive therapy (ECT) and, 432
  stimulant intoxication and, 318
Brain and neuroanatomy. *See also* Traumatic brain injury (TBI)
  in abuse and neglect, 702, 703f
  aging and, 676
  Alzheimer's disease and, 268–271, 269f
  anatomy of, 13–16, 14t, 15f, 17f
  anxiety and, 476–478, 477f
  attention deficit-hyperactivity disorder (ADHD) and, 637
  autism spectrum disorder (ASD) and, 629
  bipolar disorder and, 450
  borderline personality disorder (BPD) and, 598
  cerebellum, 14t, 16
  cerebrum, 13–14
  conduct disorder (CD) and, 654
  deep brain stimulation (DBS) and, 433
  depression and, 409–411, 410f
  diagnostic procedures used to detect altered functioning of, 32t
  diencephalon, 14t, 15
  dissociative disorders and, 542
  eating disorders and, 567
  electroconvulsive therapy (ECT) and, 417, 431–432
  frontal lobes, 14, 15f
  hypothalamus, 14t, 16
  limbic system, 15, 16, 17f
  mesencephalon, 14t, 16
  obsessive-compulsive and related disorders and, 488
  occipital lobes, 14t, 15, 15f
  panic and generalized anxiety disorders and, 480
  parietal lobes, 14t, 15, 15f
  phobias and, 483–484
  psychiatric disorders and, 31t
  psychopharmacology and, 33
  repetitive transcranial magnetic stimulation (rTMS) and, 432–433
  schizophrenia and, 367–369, 368–369f
  somatic symptom disorders and, 539
  temporal lobes, 14t, 15, 15f
  thalamus, 14t, 15–16
  topography of the mind and, 797
  Tourette's disorder and, 646
  vagus nerve stimulation (VNS) and, 433
Brain fag, 841t
Brain-reward circuitry, 302
Brainstem, 16
  Alzheimer's disease (AD) and, 270
  antipsychotics and, 80, 391
  anxiety disorders and, 477
  depression and, 410
  glycine and, 23
  Lewy bodies in, 273
  opioid peptides and, 23
  somatostatin and, 24
  substance P and, 24
  vagus nerve stimulation (VNS) and, 433
Breach of confidentiality, 54

Brexpiprazole (Rexulti), 66t
for schizophrenia, 392t
Brief mental status examination, 127, 134t
Brief psychotic disorder, 372
Bright light therapy, 433–434
Brøset Violence Checklist (BVC), 188, 188b
Brunner, Alan, 315–316
Bulimia nervosa (BN), 562
assessment of, 565–566, 566b
care plan for, 542–574t
concept care mapping for, 576, 578f
evaluation of care for, 576, 579
predisposing factors for, 566–568
treatment for, 579–581
Bullying, 224
Buprenorphine, 350–351
Bupropion (Wellbutrin), 65t, 69
for attention deficit-hyperactivity disorder (ADHD), 90, 645t
for depression, 435t
Buspirone (BuSpar), 66t, 67
for anxiety, 500t
for post-traumatic stress disorder (PTSD), 525
Butabartibal (Butisol), 88t, 309t

C

Caffeine, 301, 312, 313t
effects on the body, 318
historical perspectives on, 314
intoxication from, 318, 332t
patterns of use of, 317, 317t
withdrawal from, 319, 332t
Calcium channel blockers
mood-stabilizers and, 76t
patient and family education on, 468
Camaraderie through groups, 171
Cancer
alcohol use disorder and, 305
Cannabis/cannabinoids, 301
delirium from, 265
effects on the body, 328–329
historical perspectives on, 327–328
intoxication from, 329, 332t
medication-assisted treatment of addiction to, 351
patterns of use of, 328
for post-traumatic stress disorder (PTSD), 525–526
profile of, 326–327, 327t, 331t
schizophrenia and, 371
withdrawal from, 329
Carbamazepine (Tegretol), 464t
mood-stabilizers and, 76t
Cardiovascular system
aging and, 675
animal interaction effects on, 829–830
antipsychotics and, 80
cannabis effects on, 328
eating disorders and, 568
hallucinogen effects on, 326
opioid effects on, 323
sedative-hypnotic effects on, 311
stimulant effects on, 318
Caregivers. *See also* Family/family history
psychiatric home healthcare for, 742
role strain in, 690–691t, 746t
Carfentanil, 321t, 322
Cascara sagrada, 820t
Case management, 137–138
in community mental health centers, 740
Case managers, 138
Catapres. *See* Clonidine
Catatonia, 371, 376
Catatonic disorder, 373
Catharsis in group therapy, 173
Cathexis, 797–798
CBT. *See* Cognitive behavior therapy
Cell body, 17
Centers for Disease Control and Prevention (CDC)
on adverse childhood events (ACEs), 701
on animal-assisted therapy, 830
on autism spectrum disorder (ASD), 629
on depression, 404, 672
on obesity, 562
on suicide, 240b
on tuberculosis in homeless persons, 748
Central nervous system (CNS). *See also* Neuroendocrinology
anatomy of, 13–16, 14t, 15f, 17f
antianxiety agents and, 67
brain, 13–16, 14t, 15f, 17f
cannabis effects on, 328–329
depressants of (*See* Sedative-hypnotics)
inhalant effects on, 319–320
nerve tissue, 17–18, 18f
opioid effects on, 322–323
sedative-hypnotic effects on, 87, 311–312, 311f
stimulant effects on, 318 (*See also* Stimulants)
Cerebellum, 14t, 16
Cerebral cortex, 13
Cerebrum, 13–14, 14t
CET. *See* Cognitive enhancement therapy
Chamomile, 820t
Change, constancy of, 209
Chemically impaired nurses, 344–345
Child abuse, 707. *See also* Abuse and neglect
defined, 701
emotional, 708
physical, 707–708
physical and emotional neglect, 708
risk for delayed development related to, 717t
sexual, 708–709, 856
suspected, 49
Child Abuse Prevention and Treatment Act (CAPTA), 49, 707
Child and Adolescent Bipolar Foundation, 460
Children, 624–668. *See also* Adolescents; Attention deficit-hyperactivity disorder
adverse childhood experiences (ACEs) in, 701
anxiety disorders in, 656–660, 657–658t, 660b
attention deficit-hyperactivity disorder (ADHD) in, 29, 30, 89–92, 451–452, 635–643, 638f, 640b, 642–643t, 644f
autism spectrum disorder (ASD) in, 25–27, 29, 32, 627, 629–634, 631b, 633–634t
bipolar disorder in, 451
borderline personality disorder (BPD) and, 599
depression in, 405, 414–415, 414b
disruptive behavior disorders in, 646b, 649–655, 651b, 652–653t
dissociative identity disorder (DID) in, 535–536
dysthymia in, 405
Erikson's stage of personality development in, 801–804, 801t
Freud's stages of psychosexual development in, 798–799, 798t
grief in, 764
homeless, 749
intellectual developmental disorder in, 625–627, 626t
in military families, 777–778
persistent depressive disorder in, 405, 408b
personality development in, 588, 589t, 795–811
suicide by, 222
Sullivan's stages of personality development in, 800–801, 800t
theory of object relations and, 804–805, 804t
Tourette's disorder in, 644–649, 647–648t
treatment modalities for, 660, 662–663
trichotillomania in, 486
Chiropractic medicine, 823, 827–828, 828f
Chloral hydrate, 309t
Chlordiazepoxide (Librium), 500t
Chlordiazepoxide and fluoxetine (Limbitrol), 435t
Chlorpromazine (Thorazine), 466t
mood-stabilizers and, 77t
for schizophrenia, 391, 392t
Cholinergic neurotransmitter, 19, 21t
Christian ethics, 40
Chronic grieving, 763
Chronic pain in somatic symptom disorder, 544–545t
Cialis. *See* Tadalafil
Circadian rhythms, 16, 28–29
in psychiatric disorders, 31t
Circumstantiality, 375
Cirrhosis of the liver, 307
Cisgender identity, 848
Citalopram (Celexa), 435t
Civil law, 46
Clang associations, 375
CLAS. *See* National Standards for Culturally and Linguistically Appropriate Services in Health Care
Clinging and distancing in borderline personality disorder (BPD), 597
Clinical Institute Withdrawal Assessment of Alcohol Scale, Revised (CIWA-Ar), 334, 335–336b
Clinical judgment, 41, 49, 107
collaboration in, 255
NANDA-I on, 137
in nursing diagnosis, 133
screening tools and, 251
with suicidal patient, 226, 227, 230
Clomipramine (Anafranil), 435t

Clonazepam (Klonopin), 309t, 464t
for anxiety, 500t
mood-stabilizers and, 76t
Clonidine (Catapres), 351
for anxiety, 501
for attention deficit-hyperactivity disorder (ADHD), 645t
for Tourette's disorder, 649
Clorazepate (Tranxene), 309t
for anxiety, 500t
Clozapine (Clazaril), 66t
risk for agranulocytosis and, 83–84
for schizophrenia, 392t
Club drugs, 309t, 312
CNS. *See* Central nervous system
Cocaine, 313t, 314, 330t
delirium from, 265
effects on the body, 318
intoxication from, 318, 332t
patterns of use of, 314–315
withdrawal from, 332t
Codeine, 321t
Codependency, 345–346
Cognitive behavior therapy (CBT), 87. *See also* Behavior therapy
for anger management and aggression, 192
for anxiety, obsessive-compulsive, and related disorders, 497–498
for attention deficit-hyperactivity disorder (ADHD), 643, 663
for bipolar disorder, 460
for depression, 413, 430–431
for eating disorders, 580
for paraphilias, 858
for personality disorders, 614
for post-traumatic stress disorder (PTSD), 523
for sexual dysfunction, 864
for somatic symptom disorders, 553
for Tourette's disorder, 649, 663
Cognitive enhancement therapy (CET), 214
Cognitive factors in substance-related disorders, 302–303
Cognitive remediation therapy, 388–389
Cognitive theory
depression and, 413
phobias and, 483, 484f
post-traumatic stress disorder (PTSD) and, 513–514
Cohesiveness, group, 173
Collaborative Assessment and Management of Suicidality (CAMS) model, 230
Columbia Suicide Severity Rating Scale, 230, 230f
Common law, 46
Communication, 99–124
active listening in, 111
culture and, 108, 837
density and, 109, 837
distance and, 109, 837
feedback, 119, 121
impaired verbal, 284t, 382–383t
interpreters used for, 837, 838b
motivational interviewing in, 117–119
nontherapeutic, 111, 114–116t
nonverbal, 109–111, 111t, 116
pre-existing conditions of, 108–109
process recordings and, 119, 120t
therapeutic, 111, 112–114t
Community mental health centers, 739–740
homeless populations and, 742, 746–750
Community mental health nursing, 725–755
historical perspective on, 726–727
maturational crises in, 729–733, 734–735
primary prevention in, 727–728, 729–733
public health model and, 727–729
secondary prevention in, 728, 734–735, 736
situational crises in, 733, 735
tertiary prevention in, 728–729, 735–750
Community residential facilities, 741
Compensation, 7t
Complementary and alternative therapies (CAM), 812–834
acupressure and acupuncture, 819, 822
animal-assisted therapy and pets, 829–830, 830f
chiropractic medicine, 823, 827–828, 828f
classification of, 813, 814–817t
diet and nutrition, 822–823, 824–827t
differences between conventional health care and, 818, 819t
herbal medicine, 818–819, 820–821t
history of medicine and, 812–813
massage, 828–829
for military families, 789
most commonly used, 813, 817f
patient education on, 817–818
therapeutic touch, 828
types of, 818–830
yoga, 829, 829f
Complementary medicine, 813
Compounded rape reaction, 713
Compulsions, 485
Computed tomography (CT), 32t
for neurocognitive disorders, 278
Computerized EEG mapping, 32t
Concept care mapping, 140–141, 142f
antisocial personality disorder, 608, 612f
anxiety, obsessive-compulsive, and related disorders, 489, 496f
attention deficit-hyperactivity disorder (ADHD), 641, 644f
bipolar disorder, 457, 459f
borderline personality disorder (BPD), 600, 605f
depression, 422, 429f
dissociative disorders, 544, 552f
eating disorders, 576, 577–578f
neurocognitive disorders, 280, 285f
schizophrenia, 385, 386f
sexual dysfunction, 864, 867f
somatic symptom disorder, 544, 551f
substance use disorders, 342, 343f
Concrete thinking, 102
Conditioning and substance-related disorders, 303
Conduct disorder (CD), 652, 654–655, 656b
Conduct disturbance, adjustment disorder with, 518–519
Confabulation, 268
Confidentiality, 46–48
trust and, 102
Conscience, 796
Conscious mind, 797
Constipation, 288t
aging and, 675
CNS stimulants and, 91, 318
depression and, 421
Consultation, 135
standard of practice, 135
Continuity theory of aging, 674
Contracts, 46
Controlled response pattern, 713
Control or influence, delusions of, 374
Conversion disorder, 537–538, 538b, 539–540
Coordination of care, 135
Coping skills, 5f, 6. *See also* Ineffective coping
anxiety and, 492–493t
defensive, 610–611t
substance use disorders and, 341t
suicide risk and, 229
Corpus callosum, 13
Corrective recapitulation of primary family group, 173
Counseling
bereavement, 769
standard of practice, 136
for substance use disorders, 351–352
Countertransference, 105–106
Counting on others, 807
COVID-19, 220, 257
among homeless persons, 749
CPCs. *See* Critical pathways of care
Crashing, 318
Criminal law, 46
Crises. *See also* Stress
of anticipated life transitions, 185
balancing factors in, 184, 184f
characteristics of, 183, 183f
dispositional, 184–185
maturational and developmental, 185–186
phases in development of, 183–184, 184f
psychiatric emergencies, 186
reflecting psychopathology, 186
resulting from traumatic stress, 185
types of, 184–186
Crisis intervention, 182–204
for abuse and neglect, 718–719
for adjustment disorders, 526
for anger and aggression, 186–192, 188b, 189–191t
basic methodology for, 192–193
disaster nursing and, 194–195, 196–201t
phases of, 193–194
settings for, 192
Crisis intervention team (CIT) model, 192
Critical pathways of care (CPCs), 138, 139t

CT. *See* Computed tomography
Cultural relativity, 4
Cultural syndromes, 840, 841t
Culture, 835–846. *See also* Ethnicity and race
  assessment and, 840, 842, 843–844b
  biological variations and, 839
  communication and, 108, 837, 838b
  concepts of death and, 765, 765b
  cultural syndromes and, 840, 841t
  diagnosis and outcome identification and, 842
  environmental control and, 838–839
  evaluation and, 844
  health disparities and, 840
  nurse self-awareness and changing trends in American, 839–840
  planning and implementation and, 842
  recovery and, 207
  social organization and, 838
  space and, 837–838
  substance-related disorders and, 303
  time and, 838
Curiosity in Tidal Model, 209
Cushing's disease, 28
  depression due to, 408
Cyberbulling, 224
Cycle of battering, 705–706, 705f, 716t
Cyclothymic disorder, 448, 449b
Cymbalta. *See* Duloxetine
CYP450
  psychopharmacology and, 61, 63t
  sedative-hypnotics and, 311
Cystic fibrosis, 29
Cytokines, 30

D

Data, action, and response (DAR) format, 143–144, 144t
Date rape, 710
  drugs used in, 312, 713
DBT. *See* Dialectical behavioral therapy
Death
  advance directives for, 770
  anxiety related to, 678
  cultural concepts of, 765, 765b
  end-of-life resources for, 766, 769–770
  hospice prior to, 766, 769–770
Decisions, ethical, 42, 42f, 43b
Deep brain stimulation (DBS), 433
  for Tourette's disorder, 649
Defamation of character, 54
Defensive coping, 610–611t
  in conduct disorder (CD), 657–658t
  in oppositional defiant disorder (ODD), 652t
Defensive medicine, 253
Deficient knowledge in somatic symptom disorder, 547–548t
Dehydration, 568
Deinstitutionalization, 726, 727
  homelessness and, 747–748
Delayed development risk, 717t
Delayed ejaculation, 860, 869
Delayed or inhibited grief, 762
Delayed satisfaction, 807–808
Delirious mania, 453
Delirium, 264–265
  aging and, 678
  etiological factors with, 274, 274b
  treatment for, 287
Delirium tremens (DTs), 309
Delta-9-tetrahydrocannabinol (THC). *See* Cannabis
Delusional disorder, 372
Delusions, 374
Dementia, 265. *See also* Alzheimer's disease
  depression and, 250
  diet and, 637
  Lewy body, 272–273
  neuropeptides and, 23
Democratic leaders, 175, 175t
Dendrites, 17
Denial, 7t, 339–340t
  eating disorders and, 572–573t
Denial, in grief process, 759
Density, communication and environmental, 109, 837
Deontology, 40
Depakote. *See* Valproate
Dependent personality disorder, 594–595
Depersonalization-derealization disorder, 541–542, 542b, 554
Depressants, CNS. *See* Sedative-hypnotics
Depression, 402–444. *See also* Major depressive disorder; Seasonal affective disorder; Suicide
  adjustment disorder with, 518
  in adolescence, 415–416
  aging and, 678–679
  Alzheimer's disease and, 291
  animal interaction effects on, 830
  assessment of, 418–421, 418f, 419–420b
  attention deficit-hyperactivity disorder (ADHD) and, 639
  biological implications in, 31t
  biological theories of, 409–413, 410f
  borderline personality disorder (BPD) and, 596
  bright light therapy for, 433–434
  case study and sample care plan for, 437–438
  in childhood, 405, 414–415, 414b
  circadian rhythms and, 28
  cognitive behavior therapy (CBT) for, 430–431
  concept care mapping for, 422, 429f
  cortisol hypersecretion and, 28
  decreased gonadotropic hormones and, 28
  deep brain stimulation (DBS) for, 433
  defined, 403
  developmental implications of, 414–418, 414b
  diagnosis and outcome identification for, 421–422, 421t
  due to another medical condition, 408
  in the elderly, 404, 416–417
  electroconvulsive therapy (ECT) for, 417, 431–432
  epidemiology of, 403–405
  evaluation of care for, 422
  family therapy for, 430
  gonadotropic hormones and, 28
  in grief process, 759
  group therapy for, 428, 430
  historical perspective on, 403
  illness anxiety disorder and, 537
  link between mental illness and, 250
  as medication side effect, 411–412
  mild, 418
  moderate, 420
  in neurocognitive disorders, 291
  normal grief reactions versus symptoms of clinical, 763t
  patient and family education on, 422, 430b
  planning and implementation for, 422
  postpartum, 417–418
  predisposing factors for, 409–414, 410f
  prolactin and, 28
  psychopharmacology for, 434–437, 435t
  psychosocial theories of, 413–414
  repetitive transcranial magnetic stimulation (rTMS) for, 432–433
  secondary, 411
  severe, 420–421
  sleep disturbances and, 29
  substance/medication-induced, 408
  suicide and, 225
  treatment for, 422–437, 423–428t, 435t
  types of, 405–408, 407–408b
  vagus nerve stimulation (VNS) for, 433
  in veterans, 783–784
Depression and Bipolar Support Alliance (DBSA), 460
Deinstitutionalization, 736
Desipramine (Norpramin), 435t
Desomorphine, 321t
Desvenlafaxine (Pristiq), 65t
  for depression, 435t
Desyrel. *See* Trazodone
Developmental factors
  in borderline personality disorder (BPD), 599
  in substance-related disorders, 302
Developmental level
  communication and, 109
Developmental task theory of aging, 673–674
Dexmethylphenidate, 90
  for attention deficit-hyperactivity disorder (ADHD), 645t
Dextroamphetamine sulfate, 645t
Dextromethorphan, 324t
Diagnosis. *See also* Assessment
  abuse and neglect, 713–714
  adjustment disorders, 518–519
  anger and aggression, 186–189
  anorexia nervosa (AN), 564–565, 565b
  antisocial personality disorder, 604–608, 606b, 608t
  anxiety, 196–198t, 479–480, 488, 489b, 490t
  anxiety disorders in children, 659, 660b
  attention deficit-hyperactivity disorder (ADHD), 639, 640b
  autism spectrum disorder (ASD), 631, 631b, 632
  bipolar disorder, 452–453, 454t
  borderline personality disorder (BPD), 596–599, 597b, 599, 600t
  conduct disorder (CD), 655, 656b
  cultural concepts in, 842

Diagnosis. *See also* Assessment (*continued*)
depression, 418–421, 418f, 419–420b, 421–422, 421t
dissociative disorders, 540–542, 540–542b, 543–544, 543t
dual, 334, 337
eating disorders, 568, 570t
in elderly, 686–687
functional neurological symptom disorder (conversion disorder), 537–538, 538b
gender dysphoria, 549
illness anxiety disorder, 536–537, 537b
intellectual developmental disorder, 626–627
major depressive disorder (MDD), 407b
maladaptive grieving, 765–766
mania, 447, 447b
in military families, 785, 787–788t
neurocognitive disorders, 274–278, 275–278b, 278–279, 279t
obsessive-compulsive disorder (OCD), 488, 490t
oppositional defiant disorder (ODD), 650, 651b
panic disorder, 479
persistent depressive disorder, 408b
post-traumatic stress disorder (PTSD), 510–511
schizophrenia, 373–376, 377t
separation anxiety disorder, 660b
sexual dysfunction, 862–864
somatic symptom disorder, 536, 536b
substance use disorders, 329, 334–337, 335–336b, 337–338, 337t
of suicidal patient, 226–228, 232
Tourette's disorder, 646
trauma-related disorders, 514–515
Diagnosis-related groups (DRGs), 726
Diagnostic and Statistical Manual of Mental Disorders, Fifth Edition, Text Revision (DSM-5-TR)
on acute stress disorder, 511, 513b
on adjustment disorders, 518
on agoraphobia, 481, 481b
on anorexia nervosa (AN), 564, 565b
on antisocial personality disorder, 592, 604–606, 606b
on anxiety disorders, 6, 8
on anxiety disorders in children, 659, 660b
on attention deficit-hyperactivity disorder (ADHD), 639, 640b
on autism spectrum disorder (ASD), 627, 629, 631, 631b
on avoidant personality disorder, 594
on binge eating disorder (BED), 562, 566, 567b
on body dysmorphic disorder, 486, 486b
on bulimia nervosa (BN), 566, 566b
on caffeine and tobacco related disorders, 312
on cannabis withdrawal, 327, 329
on conduct disorder (CD), 655, 656b
on conversion disorder, 538, 538b
on cultural syndromes, 840
on delusions, 372
on dependent personality disorder, 595
on depersonalization-derealization disorder, 542, 542b
on dissociative amnesia, 540, 540b
on dissociative identity disorder, 541, 541b
on gambling disorder, 352
on gender dysphoria, 848
on hallucinogen persisting perception disorder, 326
on histrionic personality disorder, 593
on hoarding disorder, 486–487
on illness anxiety disorder, 537, 537b
on inhalant intoxication, 320
on intellectual developmental disorder, 625
on male hypoactive sexual desire disorder, 861
on manic episodes, 447
on narcissistic personality disorder, 593–594
on neurocognitive disorders, 263, 265
on obesity, 562
on obsessive-compulsive disorder, 485, 485b
on obsessive-compulsive personality disorder, 595, 596b
on oppositional defiant disorder (ODD), 649, 651b
on panic disorder, 479
on paraphilia, 853
on personality disorders, 590
on post-traumatic stress disorder (PTSD), 509, 512b, 776, 782
on psychotic disorders, 371
on schizoid personality disorder, 591
on schizophrenia, 363, 365b
on schizotypal personality disorder, 592
on seasonal depression, 405
on secondary prevention, 728
on sedative, hypnotic, or anxiolytic intoxication, 312
on sexual disorders, 848
on social anxiety disorder (SAD), 481, 482b
on somatic symptom disorders, 534, 536, 536b
on substance use disorder, 300–301
on trichotillomania, 486
Diagnostic overshadowing, 249
Dialectical behavioral therapy (DBT), 214
for eating disorders, 580
for personality disorders, 614
for suicidal patient, 235
Diazepam (Valium), 309t
for anxiety, 500t
DID. *See* Dissociative identity disorder
Diencephalon, 14t, 15
Diet and nutrition, 561–562
alcohol use disorder and, 348
for attention deficit-hyperactivity disorder (ADHD), 637, 643
complementary and alternative therapies, 822–823, 824–827t
depression and, 412
homelessness and, 749
Dietary Guidelines for Americans, 822–823, 824t
Diethyltryptamine (DET), 324t
Digital therapeutics, 525
Dimethyltryptamine, 324t
Diphenhydramine, 309t
Disaster nursing, 194
application of nursing process to, 194–195, 196–201t
Disengagement theory of aging, 674
Disequilibrium, in grief process, 759
Disorganization and despair, in grief process, 759
Displacement, 7t
Dispositional crises, 184–185
Disruptive behavior disorders, 663
conduct disorder (CD), 652, 654–655, 656b
oppositional defiant disorder (ODD), 649–652, 651b, 652–653t
Disruptive mood dysregulation disorder, 414–415, 414b, 451
Dissociative disorders, 8, 533–560
amnesia, 540, 540b, 554
assessment of, 540–542, 540–542b
concept care mapping for, 544, 552f
depersonalization-derealization disorder, 541–542, 542b, 554
diagnosis and outcome identification, 543–544, 543t
dissociative identity disorder, 535–536, 541, 541b, 554
epidemiology of, 535–536
evaluation of care for, 553
historical perspectives on, 534–535
patient and family education on, 552
planning and implementation for, 544, 544–550t
predisposing factors for, 542
treatment for, 554
Dissociative fugue, 540
Dissociative identity disorder (DID), 535–536, 541, 541b, 554
Distance, communication and, 109, 837
Distorted grief response, 762–763, 763t
Distributive justice, 41
Disturbed body image/low self-esteem
in anorexia nervosa and bulimia nervosa, 573–574t
in obesity, 575–576t
Disturbed personal identity in dissociative disorder, 549–550t
Disturbed sensory perception
in dissociative disorder, 550t
in elderly, 692–693t
in neurocognitive disorder (NCD), 282t
in schizophrenia, 378t
in somatic symptom disorder, 546–547t
Disturbed thought processes
in elderly, 689t
in neurocognitive disorder (NCD), 281t
Disulfiram (Antabuse), 347–348
Divine command ethics, 40
Dix, Dorothea, 726
DNA methylation drift, 672
Documentation, 141–145, 143–145t
electronic health records (EHRs), 54, 141, 145–146
Domestic violence. *See* Intimate partner violence (IPV)
Donepezil (Aricept), 288t

Dopamine, 21t, 22
aggression and, 703
aging and, 676
Alzheimer's disease (AD) and, 269–270
antianxiety drugs and, 67
antidepressants and, 71
anxiety disorders and, 477
attention deficit-hyperactivity disorder (ADHD) and, 637, 638
bipolar disorder and, 450
CNS stimulants and, 89
depression and, 409–410
eating disorders and, 562, 567
electroconvulsive therapy (ECT) and, 431
gambling disorder and, 353
love and, 160
obsessive-compulsive disorders (OCD) and, 488
opioid peptides and, 24
post-traumatic stress disorder (PTSD) and, 514
prolactin and, 28
schizophrenia and, 18, 367–368
somatostatin and, 24
stimulant use disorder and, 312
suicide and, 226
Dopamine hypothesis of schizophrenia, 367
Down's syndrome, 29
Doxepin, 435t
Dreaming, effects of sedative-hypnotics on, 311
Drug interactions
antipsychotics, 81t
monoamine oxidase inhibitors (MAOIs), 72, 72t
mood-stabilizing agents, 76–77t
selective serotonin reuptake inhibitors (SSRIs), 71t
tricyclic antidepressants (TCA), 71t
D-serine, 22t
Duchenne's muscular dystrophy, 29
Duloxetine (Cymbalta), 65t
for depression, 435t
Durkheim, Emile, 224
Duty to warn, 48–49
Dysthymia, 405, 408b, 420
Dystonia, 79, 84

E

Eating disorders, 561–586. *See also* Anorexia nervosa (AN); Binge eating disorder (BED); Bulimia nervosa (BN)
case study and sample care plan for, 581–582
concept care mapping for, 576, 577–578f
diagnosis and outcome identification for, 568, 570t
epidemiology of, 562
patient and family education on, 576, 579b
predisposing factors for, 566–568
real story on, 563–564
treatment for, 579–581
Echinacea, 820t
Echolalia, 375, 646
Echopraxia, 375
Ecstasy. *See* 3,4-methylenedioxyamphetamine
ECT. *See* Electroconvulsive therapy
EEG. *See* Electroencephalography
Efferent neurons, 17
Effexor. *See* Venlafaxine
Ego, 6, 796, 797t, 799
Ego defense mechanisms, 5f, 6, 7t
Ego-ideal, 796
Ego integrity versus despair stage, 801t, 803
Egoistic suicide, 225
EHRs. *See* Electronic health records
Elder abuse, 683–685, 684b, 701
suspected, 49
Elderly. *See also* Aging
assessment of, 686
benefits of pet ownership for, 830
classification of, 670
depression in, 404, 416–417
diagnosis and outcomes identification for, 686–688
economic status of, 671, 682–683
employment status of, 671
epidemiology of, 670–672, 671f
evaluation of care for, 688
grief in, 765
health status of, 672
living arrangements of, 671, 671f
long-term care for, 683
marital status of, 671
planning and implementation for, 688, 689–693t
psychiatric disorders in, 678–679
reminiscence therapy and life review with, 694b
retirement of, 682–683
sexual behavior in, 680–682, 681t
suicide by, 223, 685–686
Electra complex, 799
Electroconvulsive therapy (ECT)
for bipolar disorder, 462–463
for depression, 417, 431–432
Electroencephalography (EEG), 32t
Electrolyte disturbances
depression and, 412
eating disorders and, 568
Electronic health records (EHRs), 54, 141, 145–146
Electrophysiology and schizophrenia, 370
EMDR. *See* Eye movement desensitization and reprocessing
Emergencies, psychiatric, 186
Emergency commitments, 52
Empathy, 103–104
Employment and aging, 671
Empowerment in groups, 171
Encephalitis, 370
amnesia and, 540
Enculturation, 838
Endocrine correlation in psychiatric disorders, 31t
Endocrine system and aging, 675
End-of-life resources, 766, 769–770
Endorphins, 22t, 822
schizophrenia and, 367
Energy therapies, 817t
Engel, George, 759–760
Enkephalins, 22t
Environmental factors
aging and, 672
in anxiety disorders in children, 659
in attention deficit-hyperactivity disorder (ADHD), 637
in communication, 109
culture and, 838–839
in schizophrenia, 370–371
as situational crisis, 733
in Tourette's disorder, 646
Epilepsy, 23, 464–465t
aggression and, 702
antianxiety agents and, 68
attention deficit-hyperactivity disorder (ADHD) and, 639
cannabis-based drugs for, 328
neurocognitive disorders (NCD) and, 274
temporal lobe, 370, 542, 860
traumatic brain injury (TBI) and, 781
vagus nerve stimulation (VNS) for treatment of, 433
Erectile dysfunction, 859, 868–869
Erikson, Erik, 801–804, 801t
Erotomanic delusions, 374
Escitalopram (Lexapro), 435t
Esketamine (Spravato), 65t, 70, 325
Esophageal varices, 307
Esophagitis, 306
Estazolam, 88t, 309t
Eszopiclone (Lunesta), 88, 309t
for neurocognitive disorders, 289t
Ethical dilemmas, 40–41
Ethical egoism, 40
Ethical theory, 40
Ethics, 38–58. *See also* Legal issues
ANA code of, 39
core concepts in, 39
defined, 39
ethical dilemmas and, 40–41
ethical principles and, 41–42
model for ethical decisions, 42, 42f, 43b
in psychiatric mental health nursing, 42–45
psychopharmacology, 60–61
Ethnicity and race. *See also* Culture
defined, 835–836
demographics of, 836f
depression and, 404
health disparities and, 840
homelessness and, 746
influences on substance-related disorders, 303
suicide and, 223
Evaluation of care
abuse and neglect, 714
adjustment disorders, 520, 523
anger and aggression, 192
antisocial personality disorder, 608, 612–613
anxiety, obsessive-compulsive, and related disorders, 495
anxiety disorders in children, 660
attention deficit-hyperactivity disorder (ADHD), 641
autism spectrum disorder (ASD), 632
bipolar disorder, 457, 459
borderline personality disorder (BPD), 604

Evaluation of care (*continued*)
conduct disorder (CD), 655
crisis intervention, 194
cultural concepts in, 844
depression, 422
in disaster nursing, 195
dissociative disorders, 553
eating disorders, 576
in elderly, 688
grieving person, 766
intellectual developmental disorder, 627
for military families, 785
neurocognitive disorders, 280, 284
oppositional defiant disorder (ODD), 651–652
schizophrenia, 385
sexual dysfunction, 864
somatic symptom disorders, 553
standard of practice for, 136
substance use disorders, 342–344
suicidal patient, 241
Tourette's disorder, 646
trauma-related disorders, 517
Exaggerated grief response, 762–763, 763t
Exelon. *See* Rivastigmine
Exhibitionism, 855
Expressed response pattern, 713
Extrapyramidal symptoms (EPS), 79–80
antipsychotics and, 82t
types of, 84
Eye behavior, 110–111
Eye movement abnormalities, 376
Eye movement desensitization and reprocessing (EMDR), 523–525

F

Facial expressions, 110, 111t
Factitious disorders, 535, 538–539
Fall risk, 280t
False imprisonment, 51
Familial illnesses, 29
Family/family history. *See also* Military families; Patient and family education
antisocial personality disorder and, 607–608
anxiety disorders in children and, 659
conduct disorder (CD) and, 654–655
eating disorders and, 567–568
genograms, 177, 178f
as group, 177
oppositional defiant disorder (ODD) and, 650
recovery and, 208
somatic symptom disorders and, 539
suicide and, 224, 229, 236–240
transgender identity and, 849
Family-focused treatment (FFT), 452
Family studies
on autism spectrum disorder (ASD), 629–630
on bipolar disorder, 449–450
on depression, 409
Family therapy, 177
for abuse and neglect, 719–720
for adjustment disorders, 526
for bipolar disorder, 452, 460
for depression, 430
for eating disorders, 580
for neurodevelopmental disorders in children, 662
for post-traumatic stress disorder (PTSD), 523
for schizophrenia, 389
Family-to-Family Program, NAMI, 214
Fanapt. *See* Iloperidone
FASDs. *See* Fetal alcohol spectrum disorders
Fear, 476
of having a serious disease, 545–546t
Feedback, 119, 121
Female orgasmic dysfunction, 860–861, 869
Female sexual interest/arousal disorder, 861, 868
Female-to-male (FTM) sex reassignment surgery, 853
Fennel, 820t
Fentanyl, 321t, 322
Fetal alcohol spectrum disorders (FASDs), 307–308, 308f
Fetal solvent syndrome, 320
Fetishism, 855–856
Feverfew, 820t
Fight-or-flight response, 4–5, 19
after abuse and neglect, 718
phobias and, 483
Flakka, 313
Flashback with hallucinogens, 326
Flat affect, 376, 403
Flibanserine (Addyi), 864
Flight of ideas, 453
Flooding, 499
Flunitrazepam (Rohypnol), 309t, 312, 713
Fluoxetine (Prozac, Serafem), 70
for depression, 435t
Fluphenazine, 392t
Flurazepam, 88t, 309t
Focus Charting, 141, 143–144, 144t
Follicle-stimulating hormone (FSH), 28
Food. *See* Diet and nutrition
Food and Drug Administration (FDA), 818–819
Forebrain, 14t
Forensic nursing, 714, 717–718
4-methylmethcathinone, 324t
Frese, Fred, 384–385
Freud, Anna, 6
Freud, Sigmund, 6, 224, 542. *See also* Psychoanalytical theory
Friendship between nurse and patient, 107
Friendship-warmth touch, 110
Frontal lobes, 14, 14t, 15f
Alzheimer's disease (AD) and, 270
attention deficit-hyperactivity disorder (ADHD) and, 639
bipolar disorder and, 270
Frontotemporal neurocognitive disorder, 272
Frotteurism, 856
FSH. *See* Follicle-stimulating hormone
Functional neurological symptoms disorder, 537–538, 538b, 539–540

G

GABA. *See* Gamma-aminobutyric acid
Gabapentin (Neurontin), 465t
GAD. *See* Generalized anxiety disorder
Galactorrhea, 86
Galantamine (Razadyne), 288t
Gamblers Anonymous (GA), 353
Gambling disorder, 352–353
Gamma-aminobutyric acid (GABA), 21t, 23
benzodiazepines and, 66
in panic and generalized anxiety disorders, 480
post-traumatic stress disorder (PTSD) and, 514
schizophrenia and, 367
Gamma-hydroxybutyric acid (GHB), 309t, 312
Gastritis, 306
Gastrointestinal system
aging and, 675
hallucinogen effects on, 326
inhalant effects on, 320
opioid effects on, 323
Gender
autism spectrum disorder (ASD) and, 629
communication and, 108
defined, 848
depression and, 403–404
homelessness and, 746
suicide and, 222
Gender-affirming surgery, 853
Gender dysphoria, 848–849
in adolescents and adults, 850, 852
nursing process and, 849–850
real story on, 854–855
treatment issues with, 852–853
General adaptation syndrome, 4
General cellular stimulants, 312
Generalized amnesia, 540
Generalized anxiety disorder (GAD), 479
anxiolytics for, 499
illness anxiety disorder and, 537
theories of etiology related to, 480
Generativity versus stagnation or self-absorption stage, 801t, 803
Genetics, 29–30
abuse and neglect and, 702
aging and, 672
Alzheimer's disease and, 271
anxiety disorders in children and, 658
attention deficit-hyperactivity disorder (ADHD) and, 636–637
autism spectrum disorder (ASD), 629–630
bipolar disorder and, 449–450
borderline personality disorder (BPD) and, 598
conduct disorder (CD) and, 654
depression and, 409, 436–437
dissociative disorders and, 542
eating disorders and, 566–567
gambling disorder and, 353
intellectual developmental disorder and, 625
obsessive-compulsive and related disorders and, 487–488

panic and generalized anxiety disorders and, 480
as predisposing factor to substance-related disorders, 301–302
psychiatric disorders and, 31t
schizophrenia and, 365, 371
somatic symptom disorders and, 539
suicide and, 226
Tourette's disorder and, 645
Genital stage in psychosexual development, 798t, 799
Genitopelvic pain/penetration disorder, 861
Genitourinary syndrome of menopause, 861
Genitourinary system and aging, 675–676, 861
Genograms, 177, 178f
Genotype, 29
Genuineness, 103
Geodon. *See* Ziprasidone
Geriatrics, 670
Gerontology, 670
Geropsychiatry, 670
GH. *See* Growth hormone
GHIH. *See* Growth hormone-inhibiting hormone
Ghost sickness, 841t
GHRH. *See* Growth hormone-releasing hormone
Gift giving, 107
Ginger, 820t
Ginkgo, 820t
Ginseng, 820t
Glutamate, 21t, 23
Alzheimer's disease (AD) and, 269
dissociative disorders and, 542
post-traumatic stress disorder (PTSD) and, 514
Glutamate receptors, 70
Glycine, 21t, 23
Golden root, 820t
Gonadotropic hormones, 26t, 28
Gonadotropins, 5
Governance of groups, 171
Grandiose delusions, 374
Gravely disabled client, 53
Grief, 8–9, 756–774
aging and, 677
anticipatory, 761, 762
assessment of, 764–765
defined, 757
diagnosis and outcome identification for, 765–766
differences between normal versus maladaptive, 763–764, 763t
end-of-life resources and, 766, 769–770
evaluation of care for, 766
length of, 761–762
maladaptive, 424–425t, 516–517t, 520–522t, 527, 602–603t, 762–764, 763t
planning and implementation for, 766, 767–768t
stages of, 757–761, 758t
Group content, 172
Group facilitators, 172
Group process, 172
Groups, 170–181
defined, 171
development of, 173–174
families as, 177
functions of, 171
leadership styles and, 174–175, 175t
member roles in, 175, 176t
physical conditions influencing dynamics of, 172–173
psychodrama, 175–177
role of nurse in therapeutic, 177–178
self-help, 172, 346–347, 348b, 353, 430, 460
supportive/therapeutic, 171
task, 171
teaching, 171
therapeutic factors in, 173
types of, 171–172
Group therapy, 172
for bipolar disorder, 459–460
for depression, 428, 430
for neurodevelopmental disorders in children, 662–663
for personality disorders, 614
for post-traumatic stress disorder (PTSD), 523
for schizophrenia, 387–388
for somatic symptom disorders, 553
for substance use disorders, 352
Growth hormone (GH), 5, 26t, 27
Growth hormone-inhibiting hormone (GHIH), 27
Growth hormone-releasing hormone (GHRH), 27
Guanfacine
for attention deficit-hyperactivity disorder (ADHD), 645t
for Tourette's disorder, 649
Gustatory hallucinations, 375
Gyecomastia, 86
Gyri, 13

H

Habit reversal training, 649
Halcion. *See* Triazolam
Hallucinations, 375
antipsychotics for, 290–291
Hallucinogens, 301
delirium from, 265
effects on the body, 325–326
historical perspectives on, 324–325
intoxication from, 326
medication-assisted treatment of addiction to, 351
patterns of use of, 325
profile of, 323–324, 324t, 331t
Haloperidol (Haldol), 65t
for neurocognitive disorders, 288t
for schizophrenia, 392t
for Tourette's disorder, 648
Hamilton Anxiety Rating Scale (HAM-A), 488, 489b
Hamilton Depression Rating Scale (HDRS), 418, 419–420b
Harmony and balance, 818
Hashish. *See* Cannabis
Head trauma and Alzheimer's disease, 271
Health Insurance Portability and Accountability Act (HIPAA), 47, 47b
Health maintenance organizations (HMOs), 137–138
Health status and aging, 672
Health teaching and health promotion, 135
Hearing and aging, 676
Hepatic effects of sedative-hypnotics, 311
Hepatic encephalopathy, 307
Herbal medicine, 818–819, 820–821t
Heroin, 321t, 322
Hierarchy of needs, 3, 3f, 140
HIPAA. *See* Health Insurance Portability and Accountability Act
Histamine, 21t, 22–23
Histrionic personality disorder, 592–593
HIV/AIDS
bipolar disorder and, 449
case management for, 138
forgiveness and, 161
homeless persons and, 749
neurocognitive disorder due to, 266b, 273
substance use disorder and, 784
suicide and, 224
tuberculosis and, 749
HMOs. *See* Health maintenance organizations
Hoarding disorder, 486–487
Holistic recovery, 207
Homeless population
case study on, 751
challenges in caring for mentally ill, 748–749
community resources for, 749–750
contributing factors to mentally ill, 747–748
health-care centers and storefront clinics, 750
health issues in, 748–749
history and epidemiology of, 742
mental illness among, 747–749
shelters for, 749
Hope
recovery from, 206
Hopelessness and suicide, 225, 234t
Hops, 821t
Hormonal disturbances and depression, 412
Hospice, 766, 769–770
Hospitalization
emergency commitments, 52
gravely disabled client, 53
involuntary commitment, 51–52
involuntary outpatient commitment (IOC), 52–53
mentally ill person in need of treatment, 52
voluntary admissions, 51
Huffing, 319
Huntington's disease
depression due to, 408, 412
genetics and, 29
neurocognitive disorder due to, 273
Hwa-byung, 841t
Hydrocodone, 321t
Hydromorphone, 321t
Hydroxyzine (Vistanil), 500t

Hyperglycemia, antipsychotics and, 82t
Hypnotics. *See* Sedative-hypnotics
Hypoactive sexual desire disorder, 860, 861, 864, 867–868
Hypochondriasis. *See* Illness anxiety disorder
Hypomania, 447, 448b
  assessment of, 452
Hypotension
  antipsychotics and, 82t
  eating disorders and, 570
  from sedative-hypnotics, 311
Hypothalamic-pituitary-adrenocortical axis and depression, 411
Hypothalamic-pituitary-thyroid axis and depression, 411
Hypothalamus, 14t, 16, 27f
  aggression and, 703
  aging and, 673
  Alzheimer's disease and, 270
  anxiety disorders, 477
  appetite regulation in, 561–562
  attention deficit-hyperactivity disorder (ADHD) and, 638
  depression and, 410
  hormones, 24, 26t
  nicotine and, 318
  schizophrenia and, 368
  somatoform disorders and, 539

I

Id, 796, 797t
Ideas of reference, 374
Identification, 7t
Identity versus role confusion stage, 801t, 802–803
Illness anxiety disorder, 535, 536–537, 537b, 539–540, 545–546t
Illusions, 375
Iloperidone (Fanapt), 66t
  for schizophrenia, 392t
Imaginal desensitization, 858
Imbalanced nutrition, 571–572t
  with alcohol use disorder, 348
  with bipolar disorder, 456t
  eating disorders and (*See* Eating disorders)
  with substance use disorders, 342t
Imipramine (Tofranil), 435t
Imitative behavior in group therapy, 173
Immune system
  aging and, 672–673, 676
  implications in psychiatric illness, 30, 32
  normal response, 30
  schizophrenia and, 369
Impaired memory, 281t
  in dissociative disorder, 548–549t
Impaired social interaction, 457t, 603–604t, 633t
  in conduct disorder (CD), 657t
  gender dysphoria and, 851–852t
  in oppositional defiant disorder (ODD), 653t
  separation anxiety disorder, 662t
  in Tourette's disorder, 647–648t
Impaired verbal communication, 284t, 382–383t, 634t
Imparting of information in group therapy, 173
Implementation. *See* Planning and implementation
Implosion therapy (flooding), 499
Impulsivity, 494–495t
  aggression and, 702
  antisocial personality and, 606, 606b
  attention deficit-hyperactivity disorder (ADHD) and, 451, 635–636, 638, 646
  autism spectrum disorder (ASD) and, 632
  borderline personality disorder and, 597b, 598
  neurocognitive disorder and, 272
  suicide and, 225, 235t
Inactivated neurotransmitters, 18, 18f
Incest, 709–710
Incomprehensibility, 4
Individual psychotherapy
  for adjustment disorders, 526
  for anxiety, obsessive-compulsive, and related disorders, 495, 497
  for bipolar disorder, 459
  for eating disorders, 580
  for personality disorders, 613
  for post-traumatic stress disorder (PTSD), 785
  for schizophrenia, 387–388
  for somatic symptom disorders, 553
  standard of practice, 136
  for traumatic brain injury (TBI), 790
Industry versus inferiority stage, 801t, 802
Ineffective coping, 189t, 235t. *See also* Coping skills
  anxiety and, 492–493t
  gender dysphoria and, 851t
  separation anxiety disorder and, 661t
  somatic symptom disorder and, 544–545t
  substance use disorders and, 341t
Ineffective impulse control, 494–495t
Ineffective sexuality pattern, 866t
Inflammation
  depression and, 412–413
  trauma and, 511
Influenza, schizophrenia from, 369
Information sharing and groups, 171
Informed consent, 49–50
Inhalants, 301
  delirium from, 265
  effects on the body, 319
  intoxication from, 320, 333t
  patterns of use of, 319
  profile of, 319
  withdrawal from, 320
Inhibitory response, 18
Initiative versus guilt stage, 801t, 802
Injury risk
  with attention deficit-hyperactivity disorder (ADHD), 642t
  with bipolar disorder, 454t
  with borderline personality disorder (BPD), 601–602t
  in elderly, 689t
  with substance use disorders, 338–339t
Instillation of hope in group therapy, 173
Institute of Medicine (IOM), 39, 54, 67
  on EHR systems, 145
  Health Professions Education: A Bridge to Quality, 284, 386
  on patient-centered care, 208, 255
  Returning Home from Iraq and Afghanistan, 776
  on safety, 68
  on scope and standards of practice, 126
  on teamwork and collaboration, 537
Institutional abuse, 701
Integration, 554
Integrative health, 813
Integumentary system and aging, 675
Intellectual developmental disorder, 625–627, 626t
  assessment of, 626, 626t
  diagnoses of, 626–627
  evaluation of care for, 627
  planning and implementation for, 627, 628–629t
Intellectual functioning and aging, 677
Intellectualization, 7t
International Society of Psychiatric-Mental Health Nurses (ISPN), 39, 126
Interneurons, 17
Interpersonal learning in group therapy, 173
Interpersonal theory
  of personality, 799–801, 800t
  of suicide, 225
Interpreters, 837, 838b
Intimacy versus isolation stage, 801t, 803
Intimate distance, 109
Intimate partner violence (IPV), 701. *See also* Abuse and neglect
  assessment of, 704–707, 705f
  homelessness and, 748
Intoxication
  alcohol, 308, 332t
  caffeine, 318, 332t
  cannabis, 329, 332t
  cocaine, 318, 332t
  hallucinogen, 326
  inhalant, 320, 333t
  nicotine, 333t
  opioid, 323, 333t, 350
  phencyclidine (PCP), 326, 333t
  sedative, hypnotic, or anxiolytic, 312, 333t
  stimulant, 318, 332t, 351
  substance, 301
Introjection, 7t
Invasion of privacy, 54
Involuntary commitment, 51–52
Involuntary outpatient commitment (IOC), 52–53
IPSRT therapy, 459
IPV. *See* Intimate partner violence
Irritability
  prolactin and, 28
Isocarboxazid (Marplan), 435t
Isolation. *See* Social isolation
IS PATH WARM?, 229–230
ISPN. *See* International Society of Psychiatric-Mental Health Nurses

J

Jealous delusions, 374–375
Johnson, Larry, 422
Joint Commission on Mental Health, 726
Justice, 41–42

K

Kantianism, 40
Kava-kava, 821t
Kendra's Law, 44, 61
Ketamine, 324t
  for post-traumatic stress disorder (PTSD), 525
Koro, 841t
Korsakoff's psychosis, 306
Kratom, 321t, 322
Kübler-Ross, Elisabeth, 757

L

La bell indifference, 538
Laborit, H., 60
Laissez-faire leaders, 175, 175t
Lamborexant (Dayvigo), 88t
Lamotrigine (Lamictal), 465t
  mood-stabilizers and, 76t
Latency stage in psychosexual development, 798t, 799
Lawsuits in psychiatric nursing, 54
Leadership styles, 174–175, 175t
Learned helplessness, 413
Learning ability and aging, 677
Learning disorders and conduct disorder (CD), 654
Learning theory
  in abuse and neglect, 702–704
  depression and, 413
  obsessive-compulsive and related disorders and, 487
  phobias and, 482–483
  post-traumatic stress disorder (PTSD) and, 511
  somatic symptom disorders and, 539–540
Legal issues. *See also* Ethics
  duty to warn, 48–49
  hospitalization, 51–53
  informed consent, 49–50
  nurse practice acts, 45–46
  nursing liability, 53–55
  patient rights, 42–45, 45b
  in psychiatric mental health nursing, 46–51, 47b
  psychopharmacology, 60–61
  restraints and seclusion, 50–51
  right to privacy, 46–48, 47b
  types of law, 46
Lesbian, gay, bisexual, transgender, or questioning persons
  homelessness among, 746
  suicide by, 224
Leukopenia, 307
Levomilnacipran, 65t
Lewy body dementia, 272–273
LGBTQ. *See* Lesbian, gay, bisexual, transgender, or questioning persons
LH. *See* Luteinizing hormone
Liability, nursing, 53–55
Libel, 54
Libido, 797. *See also* Sexual function/dysfunction
  antipsychotic agent effects on, 86
  cannabis effects on, 329
  hallucinogen effects on, 326
  opioid effects on, 323
  prolactin and, 28
  sedative-hypnotic effects on, 311–312
  stimulant effects on, 318
Life change events as situational crises, 733
Life expectancy, 670
Life experiences and phobias, 484
Life review, 694b
Limbic system, 15, 16, 17f
Lisdexamfetamine (Vyvanse), 645t
Listening, active, 111
Lithium, 75–79, 76–77t, 78t
  mood-stabilizers and, 76t
Lithium carbonate, 464t
Liver
  aging and, 675
  alcoholic hepatitis and, 307
  alcohol metabolism in, 304
  antipsychotics and, 80, 92
  barbiturate use and, 311
  cirrhosis of, 307
  fight-or-flight syndrome and, 4
Living arrangements and aging, 671, 671f
Living wills, 770
Localized amnesia, 540
Long-term care, 683
Long-term memory and aging, 677
Loose associations, 375
Lorazepam (Ativan), 289t, 309t
  for anxiety, 500t
Loss, 757. *See also* Grief
Low self-esteem, 425t
  with attention deficit-hyperactivity disorder (ADHD), 642–643t
  in conduct disorder (CD), 658t
  in elderly, 691–692t
  gender dysphoria and, 852t
  in oppositional defiant disorder (ODD), 653t
Loxapine, 392t
L-tryptophan
  interactions with antianxiety agents, 68
  sleep-onset disorder and, 29
Lumateperone (Caplyta), 392t
Lunesta. *See* Eszopiclone
Lurasidone (Latuda), 66t, 466t
  for schizophrenia, 392t
Luteinizing hormone (LH), 28
Lysergic acid diethylamide (LSD), 70, 324, 324t
  patterns of use of, 325

M

Magnetic resonance imaging (MRI), 32t
  for neurocognitive disorders, 278
  schizophrenia and, 369
  for somatic symptom disorders, 539
Mahler, Margaret, 804–805, 804t
Major depressive disorder (MDD), 405, 420–421. *See also* Depression
  diagnosis of, 407b
  epidemiology of, 403–405
  genetics and, 29, 30
Major neurocognitive disorder, 265, 266b
Major tranquilizers, 391
Maladaptive grieving
  adjustment disorders and, 520–522t, 527
  chronic or prolonged grieving, 763
  delayed or inhibited grief, 762
  depression and, 424–425t
  distorted (exaggerated) grief response, 762–763, 763t
  normal versus, 763–764, 763t
  personality disorders and, 602–603t
  psychiatric home health care and, 744–745t
  trauma and, 516–517t
Male hypoactive sexual desire disorder, 861
Male-to-female (MTF) sex reassignment surgery, 853
Malpractice, 53–54
Managed care, 137–138
Mangus, Matt, 102
Mania
  acute, 452–453
  cortisol hypersecretion and, 28
  defined, 446
  delirious, 453
  diagnosis of, 447, 447b
Manipulation in borderline personality disorder (BPD), 597
Manipulative and body-based methods, 816t
MAOIs. *See* Monoamine oxidase inhibitors
Maprotiline, 435t
Marijuana. *See* Cannabis/cannabinoids
Marital rape, 710, 712
Marital status
  age and, 671
  depression and, 404–405
  suicide and, 222
Marriage as maturational crisis, 729–730, 734
Maslow, Abraham, 3, 3f
Massage, 828–829
Material boundaries, 106
Maturational crises, 185–186, 729–733, 734–735
Maudsley approach, 580
MDD. *See* Major depressive disorder
Medicaid, 683
Medicare, 683
Medication administration, 63
Medication assessment tool, 61, 61–62b
Medication-assisted treatment for substance use disorders, 348–351
Medication-induced disorders
  anxiety, 484
  bipolar disorder, 448–449
  delirium, 265
  depressive, 408
  neurocognitive, 273
  psychotic, 372
  sexual dysfunction, 861
Medulla, 14t, 16
Melancholia, 403
Melanocyte-stimulating hormone, 26t, 28
Melatonin, 29
Memantine (Namenda), 288t
Memantine, extended release + donepezil (Namzaric), 288t
Member roles in groups, 175, 176t
Membership, group, 173
Memory functioning and aging, 677

Men. *See also* Gender
communication and, 108
depression in, 403–404
genitourinary system of older, 676
sexual dysfunctions in, 859–860
sexuality and aging in, 681
sexual response cycle in, 858–859
suicide by, 222
Meningitis, 370
Menopause, 675, 680
Mental health, 2–3
Mental illness, 2–3. *See also* Schizophrenia; specific types
care for, 248–262
defined, 3–4
definition of serious, 735
homelessness and, 746, 747–749
inhalant use and, 319–320
need for education of health-care providers on, 249–250
need of treatment for, 52
nurse's role in nonpsychiatric settings, 258
referral for, 254–255, 256b
screening for, 250–254, 254b
stigmatization of, 255, 257
suicide and, 223–224, 252–253
tertiary prevention with severe and persistent, 735
trauma history and, 252
Mental status examination, 127, 134t, 275–278b
Meperidine, 321t
Mephedrone, 312
Mephobarbital, 309t
Meprobamate (Miltown, Equanil), 309t
for anxiety, 500t
Mescaline, 324t, 325
Mesencephalon, 14t, 16
Methadone, 321t, 350
Methamphetamines, 314
for attention deficit-hyperactivity disorder (ADHD), 645t
patterns of use of, 314–315
Methoxy-amphetamine (MDA), 324t
Methylone, 324t
Methylphenidate, 90
for attention deficit-hyperactivity disorder (ADHD), 645t
Midazolam (Versed), 500t
Midbrain, 14t, 16
Midlife, maturational crisis in, 731–732, 735
Migraine
delirium and, 264
dissociative disorders and, 542
mood-stabilizing agents and, 464–466t
in veterans, 780
Mild anxiety, 5f, 6
Mild cognitive impairment, 265, 266b
Mild depression, 418, 418f
Milieu therapy
for personality disorders, 614
standard of practice, 136
Military families, 775–794
adjustment of veterans in, 780
assessment of, 776–785, 782t
depression and suicide in, 783–784
diagnosis and outcome identification in, 785, 787–788t
epidemiology related to, 776
historical perspective on, 775–776
impact of deployment on, 778–779
planning, implementation, and evaluation for, 785
post-traumatic stress disorder (PTSD) and, 776, 782–783, 785
real story on, 786
spouses and children in, 777–778
substance use disorder in, 784–785
traumatic brain injury (TBI) and, 780–781, 782t, 790
treatment modalities for, 785–790, 787–789t, 788–789t
women in military and, 779–780
Mind, topography of the, 797
Mind-body interventions, 814t
Mirtazapine (Remeron), 69
for depression, 435t
for neurocognitive disorders, 289t
Mobile outreach units for homeless persons, 750
Model of Intercultural Sensitivity, 840, 842
Moderate depression, 420
Molly. *See* 3,4-methylene-dioxyamphetamine
Monoamine oxidase inhibitors (MAOIs), 65t, 68–73, 71–72t, 72t, 435t
drug interactions with, 72, 72t
Monoamines, 19, 21t, 22–23
Mood, 403, 446
in acute mania, 452–453
in delirious mania, 453
in hypomania, 452
Mood disorders
adrenocorticotropic hormone (ACTH) and, 28
circadian rhythms and, 29
conduct disorder (CD) and, 654
Mood-stabilizing agents, 73, 75–79, 76–77t, 78t
for bipolar disorder, 463–468, 464–467t
patient and family education on, 463, 468
Moral behavior, 39
Moral reform movement, 60
Morals, 39
Morphinan, 321t
Motivational interviewing, 117, 334
example, 117–119
Mourning, 8
MRI. *See* Magnetic resonance imaging
Multiple personality disorder. *See* Dissociative identity disorder (DID)
Multiple sclerosis and bipolar disorder, 449
Munchausen syndrome, 535
Musculoskeletal system and aging, 675
Myelin, 17
Myocardial infarction (MI)
antipsychotics and, 80
depression due to, 408

N

N-acetylcysteine, 350
Naloxone (Narcan), 350
Naltrexone, 350
Namenda. *See* Memantine
Namzaric. *See* Memantine, extended release + donepezil
Narcissistic personality disorder, 593–594
National Alliance on Mental Illness (NAMI), 214, 251
National Alliance to End Homelessness, 746
National Center for Complementary and Alternative Medicine (NCCAM), 813
National Certification Commission for Acupuncture and Oriental Medicine (NCCAOM), 822
National Institute of Mental Health (NIMH), 726, 735
National Intimate Partner and Sexual Violence Survey (NISVS), 701
National Mental Health Act, 726
National Standards for Culturally and Linguistically Appropriate Services in Health Care (CLAS), 840
Natural death acts, 770
Natural law theory, 40
NCCAM. *See* National Center for Complementary and Alternative Medicine
NCCAOM. *See* National Certification Commission for Acupuncture and Oriental Medicine
NCD. *See* Neurocognitive disorders
Nefazodone, 65t, 69
for depression, 435t
Negative feedback mechanism, 27
Neglect. *See* Abuse and neglect
Negligence, 53–54
Neologisms, 375
Neoplasms, 370
Nervous system. *See also* Autonomic nervous system; Central nervous system; Neurotransmitters
aging and, 676
anatomy of, 13–24
Neuroanatomy. *See* Brain and neuroanatomy
Neurochemical factors
in dissociative disorders, 542
in eating disorders, 567
in panic and generalized anxiety disorders, 480
in suicide, 226
Neurocognitive disorders (NCDs), 263–298
aging and, 678
agitation, aggression, hallucinations, thought disturbances, and wandering in, 290–291
antipsychotics and, 80
antipsychotics for, 290–291
anxiety in, 291
assessment of, 274–278, 275–278b
classified as mild or major, 265
concept care mapping for, 280, 285f
delirium, 264–265, 287
depression in, 291
due to Alzheimer's disease, 268–271, 269f, 270f
due to another medical condition, 274
due to HIV infection, 273
due to Huntington's disease, 273
due to Lewy body dementia, 272–273

due to Parkinson's disease, 273
due to prion disease, 273–274
due to traumatic brain injury, 272
etiological factors with, 274, 274b
frontotemporal, 272
immunological abnormalities and, 32
nursing diagnosis and outcome identification, 278–279, 279t
patient and family education on, 280, 286b
planning and implementation for, 280, 280t
predisposing factors for, 268–274
Quality and Safety Education for Nurses (QSEN) competencies and, 284, 286
real story on, 292–293
sleep disturbances in, 291–292, 294
substance- or medication-induced, 273
treatment for, 287–294, 288–289t
validation therapy for, 286b
vascular, 271–272
Neuroendocrinology, 24–28, 25f, 26t, 27f
aging and, 673
depression and, 411
post-traumatic stress disorder (PTSD) and, 514
Neuroglia, 17
Neurohypophysis, 24–26
Neuroleptic malignant syndrome (NMS), 72
Neuroleptics. *See* Antipsychotic agents
Neurological disorders and depression, 412
Neurons, 17–18, 18f
Neuropeptides, 22t, 23–24
Neuroscientific revolution, 13
Neuroses, 6, 8
Neurosyphilis, 370
Neurotransmitters, 18, 18f, 19, 21–22t
in Alzheimer's disease, 269
amino acids, 21–22t, 23
anxiety and, 477
bipolar disorder and, 450
cholinergic, 19, 21t
in eating disorders, 567
monoamines, 19, 21t, 22–23
neuropeptides, 22t, 23–24
in panic and generalized anxiety disorders, 480
in psychiatric disorders, 31t
psychotropics and, 64, 64f, 65–66t
schizophrenia and, 367–369, 368–369f
New Freedom Commission on Mental Health, 737–738
NIC. *See* Nursing Interventions Classification
Nicotine, 301, 312, 313t
effects on the body, 318
historical perspectives on, 314
intoxication from, 333t
patterns of use of, 317, 317t
schizophrenia and, 394
withdrawal from, 319, 333t
Nihilistic delusions, 374
NIMH. *See* National Institute of Mental Health
N-methyl-D-aspartate (NMDA) receptors, 367, 411, 525, 542, 785
NMS. *See* Neuroleptic malignant syndrome
NOC. *See* Nursing Outcomes Classification
Nonamphetamine stimulants, 313t
Noncompliance with task expectations, 643t
Noncompliance with therapy, 652t
Nonmaleficence, 41
Non-rapid eye movement (REM) sleep, 29
Nonsuicidal self-injuring behavior (NSSIB), 226–227, 253
Nontherapeutic communication, 111, 114–116t
Nonverbal communication, 109–111, 111t
SOLER nonverbal behaviors, 116
Norepinephrine, 4, 19, 21t
aggression and, 703
Alzheimer's disease (AD) and, 269, 270
anxiety disorders and, 477
attention deficit-hyperactivity disorder (ADHD) and, 638
bipolar disorder and, 450
borderline personality disorder and, 598
CNS stimulants and, 89
depression and, 409
dissociative disorders and, 542
eating disorders and, 567
love and, 160
post-traumatic stress disorder (PTSD) and, 514
psychotropics and, 64, 66
schizophrenia and, 367
sleep disturbances and, 29
stimulant use disorder and, 312
Normative influence in groups, 171
Nortriptyline (Pamelor), 288t
for depression, 435t
No-suicide contracts, 236t
NSSIB. *See* Nonsuicidal self-injuring behavior
Numbness or protest, in grief process, 759
Nuplazid. *See* Pimavanserin
Nurse-patient relationship. *See* Therapeutic relationship
phases of, 806
Nurse practice acts, 45–46
Nursing. *See also* Community mental health nursing
biopsychosocial emphasis in, 33
by chemically impaired nurse, 344–345
by codependent nurses, 346
ethical and legal issues in psychiatric mental health, 42–51
forensic, 714, 717–718
liability in, 53–55
relevance of interpersonal theory of, 801
relevance of object relations theory to, 805
relevance of Peplau's nursing model to, 809
relevance of psychoanalytic theory to, 799
role in psychopharmacology, 60–64, 61–62b, 63t
role in therapeutic groups, 177–178
role in treatment of persons with paraphilias, 858
self-disclosure in, 103, 107
Nursing diagnosis, 136–137. *See also* Diagnosis
Nursing Interventions Classification (NIC), 134, 135
Nursing Outcomes Classification (NOC), 134
Nursing process, 125–148. *See also* Assessment; Concept care mapping; Diagnosis; Evaluation of care; Outcomes identification; Planning and implementation
abuse and neglect and, 704–718
anxiety disorders in children and, 659–660
attention deficit-hyperactivity disorder (ADHD) and, 637–643
autism spectrum disorder (ASD) and, 630–632, 631b
concept care mapping in, 140–141, 142f
conduct disorder (CD) and, 655, 656b
critical pathways of care (CPCs), 138, 139t
cultural concepts in, 840–844, 843–844b
defined, 126, 126f
documentation of, 141–146, 143–145t
elderly and, 686–688
grief and, 764–766, 765b
intellectual developmental disorder, 626–627, 626t
military families and, 776–785
nursing case management in, 137–138
nursing diagnosis in, 136–137
in psychiatric setting, 138, 140
sexual dysfunction and, 862–870
standards of practice, 126–136
Tourette's disorder and, 646–649
Nutrition. *See* Diet and nutrition

O

Obesity, 562, 568, 569t, 574–576t, 579
Object constancy, 597
Object loss theory of depression, 413
Object relations theory, 804–805, 804t
Obsessions, 485
Obsessive-compulsive disorder (OCD), 485, 485b. *See also* Anxiety
biological implications in, 31t
concept care mapping for, 489, 496f
diagnosis and outcomes identification, 488, 490t
evaluation of care for, 495
patient and family education on, 489, 497b
planning and implementation for, 489, 490–495t
theories of etiology in, 487–488
Obsessive-compulsive personality disorder, 595–596, 596b
Occipital lobes, 14t, 15, 15f
O'Connor v. Donaldson, 44, 52
Oculogyric crisis, 84
ODD. *See* Oppositional defiant disorder
Oedipus complex, 799
Olanzapine (Zyprexa), 66t, 466t
mood-stabilizers and, 77t
for neurocognitive disorders, 288t
for schizophrenia, 392t

Olanzapine and fluoxetine (Symbyax), 435t, 466t
Older persons. *See* Elderly
Oleptro. *See* Trazodone
Olfactory hallucinations, 375
Ololiuqui, 324t
Operation Enduring Freedom (OEF), 776, 777
Operation Iraqi Freedom (OIF), 776, 777
Opioid peptides, 23–24
Opioids, 250, 301, 314
  delirium from, 265
  effects on the body, 322–323
  historical perspectives on, 320–321
  intoxication from, 323, 333t, 350
  medication-assisted treatment for addiction to, 350–351
  patterns of use of, 321–322
  profile of, 320, 321t
  withdrawal from, 323, 333t, 350–351
Opium, 321t
Oppositional defiant disorder (ODD), 649–652, 651b, 652–653t
Oral stage in psychosexual development, 798, 798t
Orgasmic disorders, 859, 860–862, 869–870
Orientation (introductory) phase, 104t, 105
Osteoporosis, 675
Outcomes identification
  abuse and neglect, 713–714
  adjustment disorders, 519–520
  antisocial personality disorder, 608
  anxiety, obsessive-compulsive, and related disorders, 488
  anxiety disorders in children, 659
  attention deficit-hyperactivity disorder (ADHD), 641
  autism spectrum disorder (ASD), 632
  borderline personality disorder (BPD), 599, 600t
  conduct disorder (CD), 655
  cultural concepts in, 842
  depression, 421–422
  dissociative disorders, 544
  eating disorders, 568
  in elderly, 686–688
  gender dysphoria, 549–550
  intellectual developmental disorder, 626
  maladaptive grieving, 765–766
  in military families, 785, 787–788t
  neurocognitive disorders, 278–279, 279t
  oppositional defiant disorder (ODD), 651
  schizophrenia, 376–377
  standard of practice, 133–134
  substance use disorders, 337–338
  suicidal patient, 232
  Tourette's disorder, 646
  trauma-related disorders, 514–515
Oxazepam (Serax), 289t, 309t
  for anxiety, 500t
Oxcarbazepine (Trileptal), 465t
  mood-stabilizers and, 76t
Oxycodone, 321t
Oxytocin, 25–26, 26t

P

Pacing, 376
Pain
  aging and, 677
  sexual disorders, 860, 861, 862, 870
  and symptom management in hospice care, 769
Palilalia, 646
Paliperidone (Invega), 66t
  for schizophrenia, 392t
Pamelor. *See* Nortriptyline
Pancreatitis, 307
Panic anxiety, 8, 490–492t
Panic disorder
  anxiolytics for, 499
  assessment of, 479
  biological implications in, 31t
  familial tendencies and, 29
  illness anxiety disorder and, 537
  theories of etiology related to, 480
Panic reaction with hallucinogens, 326
Paralanguage, 111
Paranoid personality disorder, 590–591
Paraphilic disorders, 853–858
Parasympathetic nervous system, 19, 20f
Parenthood
  as maturational crisis, 730–731, 734–735
  in military families, 777–778
Parietal lobes, 14t, 15, 15f
Parkinson's disease, 19, 80
  depression due to, 408, 412
  dopamine and, 22
  neurocognitive disorder due to, 263, 268, 273
  suicide and, 252
  traumatic brain injury (TBI) and, 781
Paroxetine (Paxil), 288t
  for depression, 435t
Partial hospitalization programs, 740–741
Participation skills, 808–809
Passion flower, 821t
Pathways, recovery, 207
Patient and family education
  on antidepressants, 436
  on antipsychotics, 393–394, 468
  on anxiety, obsessive-compulsive, and related disorders, 489, 497b
  on bipolar disorder, 457, 459b
  on calcium channel blockers, 468
  on complementary and alternative therapies, 817–818
  on depression, 422, 430b
  on dissociative disorders, 552
  on eating disorders, 576, 579b
  on mood stabilizers, 463, 468
  on neurocognitive disorders, 280, 286b
  on psychopharmacology, 63–64
  on schizophrenia, 385, 387b
  on sexual dysfunction, 864, 868b
  on somatic symptom disorders, 552
  on substance use disorders, 342, 344b
  on trauma-related disorders, 515, 518b
Patient Care Partnership, The, 42
Patient-centered care, 255
Patient Self-Determination Act, 45, 45b, 770
Paul Wellstone and Pete Domenici Mental Health Parity and Addictions Equity Act, 727
PCP. *See* Phencyclidine
Pedophilia, 856
Peer support in recovery, 207
Peer support specialists, 192
Pentazocine, 321t
Pentobarbital (Nembutal), 88t, 309t
Peplau, Hildegard, 805–809, 807t
Peppermint, 821t
Perception disturbances, 375
  in hypomania, 452
Perfection principle, 796
Peripheral neuropathy, 306
Perphenazine, 392t
Perphenazine and amitriptyline (Etrafon), 435t
Persecutory delusions, 374
Perseveration, 375
Persistent depressive disorder (dysthymia), 405, 408b, 420
Personal boundaries, 106
Personal distance, 109
Personality, 588, 589t, 795–811
  defined, 795
  dynamics of, 797–798
  interpersonal theory of, 799–801, 800t
  nursing model of, 805–809, 807t
  psychoanalytic theory of, 796–799, 797t, 798t
  structure of, 796–797, 797t
  temperament and, 796
  theory of objects relations and, 804–805, 804t
  theory of psychosocial development and, 801–804, 801t
Personality disorders, 587–621. *See also* Antisocial personality disorder; Avoidant personality disorder; Borderline personality disorder; Dependent personality disorder; Histrionic personality disorder; Narcissistic personality disorder; Obsessive-compulsive personality disorder; Paranoid personality disorder; Schizoid personality disorder; Schizotypal personality disorder
  case study and sample care plan for, 615–616
  clusters of, 590
  historical perspectives on, 590
  illness anxiety disorder and, 537
  personality development and, 588, 589t
  treatment for, 613–615
  types of, 590–596
Personality factors
  codependency, 345–346
  in substance-related disorders, 302
Personality theory of aging, 673
Personal wisdom in Tidal Model, 209
Person-driven recovery, 206–207
PET. *See* Positron emission tomography
Pets, 829–830, 830f
Phallic stage in psychosexual development, 798–799, 798t
Pharmacogenomics, 436–437
Pharmacological, biological and integrative therapies, 136
Pharmacological treatment for paraphilias, 857

Phencyclidine (PCP), 324, 324t
delirium from, 265
intoxication from, 326, 333t
patterns of use of, 325
withdrawal from, 333t
Phenelzine (Nardil), 435t
Phenobarbital (Luminal, Solfoton), 88t, 309t
Phenothiazines, 65t
Phenotype, 29
Phenylketonuria, 29
PHI. *See* Protected health information
Phobias, 480–482
medications for, 501
systematic desensitization for, 498
theories of etiology related to, 482–484, 484f
Photosensitivity, antipsychotics and, 82t
Physical appearance and dress, 109–110
Physical illness
bipolar disorder due to, 449
depression due to, 408
neurocognitive disorder due to, 274
schizophrenia and, 369, 370, 370b
suicide risk and, 224
Physical responses to stress, 4–5
Physician-assisted suicide, 219–220
Pibloktoq, 841t
Pimavanserin (Nuplazid), 288t
Pimozide (Orap), 392t
for Tourette's disorder, 648
Pituitary gland, 16
anterior, 26–28, 27f
hypothalamus and, 14t, 16, 27f
posterior, 24–26, 27f
Planning and implementation
abuse and neglect, 714, 715–717t
adjustment disorders, 520, 520–522t
anger and aggression, 189–191t, 189–192
antisocial personality disorder, 608, 609–611t
anxiety, obsessive-compulsive, and related disorders, 489, 490–495t
anxiety disorders in children, 659, 661–662t
attention deficit-hyperactivity disorder (ADHD), 641, 642–643t
autism spectrum disorder (ASD), 632, 633–634t
bipolar disorder, 453, 454–457t
borderline personality disorder (BPD), 599–600, 601–604t
conduct disorder (CD), 655, 657–658t
crisis intervention, 193–194
culture and, 842
depression, 422
dissociative disorders, 544, 544–550t
eating disorders, 568
for elderly, 688, 689–693t
gender dysphoria, 550, 851–852t
grieving person, 766, 767–768t
intellectual developmental disorder, 627, 628–629t
for military families, 785
neurocognitive disorders, 280, 280t
oppositional defiant disorder (ODD), 651, 652–653t
schizophrenia, 377, 378–383t, 384
sexual dysfunction, 864, 865–866t
standards of practice, 135–136
substance use disorders, 338, 338–342t
suicidal patient, 232–240, 233–235t, 236b, 237b, 240b
Tourette's disorder, 646
trauma-related disorders, 515, 515–517t
Play therapy, 663
Pleasure principle, 796
PMDD. *See* Premenstrual dysphoric disorder
PNI. *See* Psychoneuroimmunology
Pons, 14t, 16
POR. *See* Problem-oriented recording
Portal hypertension, 307
Positron emission tomography (PET), 32t
neurocognitive disorders (NCD) and, 278
schizophrenia and, 367
Posterior pituitary, 24–26, 27f
Postpartum depression, 417–418
Post-trauma syndrome, 199–201t
Post-traumatic stress disorder (PTSD), 509. *See also* Stress; Trauma
adrenocorticotropic hormone (ACTH) and, 28
assessment of, 510–511, 512b
borderline personality disorder (BPD) and, 599
grief and, 761
historical perspectives on, 509–510
treatment for, 523–526
in veterans, 776, 782–783, 785
Posturing, 376
Poverty
homelessness and, 748
as situational crisis, 733
Powerlessness, 426t, 716t
PPOs. *See* Preferred provider organizations
Prazosin (Minipress), 526
Preconscious mind, 797
Preferred provider organizations (PPOs), 138
Pregnancy and prenatal factors
alcohol use during, 307–308, 308f
attention deficit-hyperactivity disorder (ADHD) and, 637
autism spectrum disorder (ASD) and, 630
cannabis use during, 328
inhalant use during, 319–320
intellectual developmental disorder and, 625
Preinteraction phase, 104–105, 104t
Premature (early) ejaculation, 860–861, 869–870
Premenstrual dysphoric disorder (PMDD), 29, 405
Prescriptive authority and treatment, 135
Primary prevention, 727–728, 729–733
Prion disease
neurocognitive disorder due to, 273–274
Pristiq. *See* Desvenlafaxine
Privileged communication, 47
Problem, intervention, evaluation (PIE) system, 141, 144–145, 145t
Problem-oriented recording (POR), 141, 142–143, 143t
Process recordings, 119, 120t
Prochlorperazine, 392t
Prodromal syndrome, 187, 190t
Professional boundaries, 106–107
Projection, 7t
Prolactin, 26t, 28
Prolonged exposure therapy, 523
Prolonged grieving, 763
Prospective payment, 726
Prostaglandins, 367
Protected health information (PHI), 47, 47b
Protection of third parties, 48–49
Protriptyline (Vivatil), 435t
Prozac. *See* Fluoxetine
Pseudocyesis, 538
Pseudodementia, 679
Pseudoparkinsonism, 84
Psilocin, 324t
Psilocybin, 70, 324t, 325
Psychedelic drugs, 70
Psychiatric disorders in later life, 678–679
Psychiatric emergencies, 186
Psychiatric home health nursing, 741–742, 743, 744–746t
Psychiatric-Mental Health Nursing: Scope and Standards of Practice, 177, 738
Psychoactive substances, classes of, 301, 330–331t
Psychoanalytical theory, 413, 482
paraphilias and, 857
personality disorders and, 614
Psychobiology, 13
Psychodrama, 175–177
Psychodynamic theory
aggression and, 702
anxiety disorders and, 480
conversion disorder and, 539
dissociative disorders and, 542
Psychological factors
in abuse and neglect, 702–704
in aging, 677–679
in dissociative disorders, 542–543
in eating disorders, 567
in schizophrenia, 370
in somatic symptom disorders, 539
in substance-related disorders, 302–303
Psychological Recovery Model, 212–214, 215t
Psychological responses to stress
anxiety, 5–8, 5f
grief, 8–9
Psychological theories of suicide, 224–225
Psychomotor stimulants, 312
Psychoneuroimmunology (PNI)
normal immune response, 30
Psychopathology
crises reflecting, 186
role of circadian rhythms in, 28–29
Psychopharmacology, 33, 59–98. *See also* specific medications and medication types
adjustment disorders, 526–527
anxiety, obsessive-compulsive, and related disorders, 499–501, 500t
assessment in, 61, 61–62b, 63, 63t
attention deficit-hyperactivity disorder (ADHD), 641

Psychopharmacology (*continued*)
autism spectrum disorder (ASD), 632
bipolar disorder, 451–452, 463–468, 464–467t
brain and, 33
for children and adolescents, 663
controlled substance schedules, 67b
CYP450 enzymes and, 63t
depression, 434–437, 435t
eating disorders, 580–581
ethical and legal implications in, 60–61
historical perspectives on, 60
introduction to, 60
medication administration and evaluation, 63
medication mechanisms of action and, 64, 65–66t, 66
neurotransmitters and, 64, 64f, 65–66t
nursing process applied to, 66–67, 67b
obtaining drug history in, 66, 67b
patient education and, 63–64
personality disorders, 614–615
post-traumatic stress disorder (PTSD), 525–526, 785
role of nurse in, 60–64, 61–62b, 63t
schizophrenia, 391–394, 392t, 393t
somatic symptom disorders, 553–554
Tourette's disorder, 648–649
traumatic brain injury (TBI), 790
Psychosis, 8, 363, 371. *See also* Schizophrenia
brief psychotic disorder, 372
catatonic disorder due to another medical condition, 373
cortisol hypersecretion and, 28
delusional disorder, 372
due to another medical condition, 372
schizoaffective disorder, 373
schizophreniform disorder, 373
substance- and medication-induced, 372, 372b
Psychosocial development of personality, 801–804, 801t
Psychosocial factors and theories
in adjustment disorders, 519
in aging, 673–674
in bipolar disorder and schizophrenia, 451
in borderline personality disorder (BPD), 598–599
in conduct disorder (CD), 654
in depression, 413–414
sexual dysfunction, 861–862
Psychotropic medications. *See* Psychopharmacology
Psyllium, 821t
PTSD. *See* Post-traumatic stress disorder
Public distance and communication, 109
Public health model, 727–729
Pulmonary system, effects of stimulants on, 318
Purging behaviors, 565

Q

QT interval, 80, 287, 393t
Quality and Safety Education for Nurses (QSEN) competencies, 126, 135
intellectual engagement, 156
neurocognitive disorders, 284, 286
patient-centered care, 390
schizophrenia, 386–387
teamwork and collaboration, 537
Quazepam (Doral), 88t, 309t
Quetiapine (Seroquel), 66t, 467t
mood-stabilizers and, 77t
for neurocognitive disorders, 288t
for schizophrenia, 392t

R

Race. *See* Ethnicity and race
RAISE (Recovery After an Initial Schizophrenia Episode), 390–391
Ramelteon (Rozerem), 88–89, 309t
for neurocognitive disorders, 289t
Rape, 710, 712–713
rape-trauma syndrome and, 713, 715t
Rapid eye movement (REM) sleep, 29
effects of sedative-hypnotics on, 311
Rapid plasma reagin (RPR), 278
Rapport, 102
Rationalization, 7t
Razadyne. *See* Galantamine
Reaction formation, 7t
Reality principle, 796
Receptor sites, 18, 18f, 64, 64f
Recovery, 205–218
bipolar disorder, 460, 462
defined, 206
in grief process, 760
guiding principles of, 206–208
models of, 208–214
nursing interventions that assist with, 214, 215t
post-traumatic stress disorder (PTSD), 511
Psychological Recovery Model of, 212–214
schizophrenia, 390
Tidal Model of, 208–210, 215t
Wellness Recovery Action Plan (WRAP) Model of, 210–212, 215t
Reference, delusions of, 374
Referrals, 254–255, 256b
Regression, 7t, 376
Rehabilitation therapies for traumatic brain injury (TBI), 790
Relationship development. *See* Therapeutic relationship
Religion and spirituality
communication and, 108
divine command ethics and, 40
historical perspectives on suicide in, 220
in hospice care, 769
spiritual distress care plan and, 427t
suicide and, 223
Relocation stress syndrome, 527–528
Remeron. *See* Mirtazapine
Reminiscence therapy, 694b
Renal failure
delirium and, 264
inhalant abuse and, 320
neurocognitive disorder (NCD) and, 274
Renal system
inhalants effects on, 320
sedative-hypnotics effects on, 311
Reorganization, in grief process, 759
Repetitive transcranial magnetic stimulation (rTMS), 432–433
Repression, 7t
Reproductive system
aging and, 680–682, 681t
cannabis effects on, 328
Resolution of the loss, in grief process, 760
Respect, 103
recovery and, 208
in Tidal Model, 209
Respiratory system
aging and, 675
cannabis effects on, 328
hallucinogen effects on, 326
inhalants effects on, 320
sedative-hypnotics effects on, 311
Restitution, in grief process, 760
Restorative justice, 42
Restraints and seclusion, 50–51
Retirement, 682–683
maturational crisis in, 732–733, 735
Retraumatization, 718
Retribution, 42
Retrograde ejaculation, 86
Reuptake, 64
Rexulti. *See* Brexpiprazole
Right(s), 39
to the least restrictive treatment alternative, 44–45
to privacy, 46–48, 47b
to refuse treatment, 43–44
to treatment, 42–43
Risk Evaluation and Mitigation Strategy (REMS), 70, 84, 417
Risperidone (Risperdal), 66t, 467t
for autism spectrum disorder (ASD), 632
mood-stabilizers and, 77t
for neurocognitive disorders, 288t
for schizophrenia, 392t
Rivastigmine (Exelon, Exelon transdermal), 288t
Rogers, Carl, 103
Roger v. Oken, 44
Rohypnol. *See* Flunitrazepam
Romantic association between nurse and patient, 107
Rozerem. *See* Ramelteon
Russell's sign, 565

S

Safe houses/shelters, 719
Safety issues
antidepressants, 73, 74t
antipsychotics, 81, 82–83t, 89
anxiolytics, 68, 69t
mood-stabilizers, 78, 78t
suicide safety plan, 236t
Salvia divinorum, 324t, 325
SAMHSA. *See* Substance Abuse and Mental Health Services Administration
Satiation, 858
Satisfaction of needs in interpersonal theory of personality, 799
SBAR (Situation, Background, Assessment, and Recommendations) model, 54
SBIRT. *See* Screening, brief intervention, and referral to treatment

Scheibel, A., 60
Schizoaffective disorder, 373
real stories of, 406–407
Schizoid personality disorder, 591
Schizophrenia, 362–401
aging and, 679
assessment of, 373–376
biological factors in, 365–370, 368–369f, 370b
biological implications in, 31t
case study and sample care plan for, 394–395
concept care mapping for, 385, 386f
concrete thinking and, 102
current development in psychopharmacological treatment of, 86–87
defined, 363
diagnosis and outcome identification, 376–377, 377t
environmental influences on, 370–371
genetics and, 29
immune system abnormalities and, 32
patient and family education on, 385, 387b
phases of, 363–364, 365b
planning and implementation for, 377, 378–383t, 384
positive and negative symptoms of, 366b, 374–376
predisposing factors for, 365–371
prognosis with, 364
prolactin and, 28
psychological factors in, 370
psychological treatments for, 387–388
psychopharmacological treatment of, 391–394, 392t, 393t
psychotic disorders related to, 371–373, 372b
Quality and Safety Education for Nurses (QSEN) for, 386–387
real stories of, 384–385
smoking and, 394
social treatments for, 388–391
theoretical integration on, 371
toxoplasmosis and, 32
treatment for, 387–394
Schizophreniform disorder, 373
Schizotypal personality disorder, 591–592
Screening
for mental illness, 250–254, 254b
for substance use disorders, 334, 335–336b
Screening, brief intervention, and referral to treatment (SBIRT), 253
Seasonal affective disorder (SAD), 405. *See also* Depression
bright light therapy for, 433–434
circadian rhythms and, 28
Seating, group, 172
Seclusion and restraints, 50–51
Secobarbital (Seconal), 88t, 309t
Secondary depression, 411
Secondary prevention, 728, 734–735
case study on, 736
Secondary trauma, 783
Secondhand smoke, 317
Security in interpersonal theory of personality, 799
Sedation, antipsychotics and, 82t
Sedative-hypnotics, 87–89, 88t, 301
delirium from, 265
effects on the body, 87, 311–312, 311f
historical perspective on use of, 310
intoxication from, 312, 333t
for neurocognitive disorders, 292
patterns of use of, 310–311
profile of, 309–310, 309t
substance use disorder with, 309–312, 309t, 311f
withdrawal from, 312, 333t
Seizures
amnesia and, 540
conversion disorder and, 537
Selective amnesia, 540
Selective serotonin reuptake inhibitors (SSRIs), 65t, 69, 70–71, 435t
for anxiety, 499, 501
for body dysmorphic disorder, 501
drug interactions with, 71t
for eating disorders, 581
for obsessive-compulsive disorder, 501
pharmacogenomics and, 436–437
for phobic disorders, 501
for post-traumatic stress disorder (PTSD), 525, 785
for trichotillomania, 501
Selegiline transdermal system (Emsam), 435t
Self
development of concept of, 808
therapeutic use of, 101–102
Self-actualization, 3, 3f
Self-care deficit, 283t
in elderly, 690t
Self-destructive behaviors in borderline personality disorder (BPD), 597–598
Self-disclosure, 103, 107
Self-esteem, low, 425t
Self-Harm Inventory, 253, 254b
Self-help groups, 172
addiction, 349t
for adjustment disorders, 526
Alcoholics Anonymous (AA), 346–347, 348b
for bipolar disorder, 460
for depression, 430
Gamblers Anonymous (GA), 353
Self-identity maintenance and aging, 677–678
Self-mutilation risk, 633t
Self-respect, 103
Self-system in interpersonal theory of personality, 799–800
Selye, H., 4, 5
Sensory systems and aging, 676–677
Separation anxiety disorder, 656, 660b, 661–662t, 663
Separation-individuation phase of infant development, 804–805, 804t
Serafem. *See* Fluoxetine
Serax. *See* Oxazepam
Serdexmethylphenidate and dexmethylphenidate (Azstarys), 645t
Serious mental illness (SMI), 735, 737–738
among homeless persons (*See* Homeless population)
Seroquel. *See* Quetiapine
Serotonin, 21t, 22
Alzheimer's disease (AD) and, 269
attention deficit-hyperactivity disorder (ADHD) and, 638
bipolar disorder and, 450
CNS stimulants and, 89
depression and, 409
dissociative disorders and, 542
eating disorders and, 562, 567
post-traumatic stress disorder (PTSD) and, 514
schizophrenia and, 367
sleep disturbances and, 29
Serotonin-norepinephrine reuptake inhibitors (SNRIs), 65t, 69, 70–71, 71t, 435t
for anxiety, 499, 501
for phobic disorders, 501
for post-traumatic stress disorder (PTSD), 525
Serotonin syndrome, 72
Sertraline (Zoloft), 288t
for depression, 435t
Severe anxiety, 5f, 6, 8, 661t
Severe depression, 420–421
Sex, definition of, 848
Sexual abuse of a child, 708–709
incestual, 709–710
pedophilia and, 856
Sexual assault, 710
forensic nursing and, 714, 717–718
rape, 710, 712–713
rape-trauma syndrome, 713, 715t
of women in the military, 779–780
Sexual assault nurse examiner (SANE), 717
Sexual dysfunction
assessment of, 862, 863b
case study and sample care plan for, 870–871
concept care mapping for, 864, 867f
diagnosis and outcome identification, 862–864
evaluation of care for, 864
historical perspectives and epidemiology of, 859
patient and family education on, 864
planning and implementation for, 864, 865–866t
predisposing factors for, 861–862
treatment for, 864
types of, 859–860
Sexual function, 307. *See also* Libido
aging and, 680–682, 681t
cannabis effects on, 329
opioid effects on, 323
sedative-hypnotic effects on, 311–312
sexual response cycle and, 858–859
stimulant effects on, 318
Sexual harassment, 779
Sexuality, 847–875
gender dysphoria and, 848–853, 851–852t
human sexual response cycle and, 858–859
paraphilic disorders and, 853–858
sexual arousal touch and, 110

Sexually transmitted infections (STIs), 749
Sexual masochism, 856
Sexual response cycle, 858–859
Sexual sadism, 856
Shame/humiliation and suicide, 225
Shell shock, 776
Shelters
  for homeless persons, 749
  for victims of abuse, 719
Shenjing Shuairuo (neurasthenia), 841t
Shen-k'uei (or Shenkui), 841t
Shock and disbelief, in grief process, 759–760
Short-term memory and aging, 677
Sildenafil (Viagra), 868–869
Silent rape reaction, 713
Single photon emission computed tomography (SPECT), 32t
Situational crises, 733, 735
Size, group, 172–173
Skullcap, 821t
Slander, 54
Sleep
  aging and, 679
  neurocognitive disorders (NCD) and disturbances of, 291–292, 294
  sedative-hypnotic effects on, 311
Sleep-onset disorder, 29
Sleep-wakefulness cycles, 28–29
Smoking cessation, 394
SNRIs. *See* Serotonin-norepinephrine reuptake inhibitors
SOAPIE format, 142–143, 143t
Social anxiety disorder (SAD), 481, 482b
Social boundaries, 106
Social distance, 109
Social distancing, 257
Social functioning impairment, 376
Social isolation, 7t, 140, 145, 380–381t
  abuse and, 709, 719
  aging and, 265, 737, 742, 745t
  bereavement and, 759, 762
  depression and, 73, 414, 420
  military families and, 777
  personality disorders and, 591
  psychotic disorders and, 376, 380t
  self-help groups for, 172
  suicide and, 219, 227, 685
Socialization
  culture and, 838
  through groups, 171, 173
Social justice, 42
Social learning and substance-related disorders, 303
Social-polite touch, 110
Social skills training, 388
Social status and communication, 108
Social treatments for schizophrenia, 388–391
Social withdrawal, 28
  cannabis intoxication and, 329
  depression and, 415
  neurocognitive disorders (NCD) and, 268
  schizoid personality disorder and, 591
  schizophrenia and, 87, 140, 364
Socioeconomic/sociocultural factors
  in abuse and neglect, 704
  aging and, 671, 680, 682–683
  in depression, 404
  in gambling disorder and, 353
  intellectual developmental disorder and, 626
  in substance-related disorders, 303
  in suicide, 223, 225–226
SOLER nonverbal behaviors, 116
Somatic delusions, 374
Somatic symptom disorders, 8, 533–560
  assessment of, 536, 536b
  case study and sample care plan for, 555–556
  concept care mapping for, 544, 551f
  diagnosis and outcomes identification for, 543–544, 544t
  epidemiology of, 535–536
  evaluation of care for, 553
  familial tendencies and, 29
  historical perspectives on, 534–535
  patient and family education on, 552
  planning and implementation for, 544, 544–550t
  predisposing factors for, 539–540
  treatment for, 553–554
Somatization disorder and illness anxiety disorder, 537
Somatostatin, 22t, 24, 27
Sonata. *See* Zaleplon
Space and culture, 837–838
Specific phobia, 481–482, 483t
SPECT. *See* Single photon emission computed tomography
Speech, thought disturbances manifested in, 375
Speech therapy for Tourette's disorder, 649
Spiritual distress, 427t
Splitting in borderline personality disorder (BPD), 597
Spouses, military, 777–779
SSRIs. *See* Selective serotonin reuptake inhibitors
Stage of exhaustion, 4
Stage of resistance, 4
Standards of practice, 126–136
  standard 1: assessment, 126–133, 127–133b
  standard 2: diagnosis, 133
  standard 3: outcomes identification, 133–134
  standard 4: planning, 135
  standard 5: implementation, 135–136
  standard 6: evaluation, 136
Statutory law, 46
Statutory rape, 712
Stereotyping, 836
Stigmatization, 255, 257
Stimulants, 301
  for attention deficit-hyperactivity disorder, 89–92, 641
  effects on the body, 317–318
  historical perspectives on, 314
  intoxication from, 318, 332t, 351
  medication-assisted treatment of addiction to, 351
  patterns of use of, 314–315, 317, 317t
  profile of, 312–313, 313t, 330–331t
  synthetic, 313, 313t
  withdrawal from, 318–319, 332t
St. John's wort, 821t
Storefront clinics for homeless persons, 750
Stress, 508–532. *See also* Adjustment disorders; Crises; Post-traumatic stress disorder
  balancing factors in, 184, 184f
  bipolar disorder and, 451
  defined, 476, 518
  depression and, 413–414
  grief from, 8–9
  obsessive-compulsive and related disorders and, 487
  patient and family education on, 515, 518b
  physical responses to, 4–5
  psychological responses to, 5–9, 5f, 7t
  schizophrenia and, 371
  traumatic, 185
Stroke, 23
  alcohol use disorder and, 305
  amnesia and, 540
  antipsychotics and, 80
  bipolar disorder and, 449
  delirium and, 264
  depression due to, 408
  diet and, 637, 822
  psychotic symptoms and, 370
  sildenafil and, 868
Sublimation, 7t
Subluxation, 827
Substance Abuse and Mental Health Services Administration (SAMHSA), 206
  screening tools, 334
  "Zero Suicide" movement, 221
Substance-induced disorders, 301
  anxiety, 484
  bipolar disorder, 448–449
  depressive, 408
  neurocognitive, 273
  psychotic, 372, 372b
  sexual dysfunction, 861
Substance intoxication, 301
  delirium from, 265
Substance P, 22t, 24
Substance use disorders, 299–361
  adrenocorticotropic hormone (ACTH) and, 28
  aging and, 679
  alcohol, 303–309, 308f
  assessment of, 329, 334–337, 335–336b
  cannabis, 326–329, 327t
  care for, 248–262
  classes of psychoactive substances and, 301, 330–331t
  codependency and, 345–346
  concept care mapping for, 342, 343f
  conduct disorder (CD) and, 654
  counseling for, 351–352
  defined, 300–301
  diagnosis and outcomes identification, 337–338, 337t
  dual diagnosis, 334, 337
  evaluation of care for, 342–344
  group therapy for, 352
  hallucinogen, 323–326, 324t
  homelessness and, 748
  inhalant, 319–320

medication-assisted treatment for, 348–351
in military families, 784–785
motivational interviewing and, 334
in nurses, 344–345
opioid, 320–323, 321t
patient and family education on, 342, 344b
pharmacotherapy for, 347–351
planning and implementation for, 338, 338–342t
predisposing factors to, 301–303
real story on, 315–316
referral for, 254–255, 256b
role of nurse in nonpsychiatric settings, 258
screening for, 253–254, 334, 335–336b
sedative, hypnotic, or anxiolytic, 309–312, 309t, 311f
self-help groups for, 346–347, 349t
stimulant, 312–319, 313t, 317t
substance addiction, 300–301
substance intoxication, 301
substance misuse, 300
substance withdrawal, 301
treatment for, 346–352, 348b, 349t
Substance withdrawal delirium, 265
Sudden sniffing death, 320
Sufentanil, 321t, 322
Suicide, 219–246. *See also* Depression
altruistic, 225
among elderly, 685–686
analysis of suicidal crisis and, 229
anomic, 225
antipsychotics and, 89
assessment for, 226–227
biological theories of, 226
care plan for risk for, 423–424t
Columbia Suicide Severity Rating Scale, 230, 230f
cortisol hypersecretion and, 28
demographics of, 227–228
diagnosis of suicidal patient, 228, 232
eating disorders and, 570
egoistic, 225
epidemiology of, 220–221, 221t
evaluation of care for, 241
facts and myths about, 221t
five-step evaluation and triage, 237b
genetics and, 226
guiding principles for assessing risk of, 231t
historical perspectives on, 220
interpersonal theory of, 225
marital status and, 222
medical-psychiatric diagnosis of risk of, 228
neurochemical factors in, 226
no-suicide contracts, 236t
outcome identification for, 232
patient intention and, 228–229
physician-assisted, 219–220
planning and implementation for suicidal patient, 232–240, 233–235t, 236b, 237b, 240b
presenting symptoms in risk of, 229–230
protective factors against, 227b
psychological theories of, 224–225
real story on, 238–240
risk factors for, 222–224, 228f
risk for, 423–424t
safety plan, 236t
schizophrenia and, 363
screening for risk of, 252–253
sources of information related to, 240b
theories of, 224–226
three-step theory of, 225–226
toxoplasmosis and, 32
by veterans, 783–784
warning signs for, 222
Sulci, 13
Sullivan, Henry Stack, 799–801, 800t
Sundowning, 268
Superego, 796, 797t, 799
Support
in hospice care, 769
in recovery, 207
suicide risk and, 229
through groups, 171
Supportive/therapeutive groups, 171–172
role of nurse in, 177–178
Suppression, 7t
Susto, 841t
Suvorexant (Belsomra), 88t, 309t
Symbiotic phase of infant development, 804, 804t
Sympathetic nervous system, 19, 20f
Sympathy, 103
Synapses, 18, 18f
Synaptic cleft, 18
Synthetic stimulants, 313, 313t
Systematic desensitization, 498
Systemic lupus erythematosus and bipolar disorder, 449

T

Tactile hallucinations, 375
Tadalafil (Cialis), 868–869
Taijin kyofusho, 841t
Tangentiality, 375
Tarasoff v. Regents of the University of California, 48–49
Tardive dyskinesia, 79, 84
Tasimelteon (Hetlioz), 309t
Task completion and groups, 171
Task groups, 171
Taste and smell and aging, 676–677
Taylor, Sarah, 383
TBI. *See* Traumatic brain injury
Teaching groups, 171
Tegretol. *See* Carbamazepine
Temazepam (Restoril), 88t, 309t
for neurocognitive disorders, 289t
Temperament, 654, 796
anxiety disorders in children and, 659
phobias and, 484
Temperature regulation, 16
Temporal lobes, 14t, 15, 15f
Termination phase, 104t, 106
Territoriality, 109, 837
Tertiary prevention, 728–729
community residential facilities, 741
history and epidemiology in, 736–738
for individuals with severe and persistent mental illness, 735
psychiatric home health care, 741–742
treatment alternatives in, 738–742
Thalamus, 14t, 15–16
aggression and, 703
Alzheimer's disease and, 270
anxiety disorders and, 477
attention deficit-hyperactivity disorder (ADHD) and, 89, 638
depression and, 410
Theoretical perspectives on, 40
Therapeutic communication, 111, 112–114t
Therapeutic groups, 171–172
role of nurse in, 177–178
Therapeutic relationship, 100–124
boundaries in, 106–107
conditions essential to development of, 102–104
defined, 101
empathy in, 103–104
genuineness in, 103
as goal oriented, 101
nurse-patient, 101–102
phases of, 104–106, 104t
rapport in, 102
respect in, 103
standard of practice, 136
trust in, 102
Therapeutic touch, 828
Therapeutic use of self, 101–102
Thioridazine, 392t
Thiothixene (Navane), 392t
Third party, protection of, 48–49
Thirst regulation, 16
Thorazine. *See* Chlorpromazine
Thought disturbances, 374–375, 379t
antipsychotics for, 290–291
manifested in speech, 375
3,4-methylene-dioxyamphetamine (MDMA), 324, 324t
intoxication from, 326
patterns of use of, 325
for post-traumatic stress disorder (PTSD), 525
Three-step theory of suicide, 225–226
Thrombocytopenia, 307
Thyroid disorders
bipolar disorder and, 449
depression due to, 408
Thyroid-stimulating hormone (TSH), 26t, 27
aging and, 675
depression and, 411
Thyrotropic hormone, 5
Thyrotropin-releasing hormone (TRH), 27
Tidal Model, 208–210, 215t
Time
culture and, 838
in Tidal Model, 209
Tobacco. *See* Nicotine
Topiramate (Topamax), 465t
mood-stabilizers and, 76t
Torts, 46
Touch
aging and, 677
as nonverbal communication, 110
therapeutic, 828
in therapeutic relationship, 107
Tourette's disorder, 644–649, 647–648t
antipsychotics for, 80
central nervous system stimulants and, 90
Toxoplasma gondii, 32

Tramadol, 321t
Transactional model of stress and adaptation, 413–414, 451, 519
Transcendence stage, 674, 801t, 803–804
Transference, 105
Transgender identity, 848, 854–855. *See also* Gender dysphoria
Transparency in Tidal Model, 210
Transvestic disorder, 856
Tranylcypromine (Parnate), 435t
Trauma, 508–532
  addressed in recovery, 208
  Alzheimer's disease and head, 271, 272
  case study and sample care plan for, 527–528
  defined, 510
  dissociative disorders and psychological, 543
  evaluation of care for, 517
  historical perspectives on, 509–510
  patient and family education on, 515, 518b
  predisposing factors related to, 511, 513–514
  risk for, 280t
  screening for history of, 252
  as situational crisis, 733
  trauma-informed care for, 252, 510
  treatment for, 523–526
Trauma-informed care, 252, 510, 718, 719b
Traumatic brain injury (TBI), 271, 272. *See also* Brain and neuroanatomy
  bipolar disorder and, 449
  depression due to, 408
  in military veterans, 780–781, 782t, 790
Traumatic stress, crises resulting from, 185
Trazodone (Desyrel, Oleptro), 65t, 69, 70
  for depression, 435t
  for neurocognitive disorders, 289t, 291
TRH. *See* Thyrotropin-releasing hormone
Triazolam (Halcion), 88t, 309t
Trichotillomania, 486
  medications for, 501
Tricyclic antidepressants, 65t, 70–71, 71t, 435t
  drug interactions with, 71t
  for obsessive-compulsive disorder, 501
Trifluoperazine, 392t
Trigeminal nerve stimulation, 641, 643
Trileptal. *See* Oxycarbazepine
Trimipramine (Surmontil), 435t
Trintellix. *See* Vortioxetine
Triple reuptake inhibitors, 70
Trust
  abuse and, 709–710
  antipsychotics and, 81
  communication with suicidal patient and, 226, 230, 232
  in group development, 174
  in milieu therapy, 153
  neurocognitive disorders (NCD) and, 267
  paranoid personality disorder and, 590
  psychotic disorders and, 377
  rapport and, 102
  in recovery model, 207
  schizophrenia and, 140
Trust versus mistrust stage, 801–802, 801t
Tryptophan hydroxylase, 226, 409, 417
TSH. *See* Thyroid-stimulating hormone
Twin studies, 29–30
  on autism spectrum disorder (ASD), 629–630
  on bipolar disorder, 449
  on depression, 409
2,5-dimethoxy-4-methylamphetamine, 324t

U

U-47700, 321t, 322
Unconditional positive regard, 103
Unconscious mind, 797
Undoing, 7t
Universality in group therapy, 173
Utilitarianism, 40

V

Vagus nerve stimulation (VNS), 433
Valerian, 821t
Validation therapy, 286b
Valium. *See* Diazepam
Valproate (Depakote), 75, 464t
  mood-stabilizers and, 76t
Values, 7t, 39
  communication and, 108
  cultural, 107, 207, 836, 862
  ethical decision making and, 42
  in patient-centered care, 255
  process recovery and, 390
  spirituality and, 159, 161
  superego and, 796
  10 Tidal Commitments, 208–209
Vaping, 317
  THC, 327
Vardenafil (Levitra, Staxyn), 868
Vascular neurocognitive disorder, 271–272
Vasopressin, 5
Venlafaxine (Effexor), 65t
  for depression, 435t
Veracity, 42
Verapamil (Calan, Isoptin)
  barbiturates and, 88
  mood-stabilizers and, 76t
Viagra. *See* Sildenafil
Vicarious traumatization, 783
Vilazodone (Viibryd), 69
  for depression, 435t
Violence. *See* Aggression
Viral infections and schizophrenia, 369
Vision and aging, 676
Visual hallucinations, 375
Vitamins
  alcohol use disorder and, 348
  depression and, 412
  essential minerals and, 823, 825–827t
Vocal cues, 111
Voice in Tidal Model, 209
Voluntary admissions, 51
Vortioxetine (Trintellix, Brintellix), 69
  for depression, 435t
Voyeurism, 857

W

Wandering, antipsychotics for, 290–291
Waxy flexibility, 376
Wear-and-tear theory of aging, 672
Wellbutrin. *See* Bupropion
Wellness Recovery Action Plan (WRAP) Model, 210–212, 215t
Wernicke's encephalopathy, 306
Wilson's disease, 370
Withdrawal
  alcohol, 309, 332t, 349
  barbiturate, 351
  caffeine, 319, 332t
  cannabis, 329
  cocaine, 332t
  inhalant, 320
  nicotine, 319, 333t
  opioid, 323, 333t, 350–351
  phencyclidine (PCP), 333t
  sedative, hypnotic, or anxiolytic, 312, 333t
  stimulant, 318–319, 332t
  substance, 301
Women. *See also* Gender
  communication and, 108
  depression in, 403–404
  menopause in, 675, 680
  in the military, 779–780
  osteoporosis in, 675
  postpartum depression in, 417–418
  sexual dysfunctions in, 859–860
  sexuality and aging in, 680–681
  sexual response cycle in, 858–859
  suicide by, 222
  as victims of intimate partner violence (IPV), 704–707, 705f
Worden, J. William, 760–761
Word salad, 375, 377t
Working phase, 104t, 105
Wound characteristics after sexual assault, 718
WRAP Model, 210–212, 215t

X

Xanax. *See* Alprazolam

Y

Yoga, 814t, 817f, 829, 829f

Z

Zaleplon (Sonata), 88, 309t
  for neurocognitive disorders, 289t
Ziprasidone (Geodon), 66t, 467t
  mood-stabilizers and, 77t
  for schizophrenia, 392t
Zoloft. *See* Sertraline
Zolpidem (Ambien), 88, 88t, 309t
  for neurocognitive disorders, 289t
Zung Self-Rated Anxiety Scale, 488
Zung Self-Rated Depression Scale, 418
Zyprexa. *See* Olanzapine